EXPLORING MEDICAL LANGUAGE

EDITION 10

A STUDENT-DIRECTED APPROACH

Myrna LaFleur Brooks, RN, BEd
Founding President
National Association of Health Unit Coordinators
Faculty Emeritus
Maricopa County Community College District
Phoenix, Arizona

Danielle LaFleur Brooks, MEd, MA
Faculty, Medical Assisting and Allied Health Science
Community College of Vermont
Montpelier, Vermont

ELSEVIER

ELSEVIER

3251 Riverport Lane
St. Louis, Missouri 63043

EXPLORING MEDICAL LANGUAGE, A STUDENT-DIRECTED APPROACH, TENTH EDITION ISBN: 978-0-323-39645-5

Notices

Knowledge and best practice in this field are constantly changing. As new research and experience broaden our understanding, changes in research methods, professional practices, or medical treatment may become necessary.

Practitioners and researchers must always rely on their own experience and knowledge in evaluating and using any information, methods, compounds, or experiments described herein. In using such information or methods they should be mindful of their own safety and the safety of others, including parties for whom they have a professional responsibility.

With respect to any drug or pharmaceutical products identified, readers are advised to check the most current information provided (i) on procedures featured or (ii) by the manufacturer of each product to be administered, to verify the recommended dose or formula, the method and duration of administration, and contraindications. It is the responsibility of practitioners, relying on their own experience and knowledge of their patients, to make diagnoses, to determine dosages and the best treatment for each individual patient, and to take all appropriate safety precautions.

To the fullest extent of the law, neither the Publisher nor the authors, contributors, or editors, assume any liability for any injury and/or damage to persons or property as a matter of products liability, negligence or otherwise, or from any use or operation of any methods, products, instructions, or ideas contained in the material herein.

International Standard Book Number: 978-0-323-39645-5

Senior Content Strategist: Linda Woodard
Senior Content Development Manager: Luke Held
Publishing Services Manager: Julie Eddy
Senior Project Manager: Richard Barber
Design Direction: Renee Duenow

Printed in Canada

Last digit is the print number: 9 8 7 6 5 4 3

For our students,
who continue to inspire us with their dedication
to learning while balancing life's other demands.
Every page is for you.

Contents

A complete list of the tables found throughout the text is located on the very last page of the book.

Preface

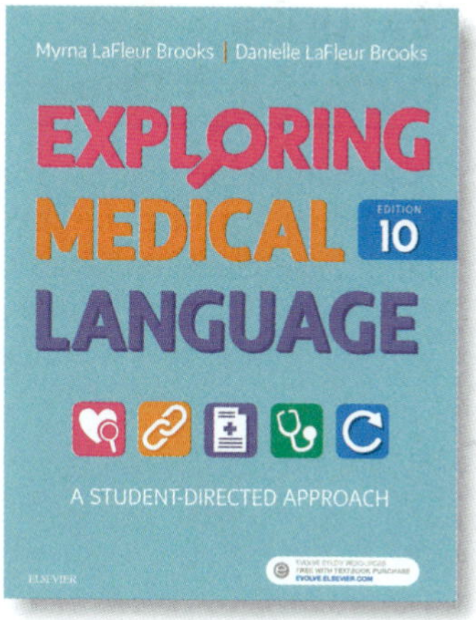

WELCOME TO THE TENTH EDITION OF *EXPLORING MEDICAL LANGUAGE*

We are excited to share this new edition of *Exploring Medical Language* with you! The tenth edition reflects knowledge we have gained working with and alongside medical terminology students and instructors over the years. In addition to updating content to reflect current use, we have refined elements of the learning system to fully engage student learning styles and enhance the development of long-term learning. Here is an overview of new and sustaining elements of our text:

New Content

- Pronunciation for anatomical terms
- Case studies with corresponding medical documentation
- New and updated term lists, diagrams, tables, and sidebar boxes
- Updated online A&P Booster
- Separate Online Gradable Quizzes for Disease and Disorder, Surgical, Diagnostic and Complementary Terms

New Instructional Strategies

- Pronunciation exercises and audio for anatomical terms
- Word part exercises directly connecting combining forms with anatomy
- Illustration exercises for suffixes and Terms NOT Built from Word Parts
- Chapter Content Quizzes
- Enhanced PowerPoint Slides with recall exercises

New Electronic Features

- Practice Student Resources on the Evolve website
- Gradable Student Resources on the Evolve website

MENU FOR PRACTICE STUDENT RESOURCES ON EVOLVE

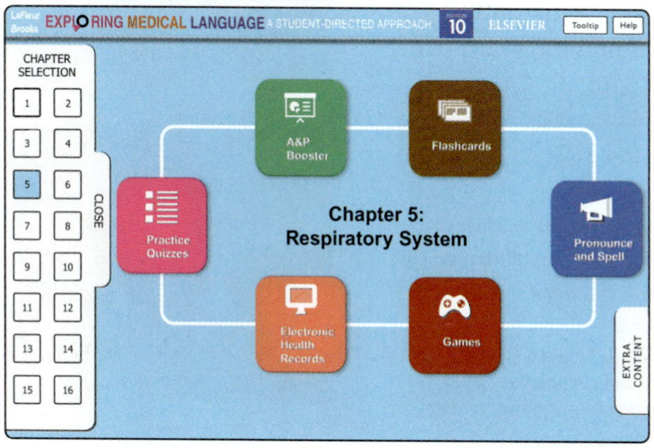

Cornerstone Features

- Paper flashcards
- Word-part learning system used to analyze, define, and build terms
- Body-system organization of content
- Term lists categorized by Terms Built from Word Parts and Terms NOT Built from Word Parts
- Subcategories of terms grouped by topic: Disease and Disorder, Surgical, Diagnostic and Complementary Terms
- Application of terms in medical documents and online EHR Modules
- Online learning opportunities aligned with the chapter objectives and exercises

Exploring Medical Language provides an effective introduction to medical language for those entering health professions as well as those in related fields, including software development, computer applications and support, insurance, law, equipment supply, pharmaceutical sales, and medical writing. Its hybrid approach of print and electronic learning tools provides a balance of hands-on and virtual experiences. A variety of ways to practice and to demonstrate learning are provided, making the textbook and companion website useful resources for a range of learning styles and classroom formats.

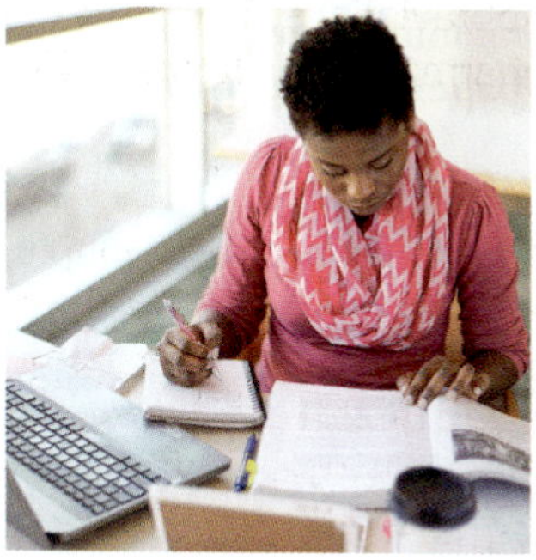

We wish you the best as you enter these pages. We remain dedicated to supporting instructors and students and invite you to follow us on our educational blog *MedTermtopics.com* and to contact us:

myrnabrooks@comcast.net
danielle.lafleurbrooks@ccv.edu

Warmly,
Myrna and Danielle

FEATURES

Outline and Objectives

Chapter introductions list sections with page numbers and student learning objectives aligned with chapter content, exercises, and assessments.

Chapter 5

Respiratory System and Introduction to Diagnostic Procedures and Tests

Objectives

Upon completion of this chapter you will be able to:

1. Pronounce organs and anatomic structures of the respiratory system.
2. Define and spell word parts related to the respiratory system.
3. Define, pronounce, and spell disease and disorder terms related to the respiratory system.
4. Define, pronounce, and spell surgical terms related to the respiratory system.

Outline

Anatomy

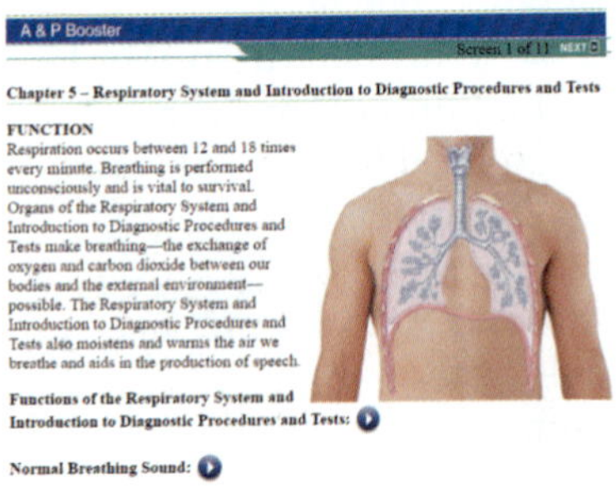

Body-system chapters introduce related anatomy and physiology (A&P). Students may supplement learning by using the **A&P Booster** available in the Practice Student Resources on the Evolve website.

NEW—**Pronunciation of organs and anatomical structures** with phonetic spelling in the textbook and audio online with Evolve Practice Student Resources.

Organs and Anatomic Structures of the Respiratory System

TERM	DEFINITION
nose (nōz)	lined with mucous membrane and fine hairs; it acts as a filter to moisten and warm the entering air
nasal septum (NĀS-el) (SEP-tum)	partition separating the right and left nasal cavities
paranasal sinuses (*par*-a-NĀ-sel) (SĪ-nus-es)	air cavities within the cranial bones that open into the nasal cavities

Word Parts

Word Part Tables present combining forms, suffixes, and prefixes related to chapter content. Textbook exercises, **paper** and **electronic flashcards,** and online activities reinforce learning.

NEW—Textbook exercises directly connecting combining forms with anatomical structures and connecting suffixes with images illustrating related medical concepts.

EXERCISE 3

Step 1: Write the definitions after the following combining forms.
Step 2: Match the descriptions on the right with the combining forms and definitions.

_____ 1. alveol/o, __________	a. tubes carrying air between the trachea and lungs
_____ 2. bronch/o, bronchi/o, __________	b. passageway for air to the bronchi from the larynx
_____ 3. pulmon/o, __________	c. spongelike organs located in the thoracic cavity
_____ 4. laryng/o, __________	d. membrane covering the lung
_____ 5. pleur/o, __________	e. lymphoid tissue located on the lateral wall at the junction of the oral cavity and oropharynx
_____ 6. thorac/o, __________	

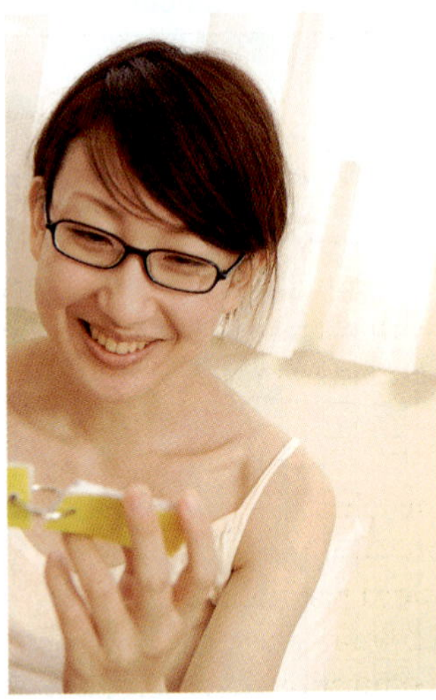

Exercise Figures

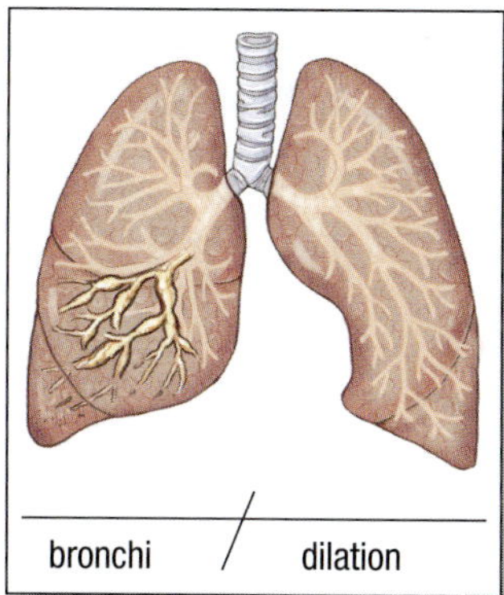

Interactive figures encourage students to apply the meaning of word parts by labeling illustrations.

Medical Terms Built From Word Parts

Students **analyze, define,** and **build** medical terms using the meaning of word parts. Learning may be extended through practice with Evolve Student Resources, including online exercises, practice quizzes, and games.

EXERCISE 13

Analyze and define the following terms by drawing slashes between word parts, writing word part abbreviations above the term, underlining combining forms, and writing combining form abbreviations below the term.

EXAMPLE: WR CV S
diaphragmat / o / cele
CF
hernia of the diaphragm

1. pleuritis ____________ ____________

7. tracheostenosis ____________ ____________

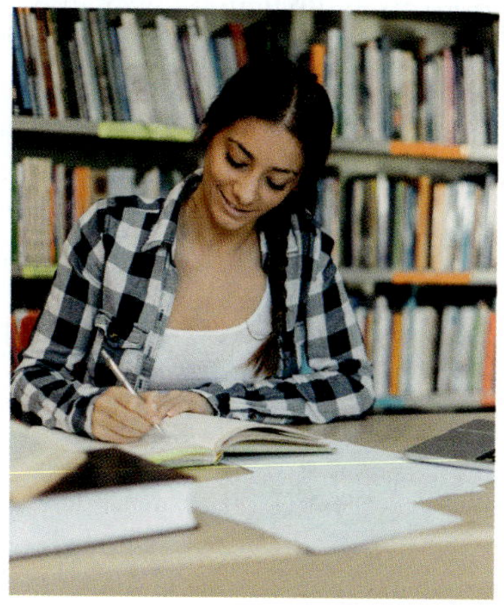

EXERCISE 14

Build disease and disorder terms for the following definitions with the word parts you have learned.

EXAMPLE: inflammation of the tonsils tonsill / itis (WR / S)

1. pain in the chest ____ / ____ (WR / S)
2. abnormal condition of fungus (infection) in the nose ____ / ____ / ____ / ____ (WR / CV / WR / S)

Medical Terms NOT Built from Word Parts

Chapters present tables of Terms NOT Built from Word Parts with corresponding illustrations and exercises.

NEW—Textbook exercises matching illustrations with medical terms NOT built from word parts. Designed to support memorization and forming connections between terms and medical concepts.

EXERCISE 15

Write the medical term pictured and defined.

1. ____________
erosion of the mucous membrane of the stomach or duodenum associated with increased secretion of acid from the stomach

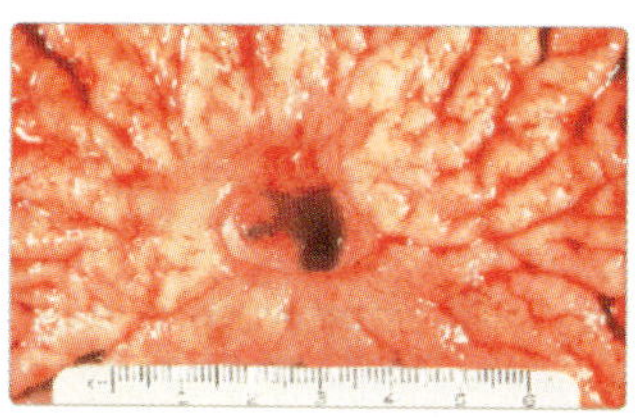

2. ____________
twisting or kinking of the intestine, causing intestinal obstruction

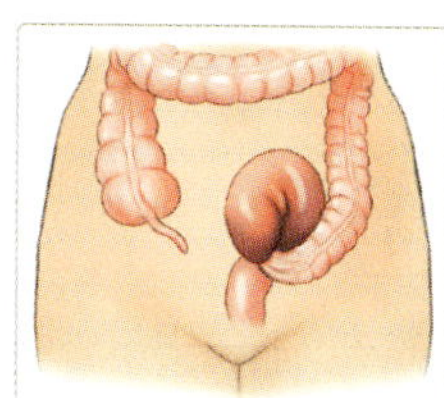

FEATURES—cont'd

Historical Perspective and Current Use

Margin boxes anchor medical language in a **historical perspective** and provide information on **current use of terms.**

> **SARCOMA**
> has been used since the time of ancient Greece to describe any fleshy tumor. Since the introduction of cellular pathology, the meaning has become **malignant connective tissue tumor.**
>
> Often, an additional word root is used to denote the type of tissue involved, such as **oste** in **osteosarcoma**, which refers to a malignant tumor of the bone.

> **INCIDENTALOMA**
> refers to a mass lesion involving an organ that is discovered unexpectedly by the use of ultrasound, computed tomography scan, or magnetic resonance imaging and has nothing to do with the patient's symptoms or primary diagnosis.

Clinical Categories and Appendices

Body-system chapters present term lists grouped by the categories of **Disease and Disorder, Surgical, Diagnostic,** and **Complementary,** the latter of which includes medical specialties, professions, signs, symptoms and other related terms. With use of additional appendices in the textbook and online, students may increase their vocabulary in the areas of Pharmacology, Health Care Delivery, Integrative Medicine, Behavioral Health, Clinical Research, Nutrition, Dentistry, and Health Information Technology.

NEW—Online Quizzes dedicated to term list categories are available in Gradable Student Resources on the Evolve website.

Quizzes >
- Quiz 1: Disease and Disorder Terms
- Quiz 2: Surgical Terms
- Quiz 3: Diagnostic Terms
- Quiz 4: Complementary Terms

Appendix N

Health Information Technology (HIT) Terms

access levels	security feature that limits access of information to the minimum necessary amount needed to perform required duties
application server provider (ASP)	external company providing computer services over a network such as an electronic health record system maintained on off-site servers (rather than locally hosted using an on-site server)
authentication	verification of the computer user or healthcare provider who is the author of the record, usually a written or electronic signature
clinical vocabulary	catalog of standardized medical terms approved to be used to describe and record health information; current clinical vocabularies in use include Systematized Nomenclature of Medicine (SNOMED), Unified Medical Language System (UMLS), and Digital Imaging and Communications in Medicine (DICOM)

Pronunciation and Spelling

Pronunciation and spelling exercises may be completed on paper or online. Students may hear terms pronounced and practice spelling online using the Practice Student Resources on the Evolve website.

NEW—Pronunciation exercises for organs and anatomical structures. Hear A&P terms pronounced online.

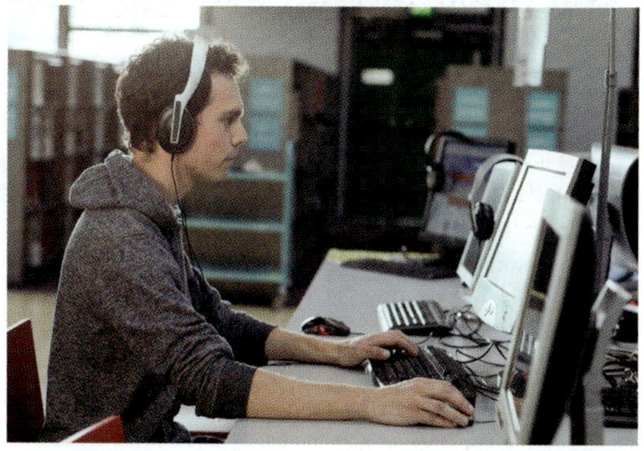

Abbreviations

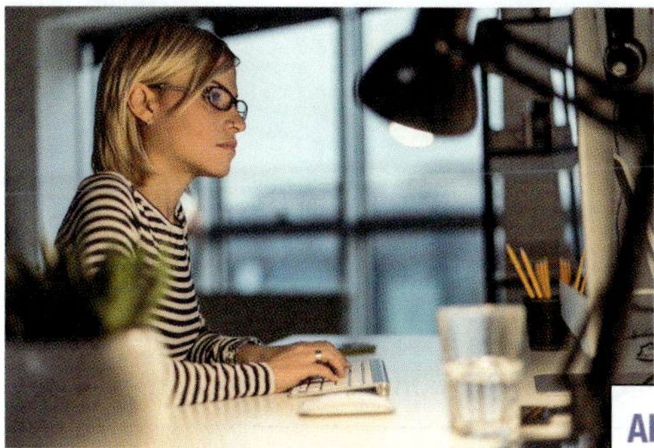

Tables introduce abbreviated medical terms related to chapter content. Textbook exercises, electronic flashcards, online exercises and practice quizzes provide practice for new learning. Students may supplement learning with additional abbreviations and error-prone abbreviations listed in Appendix E.

NEW—Online **Practice Quizzes** dedicated to abbreviations available in Practice Student Resources on the Evolve website.

Abbreviations

ABBREVIATION	TERM
ABGs	arterial blood gases
AFB	acid-fast bacilli
ARDS	acute respiratory distress syndrome

Practical Application

Students apply medical terms to case studies and medical records.

NEW—**Case Studies** and corresponding medical documentation encourage students to translate everyday language in medical language and interpret medical terms used in medical records.

EXERCISE 45 *Interact with Medical Documents and Electronic Health Records*

A. Read the report and complete it by writing medical terms on answer lines within the document. Definitions of terms to be written appear after the document.

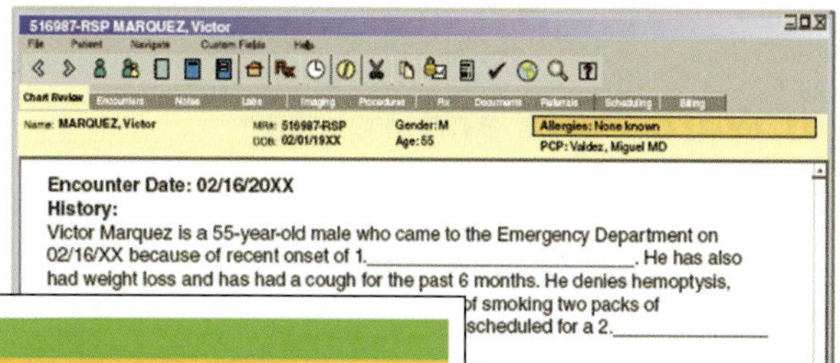

PRACTICAL APPLICATION

EXERCISE 44 *Case Study: Translate Between Everyday Language and Medical Language*

CASE STUDY: Roberta Pawlaski

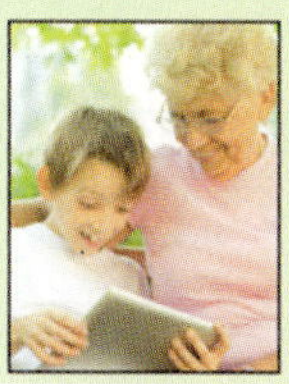

Roberta is experiencing difficulty breathing. She notices it gets worse when she tries to do chores around the house. This has been going on for about four days. She also has a cough and a runny nose. Today when she woke up she noticed that her throat was very sore. She also thinks that she might have a fever because she feels hot all over. She tried taking some over-the-counter cough medicine but this didn't seem to help. She notices when she coughs that a thick yellow mucus comes out. She hasn't had a cough like this since before she quit smoking about 10 years ago. She remembers that her grandson who stays with her after school has missed school because of a cold. She decides to call her doctor to schedule an appointment.

FEATURES—cont'd

Electronic Health Records (EHR)

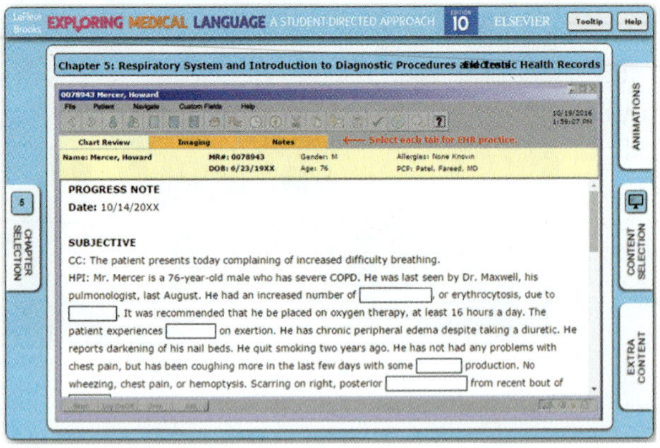

EHR Modules in Practice Student Resources on the Evolve website provide three related medical records for one patient. Students identify medical terms in context while gaining a familiarity with computer applications used in the field.

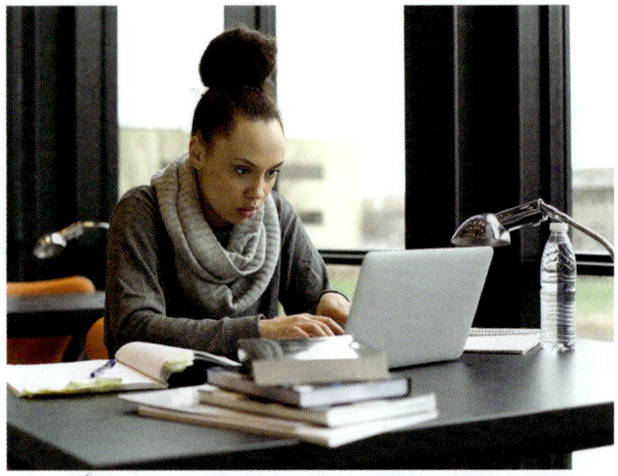

Chapter Content Quiz

NEW—Designed as a formative assessment, students can test their knowledge of chapter content by identifying medical terms used in context.

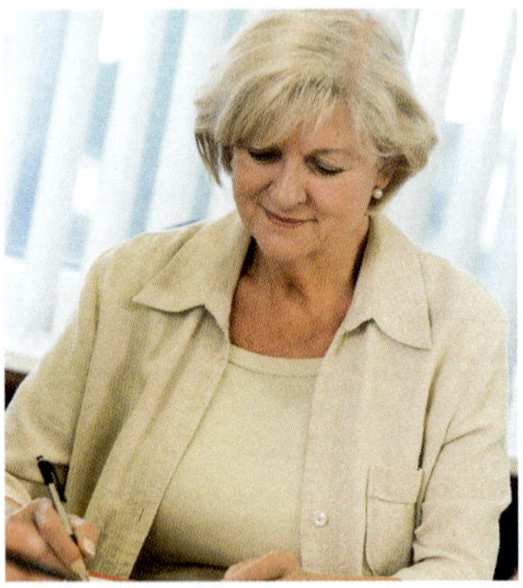

EXERCISE 47 *Chapter Content Quiz*

Test your understanding of terms and abbreviations introduced in this chapter. Circle the letter for the medical term or abbreviation related to the words in italics

1. The patient was admitted to the emergency department with a *severe nosebleed.*
   a. rhinomycosis
   b. epistaxis
   c. nasopharyngitis
2. The accident caused damage to the *larynx*, necessitating a *surgical repair.*
   a. laryngectomy
   b. laryngostomy
   c. laryngoplasty
3. Mr. Garcia was *able to breathe easier in an upright position*, so the nurse recorded that he had:
   a. orthopnea
   b. eupnea
   c. dyspnea
4. The *test on arterial blood to determine oxygen, carbon dioxide, and pH levels* indicated that the patient was *deficient in oxygen*, or had:
   a. pulse oximetry, dysphonia
   b. pulmonary functions tests, hypocapnia
   c. arterial blood gases, hypoxia

Review of Word Parts and Terms

Chapters conclude with a concise review of word parts and terms presented.

REVIEW OF WORD PARTS

Can you define and spell the following word parts?

COMBINING FORMS		PREFIXES	SUFFIXES	
adenoid/o	pharyng/o	a-	-algia	-pexy
alveol/o	phon/o			
atel/o	phren/o			

REVIEW OF TERMS

Can you define, pronounce, and spell the following terms *built from word parts?*

DISEASES AND DISORDERS	SURGICAL	DIAGNOSTIC	COMPLEMENTARY
adenoiditis	adenoidectomy	bronchoscope	acapnia
alveolitis	adenotome	bronchoscopy	alveolar
atelectasis	bronchoplasty	capnometer	anoxia

Online Evolve Resources

Evolve Resources provide multiple ways to practice and assess learning.

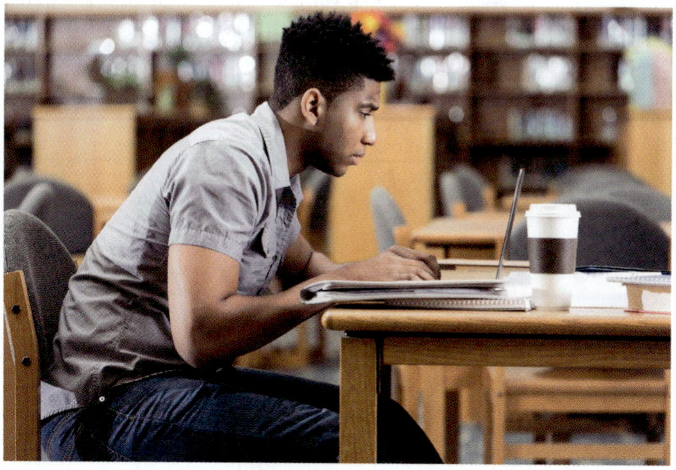

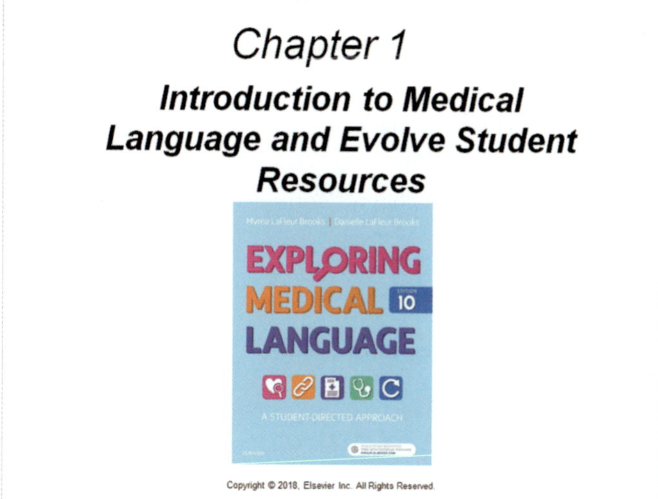

Practice Student Resources

- A&P Booster
- Word Part and Abbreviation Flashcards
- Pronounce & Spell
- Games
- Electronic Health Records
- Practice Quizzes

Mobile Resources

- Word Part and Abbreviation Flashcards
- Practice Quizzes

Gradable Student Resources

- Exercises
- Quizzes

Instructor Resources

- Course Tools
- Lesson Plans
- PowerPoints
- Test Bank

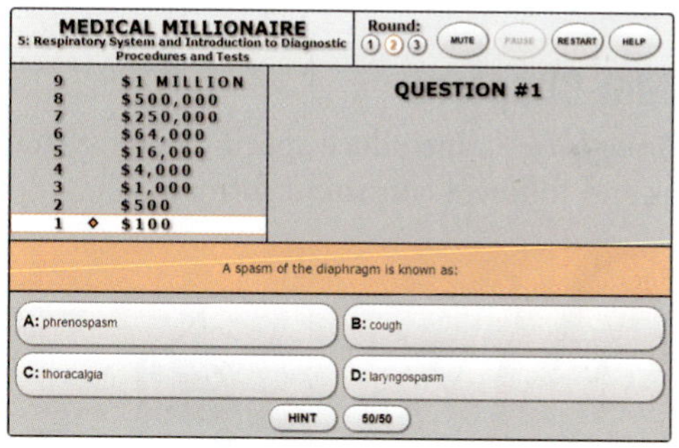

ORGANIZATION OF THE TEXTBOOK

Chapters 1 through 3 provide the foundation for building a medical vocabulary. Chapters 4 through 16 organize content by body systems, presenting related word parts, terms, and abbreviations. The textbook concludes with a series of appendices designed to extend student learning as desired.

Introductory Chapters

Chapter 1 … may be the most important chapter in the text, because you will apply the knowledge acquired here in the rest of the chapters to learn terms in an easy, quick fashion. The chapter introduces the two categories of terms—those built from word parts and those which are not; each category is accompanied by different types of exercises. Also introduced in this chapter are the **four word parts**—word root, suffix, prefix, and combining vowel, which are the basis of terms built from word parts category.

EXAMPLE **INTRAVENOUS**	WORD PART	MEANING
prefix	intra-	within
word root	ven	vein
suffix	-ous	pertaining to
term = p + wr + s	intra/ven/ous	pertaining to within a vein

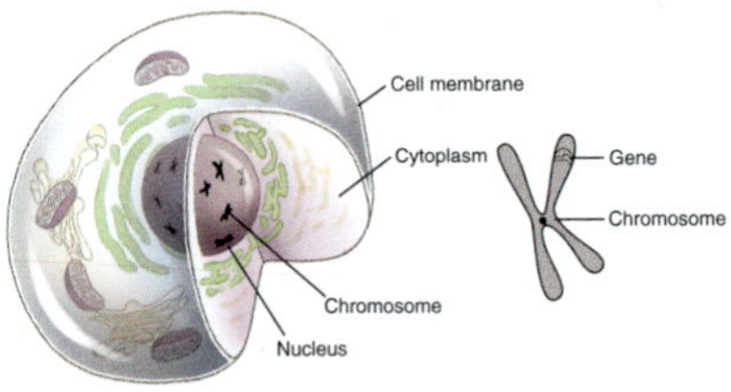

Chapter 2 … introduces **body structure** and immediately provides practice in recognizing the two categories of terms along with corresponding exercises for each. You will likely be surprised at how fast you learn the meaning and spelling of many medical terms.

Chapter 3 … introduces directional terms, planes, positions, regions, and quadrants, providing a framework for understanding the body systems and their related terms.

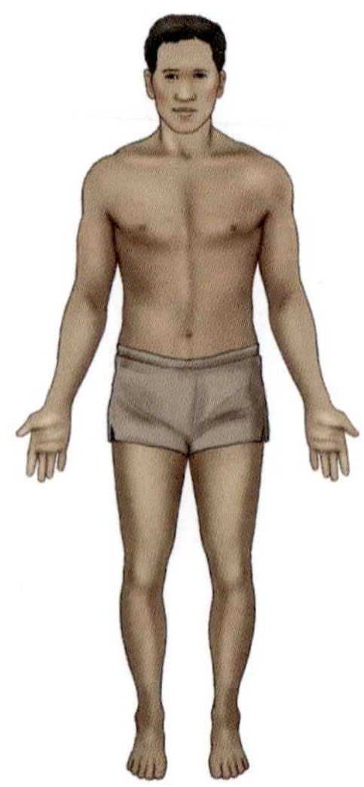

Body System Chapters

Chapters 4 through 16 … introduce specific body systems with related word parts, terms, and abbreviations and follow a consistent format.

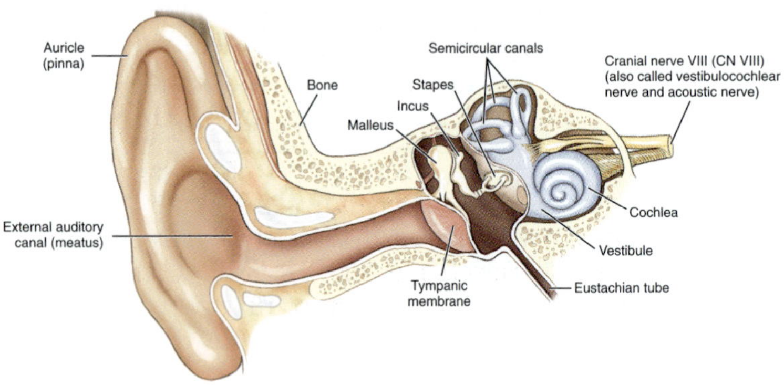

Appendices

Appendices A-F … appear in the textbook and provide an answer key for chapter exercises, directions for Student Evolve Resources, comprehensive lists of word parts and abbreviations, a list of error-prone abbreviations, and pharmacology terms.

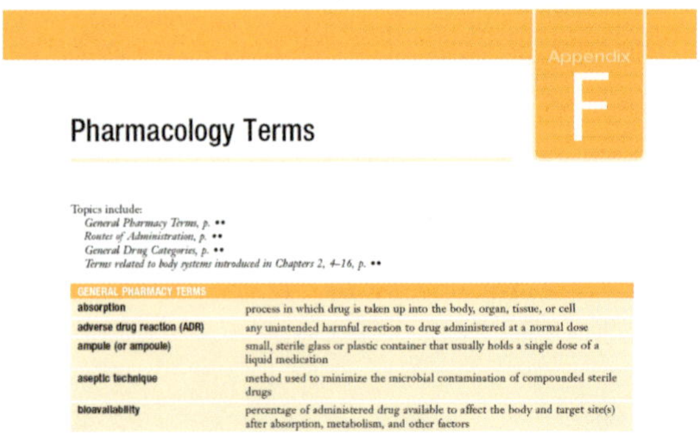
Appendix F

Pharmacology Terms

Topics include:
General Pharmacy Terms, p. ••
Routes of Administration, p. ••
General Drug Categories, p. ••
Terms related to body systems introduced in Chapters 2, 4–16, p. ••

GENERAL PHARMACY TERMS	
absorption	process in which drug is taken up into the body, organ, tissue, or cell
adverse drug reaction (ADR)	any unintended harmful reaction to drug administered at a normal dose
ampule (or ampoule)	small, sterile glass or plastic container that usually holds a single dose of a liquid medication
aseptic technique	method used to minimize the microbial contamination of compounded sterile drugs
bioavailability	percentage of administered drug available to affect the body and target site(s) after absorption, metabolism, and other factors

Appendices G-N … in Practice Student Resources on the Evolve website provide lists of additional word parts, Health Care Delivery Terms, Integrative Medicine Terms, Behavioral Health Terms, Nutrition Terms, Dental Terms, and Health Information Technology Terms. Online appendices may be found by clicking on the Extra Content tab from the main menu.

ANATOMY OF A CHAPTER

Let's take a look at the structure of body system chapter using Chapter 5 on the respiratory system as an example.

Objectives and Chapter Outline, p. 128

ANATOMY

WORD PARTS

MEDICAL TERMS

PRACTICAL APPLICATION

CHAPTER REVIEW

DEAR STUDENT

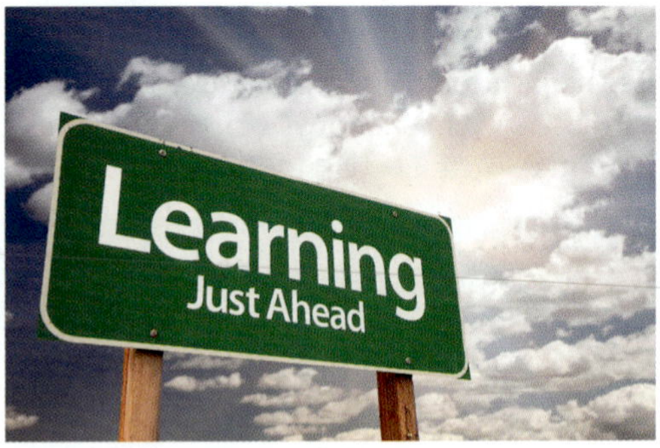

If you are reading this, you are most likely enrolled in a medical terminology course and preparing for your journey of learning medical language using this textbook. As you flip through the pages of *Exploring Medical Language* you may be thinking, "There is so much to learn. How will I do it?" or "Why are there so many exercises?"

Let us assure you that you will acquire the language in a quick and easy manner by completing chapter exercises. While it may seem daunting at first, we encourage you to be as active as possible as you read and work through chapter.

The exercises approach the terms from all angles: pronunciation, writing, defining, spelling, and application. Chapter content flows from one chapter to the next in a repetitive manner, making the best use of one's time. You may build a foundational medical vocabulary by using the textbook alone, and you may choose to extend your learning by utilizing Evolve Student Resources, which provide supplemental materials online.

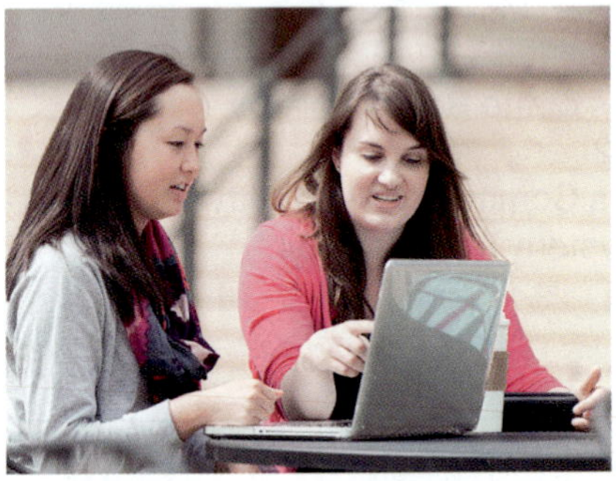

We wish you the best as you embark on this journey. You will join a select group of students who have used *Exploring Medical Language* as a textbook for over 30 years. We would like to hear of your experiences with *Exploring Medical Language*, including exercises that were most useful, suggestions for improvement, and so forth. Reach us by e-mail at the following addresses:

danielle.lafleurbrooks@ccv.edu (Danielle)
myrnabrooks@comcast.net (Myrna)

We also invite you to visit our medical terminology educational blog **MedTerm Topics** at **medtermtopics.com**. Follow the blog while you are a student and after you finish your course to help you build on your vocabulary in a fun and engaging way. Posts include quizzes, crosswords, videos, word scrambles, and introductions to emerging medical terms.

Sincerely,
Myrna and Danielle

ONLINE LEARNING RESOURCES, EVOLVE.ELSEVIER.COM

Evolve Resources provide practice activities, gradable exercises and quizzes, and resources that can be accessed from a portable device. Practice Student Resources are available to supplement your learning and scores are for student use only. If your instructor sets up a course site on Evolve and creates a gradebook, scores on Gradable Student Resources may populate your instructor's gradebook. Gradable Student Resources are available to all students whether or not your instructor chooses to record scores.

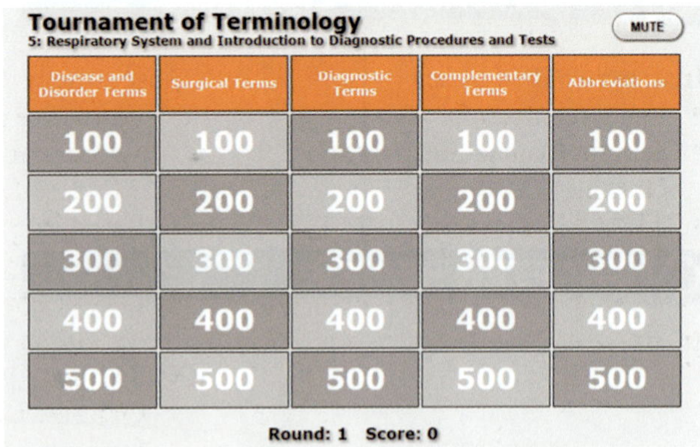

Practice Student Resources
- A&P Booster Tutorials
- Word Part and Abbreviation Flashcards
- Pronunciation and Spelling
- Electronic Health Record Modules
- Games
- Practice Quizzes
- Career Videos
- Additional Appendices with Term Lists by Medical Specialty

Mobile Resources
- Word Part and Abbreviation Flashcards
- Practice Quizzes

Gradable Student Resources
- Exercises: Word Parts, Terms Built from Word Parts, Terms NOT Built from Word Parts, and Abbreviations
- Quizzes: Disease and Disorder, Surgical, Diagnostic, and Complementary Terms

DEAR INSTRUCTOR

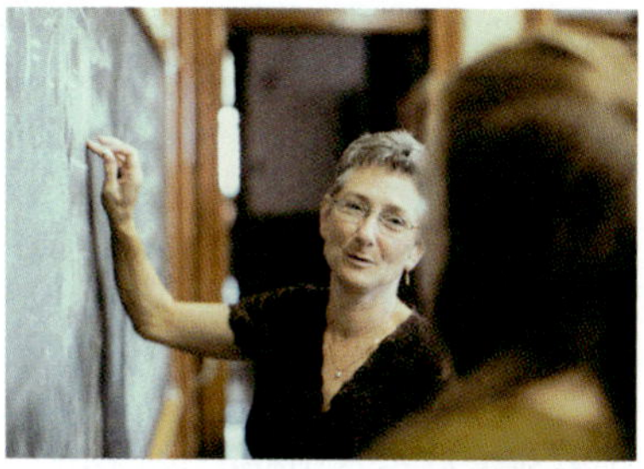

Thank you for choosing *Exploring Medical Language*! We hope you find this learning system supportive of your teaching methods and effective for your students' learning styles. With the textbook, students receive paper flashcards for word parts and access to Evolve Resources for Students. You may find the flashcards and online resources, such as pronunciation for term lists and games, useful for class activities and exam preparation.

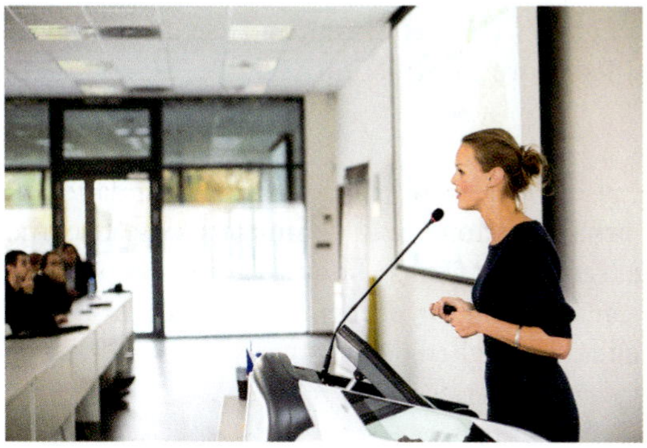

Additional teaching materials are available online at **evolve.elsevier.com** within Evolve Resources for Instructors. All resources are objective based, and we recommend beginning with the TEACH Lesson Plans for an overview of how to use the various teaching tools. The first step in accessing teaching materials is to register for the *Exploring Medical Language* 10e Evolve Resources. Please, visit evolve.elsevier.com or call 1-800-222-9570 to register.

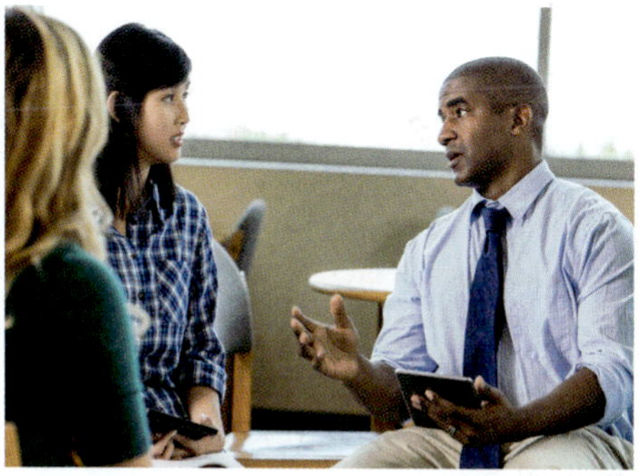

We welcome your comments and questions by email. Danielle, who currently teaches medical terminology in the traditional classroom, online, and in hybrid formats, is also happy to share ideas and materials. Contact us at

danielle.lafleurbrooks@ccv.edu
myrnabrooks@comcast.net

We also invite you to visit our medical terminology educational blog MedTerm Topics at medtermtopics.com to keep up with trends in teaching medical terminology and emerging medical language.

Looking forward to hearing from you,
Danielle and Myrna

ONLINE TEACHING RESOURCES, EVOLVE.ELSEVIER.COM

Instructor Resources
- Image Collection
- Sample Course Syllabus and Outline
- TEACH Handouts
- TEACH Lesson Plans
- TEACH PowerPoint Slides
- Test Bank

Assessment
- Formative and summative assessment plan for each lesson, TEACH Lesson Plans in Evolve Resources for Instructors
- Pretest and Posttest, TEACH Lesson Plans, in Evolve Resources for Instructors
- Practice Quizzes and Gradable Quizzes, Evolve Resources for Students
- Test Bank to build quizzes and exams, Evolve Resources for Instructors

Course Tools
- Gradebook, which populates with scores from Gradable Student Resources
- Calendar
- Discussion forums
- Assignments
- Quizzes and Exams

Using Course Tools, a course site may be created. The course will be assigned a unique ID that students will use to log in. The course may be hosted on Evolve or converted to another platform.

For assistance in registering for Evolve Resources and Course Tools, call **1-800-222-9570** or visit **evolvesupport.elsevier.com**

ADDITIONAL LEARNING AND TEACHING RESOURCES

Mosby's Medical Terminology Online

Mosby's Medical Terminology Online to accompany *Exploring Medical Language* is a great resource to supplement your textbook. This web-delivered course supplement provides a range of visual, auditory, and interactive elements to reinforce your learning and synthesize concepts presented in the text. Objective-based quizzes at the end of each section and an end-of-module exam provide you with self-testing tools. In addition, related Internet resources may be accessed by links provided throughout the program.

Instructors interested in Mosby's Medical Terminology Online, please contact your sales rep, call Faculty Support at 1-800-222-9570, or visit http://evolve.elsevier.com/LaFleur/Exploring/ for more information.

AudioTerms

The AudioTerms that accompany *Exploring Medical Language* include pronunciations and definitions. Because the AudioTerms include definitions, they are an additional tool for learning and reviewing terms. They are especially helpful when using your book is impractical, such as when you are driving in a car, walking, or doing daily chores. You may purchase the AudioTerms separately or packaged with the book for a small additional cost.

Contributors

Richard K. Brooks, MD, FACP, FACG
Internal Medicine and Gastroenterology
Mayo Clinic (retired)
Quechee, Vermont
Clinical Instructor
Geisel School of Medicine
Dartmouth College
Appendix H—Health Care Delivery Terms (Evolve website)

Catherine J. Cerulli, PhD
Director
Interwoven Healing Arts
Integrative Practitioner
University of Vermont Medical Center
Montpelier, Vermont
Appendix I—Integrative Medicine Terms (Evolve website)

Christine Costa, BS, GCM, HUC
Geriatric Care Manager
Tempe, Arizona
Appendix C—Combining Forms, Prefixes, and Suffixes Alphabetized By Word Part
Appendix D—Combining Forms, Prefixes, and Suffixes Alphabetized By Definition
Appendix E—Abbreviations
Appendix G—Additional Combining Forms, Prefixes, and Suffixes (Evolve website)
Evolve Resources (Evolve website)

Cynthia Heiss, PhD, RD
Professor
Department of Healthcare Professions
Metropolitan State University of Denver
Denver, Colorado
Appendix L—Nutrition Terms (Evolve website)

Erinn Kao, PharmD, BCNP
GE Medical
St. Louis, Missouri
Appendix F—Pharmacology Terms

Dale M. Levinsky, MD
Clinical Associate Professor
Department of Family and Community Medicine
College of Medicine
University of Arizona
Tucson, Arizona
Clinical Instructor
Pharmacy Practice-Science
College of Pharmacy
University of Arizona
Tucson, Arizona
Chapter 10—Cardiovascular, Immune, Lymphatic Systems and Blood
Chapter 11—Digestive System
Chapter 14—Musculoskeletal System
Chapter 15—Nervous System and Behavioral Health
Chapter 16—Endocrine System
Case Studies
Medical Records
Electronic Health Records (Evolve website)

Caroline M. Murphy, DDS
General Practice Dentist
Montpelier, Vermont
Appendix M—Dental Terms (Evolve website)

Bernard S. Nandiego, MD
Child Psychiatry Fellow
Child and Adolescent Psychiatry Department
University of Arizona
Tucson, Arizona
Appendix J—Behavioral Health Terms (Evolve website)

Cris E. Wells, EdD, MBA, CCRP, RT(R)(M)
Assistant Professor/Director of Interprofessional Programs and the Clinical Research Management Master of Science Program
Arizona State University, College of Nursing and Health Innovation
Phoenix, Arizona
Appendix K—Clinical Research Terms (Evolve website)

Reviewers and Advisors

Delena Kay Austin, BTIS, CMA (AAMA)
Health Science Technology Faculty
Macomb Community College
Warren, Michigan

Cynthia Ann Bjerklie, BS
Instructor
Community College of Vermont
Montpelier, Vermont

William Bohnert, MD
Past President, American Urological Association
CDI Consultant, Dignity Health
St. Joseph's Hospital
Phoenix, Arizona

Julene Bredeson, CMA (AAMA), PHN, BSN, RN
Medical Assistant Instructor
Ridgewater College
Willmar, Minnesota

Richard K. Brooks, MD, FACP, FACG
Internal Medicine and Gastroenterology
Mayo Clinic (retired)
Clinical Instructor
Geisel School of Medicine
Dartmouth College
Quechee, Vermont

Sharon A. Brooks, MSN, BA, RN
Practical Nursing Program Director
Sumner College
Portland, Oregon

Ruth Buchner, MEd
Family and Consumer Science / Health Science Educator
Chippewa Falls High School
Chippewa Falls, Wisconsin

Christine Costa, BS, GCM, HUC
Geriatric Care Manager
Tempe, Arizona

Angela Dawson-Walker, CMA, LVN
Apple Valley Unified School District
Apple Valley, California

Christopher Fields, OD
Optometrist
Fields of Vision Eye Care, Inc.
Lebanon, New Hampshire

Robert L. Fortune, MD
Cardiovascular Surgery (retired)
Scottsdale, Arizona

Janet Funk, MD
Associate Professor of Medicine & Nutritional Sciences
The University of Arizona Cancer Center
Phoenix, Arizona

Deborah Greer, MEd, RT(R)(M)
Program Director-RT Education
Penn Medicine
Philadelphia, Pennsylvania

Jane A. Hlopko, MA, RHIA
Department Chairman, Associate Professor, Health Information Technology
SUNY Broome Community College
Binghamton, New York

Colleen Horan, MD
Gynecologist and Obstetrician
Central Vermont Medical Center
Berlin, Vermont

Marjorie "Meg" Holloway, MS, RN, APRN
Instructor, Foundations of Medicine and Leader, Medicine & Healthcare Strand
Blue Valley CAPS
Overland Park, Kansas

Bradley D. Johnson, MEd, RT(R)(ARRT)
Faculty, Medical Radiography
Gateway Community College
Phoenix, Arizona

Sheri Lavadour, RN, BSN, HTP
Sumner College of Nursing, Instructor
Portland, Oregon

Dale M. Levinsky, MD
Clinical Associate Professor
Department of Family and Community Medicine
College of Medicine
University of Arizona
Tucson, Arizona
Clinical Instructor
Pharmacy Practice—Science
College of Pharmacy
University of Arizona
Tucson, Arizona

Kara Stuart Lewis, MD
Phoenix Children's Hospital
Phoenix, Arizona

Charles Machia
Billing Customer Service
University of Vermont Medical Center
Burlington, Vermont

Melody Miller, LPN
Medical Assistant Instructor
Lancaster County Career and Technology Center
Willow Street, Philadelphia

Karen O'Neill, BA
Essex Junction, Vermont

Veronique M. Parker, MBA (Healthcare Management)
Faculty
Maricopa Community Colleges
Phoenix, Arizona

Stephen M. Picca, MD
Mandl School: The College of Applied Health
New York, New York

Maynard D. Poland, MD
Internal Medicine Board—Certified
Retired:
Medical Practice & Medical Director,
Milwaukee Medical Clinic and Columbia—St. Mary's Hospitals, Milwaukee, Wisconsin
Assistant Clinical Professor, Medical College of Wisconsin
Adjunct Faculty, Edison State College, Ft. Myers, Florida

Toni L. Rodriguez, EdD, RRT, FAARC
Program Director
Respiratory Care Program
GateWay Community College
Phoenix, Arizona

Patricia L. Shinn, PhD, RN
Chair, Nursing Department
River Valley Community College
Claremont, New Hampshire

Charlene Thiessen, MEd, CMT, AHDI-F
Program Director, Medical Transcription
GateWay Community College
Phoenix, Arizona

Ann Vadala, BA
Professor, Office Administration
St. Lawrence College
Kingston, Ontario

Kari Williams, BS, DC
Program Director
Front Range Community College
Longmont, Colorado

Dokagari Woods, RN, PhD
Assistant Professor of Nursing, Undergraduate Program Director
Tarleton State University
Stephenville, Texas

Acknowledgments

We are incredibly lucky to be supported by a team of skilled professionals who worked tirelessly in creating the 10th edition of *Exploring Medical Language*. We are grateful for the time, effort, and talents of the following individuals:

Luke Held, Content Development Manager, who guided us through the revision process, all the while demonstrating exceptional patience, follow-through, and dedication. He expertly coordinated elements of production while supporting our vision for the 10th edition. His work made all elements of this project possible, and we are particularly thankful for his problem-solving and communication skills.

Linda Woodard, Content Strategist, who inspired efforts to create a full accessible learning system and who has supported the ongoing development of our work over the years. We treasure her insight and guidance.

Richard Barber, Senior Project Manager, who led the production process in a kind and thoughtful manner.

Greg Utz, Multimedia Producer, who helped us create the most effective Evolve Resources possible.

Contributors listed on page xvii and Reviewers and Advisors listed on pages xviii–xix who shared their expertise, knowledge, and precious time.

Dale Levinsky, MD, who joined us as a contributor and skillfully applied her clinical knowledge and resources to revising Chapters 10, 11, 14, 15, and 16; writing and reviewing case studies and medical records; and reviewing EHR modules and the A&P Booster on Practice Student Resources on Evolve. She generously shared her time and medical knowledge, and her work has elevated the quality of content shared in the textbook and online.

Chris Costa, who assisted with the revision of Evolve Student Resources, TEACH instructional materials, and Appendices C-F and G, as well as spending many hours searching through content with a tireless concern for accuracy. Her attention to detail, range of professional experiences, and knowledge of health care have been essential in creating effective learning tools for students and dynamic instructional materials for teachers.

Carolyn Kruse, for using her linguistic knowledge and pleasing voice for updating pronunciation, both in print and audio.

Jeanne Robertson, Medical Illustrator, whose art has brought to life many medical concepts. We have the greatest respect for her attention to detail and ability to bring beauty to technical images.

Richard K. Brooks, MD, who revised Appendix H and reviewed and assisted with revisions for all content in the text. He has been there for us every step of the way.

Winifred K. Starr (1921-1993), who was Myrna's first coauthor and whose creative contributions remain in the text today.

Faculty, who have adopted the text to use in their classrooms and have used their valuable time to give us feedback.

Students, who over the years have worn thin the pages of previous editions. Your pursuit of knowledge has been truly inspirational.

Each page of the 10th Edition is better because of your collective contributions.

Thank you.

Chapter 1

Introduction to Medical Language and Evolve Student Resources

Outline

Objectives

Upon completion of this chapter you will be able to:

1. Create an account and register on the Evolve website.
2. Describe the origins of medical language.
3. Define two categories of medical terms.
4. Identify and define the four word parts and the combining form.
5. Analyze and define medical terms.
6. Build medical terms for given definitions.

ONLINE LEARNING: EVOLVE RESOURCES FOR STUDENTS

Online learning tools are available to students through Evolve Resources hosted on the publisher's website at www.evolve.elsevier.com (Fig. 1.1). Evolve Resources provide many ways to see, hear, and practice chapter content. The platform also grades answers and gives immediate feedback to help focus study efforts. The Evolve icon ⓔ is placed throughout the text to guide you to the website at the appropriate time to maximize learning opportunities. While there are variations between chapters, generally Evolve Resources include:

Practice Student Resources
A&P Booster
Flashcards
Pronounce and Spell
Games
Electronic Health Records
Practice Quizzes

Graded Student Resources*
Word Parts
Terms Built from Word Parts
Terms NOT Built from Word Parts
Abbreviations
Quizzes

**Scores may be recorded in the gradebook if your instructor has created an Evolve course for your class.*

Mobile Resources
Flashcards
Practice Quizzes

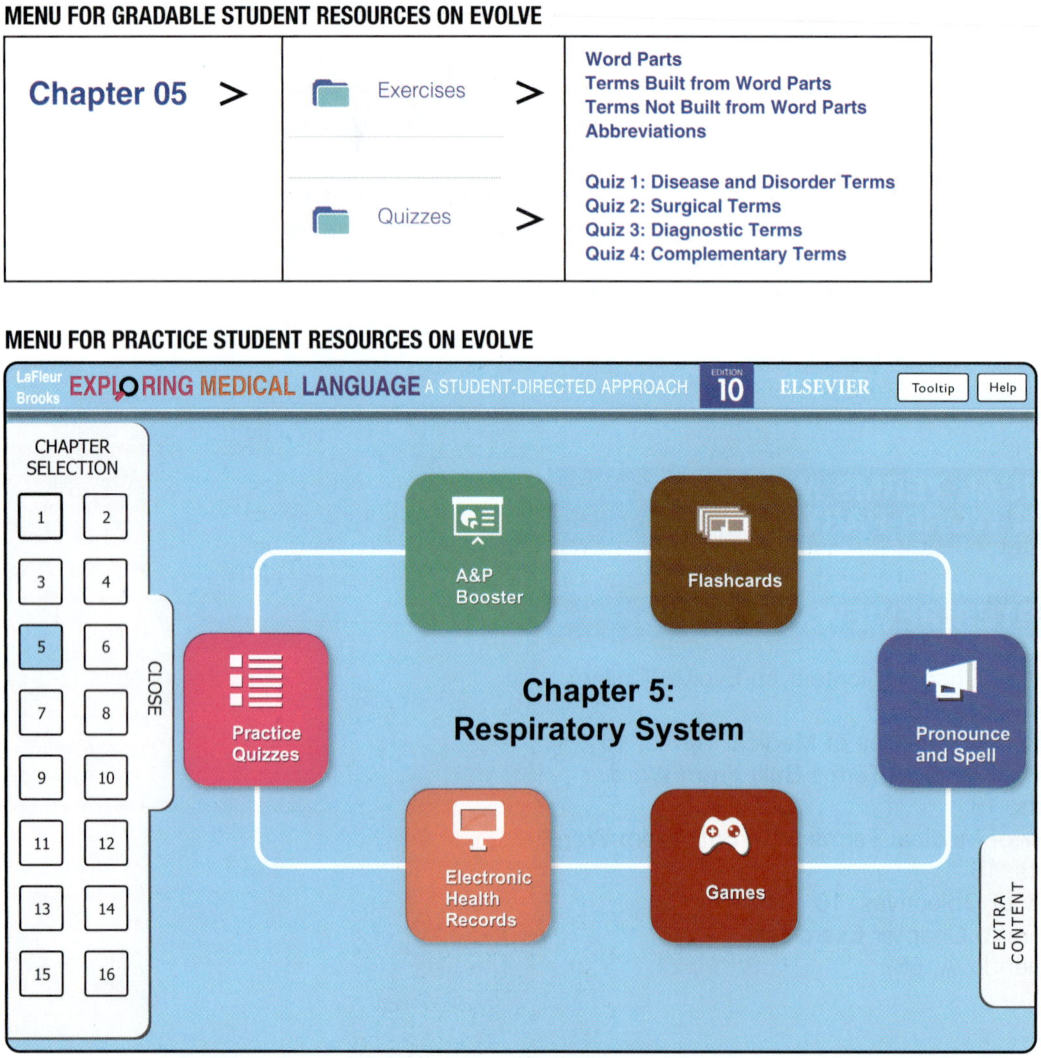

FIG. 1.1 Online menus for **Gradable Student Resources** and **Practice Student Resources** available at evolve.elsevier.com. **Career Videos** and **Appendices** of additional medical terms are available under the **Extra Content** tab.

Create an Account and Register

EXERCISE 1

Use the steps below as a starting place to create an account and register for Evolve Resources for *Exploring Medical Language, 10th edition.* Technical help may be reached by calling **1-800-222-9570**.

1. Go to evolve.elsevier.com and click on the link for students.
2. Search by author or title keyword (LaFleur Brooks or *Exploring Medical Language, 10th edition).*
3. Select Evolve Resources for *Exploring Medical Language, 10th edition.*
4. Follow the links to request the product (Evolve Resources) and to Redeem/Checkout.
5. Returning users enter Evolve username, password, and follow the links to login. New users register for an account and follow the links to continue; account information will be emailed.
6. Click the **Registered User Agreement** link located at the bottom right. Check the *Yes, I accept the Registered User Agreement* box if you agree. Follow the links to submit.
7. Follow the links to get started and access your **Resources** located on **My Evolve**.
8. Visit and bookmark evolve.elsevier.com/student for future login.

❑ Check the box when complete.

Registration steps may change as the Evolve website is updated. If difficulties arise, please:

- Call Evolve Support at **1-800-222-9570.**
- Type **evolve technical support center** in your search engine and link to the support webpage, where updated directions for registration and a video illustrating registration steps can be found.

INTRODUCTION TO MEDICAL TERMS AND MEDICAL LANGUAGE

Medical terms are words used to describe disease as well as aspects of medicine and health care. Terms built from Greek and Latin word parts, eponyms, acronyms, and modern language are types of medical terms.

Medical language or terminology is the use of medical terms to attain a standardized means of communication within the practice of medicine and in the healthcare industry. The need for fluency in medical language cannot be exaggerated.

Why are many medical terms different than words we use in everyday life? Medical language allows for clear, concise and consistent communication locally, nationally, and internationally. It enables everyone involved in medicine and health care to perform more accurately and efficiently for the patient's benefit. For example, using the medical term **osteoarthritis** (Fig. 1.2), which means **inflammation of the bone and joint,** offers a clear and concise written or verbal communication using one word instead of six. No matter the national language used, the meaning of the medical term does not change.

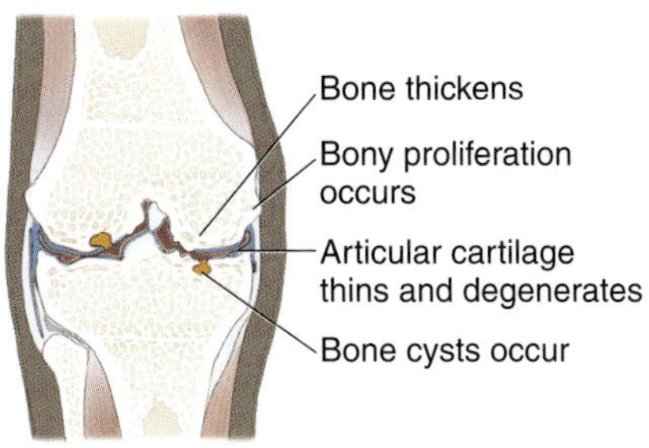

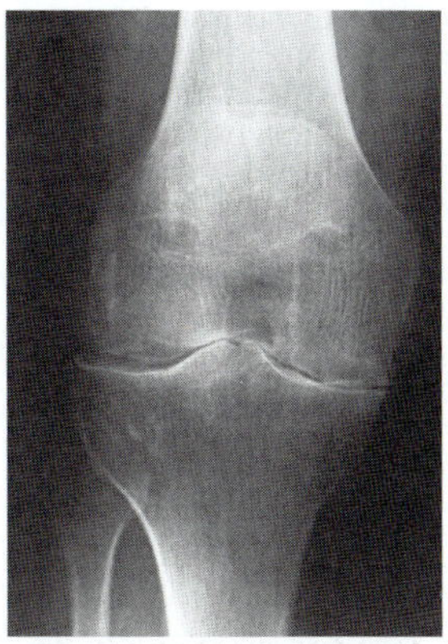

FIG. 1.2 Osteoarthritis of the knee joint, illustration and radiograph.

Origins of Medical Language

The vocabulary of medical language reflects its development over time beginning with the ancient Greeks. More than 2,000 years ago Hippocrates and Aristotle were among the first to study and write about medicine. The Romans continued the practice, adopting elements of the Greek language to use alongside Latin. The majority of terms in use today are **built from Greek and Latin word parts**. For learning purposes these terms are categorized as **Terms Built from Word Parts** in this textbook.

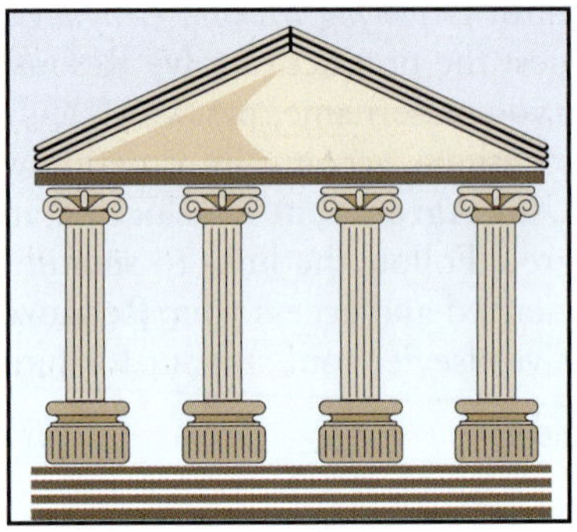

Greek and **Latin** Terms are built from word parts, such as *arthritis*.

As scientific knowledge, medical technology, and medical practice evolved so did the language of medicine, which now also includes **eponyms, acronyms, and terms from modern language**. Eponyms are terms derived from a name or place. Acronyms are terms formed from the first letters of a phrase. Modern language refers to terms from the English language, which are often descriptive of technology and procedures. For learning purposes these terms are categorized as **Terms NOT Built from Word Parts** in this textbook.

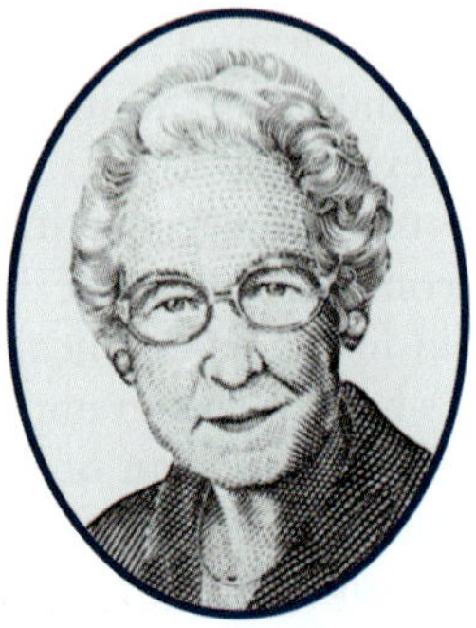

Eponyms are terms derived from the name of a person or place. Examples include **Apgar score**, named after the person who developed it, and **West Nile virus**, named after the first geographical location the virus was identified.

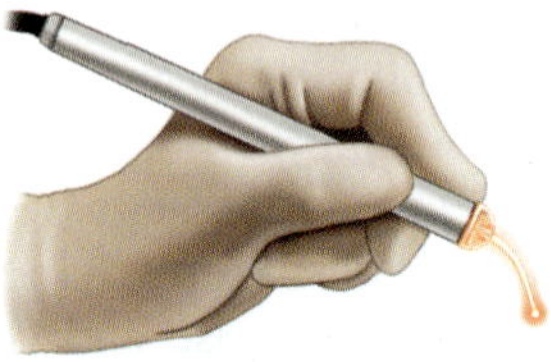

Acronyms, such as **laser** (light amplification by stimulated emission of radiation), are terms formed from the first letters of words in a phrase. Acronyms usually contain a vowel and are spoken as a whole word.

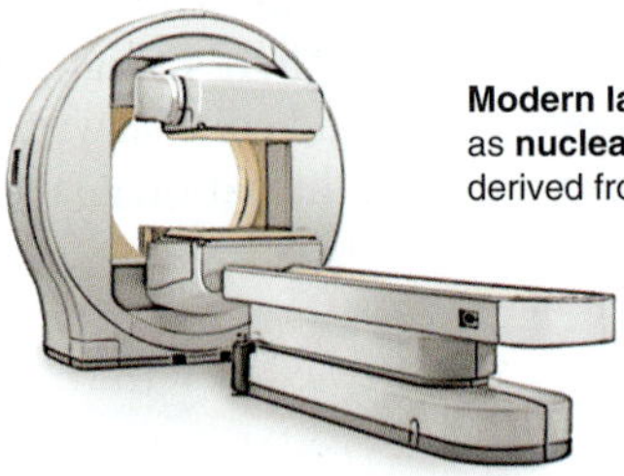

Modern language terms, such as **nuclear medicine scanner,** are derived from the English language.

VIRGINIA APGAR
an obstetric anesthesiologist born in New Jersey, developed the Apgar score in 1952 to measure the physical condition of the newborn.

EXERCISE 2

Place the letter from the first column to identify the origin of the term in the second column. You may use an answer more than once. *To check your answers to the exercises in this chapter, go to Appendix A at the back of the textbook.*

a. Greek and Latin word parts	_____ 1. West Nile virus
b. eponym	_____ 2. hepatitis
c. acronym	_____ 3. MRSA (methicillin-resistant *Staphylococcus aureus*)
d. modern language	_____ 4. posttraumatic stress disorder
	_____ 5. arthritis
	_____ 6. nuclear medicine scanner
	_____ 7. AIDS (acquired immunodeficiency syndrome)
	_____ 8. Alzheimer disease

ALZHEIMER DISEASE VS. ALZHEIMER'S DISEASE

The need for clarity and consistency in medical language has resulted in the **modern trend to eliminate the possessive form of eponyms and use instead the non-possessive form**. The non-possessive form is observed by the Association for Healthcare Documentation Integrity, the American Medical Association's Manual of Style, in most medical dictionaries, and is the style used throughout this textbook. With either use, the noun that follows is not capitalized.

Categories of Medical Terms and Learning Methods

All medical terms in the text are divided into two categories arranged according to the learning method of each (Table 1.1):

1. terms built from word parts
2. terms NOT built from word parts

Terms Built from Word Parts can be translated literally to find their meaning. Analyzing, defining, and building terms using word parts are used as learning methods. **Terms NOT Built from Word Parts** cannot be translated literally. Recalling, matching, and defining exercises are used as the learning methods.

TABLE 1.1 Categories of Medical Terms and Learning Methods

Category	Origin	Example	Learning Methods
Terms Built from Word Parts (can be translated literally to find their meaning)	1. Word parts of Greek and Latin origin placed together to form terms that can be translated literally to find their meanings	1. arthr/itis	1. Analyzing terms 2. Defining terms 3. Building terms
Terms NOT Built from Word Parts (cannot be easily translated literally to find their meaning)	1. Eponyms, terms derived from the name of a person or place 2. Acronyms, terms formed from the first letters of a phrase that can be spoken as a whole word and usually contains a vowel 3. Modern language, terms derived from the English language 4. Terms of Greek and Latin word parts that cannot be easily translated to find their meanings	1. Alzheimer disease 2. MRSA (methicillin-resistant *Staphylococcus aureus*) 3. complete blood count and differential 4. orthopedics	1. Recalling terms 2. Matching terms 3. Defining terms

EXERCISE 3

Complete the following. *To check your answers, go to Appendix A.*

Medical terms ______ ______ ______ ______ can be translated literally to find their meaning, whereas medical terms ______ ______ ______ ______ ______ cannot be easily translated literally to find their meaning.

MEDICAL TERMS BUILT FROM WORD PARTS

Terms built from word parts are composed of Greek and Latin **word roots, prefixes,** and **suffixes** and can be translated literally to find their meanings. A **combining vowel** is often added to ease pronunciation (Table 1.2 and Table 1.3). Techniques to learn these terms are **analyzing, defining,** and **building** medical terms.

Four Word Parts

Most medical terms built from word parts consist of some or all of the following components:

1. Word root
2. Prefix
3. Suffix
4. Combining vowel

WORD ROOT

The word root is the word part that is the core of the word. The word root contains the fundamental meaning of the word.

EXAMPLES

In the word	play/er, *play* is the word root.
In the medical term	arthr/itis, *arthr* (which means *joint*) is the word root.
In the medical term	hepat/itis, *hepat* (which means *liver*) is the word root.

The word root is the core of the word; therefore, each medical term contains one or more word roots.

EXERCISE 4

Complete the following. *To check your answers, go to Appendix A.*

The word root is ______.

SUFFIX

The suffix is a word part attached to the end of the word root to modify its meaning.

EXAMPLES

In the word play/er,
-er is the suffix.

In the medical term hepat/ic,
-ic (which means *pertaining to*) is the suffix.
Hepat is the word root for *liver;* therefore, *hepatic* means *pertaining to the liver.*

In the medical term hepat/itis,
-itis (which means *inflammation*) is the suffix. The medical term *hepatitis* means *inflammation of the liver.*

SUFFIXES

frequently indicate:

- **procedures,** such as -scopy, meaning visual examination, or -tomy, meaning incision
- **conditions,** such as -itis, meaning inflammation
- **diseases,** such as -oma, meaning tumor

The suffix is used to modify the meaning of a word. Most medical terms have a suffix.

EXERCISE 5

Complete the following. *To check your answers, go to Appendix A.*

The suffix is ______________________________.

PREFIX

The prefix is a word part attached to the beginning of a word root to modify its meaning.

EXAMPLES

In the word re/play,
re- is the prefix.

In the medical term sub/hepat/ic,
sub- (which means *under*) is the prefix.
Hepat is the word root for *liver,* and
-ic is the suffix for *pertaining to.* The medical term *subhepatic* means *pertaining to under the liver.*

In the medical term intra/ven/ous,
intra- (which means *within*) is the prefix, *ven* (which means *vein*) is the word root, and *-ous* (which means *pertaining to*) is the suffix. The medical term *intravenous* means *pertaining to within the vein.*

PREFIXES

often indicate:

- **number** such as bi-, meaning two
- **position,** such as sub-, meaning under
- **direction,** such as intra-, meaning within
- **time,** such as brady-, meaning slow
- **negation,** such as a-, meaning without

A prefix can be used to modify the meaning of a word. Many medical terms do not have a prefix.

EXERCISE 6

Complete the following. *To check your answers, go to Appendix A.*

The prefix is ______________________________.

COMBINING VOWEL

VOWELS
are speech sounds represented by the letters a, e, i, o, u, and sometimes y.

The combining vowel is a word part, usually an o, used to ease pronunciation. The combining vowel is:

- Placed to connect two word roots
- Placed to connect a word root and a suffix
- **Not** placed to connect a prefix and a word root

EXAMPLES

In the medical term oste/o/arthr/itis,
o is the combining vowel used between two word roots *oste* (which means bone) and *arthr* (which means joint).

In the medical term arthr/o/pathy,
o is the combining vowel used between the word root *arthr* and the suffix *-pathy* (which means *disease*).

In the medical term sub/hepat/ic,
the combining vowel is not used between the prefix *sub-* and the word root *hepat.*

> The combining vowel is used to ease pronunciation; therefore, not all medical terms have combining vowels. Medical terms introduced throughout the text that have combining vowels other than o are highlighted at their introduction.

Four Guidelines for Using Combining Vowels

Learning the four guidelines for using combining vowels will assist you in correctly spelling medical terms built from word parts. Refer to Table 1.2, as you build terms in the following chapters until the guidelines are second nature to you.

Guideline One

When connecting a word root and a suffix, a combining vowel is used if the suffix does not begin with a vowel.

EXAMPLE

In the medical term arthr/o/pathy,
the suffix *-pathy* does not begin with a vowel; therefore, a combining vowel is used.

Guideline Two

When connecting a word root and a suffix, a combining vowel is usually not used if the suffix begins with a vowel.

EXAMPLE

In the medical term hepat/ic,
the suffix *-ic* begins with the vowel *i;* therefore, a combining vowel is not used.

Guideline Three

When connecting two word roots, a combining vowel is usually used even if vowels are present at the junction.

EXAMPLE

In the medical term oste/o/arthr/itis,
o is the combining vowel used, even though the word root *oste* ends with the vowel *e,* and the word root *arthr* begins with the vowel *a.*

Guideline Four

When connecting a prefix and a word root, a combining vowel is **not** used.

EXAMPLE

In the medical term sub/hepat/ic,
the combining vowel is not used between the prefix *sub-* and the word root *hepat.*

TABLE 1.2 Guidelines for Using Combining Vowels

Combining Vowel Guidelines	Example
1. When connecting a word root and a suffix, **a combining vowel Is USED if the suffix DOES NOT BEGIN with a vowel.**	arthr/**o**/pathy
2. When connecting a word root and a suffix, **a combining vowel Is USUALLY NOT USED if the suffix BEGINS with a vowel.**	hepat/ic
3. When connecting two word roots, **a combining vowel Is USUALLY USED even if vowels are present at the junction.**	oste/**o**/arthr/itis
4. When connecting a prefix and a word root, **a combining vowel Is NOT USED.**	sub/hepat/ic

EXERCISE 7

Complete the following. *To check your answers, go to Appendix A.*

1. A combining vowel is ____
____.
2. When connecting a word root and a suffix, a combining vowel is ____________ if the suffix does not begin with a vowel.
3. When connecting a word root and a suffix, a combining vowel is usually not used if the suffix begins with a ________________.
4. When connecting two ________________, a combining vowel is usually used, even if vowels are present at the junction.
5. When connecting a prefix and a word root, a combining vowel is ____________ used.

Combining Form

A combining form is a word root with the combining vowel attached, separated by a slash. The combining form is not a word part per se; rather it is the word root and the combining vowel. *For learning purposes, word roots are presented together with their combining vowels as **combining forms** throughout the text.*

EXAMPLES

arthr/o
oste/o
ven/o

Word roots are presented as combining forms throughout the text.

EXERCISE 8

Complete the following. *To check your answers, go to Appendix A.*

A combining form is ____
____
____.

TABLE 1.3 Word Parts and Combining Form

Word Parts, Combining Form	Definition	Example
Word root	The core of the word	**hepat**/itis
Suffix	Attached at the end of a word root to modify its meaning	hepat/**itis**
Prefix	Attached at the beginning of a word root to modify its meaning	**sub**/hepatic
Combining vowel	Usually an o used to ease pronunciation	hepat/**o**/megaly
Combining form	Word root with a combining vowel attached, separated by a slash	**hepat/o**

EXERCISE 9

Match the phrases in the first column with the correct terms in the second column. *To check your answers, go to Appendix A.*

_____ 1. attached at the beginning	a. combining vowel
_____ 2. usually an *o*	b. prefix
_____ 3. all medical terms built from word parts contain at least one	c. combining form
_____ 4. attached at the end of a word root	d. word root
_____ 5. word root with combining vowel attached	e. suffix

EXERCISE 10

Answer **T** for true and **F** for false. *To check your answers, go to Appendix A.*

_____ 1. There are always prefixes at the beginning of medical terms.

_____ 2. A combining vowel is always used when connecting a word root and a suffix that begins with the letter *o*.

_____ 3. A prefix modifies the meaning of the word.

_____ 4. A combining vowel is used to ease pronunciation.

_____ 5. *I* is the most commonly used combining vowel.

_____ 6. The word root is the core of a medical term.

_____ 7. A combining vowel is used between a prefix and a word root.

_____ 8. A combining form is a word part.

_____ 9. A combining vowel is used when connecting a word root and a suffix if the suffix begins with the letter *g*.

Techniques for Learning Medical Terms Built From Word Parts

Analyzing, defining, and **building** medical terms are used in this text to learn medical terms built from word parts. You will use them many times to complete exercises in the following chapters. Refer to **Table 1.4**, p. 14, as often as needed until you become familiar with these techniques.

ANALYZING MEDICAL TERMS

To analyze medical terms, divide them into word parts and label each word part and each combining form. Follow the procedure below:

1. **Divide the term** into word parts with slashes.

   EXAMPLE: oste / o / arthr / o / pathy

2. **Label each word part** by using the following abbreviations.

   WR Word Root
   P Prefix
   S Suffix
   CV Combining Vowel

   EXAMPLE:
   WR CV WR CV S
   oste / o / arthr / o / pathy

3. **Label each combining form. Underline the word root and combining vowel, then write the abbreviation CF below the combining form.**

   EXAMPLE:
   WR CV WR CV S
   oste / o / arthr / o / pathy
   CF CF

EXERCISE 11

Analyze the following medical term. Use the Word Part List on p. 12 as a reference. *To check your answers, go to Appendix A.*

osteopathy

EXERCISE 12

Complete the following. *To check your answers, go to Appendix A.*

Three steps to analyze medical terms are:

1. ______________________________
2. ______________________________
3. ______________________________

DEFINING MEDICAL TERMS

To define medical terms, apply the meaning of each word part contained in the term.

EXERCISE 13

Define the following medical term. Use the Word Part List on p. 12 as a reference. *To check your answers, go to Appendix A.*

oste/o/arthr/o/pathy

1. Begin by defining the suffix, *-pathy*. Write the definition on the line below.
2. Move to the beginning of the term; define the word roots *oste* and *arthr*. Write the definitions on the line below, continuing the definition of the term.

oste/o/arthr/o/pathy means ________ of the ________ and ________
-pathy oste arthr

Most medical terms built from word parts can be defined by beginning with the meaning of the suffix; however, this does not always apply.

Word Part List

Word Roots	Definitions	Suffixes	Definitions	Prefixes	Definitions	Combining Vowel
arthr	joint	-itis	inflammation	intra-	within	o
hepat	liver	-ic	pertaining to	sub-	under	
ven	vein	-ous	pertaining to			
oste	bone	-pathy	disease			
		-megaly	enlargement			

EXERCISE 14

Complete the following. *To check your answers, go to Appendix A.*

To define medical terms built from word parts, ______________________________

____

EXERCISE 15

Using the Word Part List on p. 12 analyze and define the following terms. Underline the combining forms. *To check your answers, go to Appendix A.*

EXAMPLE:

WR CV WR CV S
oste / o / arthr / o / pathy
CF CF

disease of the bone and joint

1. arthritis

____

____

2. hepatitis

____

____

3. subhepatic

____

____

4. intravenous

____

____

5. arthropathy

____

____

6. osteitis

____

____

7. hepatomegaly

____

____

BUILDING MEDICAL TERMS

To build medical terms, place word parts together to form terms.

EXERCISE 16

Build the medical term for **disease of a joint.** Use the Word Part List on p. 12 as a reference, and follow the instructions below. *To check your answers, go to Appendix A.*

1. Find the word part for *disease*. Write the word part in the correct space below.
2. Find the word part for *joint*. Write the word part in the correct space below.
3. Insert the combining vowel *o* in the correct space below. (*A combining vowel is needed because the suffix does not begin with a vowel.*)

_______ / ___ / _______
WR / CV / S

EXERCISE 17

Complete the following. *To check your answers, go to Appendix A.*

To build medical terms means ____

____.

Keep in mind that the beginning of the definition usually indicates the suffix.

EXERCISE 18

Using the Word Part List on p. 12 as a reference, build medical terms for the following definitions. *To check your answers, go to Appendix A.*

EXAMPLE: **disease of a joint** arthr / o / pathy
WR / CV / S

1. inflammation of a joint _______ / _______
WR / S
2. pertaining to the liver _______ / _______
WR / S
3. pertaining to under the liver _______ / _______ / _______
P / WR / S
4. pertaining to within the vein _______ / _______ / _______
P / WR / S
5. inflammation of the bone _______ / _______
WR / S
6. inflammation of the liver _______ / _______
WR / S
7. disease of the bone and joint _______ / ___ / _______ / ___ / _______
WR / CV / WR / CV / S
8. enlargement of the liver _______ / ___ / _______
WR / CV / S

EXERCISE FIGURE A

Fill in the blanks with word parts defined to label the diagram. Refer to the Word Part List on p. 12. *To check your answers, go to Appendix A.*

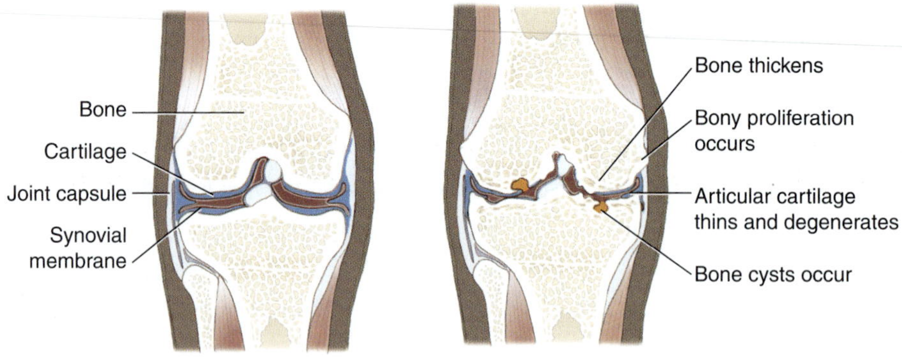

1, Normal knee joint

2, Knee joint showing

_____ / _____ / _____ / _____
bone / cv / joint / inflammation

TABLE 1.4 Techniques to Learn Medical Terms Built from Word Parts

• **Analyzing**	1. Divide medical terms into word parts	oste / o / arthr / o / pathy
	2. Label each word part	WR CV WR CV S oste / o / arthr / o / pathy
	3. Underline and label each combining form	WR CV WR CV S oste / o / arthr / o / pathy CF CF
• **Defining**	1. Apply the meaning of each word part contained in the term 2. Begin by defining the suffix, then move to the beginning of the term	WR CV WR CV S oste / o / arthr / o / pathy **disease** of the **bone** and **joint**
• **Building**	1. Place word parts together to form terms; the beginning of the definition usually indicates the suffix	**disease** of the **bone** and **joint** oste / / arthr / / pathy WR / CV / WR / CV / S
	2. Add combining vowels	oste / o / arthr / o / pathy WR / CV / WR / CV / S

At this time, do not be concerned about which word root goes first when building a term that contains two word roots. The order is usually dictated by common practice; for surgical or diagnostic terms, word roots are sometimes arranged by the order of function or by the order in which an instrument may encounter a structure. As you practice and learn, you will become accustomed to the accepted order.

MEDICAL TERMS *NOT* BUILT FROM WORD PARTS

Medical terms NOT built from word parts are terms that cannot be easily translated to find their meanings. Many varied exercises are presented in each chapter to assist in learning these terms. Origins of terms NOT built from word parts are:

1. **eponyms,** terms derived from the name of a person or place, such as Alzheimer disease and West Nile virus
2. **acronyms,** terms formed from the first letter of words in a phrase that can be spoken as a whole word and usually contains a vowel, such as MRSA (methicillin-resistant *Staphylococcus aureus*)
3. **modern language,** terms derived from the English language such as complete blood count and differential

4. **terms made up of Greek and Latin word parts that cannot be easily translated to find their meaning,** such as orthopedic. Orth/o/ped/ic is made up of three word parts: orth/o meaning straight, ped/o meaning child or foot, and -ic meaning pertaining to. Translated literally, **orthopedic** means **pertaining to a straight child or foot,** whereas its meaning as used today is a **branch of medicine dealing with the study and treatment of diseases and abnormalities of the musculoskeletal system.** As you can see, the term orthopedic cannot be translated literally to find its meaning.

EXERCISE 19

Place a check mark in the space provided to identify terms NOT built from word parts. This may be the first time you have seen some of these terms. Apply your newly acquired knowledge and see how you do. *To check your answers, go to Appendix A.*

1. ______ arthritis
2. ______ upper respiratory infection
3. ______ Lyme disease
4. ______ AIDS
5. ______ macular degeneration
6. ______ hepatitis
7. ______ nuclear medicine scanner
8. ______ malignant
9. ______ osteopathy
10. ______ Alzheimer disease

For additional practice with chapter content, go to Evolve Resources at evolve.elsevier.com and select:
Practice Student Resources > Student Resources > Chapter 1 > **Games:** Medical Millionaire
Practice Quizzes: Introduction to Medical Language

See Appendix B for instructions.

CHAPTER REVIEW

REVIEW OF CHAPTER CONTENT ON EVOLVE (ONLINE) RESOURCES

Go to evolve.elsevier.com and click on Gradable Student Resources and Practice Student Resources. Online learning activities found there can be used to review chapter content and to assess your learning of word parts, medical terms, and abbreviations. Place check marks in the boxes next to activities used for review and assessment.

GRADABLE STUDENT RESOURCES

Chapter 01 >	Exercises >	□ Analyze Medical Terms □ Build Medical Terms □ Define Medical Terms
	Quizzes >	□ Quiz 1: Introduction to Medical Language

PRACTICE STUDENT RESOURCES > STUDENT RESOURCES

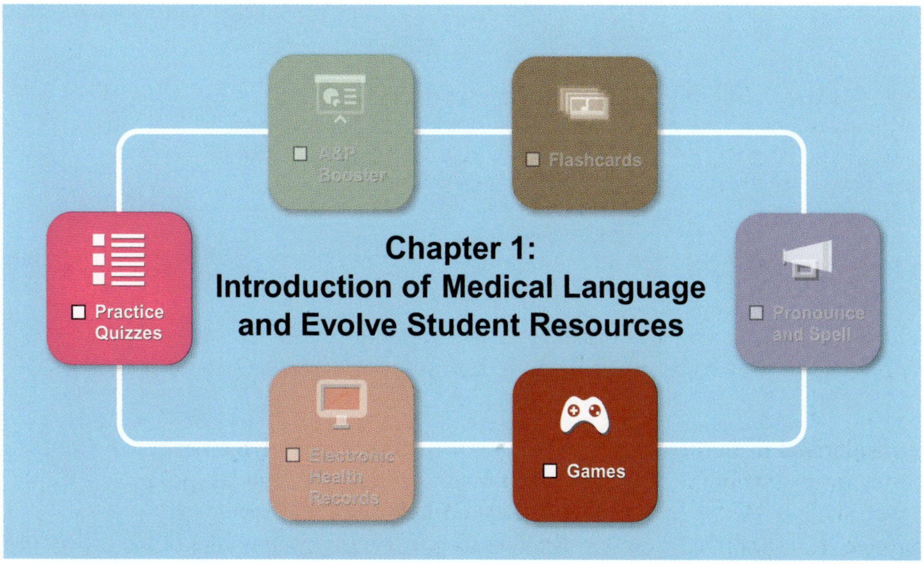

REVIEW OF CATEGORIES OF MEDICAL TERMS

Terms built from word parts—can be translated literally to find their meaning
Terms NOT built from word parts—cannot be translated literally to find their meaning

REVIEW OF MEDICAL TERMS BUILT FROM WORD PARTS

Word root—core of a word; example, **hepat**
Suffix—attached at the end of a word root to modify its meaning; example, **-ic**
Prefix—attached at the beginning of a word root to modify its meaning; example, **sub-**
Combining vowel—usually an o used between two word roots or a word root and suffix to ease pronunciation; example, hepat **o** pathy
Combining form—word root plus combining vowel separated by a slash; example, **hepat/o**
Analyzing—dividing medical terms into word parts, then labeling each word part and combining form
Defining—applying the meaning of each word part contained in the medical term to derive its meaning
Building—placing word parts together to form terms

REVIEW OF MEDICAL TERMS *NOT* BUILT FROM WORD PARTS

Eponyms—name of a person or place; examples, Apgar score and West Nile virus
Acronyms—from first letter of words, example, MRSA
Modern language—terms derived from the English language, example, complete blood count and differential
Terms made up of Greek and Latin word parts not easily translated—example, orthopedic

REVIEW OF OBJECTIVES

To complete this chapter successfully, you do not need to know what the word parts, such as *arthr*, mean. You will learn these in subsequent chapters. **It is important that you have met these objectives:**

1. Can you access the Evolve Student Resources hosted on the publisher's website evolve.elsevier.com?	yes ☐	no ☐
2. Can you describe the origins of medical language?	yes ☐	no ☐
3. Can you define two categories of medical terms?	yes ☐	no ☐
4. Can you identify and define the four word parts and combining form?	yes ☐	no ☐
5. Can you use word parts to analyze and define medical terms?	yes ☐	no ☐
6. Can you use word parts to build medical terms for a given definition?	yes ☐	no ☐

If you answered yes to these questions, you need no further practice because you will be using these concepts repeatedly as you work your way through this text. Refer to this chapter to refresh your memory as needed. Move on to Chapter 2 and begin to build your medical vocabulary so that you will be better prepared to understand and use the language of medicine.

Chapter 2

Body Structure, Color, and Oncology

Outline

Objectives

Upon completion of this chapter you will be able to:

1. Pronounce anatomic structures of the human body.
2. Define and spell word parts related to body structure, color, and oncology.
3. Define, pronounce, and spell disease and disorder oncology terms.
4. Define, pronounce, and spell body structure terms.
5. Define, pronounce, and spell complementary terms related to body structure, color, and oncology.
6. Identify and use singular and plural endings.
7. Interpret the meaning of abbreviations related to body structure and oncology.
8. Apply medical language in clinical contexts.

ANATOMY

Organization of the Body

The structure of the human body falls into the following four categories: cells, tissues, organs, and systems. Each structure is a highly organized unit of smaller structures.

STEM CELLS

Hematopoietic stem cells are immature cells found in the bone marrow and peripheral blood. They have the potential to develop into all types of blood cells. Hematopoietic stem cells for transplantation may be obtained from the patient (**autologous**), from an identical twin (**synergetic**), or from a sibling or other individual (**allogenic**).

Embryonic stem cells are derived from the earliest stage of development of the embryo and have the potential to develop into mature body cells.

Stem cell transplantation is used to treat **leukemia** (cancer involving the white blood cells), **aplastic anemia** (disease in which there is inadequate production of blood cells), **multiple myeloma** (cancer that forms tumors in the bone marrow), **lymphoma** (cancer involving lymphoid cells), and **immune deficiency disorders**.

TERM	DEFINITION
cell (sel)	basic unit of all living things (Fig. 2.1). The human body is composed of trillions of cells, which vary in size and shape according to function.
cell membrane (sel) (MEM-brān)	forms the boundary of the cell
cytoplasm (SĪ-tō-*plas*-em)	gel-like fluid inside the cell
nucleus (NŪ-klē-us)	largest structure within the cell, usually spherical and centrally located. It contains chromosomes for cellular reproduction and is the control center and source of energy production for the cell.
chromosomes (KRŌ-ma-sōms)	located in the nucleus of the cell. There are 46 chromosomes in all normal human cells, with the exception of mature sex cells, which have 23.
genes (JĒNS)	regions within the chromosome. Each chromosome has several thousand genes that determine hereditary characteristics.
DNA (D-N-A)	comprises each gene; is a genetic material that regulates the activities of the cell. DNA abbreviates deoxyribonucleic acid.
tissue (TISH-ū)	group of similar cells that performs a specific function
muscle tissue (MUS-el) (TISH-ū)	composed of cells that have a special ability to contract, usually producing movement
nervous tissue (NURV-us) (TISH-ū)	similarly specialized cells united in the performance of a particular function; found in the nerves, spinal cord, and brain. It is responsible for coordinating and controlling body activities.

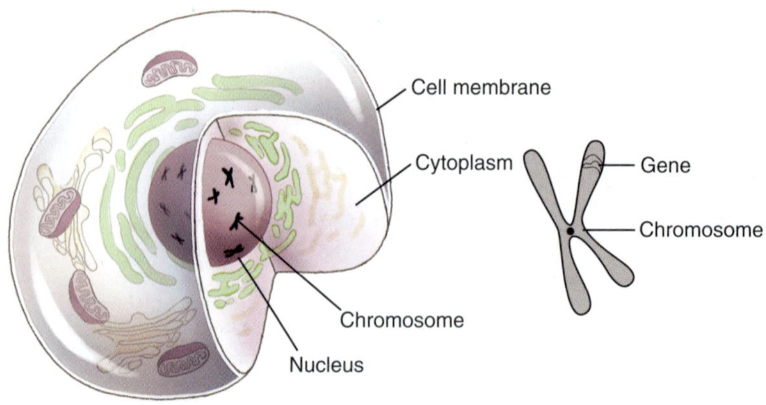

FIG. 2.1 Body cell.

CHROMOSOME is derived from the Greek **chromos**, meaning **color**, and **soma**, meaning **body**. German anatomist Waldeyer first used the term in 1888.

TERM	DEFINITION
connective tissue (ke-NEK-tiv) (TISH-ū)	connects, supports, penetrates, and encases various body structures. Adipose (fat), osseous (bone) tissues, and blood are types of connective tissue. Fibrous tissue is a type of connective tissue that provides strength and stability such as in ligaments and tendons.
epithelial tissue (*ep*-i-THĒ-lē-al) (TISH-ū)	the major covering of the external surface of the body; forms membranes that line body cavities and organs and is the major tissue in glands. Glandular tissue is designed to secrete substances such as digestive enzymes.
organ (OR-gen)	two or more types of tissues that together perform special body functions. For example, the skin is an organ composed of epithelial, connective, muscle, and nervous tissue.
viscera (VIS-er-a)	large internal organs contained in the body cavities, especially in the abdominal cavity
system (SIS-tem)	group of organs that work together to perform complex body functions. For example, the cardiovascular system consists of the heart, blood vessels, and blood. Its function is to transport nutrients and oxygen to the cells and remove carbon dioxide and other waste products (Table 2.1).

MEDICAL GENOMICS

A **genome** is the complete set of genes for all the cells of a specific organism. **Genomics** is the study of the genome and its products and interactions.

Medical genomics is the study of the genome and how it can be used to determine the cause, treatment, and prevention of disease. Medical genomics will alter twenty-first century medicine.

Gene therapy is any therapeutic procedure in which genes are intentionally introduced into human body cells to achieve gene repair, gene suppression, or gene addition. Gene therapy is still in its infancy and is currently only available in research settings. The first human gene transfer was performed on a patient with malignant melanoma in 1989.

For a list of clinical research terms, go to Evolve Resources at evolve.elsevier.com and select:
Practice Student Resources > Student Resources > **Extra Content** > Appendix K: Clinical Research Terms

See Appendix B for instructions.

TABLE 2.1 Body Systems

BODY SYSTEMS	ORGANS AND FUNCTION
INTEGUMENTARY SYSTEM	Composed of skin, nails, and glands. Forms a protective covering for the body, regulates body temperature, and helps manufacture vitamin D.
RESPIRATORY SYSTEM	Composed of nose, pharynx (throat), larynx (voice box), trachea (windpipe), bronchial tubes, and lungs. Performs respiration, which provides for the exchange of oxygen and carbon dioxide within the body.
URINARY SYSTEM	Composed of kidneys, ureters, bladder, and urethra. Removes waste material (urine) from the body, regulates fluid volume, and maintains electrolyte concentration.
REPRODUCTIVE SYSTEM	Female reproductive system is composed of ovaries, uterine tubes, uterus, vagina, and mammary glands. Male reproductive system is composed of testes, urethra, penis, prostate gland, and associated tubes. Responsible for heredity and reproduction.
CARDIOVASCULAR SYSTEM	Composed of the heart and blood vessels. Pumps and transports blood throughout the body.
LYMPHATIC SYSTEM	Composed of a network of vessels, ducts, nodes, and organs. Provides for defense against infection and drainage of extracellular fluid.

Continued

TABLE 2.1 Body Systems—cont'd

BODY SYSTEMS	ORGANS AND FUNCTION
DIGESTIVE SYSTEM	Composed of the gastrointestinal tract which includes the mouth, esophagus, stomach, small and large intestines, and anus, plus accessory organs, liver, gallbladder, and pancreas. Prepares food for use by the body cells and eliminates waste.
MUSCULOSKELETAL SYSTEM	Composed of muscle, bones, and joints. Provides movement and framework for the body, protects vital organs such as the brain, stores calcium, and produces red blood cells.
NERVOUS SYSTEM	Composed of the brain, spinal cord, and nerves. Regulates specific body activities by sending and receiving messages.
ENDOCRINE SYSTEM	Composed of glands that secrete hormones. Hormones regulate many specific body activities.

Body Cavities

The body is not a solid structure as it appears on the outside, but has five cavities (Fig. 2.2), each containing an orderly arrangement of the internal organs.

> ***A & P Booster***
> For more anatomy and physiology, go to Evolve Resources at evolve.elsevier.com and select:
> Practice Student Resources > Student Resources > Chapter 2 > **A & P Booster**
>
> See Appendix B for instructions.

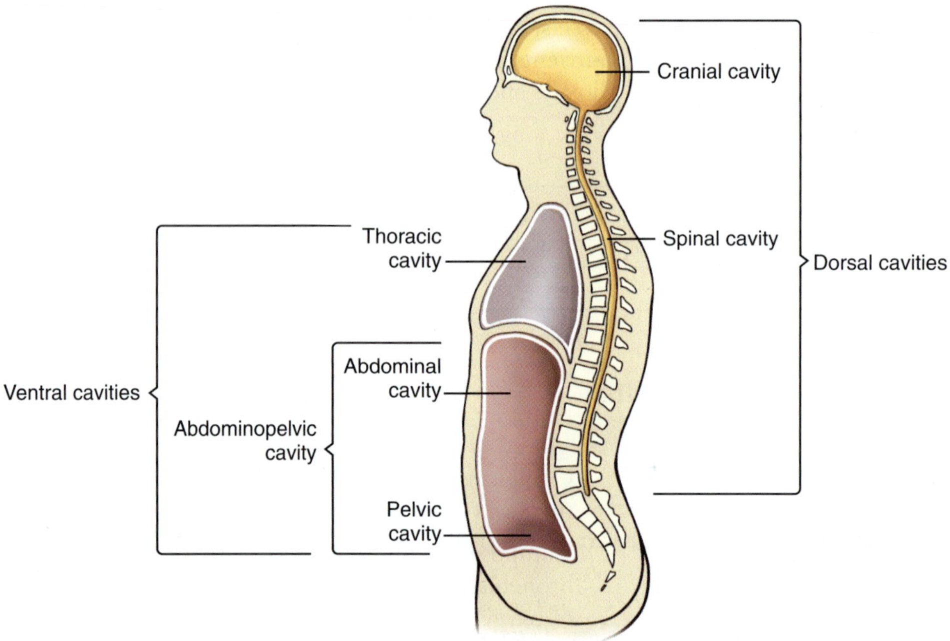

FIG. 2.2 Body cavities.

TERM	DEFINITION
cranial cavity (KRĀ-nē-al) (KAV-i-tē)	space inside the skull (cranium) containing the brain
spinal cavity (SPĪ-nal) (KAV-i-tē)	space inside the spinal column containing the spinal cord
thoracic cavity (thō-RAS-ic) (KAV-i-tē)	space containing the heart, aorta, lungs, esophagus, trachea, bronchi, and mediastinal area
abdominal cavity (ab-DOM-i-nal) (KAV-i-tē)	space containing the stomach, intestines, kidneys, adrenal glands, liver, gallbladder, pancreas, spleen, and ureters

TERM	DEFINITION
pelvic cavity (PEL-vik) (KAV-i-tē)	space containing the urinary bladder, certain reproductive organs, parts of the small and large intestine, and the anus
abdominopelvic cavity (ab-*dom*-i-nō-PEL-vik) (KAV-i-tē)	both the pelvic and abdominal cavities

EXERCISE 1

Practice saying aloud each of the Organization of the Body terms and Body Cavities. Use Table 2.2 for explanation of the pronunciation guide.

To hear the terms, go to Evolve Resources at evolve.elsevier.com and select:
Practice Student Resources > Student Resources > Chapter 2 > **Pronounce and Spell**

See Appendix B for instructions.

❑ Check the box when complete.

TABLE 2.2 Pronunciation Key

GUIDELINES	EXAMPLES
1. Words are distorted minimally to indicate proper phonetic sound.	doctor (dok-tor)
2. The macron (¯) indicates the long vowel sound.	donate (dō-nāte) **ā** as in say **ē** as in me **ī** as in spine **ō** as in no **ū** as in cute
3. Vowels with no markings should have a short sound.	medical (med-i-cal) **a** as in sad **e** as in get **i** as in sit **o** as in top **u** as in cut
4. Primary accents are indicated by capital letters; the secondary accent (which is stressed, but not as strongly as the primary accent) is indicated by italics. *There may be geographical variations in pronunciation.*	altogether (*all*-tū-GETH-er) pancreatitis (*pan*-krē-a-TĪ-tis)

WORD PARTS

Begin building your medical vocabulary by learning the word parts listed next. The list may appear long to you; however, the many exercises that follow are designed to help you understand and remember the word parts. Also, many of the word parts will be repeatedly used throughout this text.

Use the flashcards accompanying this text or electronic flashcards to assist you in memorizing the word parts for this chapter.

Reminder: the word root is the core of the word. The combining form is the word root with the combining vowel attached, separated by a vertical slash.

EPITHELIUM
originally meant **surface over the nipple**. **Epi** means **upon**, and **thela** means **nipple** (or projecting surfaces of many kinds).

Combining Forms of Body Structure

COMBINING FORM	DEFINITION
aden/o	gland
cyt/o	cell
epitheli/o	epithelium
fibr/o	fiber
hist/o	tissue
kary/o	nucleus
lip/o	fat
my/o	muscle
neur/o	nerve
organ/o	organ
sarc/o	flesh, connective tissue
system/o	system
viscer/o	internal organs

EXERCISE 2

A. Fill in the blanks with combining forms in this diagram of the organization of the body. *To check your answers for the exercises in this chapter, go to Appendix A at the back of the textbook.*

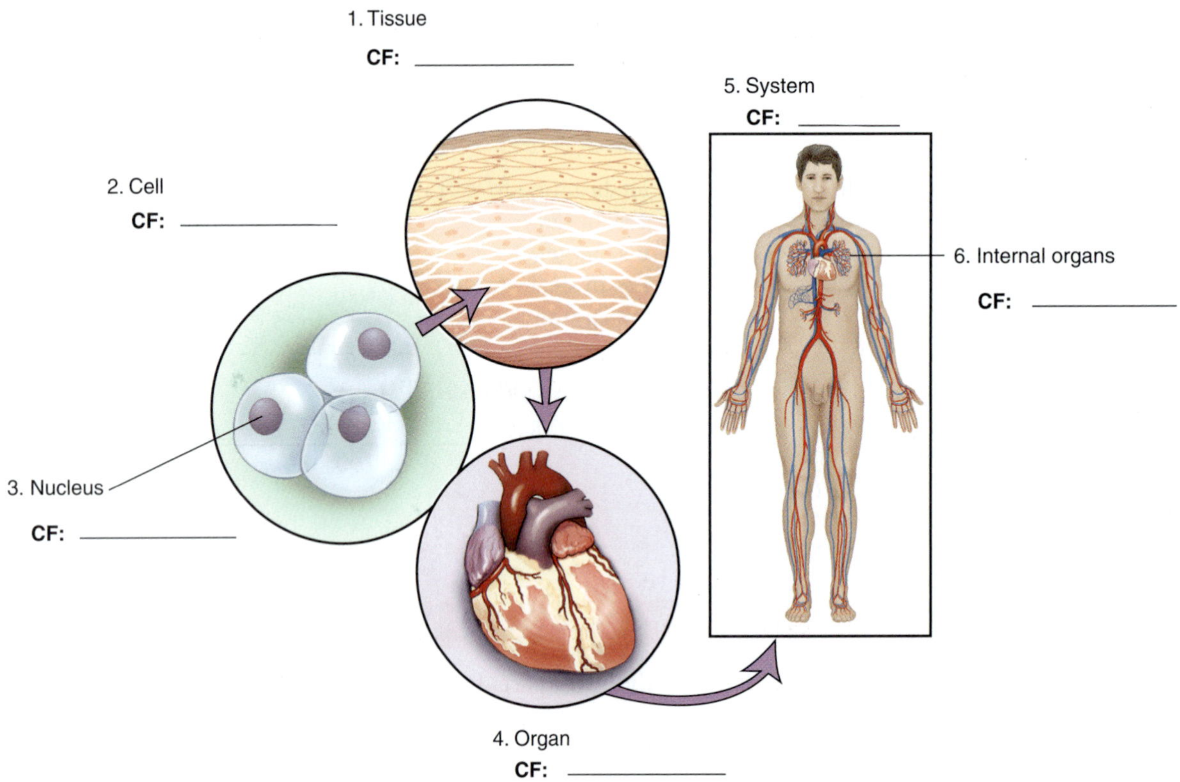

B. Fill in the blanks with combining forms in this diagram of types of tissues.

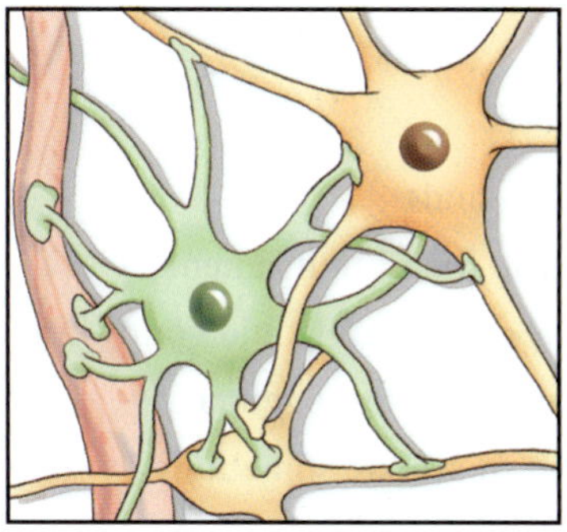

1. Nerve

CF: ______________________________

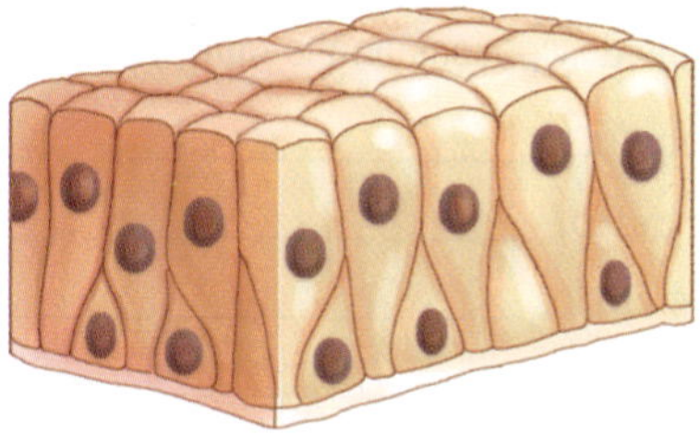

2. Epithelium

CF: ______________________________

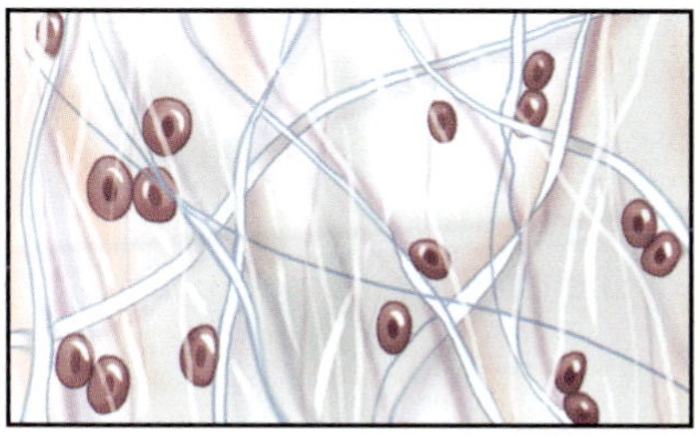

3. Connective

CF: ______________________________

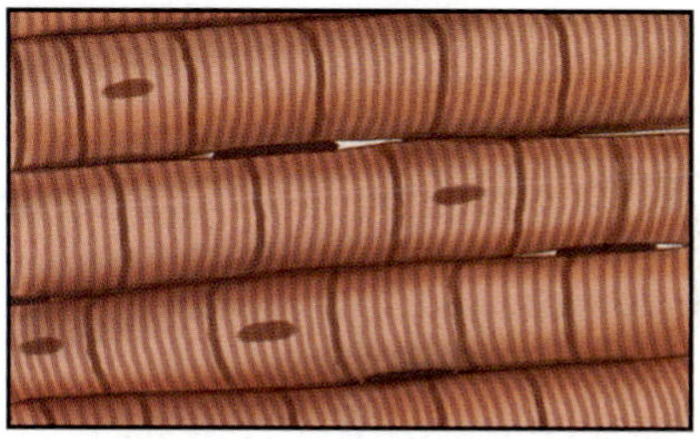

4. Muscle

CF: ______________________________

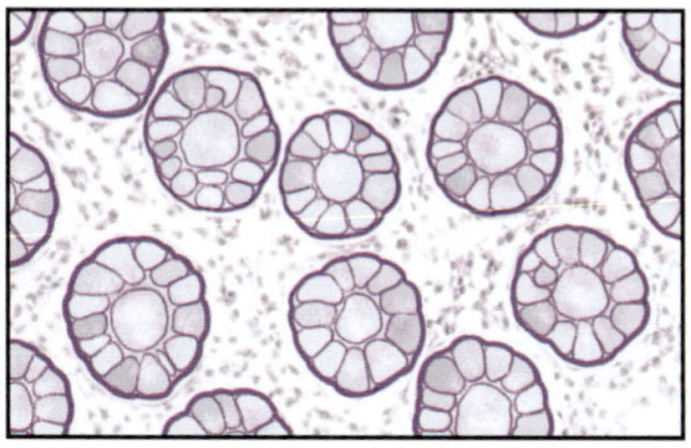

5. Gland

CF: ______________________________

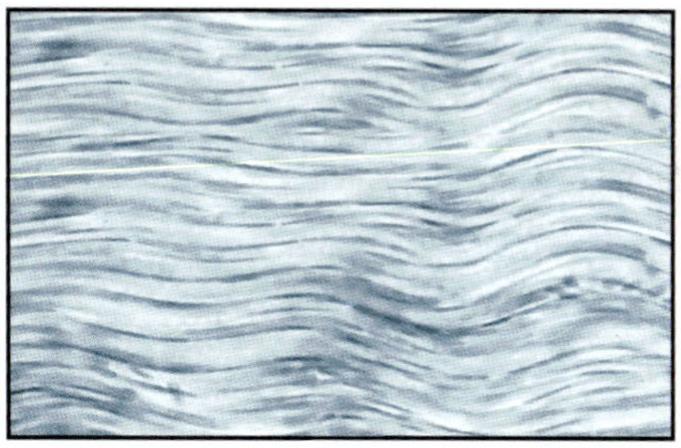

6. Fiber

CF: ______________________________

EXERCISE 3

Step 1: Write the definitions after the following combining forms.

Step 2: Match the descriptions on the right with the combining forms and definitions.

______ 1. sarc/o, ______________________	a. produces movement
______ 2. lip/o, ______________________	b. group of similar cells
______ 3. kary/o, ______________________	c. contained in body cavities
______ 4. viscer/o, ______________________	d. contains chromosomes
______ 5. cyt/o, ______________________	e. type of connective tissue
______ 6. hist/o, ______________________	f. tissue that encases various structures
______ 7. my/o, ______________________	g. basic unit of all living things

EXERCISE 4

Step 1: Write the definitions after the following combining forms.

Step 2: Match the descriptions on the right with the combining forms and definitions.

_____ 1. neur/o, ______________________

_____ 2. organ/o, ______________________

_____ 3. system/o, ______________________

_____ 4. epitheli/o, ______________________

_____ 5. fibr/o, ______________________

_____ 6. aden/o, ______________________

a. major tissue in glands

b. connective tissue found in ligaments

c. responsible for coordinating and controlling body activities

d. group of organs working together

e. tissue designed to secrete something

f. made up of at least two kinds of tissues

CANCER

Carcin and **cancer** are derived from Latin and Greek words meaning **crab**. They originated before the nature of malignant growth was understood. One explanation was that the swollen blood vessels around the diseased area looked like the claws of a crab.

Combining Forms Commonly Used With Body Structure Terms

COMBINING FORM	DEFINITION
cancer/o, carcin/o	cancer (a disease characterized by the unregulated, abnormal growth of new cells)
eti/o	cause (of disease)
gno/o	knowledge
iatr/o	physician, medicine (also means treatment)
lei/o	smooth
onc/o	tumor, mass
path/o	disease
rhabd/o	rod-shaped, striated
somat/o	body

EXERCISE 5

Write the definitions of the following combining forms.

1. onc/o ______________________
2. carcin/o ______________________
3. eti/o ______________________
4. path/o ______________________
5. somat/o ______________________
6. cancer/o ______________________
7. rhabd/o ______________________
8. lei/o ______________________
9. gno/o ______________________
10. iatr/o ______________________

EXERCISE 6

Write the combining form for each of the following.

1. disease ______________________
2. tumor, mass ______________________
3. cause (of disease) ______________________
4. cancer a. ______________________
   b. ______________________
5. body ______________________
6. smooth ______________________
7. rod-shaped, striated ______________________
8. knowledge ______________________
9. physician, medicine ______________________

Combining Forms That Describe Color

COMBINING FORM	DEFINITION
chlor/o	green
chrom/o	color
cyan/o	blue
erythr/o	red
leuk/o	white
melan/o	black
xanth/o	yellow

ERYTHR/O
Aristotle noted "two colors of blood" and applied the term **erythros** to the dark red blood.

EXERCISE 7

Write the definitions of the following combining forms.

1. cyan/o ______________________
2. erythr/o ______________________
3. leuk/o ______________________
4. xanth/o ______________________
5. chrom/o ______________________
6. melan/o ______________________
7. chlor/o ______________________

EXERCISE 8

Write the combining form for each of the following.

1. blue ______________________
2. red ______________________
3. white ______________________
4. black ______________________
5. yellow ______________________
6. color ______________________
7. green ______________________

Prefixes

PREFIX	DEFINITION
dia-	through, complete
dys-	painful, abnormal, difficult, labored
hyper-	above, excessive
hypo-	below, incomplete, deficient, under
meta-	after, beyond, change
neo-	new
pro-	before

Reminder: prefixes are placed at the beginning of word roots to modify their meanings.

EXERCISE 9

Write the definitions of the following prefixes.

1. neo- ______________________
2. hyper- ______________________
3. meta- ______________________
4. hypo- ______________________
5. dys- ______________________
6. dia- ______________________
7. pro- ______________________

EXERCISE 10

Write the prefix for each of the following.

1. new ____________________
2. above, excessive ____________________
3. below, incomplete, deficient, under ____________
4. after, beyond, change ____________________
5. painful, abnormal, difficult, labored ____________
6. through, complete ____________________
7. before ____________________

Reminder: suffixes are placed at the end of word roots to modify their meanings.

Practice two things in your dealings with disease: either help or do not harm the patient.—**Hippocrates** 460–375 BC

Suffixes

SUFFIX	DEFINITION
-al, -ic, -ous	pertaining to
-cyte	cell *(NOTE: the combining form for cell is cyt/o; the suffix for cell is -cyte, ending with an e.)*
-gen	substance or agent that produces or causes
-genic	producing, originating, causing
-logist	one who studies and treats (specialist, physician)
-logy	study of
-megaly	enlargement
-oid	resembling
-oma	tumor, swelling
-osis	abnormal condition (means *increase* when used with blood cell word roots)
-pathy	disease
-plasia	condition of formation, development, growth
-plasm	growth, substance, formation
-sarcoma	malignant tumor
-sis	state of
-stasis	control, stop, standing

The suffix -**logist** may indicate a specialist such as in **psychologist who is not a physician** or a specialist such as in **oncologist who is a physician**. For learning purposes in the text, if the specialist is a physician, it will be indicated in the definition such as **oncologist** … a **physician who studies and treats (malignant) tumors**. Also, some physicians, such as pathologists, do not treat. The definition of -logist will vary.

Some suffixes are made of a word root plus a suffix; they are presented as suffixes for ease of learning. For example, **-pathy** is made up of the word root **path** and the noun ending **-y**. When analyzing a medical term, divide the suffixes as learned. For example, **somatopathy** should be divided somat/o/pathy and **not** somat/o/path/y.

Refer to **Appendix C** and **Appendix D** for alphabetical lists of word parts and their meanings.

EXERCISE 11

A. Match the suffixes in the first column with their correct definitions in the second column.

______ 1. -osis	a. producing, originating, causing
______ 2. -pathy	b. growth, substance, formation
______ 3. -plasm	c. pertaining to
______ 4. -al, -ic, -ous	d. resembling
______ 5. -stasis	e. control, stop, standing
______ 6. -oid	f. substance that produces
______ 7. -gen	g. abnormal condition
______ 8. -sarcoma	h. state of
______ 9. -genic	i. malignant tumor
______ 10. -sis	j. disease

B. Write the suffix pictured and defined.

1. ____________________
cell

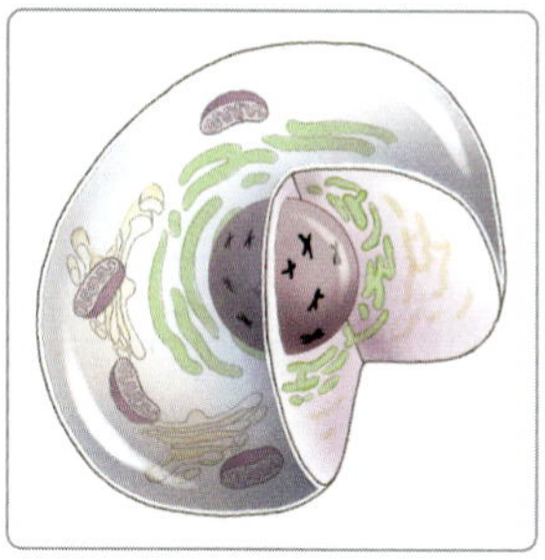

2. ____________________
condition of formation, development, growth

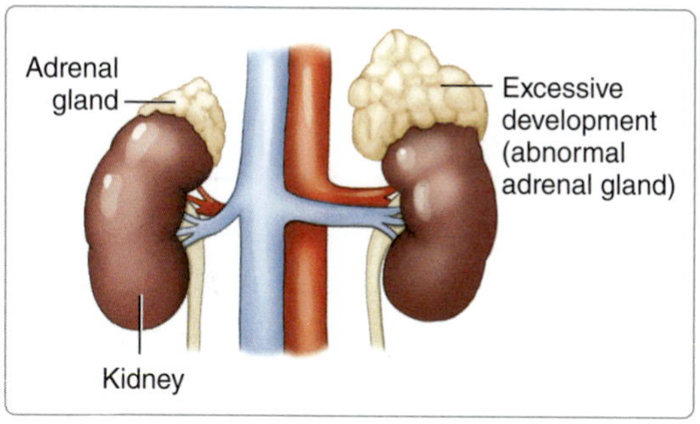

3. ____________________
one who studies and treats (specialist, physician)

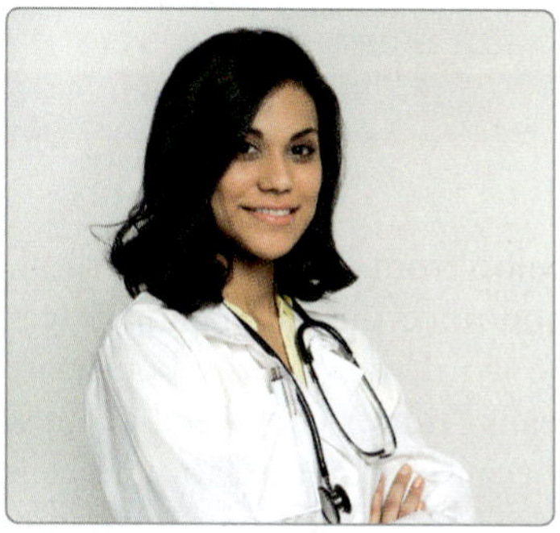

4. ____________________
study of

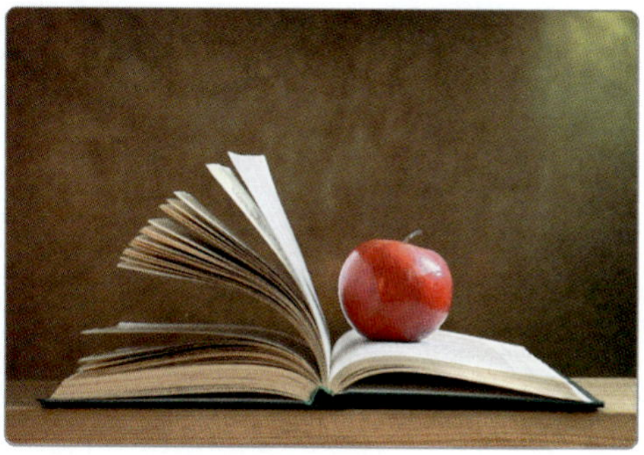

EXERCISE 11 *Pictured and Defined—cont'd*

5. ______________________

enlargement

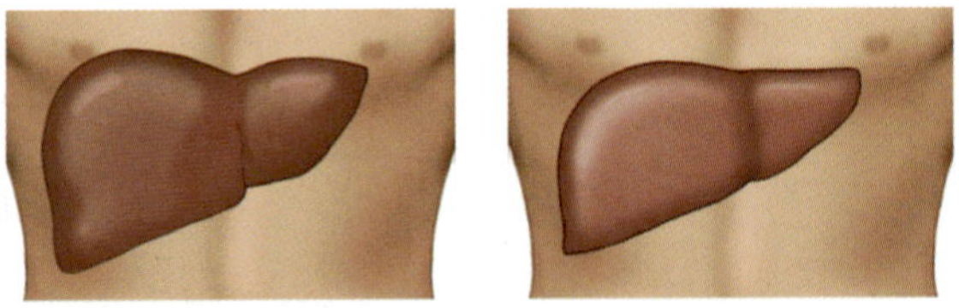

6. ______________________

tumor, swelling

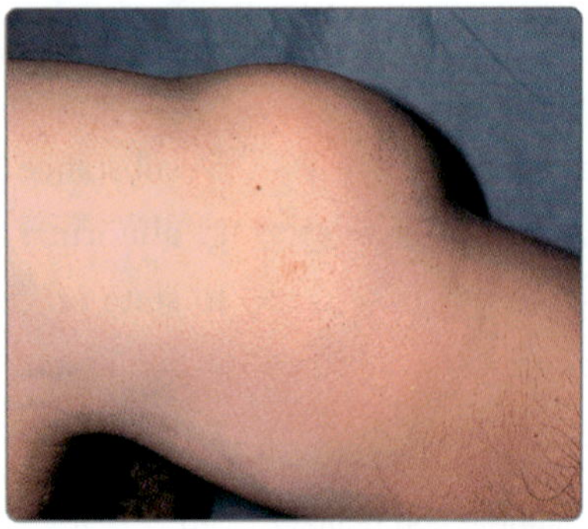

EXERCISE 12

Write the definitions of the following suffixes.

1. -logist ______________________
2. -pathy ______________________
3. -logy ______________________
4. -ic ______________________
5. -stasis ______________________
6. -cyte ______________________
7. -osis ______________________
8. -ous ______________________
9. -plasm ______________________
10. -al ______________________
11. -plasia ______________________
12. -oid ______________________
13. -gen ______________________
14. -genic ______________________
15. -oma ______________________
16. -sarcoma ______________________
17. -sis ______________________
18. –megaly ______________________

For additional practice with Word Parts, go to Evolve Resources at evolve.elsevier.com and select:
Practice Student Resources > Student Resources > Chapter 2 > **Flashcards**

See Appendix B for instructions.

MEDICAL TERMS

Oncology

Oncology is the study of tumors. Tumors can develop from excessive growth of cells from a body part. Tumors, or masses, are benign (noncancerous) or malignant (cancerous). The names of tumors are often made of the word root for the body part and the suffix **-oma,** as in the term *my/oma*, which means "tumor composed of muscle."

Oncology terms are introduced in this chapter because of their relation to cells and cell abnormalities. This is an introductory list only. **More oncology terms appear in subsequent chapters and are presented with the introduction of the related body systems.**

Disease and Disorder Oncology Terms
BUILT FROM WORD PARTS

The following terms can be translated using definitions of word parts. Further explanation is provided within parentheses as needed. *At first the list of terms may seem long to you; however, many of the word parts are repeated in many of the terms. You will soon find that knowing parts of the terms makes learning the words easy.* ***Analyzing, defining,*** *and* ***building exercises*** *are used to learn these terms.*

TERM	DEFINITION
adenocarcinoma (*ad*-e-nō-*kar*-si-NŌ-ma)	cancerous tumor of glandular tissue
adenoma (ad-e-NŌ-ma)	tumor composed of glandular tissue (benign)
carcinoma (CA) (*kar*-si-NŌ-ma)	cancerous tumor (malignant) (Exercise Figure A)
chloroma (klo-RŌ-ma)	tumor of green color (malignant, arising from myeloid tissue)
epithelioma (*ep*-i-*thē*-lē-Ō-ma)	tumor composed of epithelium (may be benign or malignant)
fibroma (fī-BRŌ-ma)	tumor composed of fiber (fibrous tissue) (benign)
fibrosarcoma (fī-brō-sar-KŌ-ma)	malignant tumor composed of fiber (fibrous tissue)
leiomyoma (*lī*-ō-mī-Ō-ma)	tumor composed of smooth muscle (benign)
leiomyosarcoma (*lī*-ō-*mī*-ō-sar-KŌ-ma)	malignant tumor of smooth muscle
lipoma (li-PŌ-ma)	tumor composed of fat (benign tumor)
liposarcoma (*lip*-ō-sar-KŌ-ma)	malignant tumor of fat
melanocarcinoma (*mel*-a-nō-*kar*-si-NŌ-ma)	cancerous black tumor (malignant)
melanoma (mel-a-NŌ-ma)	black tumor (primarily of the skin) (Exercise Figure A)
myoma (mī-Ō-ma)	tumor composed of muscle (benign)
neoplasm (NĒ-ō-plazm)	new growth (of abnormal tissue, benign or malignant)
neuroma (nū-RŌ-ma)	tumor composed of nerve (benign)
rhabdomyoma (*rab*-dō-mī-Ō-ma)	tumor composed of striated muscle (benign)
rhabdomyosarcoma (*rab*-dō-*mī*-ō-sar-KŌ-ma)	malignant tumor of striated muscle (Exercise Figure A)
sarcoma (sar-KŌ-ma)	tumor of connective tissue (such as bone or cartilage; highly malignant) (Exercise Figure A) *(NOTE: sarc/o also is presented in this chapter as a combining form.)*

TNM STAGING SYSTEM OF CANCER

AJCC (American Joint Committee on Cancer) has devised a classification widely used to stage certain types of cancer properly.

T refers to size and the extent of the primary tumor (ranked 0-4).

N denotes the involvement of the lymph nodes (ranked 0-4).

M defines whether there is metastasis (0 = none; 1 = present).

For example, T_2 N_1 M_0

T_2 refers to the primary tumor of 2 cm.

N_1 means spread of tumor to ipsilateral (same side) lymph nodes.

M_0 means no distant metastasis.

This system helps communicate the extent of cancer and is frequently cited by oncologists, surgeons, and radiation oncologists.

INCIDENTALOMA

refers to a mass lesion involving an organ that is discovered unexpectedly by the use of ultrasound, computed tomography scan, or magnetic resonance imaging and has nothing to do with the patient's symptoms or primary diagnosis.

SARCOMA

has been used since the time of ancient Greece to describe any fleshy tumor. Since the introduction of cellular pathology, the meaning has become **malignant connective tissue tumor**.

Often, an additional word root is used to denote the type of tissue involved, such as **oste** in **osteosarcoma**, which refers to a malignant tumor of the bone.

EXERCISE 13

Practice saying aloud each of the Disease and Disorder Oncology Terms Built from Word Parts. Use Table 2.2 for explanation of the pronunciation guide.

> To hear the terms, go to Evolve Resources at evolve.elsevier.com and select:
> Practice Student Resources > Student Resources > Chapter 2 > **Pronounce and Spell**
>
> See Appendix B for instructions.

❑ Check the box when complete.

EXERCISE FIGURE A

Fill in the blanks to complete labeling of these diagrams of types of cancers.

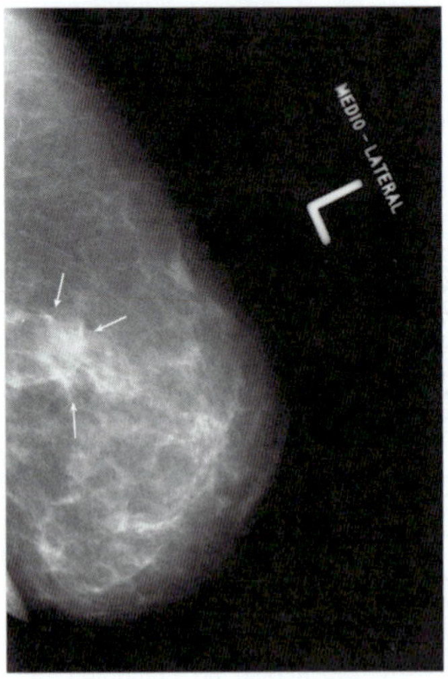

1. ____________ / ____________ of the breast
   cancer / tumor

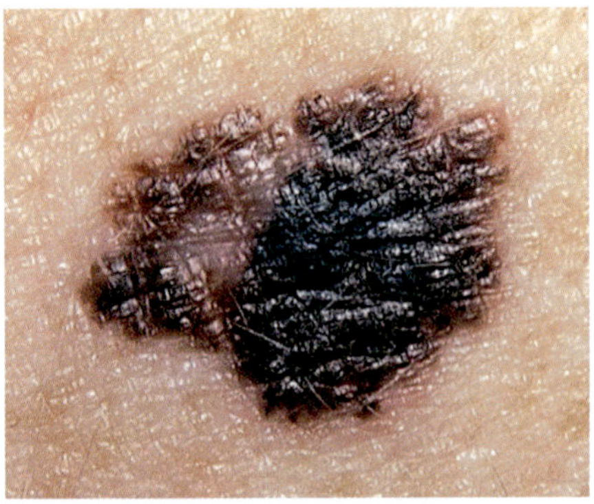

2. ____________ / ____________
   black / tumor

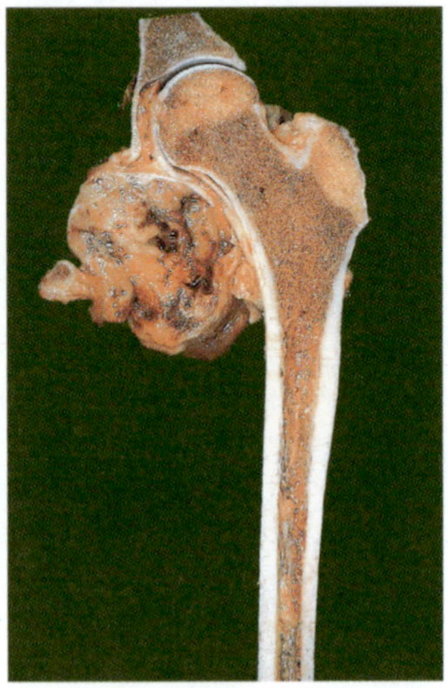

3. ____________ / ____________ of the femur
   connective tissue / tumor

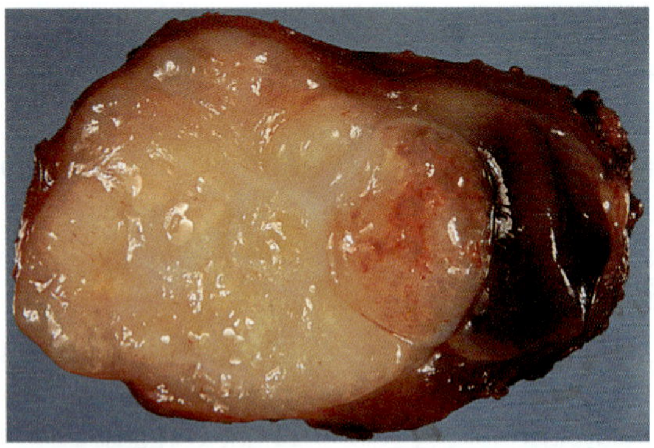

4. ____________ / cv / ____________ / cv / ____________
   striated / cv / muscle / cv / malignant tumor

EXERCISE 14

Analyze and define the following Disease and Disorder Oncology Terms by drawing slashes between word parts, writing word part abbreviations above the term, underlining combining forms, and writing combining form abbreviations below the term. Refer to Chapter 1, p. 11 to review analyzing and defining techniques. **This is an important exercise; do not skip any portion of it.**

	WR CV	WR CV	S
EXAMPLE:	lei / o /	my / o /	sarcoma
	CF	CF	

malignant tumor of smooth muscle

1. sarcoma
____
____

2. melanoma
____
____

3. epithelioma
____
____

4. lipoma
____
____

5. neoplasm
____
____

6. myoma
____
____

7. neuroma
____
____

8. carcinoma
____
____

9. melanocarcinoma
____
____

10. rhabdomyosarcoma
____
____

11. leiomyoma
____
____

12. rhabdomyoma
____
____

13. fibroma
____
____

14. liposarcoma
____
____

15. fibrosarcoma
____
____

16. adenoma
____
____

17. a d e n o c a r c i n o m a

____

____

18. c h l o r o m a

____

____

EXERCISE 15

Build Disease and Disorder Oncology Terms for the following definitions by using the word parts you have learned. If you need help, refer to Chapter 1, p. 13, to review medical term building techniques. **Once again, this is an integral part of the learning process; do not skip any part of this exercise.**

EXAMPLE: tumor composed of fat lip / oma (WR / S)

1. black tumor ______ / ______ (WR / S)
2. cancerous tumor ______ / ______ (WR / S)
3. new growth ______ / ______ (P / S(WR))

When analyzing medical terms that have a suffix containing a word root, it may appear, as in the word **neoplasm**, that the term is composed of only a prefix and a suffix. Keep in mind that the word root is embedded in the suffix and is indicated in the *Building Medical Terms* exercises by S(WR).

4. tumor composed of epithelium ______ / ______ (WR / S)
5. tumor of connective tissue ______ / ______ (WR / S)
6. cancerous black tumor ______ / ______ / ______ / ______ (WR / CV / WR / S)
7. tumor composed of nerve ______ / ______ (WR / S)
8. tumor composed of muscle ______ / ______ (WR / S)
9. malignant tumor of striated muscle ______ / ______ / ______ / ______ / ______ (WR / CV / WR / CV / S)
10. tumor composed of smooth muscle ______ / ______ / ______ / ______ (WR / CV / WR / S)
11. tumor composed of striated muscle ______ / ______ / ______ / ______ (WR / CV / WR / S)
12. malignant tumor of smooth muscle ______ / ______ / ______ / ______ / ______ (WR / CV / WR / CV / S)
13. malignant tumor of fat ______ / ______ / ______ (WR / CV / S)

14. tumor composed of fiber (fibrous tissue) ________ WR / ________ S

15. malignant tumor of fiber (fibrous tissue) ________ WR / CV / ________ S

16. tumor composed of glandular tissue ________ WR / ________ S

17. cancerous tumor of glandular tissue ________ WR / CV / ________ WR / ________ S

18. tumor of green color ________ WR / ________ S

EXERCISE 16

Spell each of the Disease and Disorder Oncology Terms built from word parts by having someone dictate them to you. Use a separate sheet of paper.

> To hear and spell the terms, go to Evolve Resources at evolve.elsevier.com and select:
> Practice Student Resources > Student Resources > Chapter 2 > **Pronounce and Spell**
>
> See Appendix B for instructions.

❑ Check the box when complete.

Body Structure Terms
BUILT FROM WORD PARTS

The following terms can be translated using definitions of word parts. Further explanation is provided within parentheses as needed. *By analyzing, defining, and building the terms in the exercises that follow, you will come to know the terms.*

TERM	DEFINITION
cytogenic (*sī*-tō-JEN-ik)	producing cells
cytoid (SĪ-toid)	resembling a cell
cytology (*sī*-TOL-o-jē)	study of cells
cytoplasm (SĪ-tō-plazm)	cell substance
dysplasia (dis-PLĀ-zha)	abnormal development (Fig. 2.6)
epithelial (*ep*-i-THĒ-lē-al)	pertaining to epithelium
erythrocyte (RBC) (e-RITH-rō-sīt)	red (blood) cell (Exercise Figure B)
erythrocytosis (e-*rith*-rō-sī-TŌ-sis)	increase in the number of red (blood) cells

EXERCISE FIGURE B

Fill in the blanks with word parts defined to label the diagram.

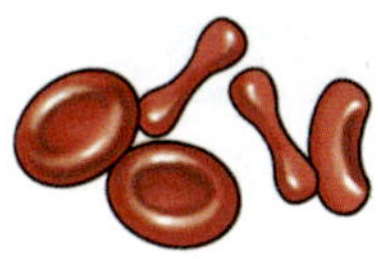

________ red / ________ cv / ________ cell(s)

EXERCISE FIGURE C

Fill in the blanks with word parts defined to label the diagram.

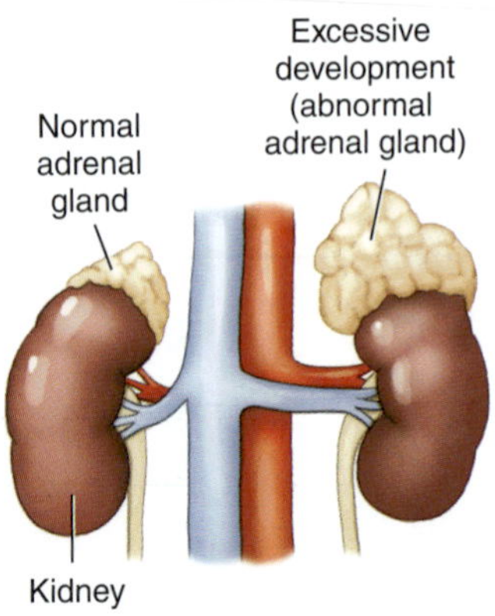

excessive / development

EXERCISE FIGURE D

Fill in the blanks with word parts defined to label the diagram.

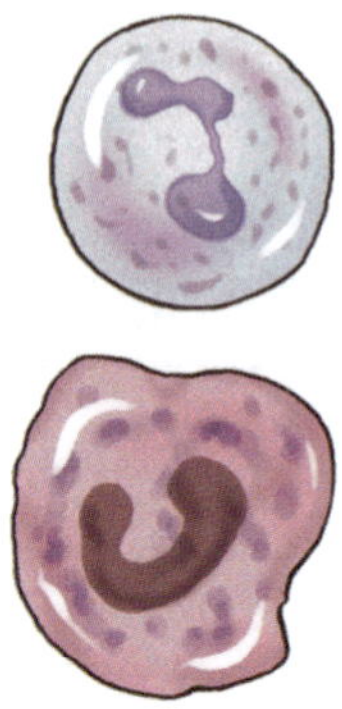

white / cv / cell(s)

Body Structure Terms—cont'd

TERM	DEFINITION
histology (his-TOL-o-jē)	study of tissue
hyperplasia (*hī*-per-PLĀ-zha)	excessive development (number of cells) (Exercise Figure C) (Fig. 2.6)
hypoplasia (hī-pō-PLĀ-zha)	incomplete development (of an organ or tissues)
karyocyte (KĀR-ē-ō-sīt)	cell with a nucleus
karyoplasm (KĀR-ē-ō-*plazm*)	substance of a nucleus
leukocyte (WBC) (LŪ-kō-sīt)	white (blood) cell (Exercise Figure D)
leukocytosis (*lū*-kō-sī-TŌ-sis)	increase in the number of white (blood) cells
lipoid (LIP-oid)	resembling fat
myopathy (mī-OP-a-thē)	disease of the muscle
neuroid (NŪ-rōyd)	resembling a nerve
organomegaly (*or*-ga-nō-MEG-a-lē)	enlargement of an organ
somatic (sō-MAT-ik)	pertaining to the body
somatogenic (*sō*-ma-tō-JEN-ik)	originating in the body (organic as opposed to psychogenic)
somatopathy (*sō*-ma-TOP-a-thē)	disease of the body
somatoplasm (sō-MAT-ō-plazm)	body substance
systemic (sis-TEM-ik)	pertaining to a (body) system (or the body as a whole)
visceral (VIS-er-al)	pertaining to the internal organs

Ellipsis is the practice of omitting an essential part of a word by common consent. Note this practice in the terms **erythrocyte** (red **blood** cell) and **leukocyte** (white **blood** cell). The word root for blood is omitted.

EXERCISE 17

Practice saying aloud each of the Body Structure Terms Built from Word Parts.

To hear the terms, go to Evolve Resources at evolve.elsevier.com and select:
Practice Student Resources > Student Resources > Chapter 2 > **Pronounce and Spell**

See Appendix B for instructions.

❑ Check the box when complete.

EXERCISE 18

Analyze and define the following Body Structure Terms by drawing slashes between word parts, writing word part abbreviations above the term, underlining combining forms, and writing combining form abbreviations below the term.

EXAMPLE:

WR CV S
cyt / o / genic
CF
producing cells

1. cytology
2. histology
3. visceral
4. karyocyte
5. karyoplasm
6. systemic
7. cytoplasm
8. somatic
9. somatogenic
10. somatoplasm
11. somatopathy
12. neuroid
13. myopathy
14. erythrocyte
15. leukocyte
16. epithelial

17. lipoid

____
____

18. hyperplasia

____
____

19. erythrocytosis

____
____

20. leukocytosis

____
____

21. hypoplasia

____
____

22. cytoid

____
____

23. dysplasia

____
____

24. organomegaly

____
____

EXERCISE 19

Build medical terms for the following body structure definitions by using the word parts you have learned.

EXAMPLE: Example: producing cells cyt / o / genic (WR / CV / S)

1. cell substance ______ / ______ / ______ (WR / CV / S)

2. substance of a nucleus ______ / ______ / ______ (WR / CV / S)

3. pertaining to the body ______ / ______ (WR / S)

4. disease of the muscle ______ / ______ / ______ (WR / CV / S)

5. body substance ______ / ______ / ______ (WR / CV / S)

6. pertaining to the internal organs ______ / ______ (WR / S)

7. originating in the body ______ / ______ / ______ (WR / CV / S)

8. disease of the body ______ / ______ / ______ (WR / CV / S)

9. red (blood) cell ____ WR / CV / S ____

10. resembling a nerve ____ WR / S ____

11. pertaining to a (body) system ____ WR / S ____

12. white (blood) cell ____ WR / CV / S ____

13. cell with a nucleus ____ WR / CV / S ____

14. resembling fat ____ WR / S ____

15. study of cells ____ WR / CV / S ____

16. excessive development (of cells) ____ P / S(WR) ____

17. resembling a cell ____ WR / S ____

18. pertaining to epithelium ____ WR / S ____

19. study of tissue ____ WR / CV / S ____

20. increase in the number of red (blood) cells ____ WR / CV / WR / S ____

21. incomplete development (of an organ or tissue) ____ P / S(WR) ____

22. increase in the number of white (blood) cells ____ WR / CV / WR / S ____

23. abnormal development ____ P / S(WR) ____

24. enlargement of an organ ____ WR / CV / S ____

EXERCISE 20

Spell each of the Body Structure Terms Built from Word Parts by having someone dictate them to you. Use a separate sheet of paper.

To hear and spell the terms, go to Evolve Resources at evolve.elsevier.com and select:
Practice Student Resources > Student Resources > Chapter 2 > **Pronounce and Spell**

See Appendix B for instructions.

❑ Check the box when complete.

Complementary Terms
BUILT FROM WORD PARTS

Complementary terms complete the vocabulary presented in the chapter by describing signs, symptoms, medical specialties, specialists, and related words. A **sign** is objective information and is detected on physical examination such as observation that the patient has cyanosis of the nail beds. A **symptom** is subjective and is evidence of disease perceived by the patient, such as stating the feeling of pain in the chest while walking.

The following terms can be translated using definitions of word parts. Further explanation is provided within parentheses as needed.

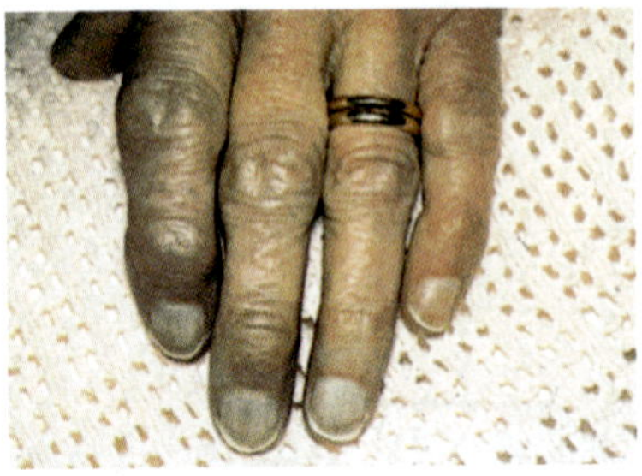

FIG. 2.3 Cyanosis in an elderly patient.

TERM	DEFINITION
cancerous (KAN-ser-us)	pertaining to cancer
carcinogen (kar-SIN-o-jen)	substance that causes cancer
carcinogenic (*kar*-sin-ō-JEN-ik)	producing cancer
cyanosis (*sī*-a-NŌ-sis)	abnormal condition of blue (bluish discoloration, especially of the skin, caused by inadequate supply of oxygen in the blood) (Fig. 2.3)
diagnosis (Dx) (*dī*-ag-NŌ-sis)	state of complete knowledge (the art of identifying a disease based on the patient's signs, symptom, and test results)
etiology (ē-tē-OL-o-jē)	study of causes (of diseases)
iatrogenic (ī-*at*-rō-JEN-ik)	produced by a physician (the unexpected results from a treatment prescribed by a physician)
iatrology (ī-a-TROL-o-jē)	study of medicine
metastasis (pl. metastases) (METS) (me-TAS-ta-sis) (me-TAS-ta-sēz)	beyond control (transfer of cells from one organ to another, as in malignant tumors) (Fig. 2.4)
oncogenic (*ong*-kō-JEN-ik)	causing tumors
oncologist (ong-KOL-o-jist)	physician who studies and treats (malignant) tumors

TERM	DEFINITION
oncology (ong-KOL-o-jē)	study of tumors (a branch of medicine concerned with the study of malignant tumors)
organic (or-GAN-ik)	pertaining to an organ
pathogenic (path-ō-JEN-ik)	producing disease
pathologist (pa-THOL-o-jist)	physician who studies diseases (examines biopsies and performs autopsies to determine the cause of disease or death)
pathology (pa-THOL-o-jē)	study of disease (a branch of medicine dealing with the study of the causes of disease and death)
prognosis (Px) (prog-NŌ-sis)	state of before knowledge (prediction of the outcome of disease based on the patient's signs, symptoms, and test results)
xanthochromic (*zan*-thō-KRŌ-mik)	pertaining to yellow color
xanthosis (zan-THŌ-sis)	abnormal condition of yellow (discoloration)

ONCOLOGY AND ONCOLOGIC

are used to name the medical specialty and healthcare nursing units devoted to the treatment and care of cancer patients.

PROGNOSIS

was used by Hippocrates to mean the same then as now: **to foretell the course of a disease**.

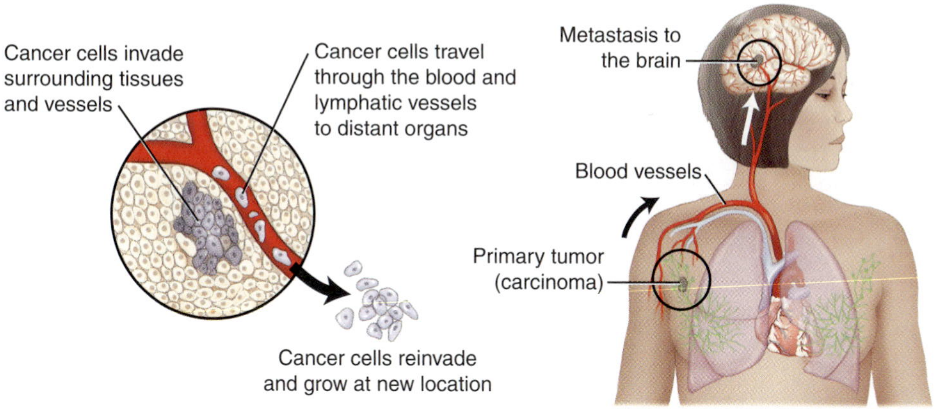

FIG. 2.4 Metastasis.

EXERCISE 21

Practice saying aloud each of the Complementary Terms Built from Word Parts.

To hear the terms, go to Evolve Resources at evolve.elsevier.com and select:
Practice Student Resources > Student Resources > Chapter 2 > **Pronounce and Spell**

See Appendix B for instructions.

❑ Check the box when complete.

EXERCISE 22

Analyze and define the following Complementary Terms by drawing slashes between word parts, writing word part abbreviations above the term, underlining combining forms, and writing combining form abbreviations below the term.

EXAMPLE:

WR CV S
path / o / genic
CF
producing disease

1. pathology

9. etiology

2. pathologist

10. xanthosis

3. metastasis

11. xanthochromic

4. oncogenic

12. carcinogen

5. oncology

13. oncologist

6. carcerous

14. prognosis

7. carcinogenic

15. organic

8. cyanosis

16. diagnosis

17. iatrogenic

____

____

18. iatrology

____

____

EXERCISE 23

Build Complementary Terms for the following definitions by using the word parts you have learned.

EXAMPLE: producing disease path / o / genic (WR / CV / S)

1. pertaining to yellow color ______ WR / CV / WR / S
2. beyond control ______ P / S(WR)
3. study of the cause (of disease) ______ WR / CV / S
4. study of tumors ______ WR / CV / S
5. study of diseases ______ WR / CV / S
6. physician who studies diseases ______ WR / CV / S
7. abnormal condition of yellow ______ WR / S
8. causing tumors ______ WR / CV / S
9. pertaining to cancer ______ WR / S
10. abnormal condition of blue ______ WR / S
11. producing cancer ______ WR / CV / S
12. substance that causes cancer ______ WR / CV / S
13. physician who studies and treats tumors ______ WR / CV / S
14. study of medicine ______ WR / CV / S

15. pertaining to an organ ______ WR / ______ S

16. state of complete knowledge ______ P / ______ WR / ______ S

17. produced by a physician ______ WR / CV / ______ S

18. state of before knowledge ______ P / ______ WR / ______ S

EXERCISE 24

Spell each of the Complementary Terms Built from Word Parts by having someone dictate them to you. Use a separate sheet of paper.

To hear and spell the terms, go to Evolve Resources at evolve.elsevier.com and select:
Practice Student Resources > Student Resources > Chapter 2 > **Pronounce and Spell**

See Appendix B for instructions.

❑ Check the box when complete.

Complementary Terms
NOT BUILT FROM WORD PARTS

Medical terms NOT built from word parts cannot be translated literally to find their meanings. The terms are learned by memorizing the whole word by using recall and spelling exercises.

The terms in this list are NOT built from word parts. The terms are commonly used in the medical world and you will need to know them. In some of the words, you may recognize a word part; however, these terms cannot be literally translated to find the meaning. New knowledge may have changed the meanings of the terms since they were coined; some terms are eponyms, some are acronyms, and some have no apparent explanation for their names. Memorization is used in the following exercises to learn the terms.

APOPTOSIS/NECROSIS

Apoptosis is a normal, beneficial cell death occurring within the body to eliminate damaged or unneeded cells. In an average adult 50-70 billion cells die each day. **Necrosis** is an abnormal, detrimental cell death caused by external conditions such as trauma, infection, or toxins.

TERM	DEFINITION
afebrile (ā-FEB-ril)	without fever
apoptosis (*ap*-op-TŌ-sis)	programmed cell death, a mechanism for cell deletion to regulate cell population, or destroy damaged or defective cells. Some cancers disrupt apoptosis; cells lose their ability to die and live indefinitely.

TERM	DEFINITION
benign (be-NĪN)	not malignant, nonrecurrent, favorable for recovery (Fig. 2.5 and Fig. 2.7)
biological therapy (bī-ō-LOJ-i-kel) (THER-a-pē)	treatment of cancer with biological response modifiers (BRM) that work with the immune system (also called **biotherapy** or **immunotherapy**) (Table 2.4)
carcinoma in situ (kar-si-NŌ-ma) (in) (SĪ-too)	cancer in the early stage before invading surrounding tissue (Fig. 2.6)
chemotherapy (chemo) (kē-mō-THER-a-pē)	treatment of cancer with drugs (Fig. 2.8)
encapsulated (en-KAP-sū-lā-ted)	enclosed within a capsule, as with benign or malignant tumors that have not spread beyond the capsule of the organ in which it originated (Fig. 2.5)
exacerbation (eg-zas-er-BĀ-shun)	increase in the severity of a disease or its symptoms

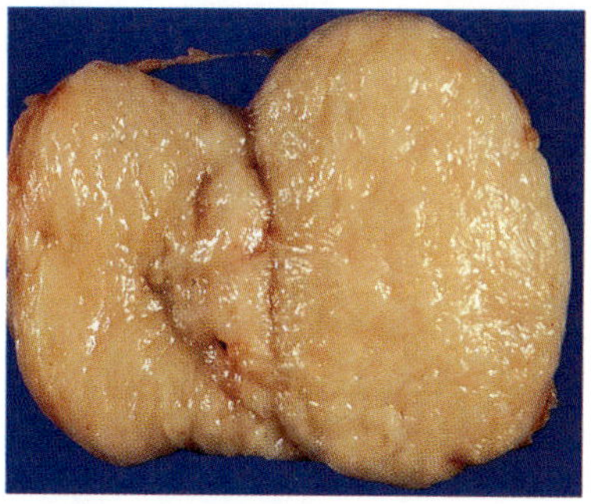

FIG. 2.5 An encapsulated benign tumor.

SITU
is from the Latin term **situs**, which means **position** or **place**. Think of **in situ** as meaning "in place" or "not wandering around."

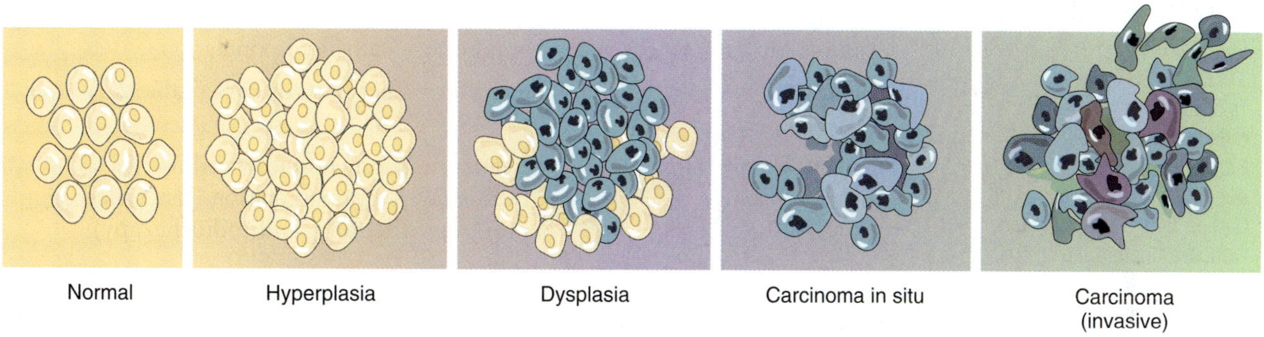

FIG. 2.6 Progression of cell growth.

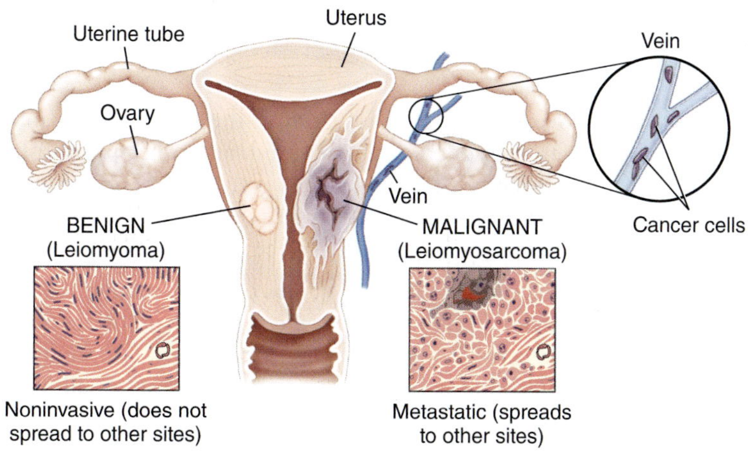

FIG. 2.7 Examples of benign and malignant tumors.

BENIGN AND MALIGNANT
Benign is derived from the Latin word root **bene**, meaning **well** or **good**, as used in **benefit** or **benefactor**. **Malignant** is derived from the Latin word root **mal** meaning **bad**, as used in **malicious**, **malaise**, **malady**, and **malign**.

Complementary Terms—cont'd

TERM	DEFINITION
febrile (FEB-ril)	having a fever
hospice (HOS-pis)	provides palliative or supportive care for terminally ill patients and their families (Table 2.3)
idiopathic (id-ē-ō-PATH-ik)	pertaining to disease of unknown origin
inflammation (in-fla-MĀ-shun)	localized protective response to injury or tissue destruction characterized by redness, swelling, heat, and pain
in vitro (in) (VĒ-trō)	outside the body or in a lab setting
in vivo (in) (VĒ-vō)	within the living body
malignant (ma-LIG-nant)	tending to become progressively worse and to cause death, as in cancer (Fig. 2.7)
morbidity (mor-BID-i-tē)	state of being diseased; incidence of illness in a population
mortality (mor-TAL-i-tē)	state of being mortal (death); incidence of the number of deaths in a population
palliative (PAL-ē-a-tiv)	providing relief but not cure (Table 2.3)
radiation therapy (XRT) (*rā*-dē-Ā-shun) (THER-a-pē)	treatment of cancer with a radioactive substance, x-ray, or radiation (also called **radiation oncology** and **radiotherapy**) (Fig. 2.9)
remission (rē-MISH-un)	improvement or absence of signs of disease

Inflammatory and inflammation are spelled with two *m's*. *Inflame* and *inflamed* have one *m*.

RADIATION THERAPIST

To see an interview with a **radiation therapist**, go to Evolve Resources at evolve.elsevier.com and select **Career Videos** located under the **Extra Content** tab on the Practice Student Resources menu. See Appendix B for instructions.

TABLE 2.3 Hospice Care/Palliative Care

THERAPY	DESCRIPTION
Hospice and Palliative Medicine	a medical subspecialty recognized by the American Board of Medical Specialties.
Hospice care	a facility or program that provides a caring environment to meet the physical and emotional needs of the terminally ill and their families. Medicare, Medicaid, and other payers offer services to patients who have a prognosis of six months or less if the disease follows its natural course, and the patient agrees to forego curative forms of treatment. A team-based palliative care approach is used in an out-of-hospital setting, usually in the patient's home.
Palliative care	provides symptom management to relieve suffering in all stages of disease and is not limited to care at the end of life. The care provided honors the patient's values and preferences throughout his or her illness. Palliative care is available to the patient at the same time as curative or life prolonging treatment. Hospice care involves palliative care; not all of palliative care is hospice care.

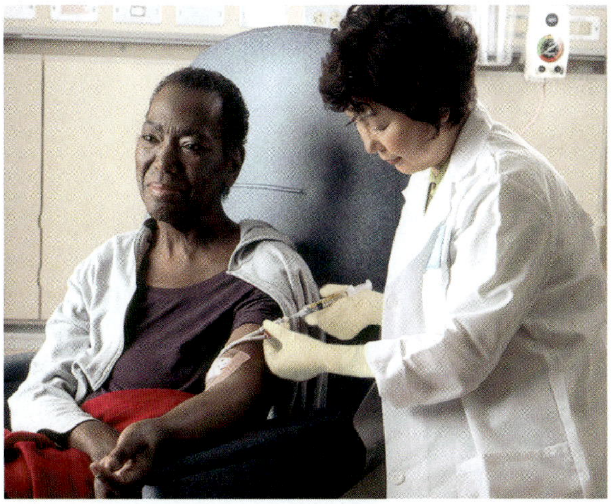

FIG. 2.8 A patient receiving intravenous chemotherapy. Chemotherapy may also be administered orally in pill form.

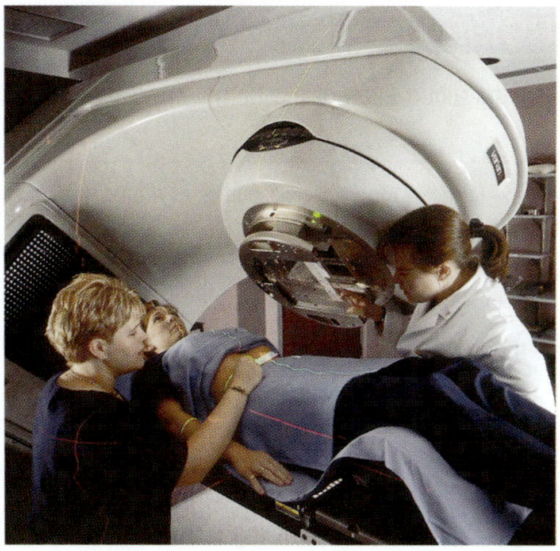

FIG. 2.9 Radiation therapist preparing the patient for radiation therapy.

TABLE 2.4 **Cancer Therapies**

THERAPY	DESCRIPTION
Neoadjuvant therapy	a cancer treatment that precedes other treatment, such as administering chemotherapy or radiation therapy to a patient before surgery.
Adjuvant chemotherapy	the use of chemotherapy after or in combination with another form of cancer treatment such as administering chemotherapy after surgery or with radiation therapy.
Brachytherapy 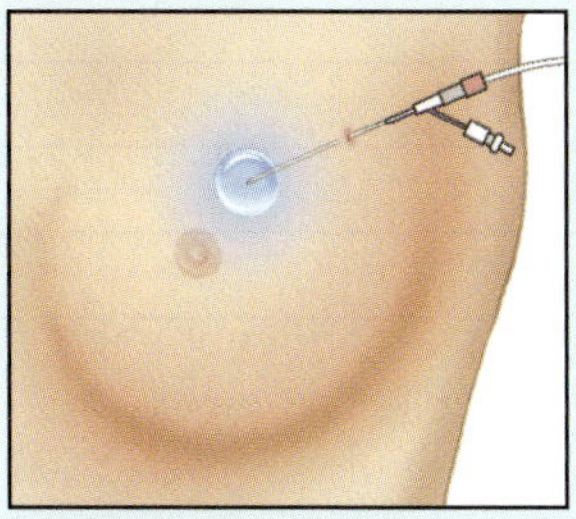	the use of radiotherapy in which the source of radiation is placed within or close to the area being treated, such as implantation of radiation sources into the breast to treat cancer (as shown in the illustration).
Biological therapy	the treatment of cancer with the use of man-made biological response modifiers (BRM) that occur naturally in the body. They alter the immune system's interaction with cancer cells to restore, direct, or boost the body's ability to fight disease. For example, an agent called **rituximab (Rituxan),** a monoclonal antibody, is used to treat some lymphomas. Other biologic agents are **thalidomide,** which is used to treat multiple myeloma, and **interferon,** which is used in the treatment of lymphomas.

EXERCISE 25

Practice saying aloud each of the Complementary Terms NOT Built from Word Parts.

To hear the terms, go to Evolve Resources at evolve.elsevier.com and select:
Practice Student Resources > Student Resources > Chapter 2 > **Pronounce and Spell**

See Appendix B for instructions.

❑ Check the box when complete.

EXERCISE 26

Write the definitions for the following terms.

1. benign ______________________________
2. malignant ______________________________
3. remission ______________________________
4. idiopathic ______________________________
5. inflammation ______________________________
6. chemotherapy ______________________________
7. radiation therapy ______________________________
8. encapsulated ______________________________
9. in vitro ______________________________
10. in vivo ______________________________
11. carcinoma in situ ______________________________
12. exacerbation ______________________________
13. palliative ______________________________
14. mortality ______________________________
15. morbidity ______________________________
16. hospice ______________________________
17. afebrile ______________________________
18. biological therapy ______________________________
19. apoptosis ______________________________
20. febrile ______________________________

EXERCISE 27

Match the complementary terms in the first column with the correct definitions in the second column. *To check your answers, go to Appendix A.*

______ 1. remission	a. outside the body or in a lab setting
______ 2. in vivo	b. disease of unknown origin
______ 3. in vitro	c. providing relief but not cure
______ 4. hospice	d. programmed cell death
______ 5. idiopathic	e. nonrecurrent, favorable for recovery
______ 6. palliative	f. absence of signs and symptoms
______ 7. apoptosis	g. palliative and supportive care
______ 8. afebrile	h. becoming progressively worse
______ 9. benign	i. within the living body
______ 10. malignant	j. without fever

EXERCISE 28

Match the complementary terms in the first column with the correct definitions in the second column. *To check your answers, go to Appendix A.*

______ 1. encapsulated	a. treatment of cancer with a radioactive substance
______ 2. biological therapy	b. state of being diseased
______ 3. radiation therapy	c. protective response to injury
______ 4. chemotherapy	d. treatment of cancer that works with the immune system
______ 5. morbidity	e. increase in severity of disease
______ 6. mortality	f. enclosed within a capsule
______ 7. febrile	g. carcinoma in the early stage
______ 8. exacerbation	h. state of being mortal (death)
______ 9. inflammation	i. treatment of cancer with drugs
______ 10. carcinoma in situ	j. having a fever

EXERCISE 29

Spell each of the Complementary Terms NOT Built from Word Parts by having someone dictate them to you.

> To hear and spell the terms, go to Evolve Resources at evolve.elsevier.com and select:
> Practice Student Resources > Student Resources > Chapter 2 > **Pronounce and Spell**
>
> See Appendix B for instructions.

❑ Check the box when complete.

Refer to **Appendix F** for pharmacology terms related to oncology.

Plural Endings for Medical Terms

In the English language plurals are formed by simply adding an "s" or "es" to the end of a word. For example, hand becomes plural by adding an "s" to form hands. Likewise, box becomes boxes by adding "es." In the language of medicine, many terms have Latin or Greek suffixes, and forming plurals for these terms is not quite as easy. Table 2.5, Common Plural Endings, lists the most common singular and plural endings used in medical terminology. When appropriate, both singular and plural endings are included in the word lists throughout the text, such as metastasis/metastases on p. 38.

Because of common usage, some plural forms of medical terms will add an "s" rather than use Greek or Latin plural endings. **Carcinomas** rather than **carcinomata** is frequently seen in medical literature.

TABLE 2.5 Common Plural Endings for Medical Terms

SINGULAR ENDINGS	SINGULAR FORMS		PLURAL ENDINGS	PLURAL FORMS	
-a	vertebra	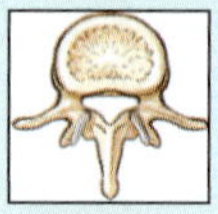	-ae	vertebr**ae**	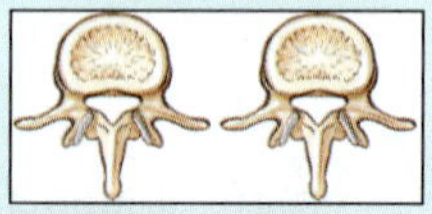
-ax	thor**ax**	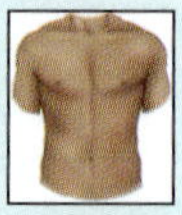	-aces	thor**aces**	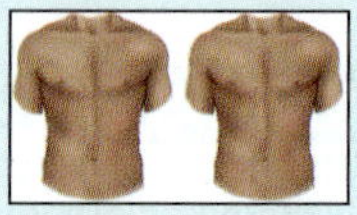
-is	test**is**	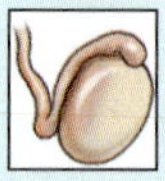	-es	test**es**	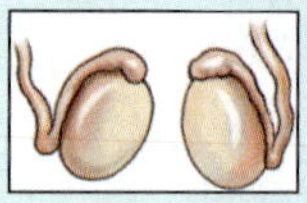
-ix	append**ix**	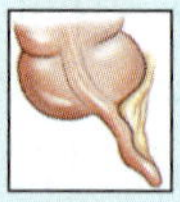	-ices	append**ices**	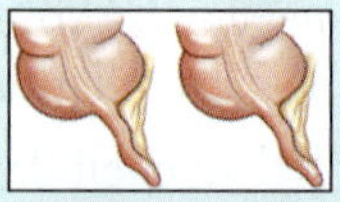
-ma	carcino**ma**	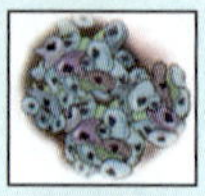	-mata	carcino**mata**	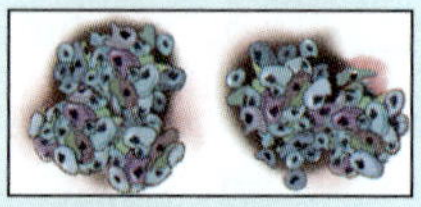
-nx	lary**nx**	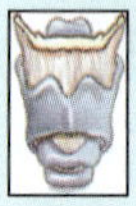	-nges	lary**nges**	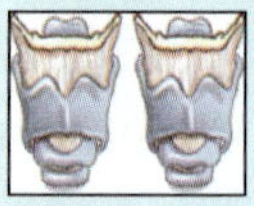
-on	gangli**on**	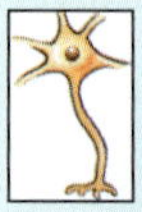	-a	gangli**a**	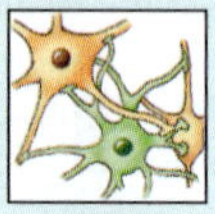
-sis	metasta**sis**	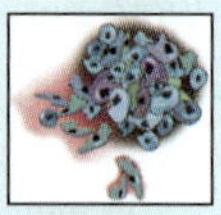	-ses	metasta**ses**	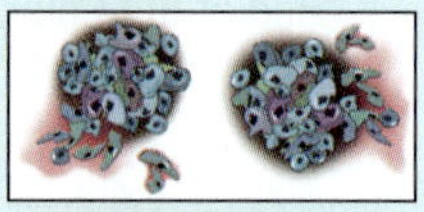
-um	ov**um**	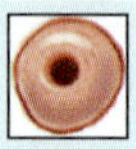	-a	ov**a**	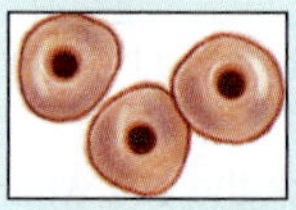
-us	fung**us**	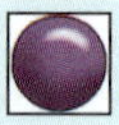	-i	fung**i**	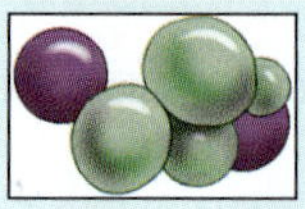
-y	biopsy	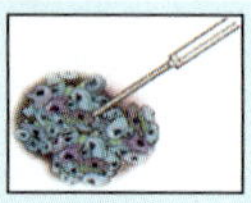	-ies	biops**ies**	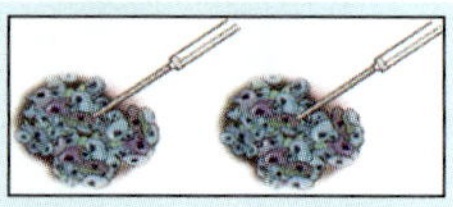

EXERCISE 30

Convert each of the following terms from singular to plural. Refer to Table 2.5, Common Plural Endings for Medical Terms, for guidance. Do not be concerned about the meaning of these terms; concentrate only on the plural endings.

1. etiology ______________________
2. staphylococcus ______________________
3. cyanosis ______________________
4. bacterium ______________________
5. nucleus ______________________
6. pharynx ______________________
7. sarcoma ______________________
8. carcinoma ______________________
9. anastomosis ______________________
10. pubis ______________________
11. prognosis ______________________
12. spermatozoon ______________________
13. fimbria ______________________
14. thorax ______________________
15. appendix ______________________

EXERCISE 31

Circle the correct singular or plural form in each sentence.

1. During a colonoscopy the gastroenterologist noted that the patient had several (**diverticula, diverticulum**) in his transverse colon.
2. Bronchogenic carcinoma was diagnosed in the patient's left (**bronchus, bronchi**).
3. Bilateral (two sides) orchiditis is inflammation of the (**testes, testis**).
4. The light brown mole with notched borders turned out to be a (**melanomata, melanoma**).
5. Multiple (**embolus, emboli**) were observed on the lung scan.
6. Many (**diagnosis, diagnoses**) of benign tumors are picked up during whole-body scanning.
7. Diagnostic studies have shown (**metastasis, metastases**) of the patient's carcinoma of the breast to both her lungs and brain.

Abbreviations

Abbreviations are frequently used verbally and in writing to communicate in the medical and healthcare setting. Abbreviations of the terms included in the chapter are listed below.

Abbreviations that are easily misinterpreted and may lead to medication errors are reported to the Institute for Safe Medication Practices. A list of these abbreviations is in **Appendix E** along with The Joint Commission's "Do Not Use" list of abbreviations.

ABBREVIATION	TERM
CA	carcinoma
chemo	chemotherapy
Dx	diagnosis
METS	metastases
Px	prognosis
RBC	red blood cell (erythrocyte)
XRT	radiation therapy
WBC	white blood cell (leukocyte)

Refer to **Appendix E** for a complete list of abbreviations.

EXERCISE 32

Write the term for each of the abbreviations in the following paragraph.

A 55-year-old woman was admitted to the oncology unit with a **Dx** ____________________ of **CA** ____________________ of the breast, **METS** ____________________ to the lung and brain. Her **Px** ____________________ was guarded. Laboratory tests, including **RBC** ____________ ____________ ____________ and **WBC** ____________ ____________ ____________ counts, were ordered. She will receive both **chemo** ________________________ and **XRT** ________________ ________________.

For additional practice with Abbreviations, go to Evolve Resources at evolve.elsevier.com and select: Practice Student Resources > Student Resources > Chapter 2 > **Flashcards:** Abbreviations

See Appendix B for instructions.

PRACTICAL APPLICATION

EXERCISE 33 *Case Study: Translate Between Everyday Language and Medical Language*

CASE STUDY: Tova Smelkinson

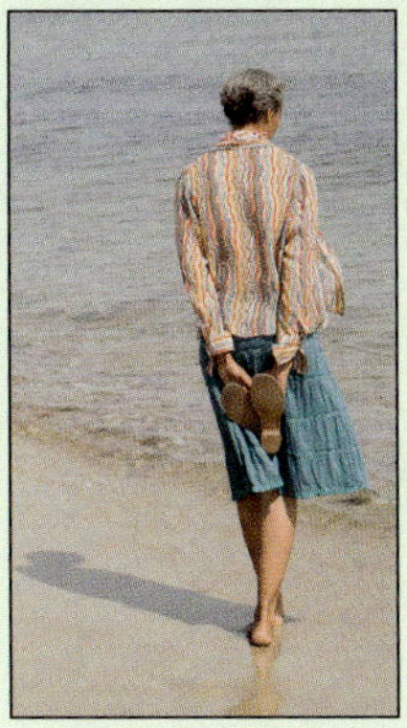

Tova has been having diarrhea. Even worse, she notices blood in it. She had this before when she was younger, and the disease was identified, but she couldn't remember the name. She recalls it was not a cancerous tumor and noted she did not have a fever. She was put on medicine and got better. It looked like a positive outcome. Now it's been going on for 3 weeks. She has pain in her belly with cramps and feels kind of full all the time. She notices she is losing weight, even though she isn't trying. She also feels more tired than usual. Tova makes an appointment with her family doctor to see if she needs to go back on medicine.

Now that you have worked through Chapter 2 on body structure, color, and oncology consider the medical terms that might be used to describe Tova's experience.

A. *Underline phrases in the case study that could be substituted with medical terms.*

B. *Write the medical term and its definition for three of the phrases you underlined.*

MEDICAL TERM	DEFINITION
1. ______________________	______________________________
	______________________________
2. ______________________	______________________________
	______________________________
3. ______________________	______________________________
	______________________________

DOCUMENTATION: Excerpt From Clinical Notation

Tova was able to see her family doctor. The following is a portion of what was noted in her clinical electronic health record (EHR):

A 54-year-old woman presented to the office with 3-week history of bloody diarrhea. She had been diagnosed with ulcerative colitis at the age of 25 years. She was referred for a colonoscopy. The examination revealed a suspicious lesion on the transverse colon. A biopsy was performed and a cytology specimen was obtained. Advanced dysplasia and inflammation were present. The pathologist made a diagnosis of carcinoma of the colon.

C. *Underline medical terms presented in Chapter 2 in the previous excerpt from Tova's medical record (EHR).*

D. *Select and define three of the medical terms you underlined.*

MEDICAL TERM	DEFINITION
1. ______________________	______________________________
	______________________________
2. ______________________	______________________________
	______________________________
3. ______________________	______________________________
	______________________________

EXERCISE 34 *Interact With Medical Documents*

A. Read the report and complete it by writing medical terms on answer lines within the document. Definitions of terms to be written appear after the document.

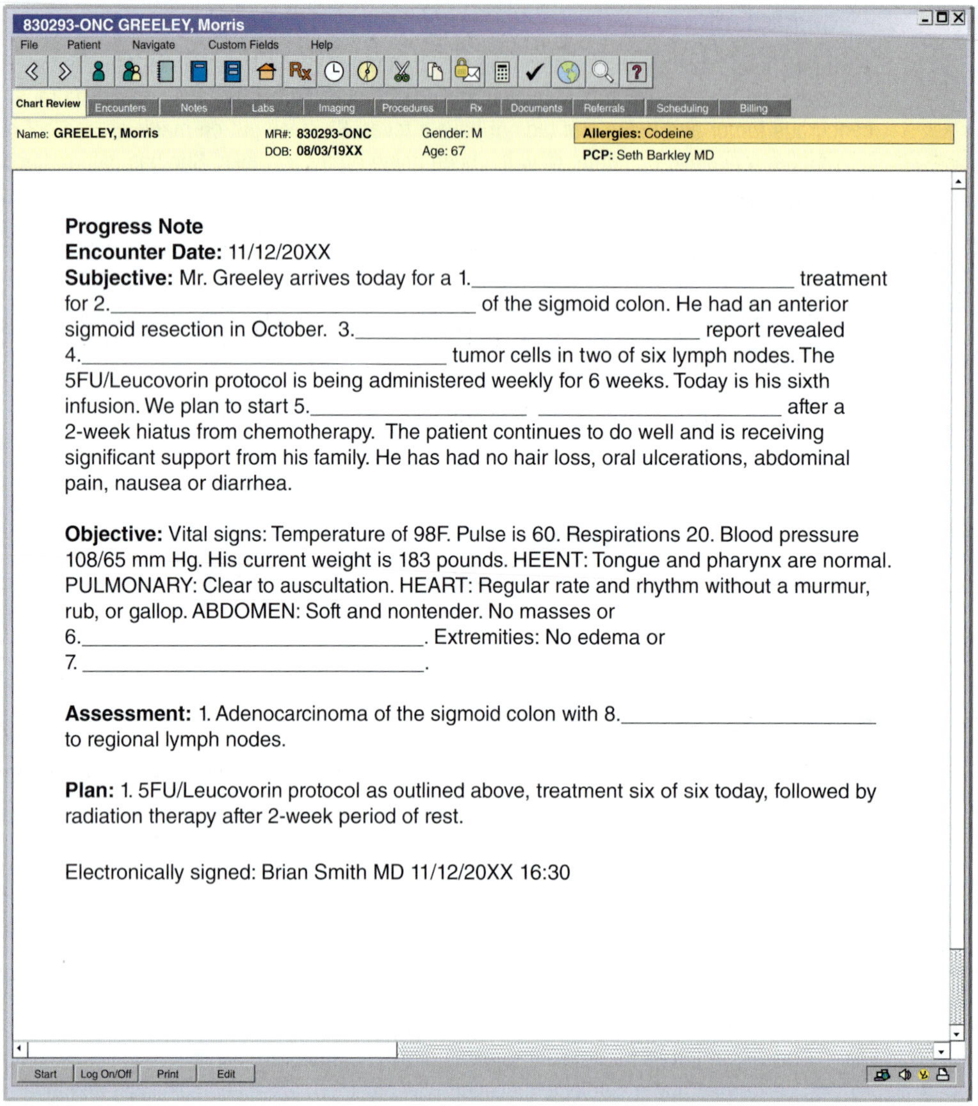

830293-ONC GREELEY, Morris

File Patient Navigate Custom Fields Help

Chart Review | Encounters | Notes | Labs | Imaging | Procedures | Rx | Documents | Referrals | Scheduling | Billing

Name: **GREELEY, Morris** MR#: **830293-ONC** DOB: **08/03/19XX** Gender: M Age: 67 **Allergies:** Codeine **PCP:** Seth Barkley MD

Progress Note
Encounter Date: 11/12/20XX
Subjective: Mr. Greeley arrives today for a 1.______________________________ treatment for 2.______________________________ of the sigmoid colon. He had an anterior sigmoid resection in October. 3.______________________________ report revealed 4.______________________________ tumor cells in two of six lymph nodes. The 5FU/Leucovorin protocol is being administered weekly for 6 weeks. Today is his sixth infusion. We plan to start 5.__________________ ____________________ after a 2-week hiatus from chemotherapy. The patient continues to do well and is receiving significant support from his family. He has had no hair loss, oral ulcerations, abdominal pain, nausea or diarrhea.

Objective: Vital signs: Temperature of 98F. Pulse is 60. Respirations 20. Blood pressure 108/65 mm Hg. His current weight is 183 pounds. HEENT: Tongue and pharynx are normal. PULMONARY: Clear to auscultation. HEART: Regular rate and rhythm without a murmur, rub, or gallop. ABDOMEN: Soft and nontender. No masses or 6.______________________________. Extremities: No edema or 7.______________________________.

Assessment: 1. Adenocarcinoma of the sigmoid colon with 8.______________________ to regional lymph nodes.

Plan: 1. 5FU/Leucovorin protocol as outlined above, treatment six of six today, followed by radiation therapy after 2-week period of rest.

Electronically signed: Brian Smith MD 11/12/20XX 16:30

Start | Log On/Off | Print | Edit

Definitions of Medical Terms to Complete the Document

Write the medical terms defined on corresponding answer lines in the document.

1. Treatment of cancer by using drugs
2. Cancerous tumor of glandular tissue
3. Study of disease
4. Tending to become progressively worse
5. Treatment of cancer by using radioactive substance, x-rays, or radiation
6. Enlargement of an organ
7. Abnormal condition of blue
8. Beyond control

B. Read the medical report and answer the questions below it.

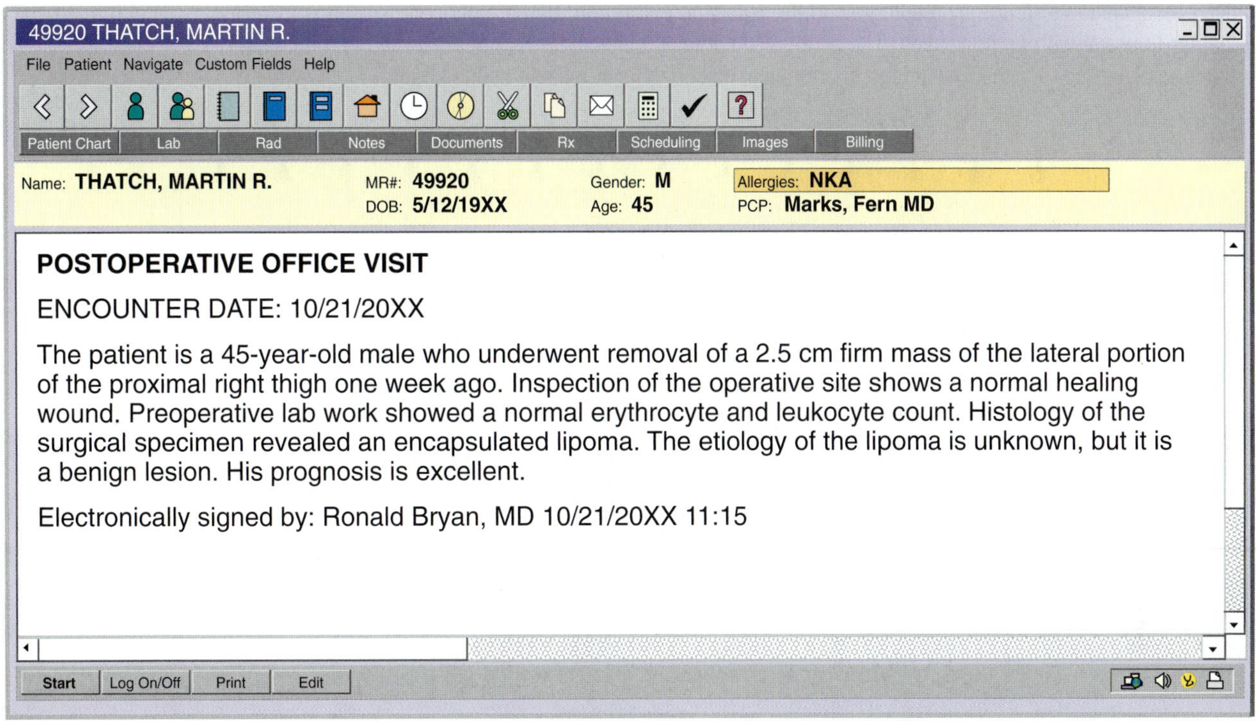

49920 THATCH, MARTIN R.

File Patient Navigate Custom Fields Help

Patient Chart | Lab | Rad | Notes | Documents | Rx | Scheduling | Images | Billing

Name: **THATCH, MARTIN R.** MR#: **49920** DOB: **5/12/19XX** Gender: **M** Age: **45** Allergies: **NKA** PCP: **Marks, Fern MD**

POSTOPERATIVE OFFICE VISIT

ENCOUNTER DATE: 10/21/20XX

The patient is a 45-year-old male who underwent removal of a 2.5 cm firm mass of the lateral portion of the proximal right thigh one week ago. Inspection of the operative site shows a normal healing wound. Preoperative lab work showed a normal erythrocyte and leukocyte count. Histology of the surgical specimen revealed an encapsulated lipoma. The etiology of the lipoma is unknown, but it is a benign lesion. His prognosis is excellent.

Electronically signed by: Ronald Bryan, MD 10/21/20XX 11:15

Start | Log On/Off | Print | Edit

Use the medical report above to answer the questions.

1. The firm mass was confirmed as a lipoma from the surgical specimen in which area of study?
   a. cell
   b. tissue
   c. blood
   d. plasma
2. The lipoma was
   a. spreading.
   b. enclosed in a capsule.
   c. inflamed.
   d. blue in color.
3. Erythr and leuk refer to the ________of cells.
   a. size
   b. shape
   c. amount
   d. color
4. Write the plural form of
   a. prognosis ________________
   b. lipoma ________________
   c. histology ________________

EXERCISE 35 *Pronounce Medical Terms in Use*

Practice pronunciation of terms by reading aloud the following paragraph. Use the phonetic spellings following medical terms from the chapter to assist with pronunciation. The script also contains medical terms not presented in the chapter. Treat them as information only or look for their meanings in a medical dictionary or a reliable online source.

A 54-year-old woman presented to the office with a 3-week history of bloody diarrhea. She had been diagnosed with ulcerative colitis at age 25 years. She was referred for a colonoscopy. The examination revealed a suspicious lesion in the transverse colon. A biopsy was performed and a **cytology** (sī-TOL-o-jē) specimen was obtained. The **pathologist** (pa-THOL-o-jist) made a **diagnosis** (dī-ag-NŌ-sis) of **carcinoma** (kar-si-NŌ-ma) of the colon. Advanced **dysplasia** (dis-PLĀ-zha) and **inflammation** (in-fla-MĀ-shun) existed in the specimen. The patient underwent surgery and was found to have no evidence of **metastasis** (me-TAS-ta-sis). Her entire colon was removed because of a high risk for developing a **malignant** (ma-LIG-nant) lesion in the remaining colon. She made an uneventful recovery and was referred to an **oncologist** (ong-KOL-o-jist) for consideration of **chemotherapy** (kē-mō-THER-a-pē). Her **prognosis** (prog-NŌ-sis) is generally positive. **Radiation therapy** (rā-dē-Ā-shun) (THER-a-pē) or **biological therapy** (bī-ō-LOJ-i-kel) (THER-a-pē) were not indicated in this case.

EXERCISE 36 *Chapter Content Quiz*

Test your understanding of terms and abbreviations introduced in this chapter. Circle the letter for the medical term or abbreviation related to the words in italics

1. Mr. Roberts was diagnosed as having a *cancerous tumor of connective tissue* or:
   a. sarcoma
   b. melanoma
   c. lipoma
2. The doctor said the tumor was *becoming progressively worse*; that is, it was:
   a. benign
   b. malignant
   c. pathogenic
3. The blood test showed an *increased amount of red blood cells*, or:
   a. erythrocytosis
   b. leukocytosis
   c. cyanosis
4. Which of the following means *pertaining to internal organs*?
   a. organic
   b. visceral
   c. systemic
5. The patient was diagnosed with a *tumor composed of fat*, or:
   a. neuroma
   b. carcinoma
   c. lipoma
6. The fatty tumor was *benign*, or:
   a. cancerous
   b. nonrecurrent
   c. recurrent
7. Substances thought to *cause cancer* are called:
   a. carcinoma
   b. carcinogenic
   c. cancerous
8. *Etiology* is the study of:
   a. causes of disease
   b. tissue disease
   c. causes of tumors
9. A *tumor* may be called:
   a. cytoplasm
   b. neoplasm
   c. karyoplasm

10. The pain *originated in the body*, or was:
    a. pathogenic
    b. oncogenic
    c. somatogenic
11. Any *disease of a muscle* is called:
    a. myoma
    b. myopathy
    c. somatopathy
12. The ultrasound revealed marked *abnormal development* on the right kidney or:
    a. hypoplasia
    b. dysplasia
    c. hyperplasia
13. The term that means *produced by a physician* is:
    a. diagnosis
    b. iatrogenic
    c. prognosis
14. The incidence of *black tumor* (primarily of the skin) is increasing.
    a. fibrosarcoma
    b. fibroma
    c. melanoma
15. The term that means *within the living body* is:
    a. in vitro
    b. in vivo
    c. encapsulated
16. Which of the following is a *malignant tumor*?
    a. sarcoma
    b. fibroma
    c. myoma
17. The term for *programmed cell death*, a natural occurrence within the body is:
    a. dysplasia
    b. xanthosis
    c. apoptosis
18. Which of the following provides *palliative and supportive care for the terminally ill* and their families?
    a. hospice
    b. palliative care
    c. therapy
19. The overall survival and acceptable *state of being diseased* justifies performing a therapeutic lymphadenectomy for nodal metastatic melanoma.
    a. mortality
    b. morbidity
    c. prognosis
20. A laboratory test was ordered for a *leukocyte* count or:
    a. WBC
    b. RBC
    c. XRT

For additional practice with chapter content, go to Evolve Resources at evolve.elsevier.com and select:
Practice Student Resources > Student Resources > Chapter 2 > **Games:** Medical Millionaire
Tournament of Terminology
Practice Quizzes: Word Parts
Terms Built from Word Parts
Terms NOT Built from Word Parts
Abbreviations

See Appendix B for instructions.

WEB LINK

For additional information on cancer visit the **National Cancer Institute** at ***http://www.nci.nih.gov***.

CHAPTER REVIEW

REVIEW OF CHAPTER CONTENT ON EVOLVE RESOURCES

Go to evolve.elsevier.com and click on Gradable Student Resources and Practice Student Resources. Online learning activities found there can be used to review chapter content and to assess your learning of word parts, medical terms, and abbreviations. Place check marks in the boxes next to activities used for review and assessment.

GRADABLE STUDENT RESOURCES

Chapter 02 >	Exercises >	☐ Analyze Medical Terms ☐ Word Parts ☐ Terms Built from Word Parts ☐ Terms Not Built from Word Parts ☐ Abbreviations ☐ Plural Endings
	Quizzes >	☐ Quiz 1: Disease and Disorder Oncology Terms ☐ Quiz 2: Body Structure Terms ☐ Quiz 3: Complementary Terms ☐ Quiz 4: Singular and Plural Endings

PRACTICE STUDENT RESOURCES > STUDENT RESOURCES

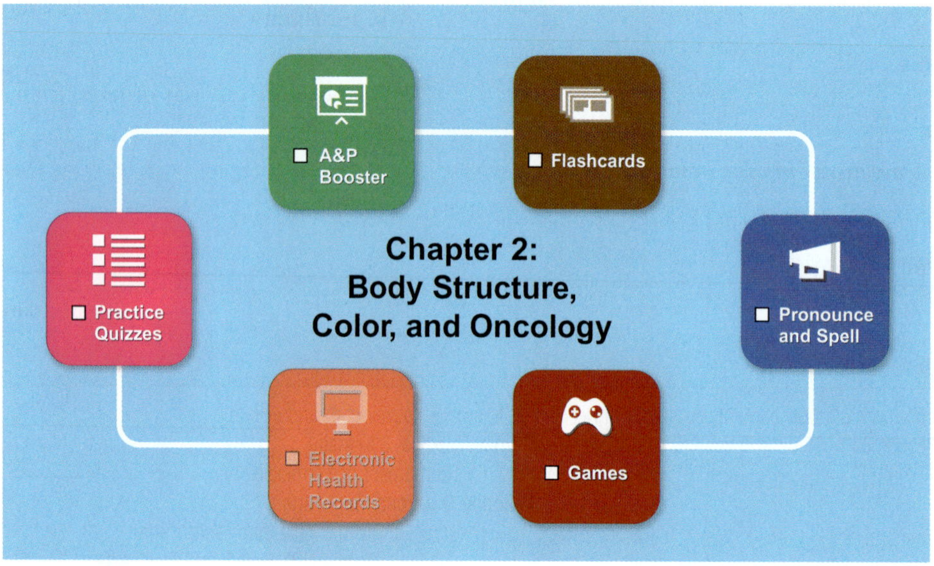

REVIEW OF WORD PARTS

Can you define and spell the following word parts?

COMBINING FORMS

aden/o	erythr/o	leuk/o	rhabd/o
cancer/o	eti/o	lip/o	sarc/o
carcin/o	fibr/o	melan/o	somat/o
chlor/o	gno/o	my/o	system/o
chrom/o	hist/o	neur/o	viscer/o
cyan/o	iatr/o	onc/o	xanth/o
cyt/o	kary/o	organ/o	
epitheli/o	lei/o	path/o	

PREFIXES	SUFFIXES		
dia-	-al	-logist	-pathy
dys-	-cyte	-logy	-plasia
hyper-	-gen	-megaly	-plasm
hypo-	-genic	-oid	-sarcoma
meta-	-ic	-oma	-sis
neo-		-osis	-stasis
pro-		-ous	

REVIEW OF TERMS

Can you define, spell, and pronounce the following terms *built from word parts*?

ONCOLOGY	BODY STRUCTURE		COMPLEMENTARY
adenocarcinoma	cytogenic	somatic	cancerous
adenoma	cytoid	somatogenic	carcinogen
carcinoma (CA)	cytology	somatopathy	carcinogenic
chloroma	cytoplasm	somatoplasm	cyanosis
epithelioma	dysplasia	systemic	diagnosis (Dx)
fibroma	epithelial	visceral	etiology
fibrosarcoma	erythrocyte (RBC)		iatrogenic
leiomyoma	erythrocytosis		iatrology
leiomyosarcoma	histology		metastasis (pl. metastases)
lipoma	hyperplasia		oncogenic
liposarcoma	hypoplasia		oncologist
melanocarcinoma	karyocyte		oncology
melanoma	karyoplasm		organic
myoma	leukocyte (WBC)		pathogenic
neoplasm	leukocytosis		pathologist
neuroma	lipoid		pathology
rhabdomyoma	myopathy		prognosis (Px)
rhabdomyosarcoma	neuroid		xanthochromic
sarcoma	organomegaly		xanthosis

Can you define, pronounce, and spell the following terms *NOT built from word parts?*

COMPLEMENTARY		
afebrile	exacerbation	malignant
apoptosis	febrile	morbidity
biological therapy	hospice	mortality
benign	idiopathic	palliative
carcinoma in situ	inflammation	radiation therapy (XRT)
chemotherapy (chemo)	in vitro	remission
encapsulated	in vivo	

INTEGRATIVE MEDICINE TERMS

According to the National Center for Complementary and Alternative Medicine (NCCAM) Institute of the National Institutes of Health (NIH), **Complementary and Alternative Medicine (CAM)** is defined as "a group of diverse medical and health care systems, practices, and products that are not generally considered part of conventional medicine."

Complementary medicine is used in conjunction with conventional medicine.

Alternative medicine is used in place of conventional medicine.

Integrative medicine is the combination of mainstream medical therapies and evidence-based CAM therapies. Use of CAM has increased dramatically in recent years as healthcare consumers search for a variety of ways to treat illness and promote wellness.

Look for **Integrative Medicine Term boxes** throughout the text.

For a complete list of integrative medicine terms, go to evolve.elsevier.com and select: Practice Student Resources > Student Resources > **Extra Content** > Appendix I, Integrative Medicine Terms

See Appendix B for instructions.

Chapter 3

Directional Terms, Planes, Positions, Regions, and Quadrants

Objectives

Upon completion of this chapter you will be able to:

1. Define and spell word parts related to directional terms.
2. Define, pronounce, and spell terms used to describe directions with respect to the body.
3. Define, pronounce, and spell terms used to describe anatomic planes.
4. Define, pronounce, and spell terms used to describe body positions.
5. Define, pronounce, and spell terms used to describe abdominopelvic regions.
6. Identify and spell the four abdominopelvic quadrants.
7. Interpret the meaning of abbreviations presented in this chapter.
8. Apply medical language in clinical contexts.

Outline

Types of body movement are presented in Chapter 14, Musculoskeletal System, on pages 576–577. Terms related to body movement are: *abduction*, *adduction*, *inversion*, *eversion*, *extension*, *flexion*, *pronation*, *supination*, and *rotation*.

ANATOMIC POSITION

When using directional terms, the body is assumed to be in the standard, neutral position of reference called the **anatomic position** (Fig. 3.1). In this position, the body is viewed as standing erect, arms at the side, palms of the hands facing forward, and feet side by side. The directional terms are the same whether the person is standing or supine (lying face up).

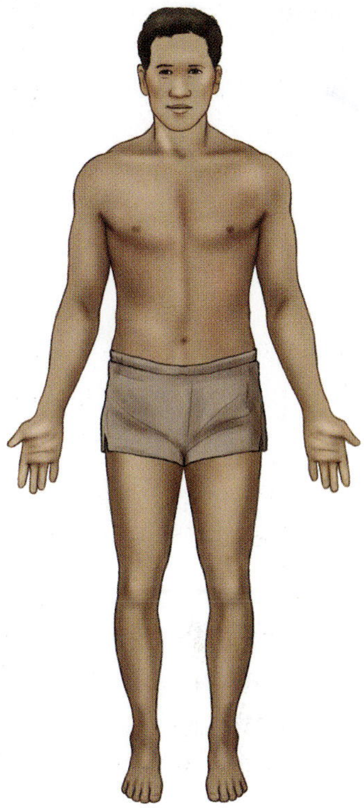

FIG. 3.1 Anatomic position.

WORD PARTS

Combining Forms of Directional Terms

Word parts you need to learn to complete this chapter are listed on the following pages. The exercises at the end of each list will help you learn their definitions and spelling.

Use the flashcards accompanying this text or electronic flashcards to assist you in memorizing the word parts for this chapter.

COMBINING FORM	DEFINITION
anter/o	front
caud/o	tail (downward)
cephal/o	head (upward)
dist/o	away (from the point of attachment of a body part)
dors/o	back
infer/o	below
later/o	side
medi/o	middle
poster/o	back, behind
proxim/o	near (the point of attachment of a body part)
super/o	above
ventr/o	belly (front)

HEAD AND TRUNK ONLY

Terms built from the combining forms **cephal/o** and **caud/o** are used to describe locations in the head and the trunk of the body.

Do not be concerned about which combining form to use for front or back. As you continue to study and use medical terms, you will become familiar with common usage of each word part.

EXERCISE 1

Write the definitions for the following combining forms. *To check your answers to the exercises in this chapter, go to Appendix A at the back of the textbook.*

1. ventr/o ______________________
2. cephal/o ______________________
3. later/o ______________________
4. medi/o ______________________
5. infer/o ______________________
6. proxim/o ______________________
7. super/o ______________________
8. dist/o ______________________
9. dors/o ______________________
10. caud/o ______________________
11. anter/o ______________________
12. poster/o ______________________

EXERCISE FIGURE A

Fill in the blanks with directional combining forms. *To check your answers, go to Appendix A.*

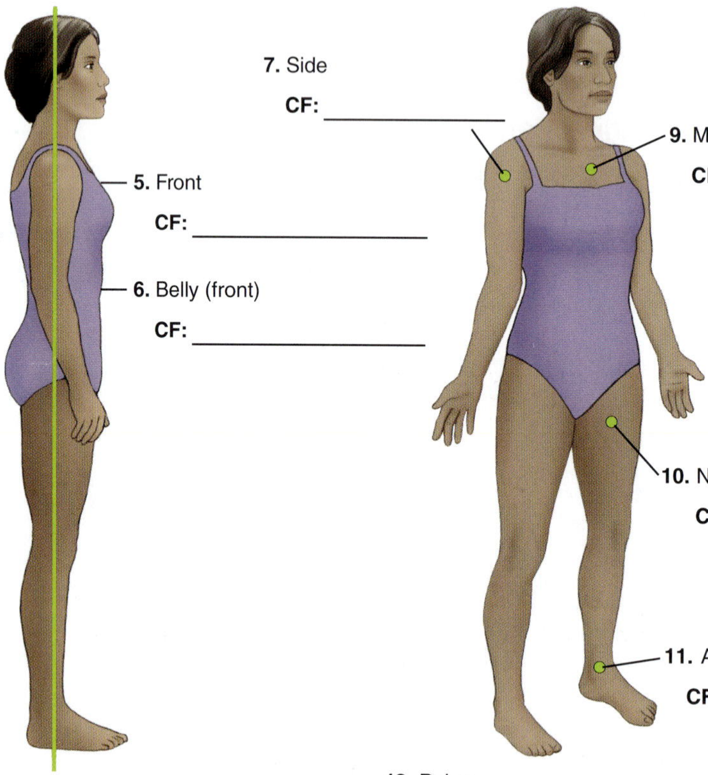

Prefixes

PREFIX	DEFINITION
bi-	two
uni-	one

Suffixes

SUFFIX	DEFINITION
-ad	toward
-ior	pertaining to

MOVEMENT

The suffix -ad used in directional terms refers to movement in a specific direction. For example, **cephal/ad** indicates movement toward the head.

Many suffixes mean **pertaining to**. You have already learned three of them in Chapter 2: **-al, -ic,** and **-ous.** You will learn more in subsequent chapters. With practice, you will learn which suffix is most commonly used with a particular word root or combining form.

Refer to **Appendix C** and **Appendix D** for alphabetical lists of word parts and their meanings.

EXERCISE 2

Match the prefixes and suffixes in the first column with their correct definitions in the second column.

_____ 1. -ad	a. one
_____ 2. -ior	b. pertaining to
_____ 3. bi-	c. toward
_____ 4. uni-	d. two

EXERCISE 3

Write the definitions of the following prefixes and suffixes.

1. -ior ______________________
2. -ad ______________________
3. bi- ______________________
4. uni- ______________________

For additional practice with Word Parts, go to Evolve Resources at evolve.elsevier.com and select: Practice Student Resources > Student Resources > Chapter 3 > **Flashcards**

See Appendix B for instructions.

MEDICAL TERMS

Directional Terms

The following terms are built from word parts you have already learned and can be translated literally to find their meanings. Further explanation of terms beyond the definition of their word parts, if needed, is included in parentheses.

TERM	DEFINITION
caudad (KAW-dad)	toward the tail (or the inferior portion of the trunk; downward)
cephalad (SEF-a-lad)	toward the head (upward)
lateral (lat) (LAT-er-al)	pertaining to a side (Fig. 3.2)
medial (med) (MĒ-dē-al)	pertaining to the middle (Fig. 3.3)
unilateral (ū-ni-LAT-er-al)	pertaining to one side (only)
bilateral (bī-LAT-er-al)	pertaining to two sides
mediolateral (*mē*-dē-Ō-LAT-er-al)	pertaining to the middle and to the side
distal (DIS-tal)	pertaining to away (from the point of attachment of a body part) (Fig. 3.4)
proximal (PROK-si-mal)	pertaining to near (to the point of attachment of a body part) (Fig. 3.4)
inferior (inf) (in-FĒR-ē-or)	pertaining to below (Fig. 3.5)

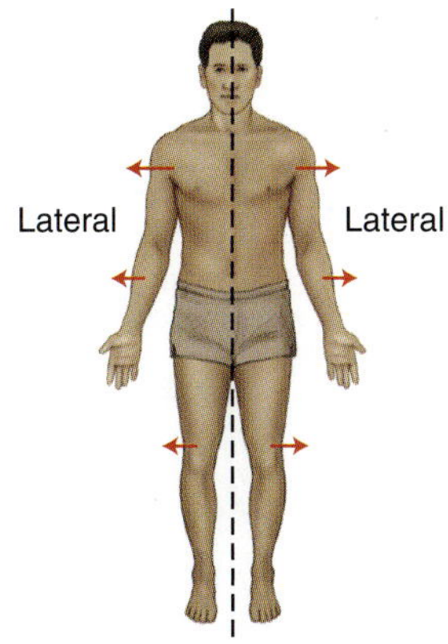

FIG. 3.2 Lateral.

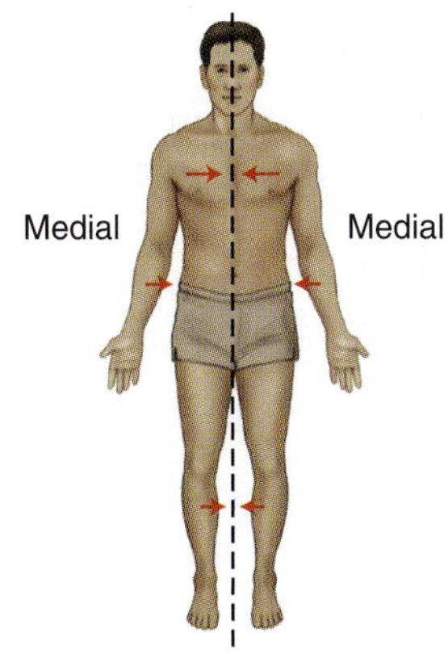

FIG. 3.3 Medial.

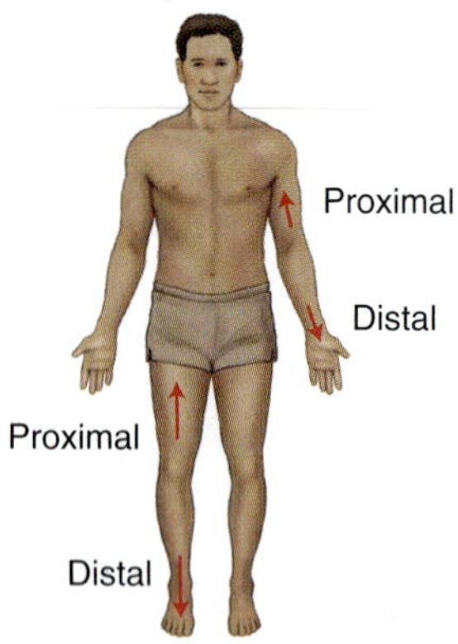

FIG. 3.4 Distal and proximal.

Directional Terms—cont'd

TERM	DEFINITION
superior (sup) (sū-PĒR-ē-or)	pertaining to above (Fig. 3.5)
caudal (KAW-dal)	pertaining to the tail (synonymous with **inferior** in human anatomy when specifying location in the trunk of the body) (Fig. 3.5)
cephalic (se-FAL-ik)	pertaining to the head (Fig. 3.5)
anterior (ant) (an-TĒR-ē-or)	pertaining to the front (Fig. 3.5)
posterior (pos-TĒR-ē-or)	pertaining to the back (Fig. 3.5)
dorsal (DOR-sal)	pertaining to the back (Fig. 3.5)
ventral (VEN-tral)	pertaining to the belly (front) (Fig. 3.5)
anteroposterior (AP) (*an*-ter-ō-pos-TĒR-ē-or)	pertaining to the front and to the back (see Exercise Figure B)
posteroanterior (PA) (*pos*-ter-ō-an-TĒR-ē-or)	pertaining to the back and to the front (see Exercise Figure B)

TABLE 3.1 Usage of Terms With Similar Meanings

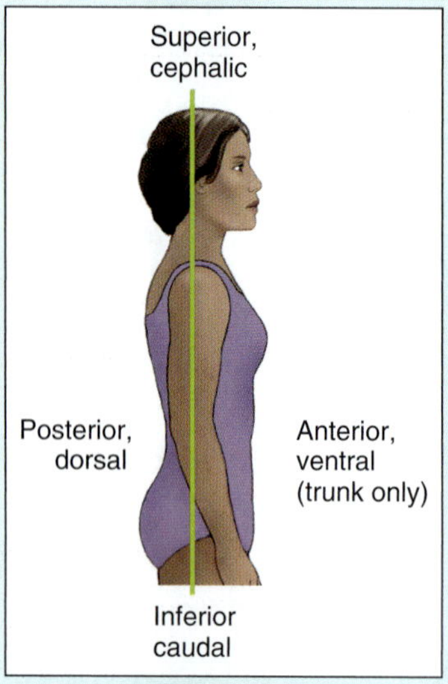

FIG. 3.5 Superior and inferior, posterior and anterior, dorsal and ventral.

SAME

When describing anatomic structures in the *head* and *trunk* of the body, the following terms are **similar** in meaning and are used interchangeably:

- **Superior** and **cephalic** describe above.
- **Inferior** and **caudal** describe below.
- **Posterior** and **dorsal** describe the back.
- **Anterior** and **ventral** (trunk only) describe the front.

DIFFERENT

Differences in uses of terms include:

- Directional terms ending with **-ior** can indicate spatial relationships of body parts to each other throughout the body. The nose is **anterior** to the ear, and the ear is **posterior** to the nose. The eye is **superior** to the mouth, and the mouth is **inferior** to the eye.
- **Ventral** describes the trunk of the body. The **ventral** cavity is located toward the belly and is made up of the thoracic and abdominopelvic cavities (Fig. 3.5). Ventral may also denote a relationship to the anterior abdominal wall. A **ventral** hernia is a hernia in the anterior abdominal wall.
- **Dorsal** describes the back of the head and trunk. The **dorsal** cavity is located in the posterior portion of the body and is made up of the cranial and spinal cavities. Dorsal also describes the surface of the hand opposite the palm and the top of the foot. The pulse palpable on the **dorsal** surface of the foot is called dorsalis pedis pulse (see p. 79).
- **Cephalic** and **caudal** apply to the head and trunk of the body only, whereas **superior** and **inferior** also apply to limbs. The ankle is **inferior** to the knee.

EXERCISE 4

Practice saying aloud each of the Directional Terms.

To hear the terms, go to Evolve Resources at evolve.elsevier.com and select:
Practice Student Resources > Student Resources > Chapter 3 > **Pronounce and Spell**

See Appendix B for instructions.

❑ Check the box when complete.

EXERCISE 5

Analyze and define the following Directional Terms by drawing slashes between word parts, writing word part abbreviations above the term, underlining combining forms, and writing combining form abbreviations below the term. *To check your answers, go to Appendix A.*

WR CV WR S
EXAMPLE: medi / o / later / al
CF
pertaining to the middle and to the side

1. cephalad

2. proximal

3. lateral

4. unilateral

5. anteroposterior

6. cephalic

7. superior

8. anterior

9. caudad

10. distal

11. medial

12. bilateral

13. posteroanterior

____

____

14. caudal

____

____

15. inferior

____

____

16. posterior

____

____

17. ventral

____

____

18. dorsal

____

____

EXERCISE 6

A. Build Directional Terms for the following definitions by using the word parts you have learned.

1. toward the head (upward) ______ / ______ (WR / S)

2. pertaining to near ______ / ______ (WR / S)

3. pertaining to away ______ / ______ (WR / S)

4. pertaining to a side ______ / ______ (WR / S)

5. pertaining to the middle ______ / ______ (WR / S)

6. toward the tail (downward) ______ / ______ (WR / S)

7. pertaining to the back and to the front ______ / ___ / ______ / ______ (WR / CV / WR / S)

8. pertaining to the middle and to the side ______ / ___ / ______ / ______ (WR / CV / WR / S)

9. pertaining to one side (only) ______ / ______ / ______ (P / WR / S)

10. pertaining to the front and to the back ______ / ___ / ______ / ______ (WR / CV / WR / S)

11. pertaining to two sides ______ / ______ / ______ (P / WR / S)

B. Write word parts to build Directional Terms.

1. ________ / ________
   above / pertaining to

2. ________ / ________
   head / pertaining to

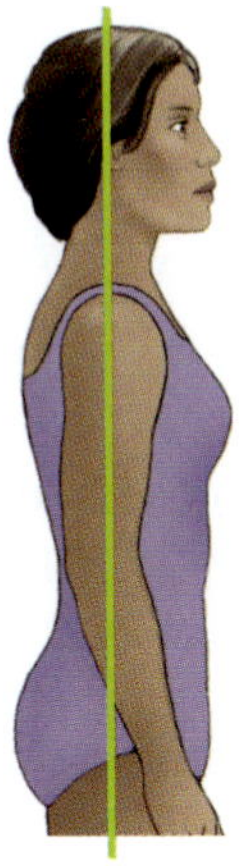

3. ________ / ________
   back / pertaining to

   ________ / ________
   back / pertaining to

6. ________ / ________
   front / pertaining to

7. ________ / ________
   belly (front) / pertaining to

4. ________ / ________
   below / pertaining to

5. ________ / ________
   tail / pertaining to

EXERCISE FIGURE B

Fill in the blanks to label the diagram.

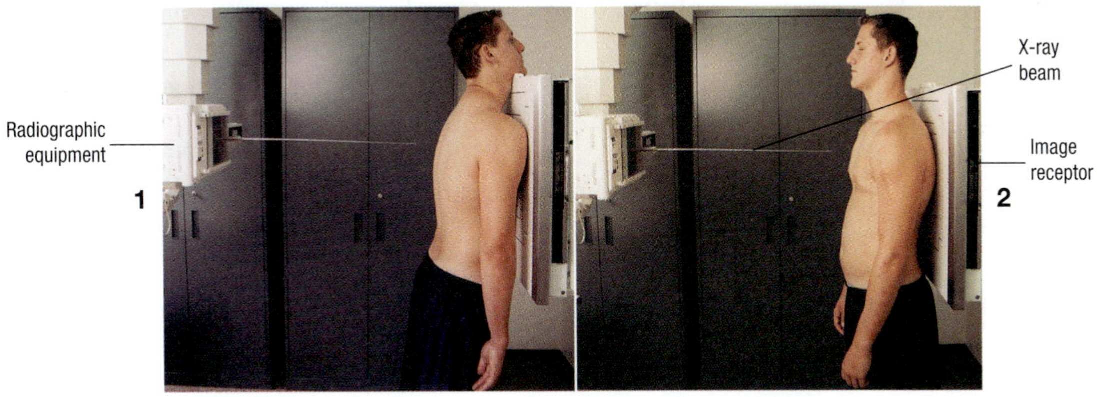

1. ________ / ____ / ________ / ________ projection
   back / cv / front / pertaining to

2. ________ / ____ / ________ / ________ projection
   front / cv / back / pertaining to

Organs and anatomy of interest closest to the image receptor are more accurately imaged. For example, a PA projection is used when the heart or other anterior structures are the focus of the study. An AP projection is used when the spine or other posterior structures are the primary focus.

EXERCISE 7

Spell each of the Directional Terms by having someone dictate them to you. Use a separate sheet of paper.

To hear and spell the terms, go to Evolve Resources at evolve.elsevier.com and select:
Practice Student Resources > Student Resources > Chapter 3 > **Pronounce and Spell**

See Appendix B for instructions.

❑ Check the box when complete.

Anatomic Planes

Planes are imaginary flat fields used as points of reference to identify or view the location of organs and anatomic structures. Anatomic planes are frequently used in diagnostic imaging and surgery. The body is assumed to be in the anatomic position unless specified otherwise (Table 3.2).

MIDLINE
is an imaginary line that separates the body, or body parts, into halves. In medical language, midline is used as a common reference point.

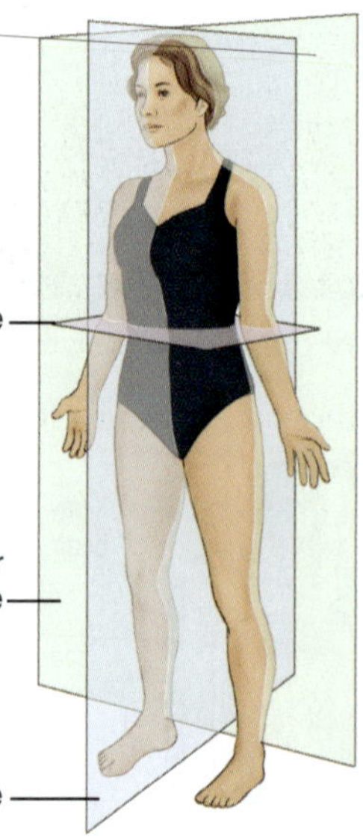

FIG. 3.6 Anatomic planes.

TERM	DEFINITION
frontal or coronal (FRON-tal) (ko-RŌN-al)	vertical plane passing through the body from side to side, dividing the body into anterior and posterior portions (Fig. 3.6)
midsagittal (mid-SAJ-i-tal)	vertical plane passing through the body from front to back at the midline, dividing the body equally into right and left halves (Fig. 3.6)
parasagittal (*par*-a-SAJ-i-tal)	vertical plane passing through the body from front to back, dividing the body into unequal left and right sides
sagittal (SAJ-i-tal)	vertical plane passing through the body from front to back, dividing the body into right and left sides (any plane parallel to the midsagittal plane)
transverse (trans-VERS)	horizontal plane dividing the body into superior and inferior portions (Fig. 3.6)

Sagittal describes vertical planes dividing the body into right and left sides. **Midsagittal** and **parasagittal** planes are both sagittal planes with the midsagittal plane dividing the body equally into halves and the parasagittal plane dividing the body into unequal sides.

EXERCISE 8

Practice saying aloud each of the Anatomic Planes.

To hear the terms, go to Evolve Resources at evolve.elsevier.com and select:
Practice Student Resources > Student Resources > Chapter 3 > **Pronounce and Spell**

See Appendix B for instructions.

❑ Check the box when complete.

TABLE 3.2 Anatomic Planes and Diagnostic Images

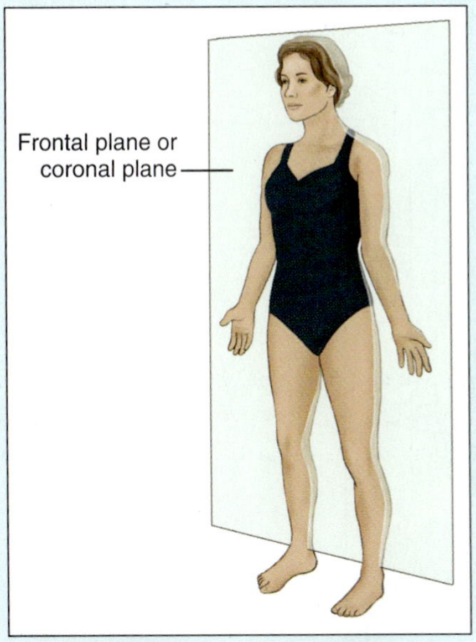

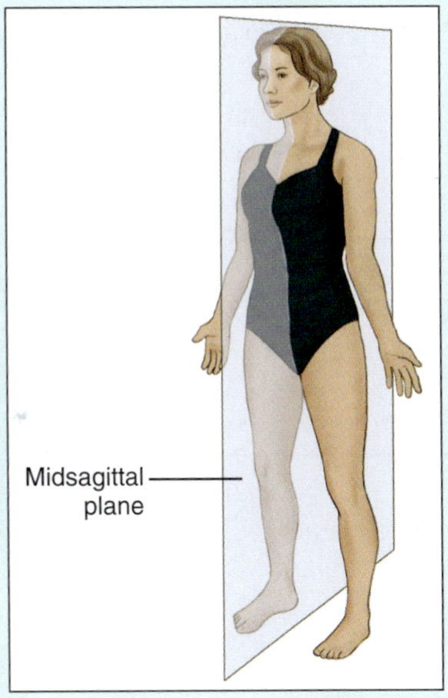

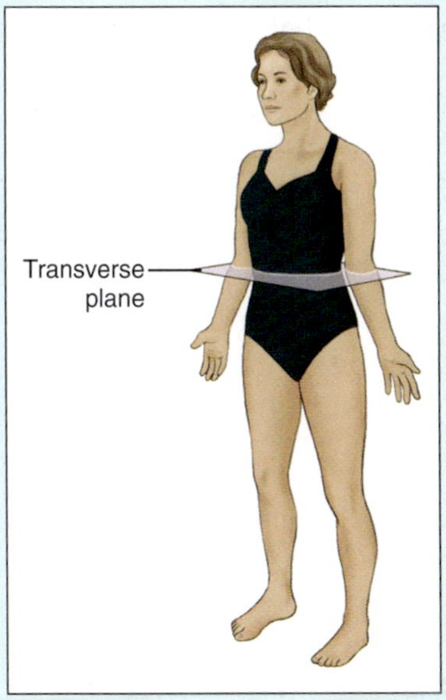

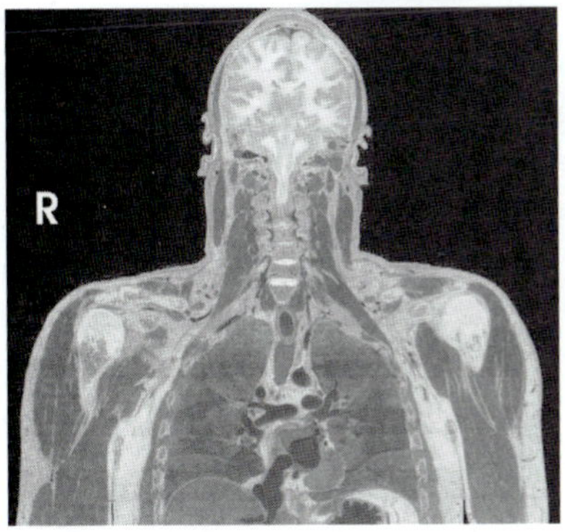

Frontal or coronal diagnostic image (MRI*)

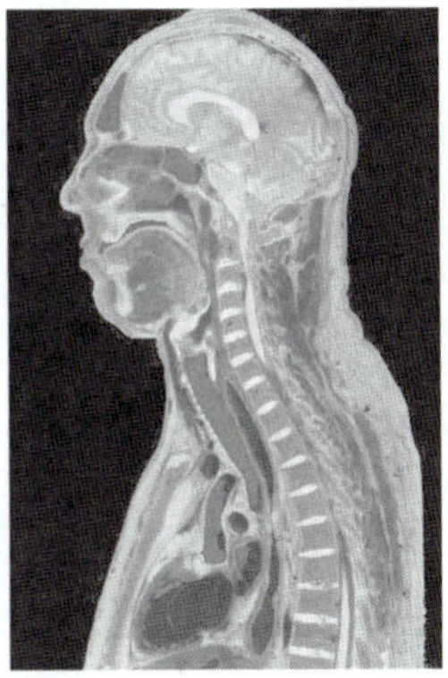

Midsagittal diagnostic image (MRI*)

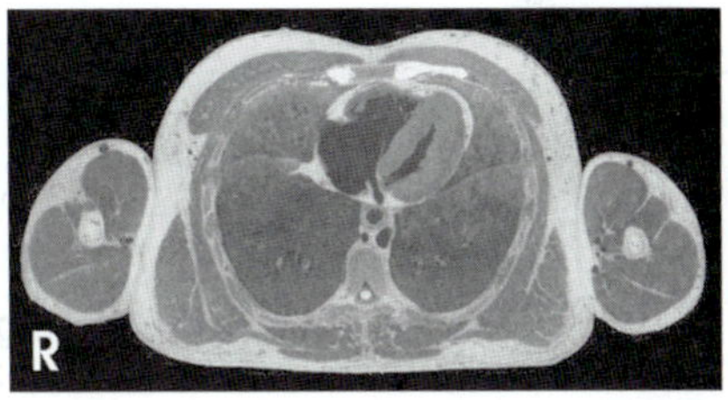

Transverse diagnostic image (MRI*)

* MRI abbreviates **magnetic resonance imaging**

EXERCISE 9

Fill in the blanks with the correct terms.

1. The plane that divides the body into superior and inferior portions is the ______________________________ plane.
2. The plane that divides the body **equally** into right and left halves is the ______________________________ plane.
3. The plane that divides the body into anterior and posterior portions is referred to as ______________________________ or ______________________________ plane.
4. Any plane that divides the body into right and left sides is referred to as a ______________________________ plane.
5. The plane that divides the body into **unequal** right and left sides is the ______________________________ plane.

EXERCISE FIGURE C

Fill in the blanks with anatomic planes.

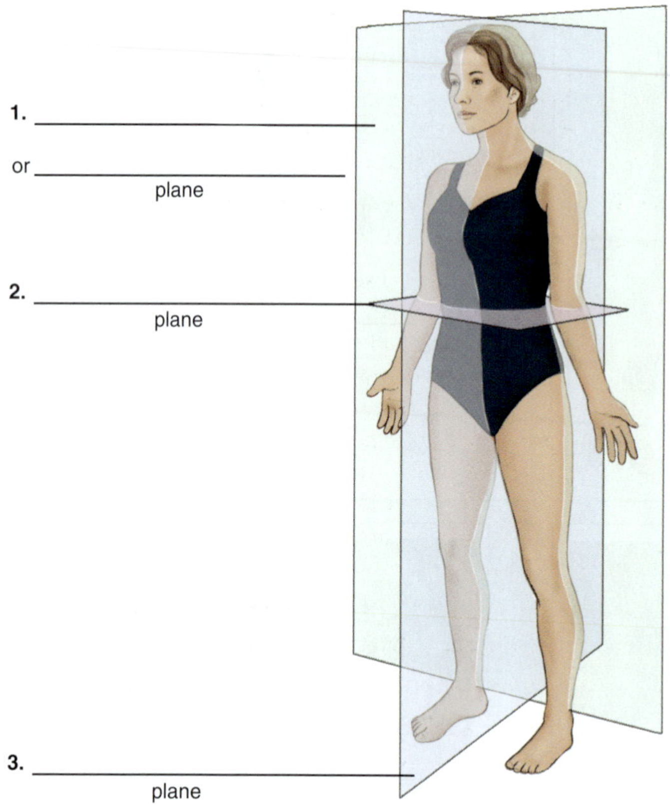

EXERCISE 10

Spell each of the Anatomic Planes by having someone dictate them to you. Use a separate sheet of paper.

> To hear and spell the terms, go to Evolve Resources at evolve.elsevier.com and select:
> Practice Student Resources > Student Resources > Chapter 3 > **Pronounce and Spell**
>
> See Appendix B for instructions.

❑ Check the box when complete.

Body Positions

Position terms are used in health care settings to communicate how the patient's body is placed for physical examination, diagnostic procedures, surgery, treatment, and recovery.

FOWLER POSITION

indicates the patient is in a sitting position with the head of the bed raised between 30° and 90°. Variations in the angle are denoted by **high Fowler**, indicating an upright position at approximately 90°; **Fowler** indicating an angle between 45° and 60°; **semi-Fowler**, 30° to 45°; and **low Fowler**, where the head is slightly elevated.

TERM	DEFINITION
Fowler position (FOW-ler) (pe-ZISH-en)	semi-sitting position with slight elevation of the knees
lateral recumbent position (LAT-er-al) (re-KUM-bent) (pe-ZISH-en)	lying on side; right and left precede the term to indicate the patient's side
lithotomy position (lith-OT-o-mē) (pe-ZISH-en)	lying on back with legs raised and feet in stirrups, hips and knees flexed, thighs abducted (away from body) and externally rotated

TERM	DEFINITION
orthopnea position (or-THOP-nē-a) (pe-ZISH-en)	sitting upright in a chair or in bed supported by pillows behind the back. Sometimes the patient tilts forward resting on a pillow supported by an overbed table (also called **orthopneic position**).
prone position (prōn) (pe-ZISH-en)	lying on abdomen, facing downward (head may be turned to one side) (also called **ventral recumbent position**)
recumbent position (rē-KUM-bent) (pe-ZISH-en)	lying down in any position (also called **decubitus position**)
Sims position (simz) (pe-ZISH-en)	lying on side in a semi-prone position with the knee drawn up toward the chest and the arm drawn behind parallel to the back. Right and left precede the term to indicate the patient's right or left side. Originally, the term specifically indicated the patient's left side; therefore, if the term Sims position is used without a description of right or left, it is assumed the patient is to be placed on the left side.
supine position (SOO-pine) (pe-ZISH-en)	lying on back, facing upward (also called **dorsal recumbent position**)
Trendelenburg position (tren-DEL-en-berg) (pe-ZISH-en)	lying on back with body tilted so that the head is lower than the feet

ORTHOPNEA POSITION

Orthopnea is built from the combining form **orth/o** meaning straight and the suffix **-pnea** meaning breathing. Patients who need to sit up straight to breathe are placed in the **orthopnea position**.

EXERCISE 11

Practice saying aloud each of the Body Positions.

To hear the terms, go to Evolve Resources at evolve.elsevier.com and select:
Practice Student Resources > Student Resources > Chapter 3 > **Pronounce and Spell**

See Appendix B for instructions.

❑ Check the box when complete.

EXERCISE 12

A. Match the body position terms in the first column with their descriptions in the second column. *To check your answers, go to Appendix A.*

_____ 1. Fowler position	a. lying on side
_____ 2. lateral recumbent position	b. lying down in any position
_____ 3. prone position	c. also called dorsal recumbent position
_____ 4. supine position	d. semi-sitting position with slight elevation of the knees
_____ 5. recumbent position	e. if "right" or "left" does not appear with the term, the patient is assumed to be placed lying on left side with right knee drawn up and with left arm drawn behind, parallel to the back
_____ 6. Sims position	f. also called ventral recumbent position

TABLE 3.3 Recumbent Positions

Recumbent position (also called **decubitus position**) is a general term indicating the patient is lying down in any position, such as supine, prone, or on one side. The specific position is indicated by additional terms.

dorsal recumbent position... lying on back; the patient is lying down facing upwards (also called **supine position**)

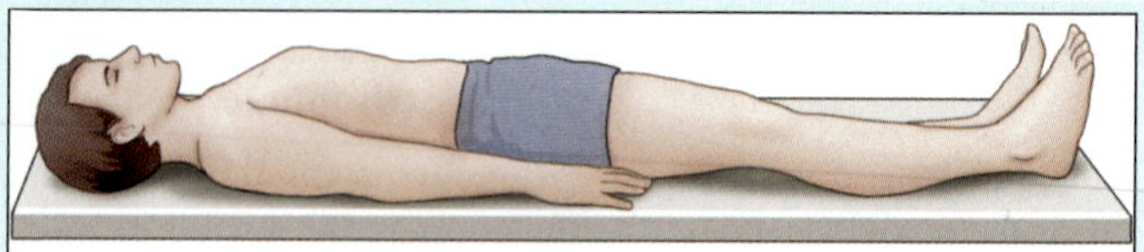

Supine

ventral recumbent position... lying face down; the patient is lying down on the belly. The face may be turned to the right or left (also called **prone position**).

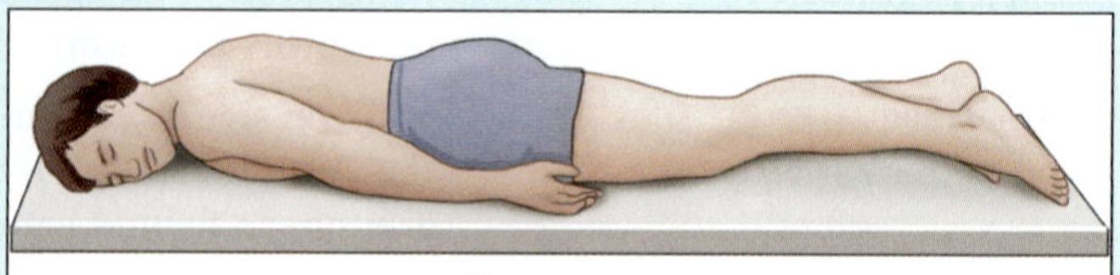

Prone

left lateral recumbent position... lying on the patient's left side; right knee may be drawn upward (also called **left lateral decubitus position, Sims position**, and **left Sims position** when knee is drawn upward)

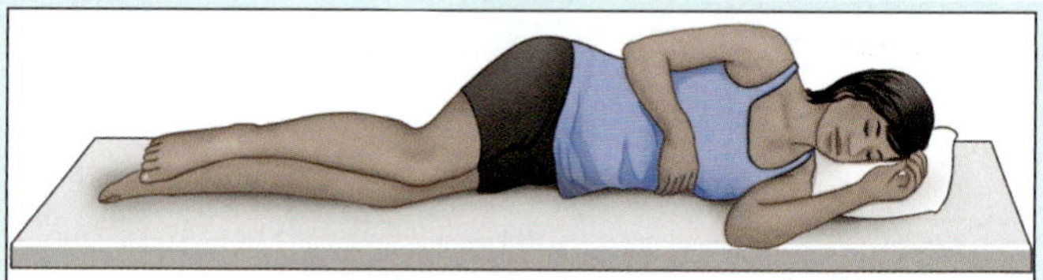

Left lateral recumbant

right lateral recumbent position... lying on the patient's right side; left knee may be drawn upward (also called **right lateral decubitus position** and **right Sims position** when knee is drawn upward)

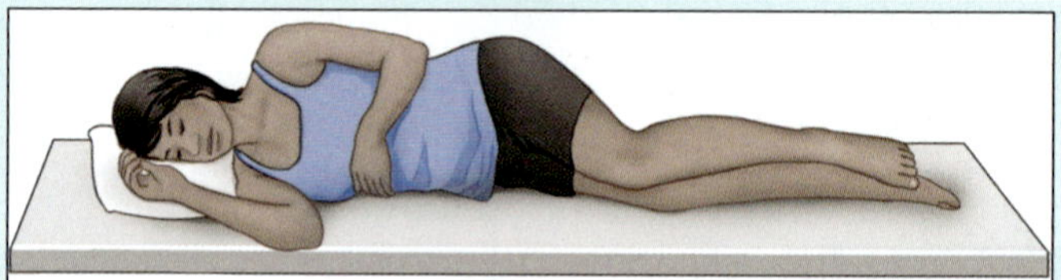

Right lateral recumbant

EXERCISE 12—*cont'd*

B. Write the patient position pictured and defined.

1. ________________ position, lying on back, facing upward (also called **dorsal recumbent position**)

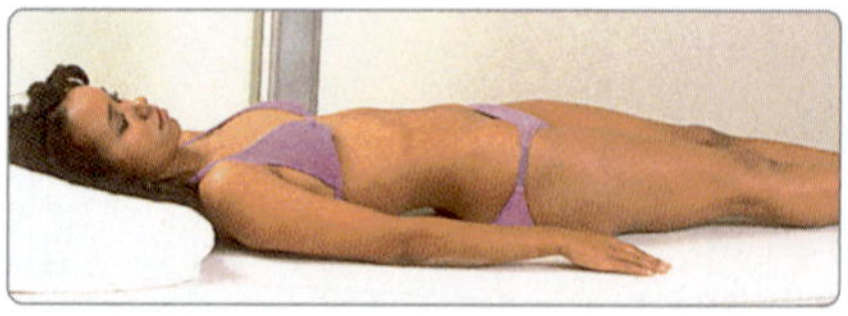

2. ________________ position, lying on abdomen, facing downward (also called **ventral recumbent position**)

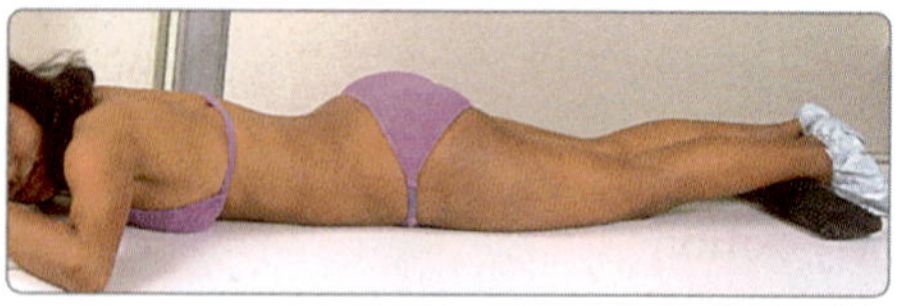

3. __________________ position, sitting upright and tilted forward resting on a pillow supported by an overbed table

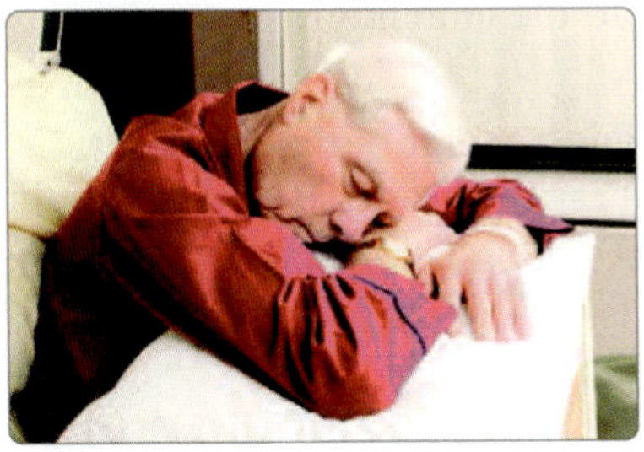

4. __________________ position, lying on back with body tilted so that the head is lower than the feet

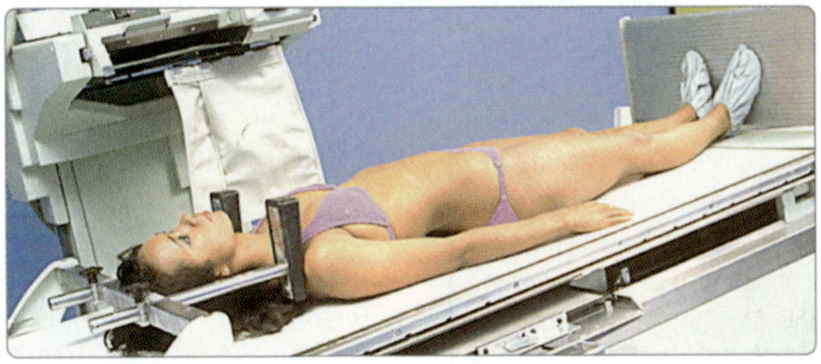

5. Modified __________________ position, lying on back with legs raised (notice legs are supported under the knees, rather than having the feet in stirrups)

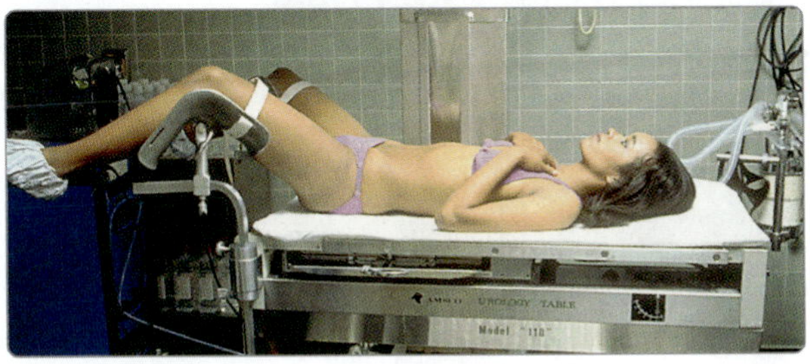

6. Modified __________________ position, lying on left side with right knee drawn up (notice the arm is placed in front, rather than behind the body)

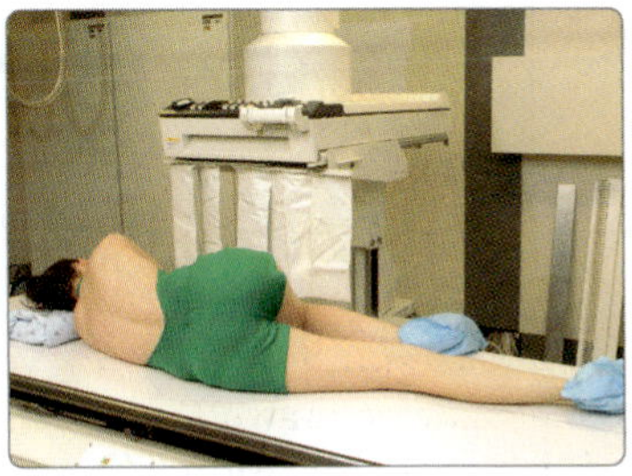

EXERCISE 13

Spell each of the Body Positions by having someone dictate them to you. Use a separate sheet of paper.

To hear and spell the terms, go to Evolve Resources at evolve.elsevier.com and select:
Practice Student Resources > Student Resources > Chapter 3 > **Pronounce and Spell**

See Appendix B for instructions.

❑ Check the box when complete.

Abdominopelvic Regions

To assist in locating medical problems with greater accuracy and for identification purposes, the abdomen and pelvis are divided into nine regions (Fig. 3.7). Abdominopelvic regions are often used in relation to physical examination and medical history to describe signs and symptoms. The number in parentheses indicates the number of regions.

TERM	DEFINITION
umbilical region (1) (um-BIL-i-kal) (RĒ-jun)	around the navel (umbilicus)
lumbar regions (2) (LUM-bar) (RĒ-junz)	to the right and left of the umbilical region, near the waist
epigastric region (1) (*ep*-i-GAS-trik) (RĒ-jun)	superior to the umbilical region

UMBILICUS
is a term derived from the Latin **umbo**, which denoted the boss, or protuberant part, of a shield. Around the first century the term was used to designate either a raised or a depressed spot in the middle of anything.

HYPOCHONDRIAC is derived from the Greek **hypo**, meaning **under**, and **chondros**, meaning **cartilage**. This ancient term was used by Hippocrates to refer to the region just below the cartilages of the ribs. In 1765, the term was first used to refer to people who experienced discomfort or painful sensations in this area but had no organic findings. Now, a person who falsely believes he or she has an illness is referred to as a **hypochondriac**.

CYBERCHONDRIA emerged in 2000 as a term describing a pattern of using Internet research to self-diagnose symptoms, fueling health anxiety and worry.

Abdominopelvic Regions—cont'd

TERM	DEFINITION
hypochondriac regions (2) (*hī*-pō-KON-drē-ak) (RĒ-junz)	to the right and left of the epigastric region
hypogastric region (1) (*hī*-pō-GAS-trik) (RĒ-jun)	inferior to the umbilical region
iliac regions (2) (IL-ē-ak) (RĒ-junz)	to the right and left of the hypogastric region, near the groin (also called **inguinal regions**)

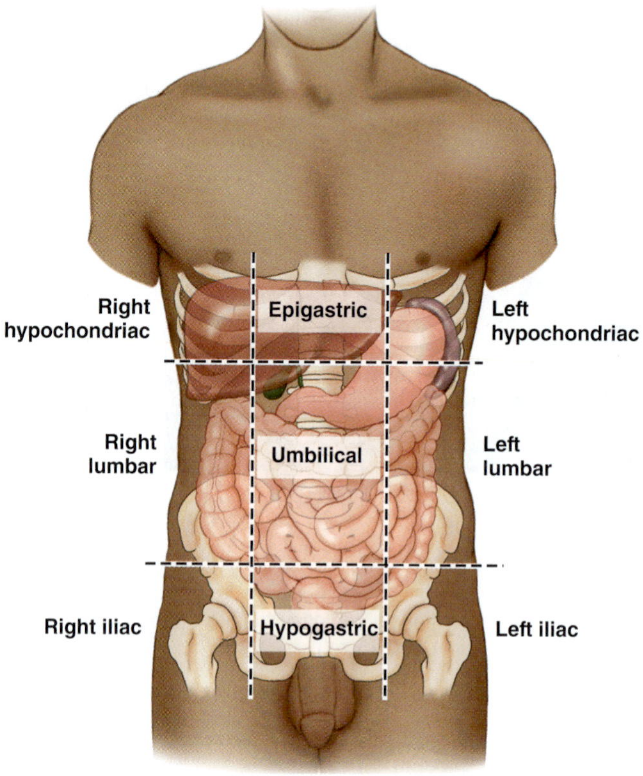

FIG. 3.7 Abdominopelvic regions. References to right and left indicate the right and left of the patient's body.

EXERCISE 14

Practice saying aloud each of the Abdominopelvic Regions.

To hear the terms, go to Evolve Resources at evolve.elsevier.com and select:
Practice Student Resources > Student Resources > Chapter 3 > **Pronounce and Spell**

See Appendix B for instructions.

❑ Check the box when complete.

EXERCISE FIGURE D

Fill in the blanks with abdominopelvic regions. To check your answers, go to Appendix A.

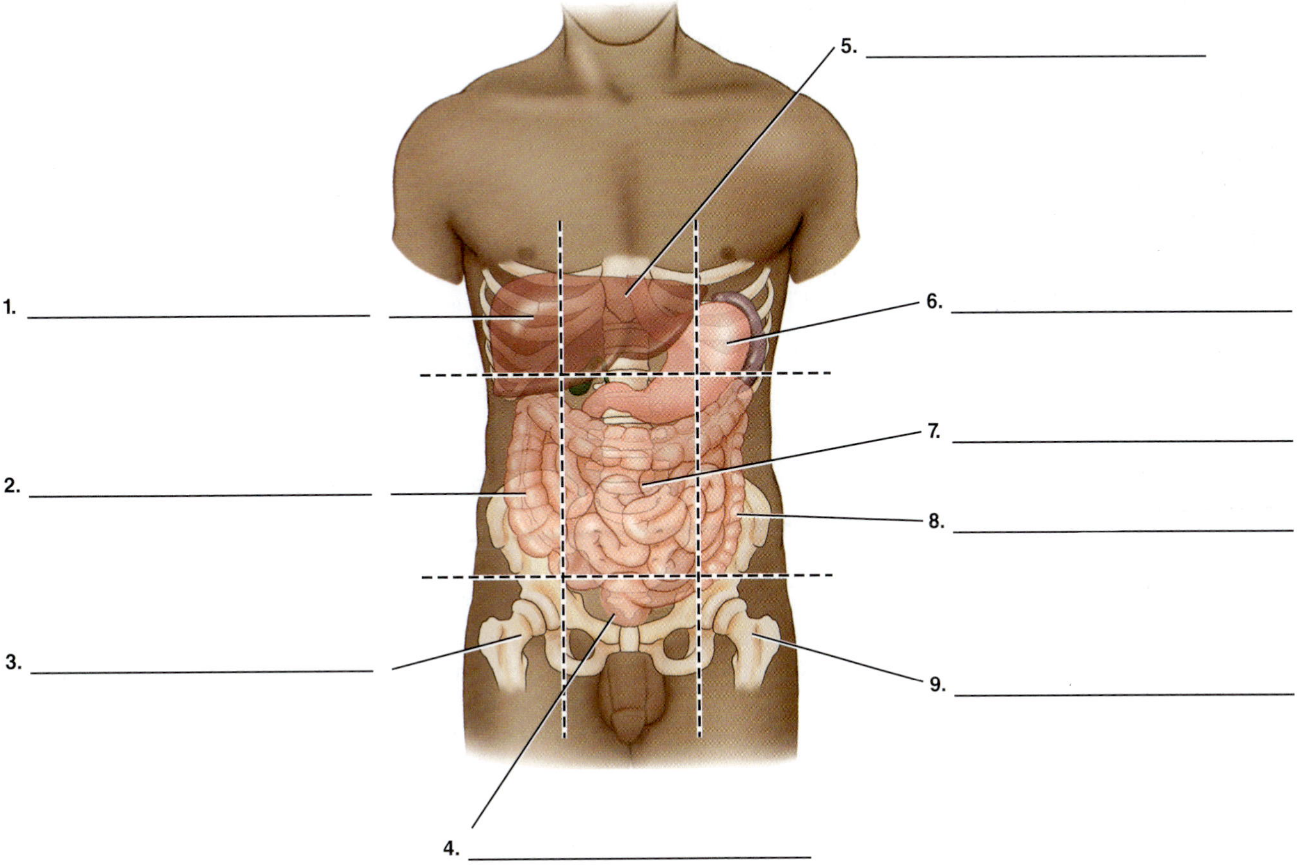

EXERCISE 15

Fill in the blanks with the correct terms.

1. The regions to the right and left of the hypogastric region, near the groin, are the ______________________ regions.
2. The ______________________ region is superior to the umbilical region.
3. Inferior to the umbilical region is the ______________________ region.
4. The ______________________ are the regions to the right and left of the epigastric region.
5. Superior to the hypogastric region is the ______________________ region.
6. To the right and the left of the umbilical region, near the waist, are the ______________________ regions.

EXERCISE 16

Match the terms in the first column with the correct definitions in the second column.

______ 1. epigastric	a. inferior to the umbilical region
______ 2. hypochondriac	b. superior to the umbilical region
______ 3. hypogastric	c. right and left of the umbilical region, near the waist
______ 4. iliac	d. right and left of the epigastric region
______ 5. lumbar	e. right and left of the hypogastric region, near the groin
______ 6. umbilical	f. inferior to the epigastric region

EXERCISE 17

Spell each of the Abdominopelvic Regions by having someone dictate them to you. Use a separate sheet of paper.

To hear and spell the terms, go to Evolve Resources at evolve.elsevier.com and select:
Practice Student Resources > Student Resources > Chapter 3 > **Pronounce and Spell**

See Appendix B for instructions.

❑ Check the box when complete.

Abdominopelvic Quadrants

The abdominopelvic area can also be divided into four quadrants by using imaginary vertical and horizontal lines that intersect at the umbilicus. These divisions are used by healthcare professionals to specify the location of pain, incisions, markings, lesions, and so forth. The quadrants provide a more general denotation than the abdominopelvic regions, and they are used in describing the location of findings from the physical examination and medical history (Fig. 3.8).

TERM	DEFINITION
right upper quadrant (RUQ) (KWOD-rant)	refers to the area encompassing the right lobe of the liver, the gallbladder, medial portion of the pancreas, and portions of the small and large intestines
left upper quadrant (LUQ) (KWOD-rant)	refers to the area encompassing the left lobe of the liver, the stomach, the spleen, lateral portion of the pancreas, and portions of the small and large intestines

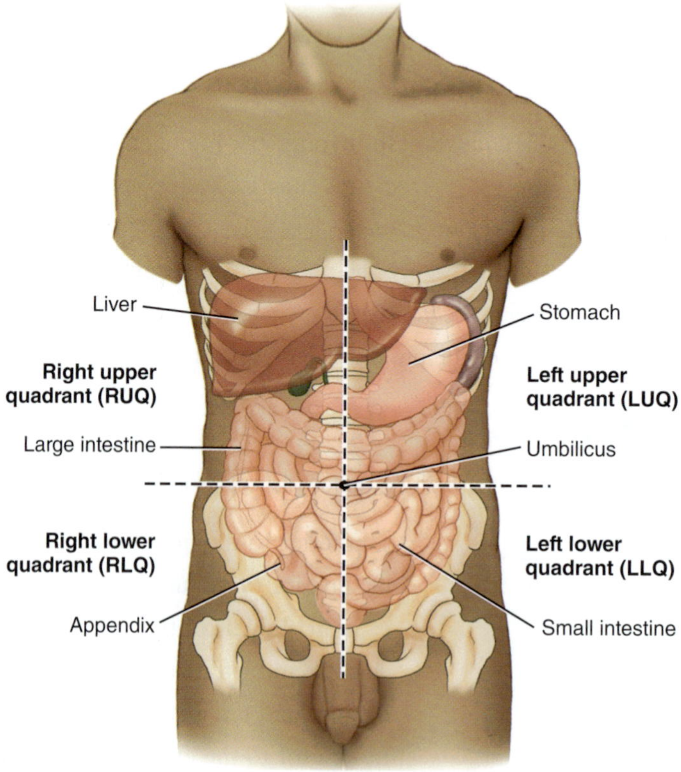

FIG. 3.8 Abdominopelvic quadrants.

TERM	DEFINITION
right lower quadrant (RLQ) (KWOD-rant)	refers to the area encompassing portions of the small and large intestines, the appendix, the right ureter, and the right ovary and uterine tube in women or the right spermatic duct in men
left lower quadrant (LLQ) (KWOD-rant)	refers to the area encompassing portions of the small and large intestines, the left ureter, and the left ovary and uterine tube in women or the left spermatic duct in men

PREVENTING WRONG-SIDE ERRORS

When facing the patient, your right and left will be opposite of the patient's right and left. Confusing the patient's right and left with the provider's right and left can lead to significant errors such as **wrong-sided surgery**.

Tips for preventing wrong-sided errors:

- Remember **"right"** and **"left"** pertain to the right and left of the patient's body.
- Avoid saying **"right"** when **"correct"** is meant.
- When a patient indicates the side choice is **"right"** confirm the response meant **"correct."**

EXERCISE 18

Write the abbreviation for the abdominopelvic quadrant associated with the following organs.
To check your answers, go to Appendix A.

_______________ 1. appendix
_______________ 2. right lobe of the liver
_______________ 3. left spermatic duct in men
_______________ 4. the stomach and the spleen
_______________ 5. right ovary and uterine tube in women
_______________ 6. gallbladder
_______________ 7. right ureter

EXERCISE FIGURE E

Fill in the blanks with abdominopelvic quadrants and the abbreviations for each.

(1) _______________
____
____
Abbrev. _______________

(2) _______________
____
____
Abbrev. _______________

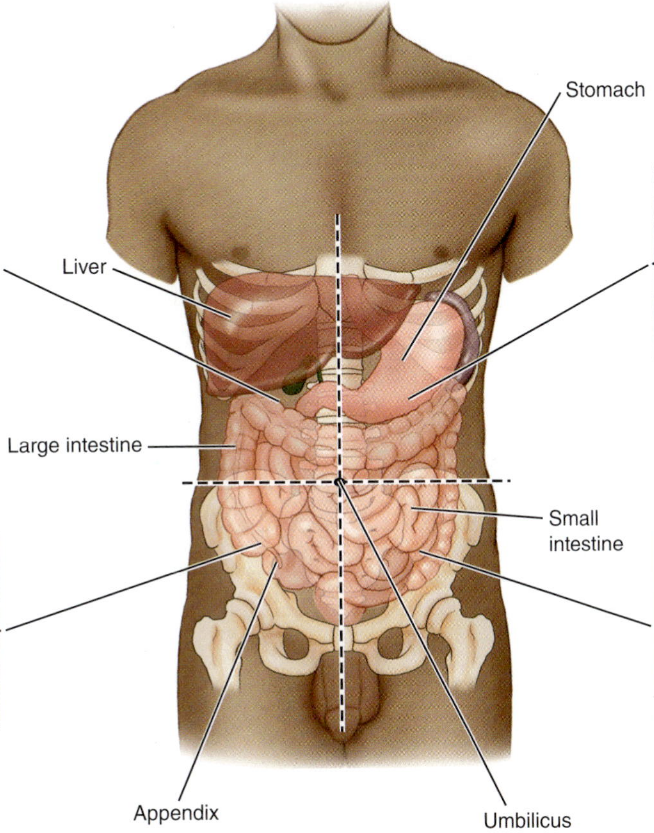

(3) _______________
____
____
Abbrev. _______________

(4) _______________
____
____
Abbrev. _______________

EXERCISE 19

Spell each of the Abdominopelvic Quadrants by having someone dictate them to you. Use a separate sheet of paper.

To hear and spell the terms, go to Evolve Resources at evolve.elsevier.com and select:
Practice Student Resources > Student Resources > Chapter 3 > **Pronounce and Spell**

See Appendix B for instructions.

❑ Check the box when complete.

Abbreviations

ABBREVIATION	TERM
ant	anterior
AP	anteroposterior
inf	inferior
lat	lateral
LLQ	left lower quadrant
LUQ	left upper quadrant
med	medial
PA	posteroanterior
RLQ	right lower quadrant
RUQ	right upper quadrant
sup	superior

For additional practice with Abbreviations, go to Evolve Resources at evolve.elsevier.com and select:
Practice Student Resources > Student Resources > Chapter 3 > **Flashcards:** Abbreviations

See Appendix B for instructions.

Refer to **Appendix E** for a complete list of abbreviations.

EXERCISE 20

Write the terms abbreviated.

1. sup ____________________
2. ant ____________________
3. inf ____________________
4. PA ____________________
5. AP ____________________
6. med ____________________
7. lat ____________________

PRACTICAL APPLICATION

EXERCISE 21 *Case Study: Translate Between Everyday Language and Medical Language*

CASE STUDY: A'idah Khalil

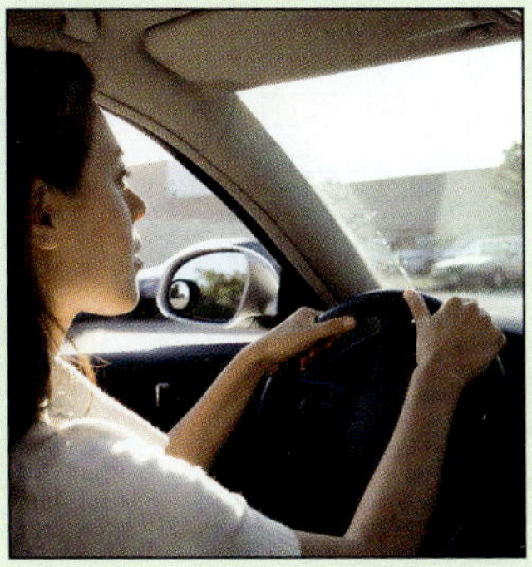

A'idah Khalil was just in a car accident, but luckily, she is awake and knows what is going on around her. The ambulance comes and the emergency team asks her where she is hurting. Her right foot hurts the most. She has pain in her upper right arm near her shoulder and notices some bleeding there. She also has some pain in her belly near the navel and in her lower back near the waist. The paramedics put her on a hard board on her back facing upward, put some kind of collar around her neck, then load her into the ambulance and take her to the hospital.

Now that you have worked through Chapter 3, consider the directional terms, positions, and regions that might be used to describe A'idah's experience. See the Review of Terms at the end of the chapter for a list of terms that might apply.

A. *Underline phrases in the case study that could be substituted with medical terms.*

B. *Write the medical term and its definition for two of the phrases you underlined.*

MEDICAL TERM	DEFINITION
1. ______________________	______________________________
	______________________________
2. ______________________	______________________________
	______________________________

DOCUMENTATION: Excerpt From Emergency Department Note

Paramedics transported A'idah to the emergency department (ED) of the nearest hospital. The following was documented in the Diagnostic Studies portion of her medical record:

Radiographs (x-rays) of the right lower extremity in the medial and lateral view identify a fracture of the calcaneus with proximal dislocation of the cuboid bone. Radiographs of the cervical spine in AP and oblique projection show no bone injury. CT scan images of the lower back reveal no significant abnormalities.

C. *Underline medical terms and abbreviations presented in Chapter 3 in the previous excerpt from A'idah's medical record. See the Review of Terms at the end of the chapter for a complete list.*

D. *Select and define two of the medical terms you underlined. To check your answers, go to Appendix A.*

MEDICAL TERM	DEFINITION
1. ______________________	______________________________
	______________________________
2. ______________________	______________________________
	______________________________

EXERCISE 22 *Interact With Medical Documents*

A. Read the report and complete it by writing medical terms on answer lines within the document. Definitions of terms to be written appear after the document.

817254-DPQ PARKER, Zoe

File Patient Navigate Custom Fields Help

Chart Review | Encounters | Notes | Labs | Imaging | Procedures | Rx | Documents | Referrals | Scheduling | Billing

Name: **PARKER, Zoe** MR#: **817254-DPQ** DOB: **03/27/19XX** Gender: F Age: 72 **Allergies:** Bees **PCP:** Means, Robert MD

Date: 3/27/20XX
Progress Note:

Mrs. Parker is here today for follow-up for degenerative joint disease of both knees and ankles. She arrived ambulatory with the assistance of a cane, walking slowly with a fairly steady gait.

On examination of the knees, there is marked crepitus that is palpable with pressure applied to the patellae with the knees flexed and extended, right greater than left. She has a range of motion from 10 degrees to 110 degrees in the right knee. Pain is evident at the end of extension at 10 degrees. The right knee is stable when stressed in an 1.____________________, valgus and varus manner.

On examination of the right ankle, there is some mild tenderness on palpation above the lateral malleolus. The right ankle moves from 0 degrees of dorsiflexsion to 25 degrees of plantar flexion. From the 2.____________________ joint line at the knee to the malleolus at the ankle, the right tib/fib is 1.5 cm shorter than the left. There is pigment change mainly on the 3.____________________ and 4.____________________ aspect of the right lower leg. There is a slight bony deformity over the 5.____________________ aspect of the mid-tibial area.

Impression:
1. Degenerative joint disease of both knees and ankles, stable.

Plan:
1. Patient is to continue on current medications unchanged.

Electronically signed: Robert Means MD on 27 March 20XX 13:30

Start | Log On/Off | Print | Edit

Definitions of Medical Terms to Complete the Document

Write the medical terms defined on corresponding answer lines in the document.

1. pertaining to the front and to the back
2. pertaining to the side
3. pertaining to the back
4. pertaining to the middle
5. pertaining to the front

B. Read the procedure documentation and answer the questions below it.

PROCEDURE FOR PALPATING ARTERIAL PULSES

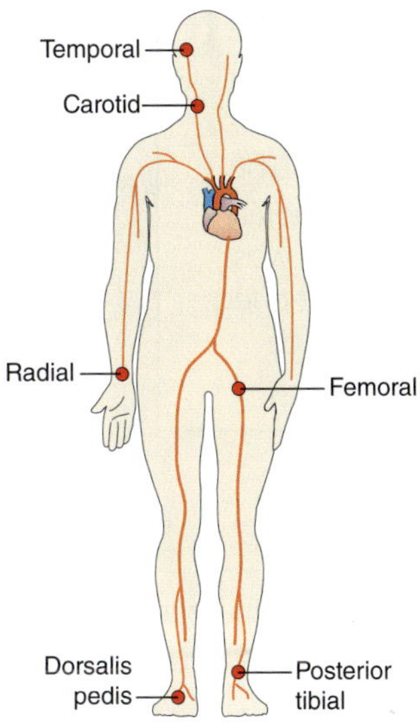

Palpate arteries with the distal pads of the first two fingers. The fingertips are used because they are the most sensitive parts of the hand. Unless contraindicated, simultaneous palpation is preferred.

Temporal: Palpate over the temporal bone on each side of the head, lateral to each eyebrow.

Carotid: Palpate the anterior edge of the sternocleidomastoid muscle, just medial and inferior to the angle of the jaw. To avoid reduction of blood flow, do not palpate right and left carotid pulses simultaneously.

Radial: Palpate lateral and anterior side of wrist, proximal to the first carpal-metacarpal junction.

Femoral: This pulse is inferior to the medial inguinal ligament; the pulse is found midway between anterior superior iliac spine and pubic tubercle.

Posterior tibial: This pulse is found posterior and slightly inferior to the medial malleolus of the ankle.

Dorsalis pedis: With the foot slightly dorsiflexed, lightly palpate the dorsal surface of the foot, just lateral to the first metatarsal.

Use the procedure documentation above to answer the questions. For questions 1-3, circle the correct answer. Use a reference source to answer question 4.

1. The **temporal pulse** is palpated
   a. just above the eyebrow.
   b. to the side of the eyebrow.
   c. below the eyebrow.
   d. to the middle of the eyebrow.
2. The **radial pulse** is palpated on the
   a. lateral and front of the wrist.
   b. lateral and back of the wrist.
   c. medial and back of the wrist.
   d. medial and front of the wrist.
3. The **femoral pulse** is located
   a. below the medial inguinal ligament.
   b. above the medial inguinal ligament.
   c. to the front of the medial inguinal ligament.
   d. to the back of the medial inguinal ligament.
4. When used with the foot, the directional term ***dorsal*** has a slightly different meaning. With the use of your medical dictionary or an online resource, describe the dorsal surface of the foot. Hint: try *dorsum* and *dorsal pedis* as search terms.
   The dorsal surface of the foot is ____________________
   ____.

EXERCISE 23 *Pronounce Medical Terms in Use*

Practice pronunciation of terms by reading aloud the following paragraph. Use the phonetic spellings following medical terms from the chapter to assist with pronunciation. The script also contains medical terms not presented in the chapter. Treat them as information only or look for their meanings in a medical dictionary or a reliable online source.

The patient presented to her physician with pain in the right **lumbar region** (LUM-bar)(RĒ-jun) and right **unilateral** (ū-ni-LAT-er-al) leg pain. The pain was felt in the **posterior** (pos-TĒR-ē -or) portion of the leg and radiated to the **distal** (DIS-tal) **lateral** (LAT-er-al) portion of the extremity. There was some **proximal** (PROK-si-mal) muscle weakness reported of the affected leg. A lumbar spine radiograph was normal. If the pain does not respond to antiinflammatory medication, she will be referred to an orthopedist.

EXERCISE 24 *Chapter Content Quiz*

Test your understanding of terms and abbreviations introduced in this chapter. For questions 1-16, circle the letter for the medical term or abbreviation related to the words in italics. For question 17, write medical terms for words in italics.

1. The plane that *divides the body into right and left sides* is a general term specifying the vertical plane running through the body from the front to back is:
   a. frontal plane
   b. transverse plane
   c. sagittal plane
2. The *midsagittal plane* more specifically describes the sagittal plane by indicating the body is divided in:
   a. half (equal portions)
   b. unequal portions
   c. anterior and posterior portions
3. Images for computed tomography (CT) scanning can be produced from the sagittal plane, the frontal plane, and the plane *dividing the body into superior and inferior portions* called the:
   a. coronal plane
   b. parasagittal plane
   c. transverse plane
4. A polyp was found in the colon *pertaining to away from the point of attachment of a body part* or ________________ to the splenic flexure.
   a. distal
   b. proximal
   c. medial
5. The drainage catheter is placed over the right *pertaining to the front* or ________________ pelvis.
   a. inferior
   b. posterior
   c. anterior
6. The incision was made at the *pertaining to above* or ________________ pole of the lesion.
   a. superior
   b. inferior
   c. lateral
7. The patient complained of *superior to umbilical region* or ________________ pain.
   a. hypochondriac region
   b. hypogastric region
   c. epigastric region
8. A *pertaining to a side* or ________________ chest radiograph displays the anatomy in the *dividing the body into right and left sides* or ________________ plane.
   a. lateral, sagittal
   b. medial, coronal
   c. bilateral, transverse
9. The patient was scheduled for an ultrasound-guided *pertaining to two (both) sides* or ________________ thoracentesis.
   a. unilateral
   b. bilateral
   c. mediolateral
10. The doctor's order indicated that the patient with dyspnea (difficulty breathing) was to be placed in the *sitting erect or upright* or ________________ position to facilitate breathing.
    a. right Sims
    b. left recumbent
    c. orthopnea

11. The patient being treated for cardiovascular shock was placed in *lying on back with the head lower than the feet* or ________________ position.
    a. Trendelenburg
    b. Fowler
    c. prone
12. Gallbladder pain is likely to be in the *abbreviated as RUQ* or ________________.
    a. lumbar region
    b. right upper quadrant
    c. upper right quadrant
13. The directional term *pertaining to the back* or ________________ is often used to describe the back of the hand or upper surface of the foot.
    a. superior
    b. anterior
    c. dorsal
14. Just before birth, the fetus shifted to a *pertaining to the head* or ________________ presentation.
    a. cephalic
    b. caudal
    c. ventral
15. A *pertaining to the tail* or ________________ epidural steroid injection may be performed to relieve chronic low back pain.
    a. dorsal
    b. caudal
    c. proximal
16. A patient who will be receiving an enema is usually placed in the left *lying on the side with the knee drawn toward the chest and the arm drawn behind* ________________ position for gravity to help the fluid flow through the sigmoid colon into the descending colon. This position may also be called left recumbent position.
    a. Fowler
    b. lithotomy
    c. Sims
17. The pathology report for the patient with a palpable right breast lump included the sections listed below. Fill in the blanks with directional terms indicated by words in italics.

    Right axillary sentinel lymph node biopsy;

    a. Right breast, ________________ margin biopsy (*pertaining to above*)
    b. Right breast, ________________ margin biopsy (*pertaining to below*)

    Right breast, deep margin biopsy;

    c. Right breast, ________________ margin biopsy (*pertaining to the middle*)
    d. Right breast, ________________ margin biopsy (*pertaining to a side*)

For additional practice with chapter content, go to Evolve Resources at evolve.elsevier.com and select:
Practice Student Resources > Student Resources > Chapter 3 > **Games:** Medical Millionaire
Tournament of Terminology
Practice Quizzes: Word Parts
Directional Terms
Planes, Positions, and Regions
Abbreviations

See Appendix B for instructions.

CHAPTER REVIEW

REVIEW OF CHAPTER CONTENT ON EVOLVE RESOURCES

Go to evolve.elsevier.com and click on Gradable Student Resources and Practice Student Resources. Online learning activities found there can be used to review chapter content and to assess your learning of word parts, medical terms, and abbreviations. Place check marks in the boxes next to activities used for review and assessment.

GRADABLE STUDENT RESOURCES

Chapter 03 >	Exercises >	□ Analyze Medical Terms □ Word Parts □ Terms Built from Word Parts □ Terms Not Built from Word Parts □ Abbreviations
	Quizzes >	□ Quiz 1: Directional Terms □ Quiz 2: Planes, Regions, Quadrants, and Positions

PRACTICE STUDENT RESOURCES > STUDENT RESOURCES

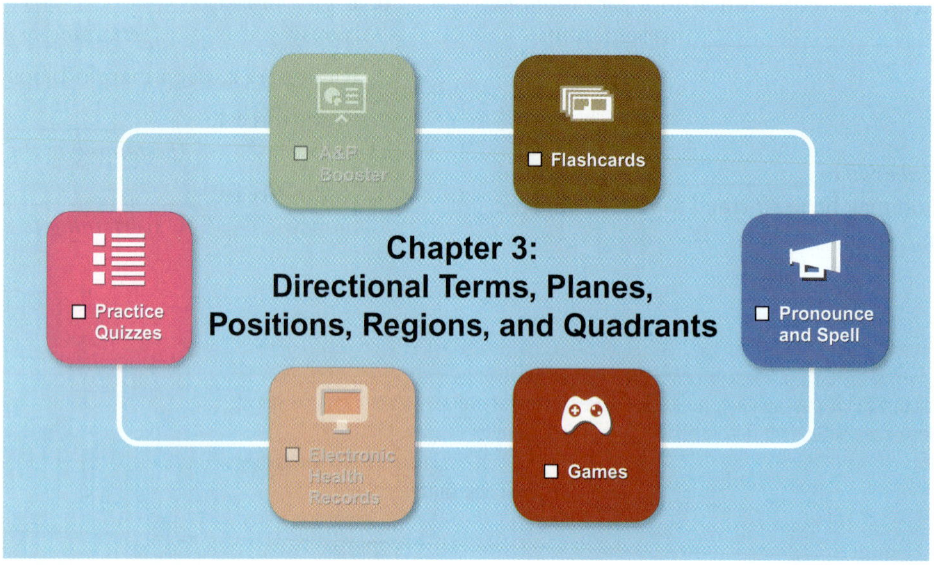

REVIEW OF WORD PARTS

Can you define and spell the following word parts?

COMBINING FORMS		PREFIXES	SUFFIXES
anter/o	medi/o	bi-	-ad
caud/o	poster/o	uni-	-ior
cephal/o	proxim/o		
dist/o	super/o		
dors/o	ventr/o		
infer/o			
later/o			

REVIEW OF TERMS

Can you define, pronounce, and spell the following terms?

DIRECTIONAL TERMS	ANATOMIC PLANES	BODY POSITIONS	ABDOMINOPELVIC REGIONS	ABDOMINOPELVIC QUADRANTS
anterior (ant)	frontal or coronal	Fowler position	epigastric region	left lower quadrant (LLQ)
anteroposterior (AP)	midsagittal	lateral recumbent position	hypochondriac regions	left upper quadrant (LUQ)
bilateral	parasagittal	lithotomy position	hypogastric region	right lower quadrant (RLQ)
caudad	sagittal	orthopnea position	iliac regions	right upper quadrant (RUQ)
caudal	transverse	prone position	lumbar regions	
cephalad		recumbent position	umbilical region	
cephalic		Sims position		
distal		supine position		
dorsal		Trendelenburg position		
inferior (inf)				
lateral (lat)				
medial (med)				
mediolateral				
posterior				
posteroanterior (PA)				
proximal				
superior (sup)				
unilateral				
ventral				

Types of body movement are presented in Chapter 14, Musculoskeletal System, on pages 576–577. Terms related to body movement are: *abduction*, *adduction*, *inversion*, *eversion*, *extension*, *flexion*, *pronation*, *supination*, and *rotation*.

Chapter 4

Integumentary System

Objectives

Upon completion of this chapter you will be able to:

1. Pronounce anatomic structures of the integumentary system.
2. Define and spell word parts related to the integumentary system.
3. Define, pronounce, and spell disease and disorder terms related to the integumentary system.
4. Define, pronounce, and spell surgical terms related to the integumentary system.
5. Define, pronounce, and spell complementary terms related to the integumentary system.
6. Interpret the meaning of abbreviations related to the integumentary system.
7. Apply medical language in clinical contexts.

Outline

ANATOMY

The integumentary system is composed of the skin, glands, hair, and nails.

INTEGUMENTARY is derived from the Latin word **teqere**, meaning to **cover.**

Function

The skin forms a protective covering for the body that, when unbroken, prevents entry of bacteria and other invading organisms. The skin also protects the body from water loss and the damaging effects of ultraviolet light. Other functions include regulation of body temperature and synthesis of vitamin D (Fig. 4.1).

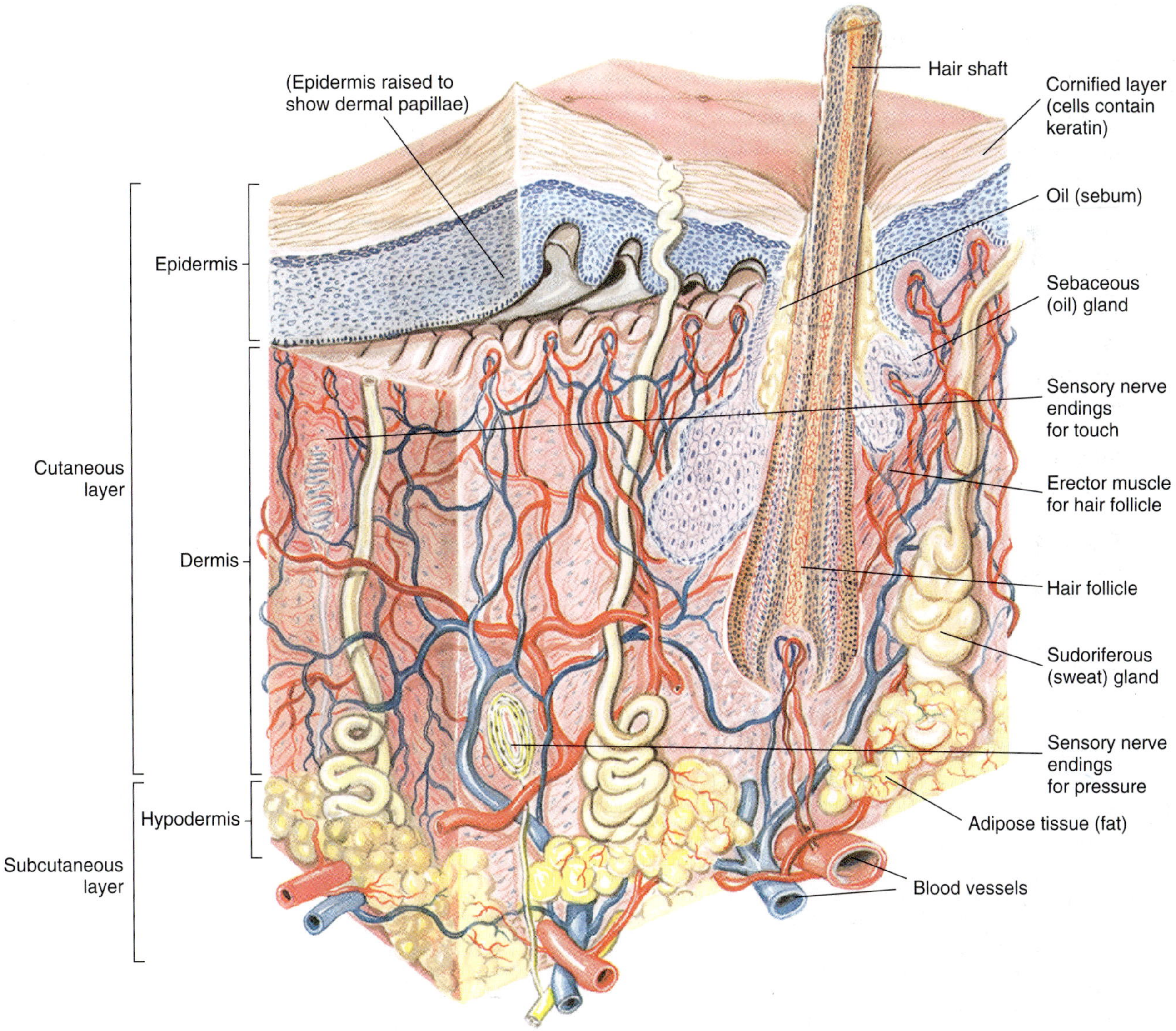

FIG. 4.1 Structure of the skin.

Anatomic Structures of the Integumentary System

TERM	DEFINITION
skin (skin)	organ covering the body; made up of layers
epidermis (ep-i-DER-mis)	outer layer of skin; protects the body from the external environment
keratin (KAR-a-tin)	scleroprotein component of the horny, or cornified, layer of the epidermis. Also, the primary component of the hair and nails
melanin (MEL-a-nin)	dark pigment produced by melanocytes; amount present determines skin color
hair (hār)	compressed, keratinized cells that arise from hair follicles, the sacs that enclose the hair fibers
nails (nālz)	horny plates made from flattened epithelial cells; found on the dorsal surface of the ends of the fingers and toes
sebaceous glands (se-BĀ-shas) (glans)	secrete sebum (oil) into the hair follicles where the hair shafts pass through the dermis
sudoriferous (sweat) glands (*soo*-da-RIF-er-as) (glans)	tiny, coiled, tubular structures that emerge through pores on the skin's surface and secrete sweat
dermis (DUR-mis)	inner layer of skin; responsible for its flexibility and mechanical strength

APPENDAGES OF THE SKIN

is a common reference to hair, nails, sudoriferous glands, and sebaceous glands, all of which derive from the epidermis.

A&P Booster

For more anatomy and physiology, go to Evolve Resources at evolve.elsevier.com and select: Practice Student Resources > Student Resources > Chapter 4 > **A&P Booster**

See Appendix B for instructions.

EXERCISE 1

Practice saying aloud each of the **Anatomic Structures**.

To hear the terms, go to Evolve Resources at evolve.elsevier.com and select: Practice Student Resources > Student Resources > Chapter 4 > **Pronounce and Spell**

See Appendix B for instructions.

❑ Check the box when complete.

WORD PARTS

Word parts you need to learn to complete this chapter are listed on the following pages. The exercises at the end of each list will help you learn their definitions and spelling.

Use the flashcards accompanying this text or electronic flashcards to assist you in memorizing the word parts for this chapter.

Combining Forms

COMBINING FORM	DEFINITION
cutane/o, derm/o, dermat/o	skin
hidr/o	sweat
kerat/o	horny tissue (keratin), hard *(Note: kerat/o is also used to refer to the cornea of the eye; see Chapter 12.)*
onych/o, ungu/o	nail
seb/o	sebum (oil)

> Do not be concerned about which **combining form** to use for **skin** or **nail**. As you continue to study and use medical terms, you will become familiar with common usage of each word part.

EXERCISE 2

Fill in the blanks with combining forms. *To check your answers, go to Appendix A at the back of the textbook.*

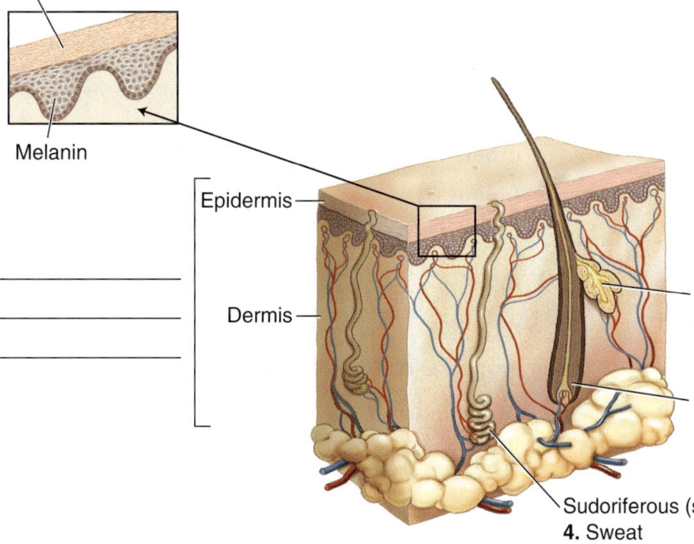

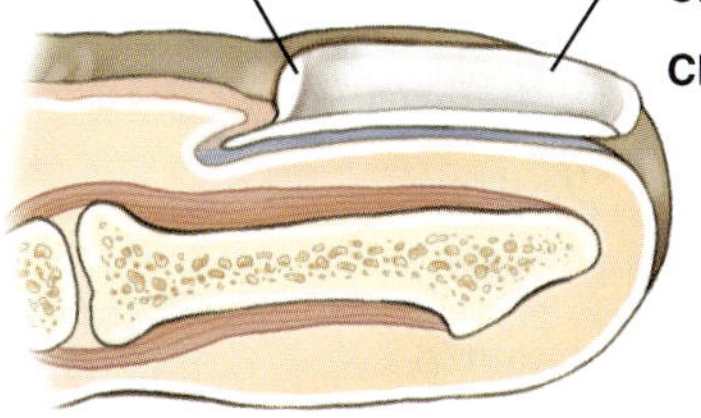

EXERCISE 3

Step 1: Write the definitions after the following combining forms.

Step 2: Match the descriptions on the right with the combining forms and definitions. Answers may be used more than once.

_____ 1. derm/o, dermat/o, ______________________________

_____ 2. seb/o, ______________________________

_____ 3. onych/o, ______________________________

_____ 4. cutane/o, ______________________________

_____ 5. kerat/o, ______________________________

_____ 6. ungu/o, ______________________________

_____ 7. hidr/o, ______________________________

a. secreted from sudoriferous glands

b. secreted from sebaceous glands

c. horny plates made from flattened epithelial cells

d. organ covering the body; made up of layers

e. scleroprotein component of the horny, or cornified, layer of the epidermis

> The prefix **bi-**, which means **two**, was presented in Chapter 3. The word root **bi** means **life**.

Combining Forms Commonly Used with Integumentary System Terms

COMBINING FORM	DEFINITION
aut/o	self
bi/o	life
coni/o	dust
crypt/o	hidden
heter/o	other
myc/o	fungus
necr/o	death (cells, body)
pachy/o	thick
rhytid/o	wrinkles
staphyl/o	grapelike clusters
strept/o	twisted chains
xer/o	dry, dryness

EXERCISE 4

Write the definitions of the following combining forms.

1. necr/o ______________________________
2. staphyl/o ______________________________
3. crypt/o ______________________________
4. pachy/o ______________________________
5. coni/o ______________________________
6. myc/o ______________________________
7. bi/o ______________________________
8. heter/o ______________________________
9. strept/o ______________________________
10. xer/o ______________________________
11. aut/o ______________________________
12. rhytid/o ______________________________

EXERCISE 5

Write the combining form for each of the following.

1. fungus ______________________________
2. death (cells, body) ______________________________
3. other ______________________________
4. dry, dryness ______________________________
5. thick ______________________________
6. twisted chains ______________________________

7. wrinkles ______________________
8. grapelike clusters ______________________
9. self ______________________
10. hidden ______________________
11. dust ______________________
12. life ______________________

Prefixes

PREFIX	DEFINITION
epi-	on, upon, over
intra-	within
para-	beside, beyond, around, abnormal
per-	through
sub-	under, below
trans-	through, across, beyond

EXERCISE 6

Write the definitions of the following prefixes.

1. sub- ______________________
2. para- ______________________
3. epi- ______________________
4. intra- ______________________
5. per- ______________________
6. trans- ______________________

EXERCISE 7

Write the prefix for each of the following.

1. within ______________________
2. under, below ______________________
3. on, upon, over ______________________
4. beside, beyond, around, abnormal ______________________
5. through ______________________
6. through, across, beyond ______________________

Suffixes

SUFFIX	DEFINITION
-a	noun suffix, no meaning
-coccus (pl. -cocci)	berry-shaped (form of bacterium)
-ectomy	excision or surgical removal
-ia	diseased or abnormal state, condition of
-itis	inflammation
-malacia	softening
-opsy	view of, viewing
-phagia	eating or swallowing
-plasty	surgical repair
-rrhea	flow, discharge
-tome	instrument used to cut

Refer to **Appendix C** and **Appendix D** for alphabetical lists of word parts and their meanings.

EXERCISE 8

A. Match the suffixes in the first column with the correct definitions in the second column.

______ 1. -a	a. softening
______ 2. -ia	b. eating or swallowing
______ 3. -malacia	c. diseased or abnormal state, condition of
______ 4. -phagia	d. flow, discharge
______ 5. -rrhea	e. noun suffix, no meaning

B. Write the suffix pictured and defined.

1. ______________________________

berry-shaped (form of bacterium)

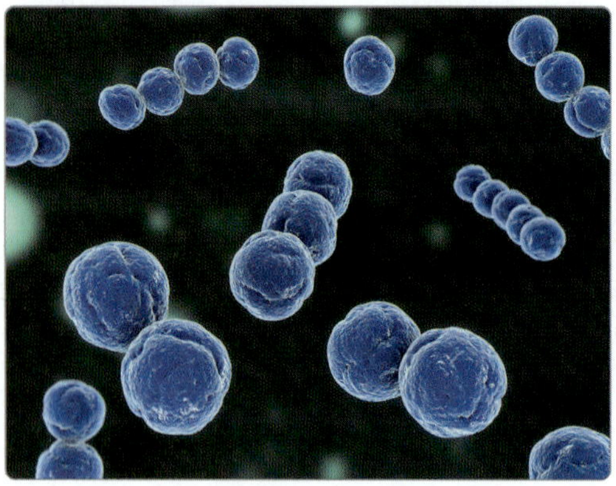

2. ______________________________

view of, viewing

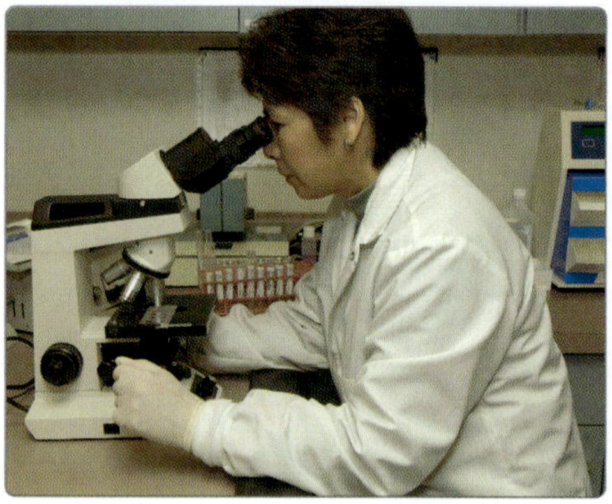

3. ______________________________

instrument used to cut

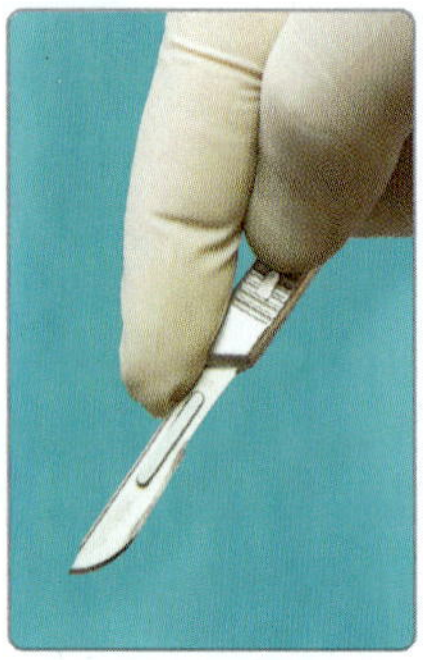

4. ______________________________

inflammation

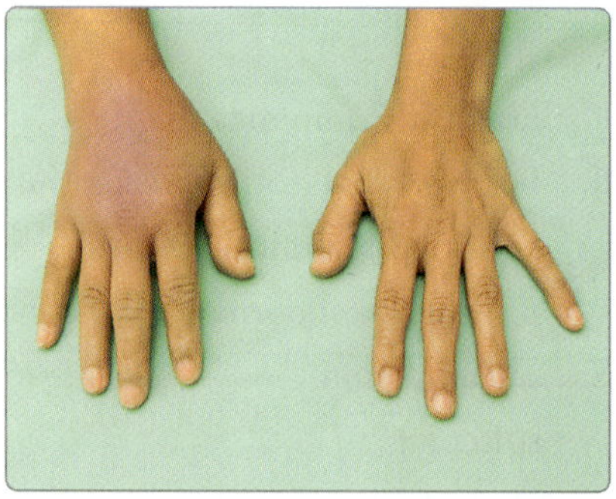

5. ______________________

surgical repair

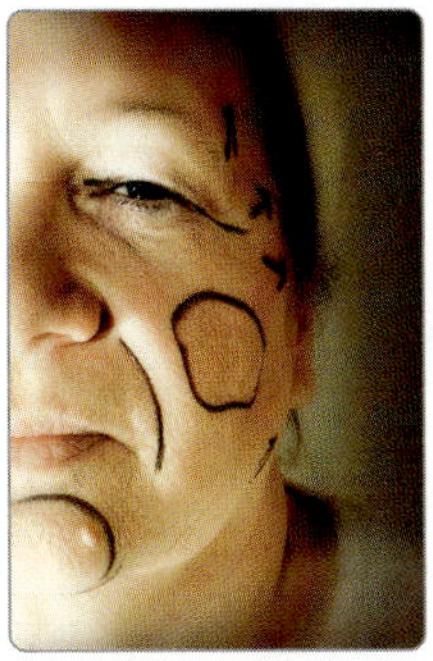

6. ______________________

excision or surgical removal

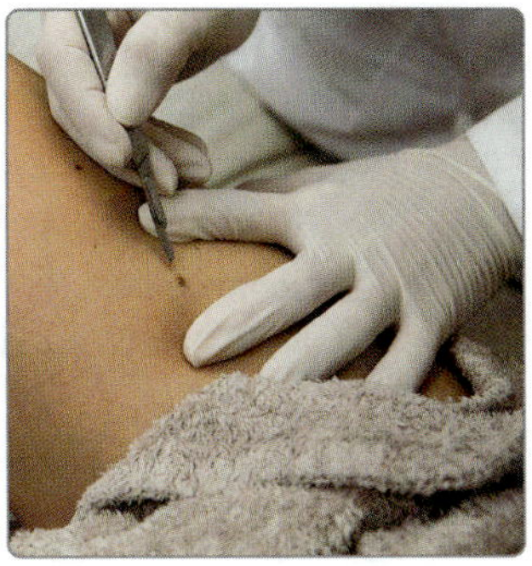

EXERCISE 9

Write the definitions of the following suffixes.

1. -plasty ______________________
2. -ectomy ______________________
3. -malacia ______________________
4. -itis ______________________
5. -tome ______________________
6. -phagia ______________________
7. -rrhea ______________________
8. -coccus ______________________
9. -opsy ______________________
10. -ia ______________________
11. -a ______________________

MEDICAL TERMS

The terms you need to learn to complete this chapter are listed on the following pages. The exercises at the end of each list will help you learn each word well enough to add it to your vocabulary.

Disease and Disorder Terms
BUILT FROM WORD PARTS

The following terms can be translated using definitions of word parts. Further explanation is provided within parentheses as needed.

TERM	DEFINITION
dermatitis (*der*-ma-TĪ-tis)	inflammation of the skin (Fig. 4.2)
dermatoconiosis (*der*-ma-tō-*kō*-nē-Ō-sis)	abnormal condition of the skin caused by dust
dermatofibroma (*der*-ma-tō-fī-BRŌ-ma)	fibrous tumor of the skin
hidradenitis (*hī*-drad-e-NĪ-tis)	inflammation of a sweat gland
keratosis (ker-a-TŌ-sis)	abnormal condition (growth) of horny tissue (keratin)

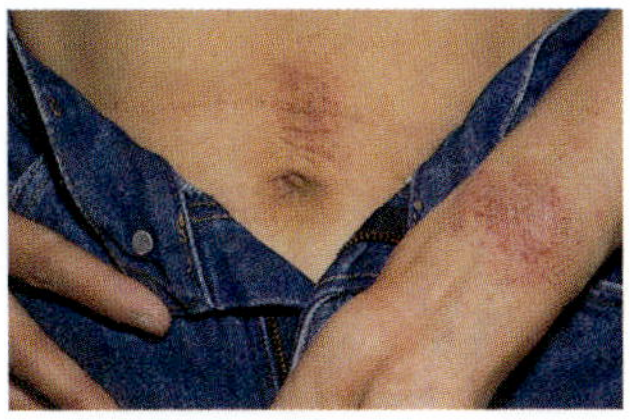

FIG. 4.2 Contact dermatitis.

Disease and Disorder Terms—cont'd

TERM	DEFINITION
leiodermia (*lī*-ō-DER-mē-a)	condition of smooth skin
onychocryptosis (*on*-i-kō-krip-TŌ-sis)	abnormal condition of a hidden nail (also called **ingrown nail**)
onychomalacia (*on*-i-kō-ma-LĀ-sha)	softening of the nails
onychomycosis (*on*-i-kō-mī-KŌ-sis)	abnormal condition of a fungus in the nails (Exercise Figure B)
onychophagia (*on*-i-kō-FĀ-ja)	eating the nails (nail biting)
pachyderma (*pak*-i-DER-ma)	thickening of the skin
paronychia (*par*-ō-NIK-ē-a)	diseased state around the nail (Exercise Figure B) *(Note: the a from para- has been dropped. The final vowel in a prefix may be dropped when the word to which it is added begins with a vowel.)*
seborrhea (seb-o-RĒ-a)	discharge of sebum (excessive)
xanthoma (zan-THŌ-ma)	yellow tumor (benign, primarily in the skin)
xeroderma (*zē*-rō-DER-ma)	dry skin (a mild form of a cutaneous disorder characterized by keratinization and noninflammatory scaling)

SEBORRHEIC

is the adjective form of **seborrhea** and means pertaining to excessive discharge of sebum.

EXERCISE FIGURE A

Fill in the blanks to label the diagrams.

1 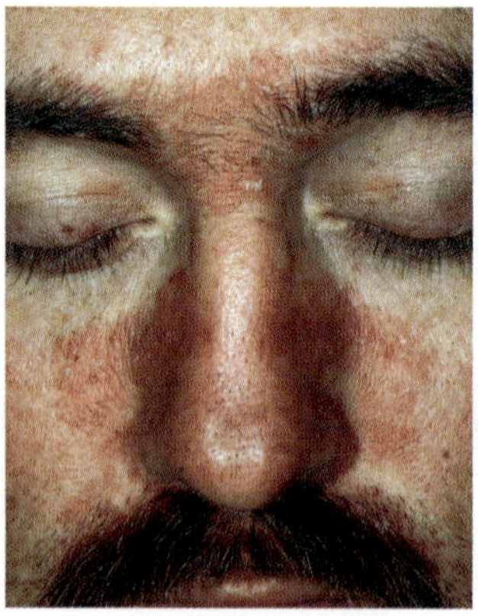

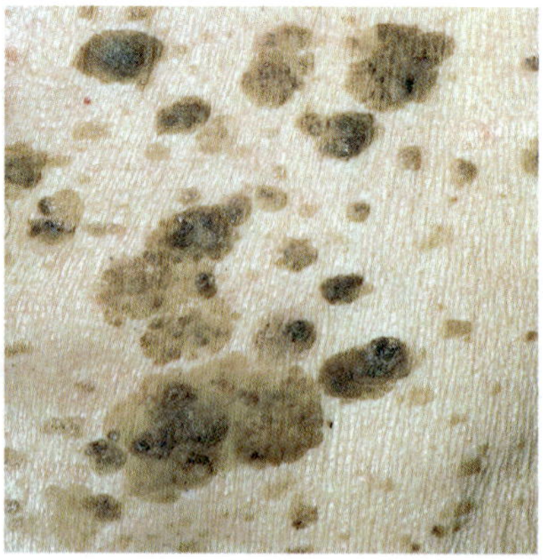 2

1. Seborrheic __________ / __________
   skin / inflammation

2. Seborrheic __________ / __________
   horny tissue / abnormal condition

EXERCISE FIGURE B

Fill in the blanks to label the diagrams.

1 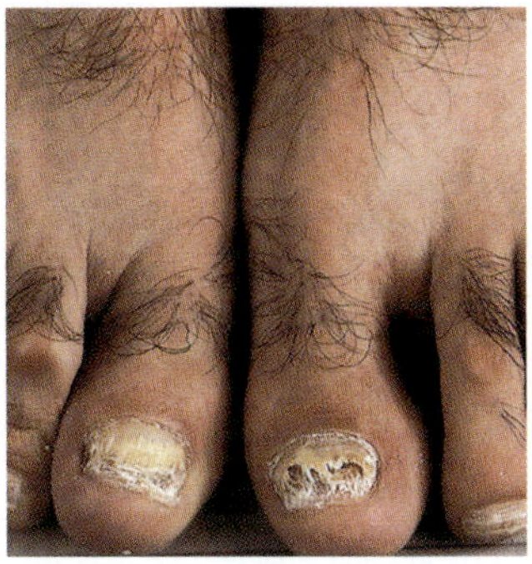

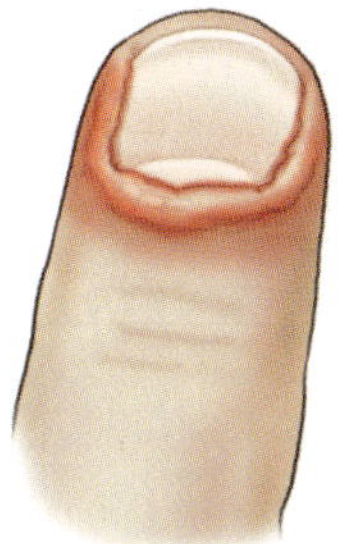 2

1. ______ / ___ / ______ / ______
   nail / cv / fungus / abnormal condition

2. ______ / ______ / ______
   around / nail / diseased state

EXERCISE 10

Practice saying aloud each of the Disease and Disorder Terms Built from Word Parts.

> To hear the terms, go to Evolve Resources at evolve.elsevier.com and select:
> Practice Student Resources > Student Resources > Chapter 4 > **Pronounce and Spell**
>
> See Appendix B for instructions.

❑ Check the box when complete.

EXERCISE 11

Analyze and define the following Disease and Disorder Terms Built from Word Parts by drawing slashes between word parts, writing word part abbreviations above the term, underlining combining forms, and writing combining form abbreviations below the term. If needed, refer to p. 11 to review analyzing and defining techniques.

EXAMPLE:

WR CV WR S
onych / o / myc / osis
CF
abnormal condition of a fungus in the nails

1. dermatoconiosis

____

____

2. hidradenitis

____

____

3. dermatitis

____

____

4. pachyderma

____

____

5. onychomalacia

____

____

6. keratosis

____

____

7. dermatofibroma

____

____

8. paronychia

____

____

9. onychocryptosis

____

____

10. seborrhea

____

____

11. onychophagia

____

____

12. xeroderma

____

____

13. leiodermia

____

____

14. xanthoma

____

____

EXERCISE 12

Build disease and disorder terms for the following definitions by using the word parts you have learned. If you need help, refer to p. 13 to review term-building techniques.

EXAMPLE: abnormal condition (growth) of horny tissue (keratin) kerat / osis (WR / S)

1. thickening of the skin ______ / ______ / ______ (WR / WR / S)

2. abnormal condition of a fungus in the nails ______ / ______ / ______ / ______ (WR / CV / WR / S)

3. discharge of sebum (excessive) ______ / ______ / ______ (WR / CV / S)

4. inflammation of the skin ______ / ______ (WR / S)

5. fibrous tumor of the skin ______ / ______ / ______ / ______ (WR / CV / WR / S)

6. softening of the nails ______ / ______ / ______ (WR / CV / S)

7. inflammation of a sweat gland ______ / ______ / ______ (WR / WR / S)

8. abnormal condition of a hidden nail ______ WR / CV / WR / S

9. abnormal condition of the skin caused by dust ______ WR / CV / WR / S

10. eating the nails ______ WR / CV / S

11. diseased state around the nail ______ P / WR / S

12. dry skin ______ WR / CV / WR / S

13. condition of smooth skin ______ WR / CV / WR / S

14. yellow tumor ______ WR / S

EXERCISE 13

Spell each of the Disease and Disorder Terms Built from Word Parts by having someone dictate them to you. Use a separate sheet of paper.

> To hear and spell the terms, go to Evolve Resources at evolve.elsevier.com and select:
> Practice Student Resources > Student Resources > Chapter 4 > **Pronounce and Spell**
>
> See Appendix B for instructions.

❑ Check the box when complete.

Disease and Disorder Terms
NOT BUILT FROM WORD PARTS

Word parts may be present in the following terms; however, their full meanings cannot be translated using definitions of word parts alone.

TERM	DEFINITION
abrasion (a-BRĀ-zhun)	scraping away of the skin by mechanical process or injury
abscess (AB-ses)	localized collection of pus
acne (AK-nē)	inflammatory disease of the skin involving the sebaceous glands and hair follicles
actinic keratosis (ack-TIN-ik) (*ker*-a-TŌ-sis)	precancerous skin condition of horny tissue formation that results from excessive exposure to sunlight. It may evolve into a squamous cell carcinoma.
albinism (AL-bi-niz-um)	congenital hereditary condition characterized by partial or total lack of pigment (melanin) in the skin, hair, and eyes

> **ABSCESS**
> is derived from the Latin **ab**, meaning **from**, and **cedo**, meaning **to go**. The tissue dies and goes away, with the pus replacing it.

> **ALBINISM**
> **Alb** is Latin word root meaning **white**. **Leuk** is the Greek word root meaning **white**.

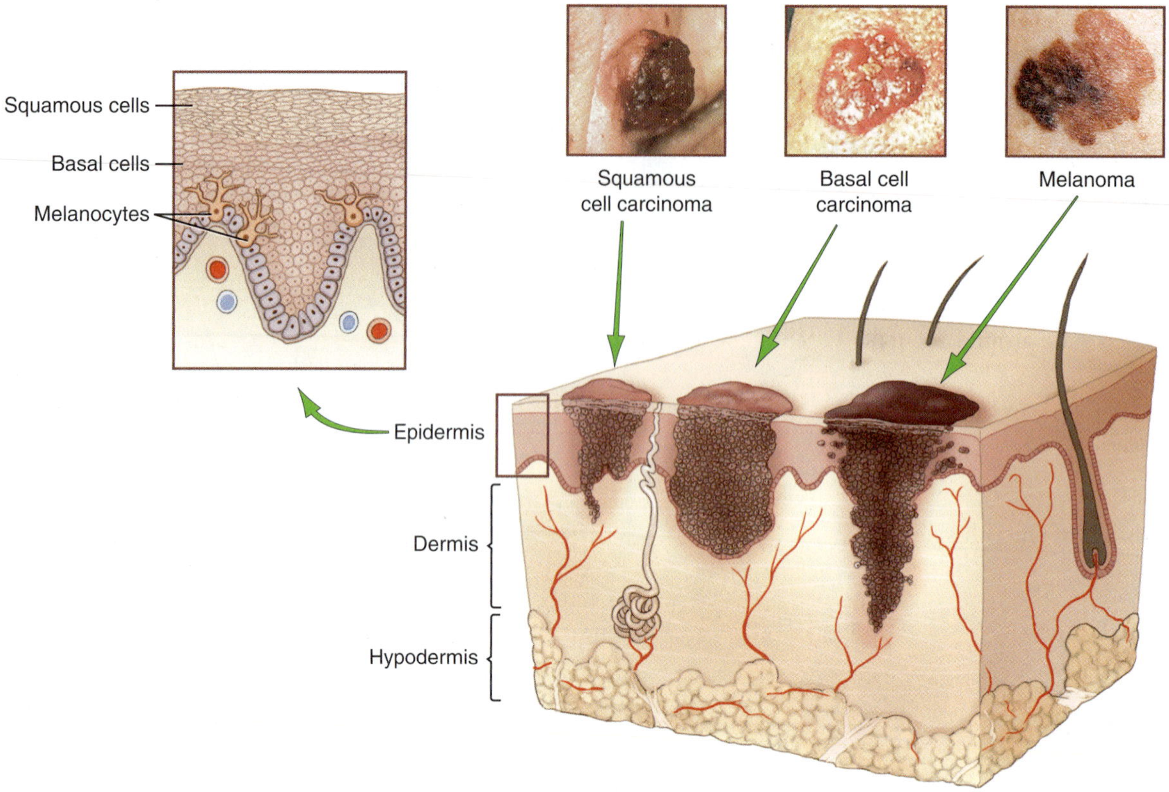

FIG. 4.3

> **CANDIDA**
> comes from the Latin **candidus**, meaning gleaming white; **albicans** is from the Latin verb **albicare**, meaning **to make white**. The growth of the fungus is white, and the infection produces a white discharge.

Disease and Disorder Terms—cont'd

TERM	DEFINITION
basal cell carcinoma (BCC) (BĀ-sal) (sel) (*kar*-si-NŌ-ma)	malignant epithelial tumor arising from the bottom layer of the epidermis called the basal layer; it seldom metastasizes, but invades local tissue and may recur in the same location. Common in individuals who have had excessive sun exposure. (Fig. 4.3)
candidiasis (*kan*-di-DĪ-a-sis)	infection of the skin, mouth (also called **thrush**), or vagina caused by the yeast-type fungus *Candida albicans*. *Candida* is normally present in the mucous membranes; overgrowth causes an infection. Esophageal candidiasis is often seen in patients with AIDS (acquired immunodeficiency syndrome).
carbuncle (KAR-bung-kl)	infection of skin and subcutaneous tissue composed of a cluster of boils (furuncles, see below) caused by staphylococcal bacteria
cellulitis (*sel*-ū-LĪ-tis)	inflammation of the skin and subcutaneous tissue caused by infection; characterized by redness, pain, heat, and swelling
contusion (kon-TŪ-zhun)	injury with no break in the skin, characterized by pain, swelling, and discoloration (also called a **bruise**)
eczema (EK-ze-ma)	noninfectious, inflammatory skin disease characterized by redness, blisters, scabs, and itching

TERM	DEFINITION
fissure (FISH-ur)	slit or cracklike sore in the skin
furuncle (FER-ung-kl)	painful skin nodule caused by staphylococcal bacteria in a hair follicle (also called a **boil**) (Fig. 4.4)
gangrene (GANG-grēn)	death of tissue caused by loss of blood supply followed by bacterial invasion (a form of necrosis)
herpes (HER-pēz)	inflammatory skin disease caused by herpes virus characterized by small blisters in clusters. Many types of herpes exist. Herpes simplex virus type 1, for example, causes fever blisters; herpes zoster, also called shingles, is characterized by painful skin eruptions that follow nerves inflamed by the virus. (see Table 4.1)
impetigo (*im*-pe-TĪ-gō)	superficial skin infection characterized by pustules and caused by either staphylococci or streptococci (see Table 4.1)
infection (in-FEK-shun)	invasion of pathogens in body tissue. An acute infection may remain localized if the body's defense mechanisms are effective or may persist to become subacute or chronic (see sidebar p. 147). A systemic infection occurs when the pathogen causing a local infection gains access to the vascular or lymphatic system and becomes disseminated throughout the body.
Kaposi sarcoma (KAP-ō-sē) (sar-KŌ-ma)	cancerous condition starting as purple or brown papules on the lower extremities that spreads through the skin to the lymph nodes and internal organs; frequently seen with AIDS
laceration (*las*-er-Ā-shun)	torn, ragged-edged wound
lesion (LĒ-zhun)	any visible change in tissue resulting from injury or disease. It is a broad term that includes sores, wounds, ulcers, and tumors.
MRSA infection (mer-SAH) (in-FEK-shun)	invasion of body tissue by methicillin-resistant *Staphylococcus aureus*, a strain of common bacteria that has developed resistance to methicillin and other antibiotics. It can produce skin and soft tissue infections and sometimes bloodstream infections and pneumonia, which can be fatal if not treated. MRSA is quite common in hospitals and long-term care facilities but is increasingly emerging as an important infection in the general population.
pediculosis (pe-*dik*-ū-LŌ-sis)	invasion into the skin and hair by lice
psoriasis (so-RĪ-a-sis)	chronic skin condition producing red lesions covered with silvery scales

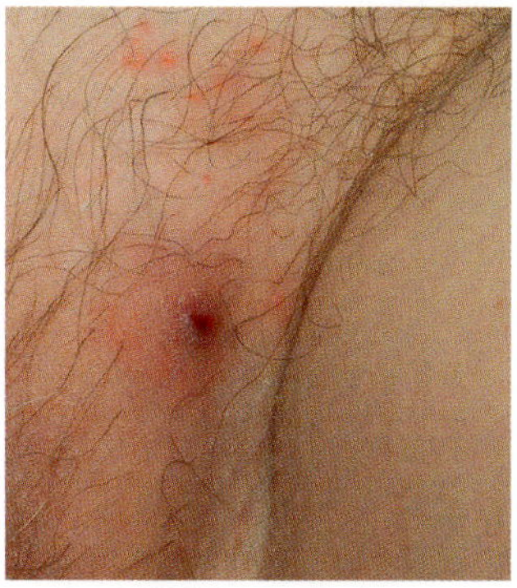

FIG. 4.4 Furuncle resulting from a *Staphylococcus aureus* infection.

HERPES

is derived from the Greek **herpo**, meaning to **creep along**. It is descriptive of the course and type of skin lesion.

TYPES OF INFECTION

Infections may be caused by a bacterium, fungus, parasite, or virus. Examples of common skin infections are:

- **Bacterial infections**—carbuncle, cellulitis, furuncle, impetigo, MRSA infection, and paronychia
- **Fungal infections**—candidiasis, tinea, and trichomycosis
- **Parasitic infections**—scabies and pediculosis
- **Viral infections**—fever blister (herpes simplex virus type 1) and shingles (herpes zoster)

TYPES OF SKIN LESIONS

Primary lesions are physical changes of the skin of pathological origin. **Secondary lesions** may result from changes in primary lesions or may be caused by injury or infection. **Vascular lesions** are related to blood vessels and include the escape of blood into the tissues (extravasation or hemorrhage). Examples of types of skin lesions include:

- **Primary lesions**—macule, papule, nodule, wheal, vesicle, pustule, and cyst
- **Secondary lesions**—cicatrix (scar), keloid, and ulcer
- **Vascular lesions**—petechia, purpura, and ecchymosis

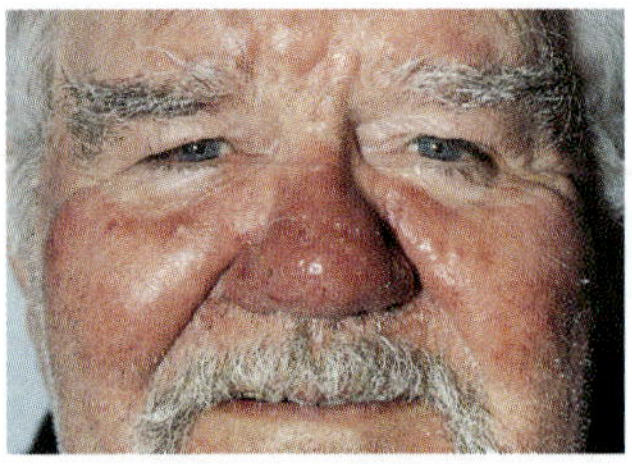

FIG. 4.5 Rosacea.

INTEGRATIVE MEDICINE TERM

Botanicals, the term used for plant-derived products, encompass the use of medicinal herbs. Studies investigating the therapeutic benefits of plant-based extract applications to skin **lesions** have demonstrated therapeutic efficacy for relieving skin discomfort and improving a number of skin conditions such as hyperpigmentation, **acne**, and premature aging.

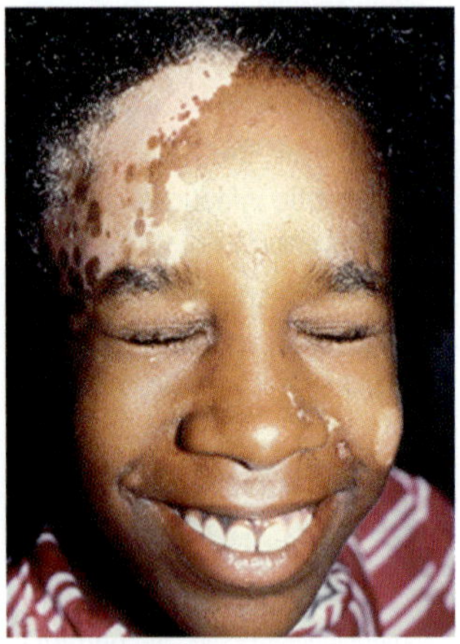

FIG. 4.6 Vitiligo.

Disease and Disorder Terms—cont'd

TERM	DEFINITION
rosacea (rō-ZĀ-shē-a)	chronic disorder of the skin that produces erythema, papules, pustules, and abnormal dilation of tiny blood vessels, usually occurring on the central area of the face in people older than 30 years (Fig. 4.5)
scabies (SKĀ-bēz)	skin infection caused by the itch mite, characterized by papule eruptions that are caused by the female burrowing into the outer layer of the skin and laying eggs. This condition is accompanied by severe itching. (Table 4.1)
scleroderma (*skle*-rō-DER-ma)	disease characterized by chronic hardening (induration) of the connective tissue of the skin and other body organs
squamous cell carcinoma (SCC) (SQWĀ-mus) (sel) (*kar*-si-NŌ-ma)	malignant growth developing from scalelike epithelial tissue of the surface layer of the epidermis; it invades local tissue and may metastasize. While most commonly appearing on the skin, SCC can occur in other parts of the body including the mouth, lips, and genitals. The most frequent cause is chronic exposure to sunlight. (Fig. 4.3)
systemic lupus erythematosus (SLE) (sis-TEM-ik) (LŪ-pus) (*e*-ri-*thē*-*ma*-TŌ-sus)	chronic inflammatory disease involving the skin, joints, kidneys, and nervous system. This autoimmune disease is characterized by periods of remission and exacerbations. It also may affect other organs.
tinea (TIN-ē-a)	fungal infection of the skin. The fungi may infect keratin of the skin, hair, and nails. Infections are classified by body regions such as *tinea capitis* (scalp), *tinea corporis* (body), and *tinea pedis* (foot). Tinea in general is also called **ringworm**, and tinea pedis specifically is also called **athlete's foot**. (Table 4.1)
urticaria (*ur*-ti-KAR-ē-a)	itchy skin eruption composed of wheals of varying sizes and shapes. Urticaria is sometimes associated with infections and with allergic reactions to food, medicine, or other agents. Other causes include internal disease, physical stimuli, and genetic disorders. (also called **hives**) (Table 4.2)
vitiligo (*vit*-i-LĪ-gō)	white patches on the skin caused by the destruction of melanocytes (Fig. 4.6)

EXERCISE 14

Practice saying aloud each of the Disease and Disorder Terms NOT Built from Word Parts.

To hear the terms, go to Evolve Resources at evolve.elsevier.com and select:
Practice Student Resources > Student Resources > Chapter 4 > **Pronounce and Spell**

See Appendix B for instructions.

❑ Check the box when complete.

TABLE 4.1 **Common Skin Infections**

DISORDER	EXAMPLES	
Impetigo (bacterial infection)	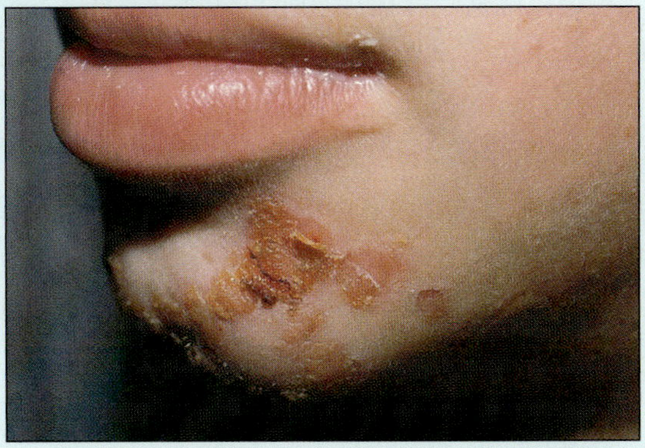	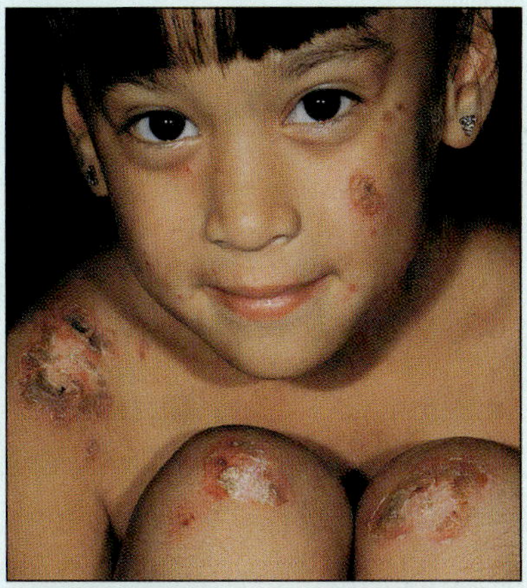
Tinea (fungal infection)	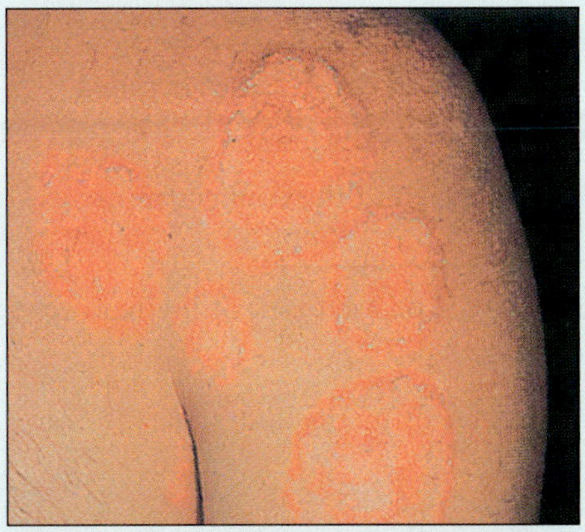 Tinea corporis (also called **ringworm**)	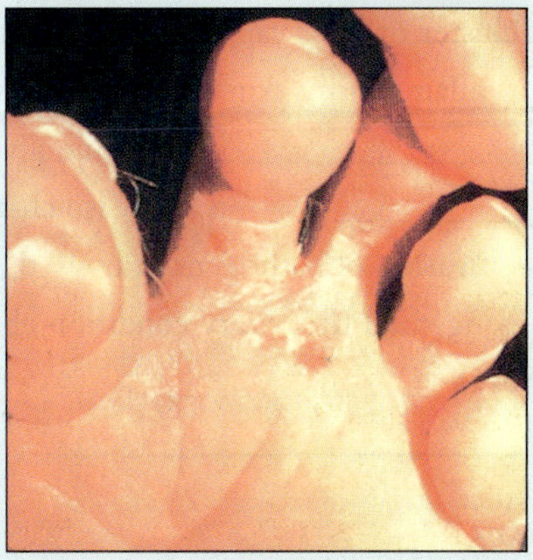 Tinea pedis (also called **athlete's foot**)
Scabies (parasitic infection)	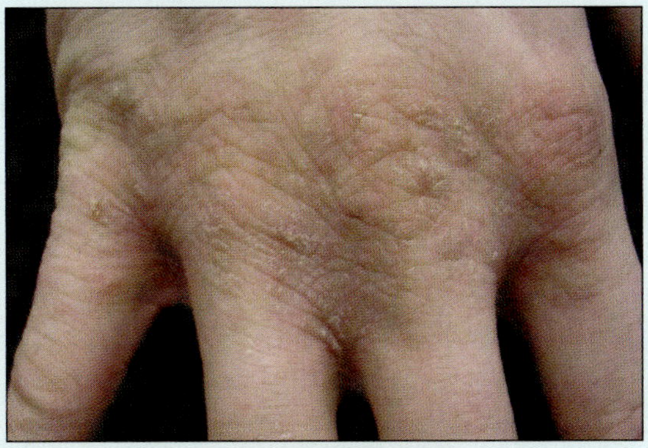	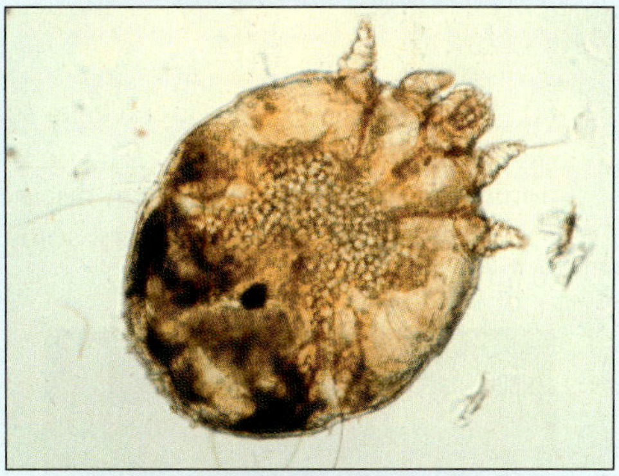 Scabies mite
Herpes zoster (also called **shingles**) (viral infection)	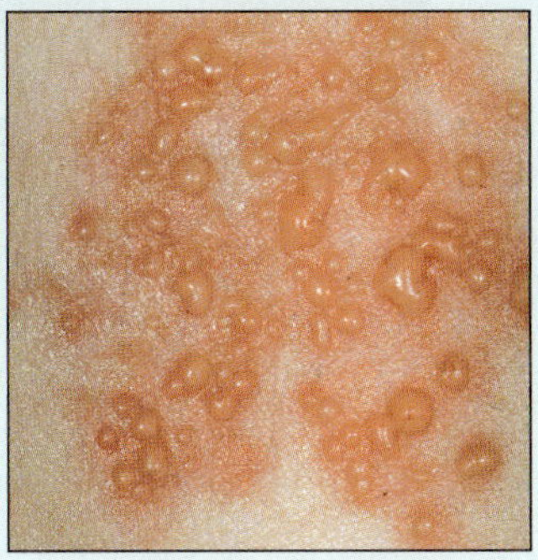	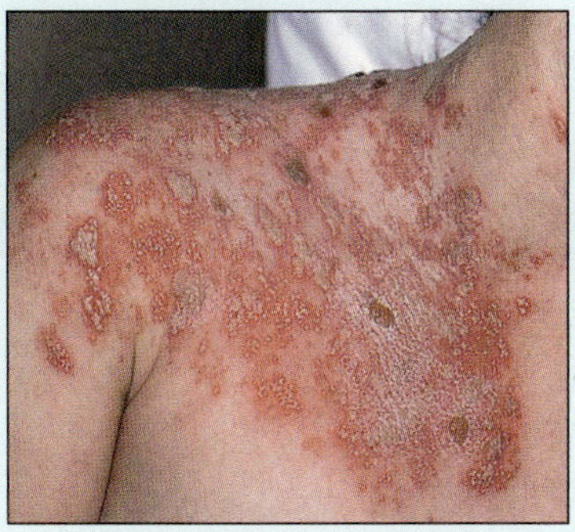

EXERCISE 15

A. Fill in the blanks with the correct disease and disorder terms.

1. A chronic inflammatory disease affecting the skin, joints, and other organs is ______________________ ______________________ ______________________.
2. A(n) ________________ is a localized collection of pus.
3. The scraping away of the skin by mechanical process or injury is called a(n) ________________.
4. ______________________ is the name given to the invasion of the skin and hair by lice.
5. An injury with no break in the skin and characterized by pain, swelling, and discoloration is called a(n) ______________________.
6. ________________ is the name given to tissue death caused by a loss of blood supply followed by bacterial invasion.
7. Any visible change in tissue resulting from injury or disease is called a ________________.
8. A cluster of boils caused by staphylococcal bacteria is a ________________.
9. An inflammatory skin disease that involves the oil glands and hair follicles is called ________________.
10. ________________ is the name given to a torn, ragged-edged wound.
11. ________________ is a disease characterized by induration of the connective tissue.
12. An invasion of pathogens in body tissue is called ________________.
13. A congenital hereditary condition characterized by partial or total lack of pigment (melanin) in the skin, hair, and eyes is ________________.
14. ________________ ________________ is an invasion of methicillin-resistant *Staphylococcus aureus* in the body tissue.

B. Write the medical term pictured and defined.

1. (a) ________________, cracklike sore in the skin caused by (b) ________________, a noninfectious inflammatory skin disease characterized by redness, blisters, scabs, and itching

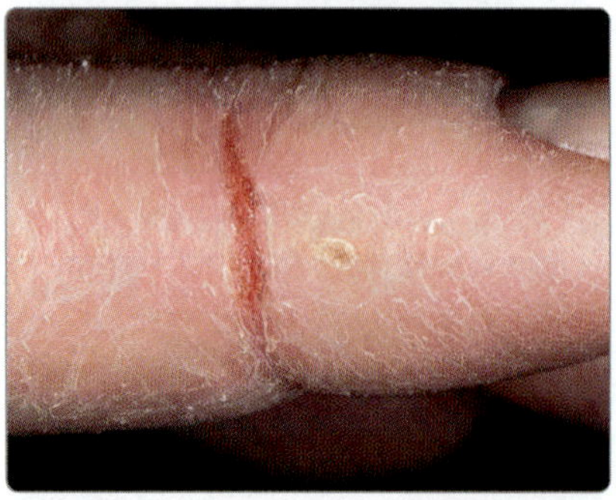

2. ________________, inflammation of the skin and subcutaneous tissue caused by infection and characterized by redness, pain, heat, and swelling

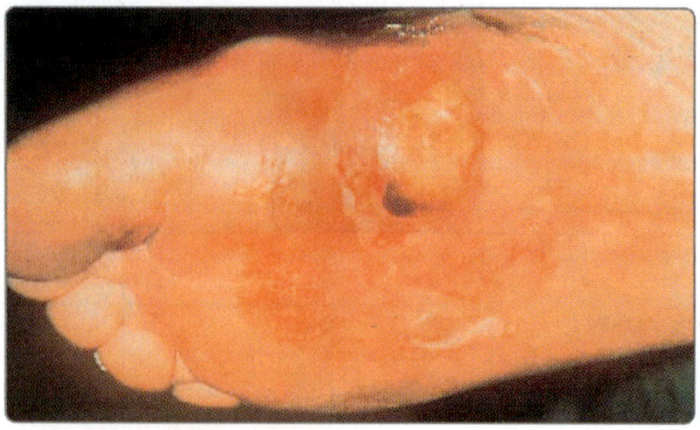

3. ____________________, chronic skin condition producing red lesions covered with silvery scales

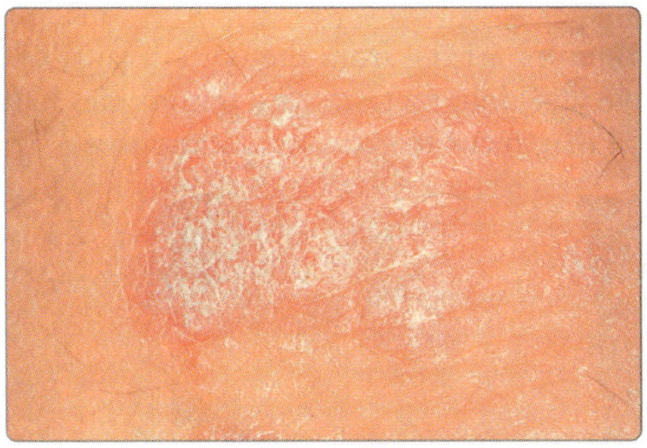

4. ____________________, inflammatory skin disease caused by a virus and characterized by small blisters

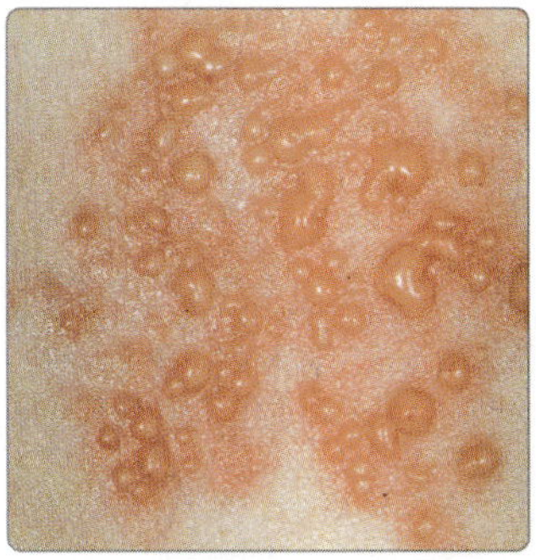

5. ____________________, fungal infection of the skin, also known as *ringworm*

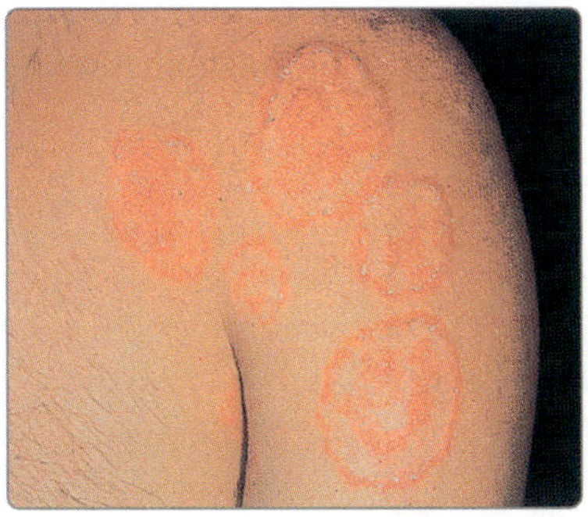

6. ____________________, cancerous condition starting as purple or brown papules on the lower extremities

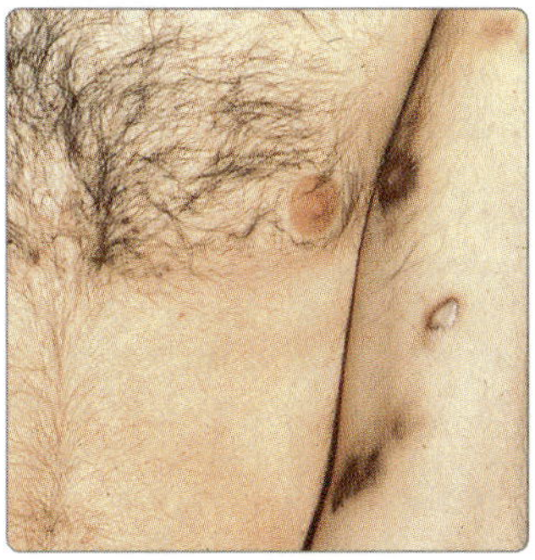

7. ____________________, horny tissue formation that results from excessive exposure to sunlight and is precancerous

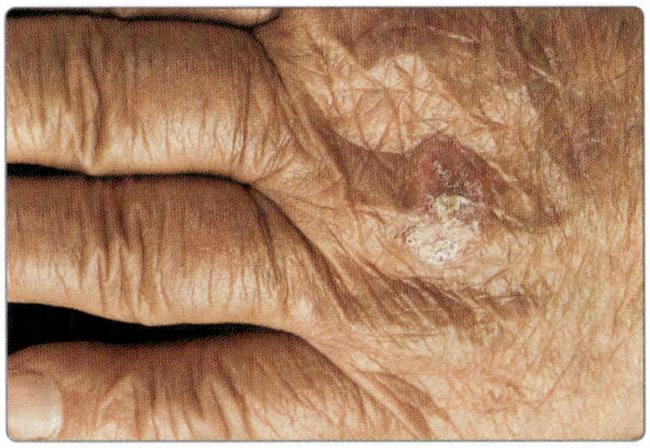

8. ____________________, painful skin nodule caused by staphylococcal bacteria in a hair follicle

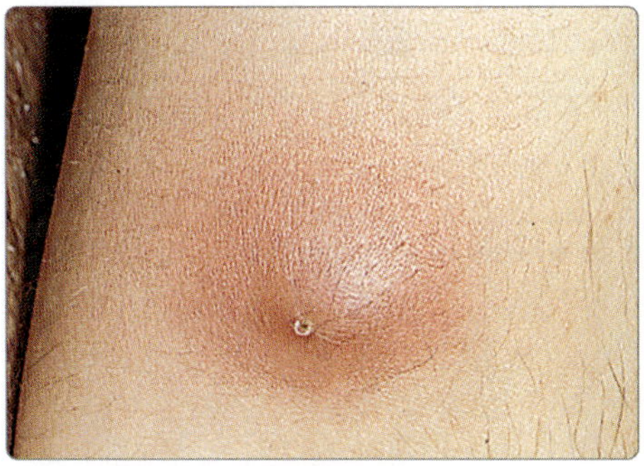

EXERCISE 15 *Pictured and Defined—cont'd*

9. ______________________________, malignant growth developing from scalelike epithelial tissue of the surface layer of the epidermis; it invades local tissue and may metastasize

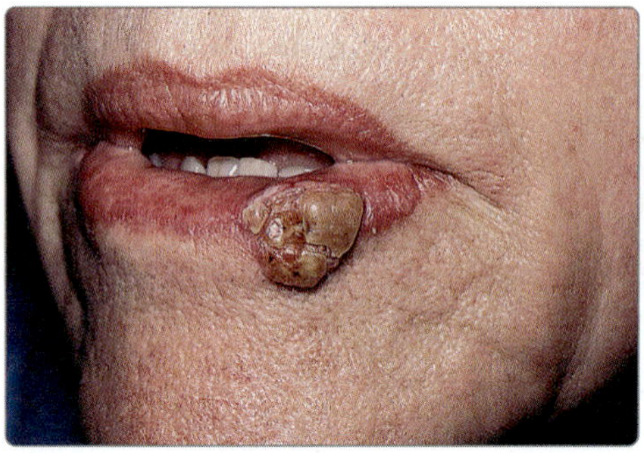

10. ______________________________, malignant epithelial tumor arising from the bottom layer of the epidermis; it seldom metastasizes, but invades local tissue and may recur in the same location

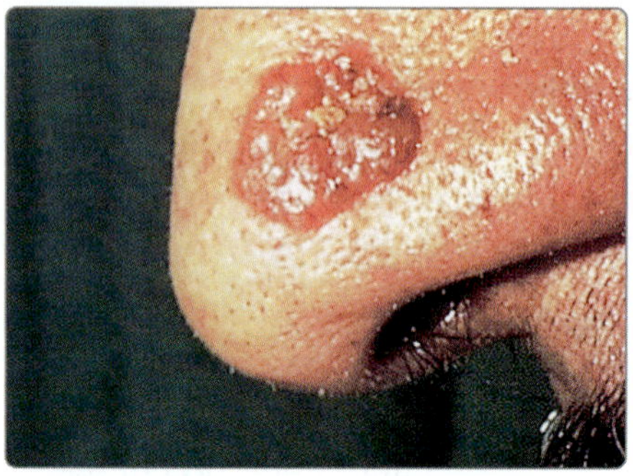

11. ______________________, superficial skin infection characterized by pustules and caused by either staphylococci or streptococci

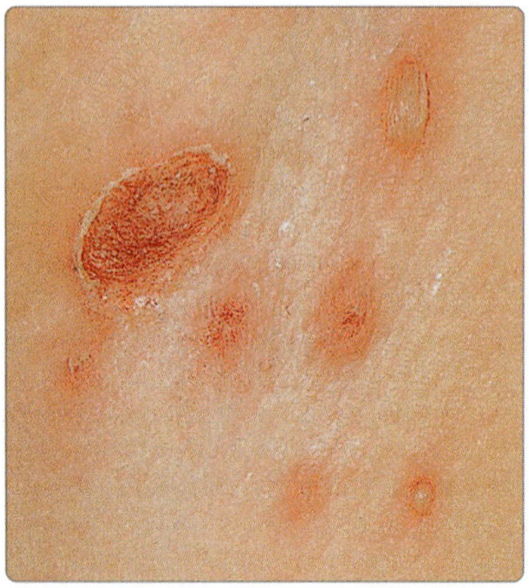

12. ______________________, skin inflammation caused by the itch mite

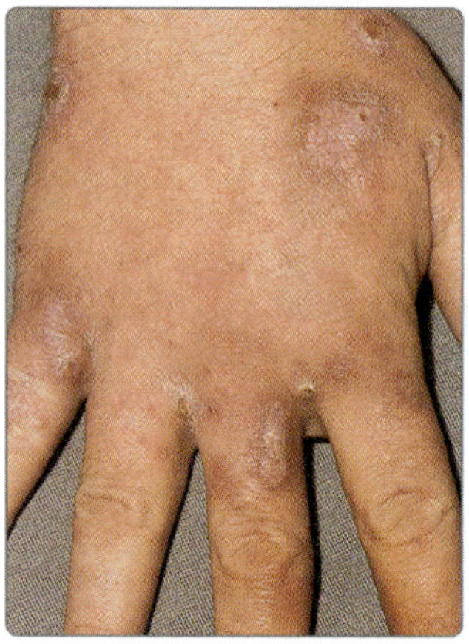

13. ______________________, itchy skin eruption composed of wheals of varying sizes and shapes

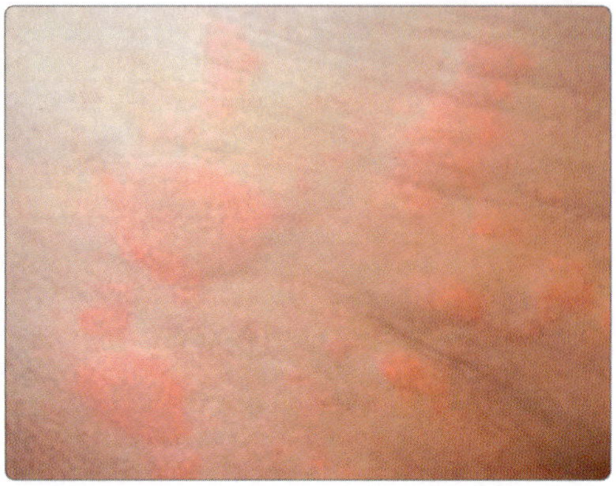

14. ______________________, infection of the skin, mouth, or vagina caused by *Candida albicans*

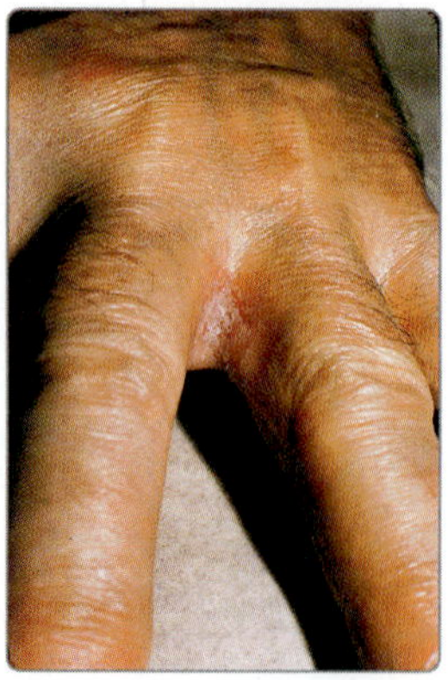

15. ____________________, white patches on the skin caused by the destruction of melanocytes

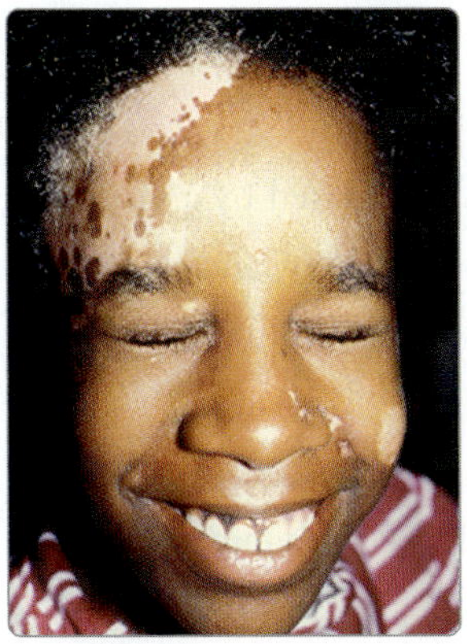

16. ____________________, chronic disorder of the skin on the central area of the face that produces erythema, papules, pustules, and abnormal dilation of tiny blood vessels

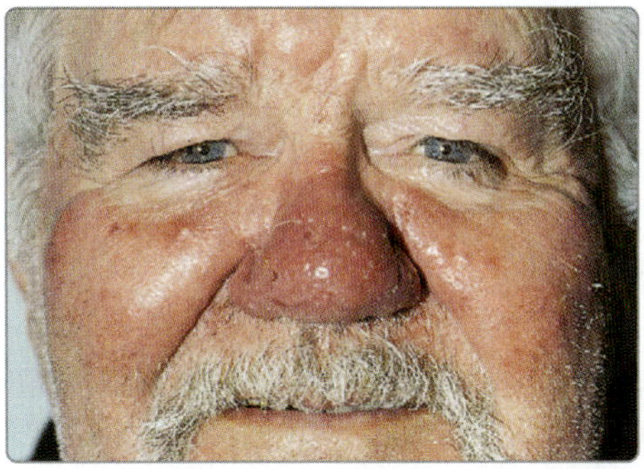

EXERCISE 16

Match the words in the first column with their correct definitions in the second column.

______	1. scleroderma	a.	death of tissue caused by loss of blood supply and entry of bacteria
______	2. abscess	b.	cracklike sore in the skin
______	3. furuncle	c.	cluster of boils
______	4. actinic keratosis	d.	chronic induration of connective tissue of the skin and other body organs
______	5. contusion	e.	noninfectious inflammatory skin disease having redness, blisters, scabs, and itching
______	6. carbuncle	f.	scraped-away skin
______	7. basal cell carcinoma	g.	involves sebaceous glands and hair follicles
______	8. fissure	h.	painful skin nodule caused by staphylococci in a hair follicle
______	9. eczema	i.	inflammation of skin and subcutaneous tissue with redness, pain, heat, and swelling
______	10. cellulitis	j.	localized collection of pus
______	11. acne	k.	injury characterized by pain, swelling, and discoloration
______	12. gangrene	l.	precancerous skin condition caused by excessive exposure to sunlight
______	13. abrasion	m.	usually occurring in the central area of the face in people older than 30 years
______	14. rosacea	n.	malignant epithelial tumor arising from the bottom layer of the epidermis; it seldom metastasizes, but invades local tissue and may recur in the same location
______	15. MRSA infection	o.	potentially serious infection caused by methicillin-resistant *Staphylococcus aureus*

EXERCISE 17

Match the words in the first column with the correct definitions in the second column.

______	1. herpes	a. skin inflammation caused by the itch mite
______	2. tinea	b. fungal infection of the skin, hair, and nails
______	3. Kaposi sarcoma	c. red lesions covered by silvery scales
______	4. vitiligo	d. inflammatory skin disease having clusters of blisters and caused by a virus
______	5. lesion	e. chronic inflammatory disease involving the skin, joints, kidney, and nervous system
______	6. pediculosis	f. cancerous condition that starts as brown or purple papules on the lower extremities
______	7. infection	g. composed of wheals
______	8. scabies	h. torn, ragged-edged wound
______	9. squamous cell carcinoma	i. superficial skin condition having pustules and caused by staphylococci or streptococci
______	10. systemic lupus erythematosus	j. characterized by lack of pigment (melanin) in the skin, hair, and eyes
______	11. impetigo	k. infection of the skin, mouth, or vagina caused by a yeast-type fungus
______	12. urticaria	l. invasion of the hair and skin by lice
______	13. candidiasis	m. visible change in tissue resulting from injury or disease
______	14. psoriasis	n. malignant growth developing from scalelike epithelial tissue of the surface layer of the epidermis; it invades local tissue and may metastasize
______	15. albinism	o. invasion of body tissue by pathogens
______	16. laceration	p. white patches on the skin caused by the destruction of melanocytes

EXERCISE 18

Spell each of the Disease and Disorder Terms NOT Built from Word Parts by having someone dictate them to you. Use a separate sheet of paper.

> To hear and spell the terms, go to Evolve Resources at evolve.elsevier.com and select:
> Practice Student Resources > Student Resources > Chapter 4 > **Pronounce and Spell**
>
> See Appendix B for instructions.

❑ Check the box when complete.

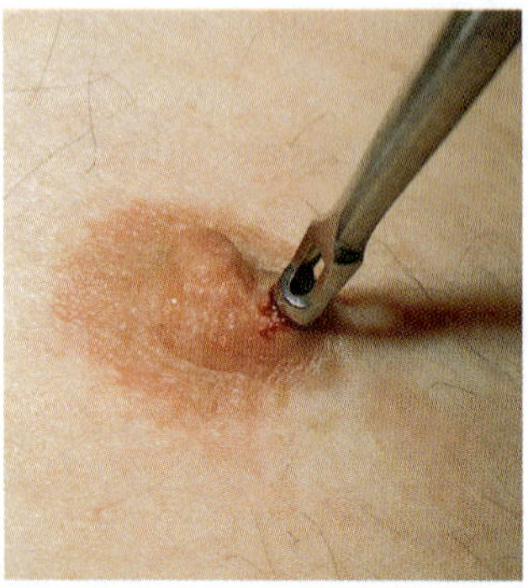

FIG. 4.7 Punch biopsy.

DERMATOME

also refers to the area of skin supplied by a specific sensory nerve root.

Surgical Terms

BUILT FROM WORD PARTS

The following terms can be translated using definitions of word parts. Further explanation is provided within parentheses as needed.

TERM	DEFINITION
biopsy (bx) (BĪ-op-sē)	view of life (the removal of living tissue from the body to be viewed under the microscope) (Fig. 4.7)
dermatoautoplasty (*der*-ma-tō-AW-tō-*plas*-tē)	surgical repair using one's own skin (skin graft) (also called **autograft**)
dermatoheteroplasty (*der*-ma-tō-HET-er-ō *plas*-tē)	surgical repair using skin from others (skin graft) (also called **allograft**)
dermatome (DER-ma-tōm)	instrument used to cut skin (in thin slices for skin grafts) *(Note: when two consonants of the same letter come together, one is sometimes dropped.)*

TERM	DEFINITION
dermatoplasty (DER-ma-tō-*plas*-tē)	surgical repair of the skin
rhytidectomy (*rit*-i-DEK-to-mē)	excision of wrinkles (also called **facelift**)
rhytidoplasty (RIT-i-dō-*plas*-tē)	surgical repair of wrinkles

BIOPSY OF THE SKIN

may be performed by the dermatologist during an office visit. Common techniques include:

- excisional biopsy removes the entire lesion along with a margin of surrounding tissue
- punch biopsy removes a cylindrical portion of tissue with a specifically designed round knife (Fig. 4.7)
- shave biopsy removes a sample of tissue with a cut parallel to the surrounding skin

EXERCISE 19

Practice saying aloud each of the Surgical Terms Built from Word Parts.

To hear the terms, go to Evolve Resources at evolve.elsevier.com and select:
Practice Student Resources > Student Resources > Chapter 4 > **Pronounce and Spell**

See Appendix B for instructions.

❑ Check the box when complete.

EXERCISE 20

Analyze and define the following Surgical Terms Built from Word Parts by drawing slashes between word parts, writing word part abbreviations above the term, underlining combining forms, and writing combining form abbreviations below the term. *Check your answers in Appendix A.*

EXAMPLE:

WR CV S
dermato / o / plasty
CF
surgical repair of the skin

1. rhytidectomy

____

____

2. biopsy

____

____

3. dermatoautoplasty

____

____

4. rhytidoplasty

____

____

5. dermatoheteroplasty

____

____

6. dermatome

____

____

EXERCISE 21

Build Surgical Terms for the following definitions by using the word parts you have learned.

EXAMPLE: surgical repair using one's own skin dermat / o / aut / o / plasty
WR / CV / WR / CV / S

1. excision of wrinkles ____________ WR / ____________ S

2. view of life (removal of living tissue from the body ____________ WR / ____________ S

3. surgical repair using skin from others ____________ WR / CV / ____________ WR / CV / ____________ S

4. surgical repair of wrinkles ____________ WR / CV / ____________ S

5. surgical repair of the skin ____________ WR / CV / ____________ S

6. instrument used to cut skin ____________ WR / ____________ S

EXERCISE 22

Spell each of the Surgical Terms Built from Word Parts by having someone dictate them to you. Use a separate sheet of paper.

To hear and spell the terms, go to Evolve Resources at evolve.elsevier.com and select:
Practice Student Resources > Student Resources > Chapter 4 > **Pronounce and Spell**

See Appendix B for instructions.

❑ Check the box when complete.

Surgical Terms
NOT BUILT FROM WORD PARTS

Word parts may be present in the following terms; however, their full meanings cannot be translated using definitions of word parts alone.

TERM	DEFINITION
cauterization (*kaw*-tur-ī-ZĀ-shun)	destruction of tissue with a hot or cold instrument, electric current, or caustic substance (also called **cautery**)
cryosurgery (*krī*-ō-SER-jer-ē)	destruction of tissue by using extreme cold, often by using liquid nitrogen (Fig. 4.8)
debridement (DA-brēd-ment)	removal of contaminated or dead tissue and foreign matter from an open wound
dermabrasion (*derm*-a-BRĀ-zhun)	procedure to remove skin scars with abrasive material, such as sandpaper
excision (ek-SIZH-en)	removal by cutting
incision (in-SIZH-en)	surgical cut or wound produced by a sharp instrument
incision and drainage (I&D) (in-SIZH-en) and (DRĀ-nij)	surgical cut made to allow the free flow or withdrawal of fluids from a lesion, wound, or cavity

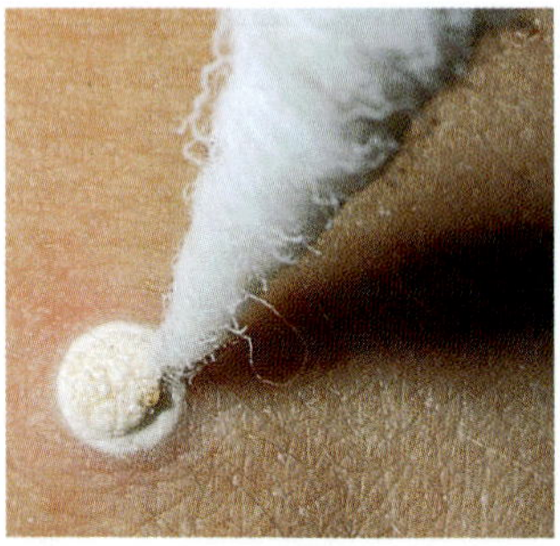

FIG. 4.8 Cryosurgery performed with a nitrogen-soaked, cotton-tipped applicator.

TERM	DEFINITION
laser surgery (LĀ-zer) (SER-jer-ē)	procedure using an instrument that emits a high-powered beam of light used to cut, burn, vaporize, or destroy tissue
Mohs surgery (mōz) (SER-jer-ē)	technique of microscopically controlled serial excisions of a skin cancer
suturing (SOO-cher-ing)	to stitch edges of a wound surgically (Fig. 4.9)

MOHS SURGERY
allows for complete tumor removal while sparing as much normal tissue as possible. Excised tissue is examined for tumor cells during the procedure. Tissue is removed until the biopsy margins are cancer free. The procedure is named after **Dr. Frederic E. Mohs**, Wisconsin, who first used the concept in 1936.

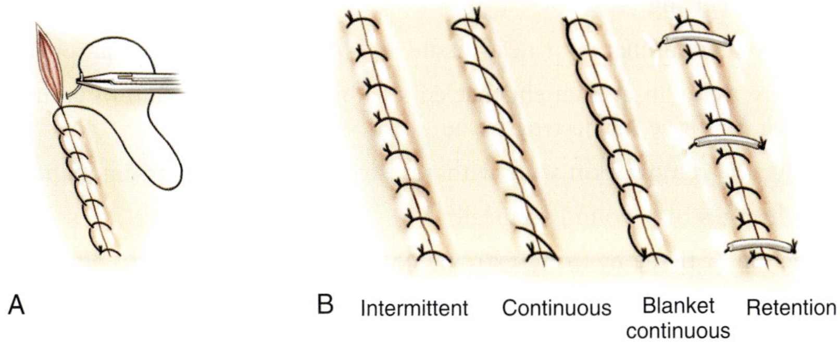

FIG. 4.9 A, Suturing. **B,** Suturing methods.

EXERCISE 23

Practice saying aloud each of the Surgical Terms NOT Built from Word Parts.

To hear the terms, go to Evolve Resources at evolve.elsevier.com and select:
Practice Student Resources > Student Resources > Chapter 4 > **Pronounce and Spell**

See Appendix B for instructions.

❑ Check the box when complete.

EXERCISE 24

Fill in the blank with the correct surgical term.

1. ________________ ________________ is a technique of microscopically controlled serial excisions used for treatment of many skin cancers.
2. A surgical cut or wound produced by a sharp instrument is called a(n) ________________________________.
3. Destruction of tissue with a hot or cold instrument, electric current, or caustic substance is called ________________.
4. ________________ is to stitch the edges of a wound surgically.
5. A surgical cut made to allow the free flow or withdrawal of fluids from a lesion, wound, or cavity is called ________________ ________________ ________________.
6. ____ is the removal of contaminated or dead tissue and foreign matter from an open wound.
7. Removal by cutting is known as ____.
8. ________________ ________________ is a procedure using an instrument that emits a high-powered beam of light used to cut, burn, vaporize, or destroy tissue.
9. The destruction of tissue by using extreme cold, often by using liquid nitrogen, is called ________________.
10. ____ is a procedure to remove skin scars with abrasive material.

EXERCISE 25

Match the terms in the first column with their correct definitions in the second column.

_____ 1. suturing
_____ 2. dermabrasion
_____ 3. laser surgery
_____ 4. incision and drainage
_____ 5. cauterization
_____ 6. excision
_____ 7. Mohs surgery
_____ 8. debridement
_____ 9. cryosurgery
_____ 10. incision

a. destruction of tissue with a hot or cold instrument, electric current, or caustic substance
b. technique of microscopically controlled serial excisions of a skin cancer
c. surgical cut or wound produced by a sharp instrument
d. surgical cut made to allow the free flow or withdrawal of fluids from a lesion, wound, or cavity
e. removal by cutting
f. removal of contaminated or dead tissue and foreign matter from an open wound
g. procedure using an instrument that emits a high-powered beam of light used to cut, burn, vaporize, or destroy tissue
h. procedure to remove skin scars with abrasive material, such as sandpaper
i. to stitch edges of a wound surgically
j. destruction of tissue by using extreme cold, often by using liquid nitrogen

EXERCISE 26

Spell each of the Surgical Terms NOT Built from Word Parts by having someone dictate them to you. Use a separate sheet of paper.

To hear and spell the terms, go to Evolve Resources at evolve.elsevier.com and select:
Practice Student Resources > Student Resources > Chapter 4 > **Pronounce and Spell**

See Appendix B for instructions.

❑ Check the box when complete.

Complementary Terms
BUILT FROM WORD PARTS

The following terms can be translated using definitions of word parts. Further explanation is provided within parentheses as needed.

TERM	DEFINITION
dermatologist (*der*-ma-TOL-o-jist)	physician who studies and treats skin (diseases)
dermatology (derm) (der-ma-TOL-o-jē)	study of the skin (branch of medicine that deals with the diagnosis and treatment of skin diseases)
epidermal (*ep*-i-DER-mal)	pertaining to upon the skin
erythroderma (e-rith-rō-DER-ma)	red skin (abnormal redness of the skin) (Exercise Figure C)
hypodermic (*hī*-pō-DER-mik)	pertaining to under the skin (Exercise Figure D)
intradermal (ID) (*in*-tra-DER-mal)	pertaining to within the skin (Exercise Figure D)
keratogenic (*ker*-a-tō-JEN-ik)	producing horny tissue
leukoderma (lū-kō-DER-ma)	white skin (white patches caused by depigmentation) (Exercise Figure C)

TERM	DEFINITION
necrosis (ne-KRŌ-sis)	abnormal condition of death (cells and tissue die because of disease)
percutaneous (*per*-kū-TĀ-nē-us)	pertaining to through the skin
staphylococcus (pl. staphylococci) (staph) (*staf*-il-ō-KOK-us) (*staf*-il-ō-KOK-sī)	berry-shaped (bacterium) in grapelike clusters (these bacteria cause many skin diseases) (Exercise Figure E)
streptococcus (pl. streptococci) (strep) (*strep*-tō-KOK-us) (*strep*-tō-KOK-sī)	berry-shaped (bacterium) in twisted chains (Exercise Figure F)
subcutaneous (subcut) (*sub*-kū-TĀ-nē-us)	pertaining to under the skin (Exercise Figure D)
subungual (sub-UNG-gwal)	pertaining to under the nail
transdermal (TD) (trans-DER-mel)	pertaining to through the skin (Exercise Figure D)
ungual (UNG-gwal)	pertaining to the nail
xanthoderma (*zan*-thō-DER-ma)	yellow skin (Exercise Figure C)
xerosis (zēr-Ō-sis)	abnormal condition of dryness (of skin, eye, or mouth)

TRANSDERMAL

usually means entering through the skin and refers to the administration of a drug applied to the skin in ointment or patch form. **Percutaneous** usually means performed through the skin, as in the insertion of a needle, catheter, or probe.

EXERCISE FIGURE C

Fill in the blanks to label the illustrations.

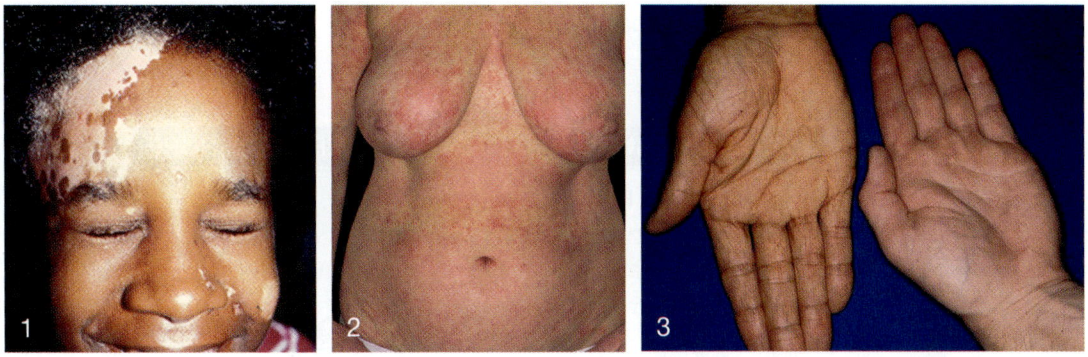

1. ______ / ______ / ______ /a as seen in vitiligo.
   white / cv / skin

2. ______ / ______ / ______ /a as seen in exfoliative dermatitis.
   red / cv / skin

3. ______ / ______ / ______ /a as seen in jaundice.
   yellow / cv / skin

EXERCISE FIGURE D

Fill in the blanks to build terms related to the routes of administration pictured below.

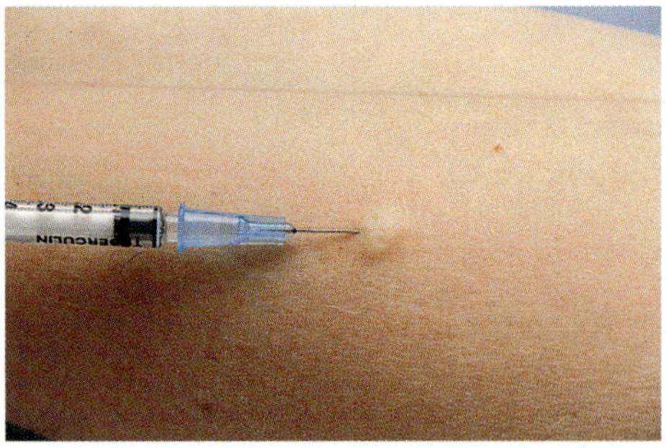

1. _____ / _____ / _____ injection
within / skin / pertaining to

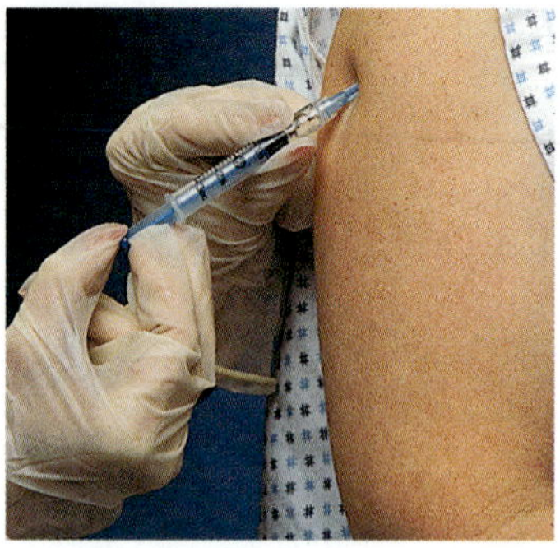

2. _____ / _____ / _____ injection
under / skin / pertaining to

using a _____ / _____ / _____ needle
under / skin / pertaining to

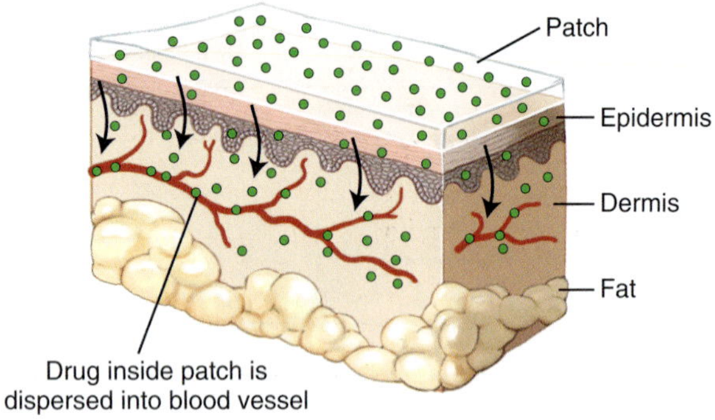

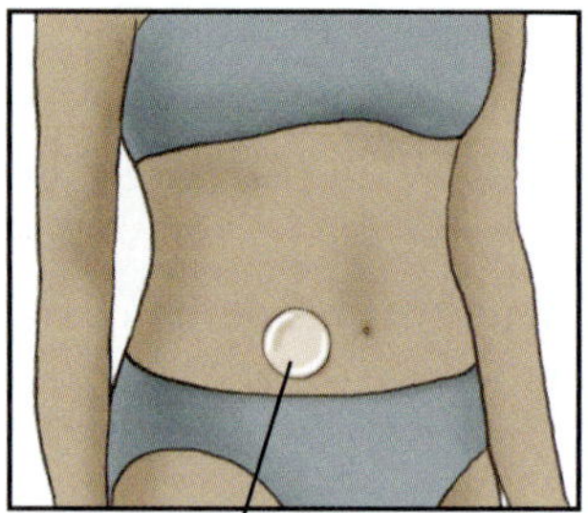

3. _____ / _____ / _____ patch
through / skin / pertaining to

EXERCISE FIGURE E

Fill in the blanks to label the diagrams.

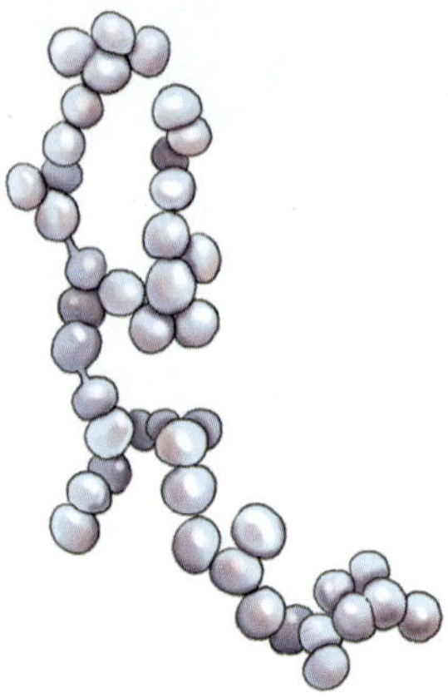

_____ / _____ / _____
grapelike clusters / cv / berry-shaped (plural)

EXERCISE FIGURE F

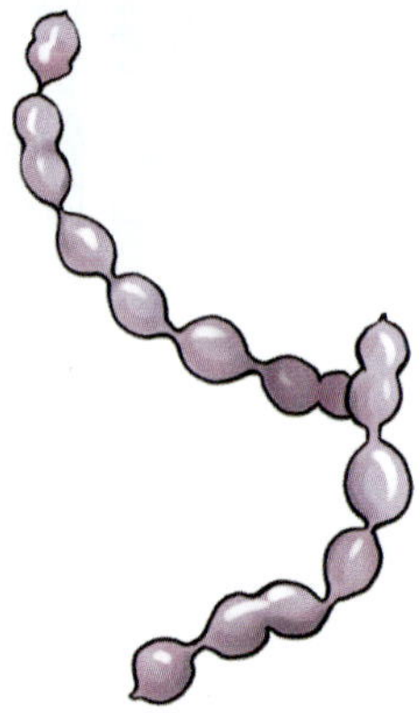

_____ / _____ / _____
twisted chains / cv / berry-shaped (plural)

EXERCISE 27

Practice saying aloud each of the Complementary Terms Built from Word Parts.

> To hear the terms, go to Evolve Resources at evolve.elsevier.com and select:
> Practice Student Resources > Student Resources > Chapter 4 > **Pronounce and Spell**
>
> See Appendix B for instructions.

❑ Check the box when complete.

EXERCISE 28

Analyze and define the following Complementary Terms Built from Word Parts by drawing slashes between word parts, writing word part abbreviations above the term, underlining combining forms, and writing combining form abbreviations below the term. *Check your answers in Appendix A.*

EXAMPLE:

P WR S
intra / derm / al
pertaining to within the skin

1. ungual

 ____
 ____

2. transdermal

 ____
 ____

3. streptococcus

 ____
 ____

4. hypodermic

 ____
 ____

5. dermatology

 ____
 ____

6. subcutaneous

 ____
 ____

7. staphylococcus

 ____
 ____

8. keratogenic

 ____
 ____

9. dermatologist

 ____
 ____

10. necrosis

 ____
 ____

11. epidermal

 ____
 ____

12. xanthoderma

 ____
 ____

13. erythroderma

____

____

14. percutaneous

____

____

15. xerosis

____

____

16. subungual

____

____

17. leukoderma

____

____

EXERCISE 29

Build complementary terms by using the word parts you have learned.

EXAMPLE: pertaining to under the skin hypo / derm / ic (P / WR / S)

1. study of the skin ______ / ______ / ______ (WR / CV / S)

2. abnormal condition of death (of cells and tissue) ______ / ______ (WR / S)

3. pertaining to the nail ______ / ______ (WR / S)

4. berry-shaped (bacterium) in grapelike clusters (singular) ______ / ______ / ______ (WR / CV / S)

5. a physician who studies and treats skin (diseases) ______ / ______ / ______ (WR / CV / S)

6. pertaining to within the skin ______ / ______ / ______ (P / WR / S)

7. pertaining to upon the skin ______ / ______ / ______ (P / WR / S)

8. pertaining to under the skin ______ / ______ / ______ (P / WR / S)

______ / ______ / ______ (P / WR / S)

9. berry-shaped (bacterium) in twisted chains (singular) ______ / ______ / ______ (WR / CV / S)

10. producing horny tissue ______ WR / ______ CV / ______ S

11. red skin ______ WR / ______ CV / ______ WR / ______ S

12. yellow skin ______ WR / ______ CV / ______ WR / ______ S

13. pertaining to through the skin ______ P / ______ WR / ______ S

______ P / ______ WR / ______ S

14. pertaining to under the nail ______ P / ______ WR / ______ S

15. white skin ______ WR / ______ CV / ______ WR / ______ S

16. abnormal condition of dryness ______ WR / ______ S

EXERCISE 30

Spell each of the Complementary Terms Built from Word Parts by having someone dictate them to you. Use a separate sheet of paper.

> To hear and spell the terms, go to Evolve Resources at evolve.elsevier.com and select:
> Practice Student Resources > Student Resources > Chapter 4 > **Pronounce and Spell**
>
> See Appendix B for instructions.

❑ Check the box when complete.

Complementary Terms

NOT BUILT FROM WORD PARTS

Word parts may be present in the following terms; however, their full meanings cannot be translated using definitions of word parts alone.

TERM	DEFINITION
alopecia (*al*-ō-PĒ-sha)	loss of hair (Fig. 4.10)
bacteria (s. bacterium) (bak-TĒR-ē-a) (bak-TĒR-ē-um)	single-celled microorganisms that reproduce by cell division and may cause infection by invading body tissue
cicatrix (SIK-a-triks)	scar
cyst (sist)	closed sac containing fluid or semisolid material (Table 4.2)

ALOPECIA
is derived from the Greek **alopex**, meaning **fox**. One was thought to bald like a mangy fox.

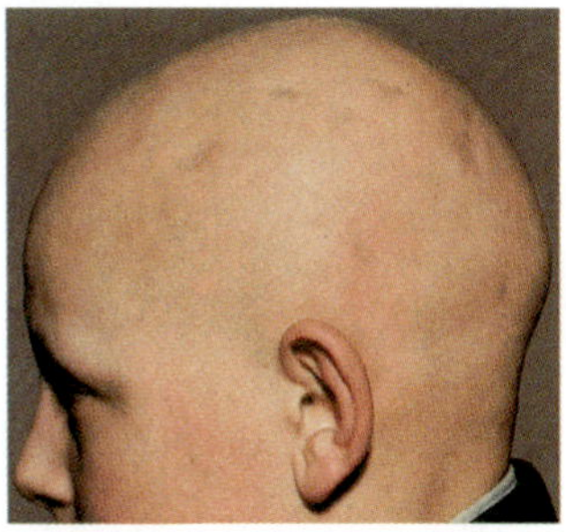

FIG. 4.10 Alopecia totalis (loss of hair from the scalp) with absence of eyelashes.

DIAPHORESIS
is derived from Greek **dia**, meaning **through**, and **phoreo**, meaning **carry**. Translated, it means the carrying through of perspiration.

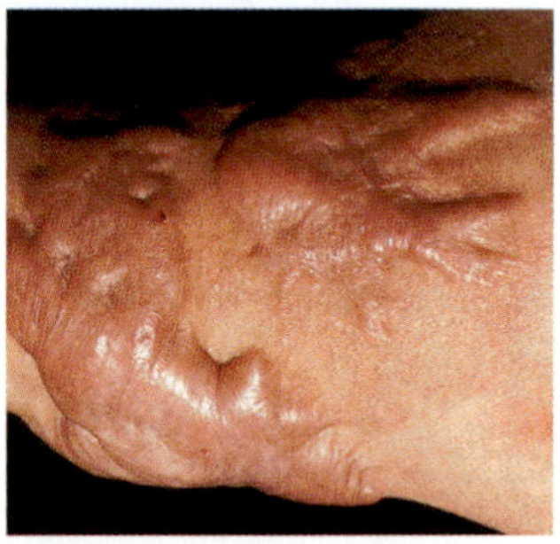

FIG. 4.11 Burn keloid.

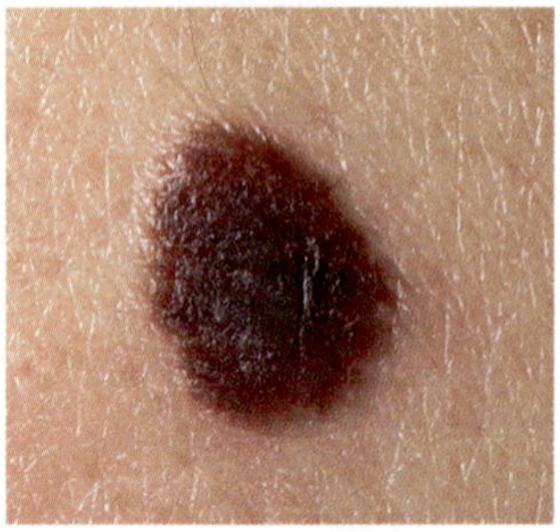

FIG. 4.12 Nevus (also called *mole*.)

PETECHIA
is originally from the Italian **petechio**, meaning **flea bite**. The small hemorrhagic spot resembles the mark made by a flea.

ECCHYMOSIS, PETECHIA, AND PURPURA
are vascular lesions related to blood vessels and the escape of blood into the skin and mucous membrane (extravasation and hemorrhage). They vary in size, with petechia being the smallest in size, up to .5 cm; purpura being the next largest, up to 1 cm; and ecchymosis being the largest, between 1 and 2 cm.

Complementary Terms—cont'd

TERM	DEFINITION
cytomegalovirus (CMV) (*sī*-to-MEG-a-lō-*vī*-rus)	herpes-type virus that usually causes disease when the immune system is compromised
diaphoresis (*dī*-a-fo-RĒ-sis)	sweating
ecchymosis (pl. ecchymoses) (*ek*-i-MŌ-sis) (*ek*-i-MŌ-sēz)	escape of blood into the skin (or mucous membrane), causing a small, flat, purple, or blue discoloration, as may occur when blood is withdrawn by a needle and syringe from an arm vein
edema (e-DĒ-ma)	puffy swelling of tissue from the accumulation of fluid
erythema (*er*-i-THĒ-ma)	redness
fungus (pl. fungi) (FUN-gus) (FUN-jī)	organism that feeds by absorbing organic molecules from its surroundings and may cause infection by invading body tissue; single-celled fungi (yeast) reproduce by budding; multicelled fungi (mold) reproduce by spore formation
induration (*in*-dū-RĀ-shun)	abnormal hard spot(s) or area of skin; may include underlying tissue
jaundice (JAWN-dis)	condition characterized by a yellow coloring of the skin, mucous membranes, and sclera (whites of the eyes) caused by the presence of bile (also called **icterus**)
keloid (KĒ-loyd)	overgrowth of scar tissue (Fig. 4.11)
leukoplakia (*lū*-kō-PLĀ-kē-a)	condition characterized by white spots or patches on mucous membrane, which may be precancerous
macule (MAK-ūl)	flat, colored spot on the skin (Table 4.2)
nevus (pl. nevi) (NĒ-vus) (NĒ-vī)	circumscribed malformation of the skin, usually brown, black, or flesh colored. A congenital nevus is present at birth and is referred to as a birthmark. (also called a **mole**) (Fig. 4.12)
nodule (NOD-ūl)	small, knotlike mass that can be felt by touch (Table 4.2)
pallor (PAL-or)	paleness
papule (PAP-ūl)	small, solid skin elevation (Table 4.2)
petechia (pl. petechiae) (pe-TĒ-kē-a) (pe-TĒ-kē-ē)	pinpoint skin hemorrhage
pressure injury (PRESH-ur) (IN-ja-rē)	damage of the skin and the subcutaneous tissue caused by prolonged pressure, often occurring in bedridden patients; the injury, which may be painful, can present as intact skin or an open ulcer. (also called **pressure ulcer** and **bedsore**; formerly called **decubitus ulcer**) (Fig. 4.14)

TABLE 4.2 Common Skin Lesions

LESION	DEFINITION	CUTAWAY SECTIONS	EXAMPLE
Macule	flat, colored spot on the skin	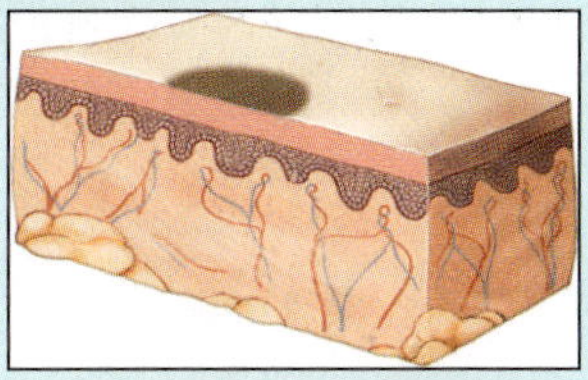	freckle
Papule	small, solid skin elevation	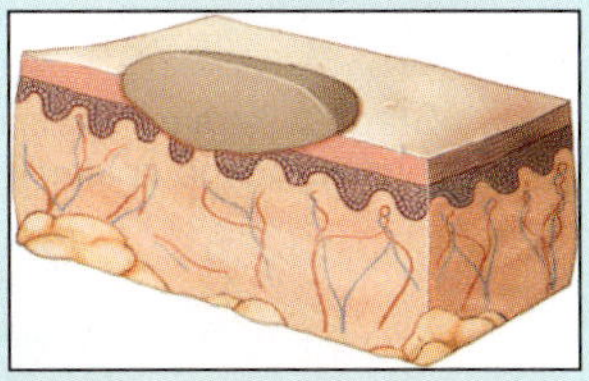	skin tag basal cell carcinoma
Nodule	small, knotlike mass	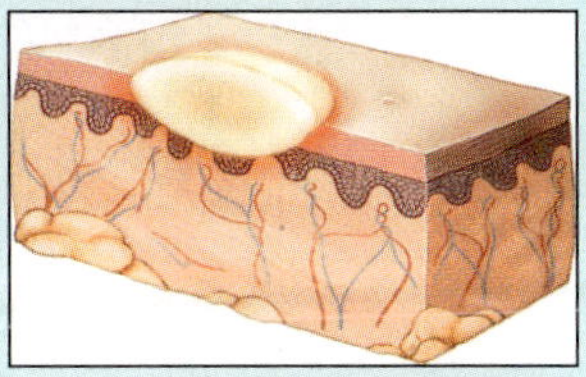	lipoma metastatic carcinoma rheumatoid nodule
Wheal	round, itchy elevation of the skin	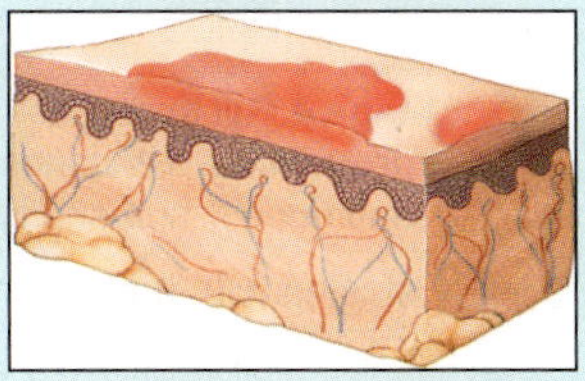	urticaria (hive)
Vesicle	small elevation of epidermis containing liquid	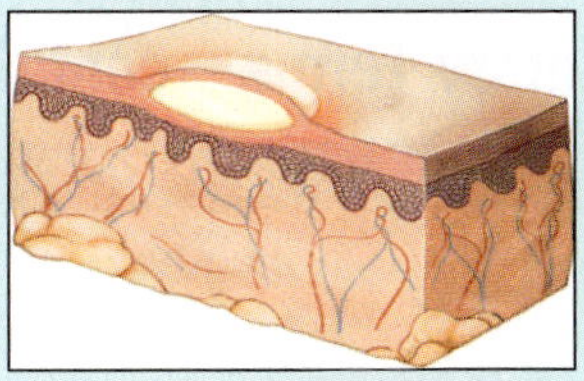	herpes zoster (shingles) herpes simplex virus type 1 contact dermatitis
Pustule	elevation of the skin containing pus	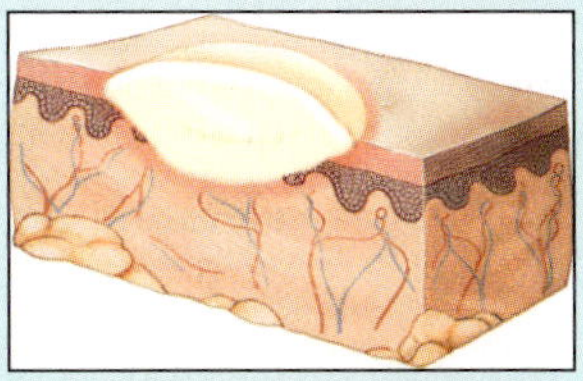	impetigo acne
Cyst	a closed sac containing fluid or semisolid material	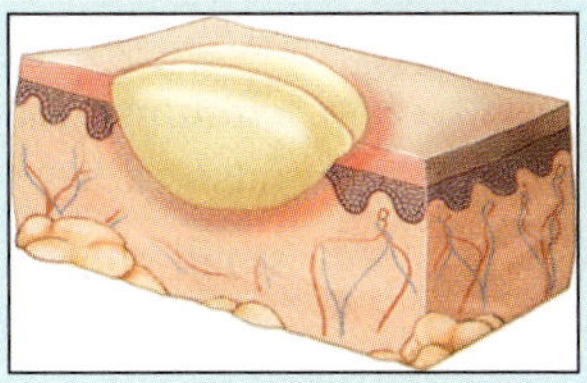	acne

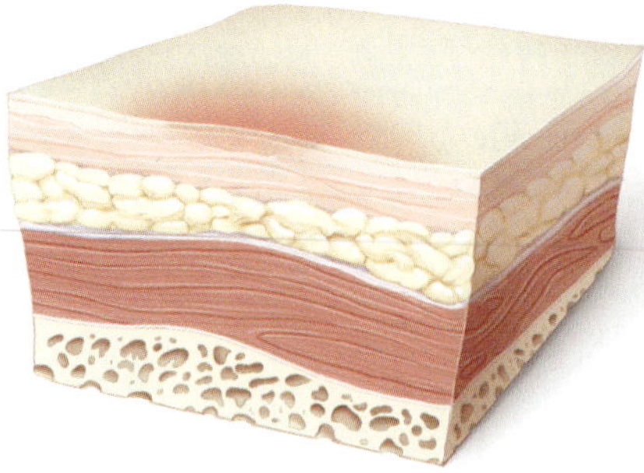

Stage 1 Nonblanching erythema, skin intact.

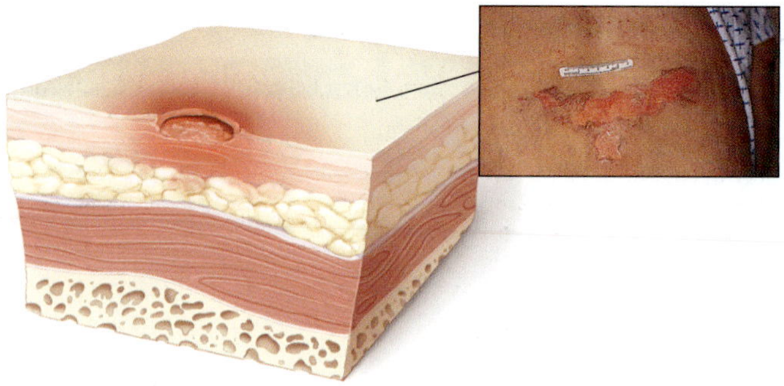

Stage 2 Partial thickness of skin loss involving the epidermis, dermis or both.

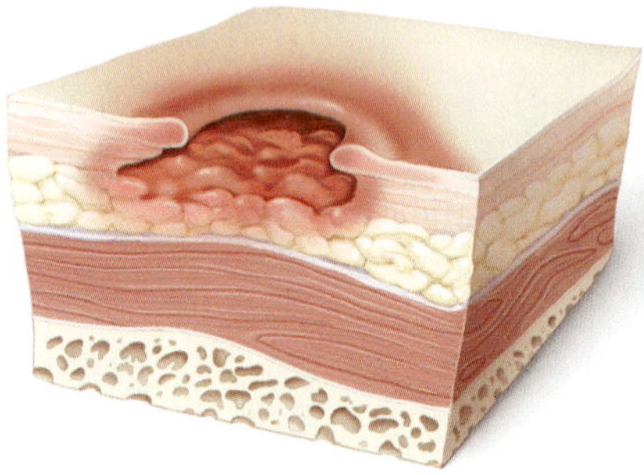

Stage 3 Full thickness of skin loss involving damage or necrosis to subcutaneous tissue.

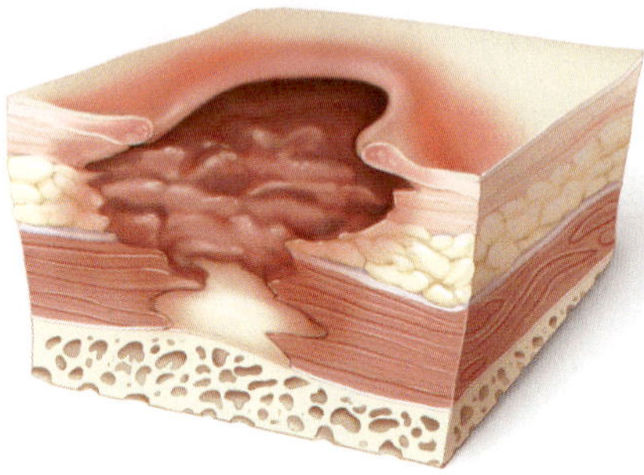

Stage 4 Full thickness of skin loss with extensive destruction, tissue necrosis, possible damage to muscle and bone tissue and other supporting structures.

FIG. 4.14 Pressure injury staging with a photograph of Stage 2.

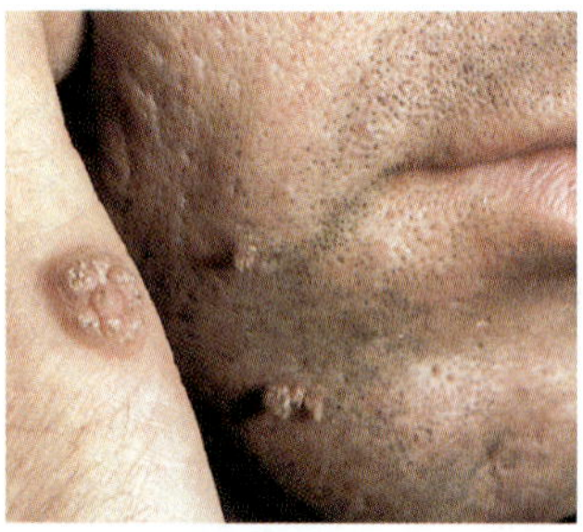

FIG. 4.13 Verruca (also called *wart.*)

Complementary Terms—cont'd

TERM	DEFINITION
pruritus (prū-RĪ-tus)	itching
purpura (PER-pū-ra)	small hemorrhages in the skin (or mucous membrane), giving a purple-red discoloration; associated with blood disorders or vascular abnormalities
pustule (PUS-tūl)	elevation of skin containing pus (Table 4.2)
ulcer (UL-ser)	erosion of the skin or mucous membrane
verruca (ver-RŪ-ka)	circumscribed cutaneous elevation caused by a virus (also called **wart**) (Fig. 4.13)
vesicle (VES-i-kl)	small elevation of the epidermis containing liquid (also called **blister**) (Table 4.2)
virus (VĪ-rus)	minute microorganism, much smaller than a bacterium, characterized by a lack of independent metabolism and the ability to replicate only within living host cells; may cause infection by invading body tissue
wheal (hwēl)	transitory, itchy elevation of the skin with a white center and a red surrounding area; a wheal is an individual urticaria (hive) lesion (Table 4.2)

Refer to **Appendix F** for pharmacology terms related to the integumentary system.

EXERCISE 31

Practice saying aloud each of the Complementary Terms NOT Built from Word Parts.

To hear the terms, go to Evolve Resources at evolve.elsevier.com and select:
Practice Student Resources > Student Resources > Chapter 4 > **Pronounce and Spell**

See Appendix B for instructions.

❑ Check the box when complete.

EXERCISE 32

Fill in the blanks with the correct terms.

1. Another name for scar is ______________________________.
2. Sweating is called ______________________________.
3. The medical term for wart is ______________________________.
4. ______________________________ is the name for a flat, colored skin spot.
5. A yellow coloring of the skin, mucous membranes, and sclera caused by the presence of bile is known as ______________________________.
6. The condition of white spots or patches on mucous membrane is called ______________________________.
7. ______________________________ is a pinpoint hemorrhage of the skin.
8. An erosion of the skin or mucous membrane is called a(n) ______________________________.
9. A(n) ______________________________ is an overgrowth of scar tissue.
10. Another name for paleness is ______________________________.
11. Small, flat, purple or blue skin discoloration caused by hemorrhage, as seen after blood has been withdrawn by needle and syringe, is referred to as ____________________.
12. Damage of the skin and subcutaneous tissue caused by prolonged pressure is a(n) ______________________________.
13. A small knotlike mass that can be felt by touch is called a(n) ______________________________.
14. A closed sac containing fluid or semisolid material is called a(n) ______________________________.
15. Itching is called ______________________________.
16. Another name for redness is ______________________________.
17. Small hemorrhages in the skin, showing a purple-red discoloration and associated with blood disorders or vascular abnormalities, is known as ______________________________.
18. ______________________________ is another name for mole.
19. Single-celled microorganisms that reproduce by cell division and may cause infection by invading body tissue are called ______________________________.
20. The term for loss of hair is ______________________________.
21. A small, solid skin elevation is called a(n) ______________________________.
22. A transitory skin elevation with a white center and a red surrounding area is a(n) ______________________________.
23. A(n) ______________________________ is a skin elevation containing pus.
24. A blister is also called a(n) ______________________________.
25. An organism that feeds by absorbing organic molecules from its surroundings and may cause infection by invading body tissue is called ______________________________.
26. A(n) ______________________________ is a minute microorganism characterized by a lack of independent metabolism and the ability to replicate only within living host cells; it also may cause infection by invading body tissue.

27. An abnormal hard spot(s) or area of skin is called ______________________.
28. ______________________ is the swelling of tissue.
29. ______________________ is a herpes-type virus.

EXERCISE 33

Match the words in the first column with their correct definitions in the second column.

_____ 1. pressure injury
_____ 2. alopecia
_____ 3. cicatrix
_____ 4. fungus
_____ 5. nodule
_____ 6. bacteria
_____ 7. diaphoresis
_____ 8. cyst
_____ 9. ecchymosis
_____ 10. erythema
_____ 11. jaundice
_____ 12. edema
_____ 13. induration

a. loss of hair
b. small, flat, purple or blue discoloration caused by blood escaping into the skin or mucous membrane
c. yellow color to the skin, mucous membranes, and sclera
d. closed sac containing fluid
e. organism that feeds by absorbing organic molecules from its surroundings and may cause infection by invading body tissue
f. small knotlike mass
g. sweating
h. swelling of tissue
i. hard spot(s) or area of skin
j. scar
k. redness
l. single-celled microorganisms that reproduce by cell division and may cause infection by invading body tissue
m. damage of the skin and the subcutaneous tissue caused by prolonged pressure

EXERCISE 34

Match the terms in the first column with their correct definitions in the second column.

_____ 1. keloid
_____ 2. leukoplakia
_____ 3. macule
_____ 4. nevus
_____ 5. pallor
_____ 6. papule
_____ 7. petechiae
_____ 8. pruritus
_____ 9. purpura
_____ 10. pustule
_____ 11. ulcer
_____ 12. verruca
_____ 13. vesicle
_____ 14. wheal
_____ 15. virus
_____ 16. cytomegalovirus

a. mole
b. itching
c. wart
d. condition of white spots or patches on mucous membranes
e. hemorrhages in the skin showing a purple-red color
f. skin elevation containing pus
g. overgrowth of scar tissue
h. small elevation of epidermis containing liquid
i. individual urticaria lesion
j. flat, colored spot on skin
k. small, solid skin elevation
l. paleness
m. minute microorganism characterized by a lack of independent metabolism and the ability to replicate only within living host cells that may cause infection by invading body tissue
n. pinpoint skin hemorrhages
o. erosion of the skin or mucous membrane
p. herpes-type virus

EXERCISE 35

Spell each of the Complementary Terms NOT Built from Word Parts by having someone dictate them to you. Use a separate sheet of paper.

To hear and spell the terms, go to Evolve Resources at evolve.elsevier.com and select:
Practice Student Resources > Student Resources > Chapter 4 > **Pronounce and Spell**

See Appendix B for instructions.

❑ Check the box when complete.

Abbreviations

ABBREVIATION	TERM
BCC	basal cell carcinoma
bx	biopsy
CMV	cytomegalovirus
CA-MRSA	community-associated MRSA infection
derm	dermatology
HA-MRSA	healthcare-associated MRSA infection
I&D	incision and drainage
ID	intradermal
MRSA	methicillin-resistant *Staphylococcus aureus*
SCC	squamous cell carcinoma
SLE	systemic lupus erythematosus
staph	staphylococcus
strep	streptococcus
subcut	subcutaneous
TD	transdermal

WEB LINK

For more information about diseases and disorders of the integumentary system and current treatments, visit the **American Academy of Dermatology** at *www.aad.org.*

Refer to **Appendix E** for a complete list of abbreviations.

EXERCISE 36

Write the meaning for each of the abbreviations in the following sentences.

1. The most common form of skin cancer is **BCC** ______________ ______________ ______________.
2. Cutaneous **CMV** ______________ infections are rarely seen in general medical practice.
3. **SLE** ______________ is a chronic relapsing disease, often with long periods of remission.
4. Long-term exposure to sunlight is by far the most frequent cause of **SCC** ______________ ______________ ______________.
5. The **bx** ______________results were negative.
6. The medication was administered by **subcut** ______________ injection.
7. **Staph** ______________ bacterium was cultured from the abscess.
8. The culture confirmed a **strep** ______________ infection of the throat.

9. **I&D** ________________ ________________ ____________________ is used to treat cutaneous abscesses, such as a furuncle.
10. Hormone replacement therapy is available by **TD** ____ administration.
11. The tuberculin test was administered by an **ID** __________________ injection.
12. The patient visited the **derm** __________________ clinic for a psoriasis follow-up visit.
13. **MRSA** __________________________ __________________________ __________________________ ___________________ infections originating in a healthcare setting are called **HA-MRSA** _______________ ________________ ____________________ ____________________, whereas MRSA infections occurring in a person who has not recently been in a healthcare setting is called **CA-MRSA** __________________ _________ __________________ __________________ __________________.

For additional practice with Abbreviations, go to Evolve Resources at evolve.elsevier.com and select: Practice Student Resources > Student Resources > Chapter 4 > **Flashcards:** Abbreviations

See Appendix B for instructions.

DERMATOLOGY, OR GIVE ME A MAN WHO CALLS A SPADE A GEOTOME

I wish the dermatologist
Were less a firm apologist
For all the terminology
That's used in dermatology
Something you or I would deem a
Redness he calls erythema;
If it's blistered, raw and warm he
Has to call it multiforme
Things to him are never simple;
Papule is his word for pimple
What's a macule, clearly stated?
Just a spot that's over-rated!
Over the skin that looks unwell
He chants Latin like a spell;
What he's labeled and obscured
Looks to him as good as cured.

Reprinted with permission from The New England Journal of Medicine, 1977; 297(12):660.

PRACTICAL APPLICATION

EXERCISE 37 *Case Study: Translate Between Everyday Language and Medical Language*

CASE STUDY: Antonne Johnson

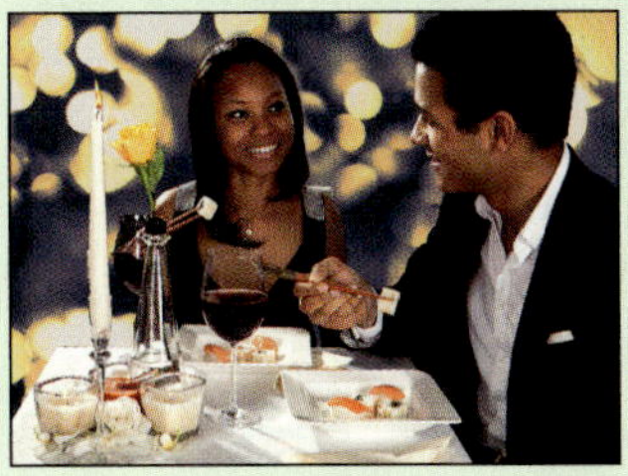

Antonne and his girlfriend were eating out when his mouth began to tingle.

"Hey, are you all right? You look pale," Sasha said.

"My stomach doesn't feel too good." This had happened before, Antonne realized, when he had eaten shellfish. Tonight he had been careful to order sushi made from fish without a shell. He signaled Sasha to call 911. In no time at all, his mouth, face, and arms felt very itchy. As she dialed, Sasha noticed his lips beginning to swell. His cheeks and arms became red and covered with tiny bumps. EMTs arrived just as it was becoming difficult for Antonne to breathe. Sasha quickly told them of Antonne's shellfish allergy.

Now that you have worked through Chapter 4 on the integumentary system, consider the medical terms that might be used to describe Antonne's experience. See the Review of Terms at the end of the chapter for a list of terms that might apply.

A. *Underline phrases in the case study that could be substituted with medical terms.*

B. *Write the medical term and its definition for three of the phrases you underlined.*

MEDICAL TERM	DEFINITION
1. ______________	______________
2. ______________	______________
3. ______________	______________

DOCUMENTATION: Excerpt from EMT Notes

CC: Patient says he is having trouble breathing.

History: Ambulance responded to a call from a young woman at a sushi restaurant on behalf of a 27-year-old male. Onset: Patient's symptoms were brought on suddenly while eating; he has experienced one previous episode of anaphylaxis. Medication: Patient has epinephrine injection. Allergies: Patient is allergic to shellfish.

Exam: BP: 90/60 mm Hg, Pulse: 120, O_2: 15L Non-rebreather mask. Pallor of face and hands is present; he appears to be experiencing pruritus and says he might vomit. Patient shows signs of edema around the lips and face and urticaria on his cheeks and arms. Upon auscultation of the lungs, wheezing is present. Assessment/Plan: Anaphylaxis: One dose of epinephrine was delivered by injection.

C. *Underline medical terms presented in Chapter 4 in the previous excerpt from Antonne's medical record. See the Review of Terms at the end of the chapter for a complete list.*

D. *Select and define three of the medical terms you underlined. To check your answers, go to Appendix A.*

MEDICAL TERM	DEFINITION
1. ______________	______________
2. ______________	______________
3. ______________	______________

EXERCISE 38 *Interact With Medical Documents*

A. Read the report and complete it by writing medical terms on answer lines within the document. Definitions of terms to be written appear after the document.

76548-INT WHARTON, Sandra L.

File Patient Navigate Custom Fields Help

Chart Review | Encounters | Notes | Labs | Imaging | Procedures | Rx | Documents | Referrals | Scheduling | Billing

Name: **WHARTON, Sandra L.** MR#: **76548-INT** DOB: **10/03/19XX** Gender: F Age: 50 **Allergies:** None known **PCP:** Spring, Lincoln MD

Encounter Date: 7/27/20XX
Operative Report:

History: The patient is a 50-year-old woman presenting to the 1.________________ clinic with concerns about a 2.________________________________ located at the 3.________________________aspect of her left eyebrow.
The patient's medical history is also significant for 4.____________________________, primarily of the scalp and ears, as well as chronic 5.____________________________, primarily of the forearms bilaterally.

Indications for Procedure:
The 6. ____ has been present for approximately 3 months. Risks, benefits, indications and expectations were discussed with the patient regarding biopsy, and she has agreed to proceed with 7.______________________________________.

Preoperative Diagnosis:
Suspicious lesion, left eyebrow.

Anesthesia: Xylocaine 1% with epinephrine.

Procedure: After written consent was obtained, the site was prepped with Betadine and draped in the usual sterile fashion. The skin was incised at the 8.____________________ pole of the lesion. The lesion was then excised, including a margin of clinically normal dermis. Specimen was submitted to 9.________________________________. The superior pole was sutured. 10.______________________________ was used to achieve hemostasis. Two A-T flaps were then constructed on superior aspect of upper left eyelid. Flaps and upper left eyelid undermined 2 to 3 mm. Flaps sutured with 6-0 Vicryl, followed by 6-0 nylon for closure. Pressure dressing was applied.

The patient tolerated the procedure well.

Postoperative Diagnosis: 11.______________________________ revealed 12.____, nodular, transected at base.

Electronically signed: William Hickman MD on 27 July 20XX 13:30

Start | Log On/Off | Print | Edit

Definitions of Medical Terms to Complete the Document

Write the medical terms defined on corresponding answer lines in the document.

1. study of skin
2. small, knotlike mass that can be felt by touch
3. pertaining to the middle
4. precancerous skin condition of horny tissue formation
5. noninfectious, inflammatory skin disease with redness, blisters, scabs, and itching
6. changes in tissue resulting from injury or disease
7. removal by cutting
8. pertaining to above
9. study of disease
10. destruction of tissue with a hot or cold instrument, electric current, or caustic substance
11. view of life
12. malignant epithelial tumor arising from the bottom layer of the epidermis

B. Read the medical report and answer the questions below it.

49785 LIGHT, Darla B.

File Patient Navigate Custom Fields Help

Chart Review | Encounters | Notes | Labs | Imaging | Procedures | Rx | Documents | Referrals | Scheduling | Billing

Name: **LIGHT, Darla B.** MR#: **49785** DOB: 6/15/19XX Sex: F Age: 29 **Allergies:** None known **PCP:** Papas, Aenea MD

PATHOLOGY REPORT

DATE/TIME COLL: Jun 12 20XX, 12:00

DATE RECEIVED: Jun 12 20XX, 16:00

DATE REPORTED: Jun 15 20XX

REPORT STATUS: FINAL REPORT

HISTORY: Previous incidence of melanoma and basal cell carcinoma, no metastases

PRE-OP DIAGNOSIS: Melanoma vs. compound nevus

PROCEDURE: Tissue biopsy

SPECIMEN: Skin biopsy, anterior, proximal right arm

GROSS DESCRIPTION: One container is received. Specimen in formalin labeled with the patient's name is a shave biopsy of gray-white hair-bearing skin measuring 0.4 × 0.3 cm in surface dimension and averaging 0.1 cm in thickness. The epidermal surface contains a symmetric, smooth, ordered, pigmented lesion measuring 0.3 cm in greatest diameter. The specimen is bisected and totally submitted.

MICROSCOPIC EXAMINATION: A microscopic examination has been performed.

DIAGNOSIS: Lesion, anterior, proximal right arm; benign compound nevus.

Electronically signed: J. Alvarez, MD, Pathologist, 6/15/20XX 10:48

Start | Log On/Off | Print | Edit

Use the medical report above to answer the questions.

1. Identify singular and plural forms of medical terms used in the pathology report. Write "p" for plural and "s" for singular next to the terms. Refer to Table 2.5 on p. 48 for plural endings.
   _____ a. melanoma
   _____ b. melanomata
   _____ c. nevi
   _____ d. nevus
   _____ e. metastasis
   _____ f. metastases
   _____ g. biopsy
   _____ h. biopsies

2. The skin biopsy was obtained from:
   a. near the shoulder on the back of the right arm
   b. near the shoulder on the front of the right arm
   c. near the wrist on the back of the right arm
   d. near the wrist on the front of the right arm

3. Use your medical dictionary or a reliable online source to find the meanings of the following terms used in the pathology report:
   a. compound ______________________________
   ____
   b. pigmented ______________________________
   ____
   c. bisected ______________________________
   ____
   d. microscopic ______________________________
   ____

EXERCISE 39 *Pronounce Medical Terms in Use*

Practice pronunciation of terms by reading aloud the following paragraph. Use the phonetic spellings following medical terms from the chapter to assist with pronunciation. The script also contains medical terms not presented in the chapter. Treat them as information only or look for their meanings in a medical dictionary or a reliable online source.

Emily visited the **dermatology** (*der*-ma-TOL-o-jē) clinic because of **pruritus** (prū-RĪ-tus) secondary to **dermatitis** (*der*-ma-TĪ-tis) involving her scalp and areas of her elbows and knees. A diagnosis of **psoriasis** (so-RĪ-a-sis) was made. **Eczema** (EK-ze-ma), **scabies** (SKĀ-bēz), and **tinea** (TIN-ē-a) were considered in the differential diagnosis. An emollient cream was prescribed. In addition the patient showed the **dermatologist** (der-ma-TOL-o-jist) the tender, discolored, thickened nail of her right great toe. Emily learned she had **onychomycosis** (*on*-i-kō-mī-KŌ-sis), for which she was given an additional prescription for an oral antifungal drug.

EXERCISE 40 *Chapter Content Quiz*

Test your understanding of terms and abbreviations introduced in this chapter. Circle the letter for the medical term or abbreviation related to the words in italics.

1. *Small hemorrhages into the tissue, giving the skin a purple-red discoloration* may be caused by blood disorders, vascular abnormalities, or trauma.
   a. pruritus
   b. purpura
   c. papule
2. Antibiotics were not prescribed for the patient who presented with fever blisters, an infection caused by *a minute microorganism characterized by a lack of independent metabolism and the ability to replicate only within living host cells.*
   a. bacteria
   b. virus
   c. fungus
3. A *technique of microscopically controlled serial excisions* was used to treat the patient's recurrent *malignant growth developing from scalelike epithelial tissue of the surface layer of the epidermis.*
   a. cryosurgery, CMV
   b. laser surgery, BCC
   c. Mohs surgery, SCC
4. The *localized collection of pus* was incised and drained.
   a. acne
   b. abscess
   c. cyst
5. A culture swab of the wound revealed *invasion of body tissue by methicillin-resistant Staphylococcus aureus.*
   a. MRSA infection
   b. herpes
   c. candidiasis
6. The patient newly diagnosed with a *chronic inflammatory disease involving the skin, joints, kidneys, and nervous system* experienced joint pain with swelling and stiffness, and a butterfly-shaped rash spread over her cheeks and the bridge of her nose.
   a. rosacea
   b. scleroderma
   c. systemic lupus erythematosus
7. *Parasitic infections* include:
   a. scabies and pediculosis
   b. candidiasis and tinea
   c. impetigo and carbuncle
8. *Death of tissue caused by loss of blood supply followed by bacterial invasion* may be evidenced by foul-smelling discharge from the infection site.
   a. gangrene
   b. pressure injury
   c. lesion

9. The medical assisting student learned the medical term for *blister* was:
   a. verruca
   b. keloid
   c. vesicle
10. *Abnormal hard spots or areas of skin* were evident in the patient diagnosed with the *disease characterized by chronic hardening of connective tissue of the skin and other organs.*
    a. lesion, psoriasis
    b. induration, scleroderma
    c. nodule, Kaposi sarcoma
11. *Eating the nails or nail biting* can damage skin around the nails and increase chances for infection.
    a. onychophagia
    b. onychomalacia
    c. onychomycosis
12. An injection given *within the skin* is described as:
    a. subcut
    b. TD
    c. ID
13. The operation for the patient who was receiving a *skin graft from her mother* was listed as:
    a. rhytidoplasty
    b. dermatoautoplasty
    c. dermatoheteroplasty
14. The *pinpoint hemorrhages* were distributed over the patient's entire body.
    a. nevi
    b. petechiae
    c. verrucae
15. Excessive *sweating* without exertion may be a symptom of a serious condition.
    a. diaphoresis
    b. edema
    c. hidradenitis
16. The nursing assistant applied lotion to the patient exhibiting signs of *dry skin.*
    a. xanthoderma
    b. xeroderma
    c. pachyderma
17. *Surgical stitching* was performed to treat the *torn, ragged edged wound.*
    a. cryosurgery, verruca
    b. suturing, laceration
    c. dermabrasion, cicatrix

For additional practice with chapter content, go to Evolve Resources at evolve.elsevier.com and select:
Practice Student Resources > Student Resources > Chapter 4 > **Games:** Medical Millionaire, Tournament of Terminology
Practice Quizzes: Word Parts, Terms Built from Word Parts, Terms NOT Built from Word Parts, Abbreviations

See Appendix B for instructions.

CHAPTER REVIEW

REVIEW OF CHAPTER CONTENT ON EVOLVE RESOURCES

Go to evolve.elsevier.com and click on Gradable Student Resources and Practice Student Resources. Online learning activities found there can be used to review chapter content and to assess your learning of word parts, medical terms, and abbreviations. Place check marks in the boxes next to activities used for review and assessment.

GRADABLE STUDENT RESOURCES

Chapter 04 >	Exercises >	□ Word Parts □ Terms Built from Word Parts □ Terms Not Built from Word Parts □ Abbreviations
	Quizzes >	□ Quiz 1: Disease and Disorder Terms □ Quiz 2: Surgical Terms □ Quiz 3: Complementary Terms

PRACTICE STUDENT RESOURCES > STUDENT RESOURCES

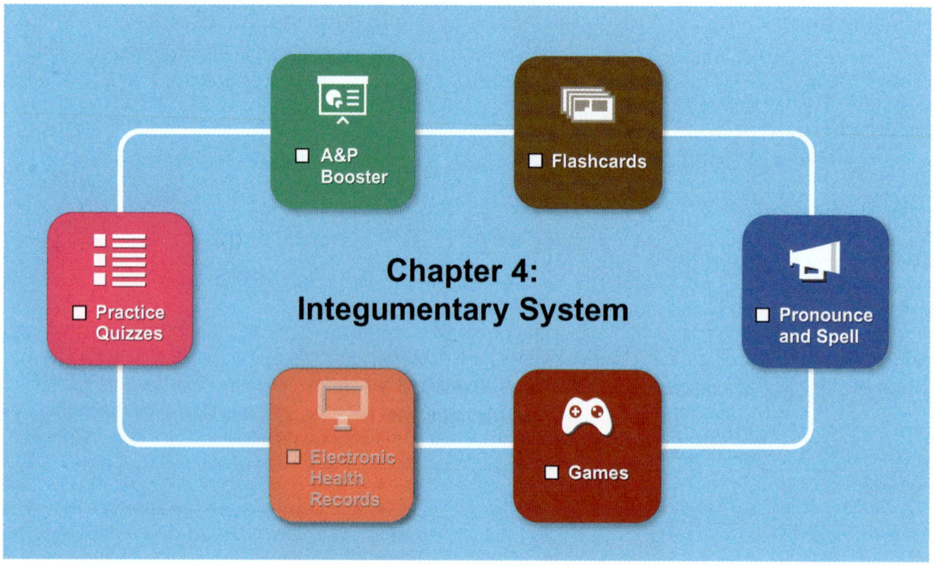

REVIEW OF WORD PARTS

Can you define and spell the following word parts?

COMBINING FORMS		PREFIXES	SUFFIXES
aut/o	myc/o	epi-	-a
bi/o	necr/o	intra-	-coccus (pl. -cocci)
coni/o	onych/o	para-	-ectomy
crypt/o	pachy/o	per-	-ia
cutane/o	rhytid/o	sub-	-itis
derm/o	seb/o	trans-	-malacia
dermat/o	staphyl/o		-opsy
heter/o	strept/o		-phagia
hidr/o	ungu/o		-plasty
kerat/o	xer/o		-rrhea
			-tome

REVIEW OF TERMS

Can you build, analyze, define, pronounce, and spell the following terms *built from word parts*?

DISEASES AND DISORDERS

dermatitis
dermatoconiosis
dermatofibroma
hidradenitis
keratosis
leiodermia
onychocryptosis
onychomalacia
onychomycosis
onychophagia
pachyderma
paronychia
seborrhea
xanthoma
xeroderma

SURGICAL

biopsy (bx)
dermatoautoplasty
dermatoheteroplasty
dermatome
dermatoplasty
rhytidectomy
rhytidoplasty

COMPLEMENTARY

dermatologist
dermatology (derm)
epidermal
erythroderma
hypodermic
intradermal (ID)
keratogenic
leukoderma
necrosis
percutaneous
staphylococcus (staph) (pl. staphylococci)
streptococcus (strep) (pl. streptococci)
subcutaneous (subcut)
subungual
transdermal (TD)
ungual
xanthoderma
xerosis

Can you define, pronounce, and spell the following terms *NOT built from word parts*?

DISEASES AND DISORDERS

abrasion
abscess
acne
actinic keratosis
albinism
basal cell carcinoma (BCC)
candidiasis
carbuncle
cellulitis
contusion
eczema
fissure
furuncle
gangrene
herpes
impetigo
infection
Kaposi sarcoma
laceration
lesion
MRSA infection
pediculosis
psoriasis
rosacea
scabies
scleroderma
squamous cell carcinoma (SCC)
systemic lupus erythematosus (SLE)
tinea
urticaria
vitiligo

SURGICAL

cauterization
cryosurgery
debridement
dermabrasion
excision
incision
incision and drainage (I&D)
laser surgery
Mohs surgery
suturing

COMPLEMENTARY

alopecia
bacteria (s. bacterium)
cicatrix
cyst
cytomegalovirus (CMV)
diaphoresis
ecchymosis (pl. ecchymoses)
edema
erythema
fungus (pl. fungi)
induration
jaundice
keloid
leukoplakia
macule
nevus (pl. nevi)
nodule
pallor
papule
petechia (pl. petechiae)
pressure injury
pruritus
purpura
pustule
ulcer
verruca
vesicle
virus
wheal

Chapter 5

Respiratory System and Introduction to Diagnostic Procedures and Tests

Objectives

Upon completion of this chapter you will be able to:

1 Pronounce organs and anatomic structures of the respiratory system.

2 Define and spell word parts related to the respiratory system.

3 Define, pronounce, and spell disease and disorder terms related to the respiratory system.

4 Define, pronounce, and spell surgical terms related to the respiratory system.

5 Define, pronounce, and spell diagnostic terms related to the respiratory system.

6 Define, pronounce, and spell complementary terms related to the respiratory system.

7 Interpret the meaning of abbreviations related to the respiratory system.

8 Apply medical language in clinical contexts.

Outline

ANATOMY

The respiratory system comprises the nose, pharynx, larynx, trachea, bronchi, and lungs. The upper respiratory tract includes the nose, pharynx, and larynx. The lower respiratory tract includes the trachea, bronchi, and lungs (Fig. 5.1).

Function

The function of the respiratory system is the exchange of oxygen (O_2) and carbon dioxide (CO_2) between the atmosphere and body cells. This process is called **respiration** or **breathing**. During **external respiration**, air containing oxygen passes through the respiratory tract, beginning with the nose, pharynx, larynx, trachea, and, finally, bronchi to the lungs (**inhalation** or **inspiration**). There, oxygen passes from the sacs in the lungs, called **alveoli**, to the blood in tiny blood vessels called **capillaries**. At the same time, carbon dioxide passes back from the capillaries to the alveoli and is expelled through the respiratory tract (**exhalation** or **expiration**) (Fig. 5.2). During internal respiration, the body cells take on **oxygen** from the blood and simultaneously give back **carbon dioxide**, a waste produced when oxygen is used to extract energy from food. The carbon dioxide is transported by the blood back to the lungs for exhalation.

RESPIRATION

is also called **breathing** or **ventilation.**

Organs and Anatomic Structures of the Respiratory System

TERM	DEFINITION
nose (nōz)	lined with mucous membrane and fine hairs; it acts as a filter to moisten and warm the entering air
nasal septum (NĀS-el) (SEP-tum)	partition separating the right and left nasal cavities
paranasal sinuses (*par*-a-NĀ-sel) (SĪ-nus-es)	air cavities within the cranial bones that open into the nasal cavities
pharynx (FAR-inks)	serves as a food and air passageway. Air enters from the nasal cavities and/or mouth and passes through the pharynx to the larynx. Food enters the pharynx from the mouth and passes into the esophagus. (also called the **throat**)
adenoids (AD-e-noids)	lymphoid tissue located on the posterior wall of the nasal cavity (also called **pharyngeal tonsils**)
tonsils (TON-sils)	lymphoid tissue located on the lateral wall at the junction of the oral cavity and oropharynx
larynx (LAR-inks)	location of the vocal cords. Air enters from the pharynx. (also called the **voice box**)
epiglottis (ep-i-GLOT-is)	flap of cartilage that automatically covers the opening of the larynx and keeps food from entering the larynx during swallowing
trachea (TRĀ-kē-a)	passageway for air to the bronchi from the larynx; (also called the **windpipe**)
bronchus (pl. bronchi) (BRONG-kus) (BRONG-ki)	one of two branches from the trachea that conducts air into the lungs, where it divides and subdivides. The branchings resemble a tree; therefore, they are referred to as a **bronchial tree.**
bronchioles (BRONG-kē-ōlz)	smallest subdivision of the bronchial tree

ADAM'S APPLE

is the largest ring of cartilage in the **larynx** and is also known as the thyroid cartilage. The name came from the belief that Adam, realizing he had sinned when he ate the forbidden fruit, was unable to swallow the apple lodged in his throat.

BRONCHI

originated from the Greek **brecho**, meaning **to pour** or **wet**. An ancient belief was that the esophagus carried solid food to the stomach and the bronchi carried liquids.

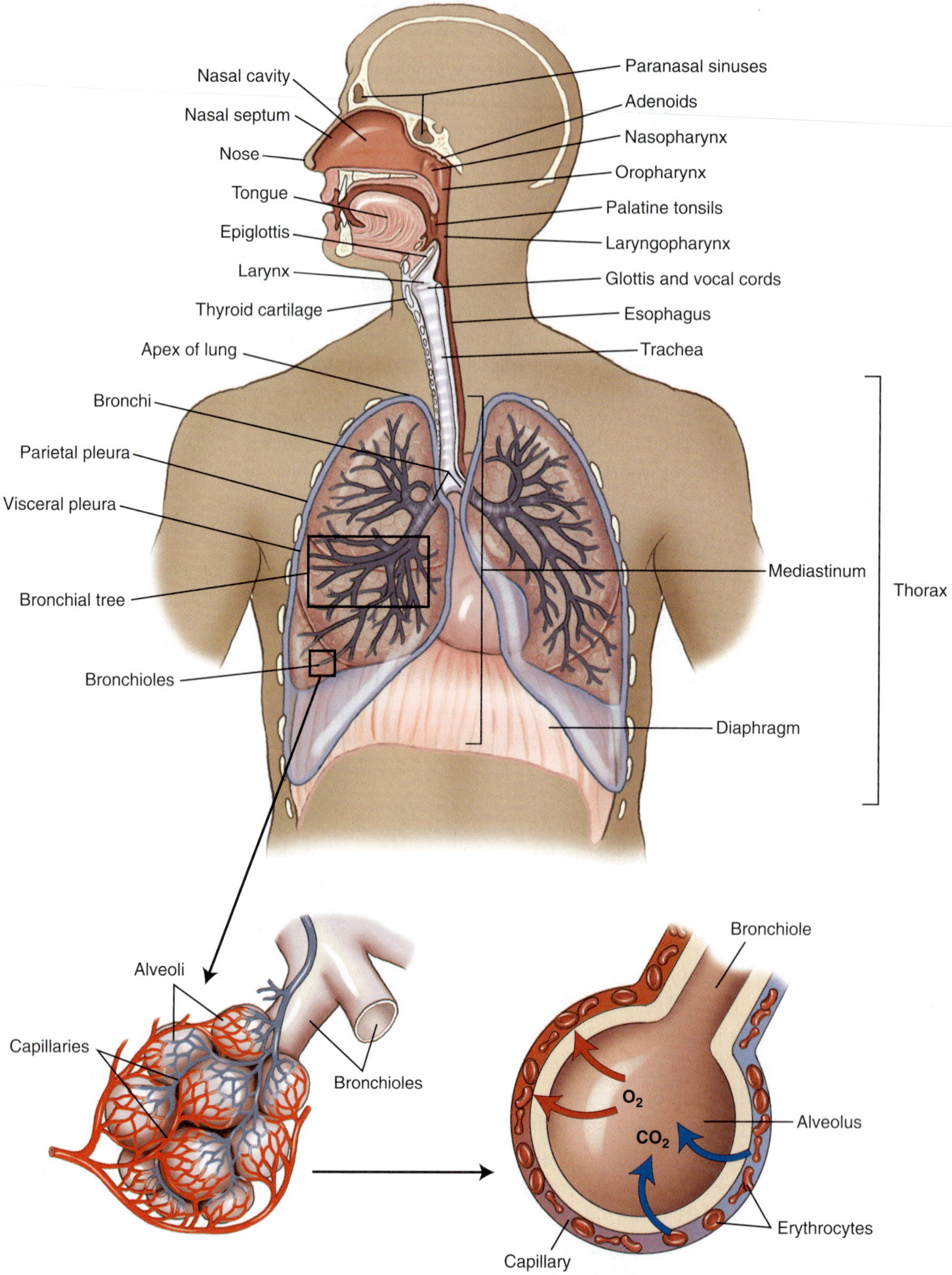

FIG. 5.1 Organs of the respiratory system.

Organs and Anatomic Structures of the Respiratory System—cont'd

TERM	DEFINITION
alveoli (s. alveolus) (al-VĒ-o-lī) (al-VĒ-o-lus)	air sacs at the end of the bronchioles. Oxygen and carbon dioxide are exchanged through the alveolar walls and the capillaries (also a term for the sockets in the jaw bones into which the teeth fit).
thorax (THOR-aks)	chest, the part of the body between the neck and the diaphragm encased by the ribs. **Thoracic cavity** is the hollow space between the neck and diaphragm.
lungs (lungs)	two spongelike organs in the thoracic cavity. The right lung consists of three lobes, and the left lung has two lobes.
pleura (PLOOR-a)	double-folded serous membrane covering each lung (visceral pleura) and lining the thoracic cavity (parietal pleura) with a small space between, called the pleural cavity, which contains serous fluid
diaphragm (DĪ-a-fram)	muscular partition that separates the thoracic cavity from the abdominal cavity. It aids in the breathing process by contracting and pulling air in, then relaxing and pushing air out.
mediastinum (*mē*-dē-a-STĪ-num)	space between the lungs. It contains the heart, esophagus, trachea, great blood vessels, and other structures.

MEDIASTINUM
literally means **to stand in the middle** because it is derived from the Latin **medius**, meaning **middle**, and **stare**, meaning **to stand**.

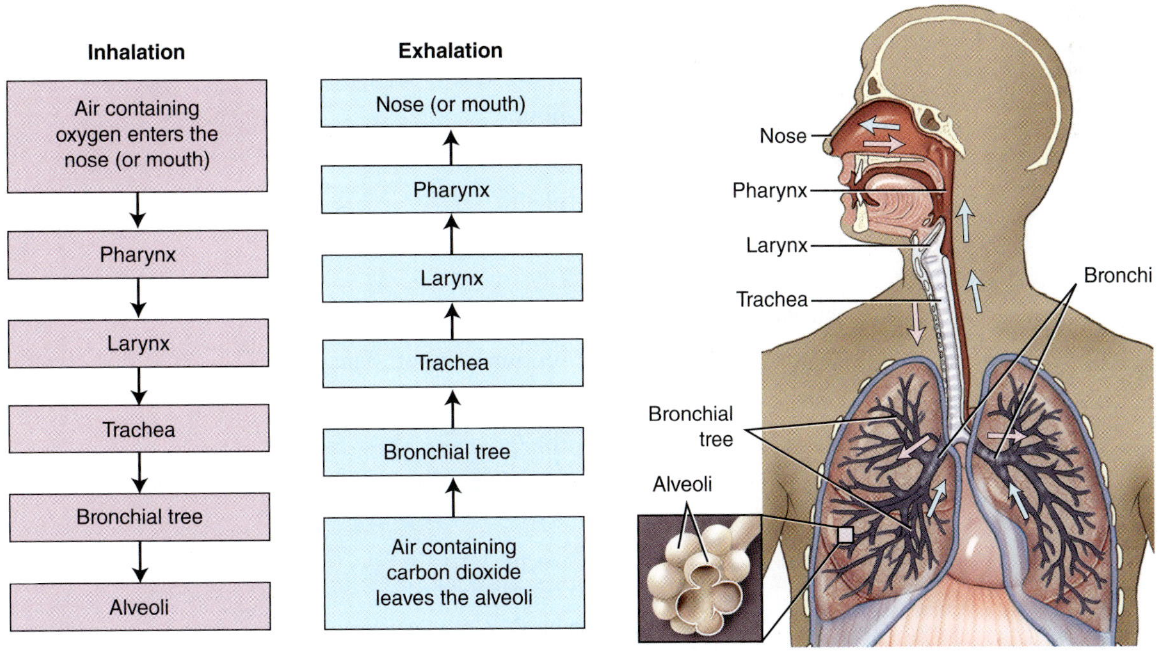

FIG. 5.2 Flow of air.

A&P Booster
For more anatomy and physiology, go to Evolve Resources at evolve.elsevier.com and select: Practice Student Resources > Student Resources > Chapter 5 > **A&P Booster**

See Appendix B for instructions.

EXERCISE 1

Practice saying aloud each of the Organs and Anatomic Structures of the Respiratory System.

To hear the terms, go to Evolve Resources at evolve.elsevier.com and select:
Practice Student Resources > Student Resources > Chapter 5 > **Pronounce and Spell**

See Appendix B for instructions.

❑ Check the box when complete.

WORD PARTS

Words parts you need to learn to complete this chapter are listed on the following pages. The exercises at the end of each list will help you learn their definitions and spelling.

Use the flashcards accompanying this text or electronic flashcards to assist you in memorizing the word parts for this chapter.

Combining Forms of the Respiratory System

COMBINING FORM	DEFINITION
adenoid/o	adenoids
alveol/o	alveolus
bronch/o, bronchi/o	bronchus
diaphragmat/o, phren/o	diaphragm
epiglott/o	epiglottis
laryng/o	larynx
lob/o	lobe
nas/o, rhin/o	nose
pharyng/o	pharynx
pleur/o	pleura
pneum/o, pneumat/o, pneumon/o	lung, air
pulmon/o	lung
sept/o	septum (wall off, fence)
sinus/o	sinus
thorac/o	thorax, chest, chest cavity
tonsill/o	tonsil *(Note: tonsil has one l, and the combining form has two ls.)*
trache/o	trachea

LOBE
literally means **the part that hangs down**, although it comes from the Greek **lobos**, meaning **capsule** or **pod**. This also applies to the lobe of an ear, the liver, or the brain.

Do not be concerned at this time about which combining form to use for terms such as *lung* or *nose* that have more than one combining form. As you continue to study and use medical terms you will become familiar with common usage of each word part.

EXERCISE 2

Fill in the blanks with combining forms in this diagram of the respiratory system. *To check your answers, go to Appendix A at the back of the textbook.*

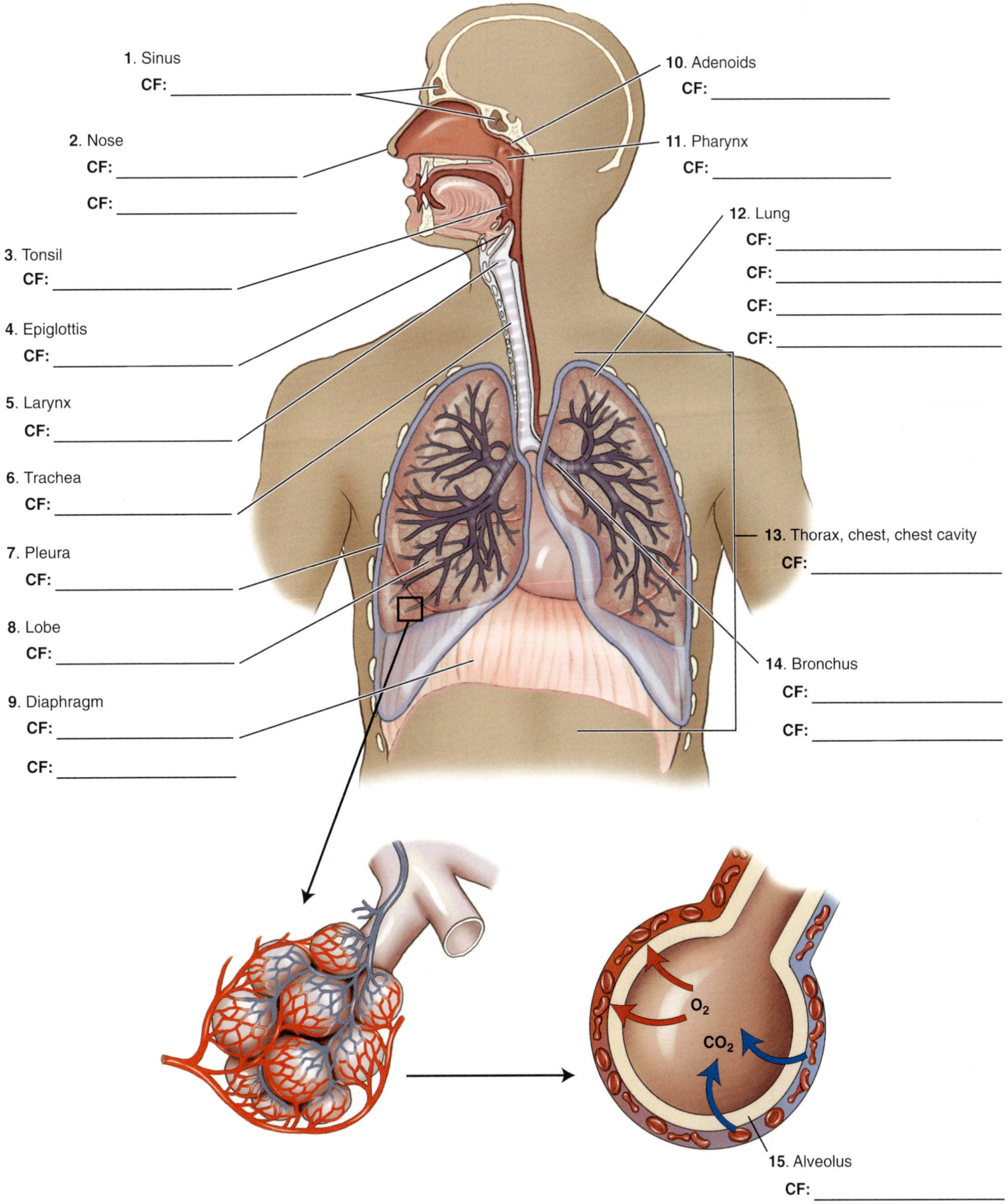

EXERCISE 3

Step 1: Write the definitions after the following combining forms.
Step 2: Match the descriptions on the right with the combining forms and definitions.

_____ 1. alveol/o, ______________________
_____ 2. bronch/o, bronchi/o, ______________________
_____ 3. pulmon/o, ______________________
_____ 4. laryng/o, ______________________
_____ 5. pleur/o, ______________________
_____ 6. thorac/o, ______________________
_____ 7. trache/o, ______________________
_____ 8. tonsil/o, ______________________
_____ 9. sinus/o, ______________________

a. tubes carrying air between the trachea and lungs
b. passageway for air to the bronchi from the larynx
c. spongelike organs located in the thoracic cavity
d. membrane covering the lung
e. lymphoid tissue located on the lateral wall at the junction of the oral cavity and oropharynx
f. air cavities within the cranial bones that open into the nasal cavities
g. location of the vocal cords
h. air sacs at the end of the bronchioles
i. the part of the body between the neck and diaphragm

EXERCISE 4

Step 1: Write the definitions after the following combining forms.
Step 2: Match the descriptions on the right with the combining forms and definitions. Answers may be used more than once.

_____ 1. adenoid/o, ______________________
_____ 2. diaphragmat/o, ______________________
_____ 3. epiglott/o, ______________________
_____ 4. lob/o, ______________________
_____ 5. nas/o, ______________________
_____ 6. pharyng/o, ______________________
_____ 7. pneumat/o, ______________________
_____ 8. pneum/o, pneumon/o, ______________________
_____ 9. rhin/o, ______________________
_____ 10. sept/o, ______________________
_____ 11. phren/o, ______________________

a. lined with mucous membrane and fine hairs; acts as a filter to moisten and warm the entering air
b. sections of a lung
c. spongelike organs located in the thoracic cavity
d. lymphoid tissue located on the posterior wall of the nasal cavity
e. flap of cartilage that keeps food out of the larynx
f. partition separating the right and left nasal cavities
g. passageway for food and air
h. separates the thoracic cavity from the abdominal cavity

Combining Forms Commonly Used with Respiratory System Terms

COMBINING FORM	DEFINITION
atel/o	imperfect, incomplete
capn/o	carbon dioxide
hem/o, hemat/o	blood
muc/o	mucus
orth/o	straight
ox/i	oxygen
phon/o	sound, voice

OXYGEN
was discovered in 1774 by Joseph Priestley. In 1775 Antoine-Laurent Lavoisier, a French chemist, noted that all the acids he knew contained oxygen. Because he thought it was an acid producer, he named it using the Greek **oxys**, meaning **sour**, and the suffix **gen**, meaning **to produce**.

COMBINING FORM	DEFINITION
py/o	pus
radi/o	x-rays, ionizing radiation
somn/o	sleep
son/o	sound
spir/o	breathe, breathing
tom/o	to cut, section, or slice

EXERCISE 5

Write the definition of the following combining forms.

1. ox/i ______________________
2. spir/o ______________________
3. muc/o ______________________
4. atel/o ______________________
5. orth/o ______________________
6. py/o ______________________
7. hem/o, hemat/o ______________________
8. somn/o ______________________
9. capn/o ______________________
10. phon/o ______________________
11. son/o ______________________
12. radi/o ______________________
13. tom/o ______________________

EXERCISE 6

Write the combining form for each of the following.

1. breathe, breathing ______________________
2. oxygen ______________________
3. imperfect, incomplete ______________________
4. straight ______________________
5. pus ______________________
6. mucus ______________________
7. blood a. ______________________
   b. ______________________
8. sleep ______________________
9. sound, voice ______________________
10. carbon dioxide ______________________
11. sound ______________________
12. x-rays, ionizing radiation ______________________
13. to cut, section, or slice ______________________

Prefixes

PREFIX	DEFINITION
a-, an-	absence of, without *(Note: an- is used when the word root begins with a vowel.)*
endo-	within *(Note: the prefix intra-, introduced in Chapter 4, also means within.)*
eu-	normal, good
poly-	many, much
tachy-	fast, rapid

EXERCISE 7

Write the definitions of the following prefixes.

1. endo- ______________________
2. a-, an- ______________________
3. eu- ______________________
4. poly- ______________________
5. tachy- ______________________

EXERCISE 8

Write the prefix for each of the following.

1. within ______________________
2. normal, good ______________________
3. absence of, without a. ______________________
   b. ______________________
4. many, much ______________________
5. fast, rapid ______________________

Suffixes

SUFFIX	DEFINITION
-algia	pain
-ar, -ary, -eal	pertaining to
-cele	hernia or protrusion
-centesis	surgical puncture to aspirate fluid (with a sterile needle)
-ectasis	stretching out, dilation, expansion
-emia	in the blood
-gram	the record, radiographic image
-graph	instrument used to record; the record
-graphy	process of recording, radiographic imaging
-meter	instrument used to measure
-metry	measurement
-pexy	surgical fixation, suspension
-pnea	breathing
-rrhagia	rapid flow of blood, excessive bleeding
-scope	instrument used for visual examination
-scopic	pertaining to visual examination
-scopy	visual examination
-spasm	sudden, involuntary muscle contraction (spasmodic contraction)
-stenosis	constriction or narrowing
-stomy	creation of an artificial opening
-thorax	chest, chest cavity
-tomy	cut into, incision

COMPARING -GRAPH, -GRAPHY, -GRAM

-graph is the instrument used to record—the machine—as in **electrocardiograph**; also means the record, as in **radiograph**.

-graphy is the process of recording, the act of setting down or registering a record, as in **radiography**.

-gram is the record (picture, radiographic image, or tracing) as in **sonogram**.

Refer to **Appendix C** and **Appendix D** for alphabetical lists of word parts and their meanings.

EXERCISE 9

Match the suffixes in the first column with their correct definitions in the second column.

______ 1. -algia	a. stretching out, dilation, expansion
______ 2. -ar, -ary, -eal	b. pertaining to visual examination
______ 3. -cele	c. pertaining to
______ 4. -rrhagia	d. hernia or protrusion
______ 5. -ectasis	e. rapid flow of blood, excessive bleeding
______ 6. -emia	f. in the blood
______ 7. -thorax	g. pain
______ 8. -stenosis	h. surgical puncture to aspirate fluid
______ 9. -spasm	i. chest, chest cavity
______ 10. -scopic	j. breathing
______ 11. -centesis	k. constriction or narrowing
______ 12. -pexy	l. sudden, involuntary muscle contraction
______ 13. -pnea	m. surgical fixation, suspension

EXERCISE 10

Write the suffix pictured and defined.

1. ______________________
instrument used for visual examination

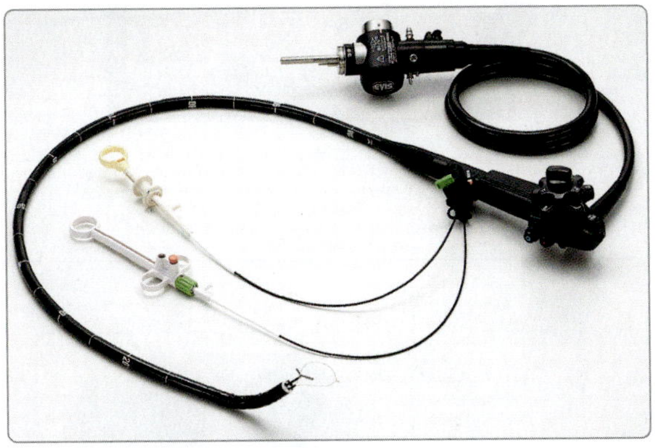

2. ______________________
visual examination

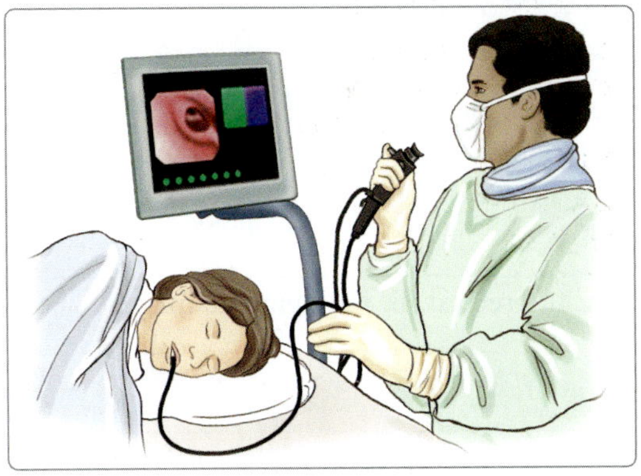

3. ______________________
cut into, incision

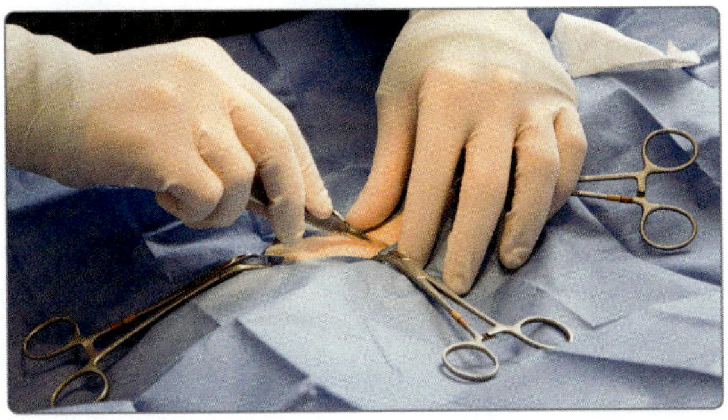

4. ______________________
creation of an artificial opening

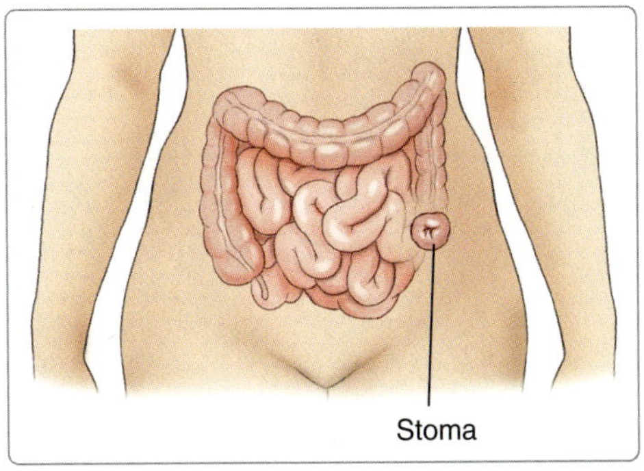

EXERCISE 10 *Pictured and Defined—cont'd*

5. ____________________
instrument used to measure

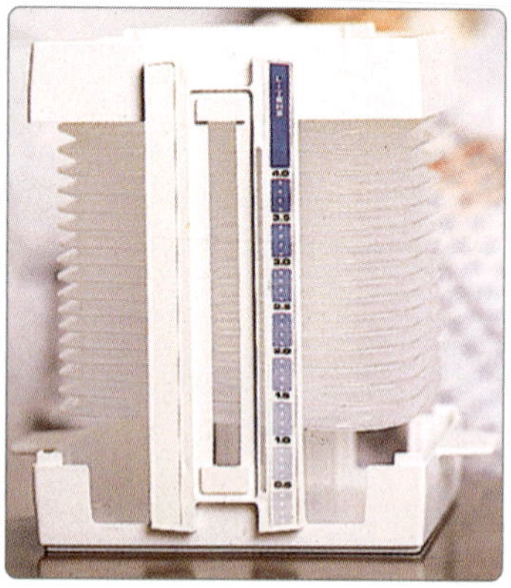

6. ____________________
measurement (use of the instrument)

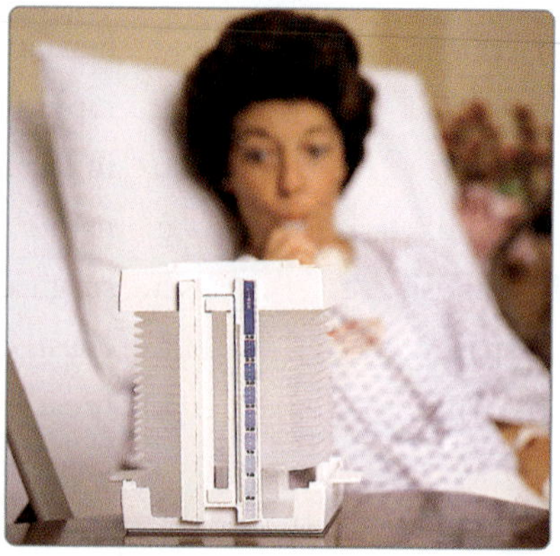

7. ____________________
instrument used to record, the record

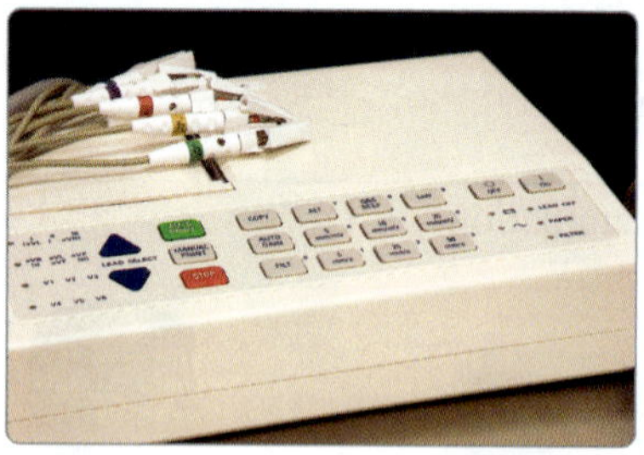

8. ____________________
process of recording, radiographic imaging

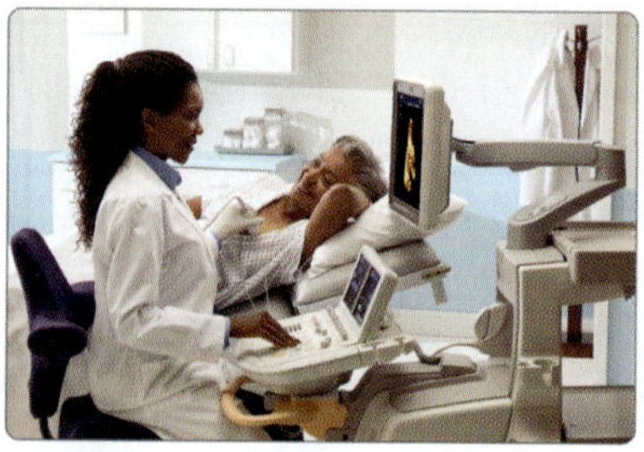

9. ____________________
A. the record, B. radiographic image

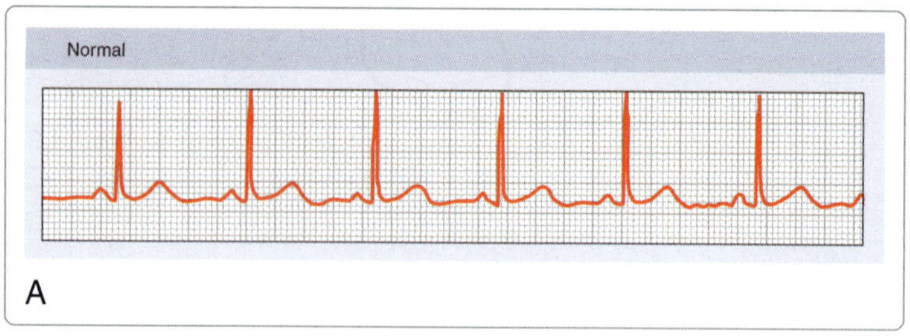

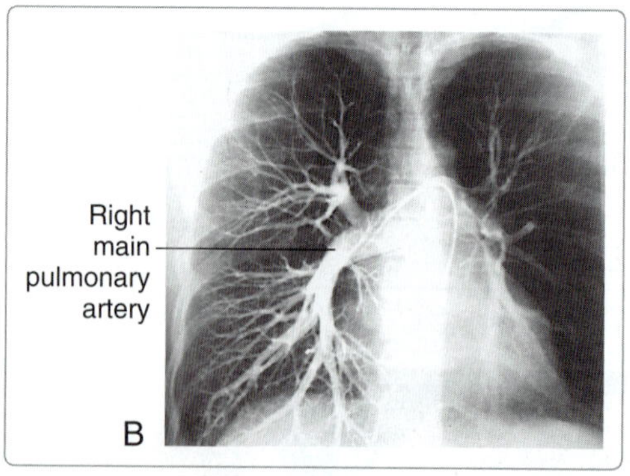

EXERCISE 11

Write the definitions of the following suffixes.

1. -thorax ____________
2. -ar, -ary, -eal ____________
3. -stenosis ____________
4. -cele ____________
5. -stomy ____________
6. -pexy ____________
7. -meter ____________
8. -spasm ____________
9. -algia ____________
10. -scopy ____________
11. -centesis ____________
12. -tomy ____________
13. -scope ____________
14. -rrhagia ____________
15. -ectasis ____________
16. -graphy ____________
17. -metry ____________
18. -emia ____________
19. -scopic ____________
20. -pnea ____________
21. -graph ____________
22. -gram ____________

For additional practice with Word Parts, go to Evolve Resources at evolve.elsevier.com and select: Practice Student Resources > Student Resources > Chapter 5 > **Flashcards**

See Appendix B for instructions.

MEDICAL TERMS

The terms you need to learn to complete this chapter are listed below and on the following pages. The exercises following each list will help you learn the definition and the spelling of each word.

Disease and Disorder Terms

BUILT FROM WORD PARTS

The following terms can be translated using definitions of word parts. Further explanation is provided within parentheses as needed.

TERM	DEFINITION
adenoiditis (*ad*-e-noyd-Ī-tis)	inflammation of the adenoids
alveolitis (*al*-vē-o-LĪ-tis)	inflammation of the alveoli (pulmonary or dental)
atelectasis (*at*-e-LEK-ta-sis)	incomplete expansion (of the lung or portion of the lung) (Fig. 5.3)
bronchiectasis (*bron*-kē-EK-ta-sis)	dilation of the bronchi (Exercise Figure A)
bronchitis (bron-KĪ-tis)	inflammation of the bronchi (Fig. 5.4)
bronchogenic carcinoma (bron-kō-JEN-ik) (*kar*-si-NŌ-ma)	cancerous tumor originating in a bronchus (also referred to as **lung cancer**) (Fig. 5.5)
bronchopneumonia (*bron*-kō-nū-MŌ-nē-a)	diseased state of the bronchi and lungs (an inflammation of the lungs that begins in the terminal bronchioles)

ATELECTASIS is derived from the Greek **ateles**, meaning **not perfect**, and **ektasis**, meaning **expansion**. It denotes an incomplete expansion of the lungs.

EXERCISE FIGURE A

Fill in the blanks to label the diagram.

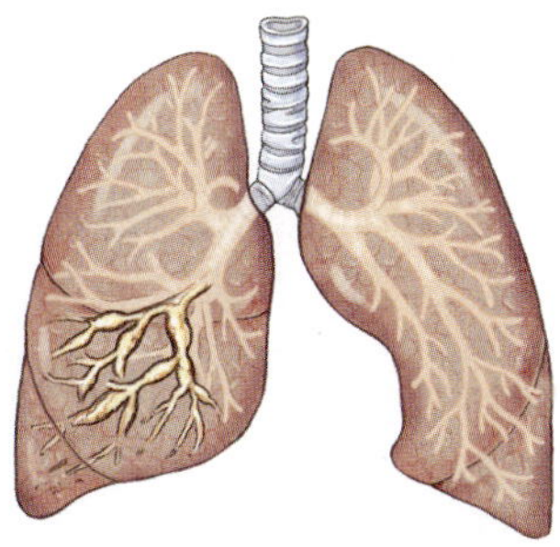

_______ bronchi / _______ dilation

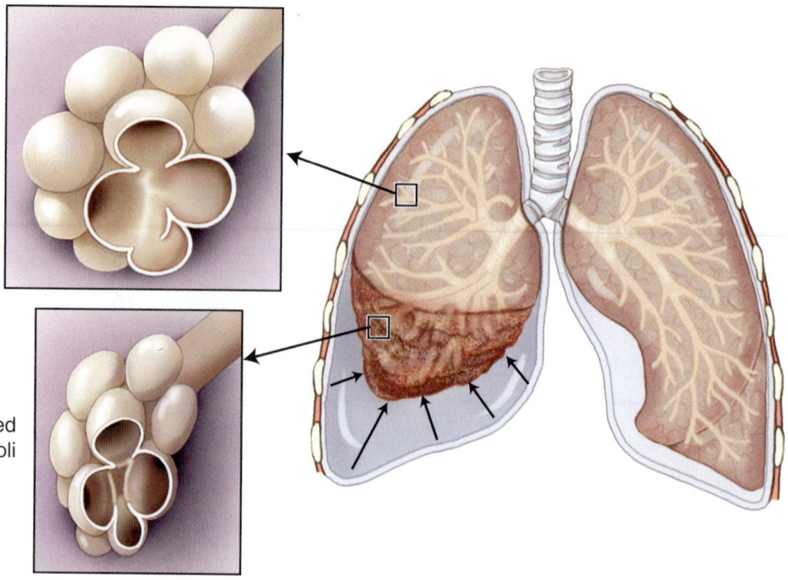

FIG. 5.3 Atelectasis showing the collapsed alveoli.

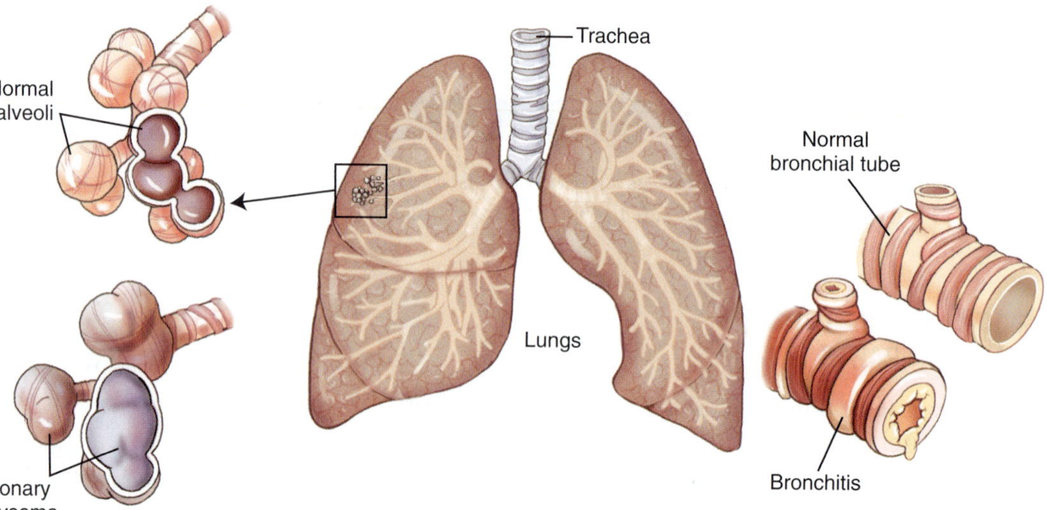

FIG. 5.4 Pulmonary emphysema and bronchitis. Chronic bronchitis and pulmonary emphysema are both components of chronic obstructive pulmonary disease (COPD).

EXERCISE FIGURE B

Fill in the blanks to label the diagram.

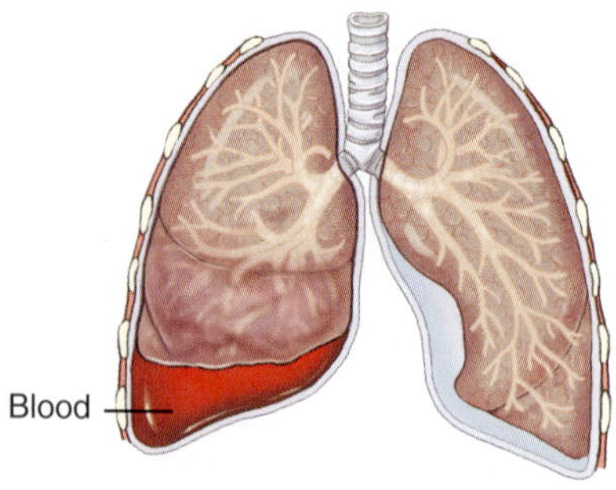

______ / ______ / ______
blood / CV / chest cavity

Disease and Disorder Terms—cont'd

TERM	DEFINITION
diaphragmatocele (*dī*-a-frag-MAT-ō-sēl)	hernia of the diaphragm
epiglottitis (*ep*-i-glo-TĪ-tis)	inflammation of the epiglottis
hemothorax (*hē*-mō-THOR-aks)	blood in the chest cavity (pleural space) (Exercise Figure B)
laryngitis (*lar*-in-JĪ-tis)	inflammation of the larynx
laryngotracheobronchitis (LTB) (la-*ring*-gō-*trā*-kē-ō-bron-KĪ-tis)	inflammation of the larynx, trachea, and bronchi (the acute form is called **croup**)

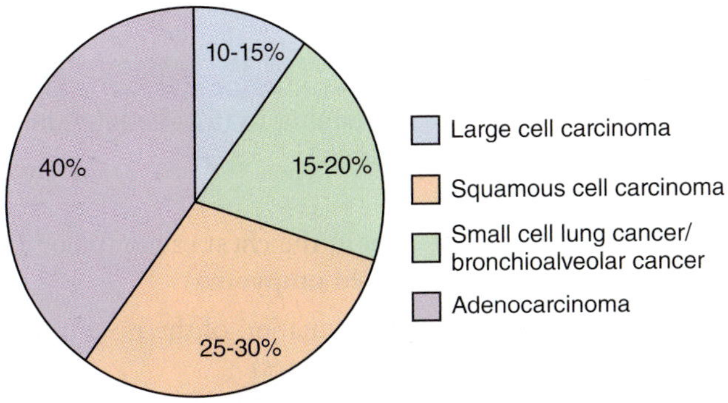

FIG. 5.5 Types of lung cancers. Lung cancer is classified as either small cell or large cell. The latter is by far the most prevalent and includes **adenocarcinoma** and **squamous cell carcinoma**. Lung cancer is one of the most common cancers in the world. It is the main cause of death due to cancer for both men and women. Smoking is the most important risk factor for the development of lung cancer. Symptoms include cough, hemoptysis, chest pain, dyspnea, fatigue, and weight loss. **Thoracentesis, bronchoscopy, chest radiograph, computed tomography (CT)**, and **positron emission tomography (PET)** scanning are used for diagnosis. Treatment includes **surgery, chemotherapy**, and **radiation**.

MESOTHELIOMA

is a rare form of cancer most common in the pleura, the sac covering the lung, and lining the thoracic cavity, and is most often caused by inhalation exposure to asbestos.

Mesothelioma also occurs in the lining of the abdominal cavity and in the lining of the heart.

TERM	DEFINITION
lobar pneumonia (LŌ-bar) (nū-MŌ-nē-a)	pertaining to the lobe(s); diseased state of the lung (infection of one or more lobes of the lung)
nasopharyngitis (*nā*-zō-*far*-in-JĪ-tis)	inflammation of the nose and pharynx
pharyngitis (*far*-in-JĪ-tis)	inflammation of the pharynx
pleuritis (plū-RĪ-tis)	inflammation of the pleura (also called **pleurisy**) (Fig. 5.6)
pneumatocele (nū-MAT-ō-sēl)	hernia of the lung (lung tissue protrudes through an opening in the chest)
pneumoconiosis (*nū*-mō-*kō*-nē-Ō-sis)	abnormal condition of dust in the lungs (pneumoconiosis is the general name given for chronic inflammatory disease of the lung caused by excessive inhalation of mineral dust. When the disease is caused by a specific dust, it is named for the dust. For example, the disease caused by silica dust is called silicosis).
pneumonia (nū-MŌ-nē-a)	diseased state of the lung (the infection and inflammation are caused by bacteria such as *Pneumococcus*, *Staphylococcus*, *Streptococcus*, and *Haemophilus*; viruses; and fungi) (see Fig. 5.13B)
pneumonitis (*nū*-mō-NĪ-tis)	inflammation of the lung
pneumothorax (*nū*-mō-THOR-aks)	air in the chest cavity (specifically, the pleural space, which causes collapse of the lung and is often a result of an open chest wound) (Exercise Figure C)

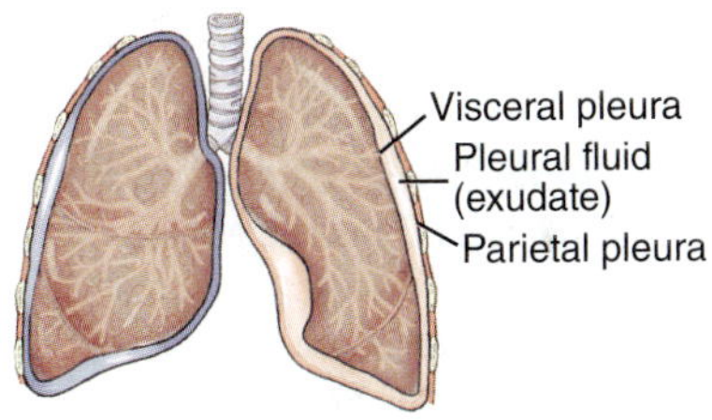

FIG. 5.6 Pleuritis, also called pleurisy.

EXERCISE FIGURE C

Fill in the blanks to label the diagram.

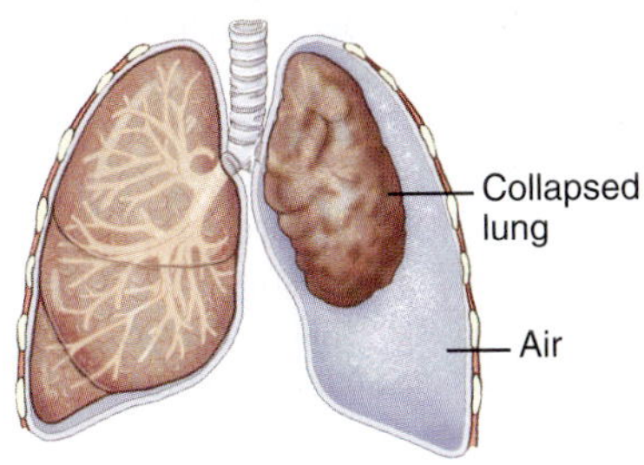

______ air / ______ CV / ______ chest cavity

Disease and Disorder Terms—cont'd

TERM	DEFINITION
pulmonary neoplasm (PUL-mō-*nar*-ē) (NĒ-ō-*plaz*-em)	pertaining to (in) the lung, new growth (tumor)
pyothorax (*pī*-ō-THOR-aks)	pus in the chest cavity (pleural space) (also called **empyema**)
rhinitis (rī-NĪ-tis)	inflammation of the nose (mucous membranes)
rhinomycosis (*rī*-nō-mī-KŌ-sis)	abnormal condition of fungus in the nose
rhinorrhagia (*rī*-nō-RĀ-ja)	rapid flow of blood from the nose (also called **epistaxis**)
sinusitis (sī-nū-SĪ-tis)	inflammation of the sinuses (Exercise Figure D)
thoracalgia (*thor*-a-KAL-ja)	pain in the chest
tonsillitis (*ton*-sil-Ī-tis)	inflammation of the tonsils
tracheitis (*trā*-kē-Ī-tis)	inflammation of the trachea
tracheostenosis (*trā*-kē-ō-sten-Ō-sis)	narrowing of the trachea

INTEGRATIVE MEDICINE TERM

Traditional Chinese medicine (TCM) is an example of a whole medical system, one of the National Center for Complementary and Alternative Medicine's (NCCAM's) five major classifications. TCM is an ancient healing system that uses herbal and nutritional therapy, acupuncture, massage, and therapeutic exercise to balance the Qi (vital energy) within the body to promote wellness and healing for body, mind, and spirit. Studies have demonstrated that a variety of TCM modalities can provide symptomatic relief and improvement in quality of life for patients with **asthma, allergic rhinitis, and other respiratory ailments.**

EXERCISE FIGURE D

Fill in the blanks to complete the labeling of the diagram.

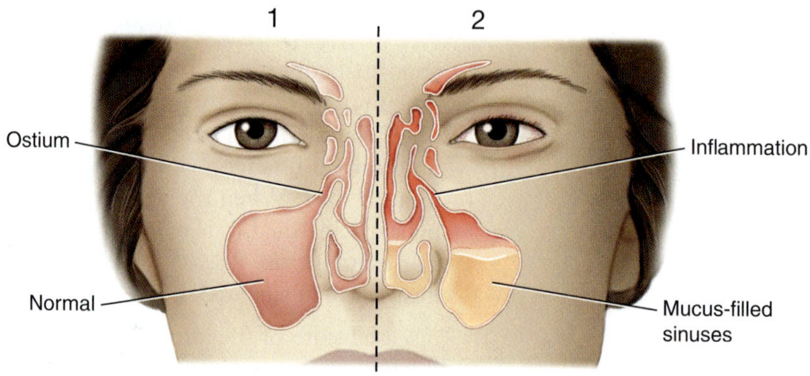

1. Normal sinuses

2. ______ / ______
sinuses / inflammation

EXERCISE 12

Practice saying aloud each of the Disease and Disorder Terms Built from Word Parts.

To hear the terms, go to Evolve Resources at evolve.elsevier.com and select:
Practice Student Resources > Student Resources > Chapter 5 > **Pronounce and Spell**

See Appendix B for instructions.

❑ Check the box when complete.

EXERCISE 13

Analyze and define the following terms by drawing slashes between word parts, writing word part abbreviations above the term, underlining combining forms, and writing combining form abbreviations below the term.

EXAMPLE:

WR CV S
diaphragmat / o / cele
CF
hernia of the diaphragm

1. pleuritis

____
____

2. nasopharyngitis

____
____

3. pneumothorax

____
____

4. sinusitis

____
____

5. atelectasis

____
____

6. rhinomycosis

____
____

7. tracheostenosis

____
____

8. epiglottitis

____
____

9. thoracalgia

____
____

10. pulmonary neoplasm

____
____

11. bronchiectasis

____
____

12. tonsillitis

____
____

13. pneumoconiosis

14. bronchopneumonia

15. pneumonitis

16. laryngitis

17. pyothorax

18. rhinorrhagia

19. bronchitis

20. pharyngitis

21. tracheitis

22. laryngotracheobronchitis

23. adenoiditis

24. hemothorax

25. lobar pneumonia

26. rhinitis

27. bronchogenic carcinoma

28. alveolitis

29. pneumonia

30. pneumatocele

EXERCISE 14

Build disease and disorder terms for the following definitions with the word parts you have learned.

EXAMPLE: inflammation of the tonsils tonsill / itis (WR / S)

1. pain in the chest ______ / ______ (WR / S)
2. abnormal condition of fungus (infection) in the nose ______ / ______ / ______ / ______ (WR / CV / WR / S)
3. pertaining to the lung; new growth (tumor) ______ / ______ (WR / S) ______ / ______ (P / S(WR))
4. inflammation of the larynx ______ / ______ (WR / S)
5. incomplete expansion (of the lung) ______ / ______ (WR / S)
6. inflammation of the adenoids ______ / ______ (WR / S)
7. inflammation of the larynx, trachea, and bronchi ______ / ______ / ______ / ______ / ______ / ______ (WR / CV / WR / CV / WR / S)
8. dilation of the bronchi ______ / ______ (WR / S)
9. inflammation of the pleura ______ / ______ (WR / S)
10. abnormal condition of dust in the lung ______ / ______ / ______ / ______ (WR / CV / WR / S)
11. inflammation of the lung ______ / ______ (WR / S)
12. inflammation of the sinuses ______ / ______ (WR / S)
13. narrowing of the trachea ______ / ______ / ______ (WR / CV / S)
14. inflammation of the nose and pharynx ______ / ______ / ______ / ______ (WR / CV / WR / S)
15. pus in the chest cavity (pleural space) ______ / ______ / ______ (WR / CV / S)

16. inflammation of the epiglottis ____ WR / ____ S

17. hernia of the diaphragm ____ WR / CV / ____ S

18. air in the chest cavity (pleural space) ____ WR / CV / ____ S

19. diseased state of the bronchi and the lungs ____ WR / CV / ____ WR / ____ S

20. rapid flow of blood from the nose ____ WR / CV / ____ S

21. inflammation of the pharynx ____ WR / ____ S

22. blood in the chest cavity (pleural space) ____ WR / CV / ____ S

23. inflammation of the trachea ____ WR / ____ S

24. inflammation of the bronchi ____ WR / ____ S

25. pertaining to the lobe(s); diseased state of the lung ____ WR / ____ S ____ WR / ____ S

26. inflammation of the nose (mucous membranes) ____ WR / ____ S

27. cancerous tumor originating in a bronchus ____ WR / CV / ____ S ____ WR / ____ S

28. inflammation of the alveoli ____ WR / ____ S

29. diseased state of the lung ____ WR / ____ S

30. hernia of the lung ____ WR / CV / ____ S

EXERCISE 15

Spell each of the Disease and Disorder Terms Built from Word Parts by having someone dictate them to you. Use a separate sheet of paper.

> To hear and spell the terms, go to Evolve Resources at evolve.elsevier.com and select:
> Practice Student Resources > Student Resources > Chapter 5 > **Pronounce and Spell**
>
> See Appendix B for instructions.

❑ Check the box when complete.

Disease and Disorder Terms
NOT BUILT FROM WORD PARTS

Word parts may be present in the following terms; however, their full meanings cannot be translated using definitions of word parts alone.

TERM	DEFINITION
acute respiratory distress syndrome (ARDS) (a-KŪT) (RES-pi-ra-*tor*-ē) (di-STRES) (SIN-drōm)	respiratory failure as a result of disease or injury. ARDS is respiratory failure in an adult. Symptoms include dyspnea, tachypnea, and cyanosis. (also called **adult respiratory distress syndrome**)
asthma (AZ-ma)	respiratory disease characterized by coughing, wheezing, and shortness of breath, caused by constriction and inflammation of airways that is reversible between attacks
chronic obstructive pulmonary disease (COPD) (KRON-ik) (ob-STRUK-tiv) (PUL-mō-*nar*-ē) (di-ZĒZ)	progressive lung disease obstructing air flow, which makes breathing difficult. Chronic bronchitis and pulmonary emphysema are the two main components of COPD. Most COPD is a result of cigarette smoking.
coccidioidomycosis (kok-*sid*-ē-*oy*-dō-mī-KŌ-sis)	fungal disease affecting the lungs and sometimes other organs of the body (also called **valley fever)**
croup (krūp)	condition resulting from acute obstruction of the larynx, characterized by a barking cough, hoarseness, and stridor. It may be caused by viral or bacterial infection, allergy, or foreign body. Occurs mainly in children. (also called **laryngotracheobronchitis**)
cystic fibrosis (CF) (SIS-tik) (fī-BRŌ-sis)	hereditary disorder of the exocrine glands characterized by excess mucus production in the respiratory tract, pancreatic deficiency, and other symptoms
deviated septum (DĒ-vē-*āt*-ed) (SEP-tum)	one part of the nasal cavity is smaller because of malformation or injury of the nasal septum
epistaxis (*ep*-i-STAK-sis)	nosebleed (also called **rhinorrhagia**)
idiopathic pulmonary fibrosis (IPF) (id-ē-ō-PATH-ik) (PUL-mō-*nar*-ē) (fī-BRŌ-sis)	chronic progressive lung disorder characterized by increasing scarring, which ultimately reduces the capacity of the lungs; etiology unknown. IPF most often affects adults over the age of 50. Smoking, pollutants, and heredity may play a role in its genesis. Symptoms include exertional dyspnea and a dry cough. Lung transplant may be indicated in severe cases; there is no cure.

INSIDIOUS/ACUTE/SUBACUTE/CHRONIC

In reference to disease:

Insidious: gradual and subtle onset of disease

Acute: sharp, sudden, short, or severe type of disease

Subacute: between acute and chronic

Chronic: disease that continues for a long time

REACTIVE AIRWAY DISEASE (RAD)

is a general term and not a specific diagnosis. It is used to describe a history of wheezing, coughing, and shortness of breath. In some people RAD may lead to **asthma**.

Disease and Disorder Terms—cont'd

INFLUENZA PANDEMIC

is the sudden outbreak of a flu that becomes very widespread, affecting a region, a continent, or the world. Examples are H1N1 swine flu and H5N1 avian flu.

TERM	DEFINITION
influenza (flu) (*in*-flū-EN-za)	highly contagious and often severe viral infection of the respiratory tract
obstructive sleep apnea (OSA) (ob-STRUK-tiv) (slēp) (AP-nē-a)	repetitive pharyngeal collapse during sleep, which leads to transient periods of apnea (absence of breathing); can produce daytime drowsiness and elevated blood pressure (Fig. 5.7)
pertussis (per-TUS-sis)	highly contagious bacterial infection of the respiratory tract characterized by an acute crowing inspiration, or whoop (also called **whooping cough**)
pleural effusion (PLŪ-ral) (e-FŪ-zhun)	fluid in the pleural space caused by a disease process or trauma
pulmonary edema (PUL-mō-*nar*-ē) (e-DĒ-ma)	fluid accumulation in the alveoli and bronchioles, most often a manifestation of heart failure
pulmonary embolism (PE) (PUL-mō-*nar*-ē) (EM-bo-liz-em)	matter foreign to the circulation, carried to the pulmonary artery and its branches, where it blocks circulation to the lungs and can be fatal if of sufficient size or number. Blood clots broken loose from the deep veins of the lower extremities are the most common source of pulmonary embolism (Fig. 5.8).
pulmonary emphysema (PUL-mō-*nar*-ē) (*em*-fi-SĒ-ma)	loss of elasticity of the alveoli resulting in distention causing stretching of the lung. As a result, the body does not receive enough oxygen. (component of COPD) (Fig. 5.4)

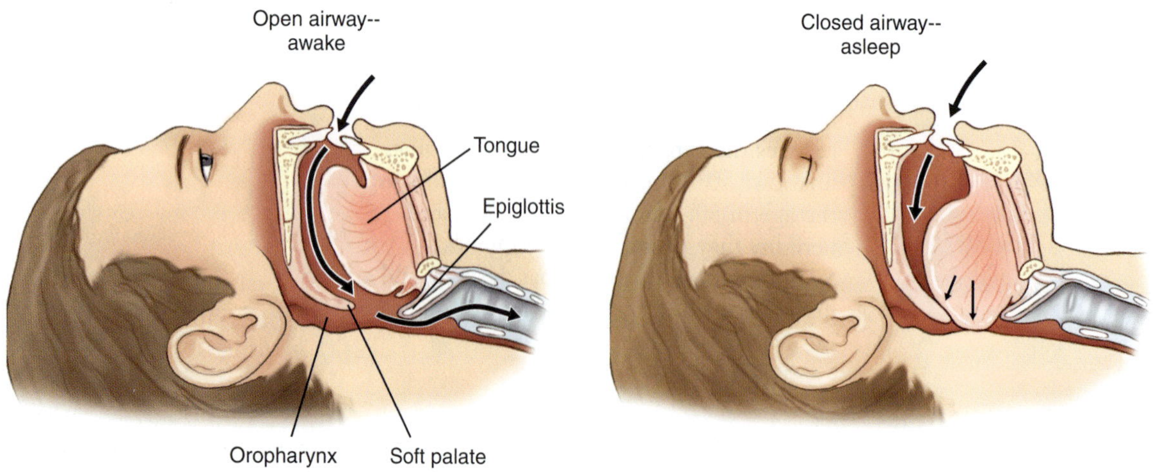

FIG. 5.7 Obstructive sleep apnea (OSA). During sleep the absence of activity of the pharyngeal muscle structure allows the airway to close. OSA is associated with increased risk for elevated blood pressure, cardiovascular disease, diabetes, and stroke. Obesity is a major risk factor and weight loss can be an effective treatment. **Polysomnography** is used to diagnose OSA. Treatment includes the use of **CPAP (continuous positive airway pressure)** during sleep and **uvulopalatopharyngoplasty (UPPP),** a surgical procedure.

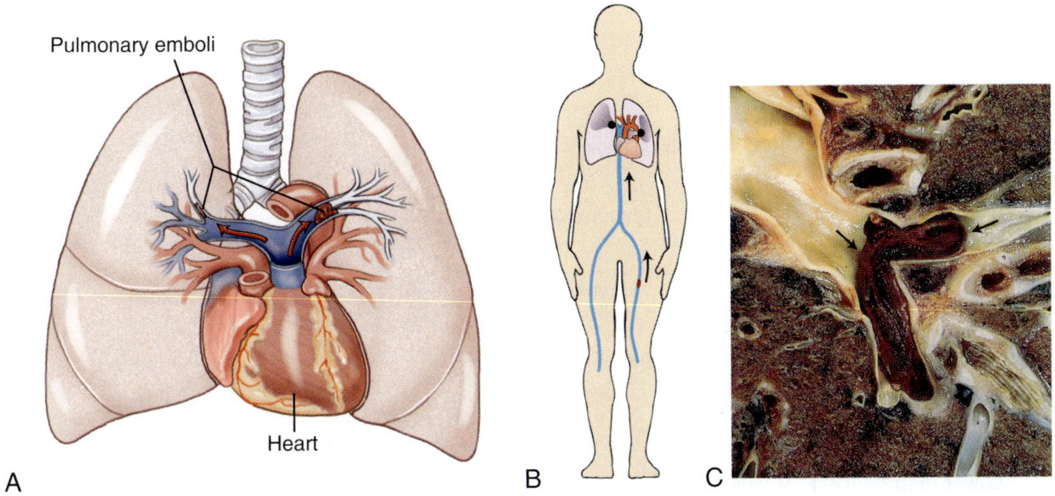

FIG. 5.8 A, Bilateral pulmonary emboli. **B,** Pulmonary emboli usually originate in the deep veins of the lower extremities. **C,** Necropsy specimen of the lung showing a large embolus.

TERM	DEFINITION
tuberculosis (TB) (tū-*ber*-kū-LŌ-sis)	infectious bacterial disease, most commonly spread by inhalation of small particles and usually affecting the lungs; may spread to other organs
upper respiratory infection (URI) (UP-er) (RES-pi-ra-*tor*-ē) (in-FEK-shun)	infection of the nasal cavity, pharynx, or larynx usually caused by a virus (commonly called a **cold**) (Fig. 5.9)

TUBERCULOSIS (TB)

is one of the most common causes of death worldwide from infectious disease, though it is preventable and curable. The risk for active TB is higher in HIV-infected persons and drug users. The development of multidrug–resistant TB is becoming a problem in treatment of the disease.

EXERCISE 16

Practice saying aloud each of the Disease and Disorder Terms NOT Built from Word Parts.

To hear the terms, go to Evolve Resources at evolve.elsevier.com and select:
Practice Student Resources > Student Resources > Chapter 5 > **Pronounce and Spell**

See Appendix B for instructions.

❑ Check the box when complete.

EXERCISE 17

Fill in the blanks with the correct terms.

1. A disease characterized by loss of elasticity of alveoli resulting in distention causing stretching of the lung is ________________ ________________.
2. ________________ ________________ is the name given to the fluid in the pleural space caused by a disease process or a trauma.
3. A fungal disease affecting the lungs is called ____.
4. ________________ ________________ is a hereditary disorder characterized by excess mucus production in the respiratory tract.
5. The medical name of a highly contagious respiratory infection commonly referred to as *flu* is ________________.

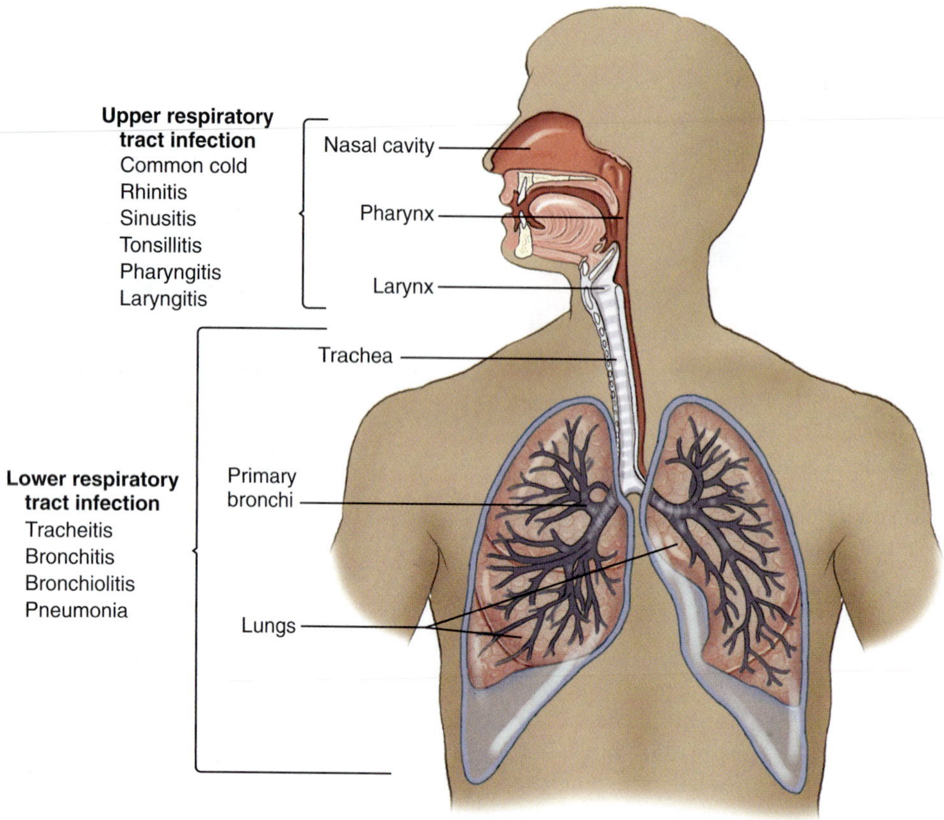

FIG. 5.9 Upper and lower respiratory tract infections.

6. Chronic bronchitis and pulmonary emphysema are two main components of ______________ ______________ ______________ ______________.
7. The medical name for the disease characterized by an acute crowing inspiration is ______________.
8. ______________ is a condition resulting from an acute obstruction of the larynx.
9. A respiratory disease characterized by shortness of breath, wheezing, and coughing is called ______________.
10. A condition in which fluid accumulates in the alveoli and bronchioles is ______________ ______________.
11. A(n) ______________ ______________ ______________ generally refers to an infection involving the nasal cavity, pharynx, or larynx, usually caused by a virus.
12. Foreign matter, such as a blood clot, carried to the pulmonary artery, where it blocks circulation to the lungs, is called a(n) ______________ ______________.
13. ______________ is another name for nosebleed.
14. A chronic progressive lung disorder that ultimately reduces the capacity of the lungs is ______________ ______________ ______________.
15. ______________ ______________ is one part of the nasal cavity that is smaller than the other because of malformation or injury.
16. The diagnosis for repetitive pharyngeal collapse is ______________ ______________ ______________.
17. An infectious bacterial disease usually affecting the lungs and caused by inhaling infected small particles is ______________.
18. ______________ ______________ ______________ ______________ is also called adult respiratory distress syndrome.

EXERCISE 18

Match the terms in the first column with the correct definitions in the second column.

_____ 1. asthma
_____ 2. chronic obstructive pulmonary disease
_____ 3. coccidioidomycosis
_____ 4. croup
_____ 5. cystic fibrosis
_____ 6. pulmonary emphysema
_____ 7. epistaxis
_____ 8. influenza
_____ 9. idiopathic pulmonary fibrosis

a. loss of elasticity of alveoli resulting in stretching of the lung
b. caused by a virus (commonly called flu)
c. hereditary disorder characterized by excess mucus in the respiratory system
d. most often caused by cigarette smoking
e. nosebleed
f. condition resulting from acute obstruction of the larynx
g. also called valley fever
h. characterized by scarring of the lung
i. caused by restriction of airways that is reversible between attacks

EXERCISE 19

Match the terms in the first column with the correct definitions in the second column.

_____ 1. pertussis
_____ 2. pleural effusion
_____ 3. pulmonary edema
_____ 4. pulmonary embolism
_____ 5. upper respiratory infection
_____ 6. deviated septum
_____ 7. obstructive sleep apnea
_____ 8. tuberculosis
_____ 9. acute respiratory distress syndrome

a. respiratory failure as a result of disease or injury
b. fluid in the pleural space
c. fluid accumulation in alveoli and bronchioles
d. whooping cough
e. foreign material, carried to the pulmonary artery, where it blocks circulation to the lungs
f. commonly called a cold
g. unequal size of nasal cavities
h. repetitive pharyngeal collapse
i. infectious bacterial disease usually affecting the lungs

EXERCISE 20

Spell each of the Disease and Disorder Terms NOT Built from Word Parts by having someone dictate them to you. Use a separate sheet of paper.

> To hear and spell the terms, go to Evolve Resources at evolve.elsevier.com and select:
> Practice Student Resources > Student Resources > Chapter 5 > **Pronounce and Spell**
>
> See Appendix B for instructions.

❑ Check the box when complete.

Surgical Terms

BUILT FROM WORD PARTS

The following terms can be translated using definitions of word parts. Further explanation is provided within parentheses as needed.

TERM	DEFINITION
adenoidectomy (*ad*-e-noyd-EK-to-mē)	excision of the adenoids (Exercise Figure E)
adenotome (AD-e-nō-*tōm*)	instrument used to cut the adenoids (Exercise Figure E) *(Note: the* oid *is missing from the word root adenoid in this term.)*
bronchoplasty (BRON-kō-*plas*-tē)	surgical repair of a bronchus
laryngectomy (*lār*-in-JEK-to-mē)	excision of the larynx
laryngoplasty (la-RING-gō-*plas*-tē)	surgical repair of the larynx
laryngostomy (*lar*-in-GOS-to-mē)	creation of an artificial opening into the larynx
laryngotracheotomy (la-*ring*-gō-*trā*-kē-OT-o-mē)	incision into the larynx and trachea
lobectomy (lō-BEK-to-mē)	excision of a lobe (of the lung) (Fig. 5.10)
pleuropexy (plū-rō-PEK-sē)	surgical fixation of the pleura
pneumonectomy (*nū*-mō-NEK-to-mē)	excision of a lung (Fig. 5.10)
rhinoplasty (RĪ-nō-*plas*-tē)	surgical repair of the nose
septoplasty (SEP-tō-*plas*-tē)	surgical repair of the (nasal) septum
septotomy (sep-TOT-o-mē)	incision into the (nasal) septum
sinusotomy (*sī*-nū-SOT-o-mē)	incision into a sinus

EXERCISE FIGURE E

Fill in the blanks to complete labeling of the diagram.

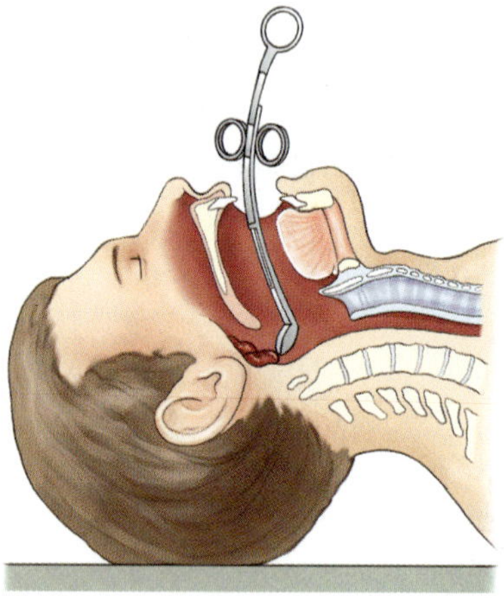

_____ / _____ performed using
adenoid / excision

a(n) _____ / _____ / _____
adenoid / cv / instrument used to cut

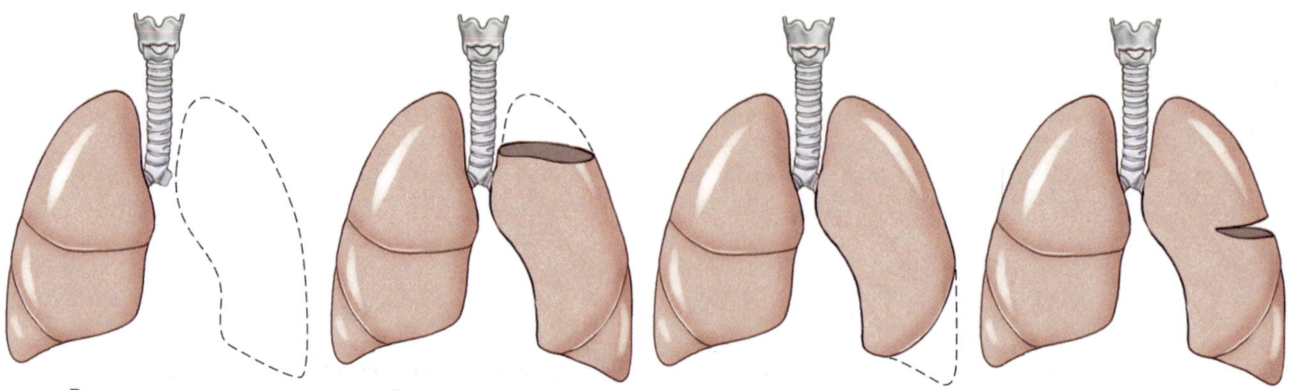

FIG. 5.10 Types of lung resection. The diagram illustrates the amount of lung tissue removed with each type of surgery.

TERM	DEFINITION
thoracocentesis (*thor*-a-kō-sen-TĒ-sis)	surgical puncture to aspirate fluid from the chest cavity (also called **thoracentesis**) (Exercise Figure F)
thoracotomy (*thor*-a-KOT-o-mē)	incision into the chest cavity (Fig. 5.11)
tonsillectomy (*ton*-sil-EK-to-mē)	excision of the tonsils
tracheoplasty (TRĀ-kē-ō-*plas*-tē)	surgical repair of the trachea
tracheostomy (*trā*-kē-OS-to-mē)	creation of an artificial opening into the trachea (Fig. 5.12)
tracheotomy (*trā*-kē-OT-o-mē)	incision into the trachea (Fig. 5.12)

CAREER VIDEOS

To see interviews with a **nurse** on a **medical-surgical unit** and a **surgical technologist**, go to Evolve Resources at evolve.elsevier.com and select **Career Videos** located under the **Extra Content** tab.

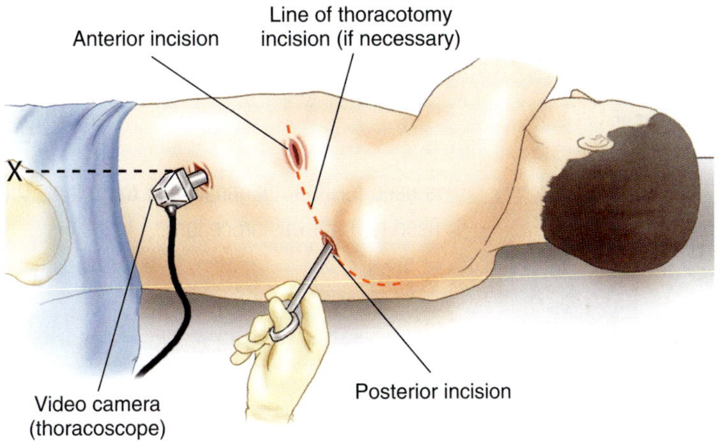

FIG. 5.11 Video-assisted thoracic surgery (VATS) is the use of a **thoracoscope** and video equipment for an endoscopic approach to diagnose and treat thoracic conditions. It often replaces the traditional **thoracotomy,** which required a large incision and greater recovery time.

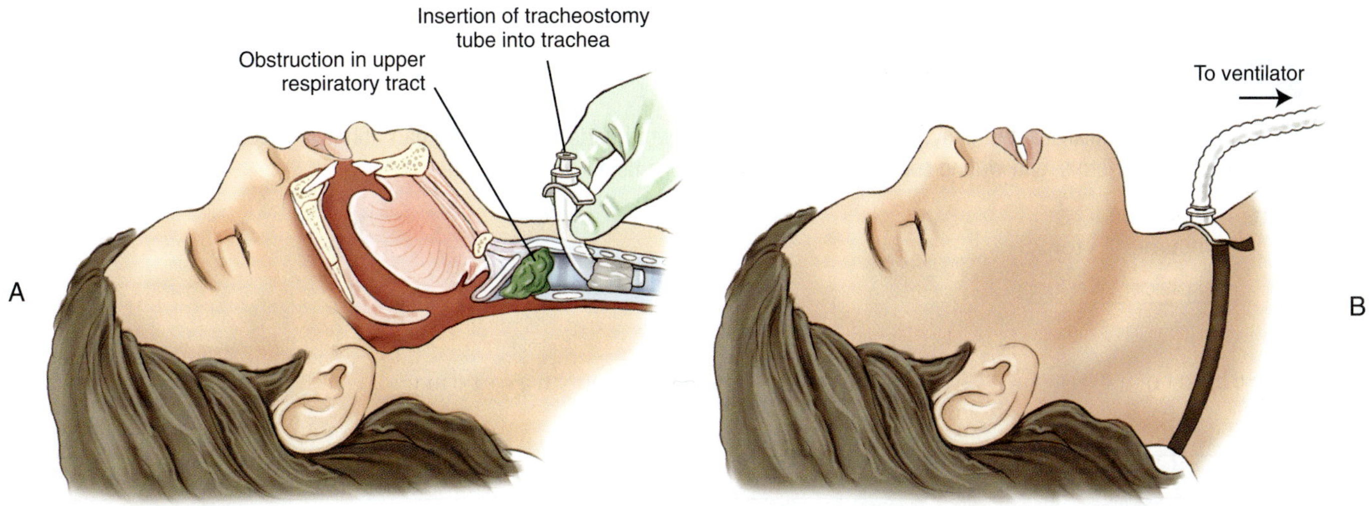

FIG. 5.12 **A,** A **tracheotomy** is performed to establish an airway when normal breathing is obstructed. If the opening needs to be maintained, a tube is inserted, creating a tracheostomy. **B,** A **tracheostomy** may be temporary, as for prolonged mechanical ventilation to support breathing or it may be permanent, as in airway reconstruction after laryngeal cancer surgery.

EXERCISE FIGURE F

Fill in the blanks to complete labeling of the diagram.

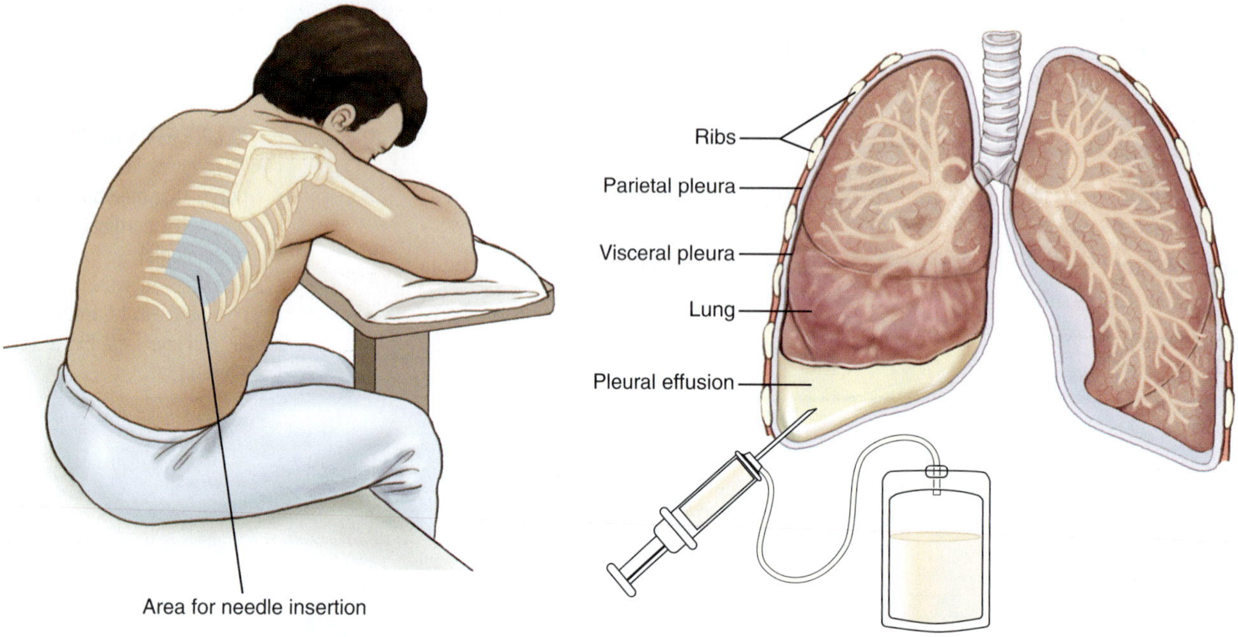

_______ / _______ / _______ is used for both diagnosis and treatment. Thoracentesis is a commonly used term for this procedure.

chest cavity / cv / surgical puncture to aspirate fluid

EXERCISE 21

Practice saying aloud each of the Surgical Terms Built from Word Parts.

To hear the terms, go to Evolve Resources at evolve.elsevier.com and select:
Practice Student Resources > Student Resources > Chapter 5 > **Pronounce and Spell**

See Appendix B for instructions.

❑ Check the box when complete.

EXERCISE 22

Analyze and define the following terms by drawing slashes between word parts, writing word part abbreviations above the term, underlining combining forms, and writing combining form abbreviations below the term.

EXAMPLE: WR S
pneumon/ectomy
excision of a lung

1. tracheotomy

____

____

2. laryngostomy

____

____

3. adenoidectomy

____

____

4. rhinoplasty

____

____

5. adenotome

____

____

6. tracheostomy

____

____

7. sinusotomy

____

____

8. laryngoplasty

____

____

9. bronchoplasty

____

____

10. lobectomy

____

____

11. laryngotracheotomy

____

____

12. tracheoplasty

____

____

13. thoracotomy

____

____

14. laryngectomy

____

____

15. thoracocentesis

____

____

16. tonsillectomy

____

____

17. pleuropexy

____

____

18. septoplasty

____

____

19. septotomy

____

____

EXERCISE 23

Build surgical terms for the following definitions by using the word parts you have learned.

EXAMPLE: surgical fixation of the pleura pleur / o / pexy
WR / CV / S

1. surgical repair of the trachea _____ WR / CV / _____ S
2. incision into the larynx and trachea _____ WR / CV / _____ WR / CV / _____ S
3. instrument used to cut the adenoids _____ WR / CV / _____ S
4. incision into the chest cavity _____ WR / CV / _____ S
5. creation of an artificial opening into the trachea _____ WR / CV / _____ S
6. excision of the tonsils _____ WR / _____ S
7. incision into the trachea _____ WR / CV / _____ S
8. surgical repair of a bronchus _____ WR / CV / _____ S
9. excision of the larynx _____ WR / _____ S
10. surgical repair of the nose _____ WR / CV / _____ S
11. incision into a sinus _____ WR / CV / _____ S
12. surgical puncture to aspirate fluid from the chest cavity _____ WR / CV / _____ S
13. excision of the adenoids _____ WR / _____ S
14. surgical repair of the larynx _____ WR / CV / _____ S
15. excision of a lobe (of the lung) _____ WR / _____ S
16. creation of an artificial opening into the larynx _____ WR / CV / _____ S

17. excision of a lung ______ WR / ______ S

18. incision into the septum ______ WR / CV / ______ S

19. surgical repair of the septum ______ WR / CV / ______ S

EXERCISE 24

Spell each of the Surgical Terms Built from Word Parts by having someone dictate them to you. Use a separate sheet of paper.

> To hear and spell the terms, go to Evolve Resources at evolve.elsevier.com and select:
> Practice Student Resources > Student Resources > Chapter 5 > **Pronounce and Spell**
>
> See Appendix B for instructions.

❑ Check the box when complete.

TABLE 5.1 Diagnostic Procedures and Tests

Diagnostic procedures are performed for use in the diagnosis, monitoring, and treatment of disease. The following is an overview of the most common types of procedures: **Diagnostic Imaging, Endoscopy,** and **Laboratory Studies.**

DIAGNOSTIC IMAGING

Diagnostic imaging is a generic term that covers **radiography, computed tomography, nuclear medicine, magnetic resonance imaging,** and **sonography.**

Radiography (x-ray) produces images of internal structures using ionizing radiation emitted from an x-ray tube. An image receptor captures the radiant energy that has been transmitted through the patient. The captured energy is digitally processed to form an image called a **radiograph**, which is stored electronically and displayed on a monitor. Radiography is performed to detect **diseases, bone fractures, or other pathology.**

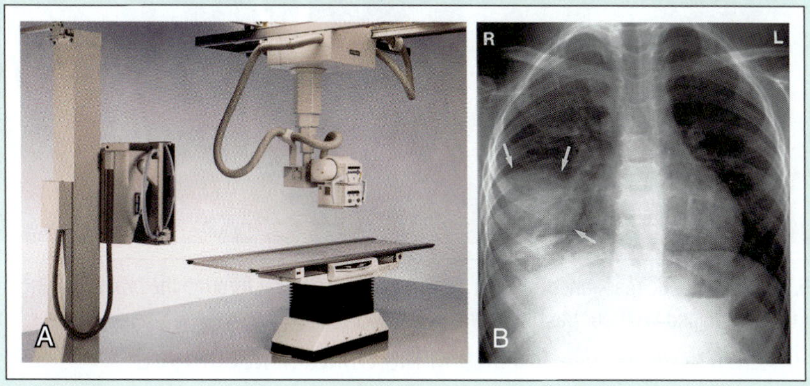

FIG. 5.13 A, Radiographic equipment and imaging table. **B,** Chest radiograph revealing pneumonia of the right lung.

X-rays were first discovered in 1895 by Wilhelm Conrad Roentgen in Germany. Because he did not understand the nature of the rays, he named them "x"-rays.

RADIOGRAPH

Radiographic image and **x-ray image** are terms used interchangeably with **radiograph**.

RADIOLOGIC AND CT TECHNOLOGISTS

To see interviews with a **radiologic technologist** and a **CT technologist**, go to Evolve Resources at evolve.elsevier.com and select **Career Videos** located under the **Extra Content** tab on the Practice Student Resources menu.

See Appendix B for instructions.

SCANNING/SCAN

Scanning means to map organs or the body with a sensing device. **Scan** is the image obtained and is often designated by the organ studied, as a **brain scan or liver scan. Scan** is the shortened form for **scintiscan,** an image created by radioisotopes.

TABLE 5.1 Diagnostic Procedures and Tests—cont'd

DIAGNOSTIC IMAGING

Computed tomography (CT) produces a series of sectional images of body organs or segments using ionizing radiation. An array of detectors collect data as the x-ray tube rotates around the patient. The data is processed by complex computer software allowing for images to be shown in transverse, sagittal, or coronal planes, as well as, 3-D reconstructions. CT is used in diagnosing **tumors, abscesses, cysts, stones, and other conditions.**

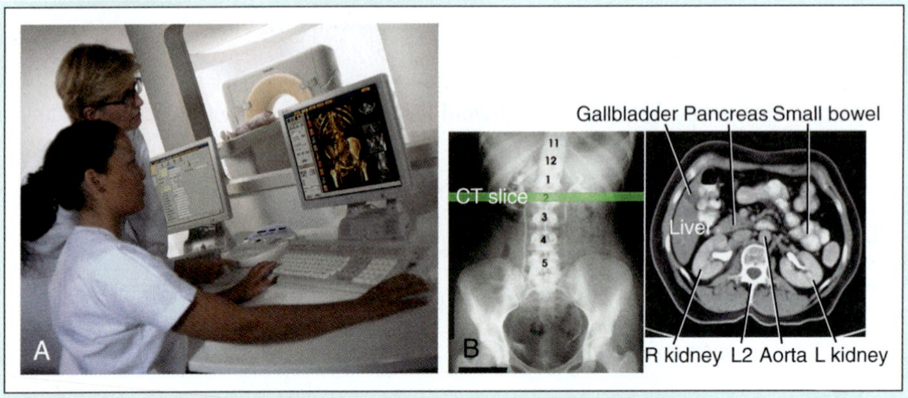

FIG. 5.14 A, Computed tomography scanner. **B,** An example of CT scan of the abdomen at level of kidneys.

CT scanners were first used in the United States in 1973.

Magnetic resonance imaging (MRI) produces images by exposing the body to high strength, computer-controlled magnetic fields (Fig. 5.15). As the magnetic field changes, the tissues of the body respond in characteristic ways. Very sensitive detectors are used to record the response of the different tissues. Computers are then used to create an image. MRI is preferred over CT to study the brain and spinal cord because it provides better detail of structure. MRI is used in detecting **tumors, bleeding, infection, injury, edema, or obstruction.** Risks of ionizing radiation are avoided by MRI scanning.

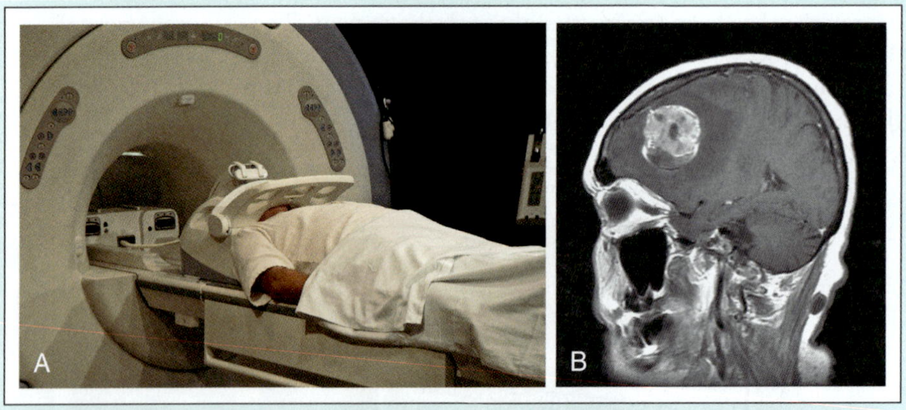

FIG. 5.15 A, Magnetic resonance scanner. **B,** Sagittal MRI section through the brain showing frontal lobe mass enhanced with contrast medium.

The first MRI scanner was installed in the Unites States in 1981.

Nuclear medicine (NM) produces images (also known as scintiscans, scans, or scintigrams) by administering radioactive material often combined with other materials to cause it to be delivered to the body part of interest (Fig. 5.16). The radioactive material and the material to which it is bound, often referred to as a **radiopharmaceutical** or **tracer**, emits energy (usually gamma rays) that is detected by a specialized camera (gamma camera). A computer translates the readings into two-dimensional images (scans) in various shades of grey or color.

DIAGNOSTIC IMAGING

The most commonly used radiopharmaceutical is **technetium-99m** or **Tc-99m,** although others including **gallium, thallium,** and **iodine** are also used and sometimes appear in the name of NM test. NM studies are used to detect abnormal function and structure of organs or of various body areas. An **nuclear medicine (NM) lung scan may be performed to detect pulmonary emboli, a bone scan to detect metastatic cancer, or a renal scan to evaluate blood flow to the kidney.** In NM the radioactive source mostly comes from within the body whereas in x-ray and computed tomography the radioactive source is from outside the body. Some NM procedures are done on blood and urine specimens that require no adminstration of a radioactive source source into the body. The risk of radiation is dependent on the dose anf radiopharmaceutical used. It can be lower than x-rays studies.

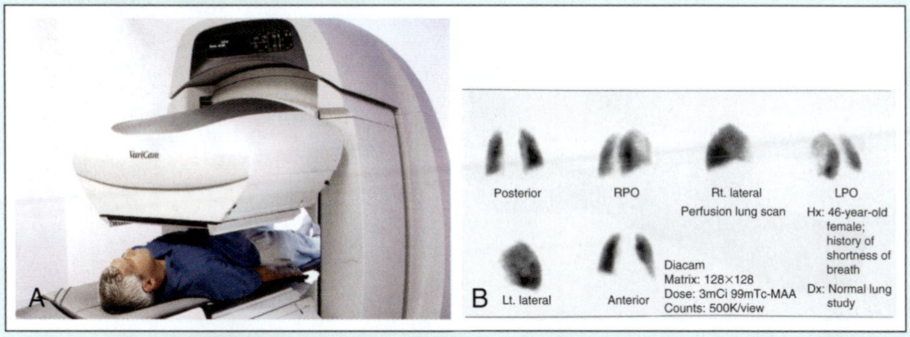

FIG. 5.16 A, Nuclear medicine scanner. **B,** Lung scan.

By 1970 most body organs could be visualized by NM procedures, and in 1971 Nuclear Medicine was officially recognized by the American Medical Association as a medical specialty.

Single-photon emission computed tomography (SPECT) is an NM technique that yields three-dimensional computer constructed images (Fig. 5.17). SPECT can be combined with CT to create a fusion imaging system that overlays the function image from a gamma camera with the anatomy of the CT images. SPECT is capable of showing blood flow through an organ and blood-deprived areas of the brain and heart. Using SPECT, the heart can be visualized from several different angles to **assess damage to cardiac tissue following a myocardial infarction (heart attack) or damage to brain tissue caused by a disruption of the normal supply of blood, which often occurs with a stroke.**

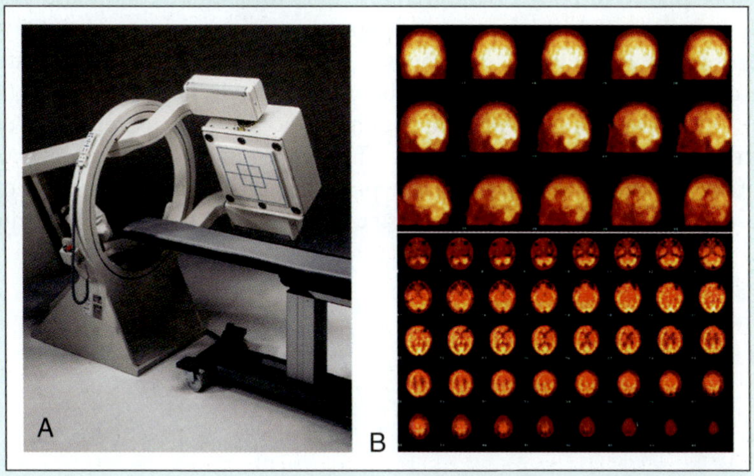

FIG. 5.17 A, SPECT camera system. **B,** Three dimensional SPECT of brain study showing a patient with left frontal lobe brain infarction. SPECT was developed in 1980.

TABLE 5.1 Diagnostic Procedures and Tests—cont'd

DIAGNOSTIC IMAGING

Positron emission tomography (PET) is a relatively new NM procedure (Fig. 5.18). Positron-emitting radioactive material is injected into the body. The positrons are picked up by a ring of detectors positioned around the body. Functional and anatomic abnormalities are demonstrated. The images can be combined with CT images to more precisely show the location of the activity in the body. PET is **used in oncology to assist in diagnosing and staging of cancer and monitoring the effects of treatment. PET is also used in neurology to assist in diagnosing Alzheimer disease.**

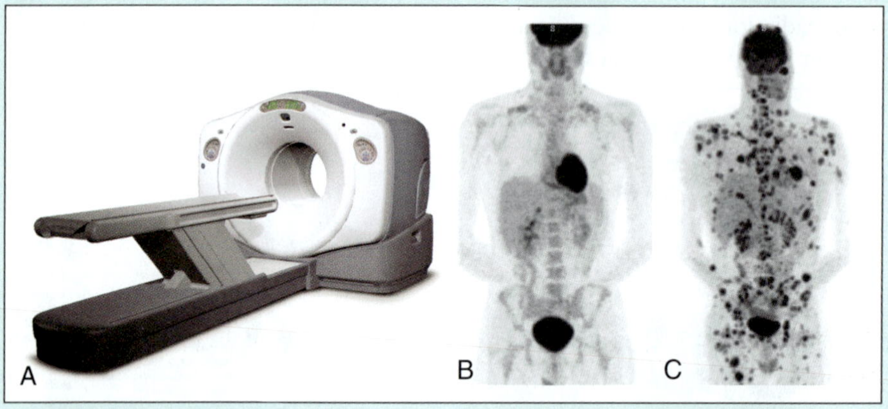

FIG. 5.18 A, A typical PET/CT scanner. **B,** PET image to evaluate a patient with a history of melanoma. Scan shows physiologic activity with no evidence of recurrence. **C,** Image six months later shows metastases throughout the body.

PET began in the 1970s as a research tool. The combination PET/CT scanner was developed in the 1990s.

ULTRASOUND OR ULTRASONOGRAPHY

are terms also used to describe sonography. Ultra- means "beyond" or "excess." The term ultrasound indicates high frequency sound waves that are beyond audible. The term sonography is used throughout this text.

Sonography, also referred to as ultrasound, produces scans using high frequency sound waves, which are beyond the range of human hearing (Fig. 5.19). A transducer (device that converts energy from one form to another), is passed over the skin of a specific body area. The transducer converts electric energy into high-frequency sound waves, which travel into the body. Some of the sound waves reflect (echo) off the internal structures back to the transducer. The echo is converted by the transducer to electrical impulses, which are transformed into visual images called sonograms. The composition and layers of different tissue types reflect sound waves differently, allowing an image to emerge. Transducers may also be placed in body cavities (endoscopic) to obtain a sonogram. For example in **transesophageal echocardiography**, the transducer is placed in the esophagus to obtain views of the heart for examining cardiac function and structure. Abdominal sonography may be used to detect **nephrolithiasis (kidney stones) or gall stones (cholelithiasis), and sonography is extensively used to evaluate the fetus during pregnancy.** The risks of ionizing radiation are eliminated by using ultrasound and in typical use, ultrasound is considered relatively harmless. It is also less expensive than MRI, CT, or NM procedures.

DIAGNOSTIC IMAGING

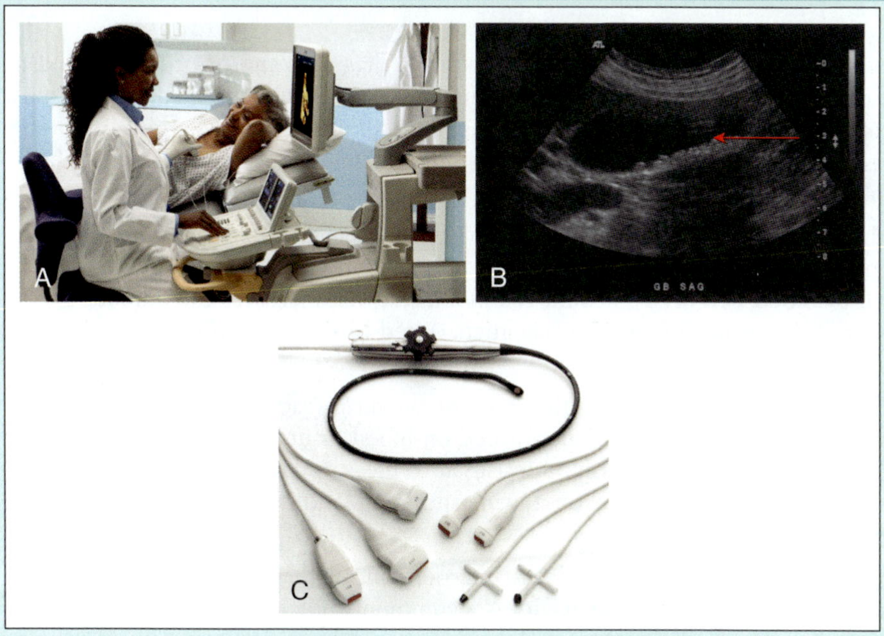

FIG. 5.19 **A,** Sonographer performing an ultrasound exam. **B,** Sagittal sonogram showing multiple small gallstones. **C,** Ultrasound transducers.

Sonography had its beginning during World War I with the development of sonar. In the 1950s anatomy ultrasound images were seen on a monitor in a series of blips. Digital systems that were introduced in the 1990s provided for images in the digital format that allowed for manipulation, viewing, and storage.

SONOGRAPHER
To see an interview with a **sonographer**, go to Evolve Resources at evolve.elsevier.com and select **Career Videos** located under the **Extra Content** tab on the Practice Student Resources menu.

See Appendix B for instructions.

ENDOSCOPY

Endoscopy is a general term for direct observation examination of a hollow body organ or cavity using a tubular instrument with a light source and a viewing lens called an endoscope (Fig. 5.20). The original endoscopes were rigid and used for direct observation. Adding lights and lenses to the endoscope allowed visualization of deeper structures. By incorporating fiberoptics and cameras, smaller flexible endoscopes were created allowing the images to be viewed on a monitor. A flexible fiberoptic scope is most often used in gastrointestinal and pulmonary endoscopy. Endoscopic procedures and instruments are named after the body part being visualized. A **bronchoscopy** means **visual examination of the bronchi**, and **bronchoscope** means **instrument used for visual examination of the bronchi**.

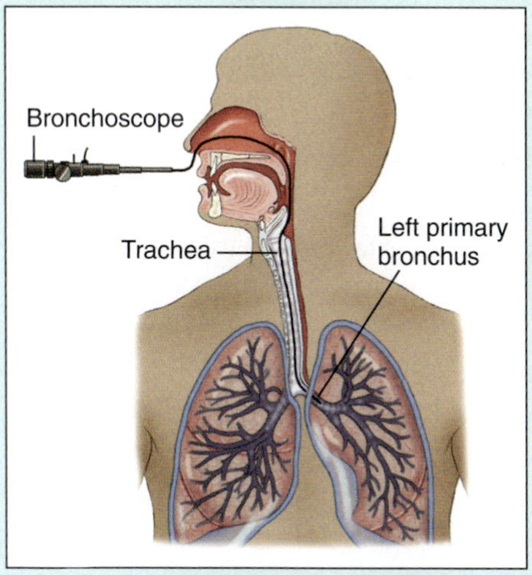

FIG. 5.20 Bronchoscopy. A bronchoscope is inserted through the nostril, pharynx, larynx, and trachea into the bronchus.

Endoscopy dates back to the time of Hippocrates (460-375 BC) who mentions using a speculum to look into the rectum. By the end of the nineteenth century cystoscopy, proctoscopy, and esophagoscopy were well established.

CLINICAL LABORATORY SCIENTIST

To see an interview with a **clinical laboratory scientist**, go to Evolve Resources at evolve.elsevier.com and select **Career Videos** located under the **Extra Content** tab on the Practice Student Resources menu.

See Appendix B for instructions.

TABLE 5.1 Diagnostic Procedures and Tests—cont'd

LABORATORY TESTS
Laboratory tests are performed to establish a diagnosis and/or prognosis, and to monitor and evaluate treatment. Specimens that are studied include blood (most common), urine, stool, sputum, sweat, wound drainage or discharge from body openings, washings, and tissue. Most studies included in this text fall into the following categories:
Hematology studies relate to the physical properties of blood such as the number of blood cells in the specimen or the clotting and bleeding factors. A **white blood cell** (WBC) count is a blood test that measures the number of white blood cells present in a specimen. A **red blood cell** (RBC) count measures the number of red blood cells.
Chemistry studies relate to the study of chemical reactions that occur in the human body and are usually performed on blood or urine specimens. **BUN** (blood urea nitrogen) is a blood test used to measure kidney function. **Urine glucose** is a test performed on a urine specimen, and is used to determine the amount of glucose in the urine.
Microbiology studies identify the microorganisms that cause disease and infection. **Culture and sensitivity** is a common study performed on almost any specimen. The specimen is placed on a medium for growth. If a pathogenic microorganism grows, it is tested for antibiotic sensitivity to determine to which antibiotics it is susceptible and those to which it is resistant. This information allows the physician to order an antibiotic that will provide the effective treatment.
Urine studies are performed on urine specimens to diagnose and monitor urinary tract disease. They are also used to detect and monitor diseases not related to the kidney such as identifying glucose in the urine, which may indicate diabetes mellitus. A **urinalysis** is the study of urine for color, clarity, degree of acidity or alkalinity, specific gravity, protein, glucose, leukocytes, and bilirubin.

SCOPE

is taken from the Greek **skopein,** which means to **see** or to **view.** It also means **observing for a purpose.** To the ancient Greeks it meant "to look out for, to monitor, or to examine."

Today the following suffixes commonly are used:

- -scope describes the instrument used to view or to examine, such as in the term endoscope.
- -scopy means visual examination, such as in the term endoscopy.
- -scopic means pertaining to visual examination, such as in the term endoscopic.

Endoscopic surgery is performed with the use of endoscopes. Most often the suffixes -**scope, -scopy,** and -**scopic** mean to **examine visually,** and that is the definition given in this text. However, the term **stethoscope** is an **instrument used for listening** to body sounds.

Diagnostic Terms

BUILT FROM WORD PARTS

The following terms can be translated using definitions of word parts. Further explanation is provided within parentheses as needed.

TERM	DEFINITION
ENDOSCOPY	
bronchoscope (BRON-kō-skōp)	instrument used for visual examination of the bronchi (Fig. 5.20)
bronchoscopy (bron-KOS-ko-pē)	visual examination of the bronchi (Fig. 5.20)
endoscope (EN-dō-skōp)	instrument used for visual examination within (a hollow organ or body cavity). (Endoscopes are used for surgical procedures as well as for viewing.)
endoscopic (*en*-dō-SKOP-ik)	pertaining to visual examination within (a hollow organ or body cavity) (used to describe the practice of performing surgeries that use endoscopes)
endoscopy (en-DOS-ko-pē)	visual examination within (a hollow organ or body cavity)

EXERCISE FIGURE G

Fill in the blanks to complete labeling of the diagram.

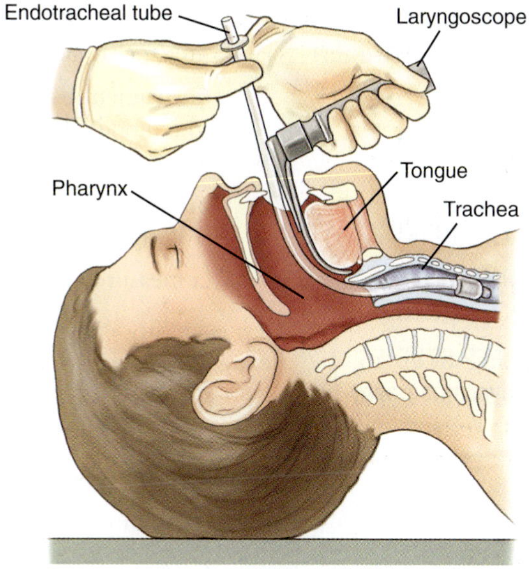

The physician is inserting a(an) ____________ / ____________ / ____________ tube,
within / trachea / pertaining to

using a(an) ____________ / ____ / ____________ to
larynx / cv / instrument used for visual examination

guide the tube into place.

TERM	DEFINITION
laryngoscope (la-RING-go-skōp)	instrument used for visual examination of the larynx (Exercise Figure G)
laryngoscopy (*lar*-in-GOS-ko-pē)	visual examination of the larynx
thoracoscope (tho-RAK-ō-skōp)	instrument used for visual examination of the chest cavity (Fig. 5.11)
thoracoscopy (*thor*-a-KOS-ko-pē)	visual examination of the chest cavity
DIAGNOSTIC IMAGING	
radiograph (RĀ-dē-ō-graph)	record of x-rays (Fig. 5.13B)
radiography (rā-dē-OG-rah-fē)	process of recording x-rays
sonogram (SON-ō-gram)	record of sound (Fig. 5.19B)
sonography (so-NOG-rah-fē)	process of recording sound (Fig. 5.19A)
tomography (to-MOG-rah-fē)	process of recording slices (anatomical cross section) (Fig. 5.14)

EXERCISE FIGURE **H**

Fill in the blanks to complete labeling of the diagram.

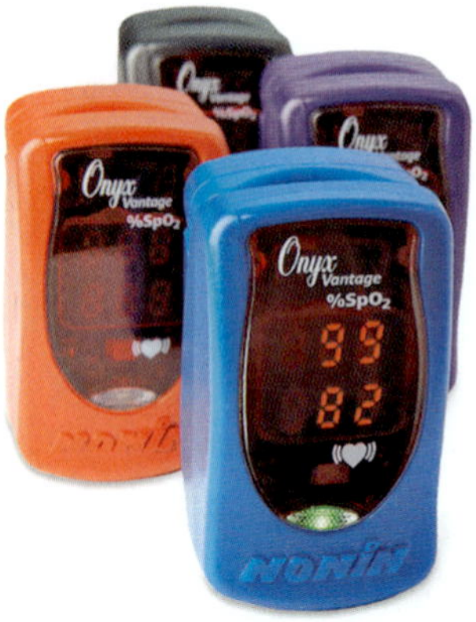

1. Pulse ______ / ______ / ______
oxygen / CV / instrument used to measure

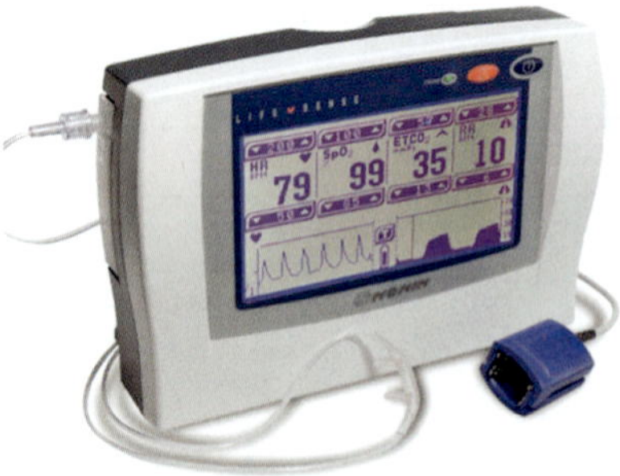

2. ______ / ______ / ______
carbon dioxide / CV / instrument used to measure

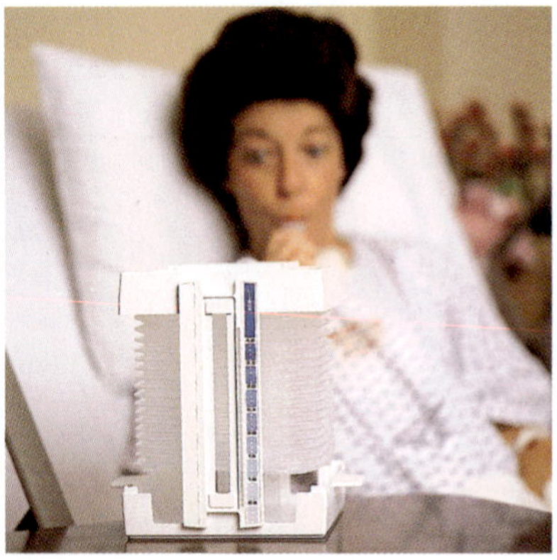

3. ______ / ______ / ______
breathing / CV / instrument used to measure

Diagnostic Terms—cont'd

TERM	DEFINITION
PULMONARY FUNCTION	
capnometer (kap-NOM-e-ter)	instrument used to measure carbon dioxide (levels in expired gas) (Exercise Figure H2)
oximeter (ok-SIM-e-ter)	instrument used to measure oxygen (saturation in the blood) (Exercise Figure H1) *(Note: the combining vowel is i.)*
spirometer (spī-ROM-e-ter)	instrument used to measure breathing (or lung volumes) (Exercise Figure H3)
spirometry (spī-ROM-e-trē)	a measurement of breathing (or air flow)
SLEEP STUDIES	
polysomnography (PSG) (*pol*-ē-som-NOG-rah-fē)	process of recording many (tests) during sleep (performed to diagnose obstructive sleep apnea [see Fig. 5.7]). Tests include **electrocardiography, electromyography, electroencephalography, air flow monitoring,** and **oximetry.**

SLEEP TECHNOLOGIST

To see an interview with a **registered sleep technologist**, go to Evolve Resources at evolve.elsevier.com and select Career Videos located under the Extra Content tab on the Practice Student Resources menu.

See **Appendix B** for instructions.

EXERCISE 25

Practice saying aloud each of the Diagnostic Terms Built from Word Parts.

To hear the terms, go to Evolve Resources at evolve.elsevier.com and select:
Practice Student Resources > Student Resources > Chapter 5 > **Pronounce and Spell**

See Appendix B for instructions.

❑ Check the box when complete.

EXERCISE 26

Analyze and define the following terms by drawing slashes between word parts, writing word part abbreviations above the term, underlining combining forms, and writing combining form abbreviations below the term.

EXAMPLE:

WR CV S
bronch / o / scopy
CF
visual examination of the bronchi

1. spirometer
2. laryngoscope
3. capnometer
4. spirometry
5. oximeter
6. laryngoscopy
7. bronchoscope
8. thoracoscope
9. endoscope
10. thoracoscopy
11. endoscopic
12. endoscopy
13. polysomnography
14. sonogram
15. sonography
16. tomography

17. radiograph

____

____

18. radiography

____

____

EXERCISE 27

Build diagnostic terms for the following definitions by using the word parts you have learned.

EXAMPLE: instrument used to measure oxygen ox / i / meter (WR / CV / S)

1. visual examination of the larynx ______ WR / CV / S
2. instrument used to measure breathing ______ WR / CV / S
3. instrument used to measure carbon dioxide ______ WR / CV / S
4. instrument used for visual examination of the larynx ______ WR / CV / S
5. visual examination of the bronchi ______ WR / CV / S
6. measurement of breathing ______ WR / CV / S
7. instrument used for visual examination of the bronchi ______ WR / CV / S
8. visual examination within (a hollow organ or body cavity ______ P / S(WR)
9. instrument used for visual examination of the chest cavity ______ WR / CV / S
10. instrument used for visual examination within (a hollow organ or body cavity) ______ P / S(WR)
11. visual examination of the chest cavity ______ WR / CV / S
12. pertaining to visual examination within (a hollow organ or body cavity) ______ P / S(WR)
13. process of recording of many (tests) during sleep ______ P / WR / CV / S

14. process of recording x-rays ______ WR / CV / ______ S

15. record of x-rays ______ WR / CV / ______ S

16. process of recording sound ______ WR / CV / ______ S

17. record of sound ______ WR / CV / ______ S

18. process of recording slices (anatomical cross sections) ______ WR / CV / ______ S

EXERCISE 28

Spell each of the Diagnostic Terms Built from Word Parts by having someone dictate them to you. Use a separate sheet of paper.

> To hear and spell the terms, go to Evolve Resources at evolve.elsevier.com and select:
> Practice Student Resources > Student Resources > Chapter 5 > **Pronounce and Spell**
>
> See Appendix B for instructions.

❑ Check the box when complete.

Diagnostic Terms
NOT BUILT FROM WORD PARTS

Word parts may be present in the following terms; however, their full meanings cannot be translated using definitions of word parts alone.

TERM	DEFINITION
DIAGNOSTIC IMAGING	
chest computed tomography (CT) scan (chest) (kom-PŪ-ted) (tō-MOG-ra-fē) (skan)	computerized radiographic images of the chest performed to diagnose tumors, abscesses, and pleural effusion (see Fig. 5.14)
chest radiograph (CXR) (chest) (RĀ-dē-ō-*graf*)	radiographic image of the chest performed to evaluate the lungs and the heart (also called a **chest x-ray**) (see Fig. 5.13)
lung ventilation/perfusion scan (VQ scan) (lung) (*ven*-ti-LĀ-shun) (per-FŪ-zhun) (skan)	two nuclear scan tests, one to measure air flow throughout the lungs (ventilation), and one to measure circulation to all areas of the lungs (perfusion). A VQ scan is used most often to help diagnose or rule out a pulmonary embolism (PE). (Fig. 5.16)
LABORATORY	
acid-fast bacilli (AFB) smear (AS-id-fast) (bah-SIL-ī) (smēr)	test performed on sputum to determine the presence of acid-fast bacilli, which cause tuberculosis

HELICAL COMPUTED TOMOGRAPHY (CT) SCAN

of the chest, also called **spiral CT scan,** is an improvement over standard CT and is the preferred study to identify pulmonary embolism. Images are continually obtained as the patient passes through the gantry, which is part of the scanner. It produces a more concise and faster image, which can be performed with one breath hold.

ACID-FAST

means not easily discolored by acid after staining.

Diagnostic Terms—cont'd

TERM	DEFINITION
sputum culture and sensitivity (C&S) (SPŪ-tum) (KUL-cher) (*sen*-si-TIV-i-tē)	test performed on sputum to determine the presence of pathogenic bacteria. Sputum is placed on a medium for growth (culture) and if pathogenic bacteria grow, is then tested for antibiotic sensitivity to identify an antibiotic that will provide the most effective treatment. C&S is used to identify the pathogen present and causing the infection.
PULMONARY FUNCTION	
arterial blood gases (ABGs) (ar-TĒ-rē-al) (blud) (GAS-es)	test performed on arterial blood to determine levels of oxygen (O_2), carbon dioxide (CO_2), and pH (acidity)
peak flow meter (PFM) (pēk) (flō) (MĒ-ter)	portable instrument used to measure air flow early in forced exhalation; helps monitor asthma and adjust medication accordingly
pulmonary function tests (PFTs) (PUL-mō-*nar*-ē) (FUNK-shun) (tests)	group of tests performed to measure breathing capacity and used to determine external respiratory function; when abnormal, they are useful in distinguishing COPD from asthma. Some tests involve the use of a spirometer.
pulse oximetry (puls) (ok-SIM-e-trē)	noninvasive method of measuring oxygen in the blood by using a device that attaches to the fingertip
OTHER	
auscultation (*aws*-kul-TĀ-shun)	the act of listening through a stethoscope for sounds within the body which are abnormal and that suggest abnormalities or disease; used for assessing and diagnosing conditions of the lungs, pleura, heart, arteries, and abdomen (Fig. 5.21).
percussion (per-KUSH-un)	the act of tapping of a body surface to determine the density of the part beneath by the sound obtained. A dull sound where normally a hollow sound would be elicited indicates displacement of air by fluid or solid waste in a body space or cavity such as in a potential pleural space (Fig. 5.22).
PPD skin test (P-P-D) (skin) (test)	test performed on individuals who have recently been exposed to tuberculosis. PPD (purified protein derivative) of the tuberculin bacillus is injected intradermally. Positive tests indicate previous exposure, not necessarily active tuberculosis (also called **TB skin test**).
stethoscope (STETH-ō-skōp)	instrument used to hear internal body sounds; used for performing auscultation and blood pressure measurement

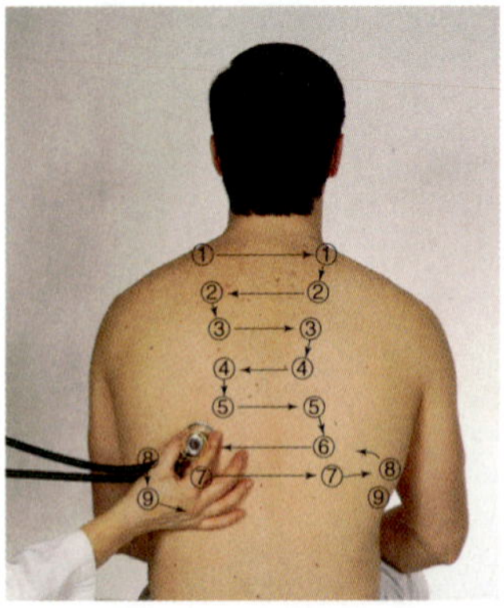

FIG. 5.21 Auscultation.

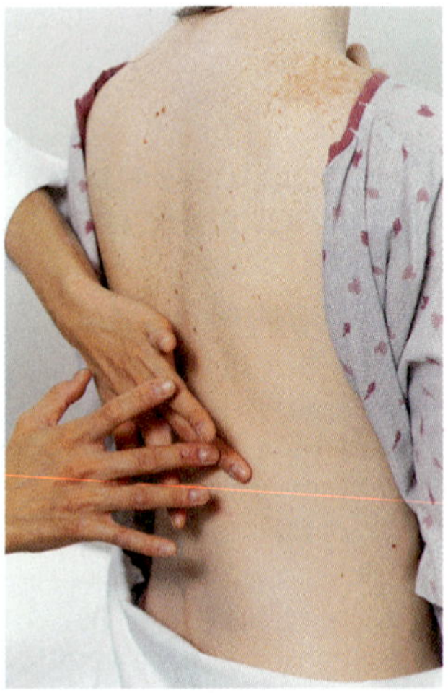
FIG. 5.22 Percussion.

EXERCISE 29

Practice saying aloud each of the Diagnostic Terms NOT Built from Word Parts.

To hear the terms, go to Evolve Resources at evolve.elsevier.com and select:
Practice Student Resources > Student Resources > Chapter 5 > **Pronounce and Spell**

See Appendix B for instructions.

❑ Check the box when complete.

EXERCISE 30

A. Fill in the blanks with the correct terms.

1. A test performed on sputum to diagnose tuberculosis is called ________________.
2. ________________ is the name of a group of tests performed on breathing capacity to determine external respiratory function or abnormalities.
3. An act that involves tapping a body surface is called ________________.
4. The act of listening for sounds which are abnormal within the body through a stethoscope is called ________________.
5. A test performed on sputum to determine the presence of pathogenic bacteria is called ________________.

B. Write the medical term pictured and defined.

1. ________________
test performed by intradermal injection on individuals who have recently been exposed to tuberculosis

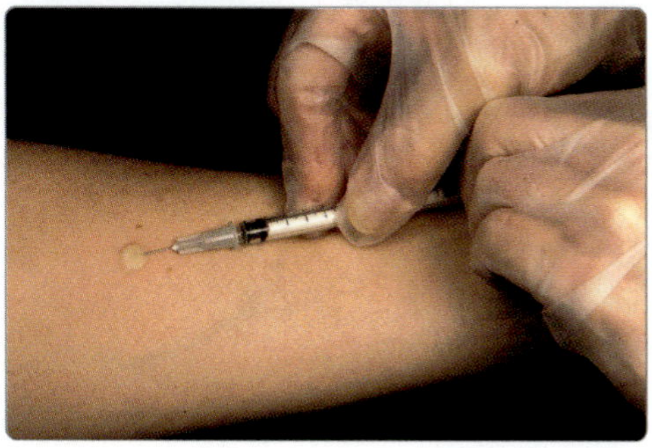

2. ________________
portable instrument used to measure air flow in forced exhalation; helps monitor asthma and adjust medication accordingly

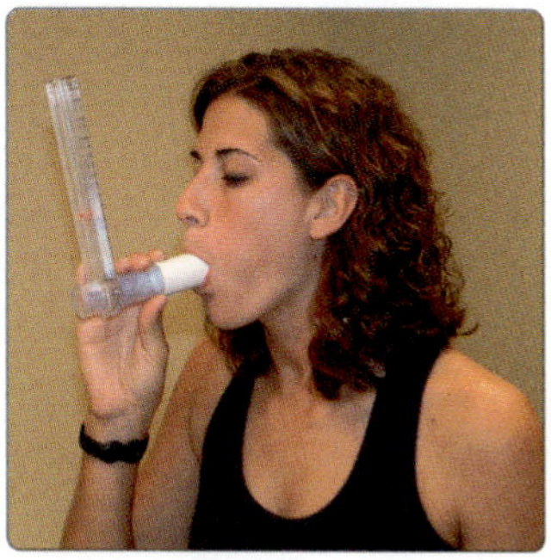

EXERCISE 30 *Pictured and Defined—cont'd*

3. ______________________________

test performed on arterial blood to determine levels of oxygen (O_2), carbon dioxide (CO_2), and pH (acidity)

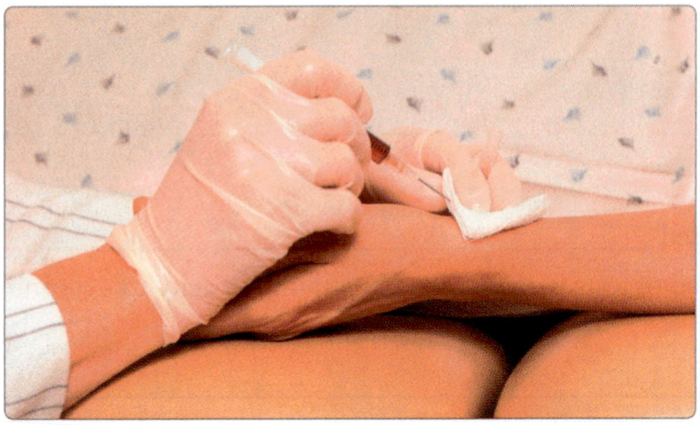

4. ______________________________

noninvasive method of measuring oxygen in the blood by using a device that attaches to the fingertip

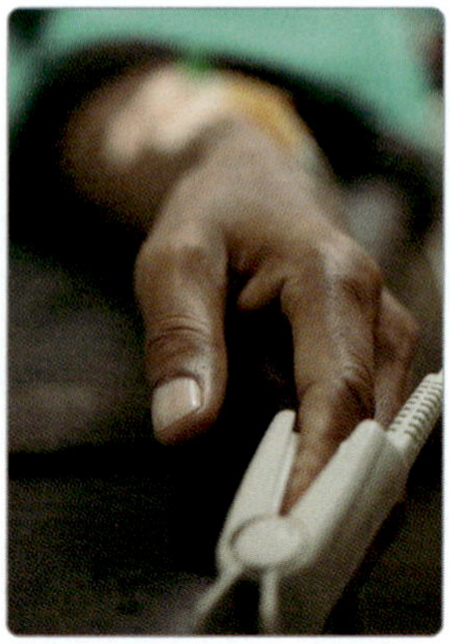

5. ______________________________

instrument used to hear internal body sounds; used for performing auscultation and blood pressure measurement

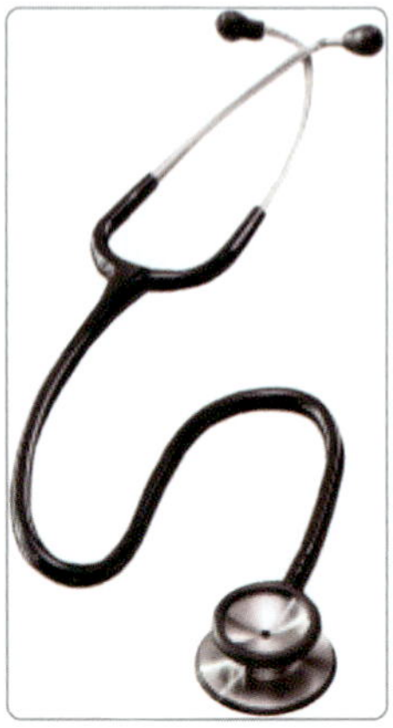

6. ______________________________

____

two nuclear scan tests used to help diagnose or rule out pulmonary embolism

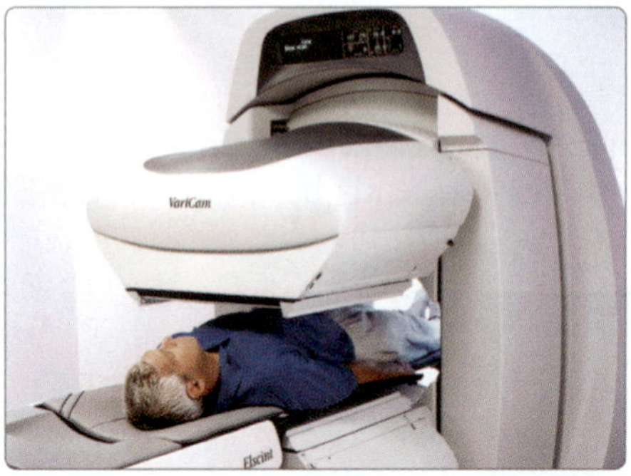

7. ______________________________

radiographic image of the chest performed to evaluate the lungs and the heart

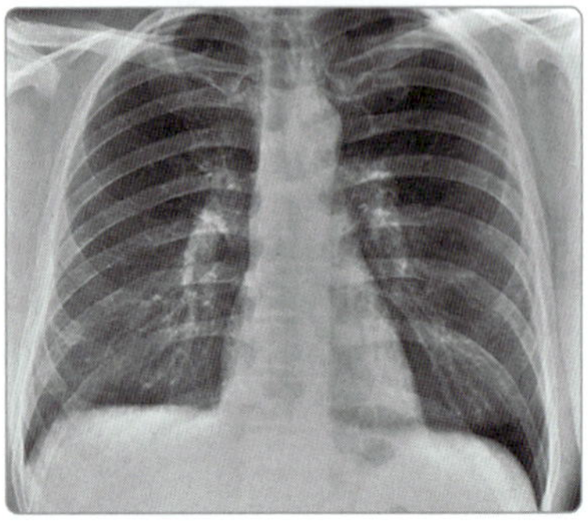

8. ______________________________

____

computerized radiographic images of the chest performed to diagnose tumors, abscesses, and pleural effusions

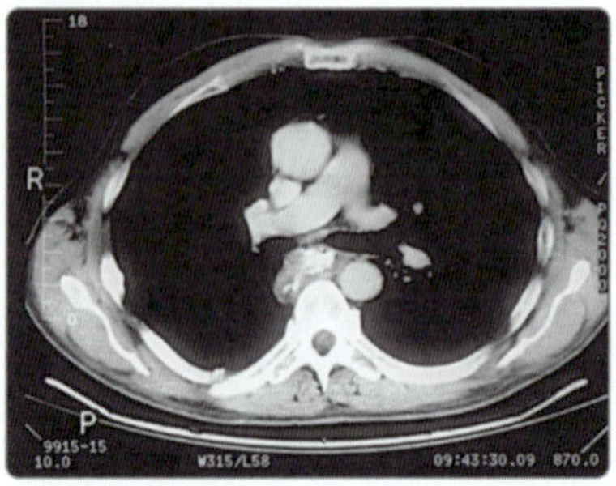

EXERCISE 31

Match the terms in the first column with their correct definitions in the second column.

_____ 1. lung ventilation/perfusion scan
_____ 2. chest radiograph
_____ 3. chest CT scan
_____ 4. acid-fast bacilli smear
_____ 5. pulse oximetry
_____ 6. arterial blood gases
_____ 7. pulmonary function tests
_____ 8. PPD skin test
_____ 9. auscultation
_____ 10. stethoscope
_____ 11. peak flow meter
_____ 12. percussion
_____ 13. sputum culture and sensitivity

a. computerized images of the chest
b. noninvasive method used to measure oxygen in the blood
c. arterial blood test used to determine levels of oxygen, carbon dioxide, and pH
d. test on sputum for tuberculosis
e. chest x-ray
f. nuclear medicine procedure used to diagnose pulmonary embolism
g. identifies which antibiotic will provide the most effective treatment
h. a group of tests performed to measure breathing capacity
i. test performed on individuals who may have been exposed to tuberculosis
j. instrument used for auscultation
k. used to help monitor asthma
l. the act of listening for sounds within the body through a stethoscope
m. the act of tapping a body surface to determine density

EXERCISE 32

Spell each of the Diagnostic Terms NOT Built from Word Parts by having someone dictate them to you. Use a separate sheet of paper.

> To hear and spell the terms, go to Evolve Resources at evolve.elsevier.com and select:
> Practice Student Resources > Student Resources > Chapter 5 > **Pronounce and Spell**
>
> See Appendix B for instructions.

❑ Check the box when complete.

Complementary Terms

BUILT FROM WORD PARTS

The following terms can be translated using definitions of word parts. Further explanation is provided within parentheses as needed.

TERM	DEFINITION
acapnia (a-CAP-nē-a)	condition of absence (less than normal level) of carbon dioxide (in the blood)
alveolar (al-VĒ-ō-lar)	pertaining to the alveolus
anoxia (a-NOK-sē-a)	condition of absence (deficiency) of oxygen
aphonia (ā-FŌ-nē-a)	condition of absence of voice
apnea (AP-nē-a)	absence of breathing

ANOXIA

literally means **without oxygen** or **absence of oxygen.** The term actually denotes an oxygen deficiency in the body tissues.

Complementary Terms—cont'd

TERM	DEFINITION
bronchoalveolar (*bron*-kō-al-VĒ-o-lar)	pertaining to the bronchi and alveoli
bronchospasm (BRON-kō-spaz-m)	spasmodic contraction of the bronchi
diaphragmatic (*dī*-a-frag-MAT-ik)	pertaining to the diaphragm (also called **phrenic**)
dysphonia (dis-FŌ-nē-a)	condition of difficult speaking (voice)
dyspnea (DISP-nē-a)	difficult breathing
endotracheal (*en*-dō-TRĀ-kē-al)	pertaining to within the trachea (see Exercise Figure F)
eupnea (ŪP-nē-a)	normal breathing
hypercapnia (*hī*-per-KAP-nē-a)	condition of excessive carbon dioxide (in the blood)
hyperpnea (*hī*-perp-NĒ-a)	excessive breathing
hypocapnia (*hī*-pō-KAP-nē-a)	condition of deficient carbon dioxide (in the blood)
hypopnea (hī-POP-nē-a)	deficient breathing
hypoxemia (*hī*-pok-SĒ-mē-a)	deficient oxygen in the blood *(Note: the o from hypo has been dropped. The final vowel in a prefix may be dropped when the word part to which it is added begins with a vowel.)*
hypoxia (hī-POK-sē-a)	condition of deficient oxygen (to the tissues) *(Note: see note for hypoxemia.)*
intrapleural (*in*-tra-PLUR-al)	pertaining to within the pleura (space between the two pleural membranes)
laryngeal (lar-IN-jē-al)	pertaining to the larynx
laryngospasm (la-RING-gō-spaz-m)	spasmodic contraction of the larynx
mucoid (MŪ-koyd)	resembling mucus
mucous (MŪ-kus)	pertaining to mucus
nasopharyngeal (*nā*-zō-fa-RIN-jē-al)	pertaining to the nose and pharynx
orthopnea (or-THOP-nē-a)	able to breathe easier in a straight (upright) position (difficulty breathing in the supine position)
phrenalgia (fre-NAL-ja)	pain in the diaphragm (also called **diaphragmalgia**)
phrenospasm (FREN-ō-spaz-m)	spasm of the diaphragm

MUCUS

is the noun that describes slimy fluid secreted by the mucous membrane. **Mucous** is the adjective that means pertaining to the mucous membrane. Pronunciation is the same for both terms.

TERM	DEFINITION
pulmonary (PUL-mō-*nar*-ē)	pertaining to the lungs
pulmonologist (*pul*-mon-OL-o-jist)	physician who studies and treats diseases of the lung
pulmonology (*pul*-mon-OL-o-jē)	study of the lung (a branch of medicine dealing with diseases of the lung)
radiologist (rā-dē-OL-o-jist)	physician who specializes in the diagnosis and treatment of disease using medical imaging (such as x-rays, computed tomography [CT], magnetic resonance imaging [MRI], nuclear medicine [NM], and sonography)
radiology (ra-dē-OL-o-jē)	study of x-rays (a branch of medicine concerned with the study and application of imaging technology including x-ray, computed tomography [CT], magnetic resonance imaging [MRI], nuclear medicine [NM], and sonography to diagnose and treat disease)
rhinorrhea (*rī*-nō-RĒ-a)	discharge from the nose (as in a cold)
tachypnea (tak-IP-nē-a)	rapid breathing
thoracic (thō-RAS-ik)	pertaining to the chest

EXERCISE 33

Practice saying aloud each of the Complementary Terms Built from Word Parts.

> To hear the terms, go to Evolve Resources at evolve.elsevier.com and select:
> Practice Student Resources > Student Resources > Chapter 5 > **Pronounce and Spell**
>
> See Appendix B for instructions.

❑ Check the box when complete.

EXERCISE 34

Analyze and define the following terms by drawing slashes between word parts, writing word part abbreviations above the term, underlining combining forms, and writing combining form abbreviations below the term.

EXAMPLE:

P WR S
hyper / capn / ia

condition of excessive carbon dioxide (in the blood)

1. laryngeal

____

____

2. eupnea

____

____

3. mucoid

____

____

4. apnea

____

____

5. hypoxia

____

____

6. laryngospasm

____

____

7. endotracheal

____

____

8. anoxia

____

____

9. dysphonia

____

____

10. bronchoalveolar

____

____

11. dyspnea

____

____

12. hypocapnia

____

____

13. bronchospasm

____

____

14. orthopnea

____

____

15. hyperpnea

____

____

16. acapnia

____

____

17. hypopnea

____

____

18. hypoxemia

____

____

19. aphonia

____

____

20. rhinorrhea

____

____

21. thoracic

____
____

22. mucous

____
____

23. nasopharyngeal

____
____

24. diaphragmatic

____
____

25. intrapleural

____
____

26. pulmonary

____
____

27. phrenalgia

____
____

28. tachypnea

____
____

29. phrenospasm

____
____

30. pulmonologist

____
____

31. pulmonology

____
____

32. alveolar

____
____

33. radiology

____
____

34. radiologist

____
____

EXERCISE 35

Build the complementary terms for the following definitions by using the word parts you have learned.

EXAMPLE: pertaining to bronchi and alveoli bronch / o / alveol / ar
WR / CV / WR / S

1. condition of deficient oxygen _______ / _______ / _______
P / WR / S

2. resembling mucus _______ / _______
WR / S

3. able to breathe easier in a straight (upright) position ______ WR / CV / ______ S

4. pertaining to within the trachea ______ P / ______ WR / ______ S

5. condition of absence of oxygen ______ P / ______ WR / ______ S

6. difficult breathing ______ P / ______ S(WR)

7. pertaining to the larynx ______ WR / ______ S

8. condition of excessive carbon dioxide (in the blood) ______ P / ______ WR / ______ S

9. normal breathing ______ P / ______ S(WR)

10. condition of absence of voice ______ P / ______ WR / ______ S

11. spasmodic contraction of the larynx ______ WR / CV / ______ S

12. condition of deficient carbon dioxide (in the blood) ______ P / ______ WR / ______ S

13. pertaining to the nose and pharynx ______ WR / CV / ______ WR / ______ S

14. pertaining to the diaphragm ______ WR / ______ S

15. condition of absence of breathing ______ P / ______ S(WR)

16. deficient oxygen in the blood ______ P / ______ WR / ______ S

17. excessive breathing ______ P / ______ S(WR)

18. spasmodic contraction of the bronchi ______ WR / CV / ______ S

19. deficient breathing ______ P / ______ S(WR)

20. condition of absence of carbon dioxide (in the blood) ______ P / ______ WR / ______ S

21. condition of difficulty in speaking (voice) ________ / ________ / ________
P / WR / S

22. discharge from the nose ________ / ___ / ________
WR / CV / S

23. pertaining to mucus ________ / ________
WR / S

24. pertaining to the chest ________ / ________
WR / S

25. pertaining to within the pleura ________ / ________ / ________
P / WR / S

26. pertaining to the lungs ________ / ________
WR / S

27. spasm of the diaphragm ________ / ___ / ________
WR / CV / S

28. rapid breathing ________ / ________
P / S(WR)

29. pain in the diaphragm ________ / ________
WR / S

30. pertaining to the alveolus ________ / ________
WR / S

31. study of the lung ________ / ___ / ________
WR / CV / S

32. physician who studies and treats diseases of the lung ________ / ___ / ________
WR / CV / S

33. physician who specializes in the use of x-rays, ultrasound, and magnetic fields in the diagnosis and treatment of disease ________ / ___ / ________
WR / CV / S

34. study of x-rays (a branch of medicine concerned with the use of x-rays, ultrasound, and magnetic fields to diagnose and treat disease) ________ / ___ / ________
WR / CV / S

EXERCISE 36

Spell each of the Complementary Terms Built from Word Parts by having someone dictate them to you. Use a separate sheet of paper.

> To hear and spell the terms, go to Evolve Resources at evolve.elsevier.com and select:
> Practice Student Resources > Student Resources > Chapter 5 > **Pronounce and Spell**
>
> See Appendix B for instructions.

❑ Check the box when complete.

Complementary Terms
NOT BUILT FROM WORD PARTS

Word parts may be present in the following terms; however, their full meanings cannot be translated using definitions of word parts alone.

TERM	DEFINITION
airway (ĀR-wā)	passageway by which air enters and leaves the lungs as well as a mechanical device used to keep the air passageway unobstructed
asphyxia (as-FIK-sē-a)	deprivation of oxygen for tissue use; suffocation
aspirate (AS-per-āt)	to withdraw fluid or suction fluid; also to draw foreign material into the respiratory tract
bronchoconstrictor (*bron*-kō-kon-STRIK-tor)	agent causing narrowing of the bronchi
bronchodilator (*bron*-kō-dī-LĀ-tor)	agent causing the bronchi to widen
crackles (KRAK-els)	discontinuous sounds heard primarily with a stethoscope during inspiration that resemble the sound of the rustling of cellophane; often heard at the base of the lung posteriorly in heart failure, pneumonia, and pulmonary fibrosis. (also called **rales**)
hyperventilation (*hī*-per-*ven*-ti-LĀ-shun)	ventilation of the lungs beyond normal body needs
hypoventilation (*hī*-pō-*ven*-ti-LĀ-shun)	ventilation of the lungs that does not fulfill the body's gas exchange needs
mucopurulent (*mū*-kō-PŪR-ū-lent)	containing both mucus and pus
mucus (MŪ-kus)	slimy fluid secreted by the mucous membranes
nebulizer (NEB-ū-lī-zer)	device that creates a mist used to deliver medication for giving respiratory treatment (Fig. 5.23)
nosocomial infection (nos-ō-KŌ-mē-al) (in-FEK-shun)	an infection acquired during hospitalization
paroxysm (PAR-ok-siz-em)	periodic, sudden attack
patent (PĀ-tent)	open, the opposite of closed or compromised, thus allowing passage of air, as in patent trachea and bronchi (can be applied to any tubular passageway in the body, as in a patent artery, allowing passage of blood)
rhonchi (RONG-kī)	low-pitched, with a snoring quality, breath sounds heard with a stethoscope suggesting secretions in the large airways

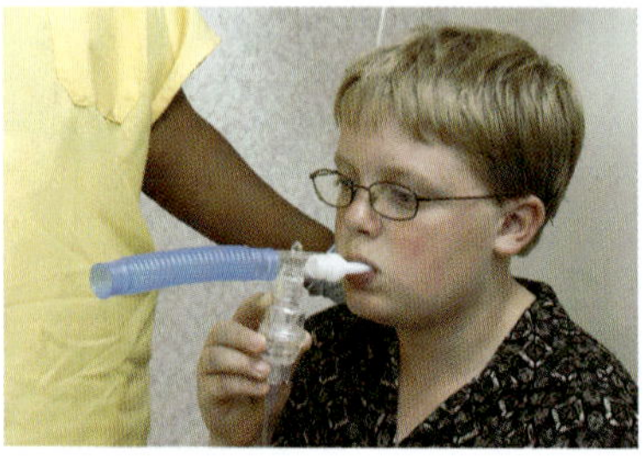

FIG. 5.23 Nebulizer.

TERM	DEFINITION
sputum (SPŪ-tum)	mucous secretion from the lungs, bronchi, and trachea expelled through the mouth
stridor (STRĪD-ir)	harsh, high-pitched breath sound heard on inspiration; indicates an acute laryngeal obstruction
ventilator (VEN-ti-*lā*-tor)	mechanical device used to assist with or substitute for breathing (Fig. 5.24)

SPUTUM

is derived from the Latin **spuere**, meaning **to spit**. In a 1693 dictionary it is defined as a "secretion thicker than ordinary spittle."

Refer to **Appendix F** for pharmacology terms related to the respiratory system.

EXERCISE 37

Practice saying aloud each of the Complementary Terms NOT Built from Word Parts.

To hear the terms, go to Evolve Resources at evolve.elsevier.com and select:
Practice Student Resources > Student Resources > Chapter 5 > **Pronounce and Spell**

See Appendix B for instructions.

❑ Check the box when complete.

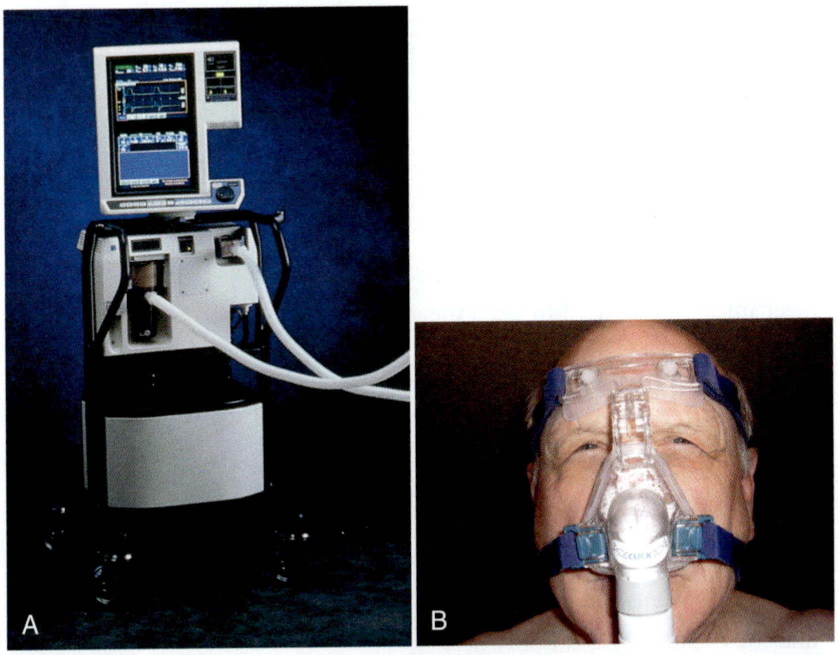

FIG. 5.24 A, Invasive ventilator. Positive pressure ventilator is applied to the patient's airway through an **endotracheal** or **tracheostomy** tube and is used when spontaneous breathing is inadequate to sustain life. **B,** CPAP (continuous positive airway pressure) is a noninvasive ventilation device used for patients who can initiate their own breathing and is often used to treat **obstructive sleep apnea**. BiPAP (bilevel positive airway pressure) not shown, is another noninvasive device that delivers two levels of pressure, one for inspiration, one for expiration whereas the CPAP machine delivers a predetermined level of pressure.

EXERCISE 38

Fill in the blanks with the correct terms.

1. Another term for ventilation of the lungs beyond normal body needs is ________________________.
2. A device that creates a mist used to deliver medication for giving respiratory treatment is a(n) ________________.
3. A(n) ________________________________ is an agent that causes the air passages to widen.
4. A patient who has difficulty breathing can be attached to a mechanical breathing device called a(n) ________________________________.
5. Another term for suffocation is ________________________________.
6. Material made up of mucous secretions from the lungs, bronchi, and trachea, expelled through the mouth, is called ________________________________.
7. To suction or withdraw fluid is to ________________________________.
8. A(n) ________________ is a mechanical device that keeps the air passageway unobstructed.
9. Harsh, high pitched, breath sound heard on inspiration is called ________________________.
10. Low-pitched breath sounds heard with a stethoscope are called ________________________.
11. Material containing both mucus and pus is referred to as being ________________________.
12. ________________ is the name given to ventilation of the lungs that does not fulfill the body's gas exchange needs.
13. An infection acquired during hospitalization is called ________________________.
14. The term that applies to a periodic, sudden attack is ________________________.
15. An airway must be kept ________________ (open) for the patient to breathe.
16. An agent that causes bronchi to narrow is called a(n) ________________________.
17. ________________ is the name given to the slimy fluid secreted by the mucous membranes.
18. Resembling the sound of rustling cellophane, ________________ may be a presenting sign in pneumonia.

EXERCISE 39

Match the terms in the first column with their correct definitions in the second column.

______ 1. airway	a. sounds that suggest secretions in the large airways
______ 2. aspirate	b. mechanical device used to keep the air passageway unobstructed
______ 3. bronchoconstrictor	c. agent that narrows the bronchi
______ 4. bronchodilator	d. discontinuous sounds heard mainly at the base of the lungs with a stethoscope during inspiration
______ 5. rhonchi	e. suffocation
______ 6. crackles	f. ventilation of the lungs beyond normal body needs
______ 7. hyperventilation	g. to draw foreign material into the respiratory tract
______ 8. asphyxia	h. agent that widens the bronchi
______ 9. stridor	i. indicates acute laryngeal obstruction

EXERCISE 40

Match the terms in the first column with their correct definitions in the second column.

______ 1. hypoventilation	a. open
______ 2. mucopurulent	b. mucous secretion from lungs, bronchi, and trachea, expelled through the mouth
______ 3. mucus	c. respiratory treatment device that sends a mist
______ 4. nebulizer	d. mechanical breathing device
______ 5. nosocomial	e. ventilation of the lungs that does not fulfill the body's gas exchange needs
______ 6. patent	f. periodic, sudden attack
______ 7. sputum	g. containing both mucus and pus
______ 8. ventilator	h. slimy fluid secreted by mucous membranes
______ 9. paroxysm	i. hospital-acquired infection

EXERCISE 41

Spell each of the Complementary Terms NOT Built from Word Parts by having someone dictate them to you. Use a separate sheet of paper.

To hear and spell the terms, go to Evolve Resources at evolve.elsevier.com and select:
Practice Student Resources > Student Resources > Chapter 5 > **Pronounce and Spell**

See Appendix B for instructions.

❑ Check the box when complete.

Abbreviations

ABBREVIATION	TERM
ABGs	arterial blood gases
AFB	acid-fast bacilli
ARDS	acute respiratory distress syndrome
C&S	culture and sensitivity
CAP	community-acquired pneumonia
CF	cystic fibrosis
CO_2	carbon dioxide
COPD	chronic obstructive pulmonary disease
CPAP	continuous positive airway pressure
CT	computed tomography
CXR	chest radiograph (chest x-ray)
flu	influenza
HAP	hospital-acquired pneumonia
IPF	idiopathic pulmonary fibrosis
LLL	left lower lobe
LTB	laryngotracheobronchitis
LUL	left upper lobe
O_2	oxygen
OSA	obstructive sleep apnea
PE	pulmonary embolism

For additional information on diseases of the lung, visit the **American Lung Association** at *www.lung.org*.

Abbreviations—cont'd

ABBREVIATION	TERM
PFM	peak flow meter
PFTs	pulmonary function tests
PSG	polysomnography
RLL	right lower lobe
RML	right middle lobe
RUL	right upper lobe
SOB	shortness of breath
TB	tuberculosis
URI	upper respiratory infection
VQ scan	lung ventilation/perfusion scan

Refer to **Appendix E** for a complete list of abbreviations.

EXERCISE 42

Write the terms abbreviated.

1. A variety of tests are used to diagnose **COPD** ____________ ____________ ____________ ____________, including:
   - **PFTs** ____________ ____________ ____________,
   - **CXR** ____________ ____________,
   - **ABGs** ____________ ____________ ____________, and
   - Chest **CT** ____________ ____________ scan.
2. **SOB** ____________ ____________ ____________ is often a symptom of COPD.
3. A. The lobes of the left lung are:
   - **LUL** ____________ ____________ ____________
   - **LLL** ____________ ____________ ____________

   B. The lobes of the right lung are **RUL** ____________ ____________ ____________
   - **RML** ____________ ____________ ____________
   - **RLL** ____________ ____________ ____________
4. **AFB** ____________ ____________ smear is used to support the diagnosis of **TB** ____________.
5. **PSG** ____________ is used to confirm the diagnosis of **OSA** ____________ ____________ ____________.
6. Respiration is the exchange of $\mathbf{O_2}$ ____________ and $\mathbf{CO_2}$ ____________ ____________ between the atmosphere and body cells.
7. Measurements obtained from using a **PFM** ____________ ____________ ____________ can be used to adjust medication for persons with asthma.

8. The etiology of **IPF** ____________ ____________ ____________ is unknown.
9. The patient had a persistent cough, hemoptysis, and fever. The chest radiograph was compatible with a pulmonary infection. The physician ordered a sputum **C&S** ____________ ____________ ____________ to determine the presence of pathogenic bacteria.
10. **HAP** ____________ ____________ ____________ is one type of nosocomial infection.
11. A **VQ scan** ______ ____________ ______ was ordered to rule out PE ____________ ____________.

EXERCISE 43

Write the terms abbreviated.

1. ARDS ____________ ____________ ____________ ____________
2. CF ____________ ____________
3. flu ____________
4. LTB ____________________________________
5. URI ____________ ____________ ____________
6. CPAP ____________ ____________ ____________ ____________
7. CAP ____________ ____________ ____________

TABLE 5.2 Common Abbreviations Used in the Respiratory Care Department within a Healthcare Facility

ABBREVIATION	TERM
BiPAP	bilevel positive airway pressure
CPT	chest physiotherapy
DPI	dry powder inhaler
HME	heat/moisture exchanger
IPPB	intermittent positive-pressure breathing
MDI	metered-dose inhaler
NIPPV	noninvasive positive-pressure ventilator
PEP	positive expiratory pressure
SVN	small-volume nebulizer
VAP	ventilator-associated pneumonia

For additional practice with Abbreviations, go to Evolve Resources at evolve.elsevier.com and select: Practice Student Resources > Student Resources > Chapter 5 > **Flashcards:** Abbreviations

See Appendix B for instructions.

PRACTICAL APPLICATION

EXERCISE 44 *Case Study: Translate Between Everyday Language and Medical Language*

CASE STUDY: Roberta Pawlaski

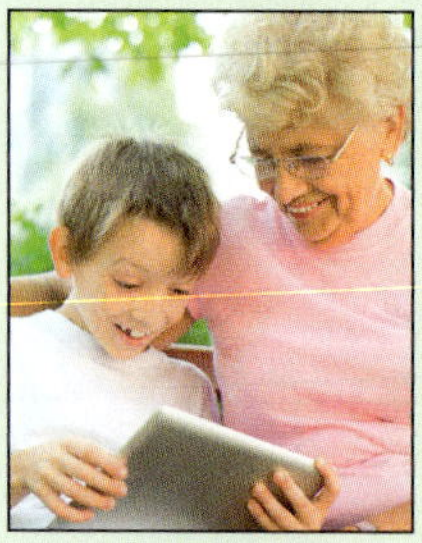

Roberta is experiencing difficulty breathing. She notices it gets worse when she tries to do chores around the house. This has been going on for about four days. She also has a cough and a runny nose. Today when she woke up she noticed that her throat was very sore. She also thinks that she might have a fever because she feels hot all over. She tried taking some over-the-counter cough medicine but this didn't seem to help. She notices when she coughs that a thick yellow mucus comes out. She hasn't had a cough like this since before she quit smoking about 10 years ago. She remembers that her grandson who stays with her after school has missed school because of a cold. She decides to call her doctor to schedule an appointment.

Now that you have worked through Chapter 5, on the respiratory system, consider the medical terms that might be used to describe Roberta's experience. See the Review of Terms at the end of the chapter for a list of terms that might apply.

A. *Underline phrases in the case study that could be substituted with medical terms.*

B. *Write the medical term and its definition for three of the phrases you underlined.*

MEDICAL TERM	DEFINITION
1. ____________________	______________________________
2. ____________________	______________________________
3. ____________________	______________________________

DOCUMENTATION: Excerpt from Hospital Admission Report

Roberta was able to see her primary care physician later that afternoon. In her electronic health record (EHR), it was noted in the Objective section of the report:

The patient is in no acute distress but exhibits dyspnea when walking. A fair amount of grey, mucoid, sputum was produced on forced cough. HEENT exam is normal except for erythema and swelling of the pharynx without exudates. Tympanic membranes are clear. There is a moderate amount of purulent rhinorrhea. The nasal mucosa is moderately swollen. Auscultation of the heart reveals a regular rhythm without a murmur, gallop, or rub. The chest is dull to percussion at the right lower base and there are crackles and rhonchi as well.

C. *Underline medical terms presented in Chapter 5 used in the previous excerpt from Roberta's medical record. See the Review of Terms at the end of the chapter for a complete list.*

D. *Select and define three of the medical terms you underlined. To check your answers, go to Appendix A.*

MEDICAL TERM	DEFINITION
1. ____________________	______________________________
2. ____________________	______________________________
3. ____________________	______________________________

EXERCISE 45 *Interact with Medical Documents and Electronic Health Records*

A. Read the report and complete it by writing medical terms on answer lines within the document. Definitions of terms to be written appear after the document.

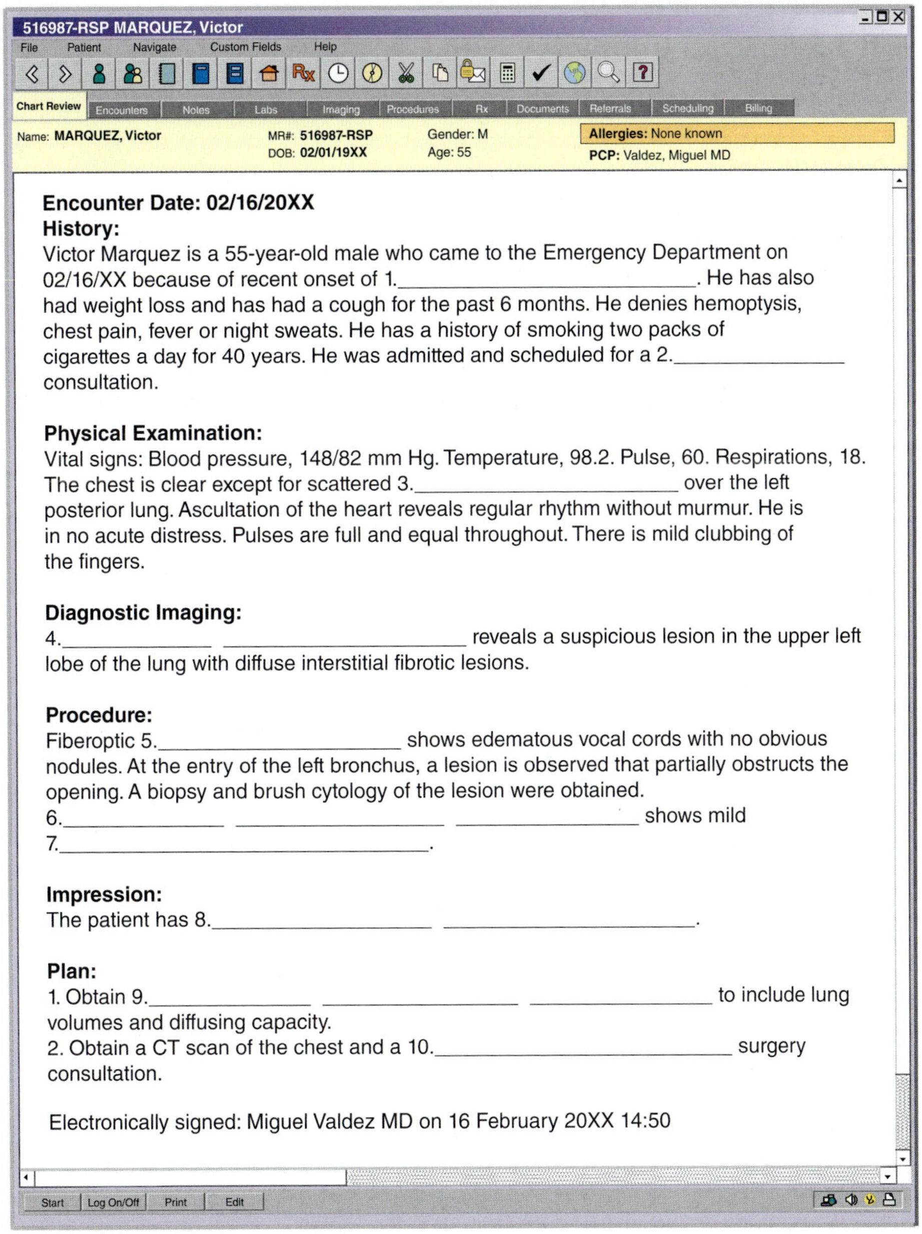

516987-RSP MARQUEZ, Victor

File Patient Navigate Custom Fields Help

Chart Review | Encounters | Notes | Labs | Imaging | Procedures | Rx | Documents | Referrals | Scheduling | Billing

Name: **MARQUEZ, Victor** MR#: **516987-RSP** DOB: **02/01/19XX** Gender: M Age: 55 **Allergies:** None known **PCP:** Valdez, Miguel MD

Encounter Date: 02/16/20XX

History:

Victor Marquez is a 55-year-old male who came to the Emergency Department on 02/16/XX because of recent onset of 1.____________________. He has also had weight loss and has had a cough for the past 6 months. He denies hemoptysis, chest pain, fever or night sweats. He has a history of smoking two packs of cigarettes a day for 40 years. He was admitted and scheduled for a 2.________________ consultation.

Physical Examination:

Vital signs: Blood pressure, 148/82 mm Hg. Temperature, 98.2. Pulse, 60. Respirations, 18. The chest is clear except for scattered 3.____________________ over the left posterior lung. Ascultation of the heart reveals regular rhythm without murmur. He is in no acute distress. Pulses are full and equal throughout. There is mild clubbing of the fingers.

Diagnostic Imaging:

4.____________ ____________________ reveals a suspicious lesion in the upper left lobe of the lung with diffuse interstitial fibrotic lesions.

Procedure:

Fiberoptic 5.____________________ shows edematous vocal cords with no obvious nodules. At the entry of the left bronchus, a lesion is observed that partially obstructs the opening. A biopsy and brush cytology of the lesion were obtained.

6.____________ ________________ _______________ shows mild 7.____________________________.

Impression:

The patient has 8.__________________ ____________________.

Plan:

1. Obtain 9.____________ ________________ _______________ to include lung volumes and diffusing capacity.
2. Obtain a CT scan of the chest and a 10.________________________ surgery consultation.

Electronically signed: Miguel Valdez MD on 16 February 20XX 14:50

Start | Log On/Off | Print | Edit

Definitions of Medical Terms to Complete the Document

Write the medical terms defined on corresponding answer lines in the document.

1. difficult breathing
2. pertaining to the lungs
3. low pitched with a snoring quality breath sounds heard with a stethoscope
4. radiographic image used to evaluate the lungs and heart
5. visual examination of the bronchi
6. test performed on arterial blood to determine the presence of oxygen, carbon dioxide, and other gases
7. deficient oxygen in the blood
8. cancerous tumor originating in the bronchus
9. group of tests performed on breathing
10. pertaining to the chest

EXERCISE 45 *Interact with Medical Documents and Electronic Health Records—cont'd*

B. Read the medical report and answer the questions below it.

7463802 FRANK, Abigail

File Patient Navigate Custom Fields Help

Chart Review | Encounters | Notes | Labs | Imaging | Procedures | Rx | Documents | Referrals | Scheduling | Billing

Name: **FRANK, Abigail** MR#: **7463802** DOB: 10/15/19XX Gender: F Age: 47 **Allergies:** Penicillan **PCP:** Irene Buchanan MD

Date: 11/16/20XX
Radiology Report: CT CHEST W/CONTRAST AT 1117 HOURS
Exam: CT OF THE CHEST
History: Cervical cancer
Technique: Multiple contiguous axial images were obtained to the chest during the uneventful infusion of **intravenous** contrast.

Findings: There has been interval decrease in size of **bilateral pulmonary metastases.** Again the largest is noted within the left lower lobe and measures 4.8 x 3.9 cm compared to 6.5 x 5.0 cm previously. Multiple smaller **lesions** within both **lungs** have decreased in size.

No significant **adenopathy** is identified. Postsurgical changes centrally within the right lower **lobe** are again noted with a surgical staple in place. There has been interval development of several patchy probably interstitial opacities within both lungs. Some are located adjacent to **metastases** that have decreased in size.

No new masses are noted. There is no pericardial or pleural effusion. The osseous structures remain within normal limits.

A left adrenal **nodule** remains essentially unchanged measuring approximately 2 cm in greatest dimension.

Impression: Interval decrease in size of **bilateral pulmonary metastases** as described following **chemotherapy** and **radiation therapy**. Development of occasional patchy predominately interstitial opacities. Given the history of **chemotherapy** and **radiation therapy** this likely reflects a postradiation or post-therapeutic **pneumonitis** or hyper-sensitivity. Additional considerations are an infectious **pneumonitis** or hemorrhage. Continued follow-up is recommended. Stable small left adrenal **nodule**.

Electronically signed: Radiologist Brian Benson DO, 11/16/20XX 14:30

Start | Log On/Off | Print | Edit

Use the medical report above to answer the questions.

_____ 1. The diagnostic imaging exam performed uses
   a. combined series of cross-sectional x-rays
   b. ionizing radiation produced by a light source
   c. mathematically constructed images and magnetic fields
   d. radiopharmaceuticals

2. **T F** Fluid is present in the pleural space.

3. **T F** Following chemotherapy and radiation, metastases in one lung was decreased.

4. **T F** The patchy interstitial opacities likely reflect a postradiation or post-therapeutic inflammation of the lung.

C. Complete the **three medical documents** within the electronic health record (EHR) on Evolve.

Topic: COPD
Documents: Progress Note, Radiology Report, Pulmonary Function Department Note

To complete the three medical records, go to Evolve Resources at evolve.elsevier.com and select:
Practice Student Resources > Student Resources > Chapter 5 > **Electronic Heath Records**

See Appendix B for instructions.

Healthcare records are stored and used in an electronic system called **Electronic Health Records (EHR)**. Electronic health records contain a collection of health information of an individual patient; the digitally formatted record can be shared through computer networks with patients, physicians, and other healthcare providers.

EXERCISE 46 *Pronounce Medical Terms in Use*

Practice pronunciation of terms by reading aloud the following paragraph. Use the phonetic spellings following medical terms from the chapter to assist with pronunciation. The script also contains medical terms not presented in the chapter. Treat them as information only or, if interested, research their meanings using a medical dictionary and reliable online sources.

A 24-year-old man visited the emergency department because of **dyspnea** (DISP-nē-a), **hyperpnea** (hī-perp-NĒ-a), and **paroxysms** (PAR-ok-sizms) of cough and the presence productive of thick, tenacious **mucus** (MŪ-kus). He had a history of **asthma** (AZ-ma) since the age of 12 years. A chest radiograph was negative for **pneumonia** (nū-MŌ-nē-a). **Arterial blood gases** (ar-TĒ-rē-al) (blud) (GAS-es) showed **hypoxemia** (hī-pok-SĒ-mē-a) but no **hypercapnia** (hī-per-KAP-nē–a). **Pulmonary function tests** (PUL-mō-ner-ē) (FUNK-shun) (tests) disclosed bronchoconstriction, which was corrected by a **bronchodilator** (*bron*-kō–dī-LĀ-tor). A **nebulizer** (NEB-ū-lī-zer) was prescribed for treatment. The asthma attack was probably precipitated by an episode of **bronchitis** (bron-KĪ-tis).

EXERCISE 47 *Chapter Content Quiz*

Test your understanding of terms and abbreviations introduced in this chapter. Circle the letter for the medical term or abbreviation related to the words in italics

1. The patient was admitted to the emergency department with a *severe nosebleed*.
   a. rhinomycosis
   b. epistaxis
   c. nasopharyngitis
2. The accident caused damage to the *larynx*, necessitating a *surgical repair*.
   a. laryngectomy
   b. laryngostomy
   c. laryngoplasty
3. Mr. Garcia was *able to breathe easier in an upright position*, so the nurse recorded that he had:
   a. orthopnea
   b. eupnea
   c. dyspnea
4. The *test on arterial blood to determine oxygen, carbon dioxide, and pH levels* indicated that the patient was *deficient in oxygen*, or had:
   a. pulse oximetry, dysphonia
   b. pulmonary functions tests, hypocapnia
   c. arterial blood gases, hypoxia

5. The physician informed the patient that a heart attack was not the cause of the *chest pain.*
   a. thoracalgia
   b. pneumothorax
   c. thoracentesis

6. The patient reported dizziness brought on by *ventilation of the lungs beyond normal bodily needs.*
   a. hyperventilation
   b. hypoventilation
   c. dysphonia

7. The physician wished the patient to have the medication given by a *device that delivers mist*, so she ordered that the treatment be given by:
   a. airway
   b. nebulizer
   c. ventilator

8. The patient with *blood in the chest cavity* was diagnosed as having:
   a. pneumothorax
   b. pleuritis
   c. hemothorax

9. After surgery, the patient had *foreign matter causing* a *block in the circulation to the pulmonary artery.*
   a. pleural effusion
   b. pulmonary edema
   c. pulmonary embolism

10. The patient was diagnosed as having *a fungal disease affecting the lung.*
    a. obstructive sleep apnea
    b. coccidioidomycosis
    c. tuberculosis

11. The physician ordered a *radiographic image of the chest* because he suspected *community-acquired pneumonia.*
    a. chest radiograph, CAP
    b. chest CT scan, CPAP
    c. bronchoscopy, HAP

12. The patient received an *intradermal injection* to determine if she had been exposed to TB.
    a. AFB
    b. ABGs
    c. PPD skin test

13. The patient was experiencing *rapid breathing.*
    a. phrenospasm
    b. tachypnea
    c. phrenalgia

14. The nurse practitioner heard *discontinuous sounds during respiration that resembled the sound of the rustling of cellophane.*
    a. stridor
    b. rhonchi
    c. crackles

15. A radiographic technician, an employee of the hospital diagnostic imaging department, uses an x-ray machine to create a *record of x-rays*, which is interpreted by *a physician who specializes in the study and application of imaging technology.*
    a. sonogram, pulmonologist
    b. radiograph, radiologist
    c. tomography, pathologist

16. The physician ordered an *AFB* smear to confirm the diagnosis of *TB.*
    a. diagnostic imaging procedure, cystic fibrosis
    b. endoscopy procedure, influenza
    c. laboratory test, tuberculosis

For additional practice with Chapter Content, go to Evolve Resources at evolve.elsevier.com and select:
Practice Student Resources > Student Resources > Chapter 5 > **Games:** Medical Millionaire, Tournament of Terminology
Practice Quizzes: Word Parts, Terms Built from Word Parts, Terms NOT Built from Word Parts, Abbreviations

See Appendix B for instructions.

C CHAPTER REVIEW

REVIEW OF CHAPTER CONTENT ON EVOLVE RESOURCES

Go to evolve.elsevier.com and click on Gradable Student Resources and Practice Student Resources. Online learning activities found there can be used to review chapter content and to assess your learning of word parts, medical terms, and abbreviations. Place check marks in the boxes next to activities used for review and assessment.

GRADABLE STUDENT RESOURCES

Chapter 05 >	Exercises >	□ Word Parts □ Terms Built from Word Parts □ Terms Not Built from Word Parts □ Abbreviations
	Quizzes >	□ Quiz 1: Disease and Disorder Terms □ Quiz 2: Surgical Terms □ Quiz 3: Diagnostic Terms □ Quiz 4: Complementary Terms

PRACTICE STUDENT RESOURCES > STUDENT RESOURCES

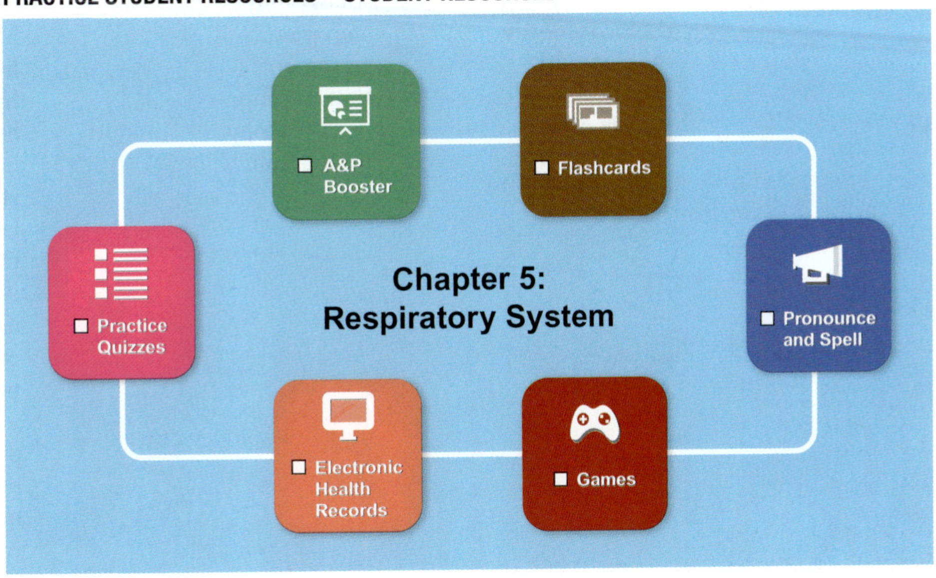

REVIEW OF WORD PARTS

Can you define and spell the following word parts?

COMBINING FORMS			PREFIXES	SUFFIXES	
adenoid/o	muc/o	py/o	a-	-algia	-pexy
alveol/o	nas/o	radi/o	an-	-ar	-pnea
atel/o	orth/o	rhin/o	endo-	-ary	-rrhagia
bronch/o	ox/i	sept/o	eu-	-cele	-scope
bronchi/o	pharyng/o	sinus/o	poly-	-centesis	-scopic
capn/o	phon/o	somn/o	tachy-	-eal	-scopy
diaphragmat/o	phren/o	son/o		-ectasis	-spasm
epiglott/o	pleur/o	spir/o		-emia	-stenosis
hem/o	pneum/o	thorac/o		-gram	-stomy
hemat/o	pneumat/o	tom/o		-graph	-thorax
laryng/o	pneumon/o	tonsill/o		-graphy	-tomy
lob/o	pulmon/o	trache/o		-meter	
				-metry	

REVIEW OF TERMS

Can you define, pronounce, and spell the following terms *built from word parts?*

DISEASES AND DISORDERS	SURGICAL	DIAGNOSTIC	COMPLEMENTARY
adenoiditis	adenoidectomy	bronchoscope	acapnia
alveolitis	adenotome	bronchoscopy	alveolar
atelectasis	bronchoplasty	capnometer	anoxia
bronchiectasis	laryngectomy	endoscope	aphonia
bronchitis	laryngoplasty	endoscopic	apnea
bronchogenic carcinoma	laryngostomy	endoscopy	bronchoalveolar
bronchopneumonia	laryngotracheotomy	laryngoscope	bronchospasm
diaphragmatocele	lobectomy	laryngoscopy	diaphragmatic
epiglottitis	pleuropexy	oximeter	dysphonia
hemothorax	pneumonectomy	polysomnography (PSG)	dyspnea
laryngitis	rhinoplasty	radiograph	endotracheal
laryngotracheobronchitis (LTB)	septoplasty	radiography	eupnea
lobar pneumonia	septotomy	sonogram	hypercapnia
nasopharyngitis	sinusotomy	sonography	hyperpnea
pharyngitis	thoracocentesis	spirometer	hypocapnia
pleuritis	thoracotomy	spirometry	hypopnea
pneumatocele	tonsillectomy	thoracoscope	hypoxemia
pneumoconiosis	tracheoplasty	thoracoscopy	hypoxia
pneumonia	tracheostomy	tomography	intrapleural
pneumonitis	tracheotomy		laryngeal
pneumothorax			laryngospasm
pulmonary neoplasm			mucoid
pyothorax			mucous
rhinitis			nasopharyngeal
rhinomycosis			orthopnea
rhinorrhagia			phrenalgia
sinusitis			phrenospasm
thoracalgia			pulmonary
tonsillitis			pulmonologist
tracheitis			pulmonology
tracheostenosis			radiologist
			radiology
			rhinorrhea
			tachypnea
			thoracic

Can you define, pronounce, and spell the following terms *NOT built from word parts?*

DISEASES AND DISORDERS	DIAGNOSTIC	COMPLEMENTARY
acute respiratory distress syndrome (ARDS)	acid-fast bacilli (AFB) smear	airway
asthma	arterial blood gases (ABGs)	asphyxia
chronic obstructive pulmonary disease (COPD)	auscultation	aspirate
coccidioidomycosis	chest computed tomography (CT) scan	bronchoconstrictor
croup	chest radiograph (CXR)	bronchodilator
cystic fibrosis (CF)	culture and sensitivity (C&S)	crackles
deviated septum	lung ventilation/perfusion scan (VQ scan)	hyperventilation
epistaxis	peak flow meter (PFM)	hypoventilation
idiopathic pulmonary fibrosis (IPF)	percussion	mucopurulent
influenza (flu)	PPD skin test	mucus
obstructive sleep apnea (OSA)	pulmonary function tests (PFTs)	nebulizer
pertussis	pulse oximetry	nosocomial infection
pleural effusion	sputum culture and sensitivity (C&S)	paroxysm
pulmonary edema	stethoscope	patent
pulmonary embolism (PE)		rhonchi
pulmonary emphysema		sputum
tuberculosis (TB)		stridor
upper respiratory infection (URI)		ventilator

Chapter 6 Urinary System

Objectives

Upon completion of this chapter you will be able to:

1. Pronounce organs and anatomic structures of the urinary system.
2. Define and spell word parts related to the urinary system.
3. Define, pronounce, and spell disease and disorder terms related to the urinary system.
4. Define, pronounce, and spell surgical terms related to the urinary system.
5. Define, pronounce, and spell diagnostic terms related to the urinary system.
6. Define, pronounce, and spell complementary terms related to the urinary system.
7. Interpret the meaning of abbreviations related to the urinary system.
8. Apply medical language in clinical contexts.

Outline

ANATOMY

Organs of the urinary system are the kidneys, ureters, bladder, and urethra (Figs. 6.1, 6.2, and 6.3).

Function

The urinary system removes waste material from the body, regulates fluid volume, maintains electrolyte concentration in the body fluid, and assists in blood pressure regulation. The kidneys secrete urine formed from water and waste materials such as urea, potassium chloride, sodium chloride, phosphates, and other elements. Urine is collected in the renal pelvis of the kidney and is transported through the ureters into the bladder, where it is stored until it can be eliminated. Urine passes from the bladder through the urethra and urinary meatus to the outside of the body (Fig. 6.4).

Organs and Anatomic Structures of the Urinary System

TERM	DEFINITION
kidneys (KID-nēz)	two bean-shaped organs located on each side of the vertebral column on the posterior wall of the abdominal cavity covered anteriorly by the parietal peritoneum. Their function is to remove waste products from the blood and to aid in maintaining water and electrolyte balances.
nephron (NEF-ron)	urine-producing microscopic structure. Approximately 1 million nephrons are located in each kidney.
glomerulus (pl. glomeruli) (glō-MER-ū-lus) (glō-MER-ū-lī)	cluster of capillaries at the entrance of the nephron. The process of filtering the blood, thereby forming urine, begins here.
renal pelvis (RĒ-nal) (PEL-vis)	funnel-shaped reservoir in the kidney that collects the urine and passes it to the ureter
hilum (HĪ-lum)	indentation on the medial side of the kidney where the renal artery, vein, and pelvis are located and the ureter leaves the kidney
ureters (Ū-re-ters)	two slender tubes, approximately 10 to 13 inches (26 to 33 cm) long, that receive the urine from the kidneys and carry it to the posterior portion of the bladder
urinary bladder (Ū-ri-nar-ē) (BLAD-er)	muscular, hollow organ that temporarily holds the urine. As it fills, the thick, muscular wall becomes thinner, and the organ increases in size.
urethra (ū-RĒ-thra)	lowest part of the urinary tract, through which the urine passes from the urinary bladder to the outside of the body. This narrow tube varies in length by sex. It is approximately 1.5 inches (3.8 cm) long in the female and approximately 8 inches (20 cm) in the male, in whom it is also part of the reproductive system. It carries seminal fluid (semen) at the time of ejaculation.
urinary meatus (Ū-ri-nar-ē) (mē-Ā-tus)	opening through which the urine passes to the outside

GLOMERULUS
is derived from the Latin **glomus,** which means **ball of thread.** It was thought that the rounded cluster of capillary loops at the nephron's entrance resembled thread in a ball.

BLADDER
is a derivative of the Anglo-Saxon **blaeddre,** meaning a **blister** or **windbag.**

MEATUS
is derived from the Latin **meare,** meaning **to pass** or **to go.** Other anatomic passages share the same name, such as the auditory meatus.

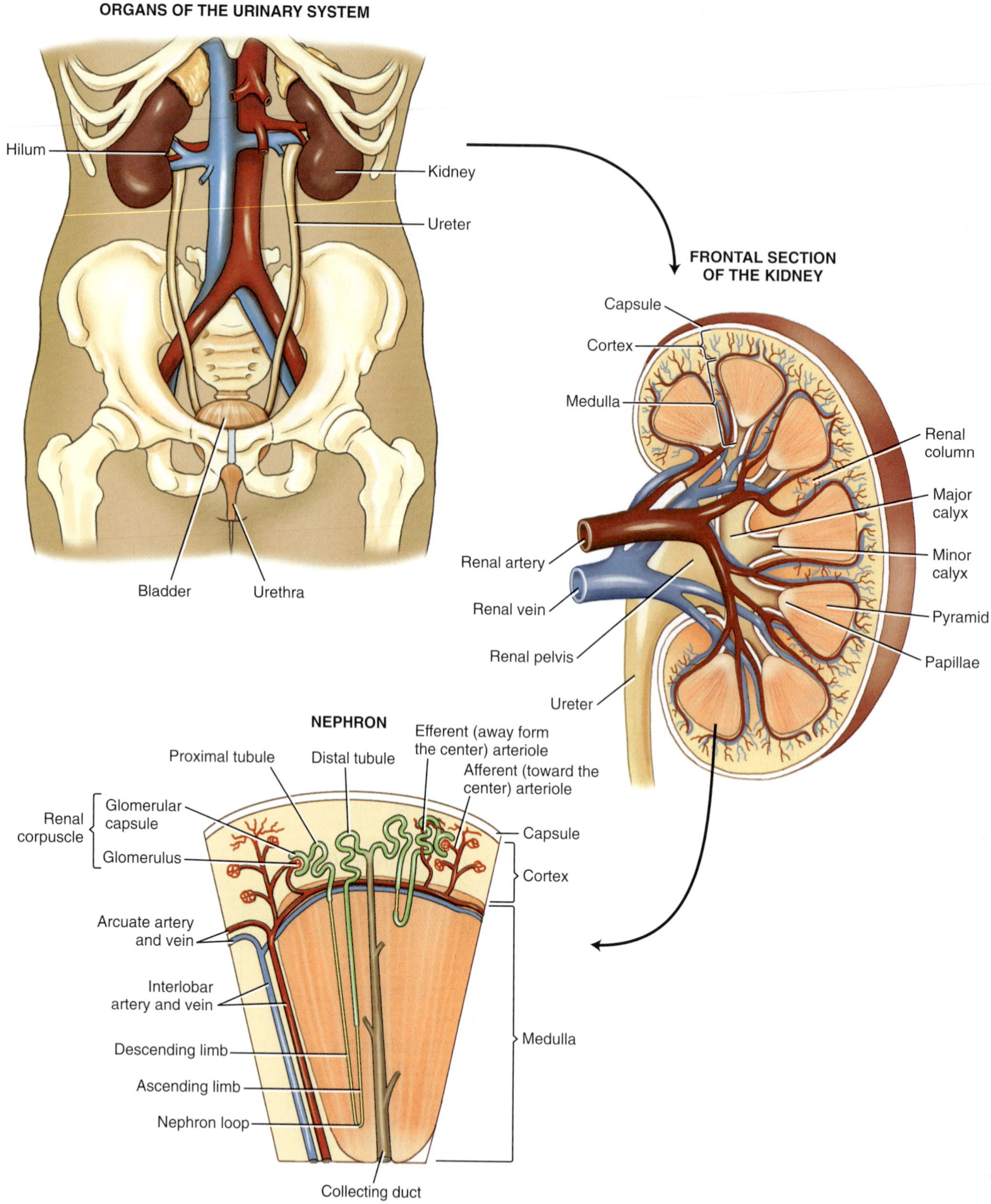

FIG. 6.1 The urinary system.

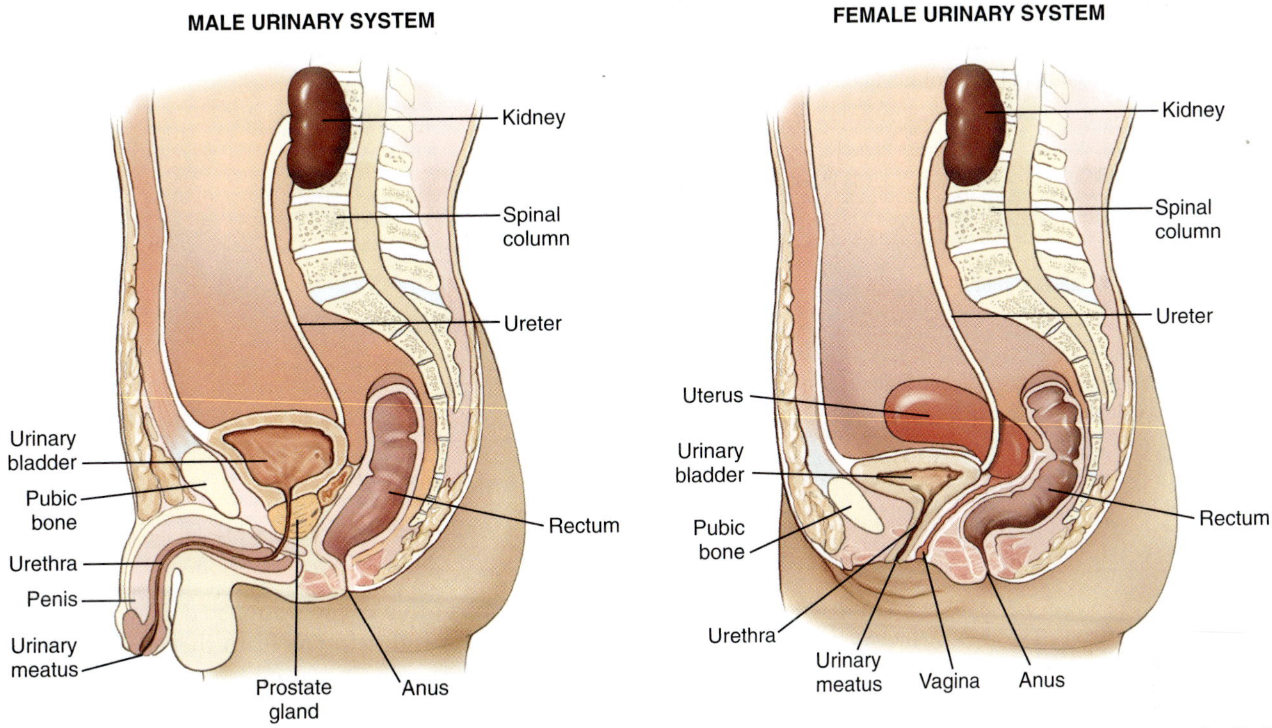

FIG. 6.2 Male and female urinary systems, sagittal view. The male urethra is approximately 8 inches (20 cm) in length compared with the female urethra, which is approximately 1.5 inches (3.8 cm) in length.

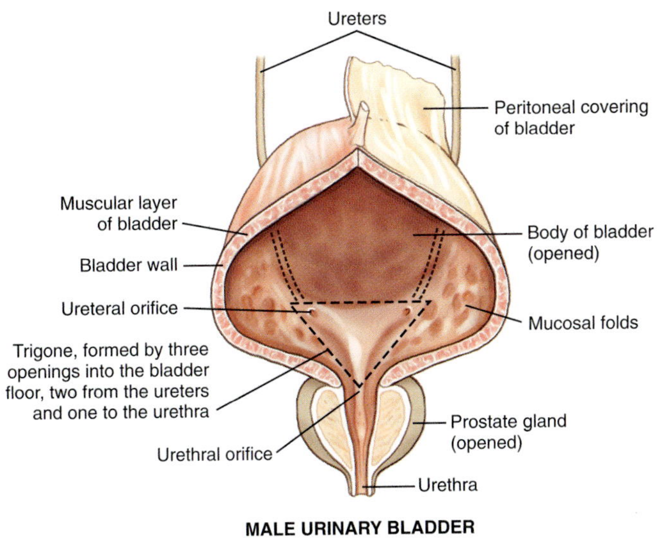

FIG. 6.3 Male urinary bladder.

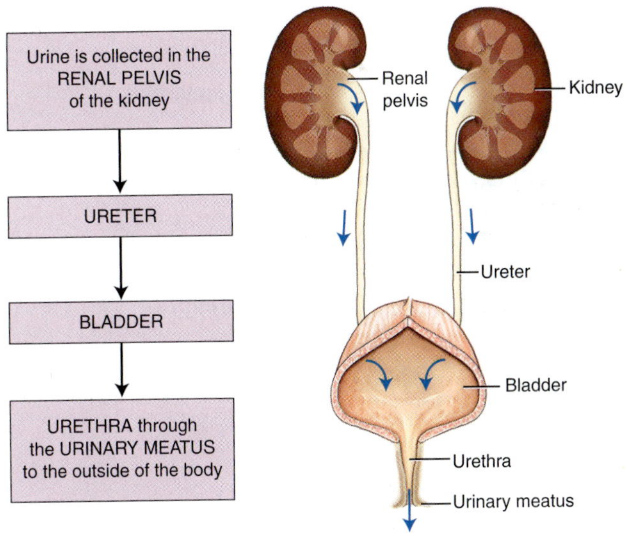

FIG. 6.4 Flow of urine.

EXERCISE 1

Practice saying aloud each of the Organs and Anatomic Structures.

To hear the terms, go to Evolve Resources at evolve.elsevier.com and select:
Practice Student Resources > Student Resources > Chapter 6 > **Pronounce and Spell**

See Appendix B for instructions.

❑ Check the box when complete.

A&P Booster
For more anatomy and physiology, go to Evolve Resources at evolve.elsevier.com and select:
Practice Student Resources > Student Resources > Chapter 6 > **A&P Booster**

See Appendix B for instructions.

WORD PARTS

Word parts you need to know to complete this chapter are listed on the following pages. The exercises at the end of each list will help you learn their definitions and spellings.

Use the flashcards accompanying this text or electronic flashcards to assist you in memorizing the word parts for this chapter.

Combining Forms of the Urinary System

COMBINING FORM	DEFINITION
cyst/o, vesic/o	bladder, sac *(Note:* cyst/o and vesic/o refer to the urinary bladder unless otherwise identified.*)*
glomerul/o	glomerulus
meat/o	meatus (opening)
nephr/o, ren/o	kidney
pyel/o	renal pelvis
ureter/o	ureter
urethr/o	urethra

PYELOS
is the Greek word for **tub-shaped vessel,** which describes the renal pelvis shape.

EXERCISE 2

A. Fill in the blanks with combining forms for this diagram of the urinary system. *To check your answers, go to Appendix A.*

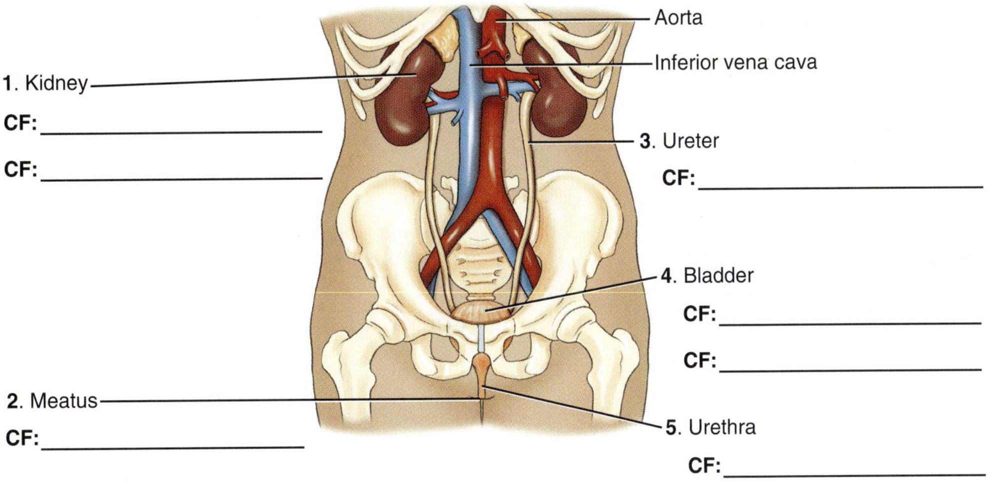

B. Fill in the blanks with combining forms to label this diagram of the internal kidney structure.

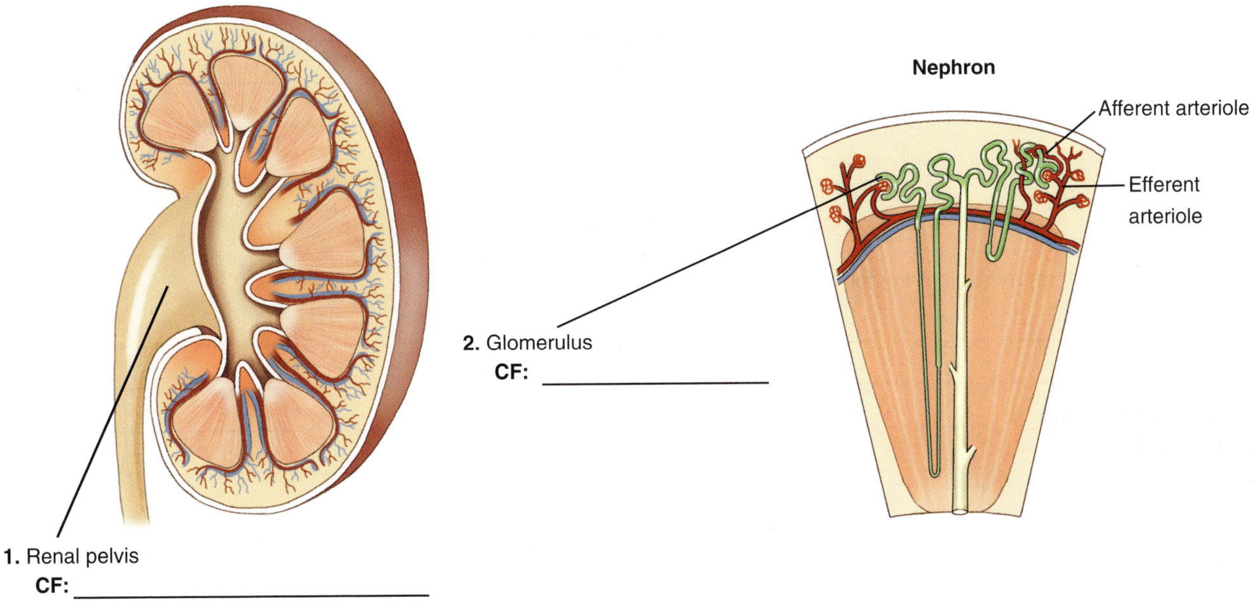

EXERCISE 3

Step 1: Write the definitions after the following combining forms.
Step 2: Match the descriptions on the right with the combining forms and definitions. Answers may be used more than once.

_____ 1. ren/o, ____________________
_____ 2. vesic/o, ____________________
_____ 3. nephr/o, ____________________
_____ 4. glomerul/o, ____________________
_____ 5. pyel/o, ____________________
_____ 6. ureter/o, ____________________
_____ 7. cyst/o, ____________________
_____ 8. meat/o, ____________________
_____ 9. urethr/o, ____________________

a. stores urine
b. outside opening through which the urine passes
c. carries urine from the kidneys to the urinary bladder
d. cluster of capillaries in the kidney where the urine begins to form
e. carries urine from the bladder to the urinary meatus
f. reservoir within the kidney that collects the urine
g. organs that remove waste products from the blood

Combining Forms Commonly Used With Urinary System Terms

COMBINING FORM	DEFINITION
albumin/o	albumin
azot/o	urea, nitrogen
blast/o	developing cell, germ cell
glyc/o, glycos/o	sugar
hydr/o	water
lith/o	stone, calculus
noct/i	night *(Note: the combining vowel is i.)*
olig/o	scanty, few
urin/o, ur/o	urine, urinary tract

EXERCISE 4

Write the definitions of the following combining forms.

1. hydr/o ____________________
2. azot/o ____________________
3. noct/i ____________________
4. lith/o ____________________
5. albumin/o ____________________
6. urin/o ____________________
7. glyc/o ____________________
8. blast/o ____________________
9. olig/o ____________________
10. ur/o ____________________
11. glycos/o ____________________

EXERCISE 5

Write the combining form for each of the following.

1. sugar a. ____________________
   b. ____________________
2. urine, urinary tract a. ____________________
   b. ____________________
3. water ____________________
4. developing cell, germ cell ____________________
5. albumin ____________________
6. night ____________________
7. urea, nitrogen ____________________
8. stone, calculus ____________________
9. scanty, few ____________________

Suffixes

SUFFIX	DEFINITION
-iasis, -esis	condition
-lysis	loosening, dissolution, separating
-ptosis	drooping, sagging, prolapse
-rrhaphy	suturing, repairing
-tripsy	surgical crushing
-uria	urine, urination

Refer to **Appendix C** and **Appendix D** for alphabetized lists of word parts and their meanings.

EXERCISE 6

A. Write the suffix pictured and defined.

1. ______________________
loosening, dissolution, separating

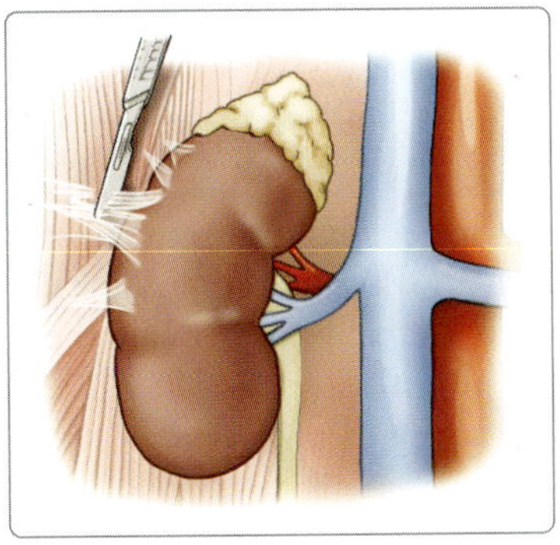

2. ______________________
drooping, sagging, prolapse

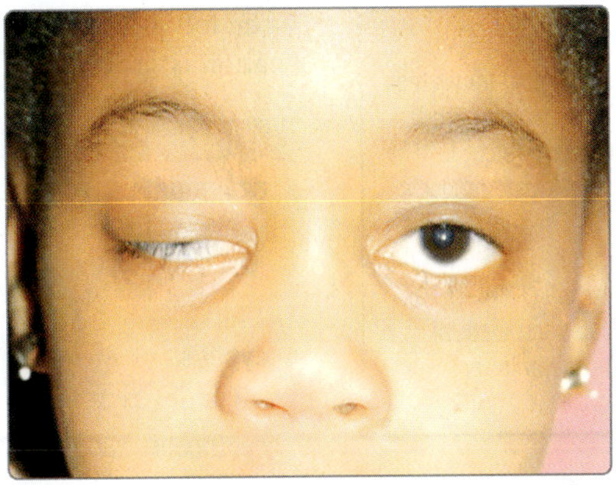

3. ______________________
surgical crushing

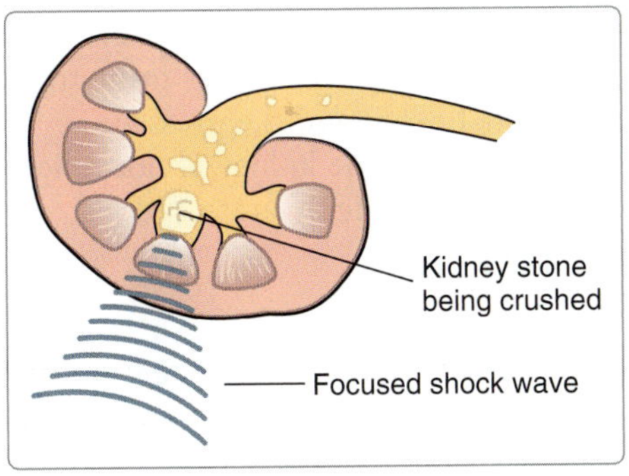

4. ______________________
suturing, repairing

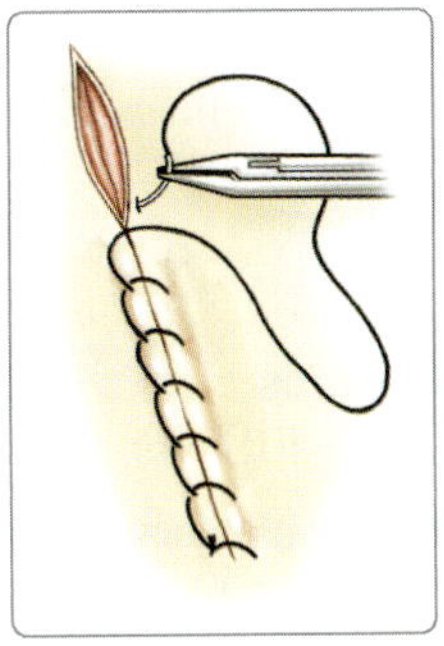

B. Write the suffix for each of the following.

1. condition ____________ , ____________
2. urine, urination ______________________

EXERCISE 7

Write the definitions of the following suffixes.

1. -rrhaphy ______________________
2. -lysis ______________________
____
3. -iasis, -esis ______________________
4. -uria ______________________
5. -ptosis ______________________
____
6. -tripsy ______________________

For additional practice with Word Parts, go to Evolve Resources at evolve.elsevier.com and select:
Practice Student Resources > Student Resources > Chapter 6 > **Flashcards**

See Appendix B for instructions.

MEDICAL TERMS

The terms you need to learn to complete this chapter are listed next. The exercises following each list will help you learn the definition and the spelling of each word.

Disease and Disorder Terms
BUILT FROM WORD PARTS

The following terms can be translated using definitions of word parts. Further explanation is provided within parentheses as needed.

TERM	DEFINITION
azotemia (*az*-ō-TĒ-mē-a)	urea in the blood (a toxic condition resulting from disease of the kidney in which waste products are in the blood that are normally excreted by the kidney); (also called **uremia**)
cystitis (sis-TĪ-tis)	inflammation of the bladder (Fig. 6.5)
cystocele (SIS-tō-sēl)	protrusion of the bladder
cystolith (SIS-tō-lith)	stone(s) in the bladder (Exercise Figure A)
glomerulonephritis (glō-*mer*-ū-lō-ne-FRĪ-tis)	inflammation of the glomeruli of the kidney
hydronephrosis (*hī*-drō-ne-FRŌ-sis)	abnormal condition of water in the kidney (obstruction of urine drainage causes urine to collect in the renal pelvis and the pressure transmitted throughout the kidney, if not relieved, can result in kidney damage)
nephritis (ne-FRĪ-tis)	inflammation of a kidney
nephroblastoma (*nef*-rō-blas-TŌ-ma)	kidney tumor containing developing (germ) cells (malignant tumor) (also called **Wilms tumor**)
nephrolithiasis (*nef*-rō-lith-Ī-a-sis)	condition of stone(s) in the kidney
nephroma (nef-RŌ-ma)	tumor of the kidney
nephromegaly (*nef*-rō-MEG-a-lē)	enlargement of a kidney
nephroptosis (*nef*-rop-TŌ-sis)	drooping kidney (also called **floating kidney** and occurs when the kidney is no longer held in place and drops out of its normal position. The kidney is normally held in position by connective and adipose tissue, so it is prone to injury, which may also cause the ureter to twist. Truck drivers and horseback riders are prone to this condition.)
pyelitis (*pī*-e-LĪ-tis)	inflammation of the renal pelvis

UREMIA
also called azotemia, translated literally is **urine in the blood;** however, the term refers to **urea** and other waste products **in the blood.** The term uremia was first used by Pierre Piorry, a French physician (1794-1879). He also created the medical terms **toxin, toxemia,** and **septicemia.**

EXERCISE FIGURE A

Fill in the blanks to label the diagram.

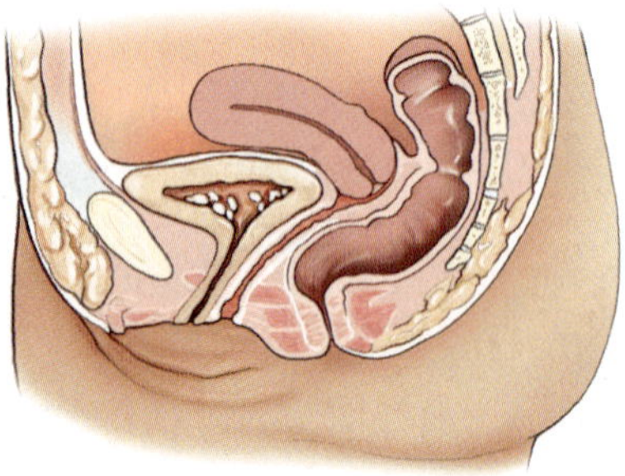

bladder / cv / stone(s)

WILMS TUMOR
also called nephroblastoma, is a rare malignancy of the kidney that primarily affects children. Named for German surgeon Dr. Max Wilms who described the disease in 1899, Wilms tumors are generally **unilateral** and can be successfully managed with appropriate surgical and oncology treatment.

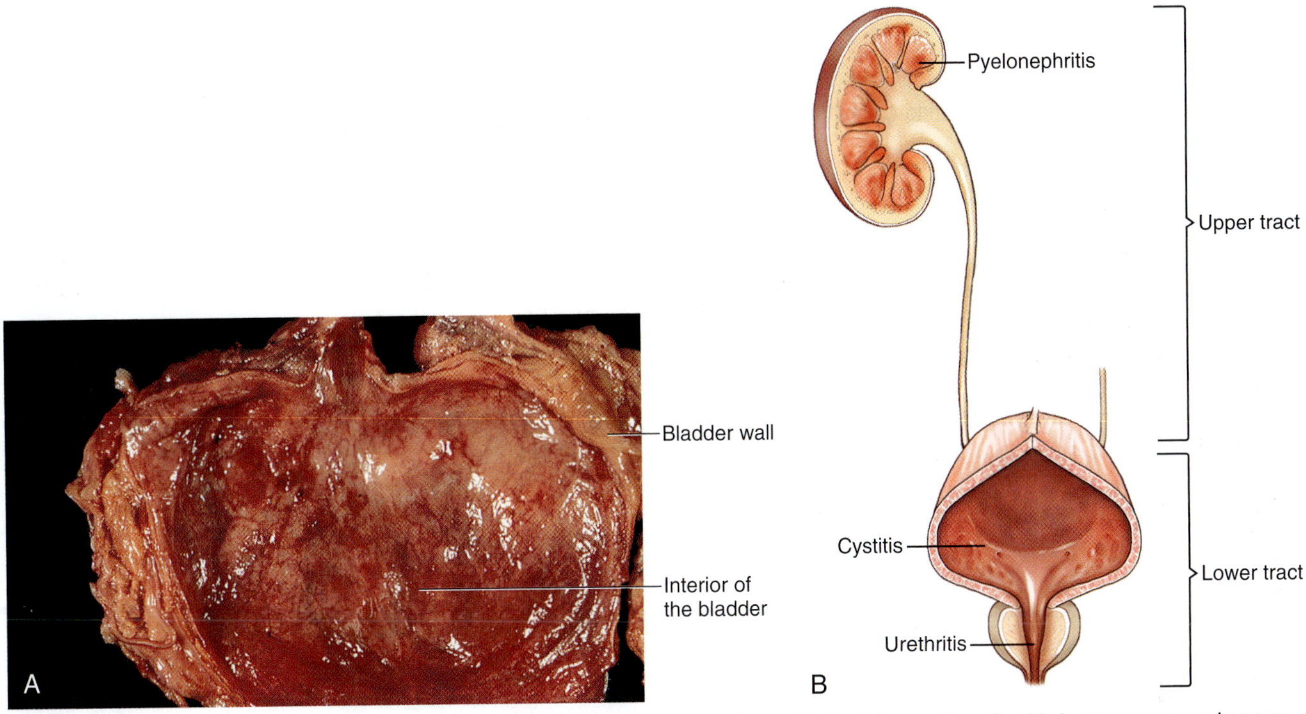

FIG. 6.5 Urinary tract infection. **A,** Acute cystitis. The swollen and red mucosa demonstrates inflammation. Cystitis is more common in women because the urethra is short, allowing easy access of bacteria to the urinary bladder. **B,** Upper and lower urinary tract infections. If cystitis is not treated promptly, the infection can spread to the kidneys, causing pyelonephritis.

TERM	DEFINITION
pyelonephritis (*pī*-e-lō-ne-FRĪ-tis)	inflammation of the renal pelvis and the kidney (Fig. 6.5B, and Fig. 6.6)
ureteritis (ū-*rē*-ter-Ī-tis)	inflammation of a ureter
ureterocele (ū-RĒ-ter-ō-*sēl*)	protrusion of a ureter (distally into the bladder)
ureterolithiasis (ū-*rē*-ter-ō-lith-Ī-a-sis)	condition of stone(s) in the ureter
ureterostenosis (ū-*rē*-ter-ō-sten-Ō-sis)	narrowing of the ureter
urethrocystitis (ū-*rē*-thrō-sis-TĪ-tis)	inflammation of the urethra and the bladder

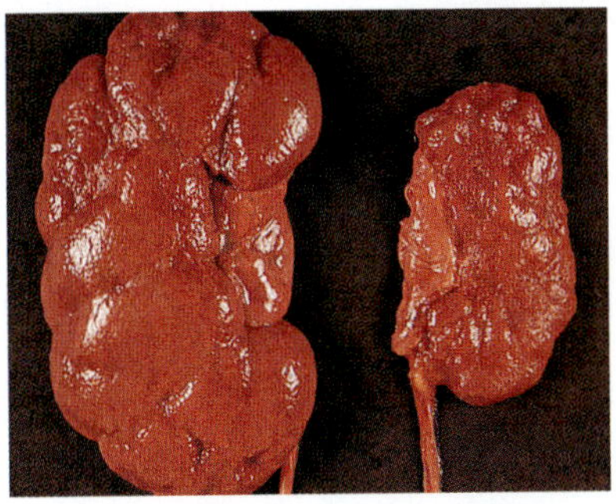

FIG. 6.6 *Kidney on left,* chronic pyelonephritis. *Kidney on right,* normal size with some scarring.

EXERCISE 8

Practice saying aloud each of the Disease and Disorder Terms Built from Word Parts.

To hear the terms, go to Evolve Resources at evolve.elsevier.com and select:
Practice Student Resources > Student Resources > Chapter 6 > **Pronounce and Spell**

See Appendix B for instructions.

❑ Check the box when complete.

EXERCISE 9

Analyze and define the following terms by drawing slashes between word parts, writing word part abbreviations above the term, underlining combining forms, and writing combining form abbreviations below the term.

EXAMPLE:

WR CV WR S
glomerul / o / nephr / itis
CF
inflammation of the glomeruli of the kidney

1. nephroma
2. cystolith
3. nephrolithiasis
4. azotemia
5. nephroptosis
6. cystocele
7. cystitis
8. pyelitis
9. ureterocele
10. hydronephrosis
11. nephromegaly
12. ureterolithiasis
13. pyelonephritis
14. ureteritis

15. nephritis

____

____

16. urethrocystitis

____

____

17. ureterostenosis

____

____

18. nephroblastoma

____

____

EXERCISE 10

Build disease and disorder terms for the following definitions with the word parts you have learned.

EXAMPLE: inflammation of the ureter ureter / itis (WR / S)

1. enlargement of the kidney ______ / ______ / ______ (WR / CV / S)
2. inflammation of the bladder ______ / ______ (WR / S)
3. inflammation of the urethra and bladder ______ / ______ / ______ / ______ (WR / CV / WR / S)
4. protrusion of the bladder ______ / ______ / ______ (WR / CV / S)
5. abnormal condition of water in the kidney ______ / ______ / ______ / ______ (WR / CV / WR / S)
6. stone(s) in the bladder ______ / ______ / ______ (WR / CV / WR)
7. inflammation of the glomeruli of the kidney ______ / ______ / ______ / ______ (WR / CV / WR / S)
8. tumor of the kidney ______ / ______ (WR / S)
9. drooping kidney ______ / ______ / ______ (WR / CV / S)
10. inflammation of a kidney ______ / ______ (WR / S)
11. condition of stone(s) in the kidney ______ / ______ / ______ / ______ (WR / CV / WR / S)

12. protrusion of a ureter ______ WR / CV / ______ S

13. inflammation of the renal pelvis ______ WR / ______ S

14. urea in the blood ______ WR / ______ S

15. narrowing of the ureter ______ WR / CV / ______ S

16. inflammation of the renal pelvis and the kidney ______ WR / CV / ______ WR / ______ S

17. condition of stone(s) in the ureter ______ WR / CV / ______ WR / ______ S

18. kidney tumor containing developing (germ) cells ______ WR / CV / ______ WR / ______ S

EXERCISE 11

Spell each of the Disease and Disorder Terms Built from Word Parts by having someone dictate them to you. Use a separate sheet of paper.

> To hear and spell the terms, go to Evolve Resources at evolve.elsevier.com and select:
> Practice Student Resources > Student Resources > Chapter 6 > **Pronounce and Spell**
>
> See Appendix B for instructions.

❑ Check the box when complete.

Disease and Disorder Terms *NOT* BUILT FROM WORD PARTS

Word parts may be present in the following terms; however, their full meanings cannot be translated using definitions of word parts alone.

TERM	DEFINITION
epispadias (*ep*-i-SPĀ-dē-as)	congenital defect in which the urinary meatus is located on the upper surface of the penis
hypospadias (*hī*-pō-SPĀ-dē-as)	congenital defect in which the urinary meatus is located on the underside of the penis. Females may also have a form of hypospadias where the urinary meatus is unusually located. (Fig. 6.7)

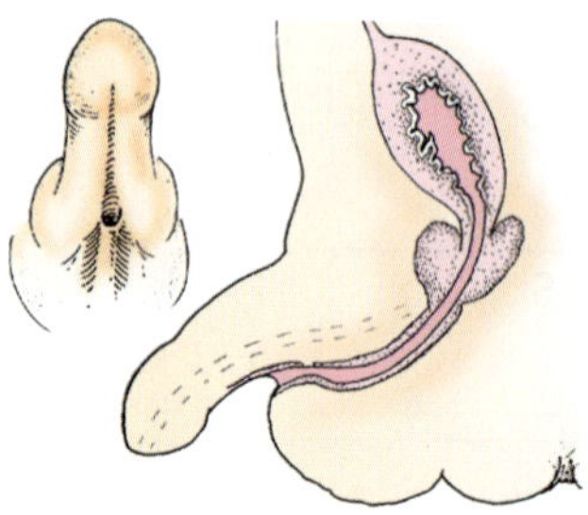

FIG. 6.7 Hypospadias.

TERM	DEFINITION
polycystic kidney disease (*pol*-ē-SIS-tik) (KID-nē) (di-ZĒZ)	condition in which the kidney contains many cysts causing progressive interference with the ability to form urine (Fig. 6.8)
renal calculus (pl. calculi) (RĒ-nal) (KAL-kū-lus), (KAL-kū-lī)	stone in the kidney
renal failure (RĒ-nal) (FĀL-ūr)	loss of kidney function resulting in its inability to remove waste products from the body and maintain electrolyte balance (Table 6.1)
renal hypertension (RĒ-nal) (*hī*-per-TEN-shun)	elevated blood pressure resulting from kidney disease
urinary retention (Ū-rin-*ār-ē*) (rē-TEN-shun)	abnormal accumulation of urine in the bladder because of an inability to urinate
urinary suppression (Ū-rin-*ār*-ē) (sū-PRESH-un)	sudden stoppage of urine formation
urinary tract infection (UTI) (Ū-rin-*ār*-ē) (trakt) (in-FEK-shun)	infection of one or more organs of the urinary tract (Fig. 6.5)

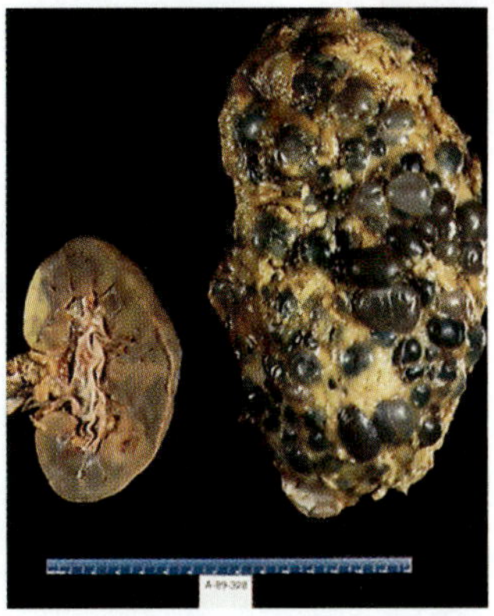

FIG. 6.8 *Kidney on left,* cross-section of normal kidney. *Kidney on right,* polycystic kidney disease.

INTEGRATIVE MEDICINE TERM

One of the renamed classifications of complimentary and alternative medicine (CAM) practices by the National Center for Complementary and Integrative Health (NCCIH) is **Natural Products**. These include therapies that use substances found in nature such as herbs, foods, probiotics, minerals, and vitamins. Positive and suggestive therapeutic effects of various natural products including, but not limited to vitamin E, cranberry extracts, saw palmetto, and Chinese herbal protocols have been documented as effective treatments of various urinary tract disorders.

EXERCISE 12

Practice saying aloud each of the Disease and Disorder Terms NOT Built from Word Parts.

To hear the terms, go to Evolve Resources at evolve.elsevier.com and select:
Practice Student Resources > Student Resources > Chapter 6 > **Pronounce and Spell**

See Appendix B for instructions.

❑ Check the box when complete.

TABLE 6.1 Renal Failure

Acute renal failure (ARF) is a rapid (less than 2 days), severe reduction in renal function resulting in a collection of metabolic waste in the body. ARF may be caused by trauma, obstruction, adverse drug reactions, or decreased blood flow (from dehydration, burns, hemorrhage, septic shock). Prompt treatment can reverse the condition and recovery can occur.

Chronic kidney disease (CKD), unlike ARF, is a progressive, irreversible, loss of renal function, and the onset of uremia. Hypertension, diabetes mellitus, and glomerulonephritis may cause CKD. Dialysis and kidney transplant are used in treating this disease, which was formerly referred to as **chronic renal failure (CRF).**

End-stage renal disease (ESRD) is what chronic kidney disease is called when kidney function is too poor to sustain life.

EXERCISE 13

Fill in the blanks with the correct terms.

1. Stone in the kidney is also called _______________ _______________.
2. The inability to urinate, which results in an abnormal amount of urine in the bladder, is known as _______________ _______________.
3. The name given to a condition in which a kidney contains many cysts is _______________ _______________ _______________.
4. _______________ is the condition in which the urinary meatus is located on the underside of the penis.
5. Elevated blood pressure resulting from kidney disease is _______________ _______________.
6. Sudden stoppage of urine formation is referred to as _______________ _______________.
7. _______________ is a condition in which the urinary meatus is located on the upper surface of the penis.
8. Infection of one or more organs of the urinary system is called _______________ _______________ _______________.
9. Loss of kidney function is called _______________ _______________.

EXERCISE 14

Match the terms in the first column with the correct definitions in the second column.

_____	1. epispadias	a. kidney with many cysts
_____	2. hypospadias	b. sudden stoppage of urine formation
_____	3. renal calculus	c. urinary meatus on the upper surface of the penis
_____	4. renal hypertension	d. kidney stone
_____	5. polycystic kidney disease	e. abnormal accumulation of urine in the bladder
_____	6. urinary retention	f. urinary meatus on the underside of the penis
_____	7. urinary suppression	g. infection of one or more organs of the urinary system
_____	8. urinary tract infection	h. characterized by elevated blood pressure
_____	9. renal failure	i. loss of kidney function

EXERCISE 15

Spell each of the Disease and Disorder Terms NOT Built from Word Parts by having someone dictate them to you. Use a separate sheet of paper.

> To hear and spell the terms, go to Evolve Resources at evolve.elsevier.com and select:
> Practice Student Resources > Student Resources > Chapter 6 > **Pronounce and Spell**
>
> See Appendix B for instructions.

❑ Check the box when complete.

Surgical Terms
BUILT FROM WORD PARTS

The following terms can be translated using definitions of word parts. Further explanation is provided within parentheses as needed.

TERM	DEFINITION
cystectomy (sis-TEK-to-mē)	excision of the bladder
cystolithotomy (*sis*-tō-li-THOT-o-mē)	incision into the bladder to remove stone(s)
cystorrhaphy (sist-OR-a-fē)	suturing the bladder
cystostomy (sis-TOS-to-mē)	creation of an artificial opening into the bladder (for urinary drainage) (Exercise Figure B)
cystotomy, vesicotomy (sis-TOT-o-mē) (*ves*-i-KOT-o-mē)	incision into the bladder
lithotripsy (LITH-ō-trip-sē)	surgical crushing of stone(s) (using shock waves) (Exercise Figure C)
meatotomy (*mē*-a-TOT-o-mē)	incision into the meatus (to enlarge it)
nephrectomy (ne-FREK-to-mē)	excision of the kidney
nephrolithotomy (*nef*-rō-li-THOT-o-mē)	incision into the kidney to remove stone(s) (Fig. 6.9)
nephrolithotripsy (*nef*-rō-LITH-o-trip-sē)	surgical crushing of stone(s) in the kidney (using shock waves) (Fig. 6.9)
nephrolysis (ne-FROL-i-sis)	separating the kidney (from other body structures)
nephropexy (NEF-rō-*peks*-ē)	surgical fixation of the kidney

EXERCISE FIGURE B

Fill in the blanks to label the diagram.

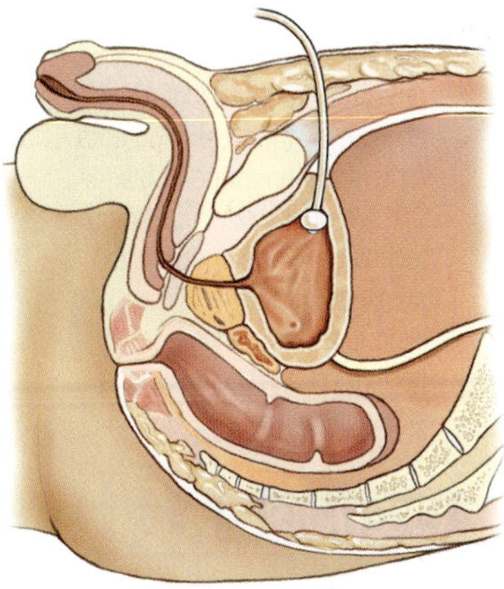

_______ / _______ / _______
bladder / cv / creation of an artificial opening

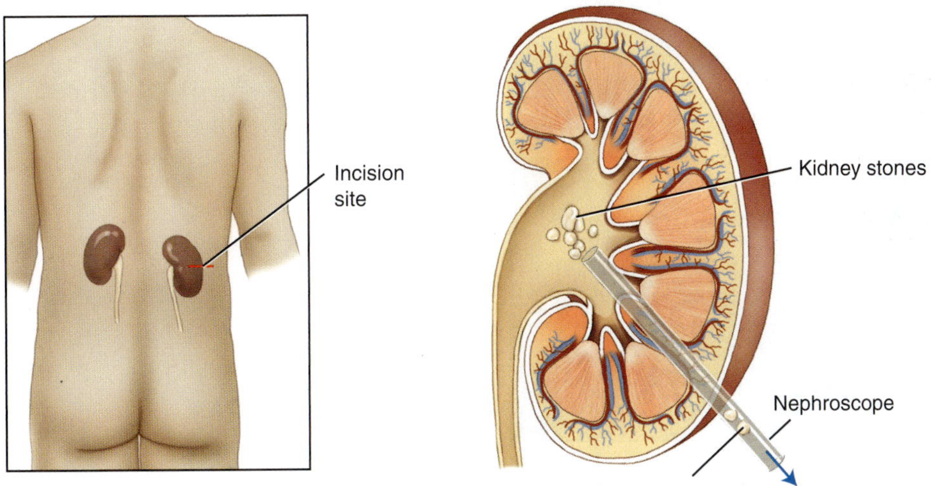

FIG. 6.9 Percutaneous nephrolithotomy or percutaneous lithotripsy uses a small incision in the back to remove medium or larger-size kidney stones. A nephroscope is passed into the kidney through the incision. In a **nephrolithotomy,** the surgeon removes the stone through the nephroscope. In a **nephrolithotripsy,** the stone is broken into fragments by a lithotripter and then removed through the nephroscope.

Surgical Terms—cont'd

TERM	DEFINITION
nephrostomy (nef-ROS-to-mē)	creation of an artificial opening into the kidney (Exercise Figure D)
pyelolithotomy (*pī*-el-ō-lith-OT-o-mē)	incision into the renal pelvis to remove stone(s) (Exercise Figure E)
pyeloplasty (PĪ-el-ō-*plas*-tē)	surgical repair of the renal pelvis
ureterectomy (ū-*rē*-ter-EK-to-mē)	excision of the ureter
ureterostomy (ū-*rē*-ter-OS-to-mē)	creation of an artificial opening into the ureter (for drainage of urine)
urethroplasty (ū-RĒ-thrō-*plas*-tē)	surgical repair of the urethra
vesicourethral suspension (*ves*-i-kō-ū-RĒ-thral) (*sus*-PEN-shun)	suspension pertaining to the bladder and urethra

STRESS INCONTINENCE

is the involuntary intermittent leakage of urine as a result of pressure, from a cough or a sneeze, on the weakened area around the urethra and bladder. The Marshall-Marchetti Krantz technique, or **vesicourethral suspension** with a midurethral sling is a suspension surgery performed on patients with stress incontinence.

EXERCISE 16

Practice saying aloud each of the Surgical Terms Built from Word Parts.

To hear the terms, go to Evolve Resources at evolve.elsevier.com and select:
Practice Student Resources > Student Resources > Chapter 6 > **Pronounce and Spell**

See Appendix B for instructions.

❑ Check the box when complete.

EXERCISE FIGURE C

Fill in the blanks to complete the labeling of the diagram.

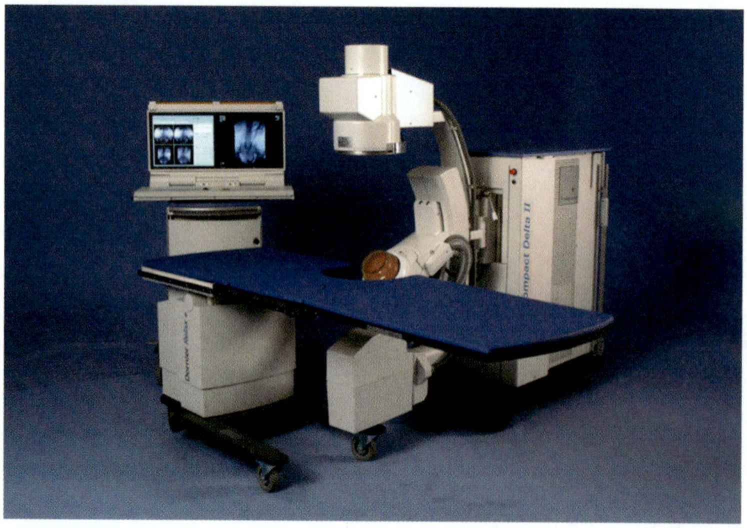

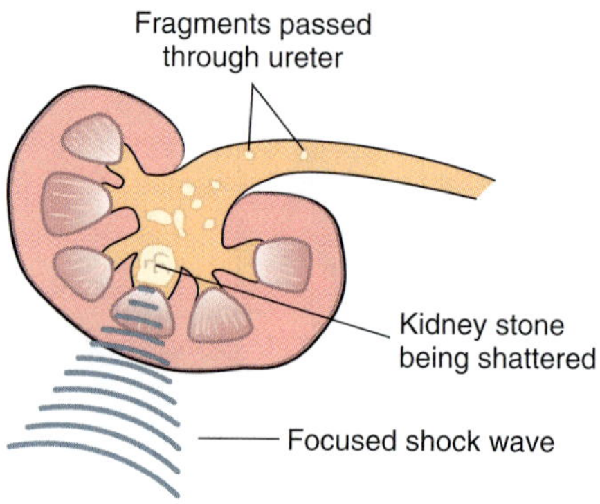

Extracorporeal shock wave ______ / ______ / ______.
stone / cv / surgical crushing

ESWL breaks down the kidney stone into fragments by shock waves from outside the body. The broken fragments are eliminated from the body with the passing of urine.

EXERCISE FIGURE D

Fill in the blanks to label the diagram.

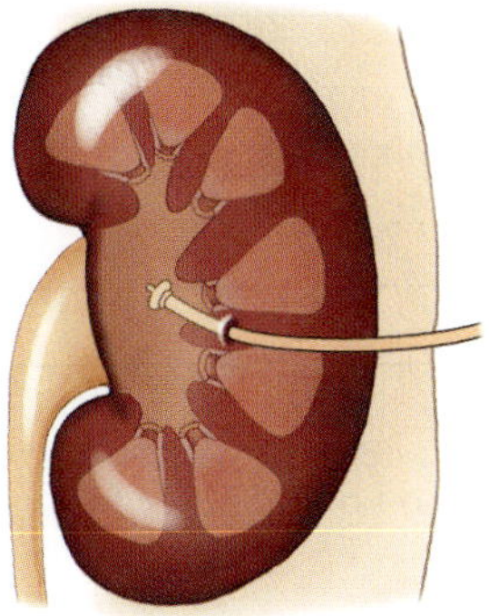

Percutaneous ________ / ____ / ________ to
kidney / cv / creation of an artificial opening

allow introduction of a catheter for urinary drainage.

EXERCISE FIGURE E

Fill in the blanks to label the diagram.

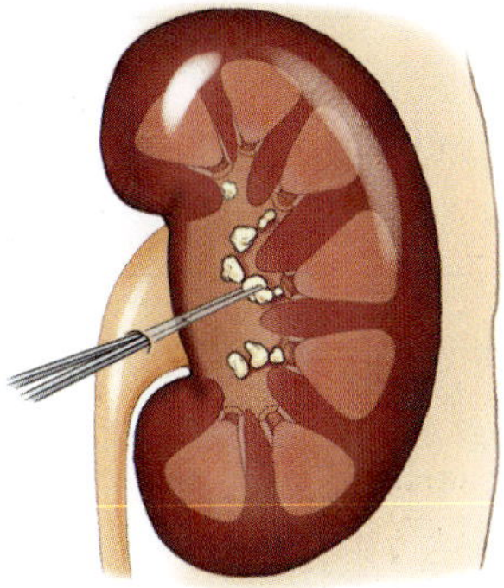

________ / ____ / ________ / ____ / ________
renal pelvis / cv / stone / cv / incision

EXERCISE 17

Analyze and define the following terms by drawing slashes between word parts, writing word part abbreviations above the term, underlining combining forms, and writing combining form abbreviations below the term.

1. vesicotomy

____

____

2. cystotomy

____

____

3. nephrostomy

____

____

4. nephrolysis

____

____

5. cystectomy

____

____

6. pyelolithotomy

____

____

7. nephropexy

____

____

8. cystolithotomy

____

____

9. nephrectomy

____

____

10. ureterectomy

____

____

11. cystostomy

____

____

12. pyeloplasty

____

____

13. cystorrhaphy

____

____

14. meatotomy

____

____

15. lithotripsy

____

____

16. urethroplasty

____

____

17. vesicourethral (suspension)

____

____

18. nephrolithotomy

____

____

19. ureterostomy

____

____

20. nephrolithotripsy

____

____

EXERCISE 18

Build surgical terms for the following definitions by using the word parts you have learned.

1. creation of an artificial opening into the ureter ______ / ______ / ______ (WR / CV / S)
2. excision of the kidney ______ / ______ (WR / S)
3. incision into the kidney to remove stone(s) ______ / ______ / ______ / ______ / ______ (WR / CV / WR / CV / S)
4. suturing the bladder ______ / ______ / ______ (WR / CV / S)
5. separating the kidney (from other structures) ______ / ______ / ______ (WR / CV / S)
6. creation of an artificial opening into the kidney ______ / ______ / ______ (WR / CV / S)
7. surgical repair of the urethra ______ / ______ / ______ (WR / CV / S)

8. excision of the bladder ______ WR / ______ S

9. incision into the meatus ______ WR / CV / ______ S

10. incision into the bladder

a. ______ WR / CV / ______ S

b. ______ WR / CV / ______ S

11. surgical repair of the renal pelvis ______ WR / CV / ______ S

12. excision of the ureter ______ WR / ______ S

13. surgical fixation of the kidney ______ WR / CV / ______ S

14. incision into the bladder to remove stone(s) ______ WR / CV / ______ WR / CV / ______ S

15. surgical crushing of a stone ______ WR / CV / ______ S

16. suspension pertaining to the bladder and urethra ______ WR / CV / ______ WR / ______ S suspension

17. creation of an artificial opening into the bladder ______ WR / CV / ______ S

18. incision into the renal pelvis to remove stone(s) ______ WR / CV / ______ WR / CV / ______ S

19. surgical crushing of stone(s) in the kidney ______ WR / CV / ______ WR / CV / ______ S

EXERCISE 19

Spell each of the Surgical Terms Built from Word Parts by having someone dictate them to you. Use a separate sheet of paper.

To hear and spell the terms, go to Evolve Resources at evolve.elsevier.com and select:
Practice Student Resources > Student Resources > Chapter 6 > **Pronounce and Spell**

See Appendix B for instructions.

❑ Check the box when complete.

Surgical Terms
NOT BUILT FROM WORD PARTS

Word parts may be present in the following terms; however, their full meanings cannot be translated using definitions of word parts alone.

EXTRACORPOREAL

means occurring outside the body.

RENAL FUNCTION REPLACEMENT THERAPIES

- Hemodialysis
- Peritoneal dialysis
- Renal transplant

TERM	DEFINITION
extracorporeal shock wave lithotripsy (ESWL) (*eks*-tra-kor-POR-ē-al) (LITH-ō-*trip*-sē)	noninvasive surgical procedure to crush stone(s) in the kidney or ureter by administration of repeated shockwaves. Stone fragments are eliminated from the body in urine. (also called **shock wave lithotripsy [SWL]**) (see Exercise Figure C).
fulguration (*ful*-gū-RĀ-shun)	destruction of living tissue with an electric spark (a method commonly used to destroy bladder growths) (Fig. 6.10)
renal transplant (RĒ-nal) (TRANS-plant)	surgical implantation of a donor kidney into a patient with inadequate renal function (Fig. 6.11)

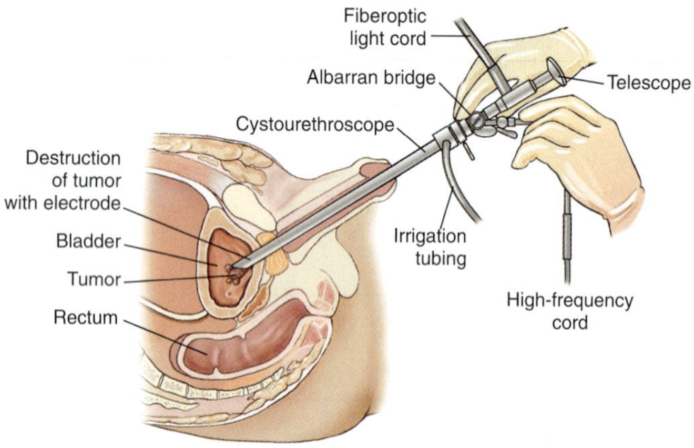

FIG. 6.10 Bladder fulguration.

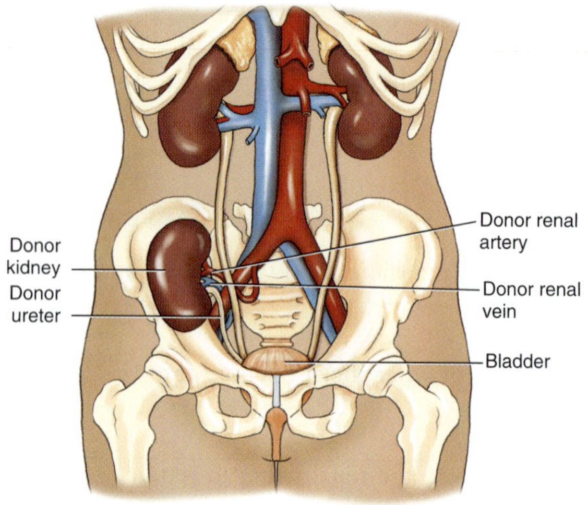

FIG. 6.11 Renal transplant showing donor kidney and blood vessels in place. Recipient's kidney is not always removed unless it is infected or is a cause of hypertension.

EXERCISE 20

Practice saying aloud each of the Surgical Terms NOT Built from Word Parts.

To hear the terms, go to Evolve Resources at evolve.elsevier.com and select:
Practice Student Resources > Student Resources > Chapter 6 > **Pronounce and Spell**

See Appendix B for instructions.

❑ Check the box when complete.

EXERCISE 21

Fill in the blanks with the correct answer.

1. The surgical implantation of a donor kidney into a patient with inadequate renal function is called ______________ ______________________________.
2. The destruction of living tissue with an electric spark is ______________________________.
3. ______________ ______________ ______________ ______________ is a noninvasive surgical procedure for removal of kidney or ureteral stones.

EXERCISE 22

Match the terms in the first column with their correct definitions in the second column.

_____ 1. fulguration	a. implantation of a donor kidney
_____ 2. renal transplant	b. used to destroy bladder growths
_____ 3. ESWL	c. also called shock wave lithotripsy

EXERCISE 23

Spell each of the Surgical Terms NOT Built from Word Parts by having someone dictate them to you. Use a separate sheet of paper.

To hear and spell the terms, go to Evolve Resources at evolve.elsevier.com and select:
Practice Student Resources > Student Resources > Chapter 6 > **Pronounce and Spell**

See Appendix B for instructions.

❑ Check the box when complete.

Diagnostic Terms
BUILT FROM WORD PARTS

The following terms can be translated using definitions of word parts. Further explanation is provided within parentheses as needed.

TERM	DEFINITION
DIAGNOSTIC IMAGING	
cystogram (SIS-tō-gram)	radiographic image of the bladder (Fig. 6.12)
cystography (sis-TOG-ra-fē)	radiographic imaging of the bladder
nephrography (ne-FROG-ra-fē)	radiographic imaging of the kidney
nephrosonography (*nef*-rō-so-NOG-ra-fē)	process of recording the kidney using sound (ultrasonography)

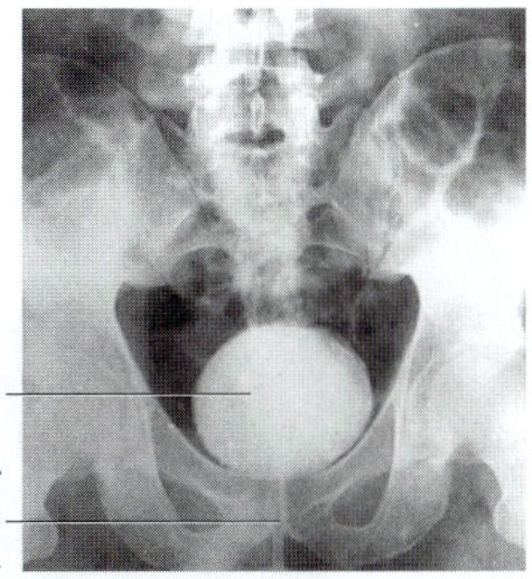

FIG. 6.12 Cystogram.

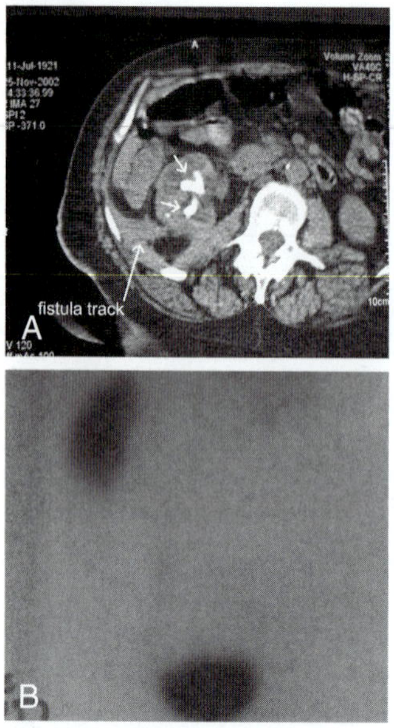

FIG. 6.13 A, CT scan of the kidney. Small arrows point to a large calculus within the renal pelvis. (transverse view)
B, Renogram. Nuclear medicine image from the same patient, showing no function of the affected kidney. (posterior view)

Diagnostic Terms—cont'd

TERM	DEFINITION
renogram (RĒ-nō-gram)	radiographic record of the kidney (a nuclear medicine test, used to evaluate kidney function); (also called **renal scan** or **nephrogram**) (Fig. 6.13B)
retrograde urogram (RET-rō-grād) (Ū-rō-gram)	radiographic image of the urinary tract (retrograde means to move in a direction opposite from normal; contrast medium is instilled into the bladder, ureter, or renal pelvis through a ureteral catheter.) (Exercise Figure F)
urogram (Ū-rō-gram)	radiographic image of the urinary tract (Fig. 6.14)
voiding cystourethrography (VCUG) (VOID-ing) (*sis*-tō-*ū*-rē-THROG-ro-fē)	radiographic imaging of the bladder and the urethra (Fig. 6.15). (Radiopaque contrast media is instilled in the bladder. Radiographic images are taken of the bladder before and during urination.)
ENDOSCOPY	
cystoscope (SIS-tō-skōp)	instrument used for visual examination of the bladder
cystoscopy (sis-TOS-ko-pē)	visual examination of the bladder (Fig. 6.16)
nephroscopy (ne-FROS-ko-pē)	visual examination of the kidney (Fig. 6.17)
ureteroscopy (ū-*rē*-ter-OS-ko-pē)	visual examination of the ureter

EXERCISE FIGURE F

Fill in the blanks to label the diagram.

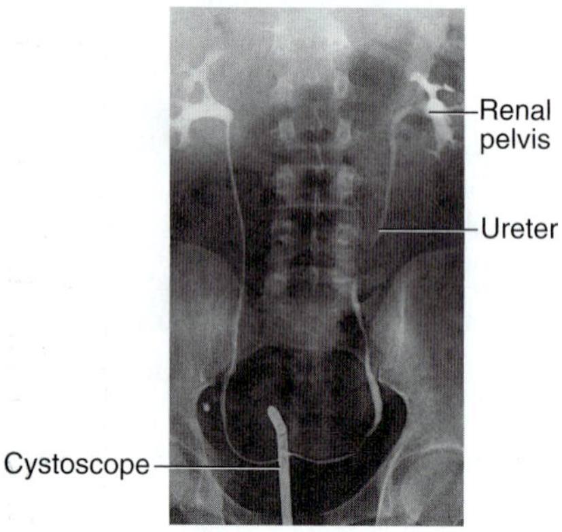

Retrograde ______/______/______.
urinary tract / cv / radiographic image.

A urethral catheter is passed by use of a cystoscope, and contrast material is injected to show urinary system structures.

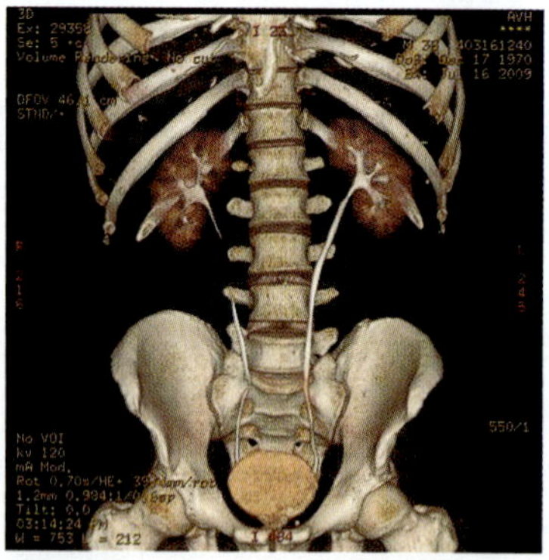

FIG. 6.14 CT urogram showing three-dimensional, reconstructed view of the kidneys, ureters, and bladder. CT urogram scans are now the primary diagnostic tool for detecting **urinary tract stones** and **perirenal infections. Intravenous urograms (IVU)** may still be used to evaluate an obstructing mass.

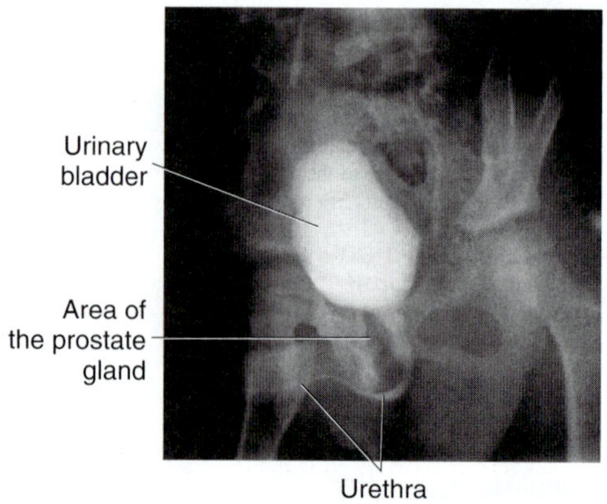

FIG. 6.15 Voiding cystourethrogram, male (lateral view).

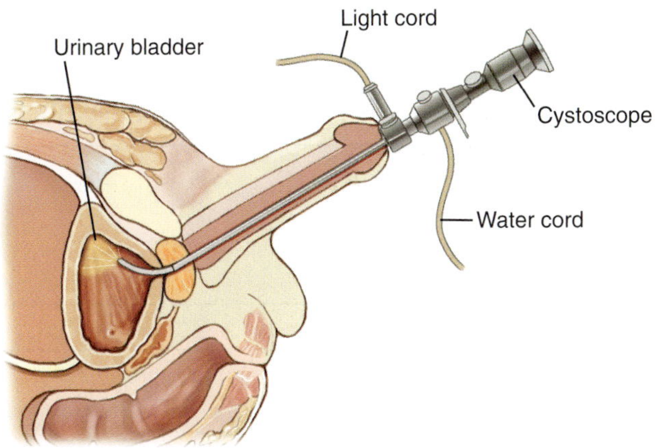

FIG. 6.16 Cystoscopy.

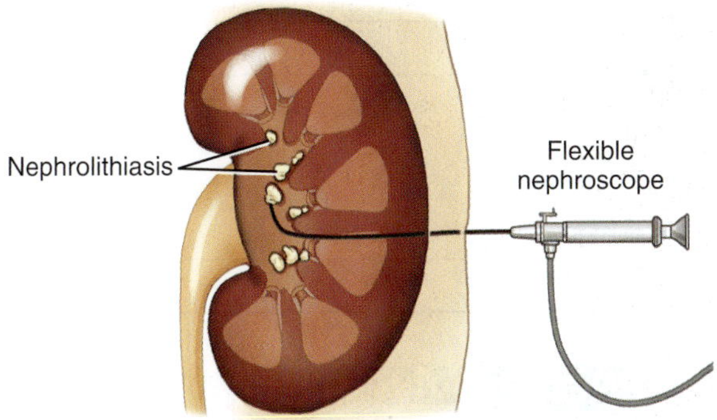

FIG. 6.17 Nephroscopy.

EXERCISE 24

Practice saying aloud each of the Diagnostic Terms Built from Word Parts.

To hear the terms, go to Evolve Resources at evolve.elsevier.com and select:
Practice Student Resources > Student Resources > Chapter 6 > **Pronounce and Spell**

See Appendix B for instructions.

❑ Check the box when complete.

EXERCISE 25

Analyze and define the following terms by drawing slashes between word parts, writing word part abbreviations above the term, underlining combining forms, and writing combining form abbreviations below the term.

1. (voiding) cystourethrography

____

____

2. cystography

____

____

3. nephrosonography

____

____

4. cystoscope

____

____

5. cystogram

____

____

6. cystoscopy

____

____

7. nephrography

____

____

8. urogram

____

____

9. (retrograde) urogram

____

____

10. renogram

____

____

11. nephroscopy

____

____

12. ureteroscopy

____

____

EXERCISE 26

Build diagnostic terms that correspond to the following definitions by using the word parts you have learned.

1. visual examination of the bladder ______ WR / CV / S
2. radiographic image of the urinary tract ______ WR / CV / S
3. process of radiographic recording the kidney using sound ______ WR / CV / WR / CV / S
4. radiographic image of the bladder ______ WR / CV / S
5. instrument used for visual examination of the bladder ______ WR / CV / S
6. radiographic imaging of the bladder and the urethra voiding ______ WR / CV / WR / CV / S
7. radiographic imaging of the bladder ______ WR / CV / S
8. radiographic record of the kidney, used to evaluate kidney function ______ WR / CV / S
9. radiographic imaging of the kidney ______ WR / CV / S
10. radiographic image of the urinary tract (with contrast medium instilled through a catheter in a direction opposite from normal) retrograde ______ WR / CV / S
11. visual examination of the kidney ______ WR / CV / S
12. visual examination of the ureter ______ WR / CV / S

EXERCISE 27

Spell each of the Diagnostic Terms Built from Word Parts by having someone dictate them to you. Use a separate sheet of paper.

To hear and spell the terms, go to Evolve Resources at evolve.elsevier.com and select:
Practice Student Resources > Student Resources > Chapter 6 > **Pronounce and Spell**

See Appendix B for instructions.

❑ Check the box when complete.

Diagnostic Terms
NOT BUILT FROM WORD PARTS

Word parts may be present in the following terms; however, their full meanings cannot be translated using definitions of word parts alone.

TERM	DEFINITION
DIAGNOSTIC IMAGING	
KUB (kidney, ureter, and bladder) (K-Ū-B)	simple radiographic image of the abdomen. It is often used to view the kidneys, ureters, and bladder to determine size, shape, and location. Also used to identify radiopaque calculi in the kidney, ureters, or bladder, or to diagnose intestinal obstruction; (also called **flat plate of the abdomen**) (Fig. 6.18)
LABORATORY	
blood urea nitrogen (BUN) (blud) (ū-RĒ-a) (NĪ-trō-jen)	blood test that measures the amount of urea in the blood. An increased BUN detects an abnormality in renal function.
creatinine (crē-AT-i-nin)	blood test that measures the amount of creatinine in the blood. An elevated amount may indicate impaired kidney function.
specific gravity (SG) (spe-SIF-ik) (GRAV-i-tē)	test performed on a urine specimen to measure the concentrating or diluting ability of the kidneys

BUN

The abbreviation BUN for blood urea nitrogen is commonly used in the healthcare setting. It is pronounced letter by letter, B-Ū-N, not as a whole word.

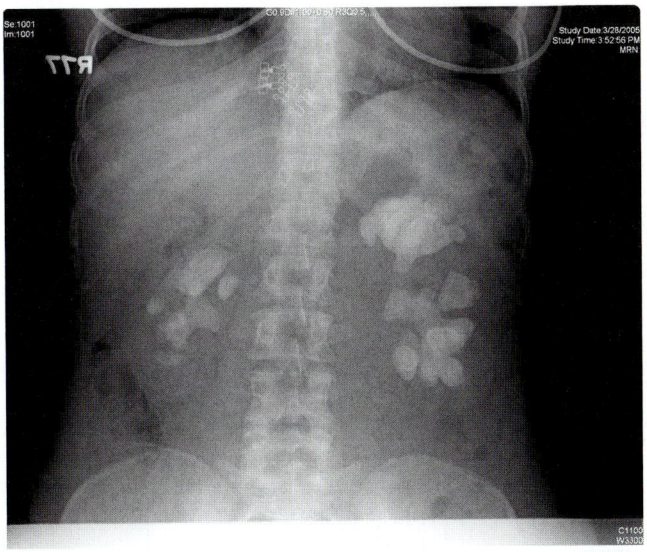

FIG. 6.18 KUB. Note the bilateral calculi that fill the renal pelvis. Due to the distinctive shape, these are called **staghorn calculi** because of the resemblance to the antlers of a stag.

Diagnostic Terms—cont'd

TERM	DEFINITION
urinalysis (UA) (ū-rin-AL-is-is)	multiple routine tests performed on a urine specimen. Visual examination and chemical analysis of a urine specimen provides screening for blood, glucose, protein, and other substances in the urine and offers a picture of overall health.

EXERCISE 28

Practice saying aloud each of the Diagnostic Terms NOT Built from Word Parts.

To hear the terms, go to Evolve Resources at evolve.elsevier.com and select:
Practice Student Resources > Student Resources > Chapter 6 > **Pronounce and Spell**

See Appendix B for instructions.

❑ Check the box when complete.

EXERCISE 29

Write the medical term pictured and defined.

1. ______________________
radiographic image of the abdomen to view kidneys, ureters, and bladder

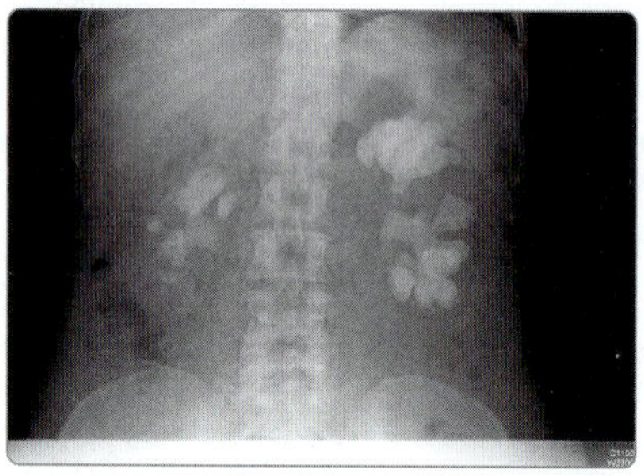

2. ______________________
multiple tests performed on a urine specimen

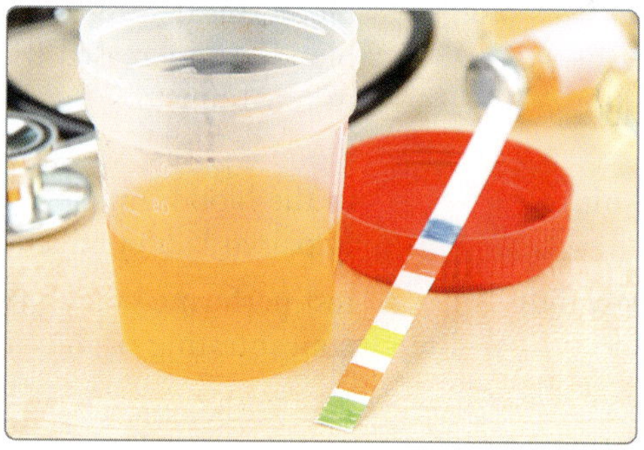

3. ______________________
A. blood test to measure the amount of urea in the blood

____
B. blood test to measure the amount of creatinine in the blood

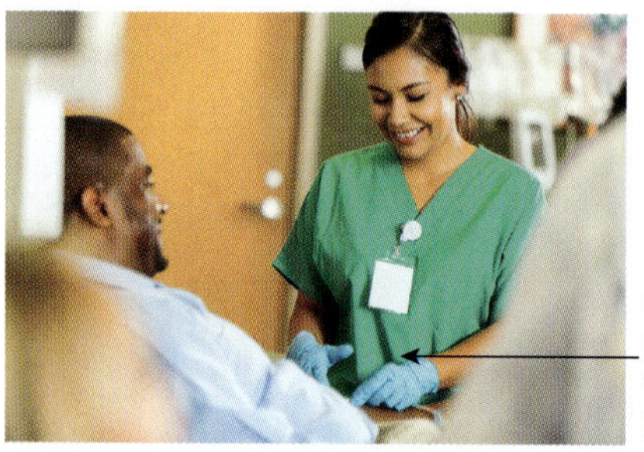

Phlebotomist preparing to withdraw a blood sample

4. ______________________
test on urine specimen to measure the concentrating and diluting abilities of the kidneys

Laboratory results

URINE
COLOR______
APPEARANCE______
PH______
SG______
ACETONE______
GLUCOSE______
BACTERIA______
WBC______
RBC______
CASTS______
OCCULT BLOOD______
OTHER______

EXERCISE 30

Match the terms in the first column with their correct definitions in the second column.

______ 1. specific gravity	a. radiographic image of the kidneys, ureters, and bladder
______ 2. blood urea nitrogen	b. blood test that measures the amount of urea in the blood
______ 3. urinalysis	c. urine test to measure concentrating or diluting abilities of the kidneys
______ 4. KUB	d. multiple routine tests performed on a urine sample
______ 5. creatinine	e. blood test that measures the amount of creatinine in the blood

EXERCISE 31

Spell each of the Diagnostic Terms NOT Built from Word Parts by having someone dictate them to you. Use a separate sheet of paper.

To hear and spell the terms, go to Evolve Resources at evolve.elsevier.com and select:
Practice Student Resources > Student Resources > Chapter 6 > **Pronounce and Spell**

See Appendix B for instructions.

❑ Check the box when complete.

Complementary Terms
BUILT FROM WORD PARTS

The following terms can be translated using definitions of word parts. Further explanation is provided within parentheses as needed.

TERM	DEFINITION
albuminuria (*al*-bū-min-Ū-rē-a)	albumin in the urine (albumin is an important protein in the blood, but when found in the urine, may indicate kidney disease; small amounts may be present in the absence of kidney disease)
anuria (an-Ū-rē-a)	absence of urine (failure of the kidney to produce urine)
diuresis (*dī*-ū-RĒ-sis)	condition of urine passing through (increased excretion of urine) *(Note: The* a *is dropped from* dia- *because uresis begins with a vowel.)*
dysuria (dis-Ū-rē-a)	difficult or painful urination
glycosuria (*glī*-kō-SŪ-rē-a)	sugar (glucose) in the urine
hematuria (*hēm*-a-TŪ-rē-a)	blood in the urine
meatal (mē-Ā-tal)	pertaining to the meatus
nephrologist (ne-FROL-o-jist)	physician who studies and treats diseases of the kidney
nephrology (ne-FROL-o-jē)	study of the kidney (a branch of medicine dealing with diseases of the kidney)
nocturia (nok-TŪ-rē-a)	night urination

DIURETICS

are medications that stimulate **diuresis** and are commonly called "water pills." Diuretics cause a marked increase in the excretion of urine and are used in the management of high blood pressure, heart failure, and edema.

Complementary Terms—cont'd

TERM	DEFINITION
oliguria (*ol*-i-GŪ-rē-a)	scanty urine (amount)
polyuria (*pol*-ē-Ū-rē-a)	much (excessive) urine
pyuria (pī-Ū-rē-a)	pus in the urine
urinary (Ū-rin-*ār*-ē)	pertaining to urine
urologist (ū-ROL-o-jist)	physician who studies and treats diseases of the urinary tract
urology (ū-ROL-o-jē)	study of the urinary tract (a branch of medicine dealing with diseases of the male and female urinary systems and the male reproductive system)

UROLOGIST/ NEPHROLOGIST

A **urologist** treats diseases of the male and female urinary system and the male reproductive system both medically and surgically. A **nephrologist** treats kidney diseases and prescribes and manages dialysis therapy.

EXERCISE 32

Practice saying aloud each of the Complementary Terms Built from Word Parts.

To hear the terms, go to Evolve Resources at evolve.elsevier.com and select:
Practice Student Resources > Student Resources > Chapter 6 > **Pronounce and Spell**

See Appendix B for instructions.

❑ Check the box when complete.

EXERCISE 33

Analyze and define the following terms by drawing slashes between word parts, writing word part abbreviations above the term, underlining combining forms, and writing combining form abbreviations below the term.

1. nocturia
____
____

2. urologist
____
____

3. oliguria
____
____

4. nephrologist
____
____

5. hematuria
____
____

6. urology
____
____

7. polyuria
____
____

8. albuminuria
____
____

9. anuria

____

____

10. diuresis

____

____

11. pyuria

____

____

12. urinary

____

____

13. glycosuria

____

____

14. dysuria

____

____

15. nephrology

____

____

16. nephrologist

____

____

EXERCISE 34

Build the complementary terms for the following definitions by using the word parts you have learned.

1. night urination ________ / ________ (WR / S)
2. scanty urine ________ / ________ (WR / S)
3. pus in the urine ________ / ________ (WR / S)
4. physician who studies and treats diseases of the urinary tract ________ / ____ / ________ (WR / CV / S)
5. much (excessive) urine ________ / ________ (P / S(WR))
6. physician who studies and treats diseases of the kidney ________ / ____ / ________ (WR / CV / S)
7. pertaining to urine ________ / ________ (WR / S)
8. blood in the urine ________ / ________ (WR / S)
9. study of the urinary tract ________ / ____ / ________ (WR / CV / S)
10. condition of urine passing through (increased excretion of urine) ________ / ________ / ________ (P / WR / S)

11. absence of urine ______ P / ______ S(WR)

12. sugar in the urine ______ WR / ______ S

13. difficult or painful urination ______ P / ______ S(WR)

14. albumin in the urine ______ WR / ______ S

15. pertaining to the meatus ______ WR / ______ S

16. study of the kidney ______ WR / CV / ______ S

EXERCISE 35

Spell each of the Complementary Terms Built from Word Parts by having someone dictate them to you. Use a separate sheet of paper.

To hear and spell the terms, go to Evolve Resources at evolve.elsevier.com and select:
Practice Student Resources > Student Resources > Chapter 6 > **Pronounce and Spell**

See Appendix B for instructions.

❑ Check the box when complete.

Complementary Terms
NOT BUILT FROM WORD PARTS

Word parts may be present in the following terms; however, their full meanings cannot be translated using definitions of word parts alone.

CATHETER
is derived from the Greek **katheter,** meaning a **thing let down.** A catheter lets down the urine from the bladder.

TERM	DEFINITION
catheter (cath) (KATH-e-ter)	flexible, tubelike device, such as a urinary catheter, for withdrawing or instilling fluids
distended (dis-TEN-ded)	stretched out (a bladder is distended when filled with urine)
electrolytes (ē-LEK-trō-lītz)	minerals in the body, such as sodium and potassium, that carry an electrolyte charge. Electrolyte balance is necessary for the body to function normally and is maintained by the kidneys.
enuresis (*en*-ū-RĒ-sis)	involuntary urination. **Nocturnal enuresis**, or bed-wetting, has been described in early literature and continues to be a problem affecting 15% to 20% of school-aged children. There is no one cause for bed wetting. **Diurnal enuresis** is daytime wetting, which may be caused by a small bladder. Various treatments are used to treat diurnal enuresis. Children generally outgrow daytime wetting.

TERM	DEFINITION
hemodialysis (HD) (*hē*-mō-dī-AL-i-sis)	procedure for removing impurities from the blood because of an inability of the kidneys to do so (Fig. 6.19)
incontinence (in-KON-ti-nens)	inability to control the bladder and/or bowels
micturate (MIK-tū-rāt)	to pass urine (also called **urinate**)
peritoneal dialysis (*pār*-i-tō-NĒ-al) (dī-AL-i-sis)	procedure for removing toxic wastes when the kidney is unable to do so; the peritoneal cavity is used as the receptacle for the fluid used in the dialysis (Fig. 6.20)
stricture (STRIK-chūr)	abnormal narrowing, such as a urethral stricture
urinal (Ū-rin-al)	receptacle for urine
urinary catheterization (Ū-rin-*ār*-ē) (*kath*-e-*ter*-i-ZĀ-shun)	passage of a catheter into the urinary bladder to withdraw urine (Exercise Figure G)
urodynamics (*ū*-rō-dī-NAM-iks)	pertaining to the force and flow of urine within the urinary tract. Urodynamic studies examine the process of voiding and test bladder tone, capacity, and pressure along with urine flow and perineal muscle function. An enlarged prostate and urethral stricture will diminish urine flow rate.
void (voyd)	to empty or evacuate waste material, especially urine

Refer to **Appendix F** for pharmacology terms related to the urinary system.

MICTURATE
is derived from the Latin **mictus,** meaning **a making of water.** The noun form of micturate is **micturition.** Note the spelling of each. **Micturition** is often misspelled as **micturation.**

EXERCISE FIGURE G

Fill in the blanks to complete labeling of the diagram.

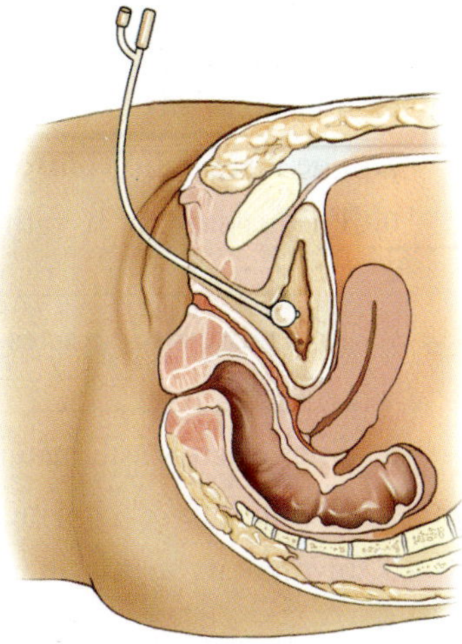

______ / ______ catheterization
urine / pertaining to

A catheter has been inserted through the urethra and urine has been drained. The balloon on the end of the catheter has been inflated to hold the catheter in the bladder for a period of time. This type of catheter is called a **retention catheter**; commonly referred to as a **Foley catheter.**

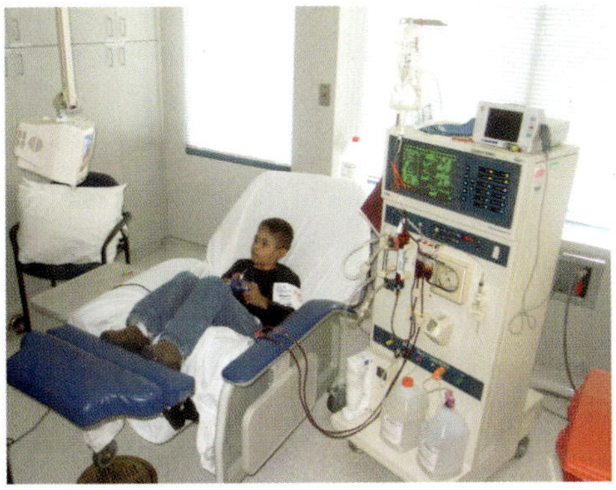

FIG. 6.19 Hemodialysis.

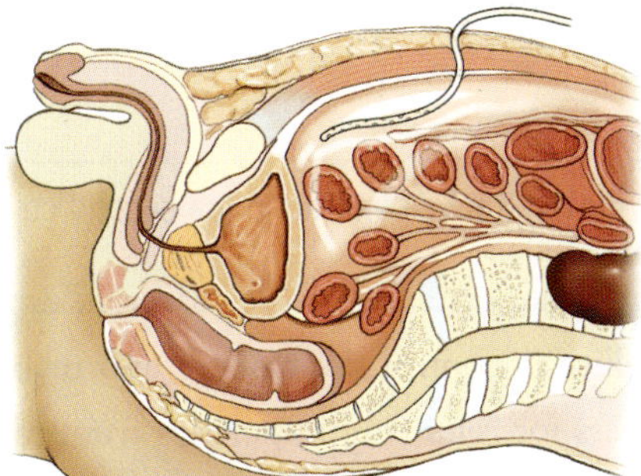

FIG. 6.20 Peritoneal dialysis. A sterile dialyzing fluid is instilled into the peritoneal cavity by gravity and dwells there for a period of time ordered by the physician. The fluid, containing the nitrogenous wastes and excess water that a healthy kidney normally removes, is drained from the cavity.

EXERCISE 36

Practice saying aloud each of the Complementary Terms NOT Built from Word Parts.

To hear the terms, go to Evolve Resources at evolve.elsevier.com and select:
Practice Student Resources > Student Resources > Chapter 6 > **Pronounce and Spell**

See Appendix B for instructions.

❑ Check the box when complete.

EXERCISE 37

Fill in the blanks with the correct terms.

1. A receptacle for urine is a(n) ______________________.
2. The procedure for removing impurities from the blood because of the inability of the kidneys to do so is called ______________________.
3. A ______________________ bladder is stretched out.
4. A flexible, tubelike device for withdrawing or instilling fluids is a(n) ______________________.
5. The inability to control the bladder and/or bowels is called ______________________.
6. The passage of a catheter into the urinary bladder to withdraw urine is a(n) ______________________ ______________________.
7. To remove toxic wastes caused by kidney insufficiency by placing dialyzing fluid in the peritoneal cavity is called ______________________ ______________________.
8. To evacuate waste material is to ______________________.
9. An abnormal narrowing is a(n) ______________________.
10. Involuntary urination is called ______________________.
11. ______________________ is another word for urinate.
12. ______________________ is the name given to the force and flow of urine.
13. ______________________ are minerals in the body such as sodium and potassium.

EXERCISE 38

Match the terms in the first column with their correct definitions in the second column.

_____ 1. catheter	a. to evacuate or empty waste material, especially urine
_____ 2. urinary catheterization	b. inability to control the bladder and/or bowels
_____ 3. distended	c. process for removing impurities from the blood when the kidneys are unable to do so
_____ 4. void	d. flexible, tubelike device for withdrawing or instilling fluids
_____ 5. hemodialysis	e. stretched out
_____ 6. incontinence	f. passage of a tubelike device into the urinary bladder to remove urine

EXERCISE 39

Match the terms in the first column with their correct definitions in the second column.

______ 1. micturate	a. to pass urine
______ 2. peritoneal dialysis	b. receptacle for urine
______ 3. stricture	c. force and flow of urine within the urinary tract
______ 4. urinal	d. use of peritoneal cavity to hold dialyzing fluid in the removal of toxic wastes
______ 5. enuresis	e. balance is necessary for the body to function normally
______ 6. urodynamics	f. involuntary urination
______ 7. electrolytes	g. abnormal narrowing

EXERCISE 40

Spell each of the Complementary Terms NOT Built from Word Parts by having someone dictate them to you. Use a separate sheet of paper.

To hear and spell the terms, go to Evolve Resources at evolve.elsevier.com and select:
Practice Student Resources > Student Resources > Chapter 6 > **Pronounce and Spell**

See Appendix B for instructions.

❑ Check the box when complete.

Abbreviations

ABBREVIATION	TERM
ARF	acute renal failure
BUN	blood urea nitrogen
cath	catheterization, catheter
CKD	chronic kidney disease
ESRD	end-stage renal disease
ESWL	extracorporeal shock wave lithotripsy
HD	hemodialysis
OAB	overactive bladder
SG	specific gravity
UA	urinalysis
UTI	urinary tract infection
VCUG	voiding cystourethrogram

EXERCISE 41

Write the terms abbreviated.

1. When imaging is used to diagnose obstructive uropathy, a KUB is usually performed first. A urogram may be used for confirming or excluding obstruction and determining its level and cause. For further examination, a **VCUG** _______________ _______________ may be performed to evaluate the posterior urethra and check for vesicoureteral reflux.
2. **SG** _______________ _______________ is one of many tests performed on the urine specimen during a **UA** _______________. It measures the concentration of particles, including water and electrolytes in the urine.
3. **BUN** _______________ _______________ _______________ is a laboratory test done on a blood sample to determine kidney function.
4. The number, size, and type of stones are important in determining if **ESWL** _______________ _______________ is the best method for treating renal calculi.
5. Bladder **cath** _______________ carries the risk of **UTI** _______________ _______________.
6. Peritoneal dialysis, **HD** _______________, and renal transplant are known as renal replacement therapies.
7. **ARF** _______________ _______________ _______________ is sudden and full recovery can occur with prompt treatment. **CKD** _______________ _______________ _______________ is irreversible and progressive. **ESRD** _______________ _______________ _______________ is when kidney function will not sustain life. A kidney transplant or renal dialysis may be used as treatment.
8. Urge incontinence is another name for **OAB** _______________ _______________ and involves a sudden, strong need to urinate. As the bladder contracts, leakage of urine occurs.

For additional practice with Abbreviations, go to Evolve Resources at evolve.elsevier.com and select: Practice Student Resources > Student Resources > Chapter 6 > **Flashcards:** Abbreviations

See Appendix B for instructions.

PRACTICAL APPLICATION

EXERCISE 42 *Case Study: Translate Between Everyday Language and Medical Language*

CASE STUDY: Tyrone Parker

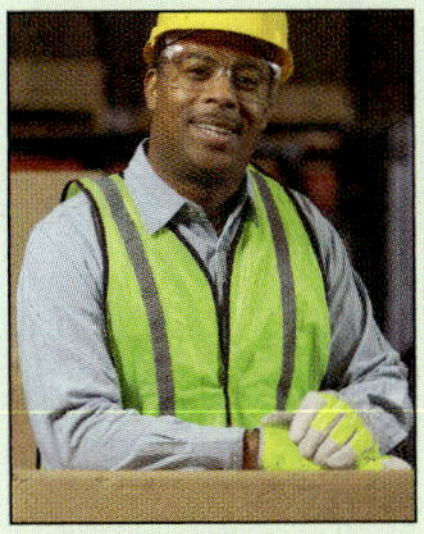

Tyrone Parker was feeling fine until about 3 days ago. He was at his job at a warehouse when he noticed pain in his back, but only on the left side. At first he thought maybe he pulled something when he was moving inventory. He took some over-the-counter pain medicine but this didn't really seem to help. In the past when he had back pain it got better after a night of sleep. When he woke up the next morning the pain was worse and it had spread into the lower part of his belly and his groin, still on the left side. He also noticed blood when he urinated. He was worried that he might have an infection of his bladder. He did not experience difficulty urinating but decided to make an appointment to see a physician who treats diseases of the urinary tract.

Now that you have worked through Chapter 6, on the urinary system, consider the medical terms that might be used to describe Tyrone's experience. See the Review of Terms at the end of the chapter for a list of terms that might apply.

A. *Underline phrases in the case study that could be substituted with medical terms.*

B. *Write the medical term and its definition for three of the phrases you underlined.*

MEDICAL TERM	DEFINITION
1. ____________________	____________________
	____________________
2. ____________________	____________________
	____________________
____________________	____________________
	____________________

DOCUMENTATION: Excerpt From the Urgent Care Visit

Tyrone decided to go to Urgent Care because he could receive care right away. The following was noted in the Subjective section of the Electronic Health Record (EHR).

The patient is a 38-year-old man who was in his usual state of good health when he began to experience left-sided flank pain accompanied by gross hematuria three days ago. He denies chills or fever. He has no prior history of renal calculi but was treated for UTI one year ago. His father had renal failure requiring hemodialysis.

C. *Underline medical terms presented in Chapter 6 in the previous excerpt from Tyrone's medical record. See the Review of Terms at the end of the chapter for a complete list.*

D. *Select and define three of the medical terms you underlined. To check your answers, go to Appendix A.*

MEDICAL TERM	DEFINITION
1. ____________________	____________________
	____________________
2. ____________________	____________________
	____________________
3. ____________________	____________________
	____________________

EXERCISE 43 *Interact With Medical Documents and Electronic Health Records*

A. Read the report and complete it by writing medical terms on answer lines within the document. Definitions of terms to be written appear after the document.

83658 OLIVER, Bruno

File Patient Navigate Custom Fields Help

Chart Review | Encounters | Notes | Labs | Imaging | Procedures | Rx | Documents | Referrals | Scheduling | Billing

Name: **OLIVER, Bruno** MR#: **7463802** DOB: **07/30/19XX** Gender: M Age: 32 **Allergies: NKDA** **PCP:** Betsy Bathilde MD

Date of Admssion: 09/20/20XX
Date of Discharge: 09/23/20XX

Discharge Summary: Bruno Oliver is a 32-year-old male, appearing his stated age, who was admitted to the hospital after presenting to the emergency department on 09/20/20XX in acute distress. He complained of intermittent pain in the right posterior lumbar area, radiating to the right flank. He has a family history of 1. ____________________ and has been treated for this condition two other times in the past 10 years.

The white blood count, hemoglobin, and hematocrit were normal. The urinalysis showed microscopic 2. ____________________ .

This patient was admitted to the 3. ____________________ Unit and was administered intravenous morphine sulfate for pain control. VITAL SIGNS: Low-grade temperature of 99.4. Initial blood pressure was 146/92 mm Hg.

A 4. ______________revealed 5. ____________________ in the region of the right renal pelvis. A 6. ____________________with a right retrograde 7. ____________________ confirmed the presence of the three stones in the right kidney. Significant ureteral obstruction was present.

A percutaneous 8. ____________________________________ was completed with no complications. A ureteral stent was inserted as was an indwelling Foley 9. __________. Drainage from the right kidney was pale yellow in 48 hours. The Foley catheter was removed 3 days postoperatively.

At discharge, the patient is voiding without difficulty. The stones were sent to the laboratory for analysis. The report indicated that they were calcium oxalate.

The patient is to follow up with his urologist in a week to have his ureteral stent removed.

Electronically signed: Evan Landis, DO 09/23/20XX 09:18

Start | Log On/Off | Print | Edit

Definitions of Medical Terms to Complete the Document

Write the medical terms defined on corresponding answer lines in the document.

1. condition of stones in the kidney
2. blood in the urine
3. study of the urinary tract
4. radiographic image of the abdomen
5. stones
6. visual examination of the bladder
7. radiographic image of the urinary tract
8. incision into the kidney to remove a stone
9. flexible, tubelike device

B. Read the medical report and answer the questions below it.

2478 HEARNE, Allen

File Patient Navigate Custom Fields Help

Chart Review | Encounters | Notes | Labs | Imaging | Procedures | Rx | Documents | Referrals | Scheduling | Billing

Name: **HEARNE, Allen** MR#: 2478 DOB: 01/01/19XX Gender: M Age: 31 **Allergies:** None **PCP:** Frank Peterson MD

Operative Report

Preoperative diagnosis: Urinary tract obstruction
Postoperative diagnosis: Ureterolithiasis
Surgery Performed: Ureteroscopy with calculus extraction

The patient, a 31-year-old previously healthy male, presented with complaints of left flank pain, oliguria, nausea, and chills. The patient denied gross hematuria. CT urogram revealed presence of a left proximal ureteral stone.

Procedure: Anesthesia was induced and the patient was then placed in the dorsal lithotomy position. The area was draped and prepared in the standard manner. Thirty mL of topical anesthesia (1% Lidocaine) was administered, and a penile clamp was applied to ensure retention. The ureteroscope was inserted, with access to the middle third of the ureter gained by passing a guidewire under fluoroscopic control. The guidewire was advanced beyond the stone, and the calculus was delivered through the ureter, engaged in a retrieval basket, and removed. The patient tolerated the procedure well and left the operating room in good condition.

Electronically signed: Martina Blancartt, MD 05/21/20XX 15:37

Start | Log On/Off | Print | Edit

Use the medical report above to answer the questions.

1. The patient presented with a complaint of
   a. difficult or painful urination.
   b. excessive urine.
   c. scanty urine.
   d. pus in the urine.
2. The presence of a ureteral stone was revealed by
   a. radiographic imaging.
   b. magnetic resonance imaging.
   c. ultrasound.
   d. computed tomography.
3. T F More than one stone was removed from the ureter.
4. Ureteroscope and ureteral are terms not included in the chapter. Using your knowledge of the meaning of word parts, define these terms.
   a. ureteral ______________________________
   b. ureteroscope ______________________________
   ____

C. Complete the **three medical documents** within the electronic health record (EHR) on Evolve.

Topic: Renal Calculus
Documents: Office Visit, Operative Report, Post-Operative Office Visit

To complete the three medical records, go to Evolve Resources at evolve.elsevier.com and select: Practice Student Resources > Student Resources > Chapter 6 > **Electronic Heath Records**

See Appendix B for instructions.

Healthcare records are stored and used in an electronic system called **Electronic Health Records (EHR)**. Electronic health records contain a collection of health information of an individual patient; the digitally formatted record can be shared through computer networks with patients, physicians, and other healthcare providers.

EXERCISE 44 *Pronounce Medical Terms in Use*

Practice pronunciation of terms by reading aloud the following paragraph. Use the phonetic spellings following medical terms from the chapter to assist with pronunciation. The script also contains medical terms not presented in the chapter. Treat them as information only or look for their meanings in a medical dictionary or a reliable online source.

A 76-year-old woman consulted with her primary care physician because of **hematuria** (*hēm*-a-TŪ-rē-a) and **dysuria** (dis-Ū-rē-a). She was referred to a **urologist** (ū-ROL-o-jist). **Urinalysis** (ū-rin-AL-is-is) disclosed 1+ albumin and mild **pyuria** (pī-Ū-rē-a) in addition to the hematuria. A spiral CT scan was obtained. Mild **nephrolithiasis** (*nef*-rō-lith-Ī-a-sis) was observed but no **hydronephrosis** (*hī*-drō-ne-FRŌ-sis). Finally a **cystoscopy** (sis-TOS-ko-pē) was performed, which showed mild **cystitis** (sis-TĪ-tis). A **urinary tract infection** (Ū-rin-*ār*-ē) (trakt) (in-FEK-shun) was diagnosed and the patient responded favorably to antibiotics. The urologist did not advise **lithotripsy** (LITH-ō-trip-sē) for the **renal calculi** (RĒ-nal) (KAL-kū-lī).

EXERCISE 45 *Chapter Content Quiz*

Test your understanding of terms and abbreviations introduced in this chapter. Circle the letter for the medical term or abbreviation related to the words in italics.

1. The patient was diagnosed with a *drooping kidney*, or:
   a. nephromegaly
   b. nephroblastoma
   c. nephroptosis
2. The patient's radiographic image showed *condition of stones in the ureter*, or a condition known as:
   a. ureterocele
   b. ureterolithiasis
   c. ureterostenosis
3. The patient was scheduled for a right ureteral pelvic junction *ESWL*, a surgical procedure to:
   a. separate tissue
   b. create an artificial opening
   c. remove a stone
4. The physician first suspected diabetes when told of the *excessive amounts of urine* voided, or:
   a. oliguria
   b. polyuria
   c. dysuria
5. The urologist told the patient with the drooping kidney that it is necessary to *secure the kidney in place* by performing a:
   a. nephropexy
   b. nephrolysis
   c. nephrolithotripsy
6. The patient had a *sudden stoppage of urine formation*, or:
   a. urinary suppression
   b. urinary retention
   c. azotemia
7. The patient was scheduled for a *radiographic image of the urinary bladder*, or:
   a. cystoscopy
   b. cystogram
   c. cystography
8. The patient's mother informed the doctor of her son's *involuntary urination*, or:
   a. diuresis
   b. dysuria
   c. enuresis
9. The patient was admitted to the hospital for *kidney and ureteral infection*, or:
   a. polycystic kidney disease
   b. urinary retention
   c. urinary tract infection
10. The nurse practitioner ordered a *UA* on the patient or:
    a. urine
    b. urinary
    c. urinalysis
11. *Albuminuria* indicates a kidney problem because of albumin in the
    a. blood
    b. urine
    c. urea
12. In the term nephrolithotripsy, *which word part indicates surgery?*
    a. first combining form
    b. second combining form
    c. suffix

13. When the bladder is *stretched out* because of urine, it is considered to be
    a. distended
    b. contracted
    c. flexible

14. *Peritoneal dialysis* is the procedure for removing which of the following when the kidney cannot do so?
    a. urine
    b. toxic waste
    c. nitrogen

15. A ureteral *stricture* means the ureter is
    a. ballooning
    b. narrowing
    c. blocked

For additional practice with chapter content, go to Evolve Resources at evolve.elsevier.com and select:
Practice Student Resources > Student Resources > Chapter 6 > **Games:** Medical Millionaire, Tournament of Terminology
Practice Quizzes: Word Parts, Terms Built from Word Parts, Terms NOT Built from Word Parts, and Abbreviations

See Appendix B for instructions.

CHAPTER REVIEW

REVIEW OF CHAPTER CONTENT ON EVOLVE RESOURCES

Go to evolve.elsevier.com and click on Gradable Student Resources and Practice Student Resources. Online learning activities found there can be used to review chapter content and to assess your learning of word parts, medical terms, and abbreviations. Place check marks in the boxes next to activities used for review and assessment.

GRADABLE STUDENT RESOURCES

Chapter 06 >	Exercises >	□ Word Parts □ Terms Built from Word Parts □ Terms Not Built from Word Parts □ Abbreviations
	Quizzes >	□ Quiz 1: Disease and Disorder Terms □ Quiz 2: Surgical Terms □ Quiz 3: Diagnostic Terms □ Quiz 4: Complementary Terms

PRACTICE STUDENT RESOURCES > STUDENT RESOURCES

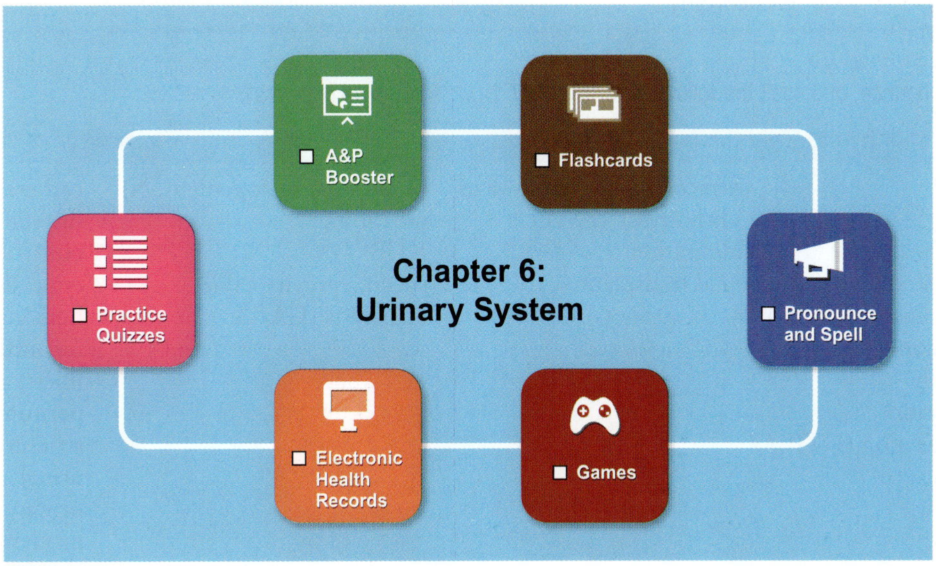

REVIEW OF WORD PARTS

Can you define and spell the following word parts?

COMBINING FORMS			SUFFIXES
albumin/o	hydr/o	ren/o	-esis
azot/o	lith/o	ureter/o	-iasis
blast/o	meat/o	urethr/o	-lysis
cyst/o	nephr/o	ur/o	-ptosis
glomerul/o	noct/i	urin/o	-rrhaphy
glyc/o	olig/o	vesic/o	-tripsy
glycos/o	pyel/o		-uria

REVIEW OF TERMS

Can you define, pronounce, and spell the following terms *built from word parts*?

DISEASES AND DISORDERS	SURGICAL	DIAGNOSTIC	COMPLEMENTARY
azotemia	cystectomy	cystogram	albuminuria
cystitis	cystolithotomy	cystography	anuria
cystocele	cystorrhaphy	cystoscope	diuresis
cystolith	cystostomy	cystoscopy	dysuria
glomerulonephritis	cystotomy	nephrography	glycosuria
hydronephrosis	lithotripsy	nephroscopy	hematuria
nephritis	meatotomy	nephrosonography	meatal
nephroblastoma	nephrectomy	renogram	nephrologist
nephrolithiasis	nephrolithotomy	retrograde urogram	nephrology
nephroma	nephrolithotripsy	ureteroscopy	nocturia
nephromegaly	nephrolysis	urogram	oliguria
nephroptosis	nephropexy	voiding cystourethrography (VCUG)	polyuria
pyelitis	nephrostomy		pyuria
pyelonephritis	pyelolithotomy		urinary
ureteritis	pyeloplasty		urologist
ureterocele	ureterectomy		urology
ureterolithiasis	ureterostomy		
ureterostenosis	urethroplasty		
urethrocystitis	vesicourethral suspension		
	vesicotomy		

Can you define, pronounce, and spell the following terms *NOT built from word parts*?

DISEASES AND DISORDERS	SURGICAL	DIAGNOSTIC	COMPLEMENTARY
epispadias	extracorporeal shock wave lithotripsy (ESWL)	blood urea nitrogen (BUN)	catheter (cath)
hypospadias	fulguration	creatinine	distended
polycystic kidney disease	renal transplant	KUB	electrolytes
renal calculus (pl. calculi)		specific gravity (SG)	enuresis
renal failure		urinalysis (UA)	hemodialysis (HD)
renal hypertension			incontinence
urinary retention			micturate
urinary suppression			peritoneal dialysis
urinary tract infection (UTI)			stricture
			urinal
			urinary catheterization
			urodynamics
			void

Chapter 7

Male Reproductive System

Outline

Objectives

Upon completion of this chapter you will be able to:

1. Pronounce organs and anatomic structures of the male reproductive system.
2. Define and spell word parts related to the male reproductive system.
3. Define, pronounce, and spell disease and disorder terms related to the male reproductive system.
4. Define, pronounce, and spell surgical terms related to the male reproductive system.
5. Define, pronounce, and spell diagnostic terms related to the male reproductive system.
6. Define, pronounce, and spell complementary terms related to the male reproductive system.
7. Interpret the meaning of abbreviations related to the male reproductive system.
8. Apply medical language in clinical contexts.

ANATOMY

The organs of the male reproductive system include the external genitalia, the penis, and scrotum, within which are contained the testes and an initial section of the vas deferens. Internally, the male pelvis includes a major portion of the vas deferens, the seminal vesicles, and the prostate gland. The penis and urethra are shared with the urinary system (Fig. 7.1).

Function

The function of the male reproductive system is to produce, sustain, and transport sperm, the male reproductive germ cells, and to secrete the hormone testosterone (Fig. 7.2).

Organs and Anatomic Structures of the Male Reproductive System

TERM	DEFINITION
testis (pl. testes) (TES-tis), (TES-tēs)	primary male sex organ, paired, oval-shaped, and enclosed in a sac called the **scrotum**. The testes produce spermatozoa (sperm cells) and the hormone testosterone. (also called **testicle**)
seminiferous tubules (*sem*-i-NIF-er-es) (TOO-bū-elz)	approximately 900 coiled tubes within the testes in which spermatogenesis occurs
sperm (spurm)	the microscopic male germ cell, which, when united with the ovum, produces a zygote (fertilized egg) that with subsequent development becomes an embryo (Fig. 7.2) (also called **spermatozoon, pl. spermatozoa**)
testosterone (tes-TOS-te-rōn)	the principal male sex hormone. Its chief function is to stimulate the development of the male reproductive organs and secondary sex characteristics such as facial hair.

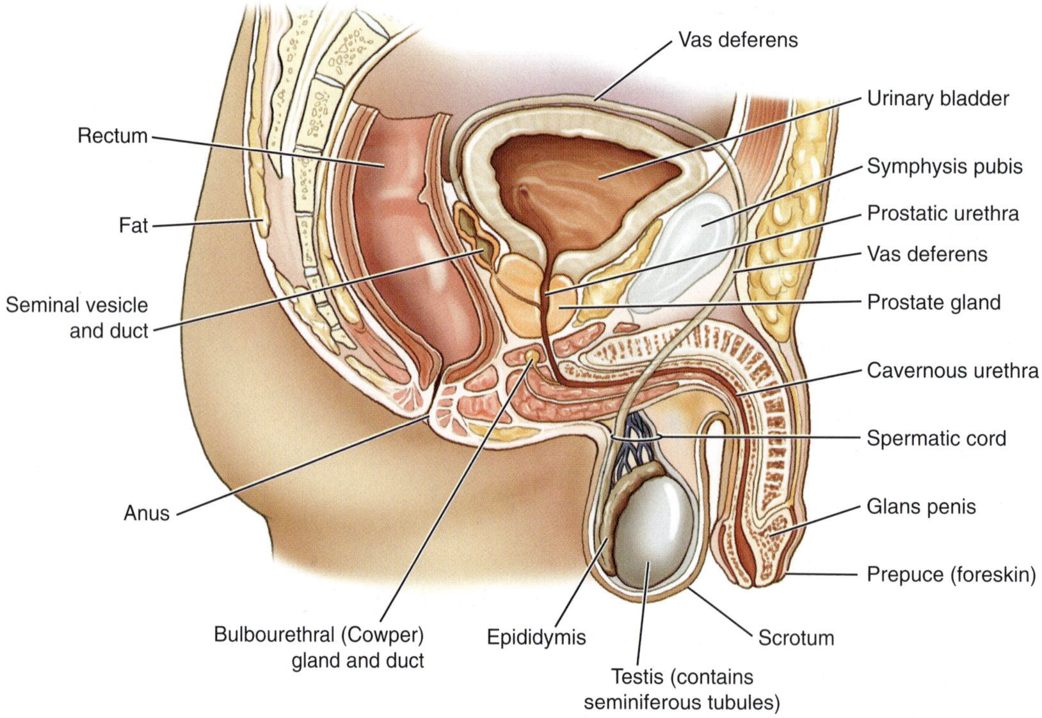

FIG. 7.1 Male reproductive organs and associated structures.

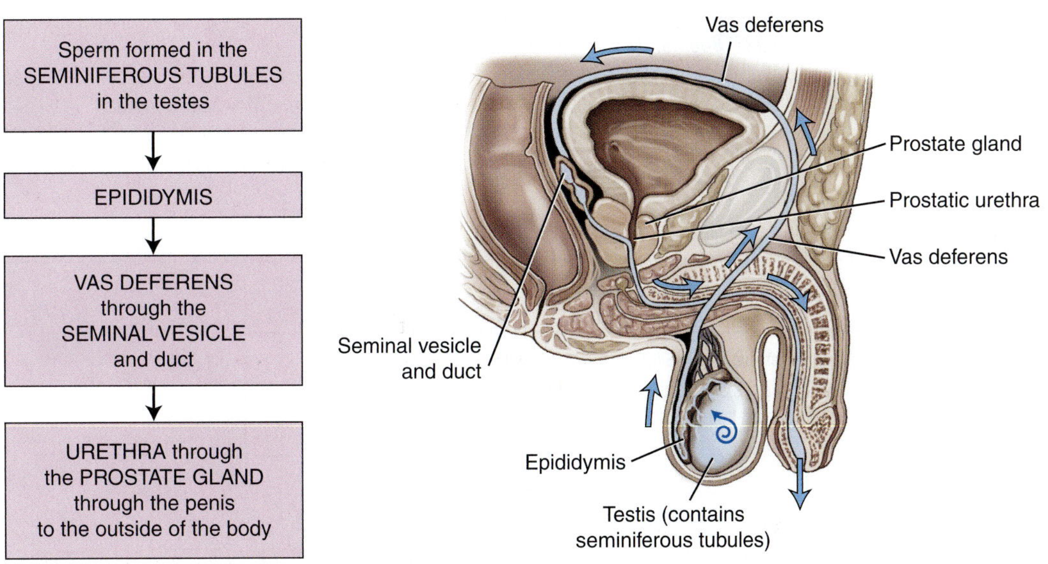

FIG. 7.2 Origination and transportation of sperm.

TERM	DEFINITION
epididymis (ep-i-DID-a-mis)	coiled tube attached to each of the testes that provides for storage, transit, and maturation of sperm; continuous with the vas deferens
vas deferens (vas) (DEF-ar-enz)	duct carrying the sperm from the epididymis to the urethra. The **spermatic cord** encloses each vas deferens with nerves, lymphatics, arteries, and veins. The urethra also connects with the urinary bladder and carries urine outside the body. A circular muscle constricts during intercourse to prevent urination. (Also called **ductus deferens**.)
seminal vesicles (SEM-e-nel) (VES-i-kelz)	two main glands located posterior to the base of the bladder that open into the vas deferens. The glands secrete a thick fluid that forms part of the semen.
prostate gland (PROS-tāt) (gland)	encircles a proximal section of the urethra. The prostate gland secretes a fluid that aids in the movement of the sperm and ejaculation.
semen (SĒ-men)	composed of sperm, seminal fluids, and other secretions
scrotum (SKRŌ-tem)	sac containing the testes and epididymis, suspended on both sides of and posterior to the penis
penis (PĒ-nis)	male organ of urination and coitus (sexual intercourse)
glans penis (glanz) (PĒ-nis)	enlarged tip on the end of the penis
prepuce (PRE-pūs)	fold of skin covering the glans penis in uncircumcised males (foreskin of the penis)
genitalia (*jen*-i-TĀ-lē-a)	reproductive organs (male or female); includes internal and external reproductive organs (also called **genitals**)
gonads (GŌ-nadz)	primary reproductive organs; testes in males, ovaries in females

PROSTATE

is derived from the Greek **pro**, meaning **before**, and **statis**, meaning **standing** or **sitting**. Anatomically it is the gland standing before the bladder.

A&P Booster
For more anatomy and physiology, go to Evolve Resources at evolve.elsevier.com and select:
Practice Student Resources > Student Resources > Chapter 7 > **A&P Booster**

See Appendix B for instructions.

EXERCISE 1

Practice saying aloud each of the Organs and Anatomic Structures.

To hear the terms, go to Evolve Resources at evolve.elsevier.com and select:
Practice Student Resources > Student Resources > Chapter 7 > **Pronounce and Spell**

See Appendix B for instructions.

❑ Check the box when complete.

WORD PARTS

Word parts you need to learn to complete this chapter are listed on the following pages. The exercises at the end of each list help you learn their definitions and spellings.

Use the flashcards accompanying this text or electronic flashcards to assist you in memorizing the word parts for this chapter.

Combining Forms of the Male Reproductive System

COMBINING FORM	DEFINITION
andr/o	male
balan/o	glans penis
epididym/o	epididymis
orchid/o, orchi/o, orch/o	testis, testicle
prostat/o	prostate gland
sperm/o, spermat/o	sperm, spermatozoon (pl. spermatozoa)
vas/o	vessel, duct (vas deferens in terms describing the male reproductive system)
vesicul/o	seminal vesicle(s)

EXERCISE 2

Fill in the blanks with combining forms for this diagram of the male reproductive system. *To check your answers, go to Appendix A.*

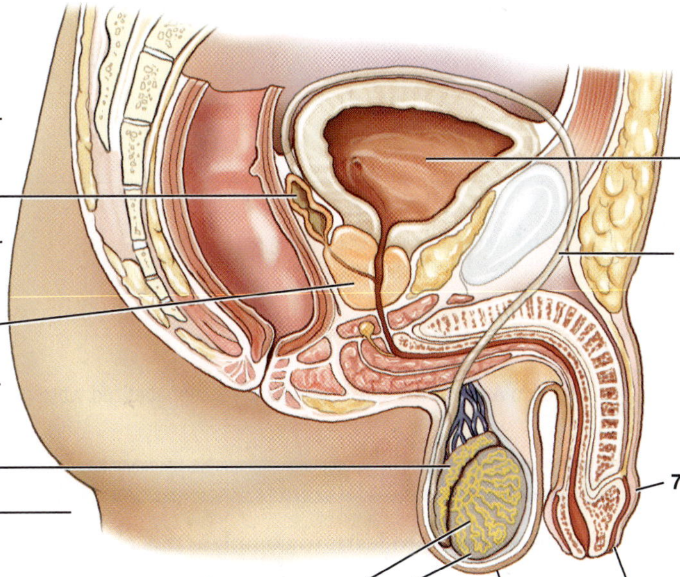

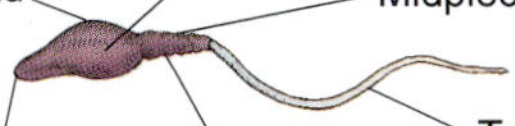

EXERCISE 3

Step 1: Write the definitions after the following combining forms.
Step 2: Match the descriptions on the right with the combining forms and definitions. Answers may be used more than once. No answer line appears for those not described in a lettered item.

_____ 1. sperm/o, ____________
_____ 2. vas/o (vas deferens), ____________
_____ 3. spermat/o, ____________
_____ 4. balan/o, ____________
_____ 5. prostat/o, ____________
_____ 6. orch/o, ____________
_____ 7. vesicul/o, ____________
_____ 8. orchi/o, ____________
_____ 9. epididym/o, ____________
_____ 10. orchid/o, ____________
11. andr/o, ____________

a. duct carrying the sperm from the epididymis to the urethra
b. enlarged tip on the end of the penis
c. two main glands located posterior to the base of the bladder that open into the vas deferens
d. primary male sex organs, paired, oval-shaped, and enclosed in a sac
e. coiled tube attached to each of the testes that provides for storage, transit, and maturation of sperm
f. encircles a proximal section of the urethra; secretes fluid that aids in the movement of the sperm and ejaculation
g. microscopic male germ cell, which, when united with the ovum, produces a zygote

Suffix

SUFFIX	DEFINITION
-ism	state of

EXERCISE 4

Write the definition for the suffix.

-ism ______________________________

For additional practice with Word Parts, go to Evolve Resources at evolve.elsevier.com and select:
Practice Student Resources > Student Resources > Chapter 7 > **Flashcards**

See Appendix B for instructions.

Refer to **Appendix C** and **Appendix D** for alphabetized word parts and their meanings.

MEDICAL TERMS

The terms you need to learn to complete this chapter are listed below. The exercises following each list will help you learn the definition and the spelling of each word.

Disease and Disorder Terms

BUILT FROM WORD PARTS

The following terms can be translated using definitions of word parts. Further explanation is provided within parentheses as needed.

TERM	DEFINITION
anorchism (an-OR-kizm)	state of absence of testis (unilateral or bilateral)
balanitis (*bal*-a-NĪ-tis)	inflammation of the glans penis (Exercise Figure A)
balanorrhea (*bal*-a-nō-RĒ-a)	discharge from the glans penis
benign prostatic hyperplasia (BPH) (be-NĪN) (pros-TAT-ik) (*hī*-per-PLĀ-zha)	excessive development pertaining to the prostate gland (nonmalignant enlargement of the prostate gland; as the gland enlarges, it causes narrowing of the urethra, which interferes with the passage of urine. Symptoms include frequency of urination, nocturia, urinary retention, and incomplete emptying of the bladder.) (also called **benign prostatic hypertrophy**) (Fig. 7.3)
cryptorchidism (krip-TOR-ki-*diz*-em)	state of hidden testis. (During fetal development, testes are located in the abdominal area near the kidneys. Before birth they move down into the scrotal sac. Failure of one or both of the testes to descend from the abdominal cavity into the scrotum before birth results in cryptorchidism.) (also called **undescended testicle** and **undescended testicles**) (Exercise Figure B)
epididymitis (*ep*-i-*did*-i-MĪ-tis)	inflammation of the epididymis

EXERCISE FIGURE A

Fill in the blanks with word parts to label the diagram.

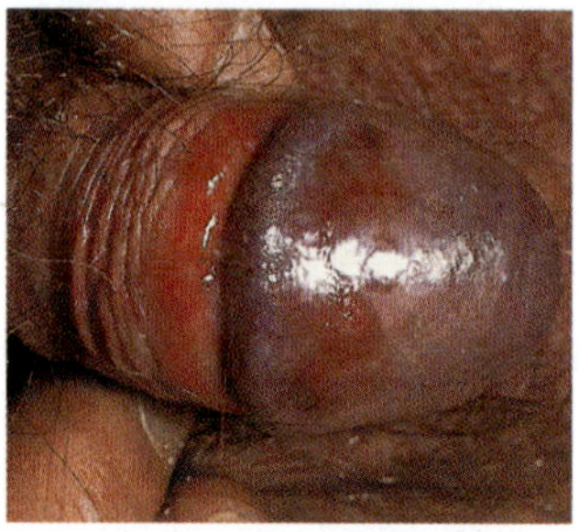

_______ / _______
glans penis / inflammation

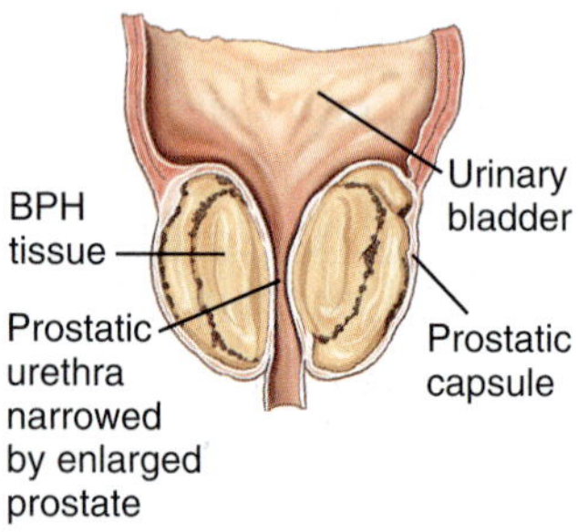

FIG. 7.3 Benign prostatic hyperplasia grows inward, causing narrowing of the urethra.

TERM	DEFINITION
orchiepididymitis (*or*-kē-*ep*-i-*did*-i-MĪ-tis)	inflammation of the testis and the epididymis
orchitis (or-KĪ-tis)	inflammation of the testis (also called **orchiditis**)
prostatitis (pros-ta-TĪ-tis)	inflammation of the prostate gland
prostatocystitis (*pros*-ta-tō-sis-TĪ-tis)	inflammation of the prostate gland and the (urinary) bladder
prostatolith (pros-TAT-ō-lith)	stone(s) in the prostate gland
prostatorrhea (pros-ta-tō-RĒ-a)	discharge from the prostate gland
prostatovesiculitis (*pros*-ta-tō-ves-*ik*-ū-LĪ-tis)	inflammation of the prostate gland and the seminal vesicles

BENIGN PROSTATIC HYPERPLASIA AND BENIGN PROSTATIC HYPERTROPHY

As the male ages, the prostate gland may undergo tissue changes called **prostatic hyperplasia**, which is the abnormal increase in the number of cells. The result is an enlarged prostate gland, referred to as **prostatic hypertrophy. Benign prostatic hyperplasia** is the correct term for the pathologic process, but **benign prostatic hypertrophy** is also currently used to describe this condition.

EXERCISE 5

Practice saying aloud each of the Disease and Disorder Terms Built from Word Parts.

To hear the terms, go to Evolve Resources at evolve.elsevier.com and select:
Practice Student Resources > Student Resources > Chapter 7 > **Pronounce and Spell**

See Appendix B for instructions.

❑ Check the box when complete.

EXERCISE FIGURE B

Fill in the blanks with word parts to label the diagram.

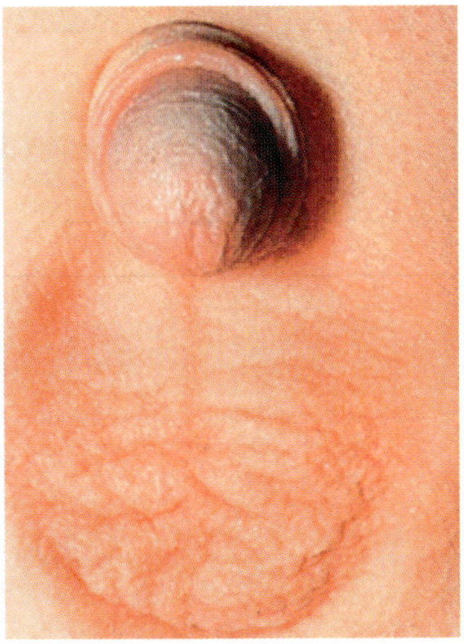

1. bilateral ______ / ______ / ______
hidden / testis / state of

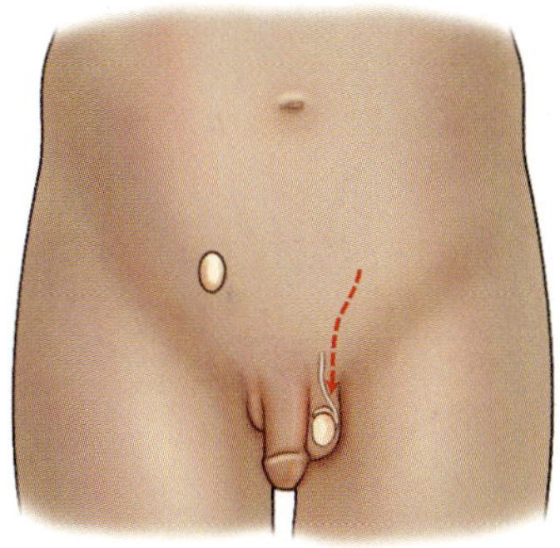

2. The *arrow* shows the path the testis takes in its descent to the scrotal sac before birth.

INTEGRATIVE MEDICINE TERM

Acupuncture is the ancient practice of inserting very thin needles into acupoints just under the skin to treat disease, increase immune response, relieve pain, and restore health. Studies suggest that acupuncture and electroacupuncture provide therapeutic benefits for men who have been diagnosed with **benign prostatic hyperplasia** and **prostate cancer**.

EXERCISE 6

Analyze and define the following terms by drawing slashes between word parts, writing word part abbreviations above the term, underlining combining forms, and writing combining form abbreviations below the term.

1. prostatolith
2. balanitis
3. orchitis
4. prostatovesiculitis
5. prostatocystitis
6. orchiepididymitis
7. prostatorrhea
8. epididymitis
9. (benign) prostatic hyperplasia
10. cryptorchidism
11. balanorrhea
12. prostatitis
13. anorchism

EXERCISE 7

Build disease and disorder terms for the following definitions with the word parts you have learned.

1. inflammation of the prostate gland and the (urinary) bladder ________ WR / CV / WR / S
2. stone(s) in the prostate gland ________ WR / CV / WR
3. inflammation of the testis ________ WR / S
4. excessive development pertaining to the prostate gland benign ________ WR / S ________ P / S(WR)
5. state of hidden testis ________ WR / WR / S
6. inflammation of the prostate gland and the seminal vesicles ________ WR / CV / WR / S
7. state of absence of testis ________ P / WR / S
8. inflammation of the prostate gland ________ WR / S
9. inflammation of the testis and the epididymis ________ WR / WR / S
10. discharge from the glans penis ________ WR / CV / S
11. inflammation of the epididymis ________ WR / S
12. inflammation of the glans penis ________ WR / S
13. discharge from the prostate gland ________ WR / CV / S

EXERCISE 8

Spell each of the Disease and Disorder Terms Built from Word Parts by having someone dictate them to you. Use a separate sheet of paper.

To hear and spell the terms, go to Evolve Resources at evolve.elsevier.com and select:
Practice Student Resources > Student Resources > Chapter 7 > **Pronounce and Spell**

See Appendix B for instructions.

❑ Check the box when complete.

Disease and Disorder Terms
NOT BUILT FROM WORD PARTS

Word parts may be present in the following terms; however, their full meanings cannot be translated using definitions of word parts alone.

ERECTILE DYSFUNCTION (ED)

Oral therapies, such as sildenafil (Viagra), vardenafil (Levitra), and tadalafil (Cialis) are currently first-line treatment for erectile dysfunction and work by relaxing smooth muscle cells and, as such, increasing the flow of blood in the genital area. Second-line treatment includes penile self-injectable drugs and vacuum devices. Surgical implantation of a penile prosthesis is available for men who cannot use or who have not responded to other treatments.

TERM	DEFINITION
erectile dysfunction (ED) (e-REK-tīl) (dis-FUNK-shun)	the inability of the male to attain or maintain an erection sufficient to perform sexual intercourse (formerly called **impotence**)
hydrocele (HĪ-drō-sēl)	fluid-filled sac around the testicle; causes scrotal swelling
phimosis (fī-MŌ-sis)	a tightness of the prepuce (foreskin of the penis) that prevents its retraction over the glans penis; it may be congenital or a result of balanitis. Circumcision is the usual treatment.
priapism (PRĪ-a-*piz-m*)	persistent abnormal erection of the penis accompanied by pain and tenderness
prostate cancer (PROS-tāt) (KAN-cer)	cancer of the prostate gland, usually occurring in men middle-aged and older (Table 7.1)
spermatocele (SPER-ma-tō-sēl)	distention of the epididymis containing an abnormal cyst-like collection of fluid and sperm cells; may cause scrotal swelling
testicular cancer (tes-TIK-ū-ler) (KAN-cer)	cancer of the testicle, usually occurring in men 15 to 35 years of age
testicular torsion (tes-TIK-ū-ler) (TOR-shun)	twisting of the spermatic cord causing decreased blood flow to the testis; occurs most often during puberty and often presents with a sudden onset of severe testicular or scrotal pain. Because of lack of blood flow to the testis, it is considered a surgical emergency.
varicocele (VAR-i-kō-*sēl*)	enlarged veins of the spermatic cord; may cause scrotal swelling

EXERCISE 9

Practice saying aloud each of the Disease and Disorder Terms NOT Built from Word Parts.

To hear the terms, go to Evolve Resources at evolve.elsevier.com and select:
Practice Student Resources > Student Resources > Chapter 7 > **Pronounce and Spell**

See Appendix B for instructions.

❑ Check the box when complete.

TABLE 7.1 Prostate Cancer

Prostate cancer is the most commonly diagnosed cancer in men and the second most common cause of cancer death among men in the United States. Approximately 95% of all cancers of the prostate are adenocarcinomas, arising from epithelial cells.

DIAGNOSTIC AND STAGING PROCEDURES

1. Digital rectal examination (DRE)
2. Prostate-specific antigen (PSA)
3. Transrectal ultrasound (TRUS)
4. Transrectal ultrasonically guided biopsy
5. MRI ultrasound fusion biopsy
6. MRI with endorectal surface coil (used for staging, not diagnosis)
7. Multiparametric MRI (used for staging, not diagnosis)

TREATMENT

Treatment depends on the stage of the prostate cancer, the age of the patient, and choices of treatment by the patient and his physician. Options include the following:

1. **Radical prostatectomy (RP)**, which may be performed by retropubic or perineal routes, laparoscopically, or with the use of robotic-assisted devices
2. **Radiation therapy**, which may be performed with an external beam or with radioactive seeds (brachytherapy)
3. **Bilateral orchiectomy** or **hormonal therapy** to reduce the production of testosterone, which fuels the growth of prostate cancer
4. **Chemotherapy**, treating cancer with drugs
5. **Active Surveillance**, with the intent to pursue active therapy if disease progresses

PROGRESSION OF PROSTATE CANCER

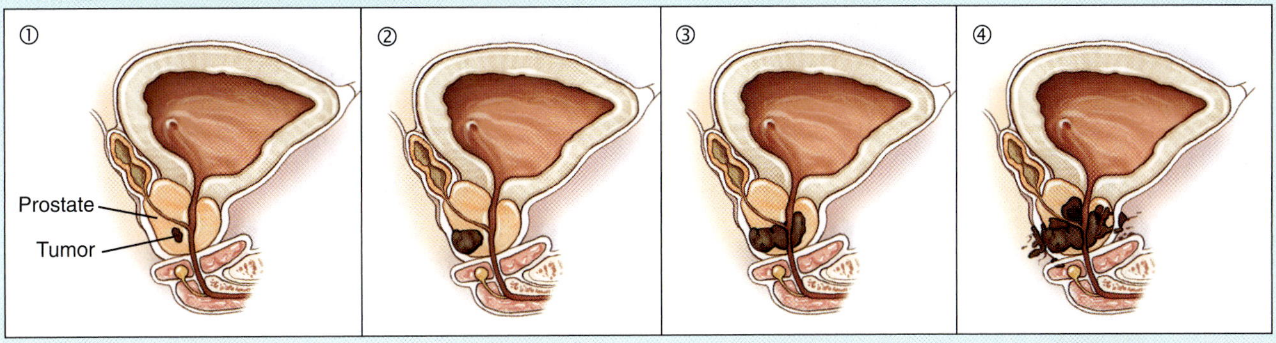

EXERCISE 10

A. Fill in the blanks with the correct terms.

1. Another way of referring to cancer of the testicle is ______________________________.
2. Inability of the man to attain or maintain an erection is called ______________________________.
3. Persistent abnormal erection is called ______________________________.
4. ______________________ is the twisting of the spermatic cord causing decreased blood flow.
5. Distention of the epididymis containing an abnormal cyst-like collection of fluid and sperm cells is called a(n) ______________________________.

EXERCISE 10—*cont'd*

B. Write the medical term pictured and defined.

1. ______________________________
enlarged veins of the spermatic cord

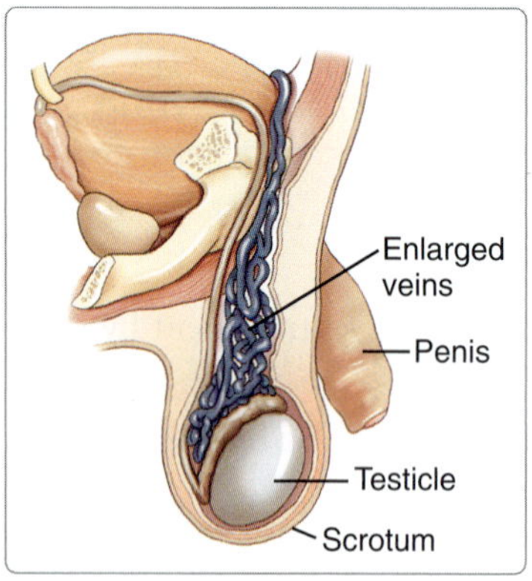

2. ______________________________
a tightness of the prepuce (foreskin of the penis) that prevents its retraction over the glans penis

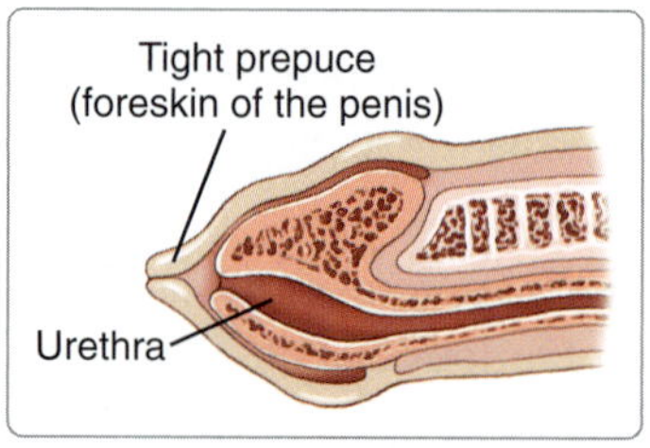

3. ______________________________
fluid-filled sac around the testicle; causes scrotal swelling

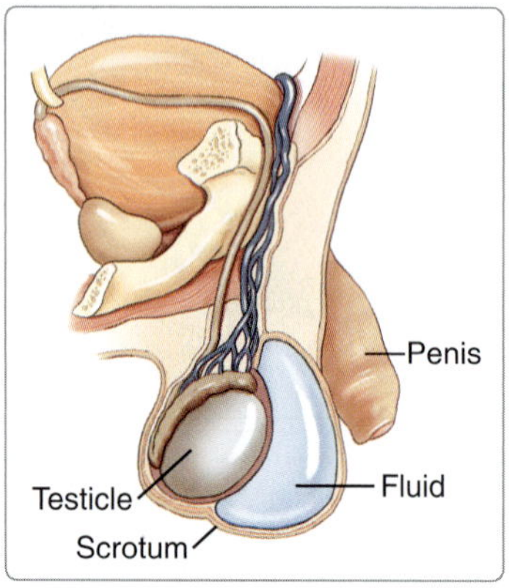

4. ______________________________
cancer of the prostate gland

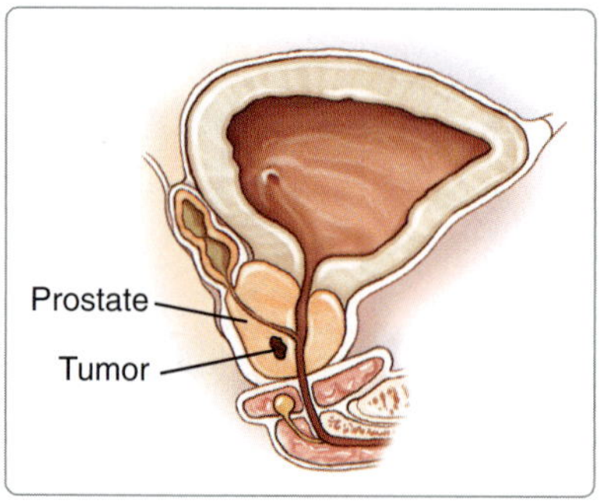

EXERCISE 11

Match the terms in the first column with the correct definitions in the second column.

______ 1. varicocele	a. fluid-filled sac around the testicle; causes scrotal swelling
______ 2. phimosis	b. inability to attain or maintain an erection
______ 3. testicular cancer	c. tightness of the prepuce
______ 4. erectile dysfunction	d. enlarged veins of the spermatic cord; may cause scrotal swelling
______ 5. hydrocele	e. cancer of the testicle
______ 6. prostate cancer	f. cancer of the prostate gland
______ 7. testicular torsion	g. distention of the epididymis containing an abnormal cyst-like collection of fluid and sperm cells
______ 8. priapism	h. persistent abnormal erection
______ 9. spermatocele	i. twisting of the spermatic cord causing decreased blood flow

EXERCISE 12

Spell each of the Disease and Disorder Terms NOT Built from Word Parts by having someone dictate them to you. Use a separate sheet of paper.

To hear and spell the terms, go to Evolve Resources at evolve.elsevier.com and select:
Practice Student Resources > Student Resources > Chapter 7 > **Pronounce and Spell**

See Appendix B for instructions.

❑ Check the box when complete.

Surgical Terms

BUILT FROM WORD PARTS

The following terms can be translated using definitions of word parts. Further explanation is provided within parentheses as needed.

TERM	DEFINITION
balanoplasty (BAL-a-nō-*plas*-tē)	surgical repair of the glans penis
epididymectomy (*ep*-i-*did*-i-MEK-to-mē)	excision of the epididymis
orchiectomy (*or*-kē-EK-to-mē)	excision of the testis (bilateral orchiectomy is called **castration**) (also called **orchidectomy**)
orchiopexy (OR-kē-ō-pek-sē)	surgical fixation of the testicle (performed to bring undescended testicle[s] into the scrotum) (also called **orchidopexy**)
orchioplasty (OR-kē-ō-*plas*-tē)	surgical repair of the testis
orchiotomy (*or*-kē-OT-o-mē)	incision into the testis (also called **orchidotomy**)
prostatectomy (*pros*-ta-TEK-to-mē)	excision of the prostate gland (Tables 7.1, 7.2, and 7.3)
prostatocystotomy (*pros*-tat-ō-sis-TOT-o-mē)	incision into the prostate gland and the (urinary) bladder
prostatolithotomy (*pros*-tat-ō-li-THOT-o-mē)	incision into the prostate gland to remove stone(s)
prostatovesiculectomy (*pros*-tat-ō-ves-*ik*-ū-LEK-to-mē)	excision of the prostate gland and the seminal vesicles
vasectomy (va-SEK-to-mē)	excision of a duct (partial excision of the vas deferens bilaterally, resulting in male sterilization [Exercise Figure C]).
vasovasostomy (*vas*-ō-vā-ZOS-to-mē)	creation of artificial openings between ducts (the severed ends of the vas deferens are reconnected in an attempt to restore fertility in men who have had a vasectomy)
vesiculectomy (ve-*sik*-ū-LEK-to-mē)	excision of the seminal vesicle(s)

EXERCISE FIGURE C

Fill in the blanks with word parts to label the diagram.

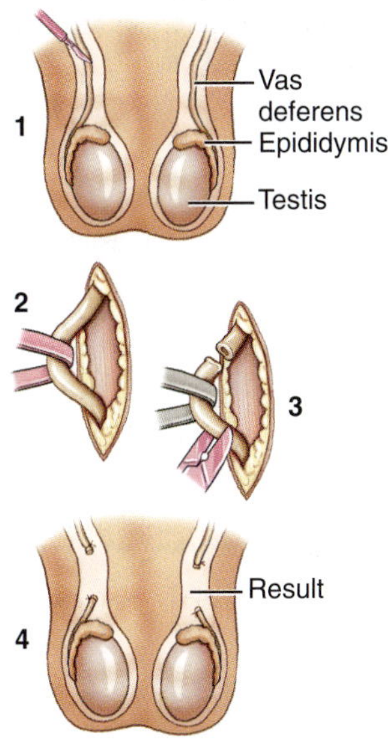

_____ / _____
duct / excision

1. incision is made into the covering of the vas deferens
2. vas deferens is exposed and ligated (tied off)
3. segment of vas deferens is excised
4. vas deferens is repositioned and skin is sutured

TABLE 7.2 Types of Prostatectomies

SIMPLE PROSTATECTOMY	RADICAL PROSTATECTOMY (RP)
The inside portion of the prostate gland is excised through an abdominal incision made above the pubic bone and through an incision in the bladder and prostate capsule.	The prostate gland with its capsule, seminal vesicles, vas deferens, and sometimes pelvic lymph nodes are excised. The procedure may be performed by various approaches, including retropubic, perineal, and laparoscopic. Retropubic and perineal approaches are performed using large, open incisions. Laparoscopic and robot-assisted surgeries use smaller incisions.
Used to treat **benign prostatic hyperplasia (BPH)**.	Used to treat **prostate cancer**.
Also called **suprapubic prostatectomy**	Also called **radical retropubic prostatectomy, laparoscopic radical prostatectomy,** and **robotic-assisted laparoscopic radical prostatectomy (RALRP)**
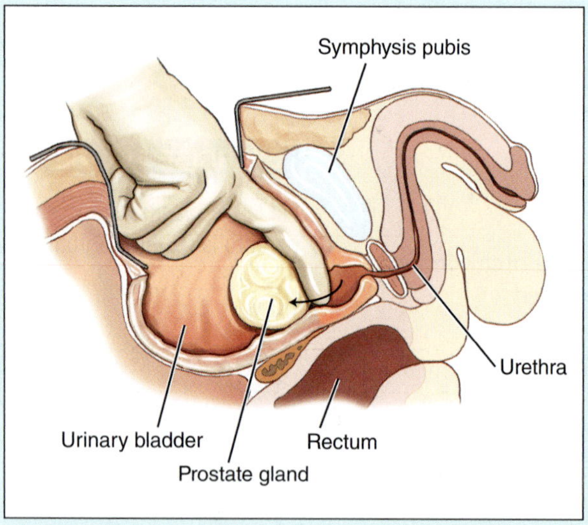	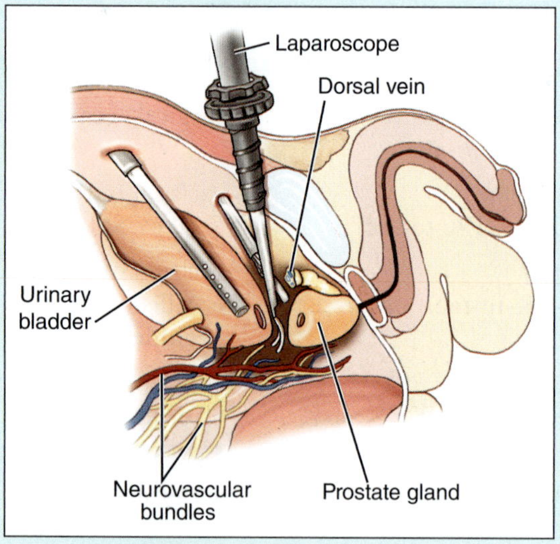
Simple prostatectomy with a suprapubic approach (large incision surgery). The surgeon approaches the prostate gland through an incision in the urinary bladder and uses a finger to remove the hyperplastic tissue.	**Radical prostatectomy** with a laparoscopic approach (small incision surgery). Laparoscopic radical prostatectomy and robotic-assisted laparoscopic radical prostatectomy (RALRP) are procedures used to treat early stages of prostate cancer.

EXERCISE 13

Practice saying aloud each of the Surgical Terms Built from Word Parts.

> To hear the terms, go to Evolve Resources at evolve.elsevier.com and select:
> Practice Student Resources > Student Resources > Chapter 7 > **Pronounce and Spell**
>
> See Appendix B for instructions.

❑ Check the box when complete.

EXERCISE 14

Analyze and define the following terms by drawing slashes between word parts, writing word part abbreviations above the term, underlining combining forms, and writing combining form abbreviations below the term.

1. vasectomy
2. prostatocystotomy
3. orchiotomy
4. epididymectomy
5. orchiopexy
6. prostatovesiculectomy
7. orchioplasty
8. vesiculectomy
9. prostatectomy
10. balanoplasty
11. vasovasostomy
12. orchiectomy
13. prostatolithotomy

EXERCISE 15

Build surgical terms for the following definitions by using the word parts you have learned.

1. excision of the testis ______ / ______
WR / S

2. surgical repair of the glans penis ______ / ______ / ______
WR / CV / S

3. incision into the prostate gland and the (urinary) bladder
_____ / _____ / _____ / _____ / _____
WR / CV / WR / CV / S

4. excision of the seminal vesicle(s)
_____ / _____
WR / S

5. incision into the prostate gland to remove stone(s)
_____ / _____ / _____ / _____ / _____
WR / CV / WR / CV / S

6. incision into the testis
_____ / _____ / _____
WR / CV / S

7. excision of the epididymis
_____ / _____
WR / S

8. surgical repair of the testis
_____ / _____ / _____
WR / CV / S

9. excision of the prostate gland
_____ / _____
WR / S

10. excision of a duct (partial excision of the vas deferens)
_____ / _____
WR / S

11. excision of the prostate gland and the seminal vesicles
_____ / _____ / _____ / _____
WR / CV / WR / S

12. surgical fixation of the testicle
_____ / _____ / _____
WR / CV / S

13. creation of artificial openings between ducts
_____ / _____ / _____ / _____ / _____
WR / CV / WR / CV / S

EXERCISE 16

Spell each of the Surgical Terms Built from Word Parts by having someone dictate them to you. Use a separate sheet of paper.

> To hear and spell the terms, go to Evolve Resources at evolve.elsevier.com and select:
> Practice Student Resources > Student Resources > Chapter 7 > **Pronounce and Spell**
>
> See Appendix B for instructions.

❑ Check the box when complete.

Surgical Terms
NOT BUILT FROM WORD PARTS

Word parts may be present in the following terms; however, their full meanings cannot be translated using definitions of word parts alone.

TERM	DEFINITION
ablation (ab-LĀ-shun)	destruction of abnormal or excessive tissue by melting, vaporizing, or eroding
circumcision (*ser*-kum-SI-zhun)	surgical removal of the prepuce (foreskin); all or part of the foreskin may be removed (Fig. 7.4)
enucleation (ē-*nū*-klē-Ā-shun)	excision of a whole organ or mass without cutting into it
hydrocelectomy (*hī*-drō-sē-LEK-to-mē)	surgical removal of a fluid-filled sac around the testicle causing scrotal swelling (hydrocele)
laser surgery (LĀ–ser) (SUR-jer-ē)	use of a focused beam of light to excise or vaporize abnormal tissue and to control bleeding; uses a variety of non-invasive and minimally invasive procedures. Two common types of laser surgery used to treat BPH are **holmium laser enucleation of the prostate gland (HoLEP)** and **photoselective vaporization of the prostate gland (PVP)**. (Table 7.3, Fig 7.5)
morcellation (*mor*-se-LĀ-shun)	cutting or grinding solid tissue into smaller pieces for removal
MRI ultrasound fusion biopsy (M-R-I) (UL-tra-sound) (FŪ-shun) (BĪ-op-sē)	combination of magnetic resonance imaging with transrectal ultrasound (TRUS) to obtain a tissue from a prostate lesion. Software merges an existing MR image with live ultrasound images. The combined, or fused, MRI-TRUS image is used to direct the biopsy needle into the area of the prostate that looked suspicious on MRI. (also called **MRI-TRUS fusion, MR-ultrasound fusion,** and **fusion guided biopsy**) (Table 7.1)
robotic surgery (rō-BOT-ik) (SUR-jer-ē)	use of small surgical instruments attached to a computer and operated by the surgeon from a console several feet from the operating table (Table 7.2, Fig. 7.6)
transurethral incision of the prostate gland (TUIP) (trans-ū-RĒ-thral) (in-SIZH-en) (PROS-tāt) (gland)	surgical procedure that widens the urethra by making a few small incisions in the bladder neck and the prostate gland. No prostate tissue is removed. TUIP may be used instead of TURP when the prostate gland is less enlarged (Table 7.3).
transurethral microwave thermotherapy (TUMT) (trans-ū-RĒ-thral) (MĪ-krō-wāv) (*ther*-mō-THER-a-pē)	treatment that eliminates excess tissue present in benign prostatic hyperplasia by using heat generated by microwave (Table 7.3)
transurethral resection of the prostate gland (TURP) (trans-ū-RĒ-thral) (rē-SEK-shun) (PROS-tāt) (gland)	surgical removal of pieces of the prostate gland tissue by using an instrument inserted through the urethra. The capsule is left intact; usually performed when the enlarged prostate gland interferes with urination (Table 7.3).

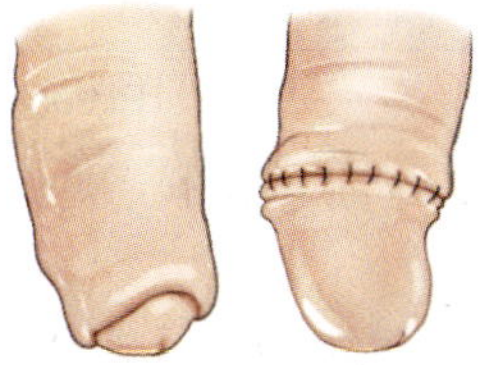

FIG. 7.4 Circumcision.

HoLEP

Holmium laser enucleation of the prostate gland (HoLEP), a minimally invasive endoscopic **laser surgery**, has demonstrated improved outcomes for patients treated for BPH. HoLEP provides a promising alternative to **transurethral resection of the prostate gland (TURP)** and suprapubic prostatectomy.

TABLE 7.3 Surgical Treatments for Benign Prostatic Hyperplasia

<table>
<tr><th>INCISIONAL SURGERIES</th><th>LASER SURGERIES</th><th>OTHER SURGICAL PROCEDURES</th></tr>
<tr><td>1. Simple prostatectomy
2. Transurethral incision of the prostate gland (TUIP)
3. Transurethral resection of the prostate gland (TURP)</td><td>1. Holmium laser enucleation of the prostate gland (HoLEP)
2. Photoselective vaporization of the prostate gland (PVP)</td><td>1. Transurethral microwave thermotherapy (TUMT)
2. Transurethral needle ablation (TUNA)</td></tr>
<tr><td>

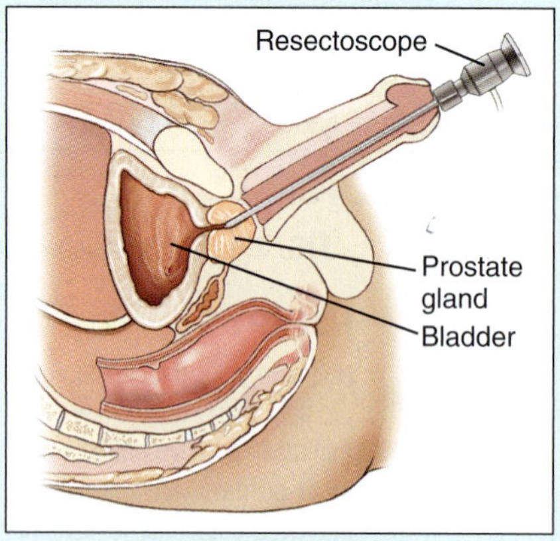

</td><td>

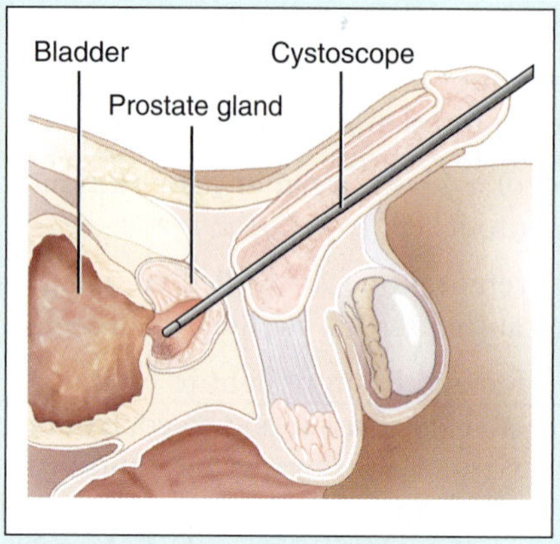

</td><td>

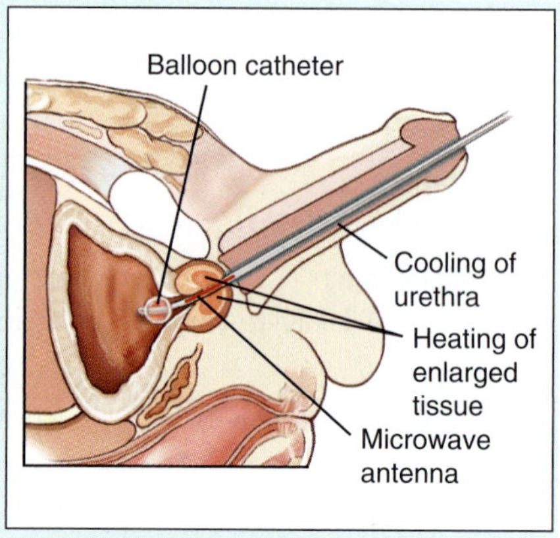

</td></tr>
<tr><td>Transurethral resection of the prostate gland (TURP) uses a resectoscope inserted through the urethra to the prostate gland. The end of the instrument is equipped to remove pieces of the enlarged prostate gland to relieve bladder outlet obstruction (BOO).</td><td>Photoselective vaporization of the prostate gland (PVP) uses a laser system operated through a cystoscope inserted through the urethra to the prostate gland. Overgrown prostate tissue is vaporized using heat generated by the laser.</td><td>Transurethral microwave thermotherapy (TUMT) destroys prostate tissue with heat from microwaves emitted by an antenna guided by a catheter, which has been inserted through the urethra. A cooling mechanism protects surrounding tissue.</td></tr>
</table>

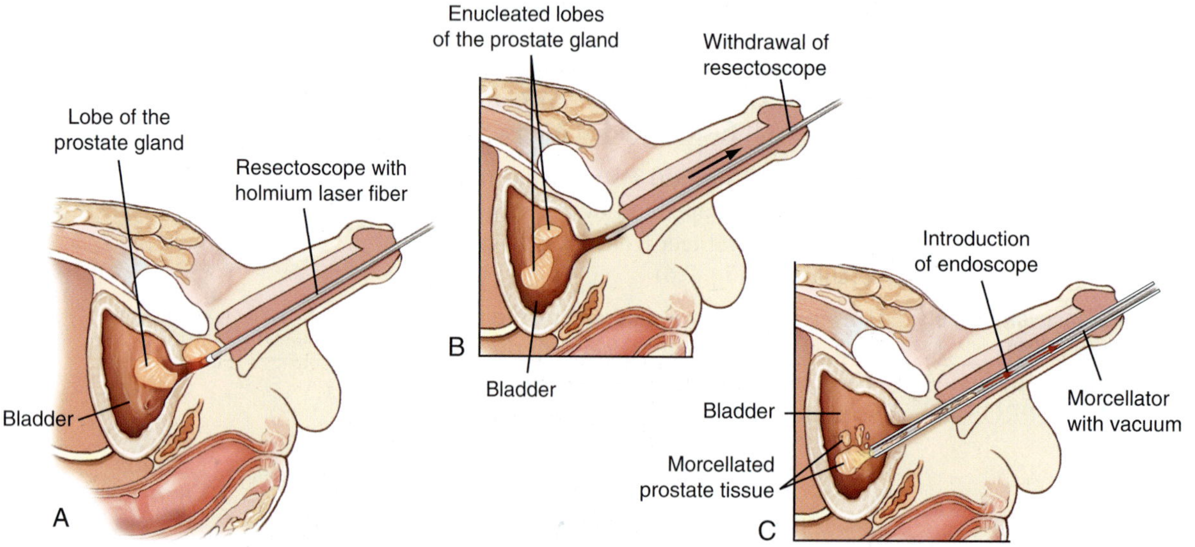

FIG. 7.5 Holmium laser enucleation of the prostate (HoLEP) is a laser surgery performed endoscopically to treat benign prostatic hyperplasia. **A,** The lobes of the prostate gland are removed intact from surrounding structures using a holmium laser. **B,** The enucleated lobes are temporarily placed in the urinary bladder. **C,** The lobes of the prostate are morcellated within the urinary bladder and removed through the endoscope using suction.

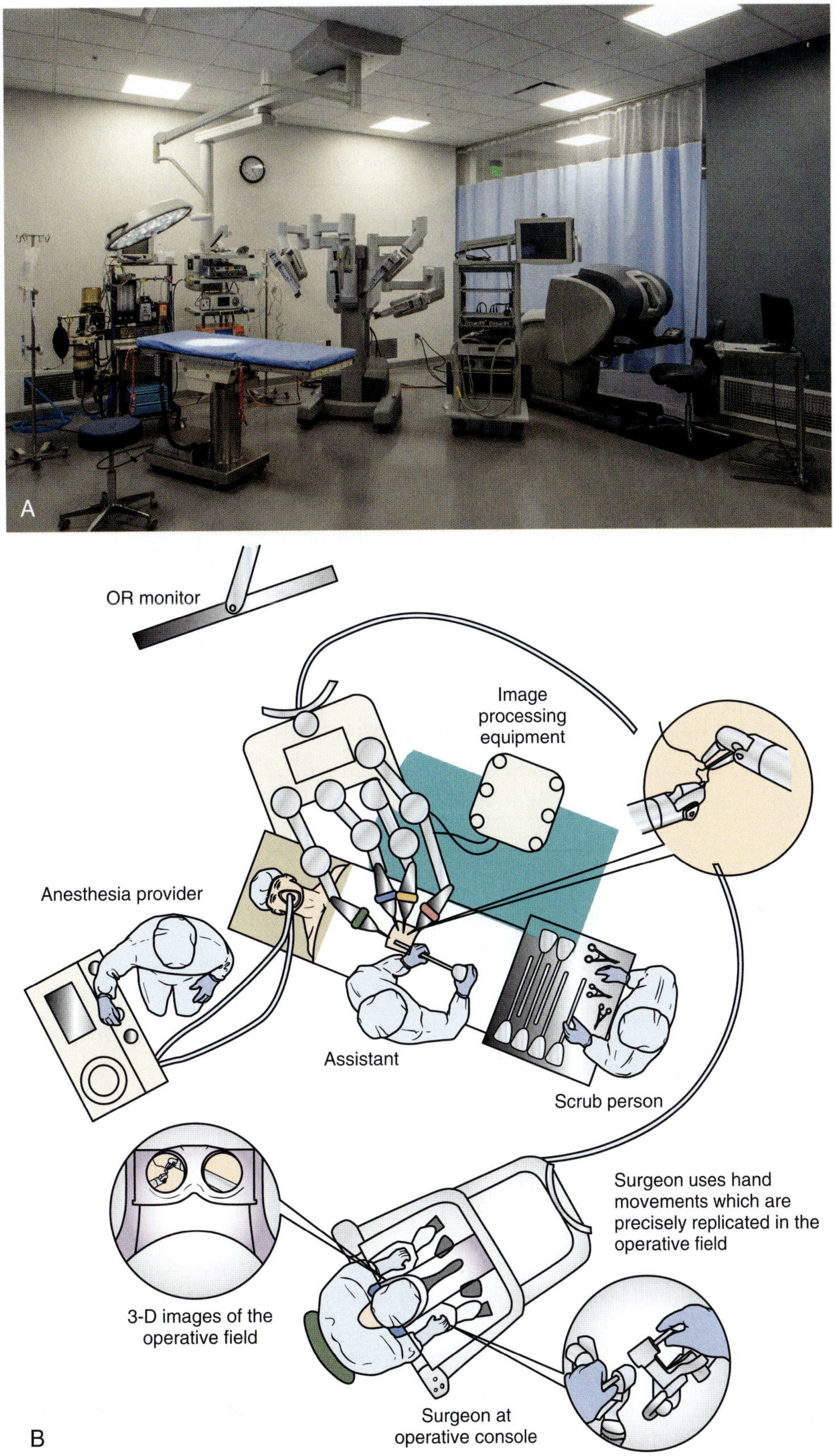

FIG. 7.6 Robotic surgery. **A,** Surgical suite. **B,** Operating room set-up for robotic-assisted laparoscopic radical prostatectomy (RALRP) with a robotic system. Note the surgeon performs the procedure at an operative console rather than hands-on surgery.

EXERCISE 17

Practice saying aloud each of the Surgical Terms NOT Built from Word Parts.

> To hear the terms, go to Evolve Resources at evolve.elsevier.com and select:
> Practice Student Resources > Student Resources > Chapter 7 > **Pronounce and Spell**
>
> See Appendix B for instructions.

❑ Check the box when complete.

EXERCISE 18

Fill in the blanks with the correct term.

1. The excision of a whole organ (such as the eye), structure (such as a lobe of the prostate gland), or mass (such as a tumor) without cutting into it is called ______________________.
2. The surgical procedure performed to remove all or part of the prepuce is called a(n) ______________________.
3. Photoselective vaporization of the prostate (PVP) is one form of ______________________, the destruction of abnormal or excessive tissue by melting, vaporizing, or eroding.
4. Surgical removal of a fluid-filled sac around the testicle causing scrotal swelling is ______________________.
5. ______________________ is a treatment for benign prostatic hyperplasia that uses heat generated by microwave.
6. A surgical procedure for benign prostatic hyperplasia that widens the urethra by making small incisions is called ______________________.
7. Pieces of prostate gland tissue are removed with an instrument during the surgical procedure called ______________________.
8. One type of ______________________, where a focused beam of light is used to excise or vaporize abnormal tissue and to control bleeding, is holmium laser enucleation of the prostate gland (HoLEP).
9. A prostatectomy may be performed using ______________________, where small surgical instruments attached to a computer are operated by the surgeon from a console several feet from the operating table.
10. Endoscopic surgeries often involve ______________________, where solid tissue is cut or ground into smaller pieces for removal.
11. Discovery of a lesion on an MRI of the prostate gland, may be followed by a(n) ______________________ ______________________ biopsy, which combines magnetic resonance imaging with transrectal ultrasound (TRUS) to guide the biopsy needle.

EXERCISE 19

Spell each of the Surgical Terms NOT Built from Word Parts by having someone dictate them to you. Use a separate sheet of paper.

> To hear and spell the terms, go to Evolve Resources at evolve.elsevier.com and select:
> Practice Student Resources > Student Resources > Chapter 7 > **Pronounce and Spell**
>
> See Appendix B for instructions.

❑ Check the box when complete.

Diagnostic Terms
NOT BUILT FROM WORD PARTS

Word parts may be present in the following terms; however, their full meanings cannot be translated using definitions of word parts alone.

TERM	DEFINITION
DIAGNOSTIC IMAGING	
multiparametric MRI (mul-TĪ-par-a-*met*-rik) (M-R-I)	magnetic resonance imaging procedure providing information of anatomic structure and physiology for the staging of prostate cancer. It uses a combination of different MRI modalities to better understand the size and extent of prostate tumors. (Table 7.1)
transrectal ultrasound (TRUS) (trans-REK-tal) (UL-tra-sound)	ultrasound procedure used to diagnose prostate cancer. Sound waves are sent and received by a transducer probe that is placed into the rectum. (Table 7.1)
LABORATORY	
prostate-specific antigen (PSA) (PROS-tāt) (spe-SIF-ik) (AN-ti-jen)	blood test that measures the level of prostate-specific antigen in the blood. Elevated test results may indicate the presence of prostate cancer, urinary or prostatic infection, or excess prostate tissue, as found in benign prostatic hyperplasia or prostatitis (Table 7.1).
semen analysis (SĒ-men) (a-NAL-i-sis)	microscopic observation of ejaculated semen, revealing the size, structure, and movement of sperm; used to evaluate male infertility and to determine the effectiveness of a vasectomy (also called **sperm count** and **sperm test**)
OTHER	
digital rectal examination (DRE) (DIJ-i-tal) (REK-tal) (eg-*zam*-i-NĀ-shun)	physical examination in which the healthcare provider inserts a gloved finger into the rectum and palpates the prostate through the rectal wall to determine the size, shape, and consistency of the gland; used to screen for BPH and prostate cancer. BPH usually presents as a uniform, nontender enlargement, whereas cancer usually presents as a stony hard nodule. (Table 7.1)

EXERCISE 20

Practice saying aloud each of the Diagnostic Terms NOT Built from Word Parts.

To hear the terms, go to Evolve Resources at evolve.elsevier.com and select:
Practice Student Resources > Student Resources > Chapter 7 > **Pronounce and Spell**

See Appendix B for instructions.

❑ Check the box when complete.

EXERCISE 21

Fill in the blanks with the correct terms.

1. A physical examination in which the healthcare provider palpates the prostate through the rectal wall to determine the size, shape, and consistency of the gland is called ______________________________.
2. A blood test that, when elevated, may indicate the presence of prostate cancer is called ______________________________.
3. A diagnostic ultrasound procedure used to obtain images of the prostate gland is called ______________________________.
4. A laboratory test for microscopic observation of ejaculated semen to evaluate male infertility is called ______________________________.
5. A magnetic resonance imaging procedure that provides structural and physiological information for the staging of prostate cancer is called ______________________________.

EXERCISE 22

Spell each of the Diagnostic Terms NOT Built from Word Parts by having someone dictate them to you. Use a separate sheet of paper.

> To hear and spell the terms, go to Evolve Resources at evolve.elsevier.com and select:
> Practice Student Resources > Student Resources > Chapter 7 > **Pronounce and Spell**
>
> See Appendix B for instructions.

❑ Check the box when complete.

Complementary Terms

BUILT FROM WORD PARTS

The following terms can be translated using definitions of word parts. Further explanation is provided within parentheses as needed.

ASPERMIA

condition of without sperm, may indicate the lack of production of spermatozoa, the lack of production of semen, or the lack of ejaculation of semen.

TERM	DEFINITION
andropathy (an-DROP-a-thē)	disease of the male (specific to the male, such as orchitis)
aspermia (a-SPER-mē-a)	condition of without sperm (or semen or ejaculation)
oligospermia (*ol*-i-gō-SPER-mē-a)	condition of scanty sperm (in the semen; may contribute to infertility)
orchialgia (*ōr*-kē-AL-ja)	pain in the testis (also called **testalgia**)
spermatolysis (*sper*-ma-TOL-i-sis)	dissolution (destruction) of sperm
transurethral (*trans*-ū-RĒ-thral)	pertaining to through the urethra

EXERCISE 23

Practice saying aloud each of the Complementary Terms Built from Word Parts.

To hear the terms, go to Evolve Resources at evolve.elsevier.com and select:
Practice Student Resources > Student Resources > Chapter 7 > **Pronounce and Spell**

See Appendix B for instructions.

❑ Check the box when complete.

EXERCISE 24

Analyze and define the following terms by drawing slashes between word parts, writing word part abbreviations above the term, underlining combining forms, and writing combining form abbreviations below the term.

1. orchialgia
____
____

2. oligospermia
____
____

3. andropathy
____
____

4. spermatolysis
____
____

5. aspermia
____
____

6. transurethral
____
____

EXERCISE 25

Build the complementary terms for the following definitions by using the word parts you have learned.

1. dissolution (destruction) of sperm ______ / ______ / ______ (WR / CV / S)

2. condition of without sperm (or semen or ejaculation) ______ / ______ / ______ (P / WR / S)

3. disease of the male ______ / ______ / ______ (WR / CV / S)

4. condition of scanty sperm (in the semen) ______ / ______ / ______ / ______ (WR / CV / WR / S)

5. pain in the testis ______ / ______ (WR / S)

6. pertaining to through the urethra ______ / ______ / ______ (P / WR / S)

EXERCISE 26

Spell each of the Complementary Terms Built from Word Parts by having someone dictate them to you. Use a separate sheet of paper.

To hear and spell the terms, go to Evolve Resources at evolve.elsevier.com and select:
Practice Student Resources > Student Resources > Chapter 7 > **Pronounce and Spell**

See Appendix B for instructions.

❑ Check the box when complete.

Complementary Terms
NOT BUILT FROM WORD PARTS

Word parts may be present in the following terms; however, their full meanings cannot be translated using definitions of word parts alone.

TERM	DEFINITION
acquired immunodeficiency syndrome (AIDS) (a-KWĪRD) (*im*-ū-nō-de-FISH-en-sē) (SIN-drōm)	advanced, chronic immune system suppression caused by human immunodeficiency virus (HIV) infection; manifested by opportunistic infections (such as candidiasis and tuberculosis), neurologic disease (peripheral neuropathy and cognitive motor impairment), and secondary neoplasms (Kaposi sarcoma)
artificial insemination (ar-ti-FISH-al) (in-*sem*-i-NĀ-shun)	introduction of washed and concentrated sperm into the female reproductive tract; used as a treatment for infertility
azoospermia (ā-*zō*-a-SPUR-mē-a)	lack of live sperm in the semen
chlamydia (kla-MID-ē-a)	sexually transmitted disease, caused by the bacterium *C. trachomatis*; sometimes referred to as a **silent STD** because many people are not aware they have the disease. Symptoms that occur when the disease becomes serious are painful urination and discharge from the penis in men and genital itching, vaginal discharge, and bleeding between menstrual periods in women.
coitus (KŌ-i-tus)	sexual intercourse between male and female
condom (KON-dum)	cover for the penis worn during coitus to prevent conception and the spread of sexually transmitted disease
ejaculation (ē-*jak*-ū-LĀ-shun)	ejection of semen from the male urethra
genital herpes (JEN-i-tal) (HER-pēz)	sexually transmitted disease caused by herpes simplex virus type 2

AZOOSPERMIA

the lack of live sperm in the semen, may be:

- **obstructive**, caused by blocked vessels or ducts;
- **nonobstructive**, caused by infection, lack of production of spermatozoa, or retrograde ejaculation where semen travels into the urinary bladder rather than exiting through the urethra.

TERM	DEFINITION
gonorrhea (gon-ō-RĒ-a)	sexually transmitted disease caused by a bacterial organism that inflames the mucous membranes of the genitourinary tract
human immunodeficiency virus (HIV) (HŪ-man) (*im*-ū-nō-de-FISH-en-sē) (VĪ-rus)	sexually transmitted disease caused by a retrovirus that infects T-helper cells of the immune system; may also be acquired in utero or transmitted through infected blood via needle sharing. Advanced HIV infection progresses to AIDS.
human papillomavirus (HPV) (HŪ-man) (*pap*-i-LŌ-ma-*vī*-rus)	sexually transmitted disease caused by viral infection; there are more than 40 types of HPV that cause benign or cancerous growths in male and female genitals (also called **genital warts**)
infertility (*in*-fer-TIL-i-tē)	reduced or absent ability to achieve pregnancy; generally defined after one year of frequent, unprotected coitus; may relate to male or female
orgasm (ŌR-gazm)	climax of sexual stimulation
puberty (PŪ-ber-tē)	period when secondary sex characteristics (such as pubic and armpit hair, deepening of voice in men, breast development in women, etc.) develop and the ability to reproduce sexually begins
sexually transmitted disease (STD) (SEK-shū-al-ē) (TRANS-mi-ted) (di-ZĒZ)	infection spread through sexual contact; STDs affect both males and females, causing damage to reproductive organs and potentially serious health consequences if left untreated (also called **sexually transmitted infection [STI]**)
sterilization (*stār*-i-li-ZĀ-shun)	procedure that prevents pregnancy, either the ability of the female to conceive or the male to induce conception
syphilis (SIF-i-lis)	infection caused by the bacterium *Treponema pallidum*. Rapidly spreads throughout the body, and if untreated becomes systemic and can progress through three stages separated by latent periods. Usually sexually transmitted, but may be acquired in utero and by direct contact with infected skin. (Fig. 7.7)
trichomoniasis (*trik*-ō-mō-NĪ-a-sis)	sexually transmitted disease caused by a one-cell organism *Trichomonas*. It infects the genitourinary tract. Men may be asymptomatic or may develop urethritis, an enlarged prostate gland, or epididymitis. Women may have vaginal itching, dysuria, and vaginal or urethral discharge.

Refer to **Appendix F** for pharmacology terms.

HUMAN PAPILLOMAVIRUS

is the cause of most cervical cancers. Some penile, vulvar, vaginal, throat, and anal cancers are also linked to **HPV** infection.

HPV is the most prevalent sexually transmitted disease and vaccines are available to protect men and women from **HPV** infection.

LIST OF MALE AND FEMALE SEXUALLY TRANSMITTED DISEASES

chlamydia
genital herpes
gonorrhea
human immunodeficiency virus
human papillomavirus
syphilis
trichomoniasis

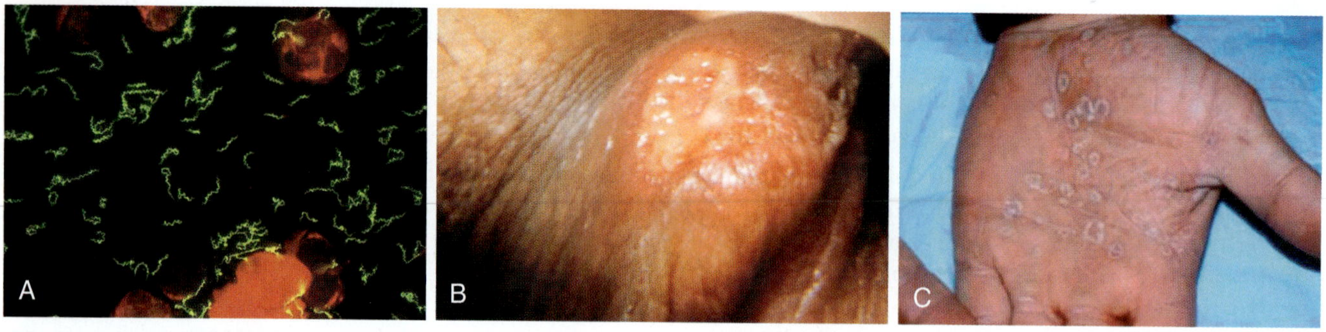

FIG. 7.7 Syphilis. **A,** *Treponema pallidum*, organism responsible for syphilis viewed microscopically. **B,** Primary syphilis, depicting a syphilitic chancre. **C,** Secondary syphilis, depicting rash on palms of hands.

EXERCISE 27

Practice saying aloud each of the Complementary Terms NOT Built from Word Parts.

To hear the terms, go to Evolve Resources at evolve.elsevier.com and select:
Practice Student Resources > Student Resources > Chapter 7 > **Pronounce and Spell**

See Appendix B for instructions.

❑ Check the box when complete.

EXERCISE 28

Match the terms in the first column with their correct definitions in the second column.

_____ 1. coitus	a. climax of sexual stimulation
_____ 2. ejaculation	b. STD caused by herpes simplex virus type 2
_____ 3. human papillomavirus	c. ejection of semen
_____ 4. genital herpes	d. lack of live sperm in the semen
_____ 5. gonorrhea	e. sexual intercourse between man and woman
_____ 6. orgasm	f. also called genital warts
_____ 7. condom	g. STD caused by a bacterium that inflames mucous membranes
_____ 8. azoospermia	h. cover for the penis worn during coitus
_____ 9. infertility	i. inability to achieve pregnancy after 1 year of unprotected coitus

EXERCISE 29

Match the terms in the first column with their correct definitions in the second column.

_____ 1. STD
_____ 2. sterilization
_____ 3. syphilis
_____ 4. puberty
_____ 5. AIDS
_____ 6. trichomoniasis
_____ 7. artificial insemination
_____ 8. chlamydia
_____ 9. HIV

a. abbreviation for infections spread through sexual contact
b. advanced, chronic immune system suppression
c. retrovirus that progresses to AIDS
d. infection caused by *Treponema pallidum*; if untreated, progresses through three stages
e. introduction of washed and concentrated sperm into the female reproductive tract
f. STD caused by a bacterium, *C. trachomatis* (silent STD)
g. procedure that prevents pregnancy, either the ability of the female to conceive, or the male to induce conception
h. STD caused by a one-cell organism, *Trichomonas*
i. period when the ability to sexually reproduce begins

EXERCISE 30

Spell each of the Complementary Terms NOT Built from Word Parts by having someone dictate them to you.

To hear and spell the terms, go to Evolve Resources at evolve.elsevier.com and select:
Practice Student Resources > Student Resources > Chapter 7 > **Pronounce and Spell**

See Appendix B for instructions.

❑ Check the box when complete.

Abbreviations

ABBREVIATION	TERM
AIDS	acquired immunodeficiency syndrome
BOO	bladder outlet obstruction
BPH	benign prostatic hyperplasia
DRE	digital rectal examination
ED	erectile dysfunction
HIV	human immunodeficiency virus
HoLEP	holmium laser enucleation of the prostate gland
HPV	human papillomavirus
LUTS	lower urinary tract symptoms
PSA	prostate-specific antigen
PVP	photoselective vaporization of the prostate gland
RP	radical prostatectomy
STD	sexually transmitted disease
STI	sexually transmitted infection
TRUS	transrectal ultrasound

WEB LINK

For more information on a spectrum of topics related to the male reproductive system, visit the National Institutes of Health at www.health.nih.gov and click on Men's Health.

Abbreviations—cont'd

ABBREVIATION	TERM
TUIP	transurethral incision of the prostate gland
TUMT	transurethral microwave thermotherapy
TURP	transurethral resection of the prostate gland

Refer to **Appendix E** for a complete list of abbreviations.

EXERCISE 31

Write the term abbreviated.

1. The patient experienced **LUTS** ______________________________ ______________ caused by **BOO** ______________________________.
2. The physician performed a **DRE** ______________________________ on the patient to assist in diagnosing **BPH** ______________________________.
3. Surgical treatments for BPH include:
   TUIP ______________________________ of the prostate gland
   TURP ______________________________ of the prostate gland
   TUMT ______________________________
   PVP ______________________________ of the prostate gland
   HoLEP ______________________________ of the prostate gland
4. **HIV** ______________________________ is a type of retrovirus that causes **AIDS** ______________________________.
5. **HPV** ______________________________ causes female and male genital warts and most cervical cancers.
6. **STI** ______________________________ is another name for **STD** ______________________________.
7. **PSA** ______________________________ is a laboratory test used to diagnose cancer of the prostate.
8. **RP** ______________________________ is a surgical procedure to treat prostate cancer.
9. **ED** ______________________________ was formerly referred to as impotence.
10. **TRUS** ______________________________, used in the diagnosis of prostate cancer, provides imaging of the prostate gland and is used as a guide for biopsy of the prostate.

For additional practice with Abbreviations, go to Evolve Resources at evolve.elsevier.com and select: Practice Student Resources > Student Resources > Chapter 7 > **Flashcards: Abbreviations**

See Appendix B for instructions.

PRACTICAL APPLICATION

EXERCISE 32 *Case Study: Translate Between Everyday Language and Medical Language*

CASE STUDY: Jimmie Zeller

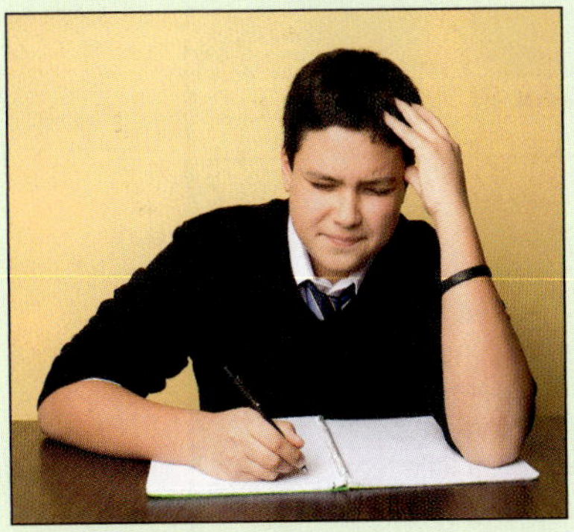

Jimmie, a 15-year-old male, is in the Emergency Department (ED) because of pain in his testicle that started about 6 hours ago. The pain started suddenly, he felt nauseated, and vomited twice. The ED physician examined him and found that his scrotum was swollen, and the painful testicle was higher than the other. A Doppler ultrasound was performed and the findings suggested twisting of the spermatic cord with decreased blood flow to the testis. A surgeon was called immediately to examine Jimmie, since this condition requires immediate surgical fixation of the testis or even surgical removal of the testis. The surgeon examined him quickly, and took him immediately to the operating room, since she knew that the risk of reduced or absent ability to achieve pregnancy increases when this condition is left untreated.

Now that you have worked through Chapter 7 on the male reproductive system, consider the medical terms that might be used to describe Jimmie's experience. See the Review of Terms at the end of the chapter for a list of terms that might apply.

A. *Underline phrases in the case study that could be substituted with medical terms.*

B. *Write the medical term and its definition for three of the phrases you underlined.*

MEDICAL TERM	DEFINITION
1. ______________________	______________________________
2. ______________________	______________________________
3. ______________________	______________________________

DOCUMENTATION: Excerpt From Operative Note

This 15-year-old male presented to the Emergency Department with orchialgia and a swollen scrotum of approximately 6 hours duration. A Doppler ultrasound was suspicious for testicular torsion and my examination was also highly suggestive of this. He was brought to the operating room for surgical exploration. The patient and his mother received informed consent in which the possibilities of orchiectomy and future infertility were addressed. After appropriate anesthesia and sterile preparation of the surgical field were performed, a transscrotal approach was used to bring the affected testicle into the operative field. Testicular torsion was confirmed and the spermatic cord was detorsed until no twists were visible. Orchiopexy was then performed on both testes using permanent sutures.

C. *Underline medical terms presented in Chapter 7 used in the previous excerpt from Jimmie's medical record. See the Review of Terms at the end of the chapter for a complete list*

D. *Select and define three of the medical terms you underlined. To check your answers, go to Appendix A.*

MEDICAL TERM	DEFINITION
1. ______________________	______________________________
2. ______________________	______________________________
3. ______________________	______________________________

EXERCISE 33 *Interact With Medical Documents and Electronic Health Records*

A. Read the report and complete it by writing medical terms on answer lines within the document. Definitions of terms to be written appear after the document.

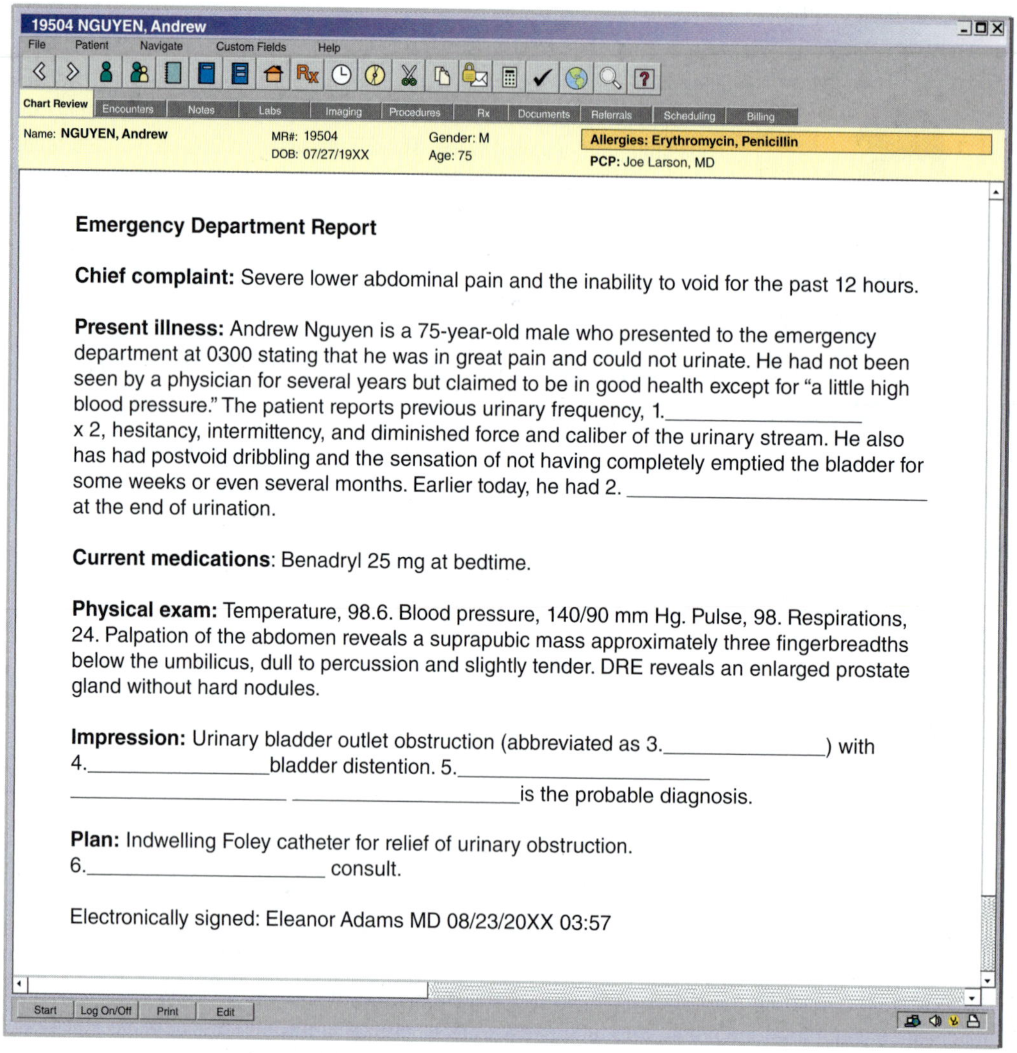

19504 NGUYEN, Andrew

File Patient Navigate Custom Fields Help

Chart Review | Encounters | Notes | Labs | Imaging | Procedures | Rx | Documents | Referrals | Scheduling | Billing

Name: **NGUYEN, Andrew** MR#: 19504 DOB: 07/27/19XX Gender: M Age: 75 **Allergies: Erythromycin, Penicillin** **PCP:** Joe Larson, MD

Emergency Department Report

Chief complaint: Severe lower abdominal pain and the inability to void for the past 12 hours.

Present illness: Andrew Nguyen is a 75-year-old male who presented to the emergency department at 0300 stating that he was in great pain and could not urinate. He had not been seen by a physician for several years but claimed to be in good health except for "a little high blood pressure." The patient reports previous urinary frequency, 1.__________________ x 2, hesitancy, intermittency, and diminished force and caliber of the urinary stream. He also has had postvoid dribbling and the sensation of not having completely emptied the bladder for some weeks or even several months. Earlier today, he had 2. ____________________________ at the end of urination.

Current medications: Benadryl 25 mg at bedtime.

Physical exam: Temperature, 98.6. Blood pressure, 140/90 mm Hg. Pulse, 98. Respirations, 24. Palpation of the abdomen reveals a suprapubic mass approximately three fingerbreadths below the umbilicus, dull to percussion and slightly tender. DRE reveals an enlarged prostate gland without hard nodules.

Impression: Urinary bladder outlet obstruction (abbreviated as 3.______________) with 4.________________bladder distention. 5._______________________ ____________________ ____________________is the probable diagnosis.

Plan: Indwelling Foley catheter for relief of urinary obstruction.
6.______________________ consult.

Electronically signed: Eleanor Adams MD 08/23/20XX 03:57

Start | Log On/Off | Print | Edit

Definitions of Medical Terms to Complete the Document

Write the medical terms defined on corresponding answer lines in the document.

1. night urination
2. blood in the urine
3. abbreviation for bladder outlet obstruction
4. pertaining to urine
5. nonmalignant excessive development pertaining to the prostate gland (enlargement of the prostate gland)
6. study of the urinary tract

B. Read the medical report and answer the questions below it.

Michigan Oncology Group
44976 East Lincoln
Detroit, MI 97654

January 23, 20XX

Kathryn S. Marcus, MD
Internal Medicine Services
2301 North Brinkley
Detroit, MI 97654

Re: Brindley, Javier
DOB: 08/24/19XX

Dear Dr. Marcus:

It is now three years since this patient had brachytherapy using radioactive seeds for his T2a, Gleason 5 prostate cancer. He continues to experience nocturia and some erectile dysfunction with a prostate obstruction score of 3.

His weight is stable at 209 pounds and blood pressure is 122/82 mm Hg. He has no adenopathy. DRE reveals a smooth prostate with no nodules. There is a slight asymmetry with greater prominence on the right side. The PSA remains 0.1 as of August 20, 20XX.

He is doing well and is likely cured of his cancer. I would like to continue seeing him on a yearly basis with a repeat PSA. He will continue seeing you as needed.

Joseph P. Potter, MD
JPP/bko

Use the medical report above to answer the questions.

1. In addition to erectile dysfunction, the patient's symptoms include:
   a. pus in the urine
   b. excessive urine
   c. night urination
   d. blood in the urine
2. Brachytherapy using radioactive seeds was used to treat:
   a. benign prostatic hyperplasia
   b. prostate cancer
   c. erectile dysfunction
3. Which diagnostic test revealed "a smooth prostate"?
   a. transrectal ultrasound
   b. prostate-specific antigen
   c. digital rectal examination
4. Three years after treatment, the patient:
   a. appears to be cancer free
   b. shows disease progression
   c. has been recommended for a radical prostatectomy

C. Complete the **three medical documents** within the electronic health record (EHR) on Evolve.

Topic: Prostate Cancer
Documents: Office Visit, Pathology Report, Progress Note

To complete the three medical records, go to Evolve Resources at evolve.elsevier.com and select:
Practice Student Resources > Student Resources > Chapter 7 > **Electronic Heath Records**

See Appendix B for instructions.

EXERCISE 34 *Pronounce Medical Terms in Use*

Practice pronunciation of terms by reading aloud the following paragraph. Use the phonetic spellings following medical terms from the chapter to assist with pronunciation. The script also contains medical terms not presented in the chapter. Treat them as information only or look for their meanings in a medical dictionary or a reliable online source.

A 62-year-old male was found to have an elevated **prostate-specific antigen** (PROS-tāt) (spe-SIF-ik) (AN-ti-jen) test during a routine physical examination. At the age of 42 years he underwent a **vasectomy** (va-SEK-to-mē). The patient denies having nocturia or any significant change in his urinary stream. **Digital rectal examination** (DIJ-i-tal) (REK-tal) (eg-*zam*-i-NĀ-shun) revealed a mildly enlarged prostate gland with a 1.0 cm stony hard nodule of the right lobe. The urologist performed a **transrectal ultrasound** (trans-REK-tal) (UL-tra-sound) and biopsy. A diagnosis of adenocarcinoma of the prostate was made. The patient elected to undergo a robot-assisted radical **prostatectomy** (*pros*-ta-TEK-to-mē). Urinary incontinence complicated his postoperative course but this lasted for only 3 months. No **erectile dysfunction** (e-REK-tīl) (dis-FUNK-shun) was reported. His prognosis for full recovery should be excellent.

EXERCISE 35 *Chapter Content Quiz*

Test your understanding of terms and abbreviations introduced in this chapter. Circle the letter for the medical term or abbreviation related to the words in italics.

1. *Inflammation of the testis* is often caused by a bacterial or viral infection.
   a. orchitis
   b. epididymitis
   c. prostatitis
2. The medical term for *discharge from the glans penis* is:
   a. balanitis
   b. balanorrhea
   c. balanorrhaphy
3. Radical *excision of the prostate gland* is used to treat prostate cancer.
   a. prostatectomy
   b. orchiectomy
   c. epididymectomy
4. HoLEP and PVP are surgical procedures used to treat *nonmalignant enlargement of the prostate gland.*
   a. anorchism
   b. testicular cancer
   c. benign prostatic hyperplasia
5. *State of hidden testicles* is an associated risk factor for the development of *cancer of the testicle.*
   a. cryptorchidism, testicular cancer
   b. anorchism, testicular torsion
   c. prostatitis, prostate cancer
6. *Inflammation of the testis and the epididymis* may be caused by an STI.
   a. prostatocystitis
   b. prostatovesiculitis
   c. orchiepididymitis
7. *A fluid-filled sac around the testicle causing scrotal swelling* is common in newborns.
   a. spermatocele
   b. hydrocele
   c. varicocele
8. *Surgical repair of the glans penis* is performed to correct anterior hypospadias.
   a. balanoplasty
   b. orchioplasty
   c. prostatocystotomy
9. The surgical procedure circumcision is the removal of all or part of the *foreskin.*
   a. glans penis
   b. testes
   c. prepuce
10. A surgical procedure that *destroys abnormal or excessive tissue by melting, vaporizing, or eroding* utilizes:
    a. morcellation
    b. enucleation
    c. ablation

11. The abbreviation for the *ultrasound procedure used to diagnose prostate cancer* with use of a transducer probe placed in the rectum is:
    a. TUMT
    b. TRUS
    c. PSA

12. Sudden onset of *pain in the testis* can be a symptom of *twisting of the spermatic cord.*
    a. orchialgia, testicular torsion
    b. aspermia, anorchism
    c. prostatolith, prostatolithotomy

13. A *microscopic observation of ejaculated semen* was ordered after the patient's *excision of a duct (vas deferens)* to evaluate the success of the procedure.
    a. prostate-specific antigen, prostatovesiculectomy
    b. digital rectal examination, vasovasostomy
    c. semen analysis, vasectomy

14. Upon diagnosis of an intratesticular mass, a radical inguinal *excision of the testis* was recommended as a diagnostic and therapeutic procedure.
    a. orchiectomy
    b. prostatectomy
    c. vasectomy

15. The term meaning *reduced or absent ability to achieve pregnancy* does not mean complete inability to create offspring.
    a. erectile dysfunction
    b. sterilization
    c. infertility

16. *Condition of scanty* sperm and *lack of live sperm in* semen are terms frequently used in discussions of male infertility.
    a. oligospermia, azoospermia
    b. spermatolysis, andropathy
    c. chlamydia, syphilis

For additional practice with chapter content, go to Evolve Resources at evolve.elsevier.com and select:
Practice Student Resources > Student Resources > Chapter 7 > **Games:** Medical Millionaire, Tournament of Terminology
Practice Quizzes: Word Parts, Terms Built from Word Parts, Terms NOT Built from Word Parts, Abbreviations

See Appendix B for instructions.

CHAPTER REVIEW

REVIEW OF CHAPTER CONTENT ON EVOLVE RESOURCES

Go to evolve.elsevier.com and click on Gradable Student Resources and Practice Student Resources. Online learning activities found there can be used to review chapter content and to assess your learning of word parts, medical terms, and abbreviations. Place check marks in the boxes next to activities used for review and assessment

GRADABLE STUDENT RESOURCES

Chapter 07 >	Exercises >	□ Word Parts □ Terms Built from Word Parts □ Terms Not Built from Word Parts □ Abbreviations
	Quizzes >	□ Quiz 1: Disease and Disorder Terms □ Quiz 2: Surgical Terms □ Quiz 3: Complementary Terms

PRACTICE STUDENT RESOURCES > STUDENT RESOURCES

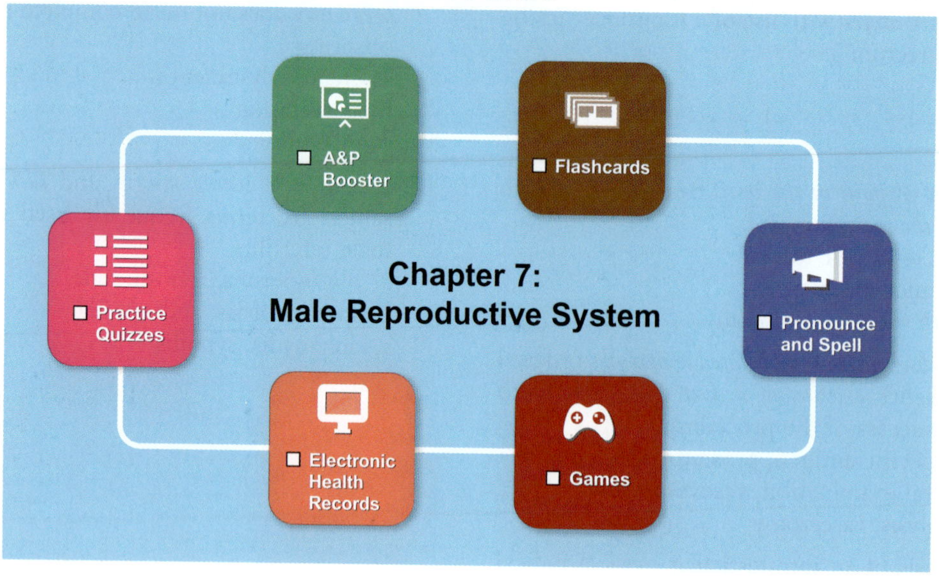

REVIEW OF WORD PARTS

Can you define and spell the following word parts?

COMBINING FORMS		SUFFIX
andr/o	prostat/o	-ism
balan/o	sperm/o	
epididym/o	spermat/o	
orch/o	vas/o	
orchi/o	vesicul/o	
orchid/o		

REVIEW OF TERMS

Can you define, pronounce, and spell the following terms *built from word parts*?

DISEASES AND DISORDERS	SURGICAL	COMPLEMENTARY
anorchism	balanoplasty	andropathy
balanitis	epididymectomy	aspermia
balanorrhea	orchiectomy	oligospermia
benign prostatic hyperplasia (BPH)	orchiopexy	orchialgia
cryptorchidism	orchioplasty	spermatolysis
epididymitis	orchiotomy	transurethral
orchiepididymitis	prostatectomy	
orchitis	prostatocystotomy	
prostatitis	prostatolithotomy	
prostatocystitis	prostatovesiculectomy	
prostatolith	vasectomy	
prostatorrhea	vasovasostomy	
prostatovesiculitis	vesiculectomy	

Can you define, pronounce, and spell the following terms *NOT built from word parts*?

DISEASES AND DISORDERS	SURGICAL	DIAGNOSTIC	COMPLEMENTARY
erectile dysfunction (ED) hydrocele phimosis priapism prostate cancer spermatocele testicular cancer testicular torsion varicocele	ablation circumcision enucleation hydrocelectomy laser surgery morcellation MRI ultrasound fusion biopsy robotic surgery transurethral incision of the prostate gland (TUIP) transurethral microwave thermotherapy (TUMT) transurethral resection of the prostate gland (TURP)	digital rectal examination (DRE) multiparametric MRI prostate-specific antigen (PSA) semen analysis transrectal ultrasound (TRUS)	acquired immunodeficiency syndrome (AIDS) artificial insemination azoospermia chlamydia coitus condom ejaculation genital herpes gonorrhea human immunodeficiency virus (HIV) human papillomavirus (HPV) infertility orgasm puberty sexually transmitted disease (STD) sterilization syphilis trichomoniasis

Chapter 8

Female Reproductive System

Objectives

Upon completion of this chapter you will be able to:

1. Pronounce organs and anatomic structures of the female reproductive system.
2. Define and spell word parts related to the female reproductive system.
3. Define, pronounce, and spell disease and disorder terms related to the female reproductive system.
4. Define, pronounce, and spell surgical terms related to the female reproductive system.
5. Define, pronounce, and spell diagnostic terms related to the female reproductive system.
6. Define, pronounce, and spell complementary terms related to the female reproductive system.
7. Interpret the meaning of abbreviations related to the female reproductive system.
8. Apply medical language in clinical contexts.

Outline

ANATOMY

Externally, the female reproductive system consists of the vulva, clitoris, and mammary glands. Internally, this system consists of the vagina, uterus, uterine tubes, and ovaries (Fig. 8.1).

Function

The female reproductive system comprises external and internal organs, glands, and structures and is responsible for supporting conception and pregnancy. As the female matures throughout her lifespan, this system develops and changes based on the influence of hormones produced by the ovaries. Estrogen and progesterone are female hormones essential for sexual maturation and the overall health of the female. These hormones affect the structure and function of the integumentary, urinary, cardiac, musculoskeletal, and neurologic systems.

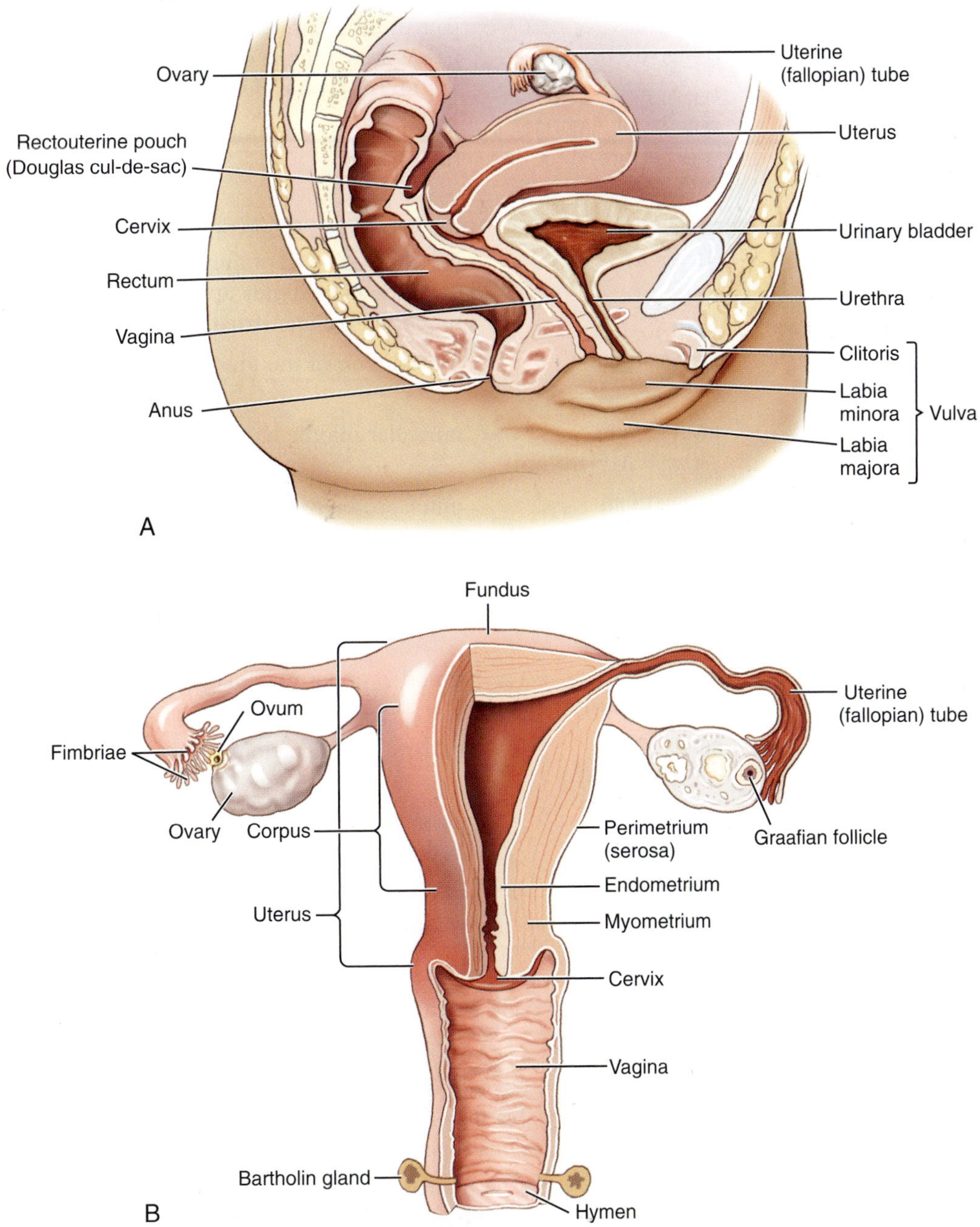

FIG. 8.1 Female reproductive organs. **A,** Sagittal view. **B,** Frontal view.

Internal Organs and Anatomic Structures of the Female Reproductive System

TERM	DEFINITION
ovaries (Ō-var-ēs)	almond-shaped organs located in the pelvic cavity; form and store egg cells (ova) and produce the hormones estrogen and progesterone
ovum (pl. ova) (Ō-vum) (Ō-va)	female egg cell
graafian follicles (GRA-fē-en) (FOL-i-kels)	100,000 microscopic sacs that make up a large portion of the ovaries. Each follicle contains an immature ovum. Normally one graafian follicle develops to maturity monthly between puberty and menopause. It moves to the surface of the ovary and releases the ovum, which passes into the uterine tube.
uterine tubes (Ū-ter-in) (toobz)	pair of tubes attached to the uterus that provide a passageway for the ovum to move from the ovary to the uterus (also called **fallopian tubes**)
fimbria (pl. fimbriae) (FIM-brē-a) (FIM-brē-ā)	finger-like projection at the free end of the uterine tube
uterus (Ū-ter-us)	pear-sized and shaped muscular organ that lies in the pelvic cavity, except during pregnancy when it enlarges and extends up into the abdominal cavity. Its functions are menstruation, pregnancy, and labor.
endometrium (en-dō-MĒ-trē-um)	inner lining of the uterus
myometrium (*mī*-ō-MĒ-trē-um)	muscular middle layer of the uterus
perimetrium (*per*-i-MĒ-trē-um)	outer protective layer of the uterus that secretes watery serous fluid to reduce friction (also called **uterine serosa**)
corpus (KŌR-pus)	large central portion of the uterus
fundus (FUN-dus)	rounded upper portion of the uterus
cervix (Cx) (SER-vicks)	narrow lower portion of the uterus
vagina (va-JĪ-nah)	passageway between the uterus and the outside of the body
hymen (HĪ-men)	fold of membrane found near the opening of the vagina

THE GRAAFIAN FOLLICLE
is named for Dutch anatomist Reinier de Graaf, who discovered the sac in 1672.

THE FALLOPIAN TUBE
was named in honor of Gabriele Fallopius, 1523-1562, because he described it in his works. Fallopius also gave the **vagina** and the **placenta** their names.

External Female Reproductive Structures

TERM	DEFINITION
vulva (VUL-va)	external genitals of the female, including the mons pubis, labia majora, labia minora, clitoris, urinary meatus, and vaginal opening
perineum (*per*-i-NĒ-um)	pelvic floor in both the male and female. In females it refers to the area between the vaginal opening and the anus.

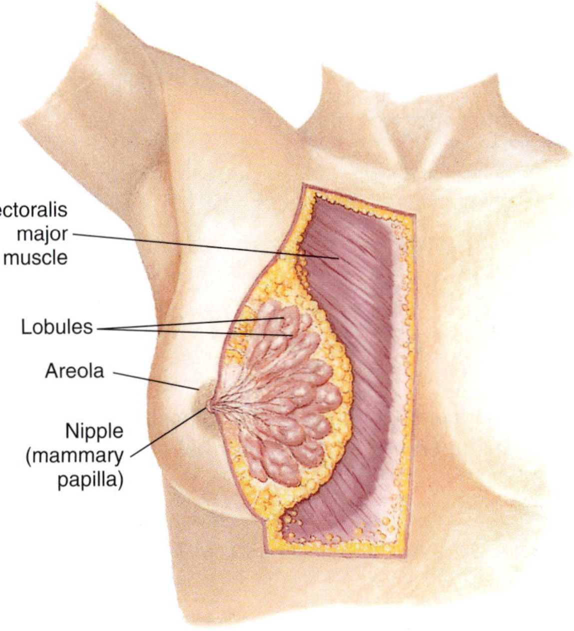

FIG. 8.2 Female breast.

Glands of the Female Reproductive System

TERM	DEFINITION
Bartholin glands (BAR-tō-lin) (glans)	pair of mucus-producing glands located on each side of the vagina, just above the vaginal opening
breasts (brests)	milk-producing glands. Each breast consists of 15 to 20 divisions or lobules. (also called **mammary glands**) (Fig. 8.2)
mammary papilla (MAM-a-rē) (pa-PIL-a)	breast nipple
areola (a-RĒ-ō-la)	pigmented area around the breast nipple

BARTHOLIN GLANDS were described by Caspar Bartholin, a Danish anatomist, in 1675.

A&P Booster
For more anatomy and physiology, go to Evolve Resources at evolve.elsevier.com and select: Practice Student Resources > Student Resources > Chapter 8 > **A&P Booster**

See Appendix B for instructions.

EXERCISE 1

Practice saying aloud each of the Organs and Anatomic Structures for the Female Reproductive System.

To hear the terms, go to Evolve Resources at evolve.elsevier.com and select:
Practice Student Resources > Student Resources > Chapter 8 > **Pronounce and Spell**

See Appendix B for instructions.

❑ Check the box when complete.

WORD PARTS

Word parts you need to learn to complete this chapter are listed on the following pages. The exercises at the end of each list will help you learn their definitions and spellings.

Use the flashcards accompanying this text or the electronic flashcards to assist you in memorizing the word parts for this chapter.

Combining Forms of the Female Reproductive System

COMBINING FORM	DEFINITION
arche/o	first, beginning
cervic/o, trachel/o	cervix
colp/o, vagin/o	vagina
endometri/o	endometrium
episi/o, vulv/o	vulva
gynec/o, gyn/o	woman
hymen/o	hymen
hyster/o, metr/o	uterus
mamm/o, mast/o	breast
men/o	menstruation
oophor/o	ovary
pelv/i	pelvis, pelvic bones, pelvic cavity
perine/o	perineum
salping/o	uterine tube (fallopian tube) (Fig. 8.3)

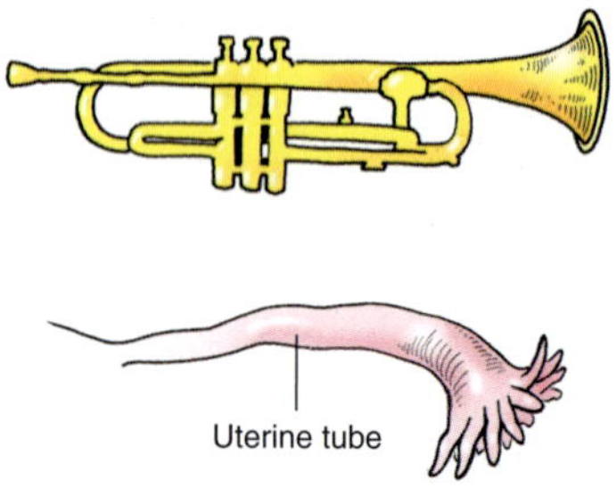

FIG. 8.3 Salpinx is derived from the Greek term for trumpet. The term was used for the uterine tubes because of their trumpet-like shape.

EXERCISE 2

A. Fill in the blanks with combining forms in this diagram of internal female reproductive organs and anatomic structures. *To check your answers for the exercises in this chapter, go to Appendix A.*

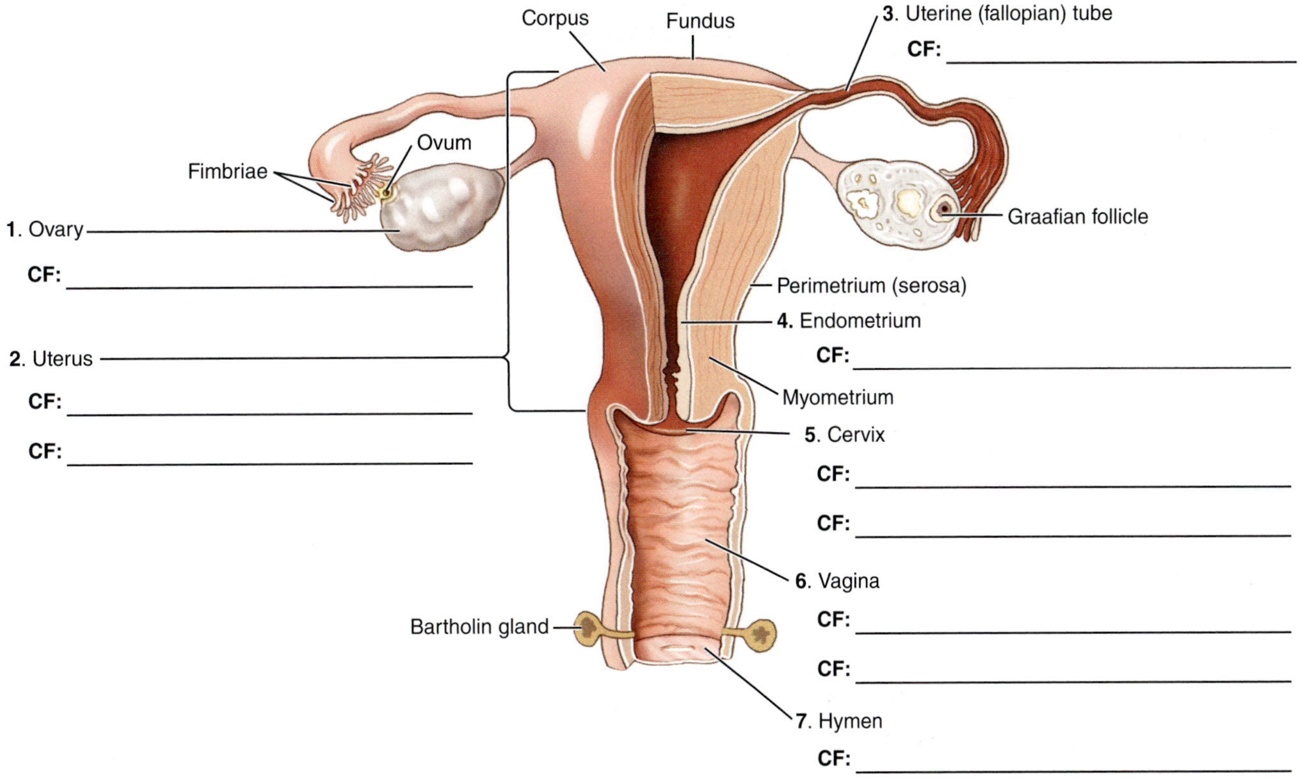

B. Fill in the blanks with combining forms in this diagram of external female reproductive organs and anatomic structures.

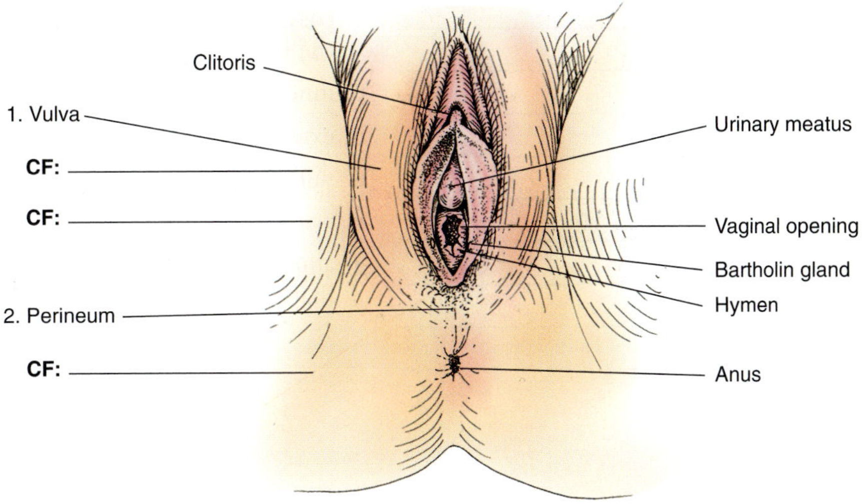

C. Write the combining form defined

1. menstruation ______________________________
2. woman a. ______________________, b. ______________________
3. first, beginning______________________________
4. breast a. ______________________, b. ______________________
5. pelvis______________________________

EXERCISE 3

Step 1: Write the definitions after the following combining forms.
Step 2: Match the descriptions on the right with the combining forms and definitions. Answers may be used more than once; no answer line appears for those not described in a lettered item.

_____ 1. salping/o, ______________________
_____ 2. metr/o, ______________________
_____ 3. perine/o, ______________________
_____ 4. cervic /o, ______________________
_____ 5. colp/o, ______________________
_____ 6. trachel/o, ______________________
_____ 7. mamm/o, ______________________
8. arche/o, ______________________
9. pelv/i, ______________________

a. pelvic floor in male and female anatomy
b. passageway between the uterus and the outside of the body
c. narrow lower portion of the uterus
d. milk-producing glands
e. pear-sized and shaped muscular organ
f. passageway for ovum to move from the ovary to the uterus

EXERCISE 4

Step 1: Write the definitions after the following combining forms.
Step 2: Match the descriptions on the right with the combining forms and definitions. Answers may be used more than once; no answer line appears for those not described in a lettered item.

_____ 1. vagin/o, ______________________
_____ 2. hymen/o, ______________________
_____ 3. episi/o, ______________________
_____ 4. hyster/o, ______________________
_____ 5. mast/o, ______________________
_____ 6. oophor/o, ______________________
_____ 7. vulv/o, ______________________
_____ 8. endometri/o, ______________________
9. men/o, ______________________
10. gynec/o, gyn/o, ______________________

a. fold of membrane near the opening of the vagina
b. passageway between the uterus and the outside of the body
c. inner lining of the uterus
d. external genitals of the female
e. milk-producing glands
f. pear-sized and shaped muscular organ
g. almond-shaped organ located in the pelvic cavity that produce and store female reproductive cells

Prefix and Suffixes

PREFIX	DEFINITION
peri-	surrounding (outer)
SUFFIX	**DEFINITION**
-cleisis	surgical closure
-salpinx	uterine tube (fallopian tube) (Fig. 8.3)

Refer to **Appendix C** and **Appendix D** for alphabetized word parts and their meanings.

EXERCISE 5

Write the prefix or suffix for each of the following.

1. uterine tube ____________________
2. surrounding ____________________
3. surgical closure ____________________

EXERCISE 6

Write the definitions of the following prefix and suffixes.

1. -salpinx ____________________
2. peri- ____________________
3. -cleisis ____________________

For additional practice with Word Parts, go to Evolve Resources at evolve.elsevier.com and select: Practice Student Resources > Student Resources > Chapter 8 > **Flashcards**

See Appendix B for instructions.

MEDICAL TERMS

The terms you need to learn to complete this chapter are listed on the following pages. The exercises following each list will help you learn the definition and spelling of each word.

Disease and Disorder Terms

BUILT FROM WORD PARTS

The following terms can be translated using definitions of word parts. Further explanation is provided within parentheses as needed.

TERM	DEFINITION
amenorrhea (a-*men*-ō-RĒ-a)	absence of menstrual flow
Bartholin adenitis (BAR-tō-lin) (*ad*-e-NĪ-tis)	inflammation of the Bartholin gland (also called **bartholinitis**)
cervicitis (*ser*-vi-SĪ-tis)	inflammation of the cervix (Fig. 8.7)
dysmenorrhea (dis-*men*-ō-RĒ-a)	painful menstrual flow

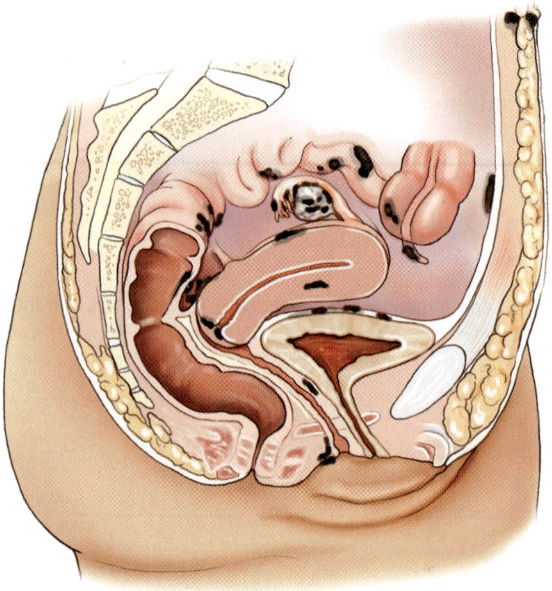

FIG. 8.4 Endometriosis. Spots indicate common sites of endometrial deposits.

Disease and Disorder Terms—cont'd

TERM	DEFINITION
endometriosis (*en*-dō-*mē*-trē-Ō-sis)	abnormal condition of the endometrium (endometrial tissue grows outside of the uterus in various areas in the pelvic cavity, including ovaries, uterine tubes, intestines, and uterus) (Fig. 8.4)
endometritis (*en*-dō-mē-TRĪ-tis)	inflammation of the endometrium (Fig. 8.7)
hematosalpinx (*hem*-a-tō-SAL-pinks)	blood in the uterine tube
hydrosalpinx (*hī*-drō-SAL-pinks)	water in the uterine tube (Exercise Figure D)
mastitis (*mas*-TĪ-tis)	inflammation of the breast
menometrorrhagia (*men*-ō-*met*-rō-RĀ-jea)	excessive bleeding from the uterus at menstruation (and between menstrual cycles; heavy and irregular bleeding)
menorrhagia (*men*-ō-RĀ-jea)	excessive bleeding at menstruation (heavy bleeding in regular, cyclical pattern)
metrorrhagia (*mē*-trō-RĀ-jea)	excessive bleeding from the uterus (irregular, out-of-cycle bleeding ranging from heavy to light, including spotting)
myometritis (*mī*-o-me-TRĪ-tis)	inflammation of the uterine muscle (myometrium)
oligomenorrhea (*ol*-i-gō-*men*-ō-RĒ-a)	scanty menstrual flow (infrequent menstrual flow)
oophoritis (*ō*-of-o-RĪ-tis)	inflammation of the ovary

ABNORMAL UTERINE BLEEDING (AUB)

is irregular bleeding in the absence of pregnancy. **Menometrorrhagia, menorrhagia,** and **metrorrhagia** are some types of AUB.

TERM	DEFINITION
perimetritis (*per*-i-me-TRĪ-tis)	inflammation surrounding the uterus (perimetrium)
pyosalpinx (*pī*-ō-SAL-pinks)	pus in the uterine tube
salpingitis (*sal*-pin-JĪ-tis)	inflammation of the uterine tube (Exercise Figure A and Fig. 8.7)
salpingocele (sal-PING-gō-sēl)	hernia of the uterine tube
vaginitis (*vaj*-i-NĪ-tis)	inflammation of the vagina (Fig. 8.7)
vaginosis (*vaj*-i-NŌ-sis)	abnormal condition of the vagina (caused by a bacterial imbalance) (also called **bacterial vaginosis**)
vulvovaginitis (*vul*-vō-*vaj*-i-NĪ-tis)	inflammation of the vulva and vagina

EXERCISE FIGURE A

Fill in the blanks with word parts to label the diagram.

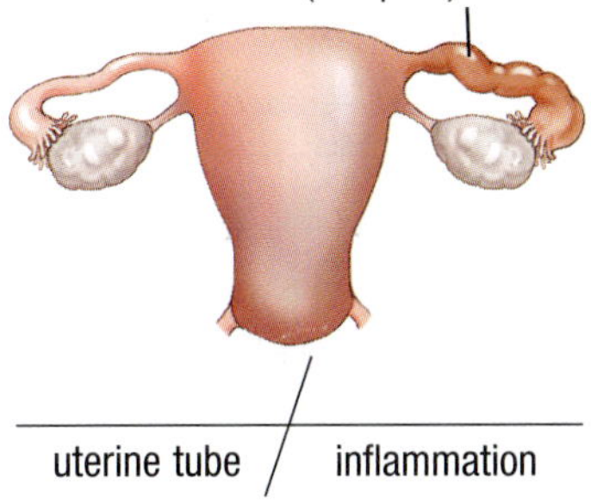

EXERCISE 7

Practice saying aloud each of the Disease and Disorder Terms Built from Word Parts.

To hear the terms, go to Evolve Resources at evolve.elsevier.com and select:
Practice Student Resources > Student Resources > Chapter 8 > **Pronounce and Spell**

See Appendix B for instructions.

❑ Check the box when complete.

EXERCISE 8

Analyze and define the following disease and disorder terms.

1. endometriosis
____
____

2. cervicitis
____
____

3. hydrosalpinx
____
____

4. hematosalpinx
____
____

5. metrorrhagia
____
____

6. oophoritis
____
____

7. (Bartholin) adenitis
____
____

8. vulvovaginitis
____
____

9. salpingocele

____

____

10. menometrorrhagia

____

____

11. amenorrhea

____

____

12. dysmenorrhea

____

____

13. mastitis

____

____

14. perimetritis

____

____

15. myometritis

____

____

16. endometritis

____

____

17. pyosalpinx

____

____

18. vaginosis

____

____

19. salpingitis

____

____

20. vaginitis

____

____

21. menorrhagia

____

____

22. oligomenorrhea

____

____

EXERCISE 9

Build disease and disorder terms for the following definitions with the word parts you have learned.

1. inflammation of the breast ______ / ______ (WR / S)
2. excessive bleeding from the uterus (irregular, out of cycle bleeding ranging from heavy to light or spotting) ______ / ______ / ______ (WR / CV / S)
3. inflammation of the uterine tube ______ / ______ (WR / S)
4. inflammation of the vulva and vagina ______ / ______ / ______ / ______ (WR / CV / WR / S)

5. absence of menstrual flow — P / WR / CV / S

6. inflammation of the cervix — WR / S

7. inflammation of (Bartholin) gland — Bartholin WR / S

8. water in the uterine tube — WR / CV / S

9. painful menstrual flow — P / WR / CV / S

10. blood in the uterine tube — WR / CV / S

11. inflammation of the vagina — WR / S

12. excessive bleeding from the uterus at menstruation (and between cycles; heavy and irregular bleeding) — WR / CV / WR / CV / S

13. inflammation of the ovary — WR / S

14. hernia of the uterine tube — WR / CV / S

15. inflammation surrounding the uterus (outer layer) — P / WR / S

16. inflammation of the endometrium — WR / S

17. abnormal condition of the vagina (caused by a bacterial imbalance) — WR / S

18. inflammation of the uterine muscle — WR / CV / WR / S

19. pus in the uterine tube — WR / CV / S

20. abnormal condition of the endometrium (endometrial tissue grows outside of the uterus in various areas of the pelvic cavity) — WR / S

21. scanty menstrual flow (infrequent menstrual flow) — WR / CV / WR / CV / S

22. excessive bleeding at menstruation (heavy bleeding in regular, cyclical pattern) — WR / CV / S

EXERCISE 10

Spell each of the Disease and Disorder Terms Built from Word Parts by having someone dictate them to you. Use a separate sheet of paper.

To hear and spell the terms, go to Evolve Resources at evolve.elsevier.com and select:
Practice Student Resources > Student Resources > Chapter 8 > **Pronounce and Spell**

See Appendix B for instructions.

❑ Check the box when complete.

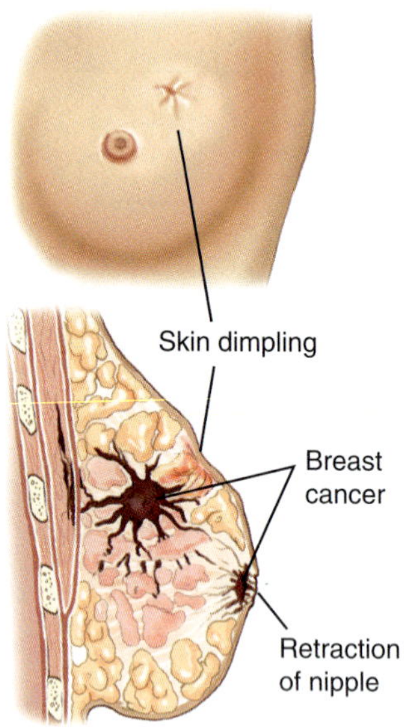

FIG. 8.5 Clinical signs of breast cancer.

HPV VACCINE

The Food and Drug Administration (FDA) approved a vaccine for human papillomavirus (HPV) in 2006, directly impacting the prevention of **cervical cancer**. The vaccine is highly effective in protecting against several forms of HPV as long as it is administered before a male or female becomes sexually active. Because vaccination does not combat all strains of HVP and is not 100% effective, periodic cervical cancer screening is strongly recommended.

Disease and Disorder Terms
NOT BUILT FROM WORD PARTS

Word parts may be present in the following terms; however, their full meanings cannot be translated using definitions of word parts alone.

TERM	DEFINITION
adenomyosis (*ad*-e-nō-mī-Ō-sis)	growth of endometrium into the muscular portion of the uterus
breast cancer (brest) (KAN-cer)	malignant tumor of the breast (Fig. 8.5)
cervical cancer (SER-vi-kal) (KAN-cer)	malignant tumor of the cervix, which progresses from cervical dysplasia to carcinoma. Its cause is linked to human papillomavirus (HPV) infection.
endometrial cancer (*en*-dō-MĒ-trē-al) (KAN-cer)	malignant tumor of the endometrium (also called **uterine cancer**) (Fig. 8.6)
fibrocystic breast changes (FCC) (*fī*-brō-SIS-tik) (brest) (CHĀN-jiz)	fibrosis, benign cysts, and pain or tenderness in one or both breasts; thought to be caused by monthly hormonal changes (also called **fibrocystic breasts**; formerly called **fibrocystic breast disease**)
ovarian cancer (ō-VAR-ē-an) (KAN-cer)	malignant tumor of the ovary
pelvic inflammatory disease (PID) (PEL-vik) (in-FLAM-a-*tor*-ē) (di-ZĒZ)	inflammation of some or all of the female pelvic organs; can be caused by many different pathogens. If untreated, the infection may spread upward from the vagina, involving the uterus, uterine tubes, ovaries, and other pelvic organs. An ascending infection may result in infertility and, in acute cases, fatal septicemia (Fig. 8.7).
polycystic ovary syndrome (PCOS) (*pol*-ē-SIS-tik) (Ō-vah-rē) (SIN-drōm)	condition typically characterized by hormonal imbalances, ovulatory dysfunction, and multiple ovarian cysts; symptoms can include irregular menstruation, acne, excess facial and body hair, and infertility. People with this condition have increased risks of cardiovascular disease, obesity, and glucose intolerance.

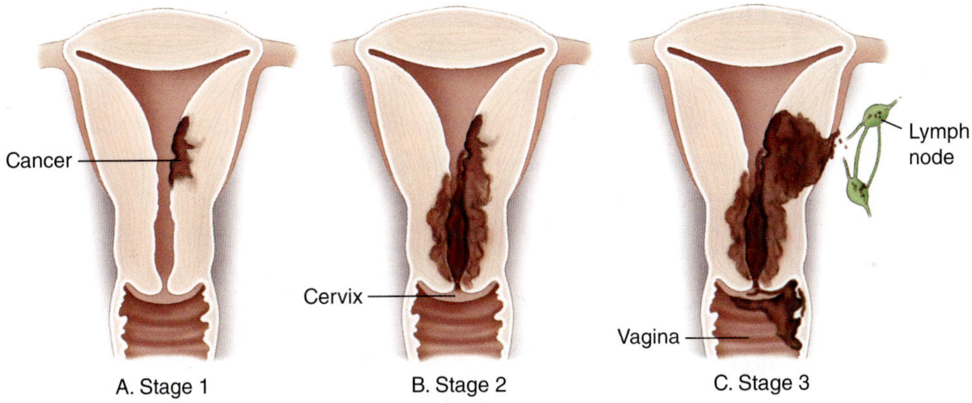

FIG. 8.6 Endometrial cancer. **A,** Stage 1: Confined to the endometrium. **B,** Stage 2: Spread into support structures of the cervix from the body of the uterus. **C,** Stage 3: Spreads to other organs such as the vagina.

INTEGRATIVE MEDICINE TERM

Massage therapy is the manual manipulation of soft tissue, incorporating stroking, kneading, and percussion motions. Studies have shown that massage therapy is useful as a supportive measure to improve quality of life during cancer treatment by reducing physical and emotional side effects associated with treatment.

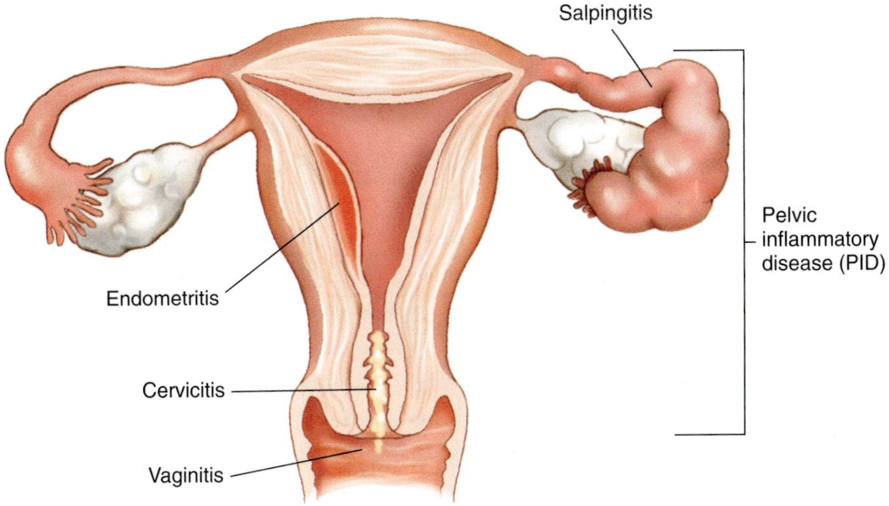

FIG. 8.7 Ascending infection of the female reproductive system as seen in pelvic inflammatory disease.

TERM	DEFINITION
toxic shock syndrome (TSS) (TOK-sik) (shok) (SIN-drōm)	severe illness characterized by high fever, rash, vomiting, diarrhea, and myalgia, followed by hypotension and, in severe cases, shock and death; usually affects menstruating women using tampons; caused by *Staphylococcus aureus* and *Streptococcus pyogenes*
uterine fibroid (Ū-ter-in) (FĪ-broyd)	benign tumor of the uterine muscle (also called **myoma of the uterus** or **leiomyoma**)
uterine prolapse (Ū-ter-in) (prō-LAPS)	downward displacement of the uterus into the vagina
vaginal fistula (VAJ-i-nal) (FIS-tū-la)	abnormal opening between the vagina and another organ, such as the urinary bladder, colon, or rectum (Table 8.1)

TABLE 8.1 Types and Causes of Vaginal Fistulas

TYPES	CAUSES	ILLUSTRATION
• **Vesicovaginal Fistula,** abnormal opening between the urinary bladder and the vagina • **Colovaginal Fistula,** abnormal opening between the vagina and colon (large intestine) • **Rectovaginal Fistula,** abnormal opening between the vagina and rectum	• Gynecological surgery, including hysterectomy and caesarean section • Inflammatory bowel disease, including Crohn disease and colitis • Diverticulitis • Malignancies in the pelvic region • Radiation therapy for pelvic cancers • Injuries during childbirth (occurs more frequently in developing countries where access to medical care may be limited)	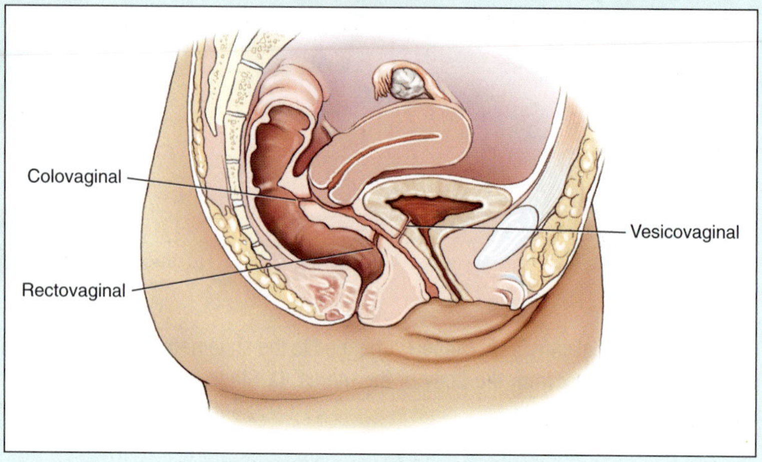 Types of vaginal fistulas: vesicovaginal, colovaginal, and rectovaginal.

EXERCISE 11

Practice saying aloud each of the Disease and Disorder Terms NOT Built from Word Parts.

To hear the terms, go to Evolve Resources at evolve.elsevier.com and select:
Practice Student Resources > Student Resources > Chapter 8 > **Pronounce and Spell**

See Appendix B for instructions.

❑ Check the box when complete.

EXERCISE 12

Fill in the blanks with the correct definitions.

1. uterine prolapse ______________________________
2. pelvic inflammatory disease ______________________________
3. vaginal fistula ______________________________
4. uterine fibroid ______________________________
5. polycystic ovary syndrome ______________________________
6. adenomyosis ______________________________

7. toxic shock syndrome ______________________________

____

8. fibrocystic breast changes ______________________________

____

9. ovarian cancer ______________________________

10. breast cancer ______________________________

11. cervical cancer ______________________________

12. endometrial cancer ______________________________

EXERCISE 13

A. Write the term for each of the following.

1. growth of endometrium into the muscular portion of the uterus ______________
2. severe illness usually affects menstruating women using tampons ______________ ______________ ______________
3. fibrosis, benign cysts, and pain or tenderness in one or both breasts ______________ ______________ ______________
4. hormonal imbalance characterized by multiple cysts on ovaries, difficulty in releasing mature female egg cells, and menstrual irregularities ______________ ______________ ______________
5. malignant tumor of the ovaries ______________ ______________
6. malignant tumor of the cervix ______________ ______________

B. Write the medical term pictured and defined.

1. ______________________________
downward placement of the uterus into the vagina

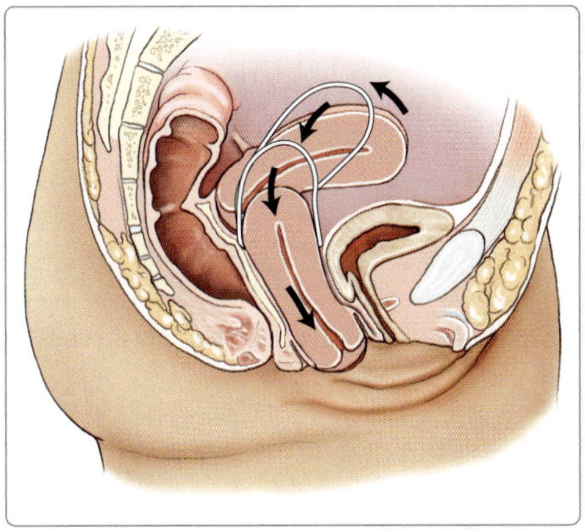

2. ______________________________
benign tumor of the uterine muscle

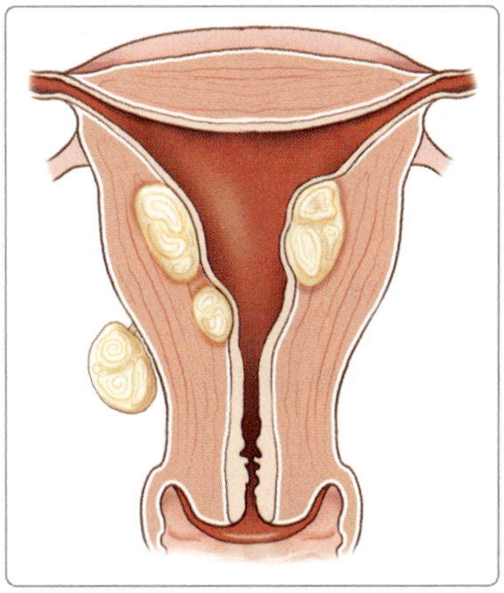

EXERCISE 13 *Pictured and Defined—cont'd*

3. ______________________________
malignant tumor of the endometrium

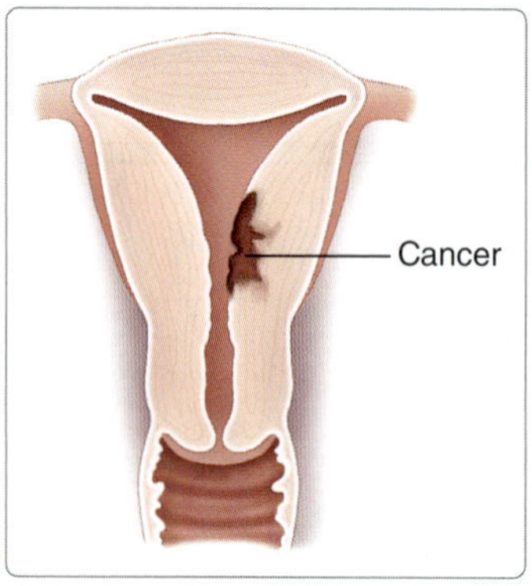

4. ______________________________
malignant tumor of the breast

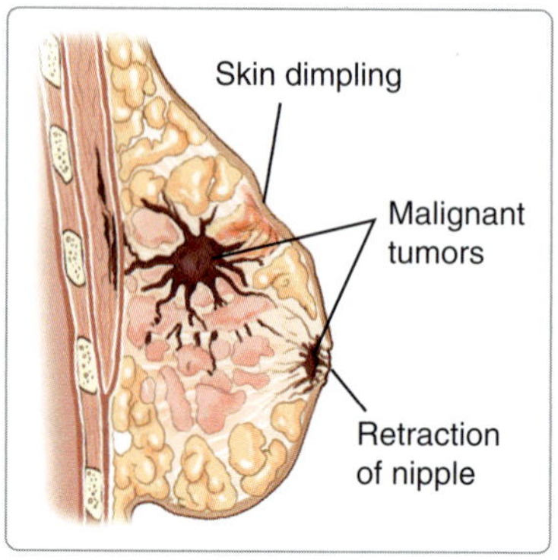

5. ______________________________
inflammation of some or all of the female pelvic organs

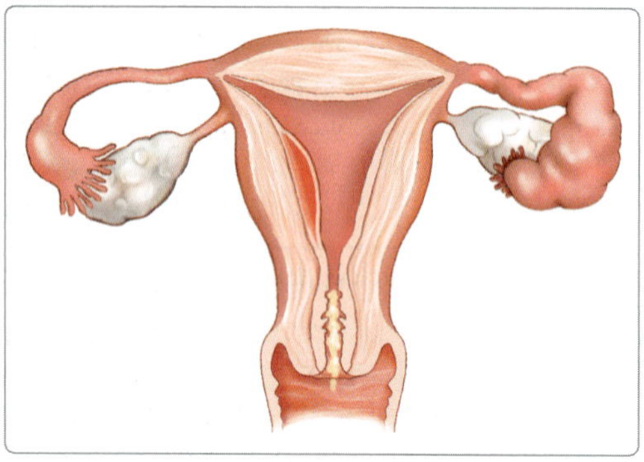

6. ______________________________
abnormal opening between the vagina and another organ, such as the urinary bladder, colon, or rectum

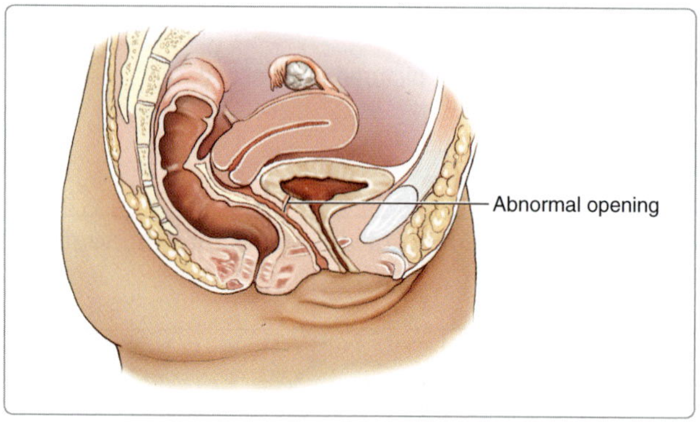

EXERCISE 14

Spell each of the Disease and Disorder Terms NOT Built from Word Parts by having someone dictate them to you. Use a separate sheet of paper.

To hear and spell the terms, go to Evolve Resources at evolve.elsevier.com and select:
Practice Student Resources > Student Resources > Chapter 8 > **Pronounce and Spell**

See Appendix B for instructions.

❑ Check the box when complete.

Surgical Terms
BUILT FROM WORD PARTS

The following terms can be translated using definitions of word parts. Further explanation is provided within parentheses as needed.

TERM	DEFINITION
colpocleisis (*kol*-pō-KLĪ-sis)	surgical closure of the vagina
colpoperineorrhaphy (kol-pō-*per*-i-nē-OR-a-fē)	suturing of the vagina and the perineum (performed to mend perineal vaginal tears)
colpoplasty (KOL-pō-*plas*-tē)	surgical repair of the vagina
colporrhaphy (kol-POR-a-fē)	suturing of the vagina (wall of the vagina)
episioperineoplasty (e-*piz*-ē-ō-*per*-i-NĒ-o-*plas*-tē)	surgical repair of the vulva and the perineum
episiorrhaphy (e-*piz*-ē-OR-a-fē)	suturing of (a tear in) the vulva
hymenectomy (*hī*-men-EK-to-mē)	excision of the hymen
hymenotomy (*hī*-men-OT-o-mē)	incision into the hymen
hysterectomy (*his*-te-REK-to-mē)	excision of the uterus (Table 8.2, Exercise Figure B, Fig. 8.8)
hysteropexy (HIS-ter-ō-*pek*-sē)	surgical fixation of the uterus
hysterosalpingo-oophorectomy (*his*-ter-ō-sal-*ping*-gō-ō-*of*-o-REK-to-mē)	excision of the uterus, uterine tubes, and ovaries (Exercise Figure B)
mammoplasty (MAM-ō-*plas*-tē)	surgical repair of the breast (performed to enlarge or reduce in size, and to reconstruct after removal of a tumor) (Fig. 8.9)
mastectomy (mas-TEK-to-mē)	surgical removal of the breast (Table 8.3, Fig. 8.9)
mastopexy (MAS-tō-pek-sē)	surgical fixation of the breast (performed to lift sagging breast tissue or to create symmetry) (Fig. 8.9)

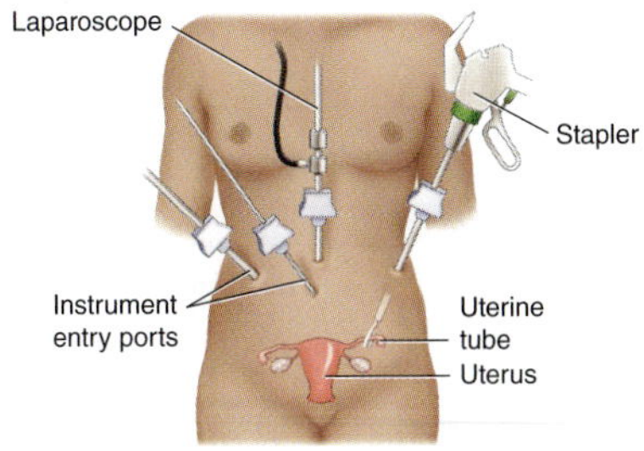

FIG. 8.8 Operative setup for laparoscopically-assisted vaginal hysterectomy (LAVH). Laparoscopic surgery is performed using a fiberoptic laparoscope, a type of endoscope. The laparoscope is inserted into the abdominopelvic cavity through a tiny incision near the umbilicus, allowing direct observation of the pelvic organs and structures. Three or four additional tiny incisions may be made to accommodate other instruments and devices. Numerous gynecological surgeries can be performed laparoscopically, including **hysterectomy, hysteropexy, myomectomy, oophorectomy, salpingectomy, salpingostomy,** and **tubal ligation.**

TABLE 8.2 Types of Hysterectomies

Total hysterectomy	Excision of the entire uterus, including the cervix; can be performed abdominally, vaginally, or laparoscopically
Subtotal hysterectomy	Excision of the upper part of the uterus leaving the cervix in place; can be performed abdominally or laparoscopically (also called **supracervical hysterectomy**)
Radical hysterectomy	Excision of the entire uterus, upper portion of the vagina, and surrounding tissues; performed abdominally

EXERCISE FIGURE B

Fill in the blanks with word parts to label the diagram.

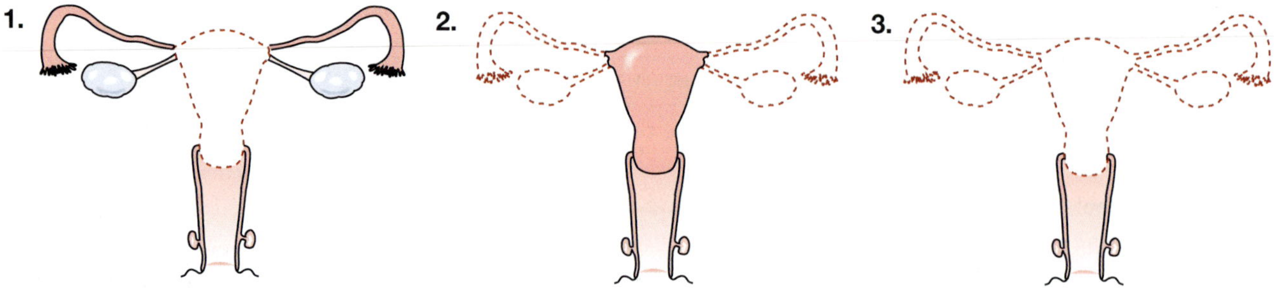

1. Total ______ / ______
   uterus / excision

2. Bilateral ______ / ______ / - ______ / ______
   uterine tube / cv / ovary / excision

3. ______ / ______ / ______ / ______ / - ______ / ______
   uterus / cv / uterine tube / cv / ovary / excision

Surgical Terms—cont'd

TERM	DEFINITION
oophorectomy (*ō*-of-o-REK-to-mē)	excision of the ovary
perineorrhaphy (*per*-i-nē-OR-a-fē)	suturing of (a tear in) the perineum
salpingectomy (*sal*-pin-JEK-to-mē)	excision of the uterine tube
salpingo-oophorectomy (sal-*ping*-gō-ō-*of*-o-REK-to-mē)	excision of the uterine tube and the ovary (Exercise Figure B)
salpingostomy (*sal*-ping-GOS-to-mē)	creation of an artificial opening in the uterine tube (performed to restore patency)
trachelectomy (*trā*-ke-LEK-to-mē)	excision of the cervix (also called **cervicectomy**)
trachelorrhaphy (trā-ke-LŌR-a-fē)	suturing of the cervix (also called **cervical cerclage**)
vulvectomy (vul-VEK-to-mē)	excision of the vulva

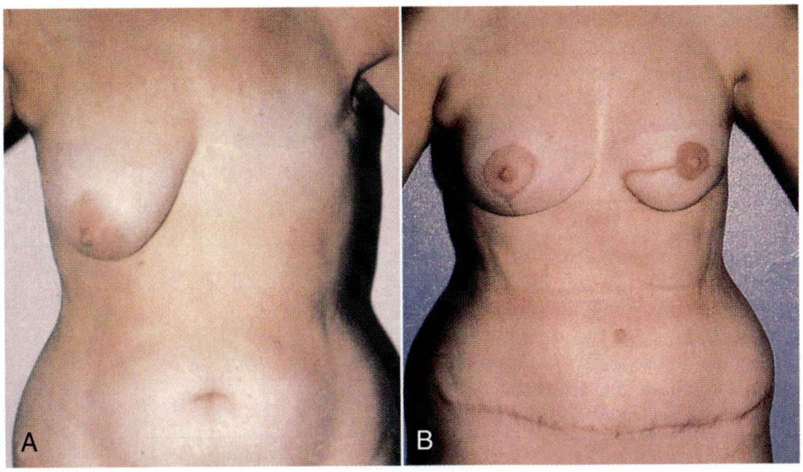

FIG. 8.9 Breast surgery and reconstruction. **A,** Left breast shows modified radical mastectomy scar. **B,** Left breast shows mammoplasty by TRAM (transverse rectus abdominis muscle) reconstruction (note the extensive lower abdominal scar, repositioned navel, and reconstructed nipple) and right mastopexy.

TYPES OF MAMMOPLASTY

- **Implant** uses a silicone or saline implant to create a breast.
- **Flap reconstruction** uses the patient's muscle or fat and surrounding tissue that is surgically transferred to the chest to create a breast mound (Fig. 8.9B).

TABLE 8.3 Types of Surgeries Performed to Treat Malignant Breast Tumors

Radical mastectomy	Removal of breast tissue, nipple, lymph nodes, and underlying chest wall muscle; also called **Halsted mastectomy** (rarely performed)
Modified radical mastectomy	Removal of breast tissue, nipple, and lymph nodes (Fig. 8.9A)
Simple mastectomy	Removal of breast tissue and nipple (also called **total mastectomy**)
Subcutaneous mastectomy	Removal of breast tissue only, preserving the overlying skin, nipple and areola (also called **nipple-sparing mastectomy**)
Segmental mastectomy	Removal of a quadrant, or wedge, of breast tissue (also called **quadrantectomy)**
Lumpectomy	Removal of the cancerous lesion along with a margin of surrounding healthy breast tissue (also called **partial mastectomy** or **breast-conserving surgery**)

EXERCISE 15

Practice saying aloud each of the Surgical Terms Built from Word Parts.

To hear the terms, go to Evolve Resources at evolve.elsevier.com and select:
Practice Student Resources > Student Resources > Chapter 8 > **Pronounce and Spell**

See Appendix B for instructions.

❑ Check the box when complete.

EXERCISE 16

Analyze and define the following surgical terms.

1. colporrhaphy
2. colpoplasty
3. episiorrhaphy
4. hymenotomy
5. hysteropexy
6. vulvectomy
7. perineorrhaphy
8. salpingostomy
9. salpingo-oophorectomy
10. oophorectomy
11. mastectomy
12. salpingectomy
13. trachelectomy
14. colpoperineorrhaphy
15. episioperineoplasty
16. hymenectomy

17. hysterosalpingo-oophorectomy

18. hysterectomy

19. mammoplasty

20. mastopexy

21. trachelorrhaphy

22. colpocleisis

EXERCISE 17

Build surgical terms for the following definitions by using the word parts you have learned.

1. suturing of the vagina
   WR / CV / S

2. excision of the cervix
   WR / S

3. suturing of the vulva
   WR / CV / S

4. surgical repair of the vulva and perineum
   WR / CV / WR / CV / S

5. surgical repair of the vagina
   WR / CV / S

6. suturing of the vagina and perineum
   WR / CV / WR / CV / S

7. excision of the uterus, ovaries, and uterine tubes
   WR / CV / WR / CV / - WR / S

8. surgical fixation of the uterus
   WR / CV / S

9. excision of the hymen
   WR / S

10. incision into the hymen
    WR / CV / S

11. excision of the uterus ______ WR / ______ S

12. excision of the ovary ______ WR / ______ S

13. surgical removal of the breast ______ WR / ______ S

14. excision of the uterine tube ______ WR / ______ S

15. suturing of the perineum ______ WR / ______ CV / ______ S

16. excision of the uterine tube and the ovary ______ WR / ______ CV / - ______ WR / ______ S

17. creation of an artificial opening in the uterine tube ______ WR / ______ CV / ______ S

18. excision of the vulva ______ WR / ______ S

19. surgical repair of the breast ______ WR / ______ CV / ______ S

20. surgical fixation of the breast ______ WR / ______ CV / ______ S

21. suturing of the cervix ______ WR / ______ CV / ______ S

22. surgical closure of the vagina ______ WR / ______ CV / ______ S

EXERCISE 18

Spell each of the Surgical Terms Built from Word Parts by having someone dictate them to you. Use a separate sheet of paper.

To hear and spell the terms, go to Evolve Resources at evolve.elsevier.com and select:
Practice Student Resources > Student Resources > Chapter 8 > **Pronounce and Spell**

See Appendix B for instructions.

❑ Check the box when complete.

Surgical Terms

NOT BUILT FROM WORD PARTS

Word parts may be present in the following terms; however, their full meanings cannot be translated using definitions of word parts alone.

TERM	DEFINITION
anterior and posterior colporrhaphy (A&P repair) (an-TĒR-ē-or) (pos-TĒR-ē-or) (kol-POR-a-fē)	surgical repair of a weakened vaginal wall to correct a cystocele (protrusion of the bladder against the anterior wall of the vagina) and a rectocele (protrusion of the rectum against the posterior wall of the vagina) (Exercise Figure C)
conization (*kon*-i-ZĀ-shun)	surgical removal of a cone-shaped area of the cervix; used in the treatment for noninvasive cervical cancer. Types of conization include loop electrosurgical excision (LEEP), cryosurgery (cold knife conization), and laser ablation. (also called **cone biopsy**)
dilation and curettage (D&C) (dī-LĀ-shun) (kū-re-TAHZH)	surgical procedure to widen the cervix and remove contents from the uterus using a curette, an instrument for scraping or suctioning; the procedure can be diagnostic or therapeutic (Fig. 8.10)
endometrial ablation (*en*-dō-MĒ-trē-al) (ab-LĀ-shun)	procedure to destroy or remove the endometrium by use of laser, electrical, or thermal energy; used to treat abnormal uterine bleeding (Fig. 8.11)

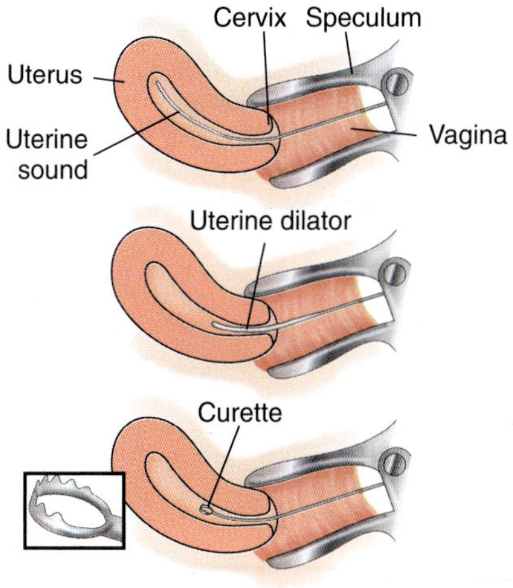

FIG. 8.10 Dilation and curettage (D&C) using a scraping or sharp curette.

EXERCISE FIGURE C

Fill in the blanks to complete the labeling of the diagrams.

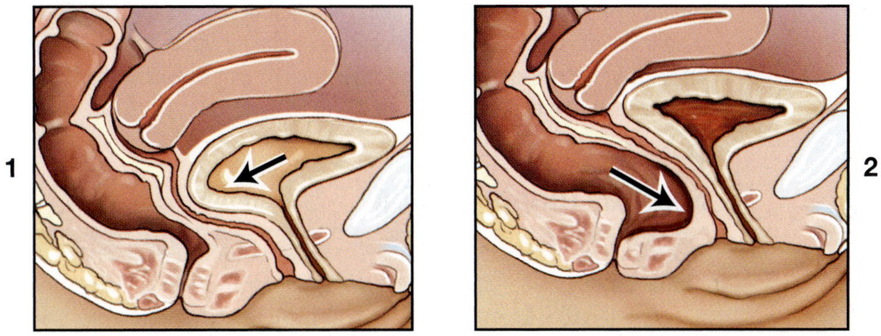

Anterior and posterior ____________ / ____ / ____________ corrects the conditions of:
vagina / cv / suturing

1. ____________ / ____ / ____________
bladder / cv / protrusion

2. Rectocele

ABLATION
is from the Latin **ablatum**, meaning **to carry away**. In surgery **ablation** means **excision or eradication**, especially by cutting with laser or electrical energy.

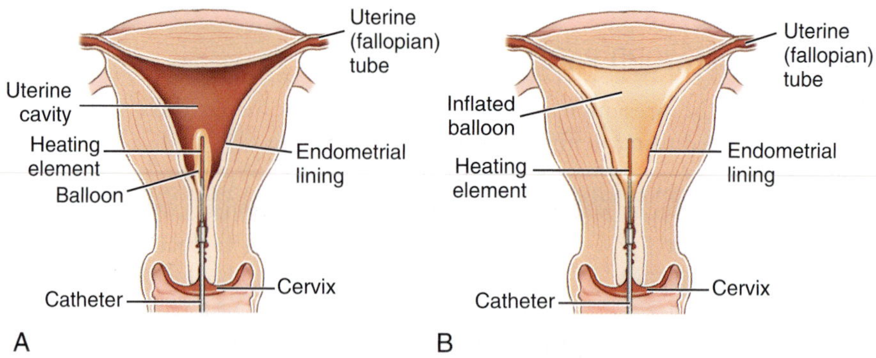

FIG. 8.11 Endometrial ablation using thermal energy. **A,** The balloon catheter (deflated) is inserted through the cervix into the uterine cavity. **B,** The balloon is inflated with a solution of 5% dextrose and water and heated to 87°C for 8 minutes, ablating the endometrial lining.

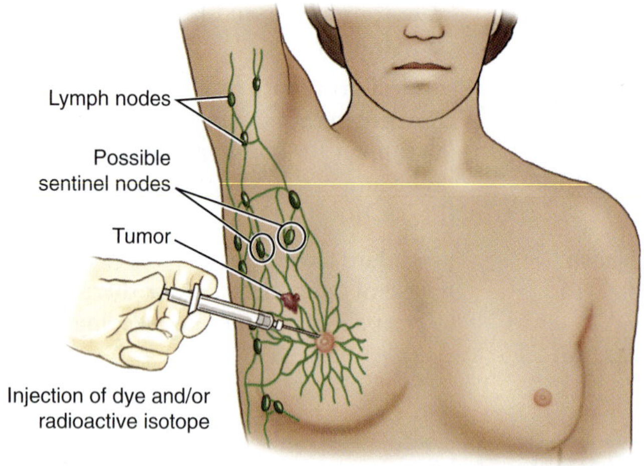

FIG. 8.12 Preparation for sentinel lymph node biopsy. The process of identifying the sentinel node(s) is performed in the nuclear medicine department of radiology. The biopsy is performed in surgery. The sentinel lymph node biopsy procedure was first developed for patients with melanoma. It is now also used to determine metastasis of breast cancer to the lymph nodes. Previously, surgeons would remove 10 to 20 lymph nodes to determine the spread of cancer, which often caused lymphedema and painful and swelling of the affected arm.

Surgical Terms—cont'd

TERM	DEFINITION
laparoscopy (*lap*-a-ROS-ko-pē)	visual examination of the abdominopelvic cavity, accomplished by inserting a laparoscope through a tiny incision near the umbilicus. Numerous female reproductive system surgeries are performed with this technique. (also called **laparoscopic surgery**) (Fig. 8.8)
myomectomy (*mī*-ō-MEK-to-mē)	excision of a uterine fibroid (myoma)
sentinel lymph node biopsy (SEN-tin-el) (limf) (nōd) (BĪ-op-sē)	injection of blue dye and/or radioactive isotope used to identify the sentinel lymph node(s), the first in the axillary chain and most likely to contain metastasis of breast cancer. The nodes are removed and microscopically examined. If the nodes closest to the cancer (called "sentinel nodes") are negative, additional nodes are not removed. (Fig. 8.12).

TYPES OF BREAST BIOPSY

- **Directed breast biopsy** uses mammography, sonography, or magnetic resonance (MR) images to guide a biopsy needle.
- **Surgical breast biopsy** involves making an incision to remove a palpable breast lesion (also called **open** or **incisional biopsy**).
- **Wire localization biopsy** combines both modalities and uses radiographic guidance to place a thin, flexible wire directly into a breast lesion. The lesion is removed surgically with the wire intact.

TERM	DEFINITION
stereotactic breast biopsy (*ster*-ē-ō-TAK-tik) (brest) (BĪ-op-sē)	technique that combines mammography and computer-assisted biopsy to obtain tissue from a breast lesion (Fig. 8.13)
tubal ligation (TOO-bul) (lī-GĀ-shun)	surgical closure of the uterine tubes for sterilization; tubes may be cut and tied (ligated), cut and cauterized, or closed off with a clip, clamp, ring, or band (also called **tubal sterilization** and **female surgical sterilization**) (Fig. 8.14)
uterine artery embolization (UAE) (Ū-ter-in) (AR-ter-ē) (*em*-be-li-ZĀ-shun)	placement of small gelatin beads into uterine arteries to stop blood flow supplying uterine fibroids or to stop severe hemorrhage after childbirth; performed by an interventional radiologist (also called **uterine fibroid embolization** when used to treat uterine fibroids)

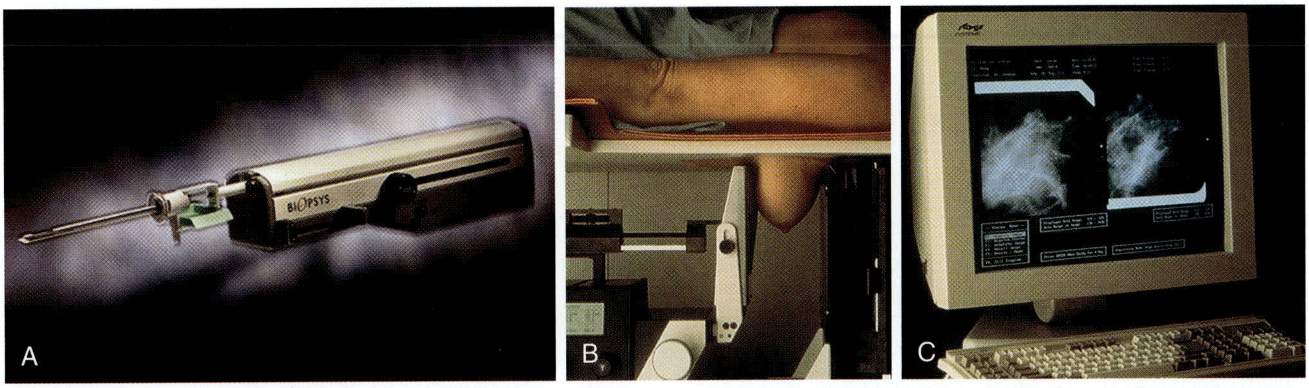

FIG. 8.13 Stereotactic breast biopsy, which is used for nonpalpable lesions that are visible on mammography. The patient is placed prone on a special table with the breast suspended through an opening. The breast is placed in a mammography machine under the table, which produces a digital mammography image that identifies the exact location of the lesion. The biopsy instrument is guided by a radiologist or surgeon. **A,** The stereotactic needle is used to obtain the specimen for biopsy. **B,** The patient is positioned for stereotactic breast biopsy. **C,** The mammogram appears digitally and is used to determine the placement of the biopsy needle.

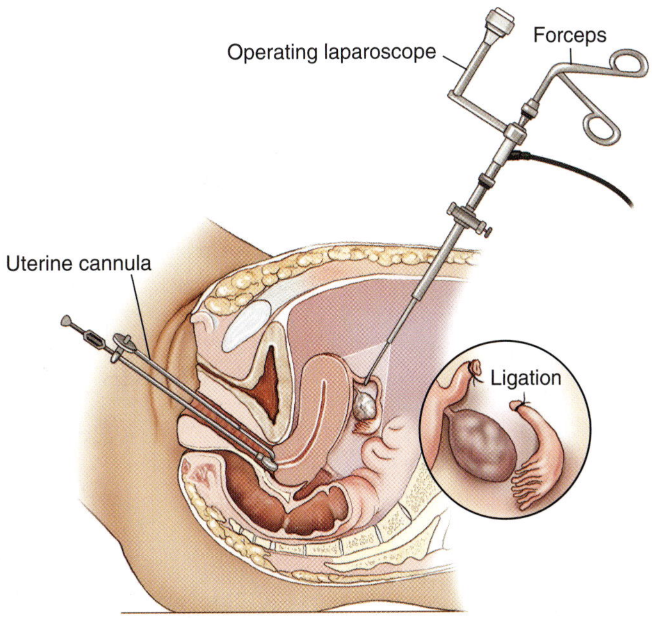

FIG. 8.14 Laparoscopic tubal sterilization.

EXERCISE 19

Practice saying aloud each of the Surgical Terms NOT Built from Word Parts.

> To hear the terms, go to Evolve Resources at evolve.elsevier.com and select:
> Practice Student Resources > Student Resources > Chapter 8 > **Pronounce and Spell**
>
> See Appendix B for instructions.

❑ Check the box when complete.

EXERCISE 20

Fill in the blanks with the correct term.

1. A surgical procedure used for sterilization of women is ____________ ______________________.
2. The surgery used to repair a cystocele and rectocele is a(n) ______________ and ______________ ______________.
3. D&C is the abbreviation for ____________ and ______________________.
4. ____________ ____________ ____________ is a technique used to obtain tissue from a breast lesion.
5. Excision of a uterine fibroid is called ______________________.
6. A procedure to destroy endometrium by laser, electrical, or thermal energy is called ______________ ______________.
7. A procedure used to treat uterine fibroids by blocking the blood supply is called ______________ ______________ ______________.
8. Surgical removal of a cone-shaped area of the cervix is called ______________________.
9. A procedure to identify metastasis of breast cancer in the axillary lymph nodes for biopsy is called ____________ ____________ ____________ ____________.
10. A surgical procedure performed through a tiny incision near the umbilicus is called ______________ or ______________ ______________.

EXERCISE 21

Match the surgical procedures in the first column with the corresponding organs in the second column. You may use the answers in the second column more than once.

_____ 1. dilation and curettage	a. uterine tubes
_____ 2. laparoscopic surgery for sterilization	b. vagina
_____ 3. tubal ligation	c. uterus
_____ 4. anterior and posterior colporrhaphy repair	d. ovaries
_____ 5. myomectomy	e. vulva
_____ 6. stereotactic breast biopsy	f. mammary glands
_____ 7. conization	g. lymph nodes
_____ 8. endometrial ablation	h. cervix
_____ 9. sentinel lymph node biopsy	
_____ 10. uterine artery embolization	

EXERCISE 22

Spell each of the Surgical Terms NOT Built from Word Parts by having someone dictate them to you. Use a separate sheet of paper.

To hear and spell the terms, go to Evolve Resources at evolve.elsevier.com and select:
Practice Student Resources > Student Resources > Chapter 8 > **Pronounce and Spell**

See Appendix B for instructions.

❑ Check the box when complete.

Diagnostic Terms

BUILT FROM WORD PARTS

The following terms can be translated using definitions of word parts. Further explanation is provided within parentheses as needed.

TERM	DEFINITION
DIAGNOSTIC IMAGING	
hysterosalpingogram (HSG) (*his*-ter-ō-*sal*-PING-gō-gram)	radiographic image of the uterus and uterine tubes (after an injection of a contrast agent) (Exercise Figure D)
mammogram (MAM-ō-gram)	radiographic image of the breast (Fig. 8.15)

EXERCISE FIGURE D

Fill in the blanks to complete the labeling of the diagram.

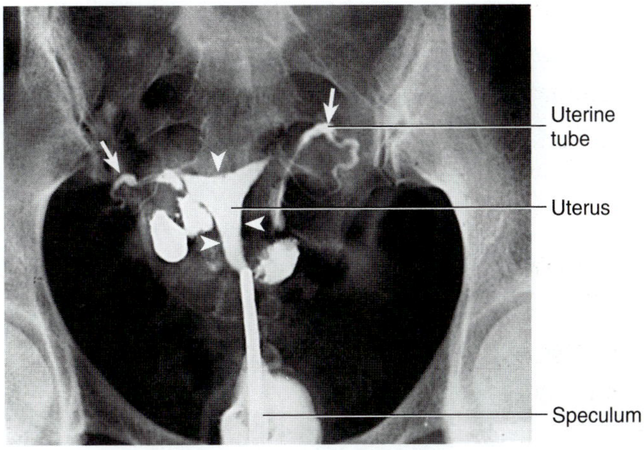

The ______ / ______ / ______ / ______ / ______ reveals bilateral ______ / ______ / ______.
uterus / cv / uterine tube / cv / radiographic image; water / cv / uterine tube

Liquid contrast medium is injected through the vagina and is used to outline the uterus and uterine tubes before the radiographic image is made. This procedure usually is performed to determine whether obstructions exist in the uterine tubes causing infertility.

Diagnostic Terms—cont'd

TERM	DEFINITION
mammography (ma-MOG-ra-fē)	radiographic imaging of the breast (also called **digital mammography** when images are obtained electronically and viewed on a computer) (Fig. 8.15)
sonohysterography (SHG) (*son*-ō-*his*-ter-OG-ra-fē)	process of recording the uterus by use of sound (an ultrasound procedure; saline solution is injected into the uterine cavity, during transvaginal sonography. It is used preoperatively to assess polyps, myomas, and adhesions.) (also called **hysterosonography**)
ENDOSCOPY	
colposcope (KOL-pō-skōp)	instrument used for visual examination of the vagina (and cervix)
colposcopy (kol-POS-ko-pē)	visual examination (with a magnified view) of the vagina (and cervix)
hysteroscope (HIS-ter-ō-skōp)	instrument used for visual examination of the uterus (uterine cavity)
hysteroscopy (*his*-ter-OS-ko-pē)	visual examination of the uterus (uterine cavity)
pelviscopic (pel-vi-SKOP-ik)	pertaining to visual examination of the pelvic cavity (female reproductive organs)
pelviscopy (pel-VIS-ku-pē)	visual examination of the pelvic cavity (female reproductive organs) (also called **gynecologic laparoscopy**)

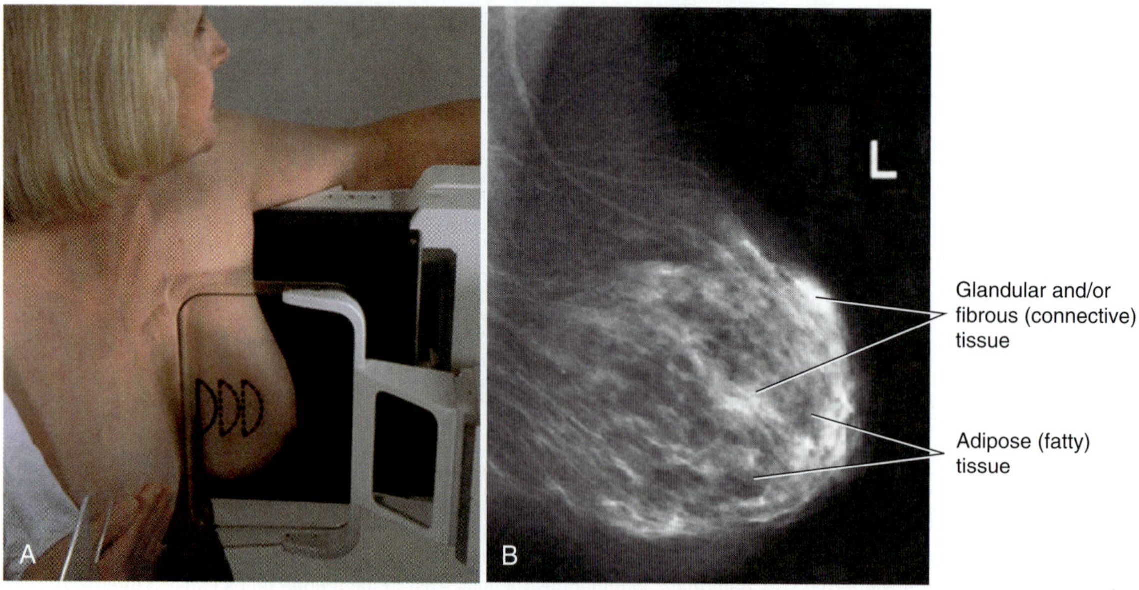

FIG. 8.15 A, Mammography. **B,** Mammogram.

EXERCISE 23

Practice saying aloud each of the Diagnostic Terms Built from Word Parts.

To hear the terms, go to Evolve Resources at evolve.elsevier.com and select:
Practice Student Resources > Student Resources > Chapter 8 > **Pronounce and Spell**

See Appendix B for instructions.

❑ Check the box when complete.

EXERCISE 24

Analyze and define the following diagnostic terms.

1. colposcopy

____
____

2. mammogram

____
____

3. colposcope

____
____

4. hysteroscopy

____
____

5. hysterosalpingogram

____
____

6. pelviscopic

____
____

7. pelviscopy

____
____

8. mammography

____
____

9. hysteroscope

____
____

10. sonohysterography

____
____

EXERCISE 25

Build diagnostic terms that correspond to the following definitions by using the word parts you have learned.

1. radiographic image of the uterus and uterine tubes
   ______ WR / CV / ______ WR / CV / ______ S
2. visual examination of the vagina (and cervix)
   ______ WR / CV / ______ S
3. instrument used for visual examination of the vagina (and cervix)
   ______ WR / CV / ______ S
4. visual examination of the uterus
   ______ WR / CV / ______ S
5. radiographic image of the breast
   ______ WR / CV / ______ S
6. pertaining to visual examination of the pelvic cavity (female reproductive organs)
   ______ WR / CV / ______ S
7. visual examination of the pelvic cavity (female reproductive organs)
   ______ WR / CV / ______ S
8. instrument used for visual examination of the uterus
   ______ WR / CV / ______ S
9. radiographic imaging of the breast
   ______ WR / CV / ______ S
10. process of recording the uterus with sound
    ______ WR / CV / ______ WR / CV / ______ S

EXERCISE 26

Spell each of the Diagnostic Terms Built from Word Parts by having someone dictate them to you. Use a separate sheet of paper.

> To hear and spell the terms, go to Evolve Resources at evolve.elsevier.com and select:
> Practice Student Resources > Student Resources > Chapter 8 > **Pronounce and Spell**
>
> See Appendix B for instructions.

❑ Check the box when complete.

Diagnostic Terms

NOT BUILT FROM WORD PARTS

Word parts may be present in the following terms; however, their full meanings cannot be translated using definitions of word parts alone.

TERM	DEFINITION
DIAGNOSTIC IMAGING	
transvaginal sonography (TVS) (trans-VAJ-i-nal) (so-NOG-ra-fē)	ultrasound procedure that uses a transducer placed in the vagina to obtain images of the ovaries, uterus, cervix, uterine tubes, and surrounding structures; used to diagnose masses such as ovarian cysts or tumors, to monitor pregnancy, and to evaluate ovulation for the treatment of infertility (Fig. 8.16)
LABORATORY	
CA-125 test (C-A-1-25) (test)	blood test primarily used to monitor treatment for ovarian cancer and to detect recurrence once treatment is complete. CA-125 (cancer antigen 125) is a protein found on the surface of most ovarian cancer cells and is released into the bloodstream. Elevated amounts of CA-125 in the blood may indicate the presence of ovarian cancer. (also called **CA-125** and **CA 125 tumor marker**)
HPV test (H-P-V) (test)	cytological study of cervical and vaginal secretions to detect high-risk forms of the human papillomavirus (HPV) that can cause abnormal cervical cells and cervical cancer; used for cervical cancer screening
Pap test (pap) (test)	cytological study of cervical and vaginal secretions to detect abnormal and cancerous cells; primarily used for cervical cancer screening (also called **Papanicolaou** [*pap*-a-NIK-kō-lā-oo] **test**; formerly called **Pap smear**) (Fig. 8.17)

PAP TEST
is named after Dr. George N. Papanicolaou (1883-1962), a Greek physician practicing in the United States, who developed the cell smear method for the diagnosis of cancer in 1943. Though the smear method could be used to sample cells from any organ, it has been commonly used on cervical and vaginal secretions to detect cervical cancer. In 1966 the FDA approved a liquid-based screening system, which improved the detection of squamous intraepithelial lesions. With use of the liquid-based method surpassing use of the smear method, the procedure is more commonly called a Pap test, rather than a Pap smear.

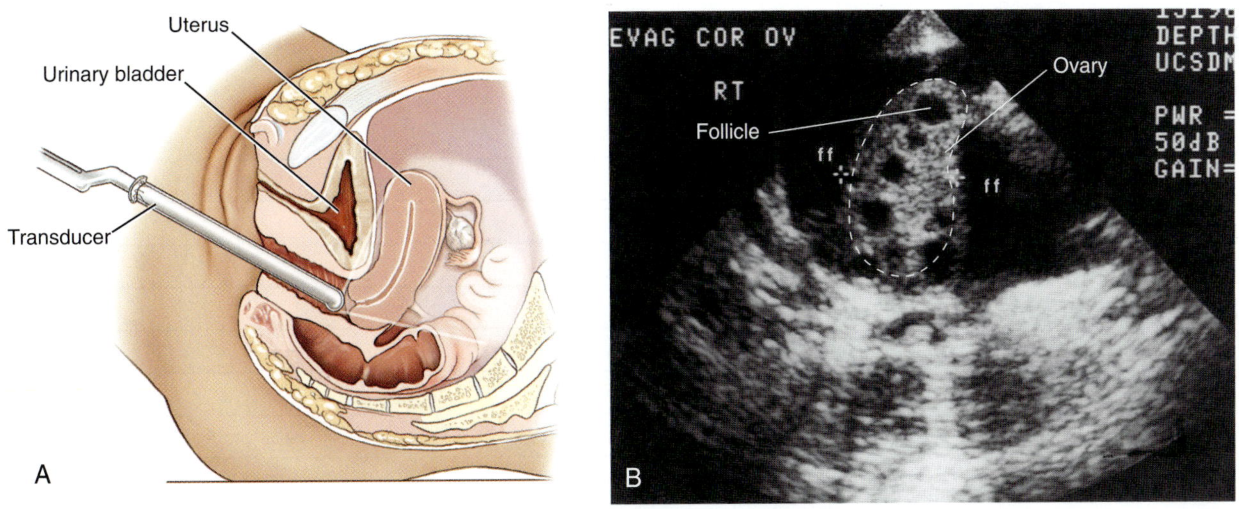

FIG. 8.16 Transvaginal sonography. A, Transducer placed in the vagina. **B,** Transvaginal coronal image of the right ovary with multiple follicles, showing free fluid surrounding the ovary.

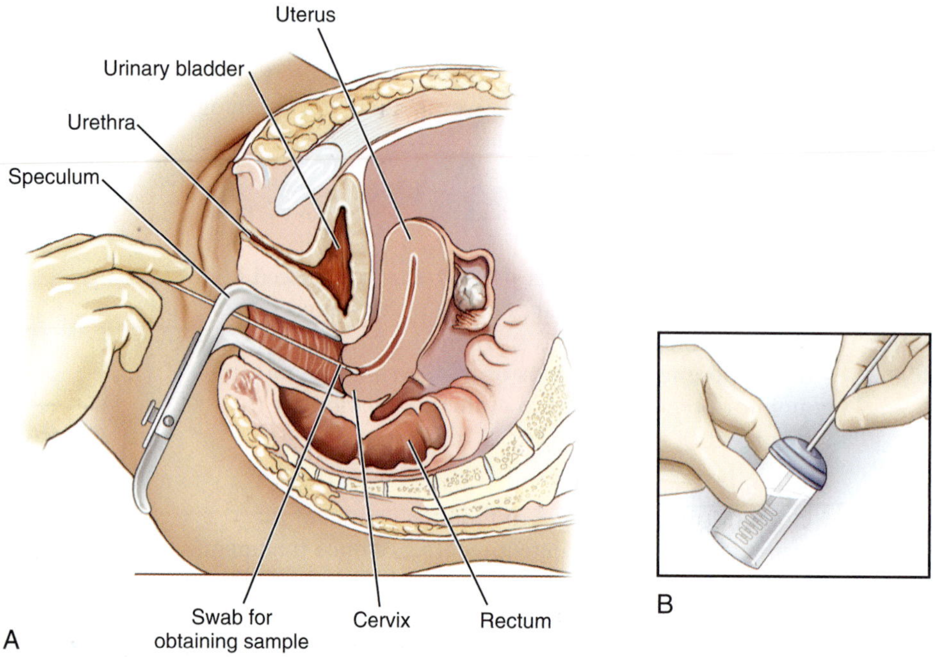

FIG. 8.17 Collection of cervical and vaginal secretions for the Pap test and the HPV test. **A,** Obtaining the specimen. **B,** Dispersion of cells in the vial filled with a liquid medium. In the laboratory, the specimen is transferred to slides for cytological study and can be used for the Pap test and HPV test.

EXERCISE 27

Practice saying aloud each of the Diagnostic Terms NOT Built from Word Parts.

To hear the terms, go to Evolve Resources at evolve.elsevier.com and select:
Practice Student Resources > Student Resources > Chapter 8 > **Pronounce and Spell**

See Appendix B for instructions.

❑ Check the box when complete.

EXERCISE 28

A. Write the correct definition on the line.

1. Pap test ______________________________

____

2. transvaginal sonography ______________________________

____

3. CA-125 test ______________________________

____

4. HPV test ______________________________

____

B. Write the term for each of the following.

1. Lab tests for cervical cancer screening include:
   a. _____________ _______________ , the cytological study of cervical and vaginal secretions to detect abnormal and cancerous cells
   b. _____________ _______________ , the cytological study of cervical and vaginal secretions to detect high-risk forms of the human papillomavirus
2. blood test used to monitor treatment for ovarian cancer and to detect recurrence _____________ _____________
3. obtains images of the ovaries, uterus, cervix, uterine tubes, and surrounding structures _____________________ _____________________

EXERCISE 29

Spell each of the Diagnostic Terms NOT Built from Word Parts by having someone dictate them to you. Use a separate sheet of paper.

To hear and spell the terms, go to Evolve Resources at evolve.elsevier.com and select:
Practice Student Resources > Student Resources > Chapter 8 > **Pronounce and Spell**

See Appendix B for instructions.

❑ Check the box when complete.

Complementary Terms

BUILT FROM WORD PARTS

The following terms can be translated using definitions of word parts. Further explanation is provided within parentheses as needed.

TERM	DEFINITION
endocervical (*en*-dō-SER-vi-kal)	pertaining to within the cervix
gynecologist (*gīn*-ek-OL-o-jist)	physician who studies and treats diseases of women (female reproductive system)
gynecology (GYN) (*gīn*-ek-OL-o-jē)	study of women (branch of medicine dealing with health and diseases of the female reproductive system)
gynopathic (*gīn*-ō-*PATH*-ik)	pertaining to (reproductive system) diseases of women
leukorrhea (*lū*-kō-RĒ-a)	white discharge (from the vagina)
mastalgia (mas-TAL-ja)	pain in the breast
menarche (me-NAR-kē)	beginning of menstruation (specifically, first menstrual period)
vaginal (VAJ-i-nal)	pertaining to the vagina
vesicovaginal (*ves*-i-kō-VAJ-i-nal)	pertaining to the (urinary) bladder and the vagina
vulvovaginal (*vul*-vō-VAJ-i-nal)	pertaining to the vulva and vagina

EXERCISE 30

Practice saying aloud each of the Complementary Terms Built from Word Parts.

To hear the terms, go to Evolve Resources at evolve.elsevier.com and select:
Practice Student Resources > Student Resources > Chapter 8 > **Pronounce and Spell**

See Appendix B for instructions.

❑ Check the box when complete.

EXERCISE 31

Analyze and define the following complementary terms.

1. gynecologist
____
____
2. gynecology
____
____
3. vulvovaginal
____
____
4. mastalgia
____
____
5. menarche
____
____
6. leukorrhea
____
____
7. gynopathic
____
____
8. vesicovaginal
____
____
9. vaginal
____
____
10. endocervical
____
____

EXERCISE 32

Build complementary terms that correspond to the following definitions by using the word parts you have learned.

1. white discharge (from the vagina) ________ / ____ / ________
WR / CV / S

2. beginning of menstruation ________ / ________
WR / WR

3. pain in the breast ______ WR / ______ S

4. pertaining to the vulva and vagina ______ WR / CV / ______ WR / ______ S

5. physician who studies and treats diseases of women ______ WR / CV / ______ S

6. study of women (branch of medicine dealing with health and diseases of the female reproductive system) ______ WR / CV / ______ S

7. pertaining to the (urinary) bladder and the vagina ______ WR / CV / ______ WR / ______ S

8. pertaining to (reproductive system) diseases of women ______ WR / CV / ______ WR / ______ S

9. pertaining to the vagina ______ WR / ______ S

10. pertaining to within the cervix ______ P / ______ WR / ______ S

EXERCISE 33

Spell each of the Complementary Terms Built from Word Parts by having someone dictate them to you. Use a separate sheet of paper.

> To hear and spell the terms, go to Evolve Resources at evolve.elsevier.com and select:
> Practice Student Resources > Student Resources > Chapter 8 > **Pronounce and Spell**
>
> See Appendix B for instructions.

❑ Check the box when complete.

Complementary Terms

NOT BUILT FROM WORD PARTS

Word parts may be present in the following terms; however, their full meanings cannot be translated using definitions of word parts alone.

TERM	DEFINITION
anovulation (*an*-ov-ū-LĀ-shun)	absence of ovulation
contraception (KON-tra-*sep*-shen)	intentional prevention of conception (pregnancy) (also called **birth control [BC]**) (Fig. 8.18)

METHODS OF CONTRACEPTION

Numerous contraceptive methods exist, including:

- barrier (condoms)
- chemical (spermicides)
- oral pharmaceutical (birth control pill)
- long-acting reversible contraception (LARC), including an intrauterine device (IUD), intrauterine system (IUS), implant, and injection

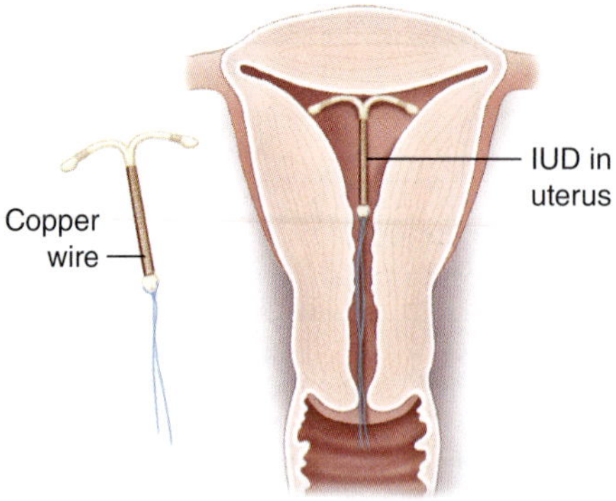

FIG. 8.18 Intrauterine device (IUD). Inserted through the cervix, this T-shaped device provides long-term contraception by changing the intrauterine environment.

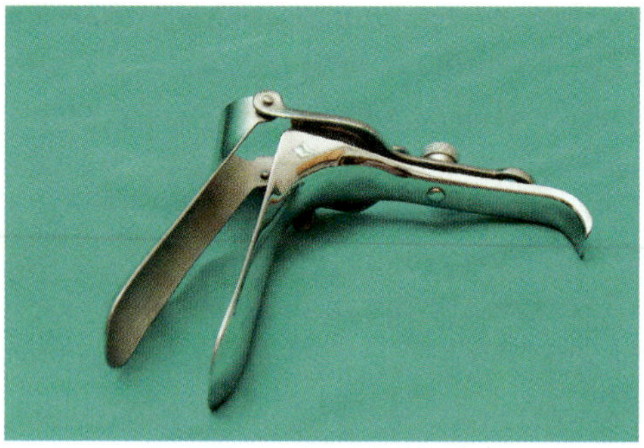

FIG. 8.19 Vaginal speculum.

PELVIC ORGAN PROLAPSE (POP)

is the abnormal downward displacement of pelvic organs, including the urinary bladder, uterus, and vagina. Pelvic organs may slip out of place when supporting muscles and ligaments are damaged or weakened from childbirth, gynecological surgery, and menopause.

Complementary Terms—cont'd

TERM	DEFINITION
dyspareunia (*dis*-pa-RŪ-nē-a)	difficult or painful intercourse
fistula (FIS-tū-la)	abnormal passageway between two organs or between an internal organ and the body surface
hormone replacement therapy (HRT) (HŌR-mōn) (RĒ-plās-ment) (THER-a-pē)	replacement of hormones, estrogen and progesterone, to treat symptoms associated with menopause
menopause (MEN-o-pawz)	cessation of menstruation, usually around the ages of 48 to 53 years; may be induced at an earlier age surgically (bilateral oophorectomy) or medically (side effect of chemotherapy treatment)
oligoovulation (*ol*-i-gō-OV-ū-LĀ-shun)	infrequent ovulation
ovulation (OV-ū-LĀ-shun)	release of an ovum from a mature graafian follicle
premenstrual syndrome (PMS) (prē-MEN-stroo-al) (SIN-drōm)	syndrome involving physical and emotional symptoms occurring up to 10 days before menstruation. Symptoms include nervous tension, irritability, mastalgia, edema, and headache.
prolapse (prō-LAPS)	displacement of an organ or anatomic structure from its normal position (also called **ptosis**)
speculum (SPEK-ū-lum)	instrument for opening a body cavity to allow visual inspection (Fig. 8.19)

Refer to **Appendix F** for pharmacology terms related to the female reproductive system.

EXERCISE 34

Practice saying aloud each of the Complementary Terms NOT Built from Word Parts.

> To hear the terms, go to Evolve Resources at evolve.elsevier.com and select:
> Practice Student Resources > Student Resources > Chapter 8 > **Pronounce and Spell**
>
> See Appendix B for instructions.

❑ Check the box when complete.

EXERCISE 35

Write the definitions of the following terms.

1. menopause ____________________
2. dyspareunia ____________________
3. fistula ____________________
____
4. premenstrual syndrome ____________________
____
5. speculum ____________________
____
6. hormone replacement therapy ____________________
____
7. prolapse ____________________
____
8. contraception ____________________
9. ovulation ____________________
10. oligoovulation ____________________
11. anovulation ____________________

EXERCISE 36

Write the term for each of the following.

1. abnormal passageway ____________________
2. release of an ovum from a mature graafian follicle ____________________
3. painful intercourse ____________________
4. cessation of menstruation ____________________
5. syndrome involving physical and emotional symptoms ____________________
6. instrument for opening a body cavity ____________________
7. replacement of hormones to treat symptoms associated with menopause ____________________
8. intentional prevention of conception ____________________
9. displacement of an organ or anatomic structure from its normal position ____________________
10. absence of ovulation ____________________
11. infrequent ovulation ____________________

EXERCISE 37

Spell each of the Complementary Terms NOT Built from Word Parts by having someone dictate them to you. Use a separate sheet of paper.

> To hear and spell the terms, go to Evolve Resources at evolve.elsevier.com and select:
> Practice Student Resources > Student Resources > Chapter 8 > **Pronounce and Spell**
>
> See Appendix B for instructions.

❑ Check the box when complete.

WEB LINK

For more information on a spectrum of topics related to breast health and the female reproductive system, visit the National Institutes of Health at *www.nlm.nih.gov/medlineplus/womenhealth.html* and click on Women's Health.

Abbreviations

ABBREVIATION	TERM
A&P repair	anterior and posterior colporrhaphy
BC	birth control
Cx	cervix
D&C	dilation and curettage
FCC	fibrocystic breast changes
GYN	gynecology
HRT	hormone replacement therapy
HSG	hysterosalpingogram
IUD	intrauterine device
IUS	intrauterine system
LAVH	laparoscopically-assisted vaginal hysterectomy
PCOS	polycystic ovary syndrome
PID	pelvic inflammatory disease
PMS	premenstrual syndrome
SHG	sonohysterography
TAH/BSO	total abdominal hysterectomy/bilateral salpingo-oophorectomy
TLH	total laparoscopic hysterectomy
TSS	toxic shock syndrome
TVH	total vaginal hysterectomy
TVS	transvaginal sonography
UAE	uterine artery embolization

Refer to **Appendix E** for a complete list of abbreviations.

EXERCISE 38

Write the meaning for each of the abbreviations in the following sentences.

1. To repair a cystocele and rectocele the patient is scheduled in surgery for an **A&P repair** ______________ & ______________ ______________.
2. Following a **TAH/BSO** ______________ ______________ ______________ and ______________ ______________ ______________ the gynecologist prescribed **HRT** ______________ ______________ ______________ for the patient to take for 3 months after surgery.
3. **SHG** ______________ and **TVS** ______________ ______________ are diagnostic ultrasound procedures used to assist in diagnosing diseases and disorders of the female reproductive organs.
4. When performing a **TVH** ______________ ______________ ______________ the surgeon removes the uterus through the vagina without a surgical incision into the abdomen. During a(n) **LAVH** ______________ ______________ ______________ ______________ the surgeon uses a fiberoptic laparoscope inserted through a tiny incision near the umbilicus to visualize the uterus and guide removal through the vagina. In a **TLH** ______________ ______________ ______________, morcellation is used to remove the uterus through the laparoscope.
5. **D&C** ______________ & ______________ is the dilation of the **Cx** ______________ and scraping of the endometrium.
6. **FCC** ______________ ______________ ______________ is the most common breast problem of women in their 20s.
7. A female patient with probable **PID** ______________ ______________ ______________ was referred to the **GYN** ______________ clinic for evaluation and care.
8. The medical management of **PMS** ______________ ______________ emphasizes the relief of symptoms.
9. **UAE** ______________ ______________ ______________ offers a minimally invasive treatment option for some women with symptomatic uterine fibroids.
10. For long-acting reversible contraception, the female patient considered an **IUD** ______________ ______________ and **IUS** ______________ ______________ either of which would be inserted by a gynecologist. While these methods of **BC** ______________ ______________ are effective in preventing pregnancy, they do not protect against sexually transmitted infections.
11. A diagnosis of **PCOS** ______________ ______________ ______________ may be made if two of the following criteria are met: 1) chronic anovulation, 2) hyperandrogenism (excessive secretion of androgens with clinical or biological manifestations), and 3) polycystic ovaries.

For additional practice with Abbreviations, go to Evolve Resources at evolve.elsevier.com and select: Practice Student Resources > Student Resources > Chapter 8 > **Flashcards:** Abbreviations

See Appendix B for instructions.

PRACTICAL APPLICATION

EXERCISE 39 *Case Study: Translate Between Everyday Language and Medical Language*

CASE STUDY: Cindy Collier and Rajive Modi

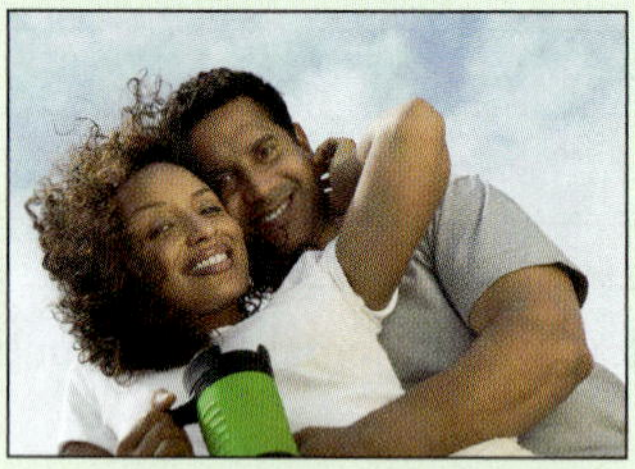

Cindy and Rajive want to have a baby. They have been trying for over a year to get pregnant, but it hasn't happened. Cindy worries something is wrong. Even though she has her period every month, menstruating is very painful, and she bleeds a lot. She often has pain low in her belly. She had sexual partners before Rajive, and she is worried that one may have given her a disease. Rajive is also concerned, and wonders if something might be wrong with him that is keeping Cindy from getting pregnant. When he was born only one of his testicles was down, and they had to do surgery to fix the other one. He hasn't had any problems since then. He had partners before Cindy, and he is worried that he may have passed something on to her.

Now that you have worked through Chapters 7 and 8 on the reproductive systems, consider the medical terms that might be used to describe Cindy and Rajive's experience. See the Review of Terms at the end of Chapters 7 and 8 for a list of terms that might apply.

A. *Underline phrases in the case study that could be substituted with medical terms.*

B. *Write the medical term and its definition for three of the phrases you underlined.*

MEDICAL TERM	DEFINITION
1. ______________	______________
2. ______________	______________
3. ______________	______________

DOCUMENTATION: Excerpt from Infertility Clinic Consultation

Cindy, a 31-year-old female, and her husband Rajive, a 32-year-old male, present for workup and treatment for infertility. They have been trying to conceive for 14 months. Rajive: past medical history is significant for cryptorchidism at birth, which was repaired by orchidopexy at age 2. Cindy: menarche at 14, symptoms of dysmenorrhea and menorrhagia, both of which have worsened since discontinuing birth control pills. She had a normal Pap test approximately 1 year ago.

Diagnostic Studies: A complete blood count (CBC) was ordered as well as serum tests for thyroid-stimulating hormone (TSH), follicle-stimulating hormone (FSH), and prolactin level (PRL). A urine pregnancy test was negative.

Impression: Primary infertility; cause undetermined. Possible cervicitis caused by chlamydia and possible pelvic inflammatory disease.

Recommendation: We will await culture results and treat both partners with antibiotics if necessary. If labs are normal, we will proceed with a semen analysis for Rajive. We should consider a hysterosalpingogram (HSG) for Cindy based on her history and physical exam findings.

C. *Underline medical terms presented in Chapters 7 and 8 used in the previous excerpt from the infertility consultation. See the Review of Terms at the end of the chapter for a complete list.*

D. *Select and define three of the medical terms you underlined. To check your answers, go to Appendix A.*

MEDICAL TERM	DEFINITION
1. ______________	______________
2. ______________	______________
3. ______________	______________

EXERCISE 40 *Interact With Medical Documents and Electronic Health Records*

A. Read the report and complete it by writing medical terms on answer lines within the document. Definitions of terms to be written appear after the document.

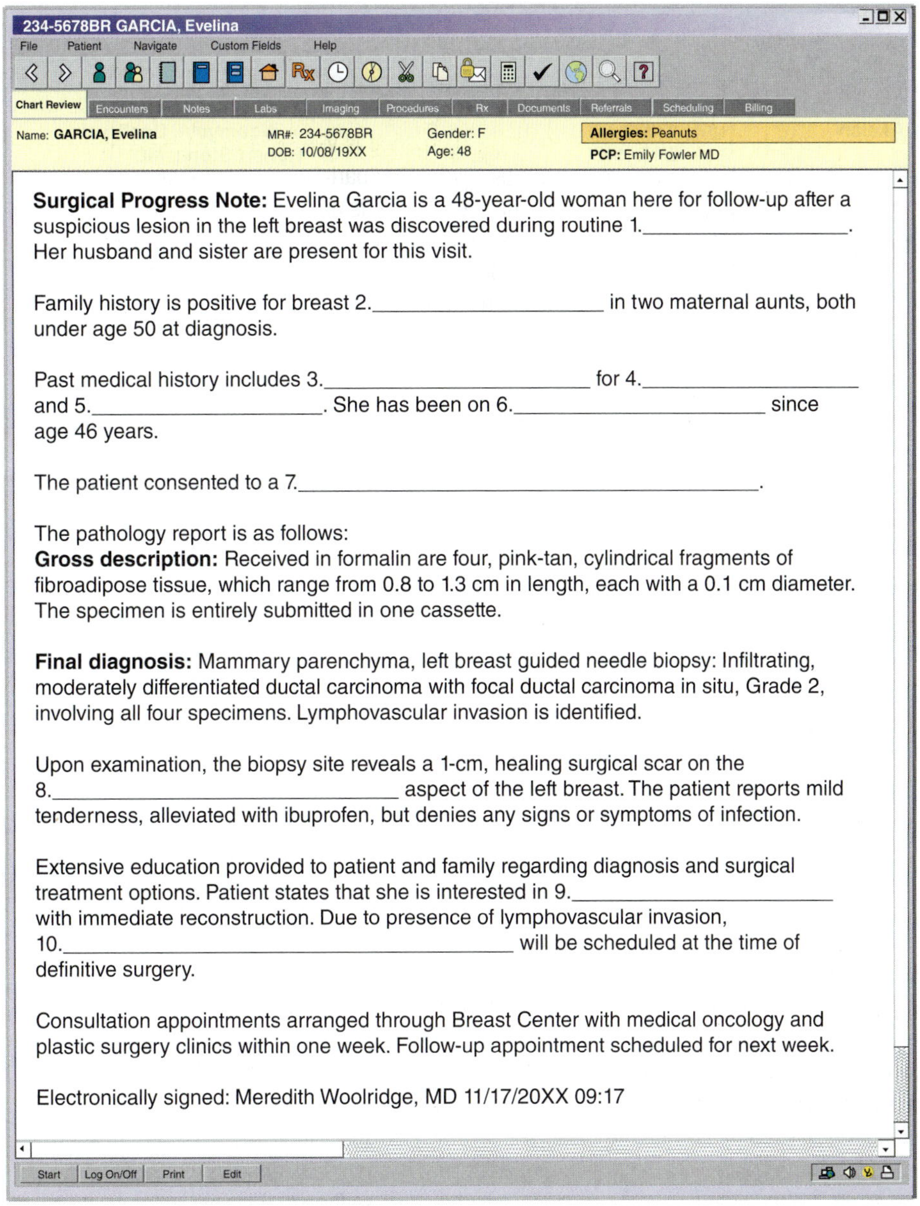

234-5678BR GARCIA, Evelina

File Patient Navigate Custom Fields Help

Chart Review | Encounters | Notes | Labs | Imaging | Procedures | Rx | Documents | Referrals | Scheduling | Billing

Name: **GARCIA, Evelina** MR#: 234-5678BR DOB: 10/08/19XX Gender: F Age: 48 **Allergies:** Peanuts **PCP:** Emily Fowler MD

Surgical Progress Note: Evelina Garcia is a 48-year-old woman here for follow-up after a suspicious lesion in the left breast was discovered during routine 1.__________________. Her husband and sister are present for this visit.

Family history is positive for breast 2.____________________ in two maternal aunts, both under age 50 at diagnosis.

Past medical history includes 3.______________________ for 4.__________________ and 5.____________________. She has been on 6.______________________ since age 46 years.

The patient consented to a 7.____.

The pathology report is as follows:
Gross description: Received in formalin are four, pink-tan, cylindrical fragments of fibroadipose tissue, which range from 0.8 to 1.3 cm in length, each with a 0.1 cm diameter. The specimen is entirely submitted in one cassette.

Final diagnosis: Mammary parenchyma, left breast guided needle biopsy: Infiltrating, moderately differentiated ductal carcinoma with focal ductal carcinoma in situ, Grade 2, involving all four specimens. Lymphovascular invasion is identified.

Upon examination, the biopsy site reveals a 1-cm, healing surgical scar on the 8.______________________________ aspect of the left breast. The patient reports mild tenderness, alleviated with ibuprofen, but denies any signs or symptoms of infection.

Extensive education provided to patient and family regarding diagnosis and surgical treatment options. Patient states that she is interested in 9.______________________ with immediate reconstruction. Due to presence of lymphovascular invasion, 10.____ will be scheduled at the time of definitive surgery.

Consultation appointments arranged through Breast Center with medical oncology and plastic surgery clinics within one week. Follow-up appointment scheduled for next week.

Electronically signed: Meredith Woolridge, MD 11/17/20XX 09:17

Start | Log On/Off | Print | Edit

Definitions of Medical Terms to Complete the Document

Write the medical terms defined on corresponding answer lines in the document.

1. radiographic imaging of the breast
2. cancerous tumor
3. excision of the uterus
4. growth of endometrium into the muscular portion of the uterus
5. abnormal condition in which endometrial tissue occurs in various areas of the pelvic cavity
6. abbreviation for replacement of hormones to treat menopause
7. combines mammography and computer-assisted biopsy to obtain tissue from a breast lesion
8. pertaining to the middle and to (one) side
9. surgical removal of a breast
10. an injection of blue dye and/or radioactive isotope used to identify the first in the axillary chain and most likely to contain metastasis of breast cancer

EXERCISE 40 *Interact With Medical Documents and Electronic Health Records—cont'd*

B. Read the medical report and answer the questions below it.

47820 CARLSON, AKELAH

File Patient Navigate Custom Fields Help

Patient Chart | Lab | Rad | Notes | Documents | Rx | Scheduling | Images | Billing

Name: **CARLSON, Akelah** MR#: **47820** DOB: **2/15/19XX** Gender: **F** Age: **37** Allergies: **Neomycin, Bacitracin** PCP: **Robert Stone, MD**

CHART NOTE

ENCOUNTER DATE: 11/13/20XX

HISTORY: This 37-year-old gravida 2 para 2 woman was referred by her primary care provider. She complains of fullness in the pelvic region and menometrorrhagia. She admits to frequency and urgency of urination. Also, she complains of fatigue. The patient's last menstrual period was two weeks ago. Her mother was treated for ovarian cancer.

PHYSICAL EXAMINATION: Upon bimanual pelvic examination, an ill-defined mass was palpable on left lateral portion of the uterus.

DIAGNOSTIC STUDIES: Pap test results showed normal cytology. CA-125 test results were normal. Transvaginal sonography confirmed the presence of a pedunculated uterine fibroid. The uterine tubes and ovaries were normal.

IMPRESSION: Uterine fibroids.

RECOMMENDATION: We discussed the benefits of having a vaginal hysterectomy with bilateral salpingo-oophorectomy in view of her mother's history of ovarian cancer. The patient declined this approach because of the desire to have another child. A laparoscopic myomectomy is therefore recommended.

Electronically signed by: Elizabeth Fuller, MD 11/14/20XX 15:34

Start | Log On/Off | Print | Edit

Use the medical report above to answer the questions.

1. The patient's symptoms include:
   a. absence of menstrual flow
   b. scanty menstrual flow
   c. increased amount of menstrual flow during menses and bleeding between periods
   d. painful menstruation
2. The CA-125 diagnostic study was used to detect the presence of:
   a. ovarian cancer
   b. cervical cancer
   c. endometrial cancer
   d. endometriosis
3. The recommended procedure, a myomectomy, will entail the surgical excision of:
   a. the breast
   b. the uterus
   c. ovarian cancer
   d. uterine fibroids

C. Complete the **three medical documents** within the electronic health record (EHR) on Evolve.

Topic: Invasive Ductal Carcinoma
Documents: Gynecology Clinic Visit, Radiology Final Report, Pathology Final Diagnosis

To complete the three medical records, go to Evolve Resources at evolve.elsevier.com and select:
Practice Student Resources > Student Resources > Chapter 8 > **Electronic Heath Records**

See Appendix B for instructions.

EXERCISE 41 *Pronounce Medical Terms in Use*

Practice pronunciation of terms by reading aloud the following paragraphs. Use the phonetic spellings following medical terms from the chapter to assist with pronunciation. The script also contains medical terms not presented in the chapter. Treat them as information only or look for their meanings in a medical dictionary or a reliable online source.

CANCERS OF THE FEMALE REPRODUCTIVE SYSTEM

Breast Cancer

The breast is the most common site of cancer in women. More than 80% of **breast cancer** (brest) (KAN-cer) is infiltrating ductal cancer (IDC), which originates in the mammary ducts. The rate of growth depends on hormonal influences. As long as the cancer remains in the duct, it is considered noninvasive and is called *ductal carcinoma in situ (DCIS).*

Mammography (ma-MOG-ra-fē) is the most common method used for diagnosing cancer of the breast. Confirmation is done with a biopsy obtained by conventional surgery or guided breast biopsy, such as **stereotactic breast biopsy** (ster-ē-ō-TAK-tik) (brest) (BĪ-op-sē).Treatment may include lumpectomy, **mastectomy** (mas-TEK-to-mē),chemotherapy, radiation therapy, and hormonal therapy.

Cervical Cancer

In many regions of the world **cervical cancer** (SER-vi-kal) (KAN-cer) is the leading cause of death in women. Cervical cancer resembles and results from a sexually transmitted disease, a feature that distinguishes it from other cancers. Abnormal **vaginal** (VAJ-i-nal) bleeding is the most common symptom. **Pap test** (pap) (test) followed by **colposcopy** (kol-POS-ko-pē) biopsy is used to diagnose this disease Surgical treatment options are **conization** (*kon*-i-ZĀ-shun), such as LEEP, and **hysterectomy** (his-te-REK-to-mē). Chemotherapy and radiation therapy may also be used. A vaccine for human papillomavirus is now available and can be used for the prevention of cervical cancer.

Endometrial Cancer

Currently 75% of women diagnosed with **endometrial cancer** (en-dō -MĒ-trē -al) (KAN-cer) are postmenopausal. Inappropriate bleeding is a warning sign; hence early diagnosis is common. Pelvic examination, Pap smear, and endometrial sampling are used to diagnose this disease. Treatment is **hysterosalpingo-oophorectomy** (*his*-ter-ō-sal-*ping*-gō -ō-*of*-o-REK-to-mē), which may be followed by chemotherapy and radiation therapy. Laparoscopic -assisted **vaginal hysterectomy** (VAJ-i-nal) (*his*-te-REK-to-mē) may also be used.

Ovarian Cancer

Ovarian cancer (ō -VAR-ē-an) (KAN-cer) is the ninth most common form of cancer in women, yet it is the most challenging to diagnose and causes more deaths than any other cancer of the female reproductive system. Early symptoms are often absent or associated with other problems; thus early diagnosis is uncommon. Early symptoms include abdominal discomfort and bloating; later stages include abdominal or pelvic pain and urinary or menstrual irregularities. **CA-125 test** (C-A-1-25) (test) and **transvaginal sonography** (trans-VAJ-i-nal) (so-NOG-ra-fē) are used in diagnosing this disease. Treatment is total abdominal **hysterectomy** (*his*-te-REK-to-mē) and bilateral **salpingo-oophorectomy** (sal-ping-gō-ō-*of*-o-REK-to-mē) and removal of as much additional involved tissue as possible, including lymph nodes in the pelvic area. Chemotherapy is usually prescribed following surgery.

EXERCISE 42 *Chapter Content Quiz*

Test your understanding of terms and abbreviations introduced in this chapter. Circle the letter for the medical term or abbreviation related to the words in italics.

1. A severe illness that *may affect menstruating women after using tampons* is abbreviated as:
   a. TSS
   b. TVS
   c. TVH
2. The term meaning *inflammation of the mucous-producing gland(s) on each side of the vagina just above the opening* refers to inflammation of the gland without the formation of an abscess.
   a. cervicitis
   b. vulvovaginitis
   c. Bartholin adenitis
3. *Inflammation of the breast*, is an infection characterized by *pain in the breast*, edema, warmth, and erythema and most commonly occurs with breast-feeding.
   a. mastitis, mastalgia
   b. myometritis, mastopexy
   c. perimetritis, mammoplasty
4. Bilateral *water in the uterine tube* indicates both uterine tubes are blocked by watery liquid and can be a cause of female infertility.
   a. salpingocele
   b. hematosalpinx
   c. hydrosalpinx
5. Symptoms of *growth of the endometrium into the muscular portion of the uterus* include dysmenorrhea, menorrhagia, and *difficult or painful intercourse.*
   a. endometriosis, mastalgia
   b. adenomyosis, dyspareunia
   c. myometritis, amenorrhea
6. Monthly hormonal changes may cause *fibrosis, benign cysts, and mastalgia in one or both breasts.*
   a. FCC
   b. PMS
   c. PID
7. Cryosurgery, laser ablation, and LEEP are various surgical techniques performed to *remove a cone-shaped area of the cervix.*
   a. colporrhaphy
   b. conization
   c. myomectomy
8. The *surgical procedure to widen the cervix and remove contents from the uterus* can be used for treatment and for diagnostics.
   a. CX
   b. D&C
   c. SHG
9. A *surgical repair of the breast* to reduce size is called reduction:
   a. mammoplasty
   b. mammogram
   c. mastectomy
10. Partial *surgical closure of the vagina* may be used to treat vaginal prolapse for patients who are not candidates for more complex reconstructive surgeries and who are no longer sexually active.
    a. colpocleisis
    b. episiorrhaphy
    c. trachelorrhaphy
11. In *total excision of the uterus performed laparoscopically*, the uterus, including the cervix, is morcellated and withdrawn through the laparoscope.
    a. TAH/BSO
    b. TLH
    c. TVH
12. The *instrument used for visual examination of the uterus* is a thin, lighted device inserted through the vagina that transmits images of the inside of the uterus to a computer screen.
    a. hysteroscope
    b. colposcope
    c. pelviscopy
13. The *cytological study of cervical and vaginal secretions to detect high-risk forms of the human papillomavirus* is a lab test conducted to screen for cervical cancer.
    a. CA-125 test
    b. Pap test
    c. HPV test
14. *Infrequent release of an ovum from a mature graafian follicle* generally refers to having 8 or fewer menstrual cycles in one year.
    a. ovulation
    b. oligoovulation
    c. anovulation
15. A *vesicovaginal fistula* is an abnormal passage way between the vagina and the:
    a. rectum
    b. urinary bladder
    c. vulva
16. The *instrument used to open* the vagina to conduct a pelvic exam is called:
    a. speculum
    b. hysteroscope
    c. colposcope

CHAPTER REVIEW

REVIEW OF CHAPTER CONTENT ON EVOLVE RESOURCES

Go to evolve.elsevier.com and click on Gradable Student Resources and Practice Student Resources. Online learning activities found there can be used to review chapter content and to assess your learning of word parts, medical terms, and abbreviations. Place check marks in the boxes next to activities used for review and assessment.

GRADABLE STUDENT RESOURCES

Chapter 08 >	Exercises >	☐ Word Parts ☐ Terms Built from Word Parts ☐ Terms Not Built from Word Parts ☐ Abbreviations
	Quizzes >	☐ Quiz 1: Disease and Disorder Terms ☐ Quiz 2: Surgical Terms ☐ Quiz 3: Diagnostic Terms ☐ Quiz 4: Complementary Terms

PRACTICE STUDENT RESOURCES > STUDENT RESOURCES

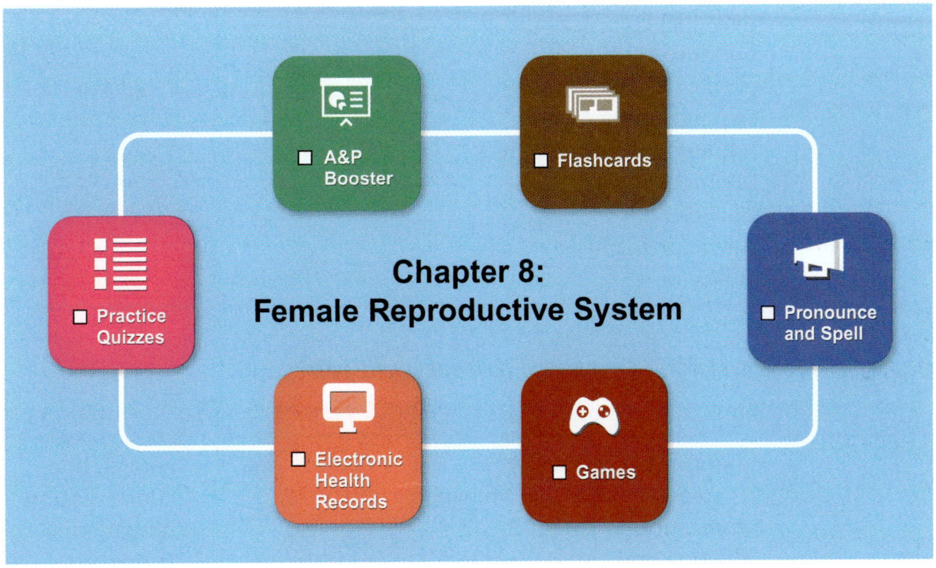

REVIEW OF WORD PARTS

Can you define and spell the following word parts?

COMBINING FORMS		PREFIX	SUFFIXES
arche/o	men/o	peri-	-clesis
cervic/o	metr/o		-salpinx
colp/o	oophor/o		
endometri/o	pelv/i		
episi/o	perine/o		
gyn/o	salping/o		
gynec/o	trachel/o		
hymen/o	vagin/o		
hyster/o	vulv/o		
mamm/o			
mast/o			

REVIEW OF TERMS

Can you build, analyze, define, pronounce, and spell the following terms *built from word parts*?

DISEASES AND DISORDERS	SURGICAL	DIAGNOSTIC	COMPLEMENTARY
amenorrhea	colpocleisis	colposcope	endocervical
Bartholin adenitis	colpoperineorrhaphy	colposcopy	gynecologist
cervicitis	colpoplasty	hysterosalpingogram (HSG)	gynecology (GYN)
dysmenorrhea	colporrhaphy	hysteroscope	gynopathic
endometriosis	episioperineoplasty	hysteroscopy	leukorrhea
endometritis	episiorrhaphy	mammogram	mastalgia
hematosalpinx	hymenectomy	mammography	menarche
hydrosalpinx	hymenotomy	pelviscopic	vaginal
mastitis	hysterectomy	pelviscopy	vesicovaginal
menometrorrhagia	hysteropexy	sonohysterography (SHG)	vulvovaginal
menorrhagia	hysterosalpingo-oophorectomy		
metrorrhagia	mammoplasty		
myometritis	mastectomy		
oligomenorrhea	mastopexy		
oophoritis	oophorectomy		
perimetritis	perineorrhaphy		
pyosalpinx	salpingectomy		
salpingitis	salpingo-oophorectomy		
salpingocele	salpingostomy		
vaginitis	trachelectomy		
vaginosis	trachelorrhaphy		
vulvovaginitis	vulvectomy		

Can you define, pronounce, and spell the following terms *NOT built from word parts*?

DISEASES AND DISORDERS	SURGICAL	DIAGNOSTIC	COMPLEMENTARY
adenomyosis	anterior and posterior colporrhaphy (A&P repair)	CA-125 test	anovulation
breast cancer	conization	HPV test	contraception
cervical cancer	dilation and curettage (D&C)	Pap test	dyspareunia
endometrial cancer	endometrial ablation	transvaginal sonography (TVS)	fistula
fibrocystic breast changes (FCC)	laparoscopy		hormone replacement therapy (HRT)
ovarian cancer	myomectomy		menopause
pelvic inflammatory disease (PID)	sentinel lymph node biopsy		oligoovulation
polycystic ovary syndrome (PCOS)	stereotactic breast biopsy		ovulation
toxic shock syndrome (TSS)	tubal ligation		premenstrual syndrome (PMS)
uterine fibroid	uterine artery embolization (UAE)		prolapse
uterine prolapse			speculum
vaginal fistula			

Chapter 9

Obstetrics and Neonatology

Outline

Objectives

Upon completion of this chapter you will be able to:

1. Pronounce organs and anatomic structures relating to pregnancy.
2. Define and spell word parts related to obstetrics and neonatology.
3. Define, pronounce, and spell disease and disorder terms related to obstetrics and neonatology.
4. Define, pronounce, and spell surgical and diagnostic terms related to obstetrics.
5. Define, pronounce, and spell complementary terms related to obstetrics and neonatology.
6. Interpret the meaning of abbreviations related to obstetrics and neonatology.
7. Apply medical language in clinical contexts.

ANATOMY

Obstetrics is the branch of medicine that deals with childbirth and the care of the mother before, during, and after birth. **Neonatology** is the branch of medicine that deals with the diagnosis and treatment of disorders of the newborn.

Terms Relating to Pregnancy

TERM	DEFINITION
gamete (GAM-ēt)	mature germ cell, either sperm (male) or ovum (female)
conception (kon-SEP-shun)	beginning of pregnancy, when the sperm enters the ovum. Conception normally occurs in the uterine tubes. (also called **fertilization**) (Fig. 9.1A)
zygote (ZĪ-gōt)	cell formed by the union of the sperm and the ovum
embryo (EM-brē-ō)	unborn offspring in the stage of development from implantation of the zygote to the end of the eighth week of pregnancy. This period is characterized by rapid growth of the embryo.
fetus (FĒ-tus)	unborn offspring from the beginning of the ninth week of pregnancy until birth (Fig. 9.2)
gestation (jes-TĀ-shun)	development of a new individual from conception to birth (also called **pregnancy**)
gestation period (jes-TĀ-shun) (PĒR-ē-ed)	duration of pregnancy; normally 38 to 42 weeks, which can be divided into three equal periods, called *trimesters*
implantation (*im*-plan-TĀ-shun)	embedding of the zygote in the uterine lining. The process normally begins about 7 days after fertilization and continues for several days. (Fig. 9.1A)

SKIN CHANGES THAT OCCUR THROUGHOUT PREGNANCY

- **striae gravidarum**: "stretch marks" occurring on the abdomen, breast, buttocks, and thighs from weakening of elastic tissues
- **linea nigra**: dark medial line extending from the pubis upward
- **chloasma**: hyperpigmentation of blotchy brown macules usually evenly distributed over the cheeks and forehead

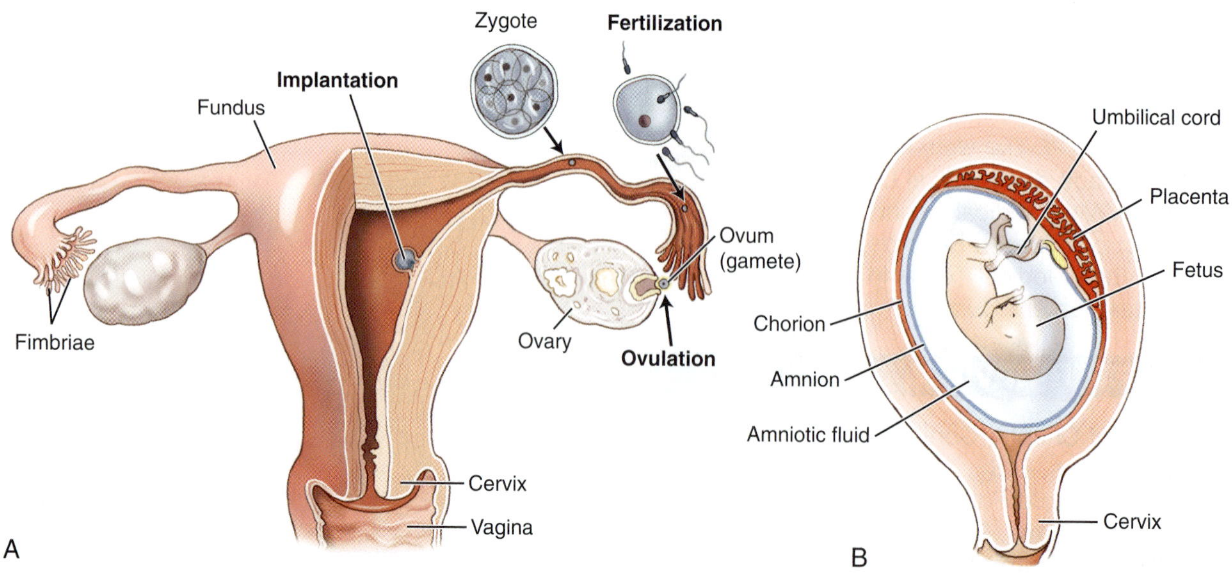

FIG. 9.1 **A,** Ovulation, fertilization, and implantation. **B,** Development of the fetus.

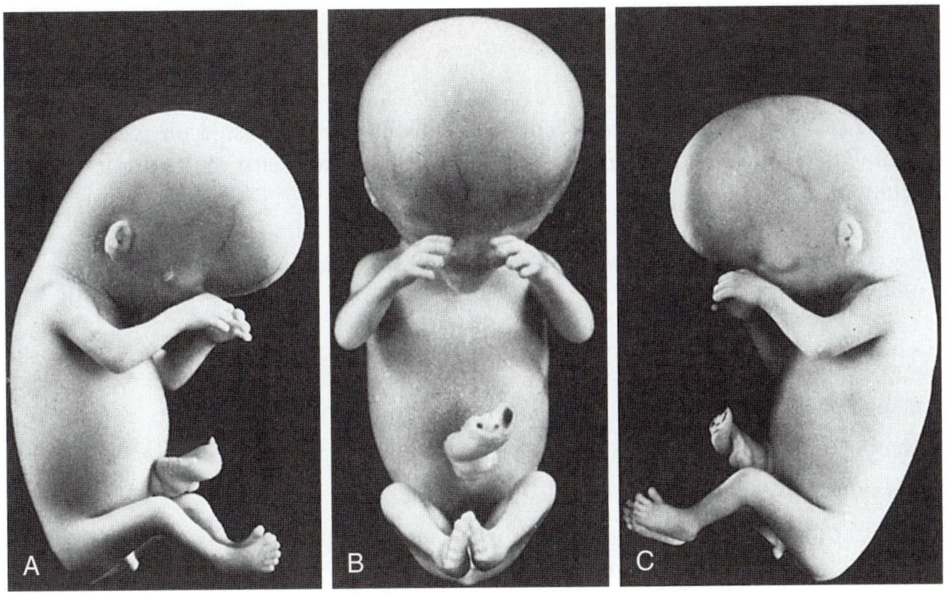

FIG. 9.2 Human male fetus at 68 days (1.85 inches, 47 mm). **A,** Right. **B,** Frontal. **C,** Left.

TERM	DEFINITION
placenta (pla-SEN-ta)	structure that grows on the wall of the uterus during pregnancy and allows for nourishment of the fetus (commonly referred to as **afterbirth**) (Fig. 9.1B)
amniotic sac (*am*-nē-OT-ic) (sak)	membranous bag that surrounds the fetus before delivery (also called **amnionic sac** and commonly referred to as **bag of waters**) (Fig. 9.1B)
chorion (KOR-ē-on)	outermost layer of the fetal membrane
amnion (*am*-nē-ON)	innermost layer of the fetal membrane
amniotic fluid (*am*-nē-OT-ic) (flu-id)	fluid within the amniotic sac, which surrounds the fetus (also called **amnionic fluid**)
umbilicus (um-BIL-i-cus)	navel (belly button); marks the site of attachment of the umbilical cord to the fetus

A&P Booster

For more anatomy and physiology, go to Evolve Resources at evolve.elsevier.com and select:
Practice Student Resources > Student Resources > Chapter 9 > **A&P Booster**

See Appendix B for instructions.

EXERCISE 1

Practice saying aloud each of the Terms Relating to Pregnancy.

To hear the terms, go to Evolve Resources at evolve.elsevier.com and select:
Practice Student Resources > Student Resources > Chapter 9 > **Pronounce and Spell**

See Appendix B for instructions.

❑ Check the box when complete.

WORD PARTS

Combining Forms of Obstetrics and Neonatology

Word parts you need to learn to complete this chapter are listed on the following pages. The exercises at the end of each list will help you learn their definitions and spelling.

Use the flashcards accompanying this text or electronic flashcards to assist you in memorizing the word parts for this chapter.

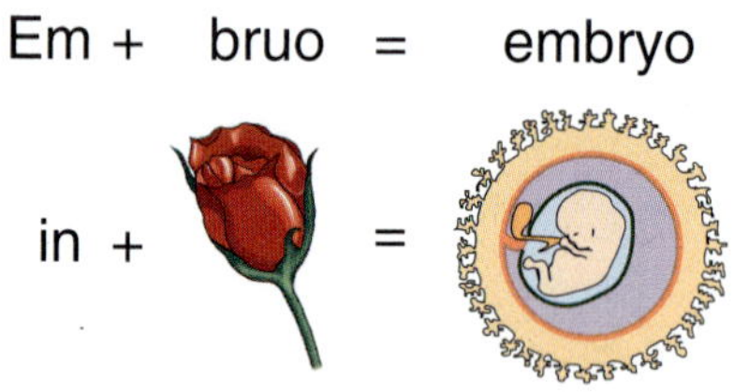

FIG. 9.3 ***Embryo*** comes from the Greek ***em,*** meaning "in," plus ***bruo,*** meaning "to bud" or "to shoot."

PUERPER is made up of two Latin word roots: **puer,** meaning **child,** and **per**, meaning **through.**

COMBINING FORM	DEFINITION
amni/o, amnion/o	amnion, amniotic fluid
chori/o	chorion
embry/o	embryo (Fig. 9.3)
fet/o, fet/i	fetus, unborn offspring *(Note: both* i *and* o *may be used as combining vowels with* fet/.*)*
gravid/o	pregnancy
lact/o	milk
nat/o	birth
omphal/o	umbilicus, navel
par/o, part/o	bear, give birth to, labor, childbirth
puerper/o	childbirth

EXERCISE 2

A. Fill in the blanks with combining forms in this diagram of fetal development. *To check your answers, go to Appendix A.*

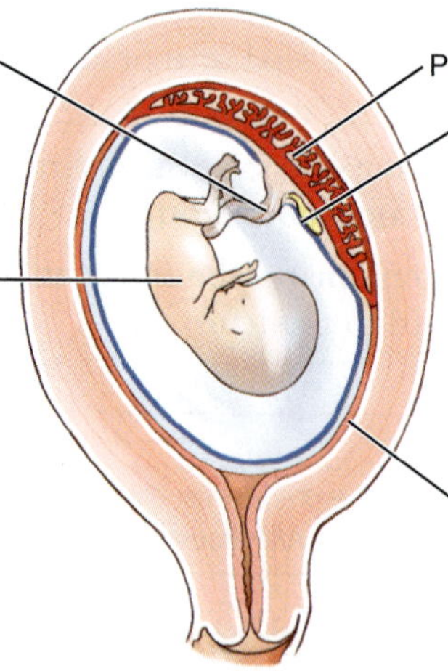

1. Umbilicus
   CF: ______________________
2. Fetus
   CF: ______________________
   CF: ______________________
3. Amnion, amniotic fluid
   CF: ______________________
   CF: ______________________
4. Chorion
   CF: ______________________

B. Write the combining form for each of the following terms.

1. childbirth ______________________
2. bear, give birth to, labor, childbirth a. ______________________ b. ______________________
3. pregnancy ______________________
4. embryo ______________________
5. birth ______________________
6. umbilicus, navel ______________________

EXERCISE 3

A. Step 1: Write the definitions after the following combining forms.
Step 2: Match the descriptions on the right with the combining forms and definitions. Answers may be used more than once.

_____ 1. amni/o, ____________________
_____ 2. embry/o, ____________________
_____ 3. omphal/o, ____________________
_____ 4. amnion/o, ____________________
_____ 5. fet/o, fet/i, ____________________
_____ 6. chori/o, ____________________

a. outermost layer of the fetal membrane
b. implantation of the zygote through eight weeks of pregnancy
c. nine weeks of pregnancy to birth
d. innermost layer of fetal membrane; fluid surrounding the fetus
e. site of the umbilical cord attachment to the fetus

B. Write the definitions of the following combining forms.

1. lact/o ____________________
2. par/o, part/o ____________________
3. puerper/o ____________________
4. gravid/o ____________________
5. nat/o ____________________

Combining Forms Commonly Used in Obstetrics and Neonatology

COMBINING FORM	DEFINITION
cephal/o	head
esophag/o	esophagus (tube leading from the throat to the stomach) (see Fig. 11.1)
prim/i	first *(Note: the combining vowel is* i.*)*
pseud/o	false
pylor/o	pylorus, pyloric sphincter (see Fig. 11.2)
terat/o	malformations

TERAT/O
is translated literally as **monster**; however, in terms containing terat/o relating to obstetrics, terat/o refers to malformations or abnormal development.

EXERCISE 4

Write the definition of the following combining forms.

1. prim/i ____________________
2. pylor/o ____________________
3. cephal/o ____________________
4. esophag/o ____________________
5. pseud/o ____________________
6. terat/o ____________________

EXERCISE 5

Write the combining form for each of the following.

1. head ____________________
2. pylorus, pyloric sphincter ____________________
3. false ____________________
4. esophagus ____________________
5. first ____________________
6. malformations ____________________

Prefixes

PREFIX	DEFINITION
ante-, pre-	before
micro-	small
multi-	many
nulli-	none
post-	after

EXERCISE 6

Write the definitions of the following prefixes.

1. post- ____________
2. multi- ____________
3. nulli- ____________
4. micro- ____________
5. ante- ____________
6. pre- ____________

EXERCISE 7

Write the prefix for each of the following definitions.

1. none ____________
2. small ____________
3. many ____________
4. before a. ____________
   b. ____________
5. after ____________

Suffixes

SUFFIX	DEFINITION
-amnios	amnion, amniotic fluid
-cyesis	pregnancy
-e	noun suffix, no meaning
-is	noun suffix, no meaning
-rrhexis	rupture
-tocia	birth, labor
-um	noun suffix, no meaning
-us	noun suffix, no meaning

-RRHEXIS

is the last of the four **-rrh** suffixes to be learned. The other three introduced in earlier chapters are:

- **-rrhea** – flow or discharge
- **-rrhagia** – rapid flow of blood, excessive bleeding
- **-rrhaphy** – suturing, repairing

The noun suffix **-a,** introduced in Chapter 4, also has no meaning.

Refer to **Appendix C** and **Appendix D** for alphabetized word parts and their meanings.

EXERCISE 8

Write the definitions of the following suffixes.

1. -rrhexis ____________
2. -tocia ____________
3. -cyesis ____________
4. -amnios ____________

EXERCISE 9

Write the suffix pictured and defined.

1. ______________________
birth, labor

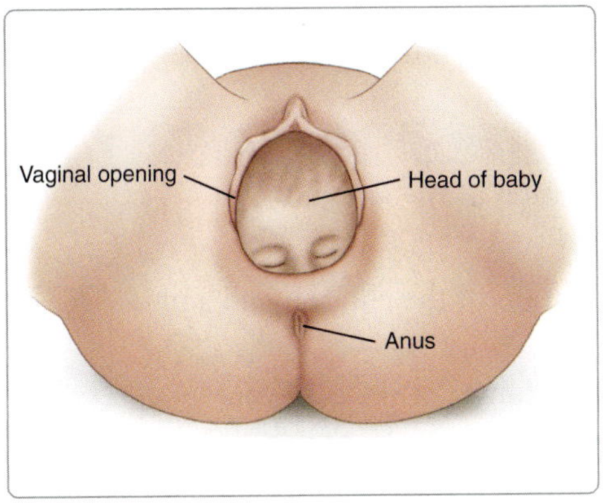

2. ______________________
rupture

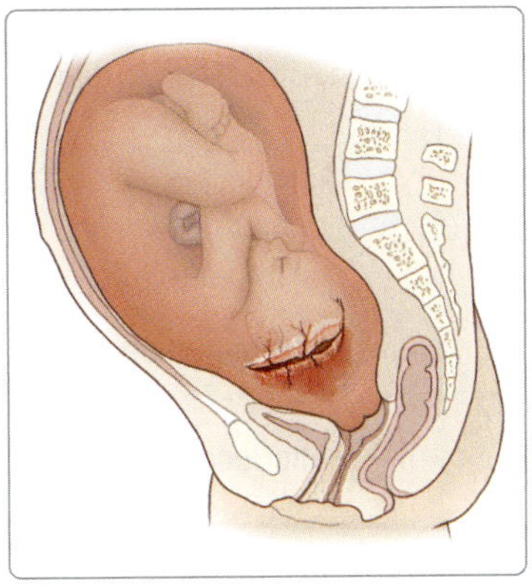

3. ______________________
pregnancy

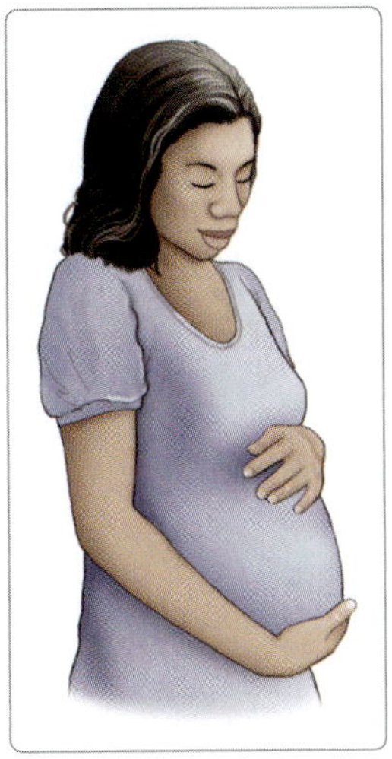

4. ______________________
amnion, amniotic fluid

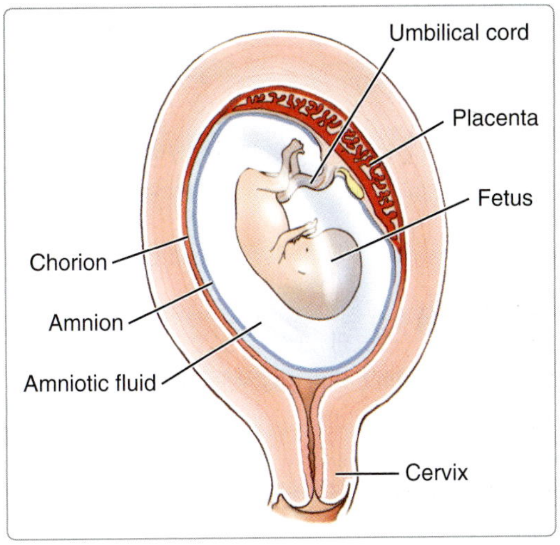

EXERCISE 10

Write the noun suffixes introduced in this chapter that have no meaning.

1. ______________________
2. ______________________
3. ______________________
4. ______________________

For additional practice with Word Parts, go to Evolve Resources at evolve.elsevier.com and select: Practice Student Resources > Student Resources > Chapter 9 **Flashcards**

See Appendix B for instructions.

MEDICAL TERMS

The terms you need to learn to complete this chapter are listed next. The exercises following each list will help you learn the definition and the spelling of each word.

Obstetric Disease and Disorder Terms

BUILT FROM WORD PARTS

The following terms can be translated using definitions of word parts. Further explanation is provided within parentheses as needed.

TERM	DEFINITION
amnionitis (*am*-nē-ō-NĪ-tis)	inflammation of the amnion
chorioamnionitis (*kor*-ē-ō-*am*-nē-ō-NĪ-tis)	inflammation of the chorion and amnion
choriocarcinoma (*kor*-ē-ō-*kar*-si-NŌ-ma)	cancerous tumor of the chorion
dystocia (dis-TŌ-sha)	difficult labor (obstructed or prolonged; causes may be from maternal factors, such as ineffective uterine contractions and abnormal pelvic shape, or from fetal causes, such as large size and abnormal birth presentation)
hysterorrhexis (*his*-ter-ō-REK-sis)	rupture of the uterus
oligohydramnios (*ol*-i-gō-hī-DRAM-nē-os)	scanty amnion water (less than the normal amount of amniotic fluid; 500 mL or less)
polyhydramnios (*pol*-ē-hī-DRAM-nē-os)	much amnion water (more than the normal amount of amniotic fluid; 2000 mL or more) (also called **hydramnios**)

INTEGRATIVE MEDICINE TERM

Acupressure is the ancient practice of applying finger pressure to specific acupoints on the body to preserve and restore health. Studies suggest that acupressure on specific acupoints may be a useful treatment for relieving symptoms experienced by women with hyperemesis gravidarum, reduce early-pregnancy nausea, and reduce the duration and severity of pain during labor.

EXERCISE 11

Practice saying aloud each of the Obstetric Disease and Disorder Terms Built from Word Parts.

To hear the terms, go to Evolve Resources at evolve.elsevier.com and select:
Practice Student Resources > Student Resources > Chapter 9 > **Pronounce and Spell**

See Appendix B for instructions.

❑ Check the box when complete.

EXERCISE 12

Analyze and define the following disease and disorder terms.

1. chorioamnionitis

____

____

2. choriocarcinoma

____

____

3. dystocia

____

____

4. amnionitis

____

____

5. hysterorrhexis

____

____

6. oligohydramnios

____

____

7. polyhydramnios

____

____

EXERCISE 13

Build disease and disorder terms for the following definitions by using the word parts you have learned.

1. cancerous tumor of the chorion ______ / ______ / ______ / ______
   WR / CV / WR / S
2. inflammation of the amnion ______ / ______
   WR / S
3. inflammation of the chorion and amnion ______ / ______ / ______ / ______
   WR / CV / WR / S
4. difficult labor ______ / ______
   P / S(WR)
5. rupture of the uterus ______ / ______ / ______
   WR / CV / S
6. scanty amnion water (less than normal amniotic fluid) ______ / ______ / ______ / ______
   WR / CV / WR / S
7. much amnion water (more than normal amniotic fluid) ______ / ______ / ______
   P / WR / S

EXERCISE 14

Spell each of the Obstetric Disease and Disorder Terms Built from Word Parts by having someone dictate them to you. Use a separate sheet of paper.

> To hear and spell the terms, go to Evolve Resources at evolve.elsevier.com and select:
> Practice Student Resources > Student Resources > Chapter 9 > **Pronounce and Spell**
>
> See Appendix B for instructions.

❑ Check the box when complete.

Obstetric Disease and Disorder Terms
NOT BUILT FROM WORD PARTS

Word parts may be present in the following terms; however, their full meanings cannot be translated using definitions of word parts alone.

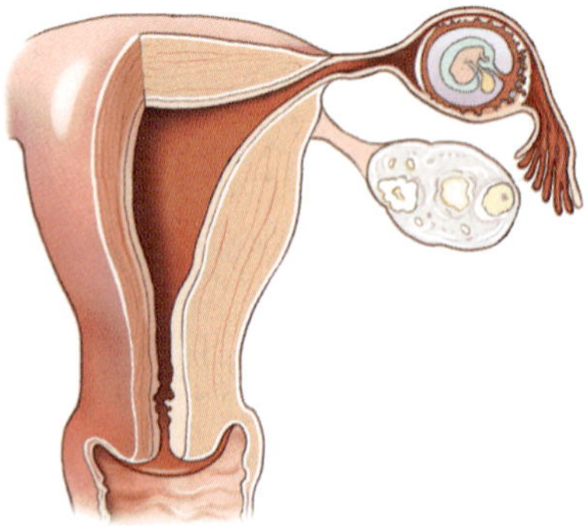

FIG. 9.4 Ectopic pregnancy.

TERM	DEFINITION
abortion (AB) (a-BŌR-shun)	termination of pregnancy by the expulsion from the uterus of an embryo or fetus before viability, usually before 20 weeks of gestation. Spontaneous abortion is the termination of pregnancy that occurs naturally and is commonly referred to as *miscarriage*. Induced abortion is the intentional termination of pregnancy by surgical or medical intervention.
abruptio placentae (ab-RUP-shē-ō) (pla-SEN-tē)	premature separation of the placenta from the uterine wall (Fig. 9.5A)
eclampsia (e-KLAMP-sē-a)	severe complication and progression of preeclampsia characterized by convulsion (see *preeclampsia* later). Eclampsia is a potentially life-threatening disorder.
ectopic pregnancy (ek-TOP-ik) (PREG-nan-sē)	pregnancy occurring outside the uterus, commonly in the uterine tubes (Fig. 9.4)
placenta previa (pla-SEN-ta) (PRĒ-vē-a)	abnormally low implantation of the placenta on the uterine wall completely or partially covering the cervix. (Dilation of the cervix can cause separation of the placenta from the uterine wall, resulting in bleeding. With severe hemorrhage, a cesarean section is necessary to save the mother and baby's life.) (Fig. 9.5B)
preeclampsia (prē-ē-KLAMP-sē-a)	abnormal condition encountered during pregnancy or shortly after delivery characterized by high blood pressure and proteinuria, but with no convulsions. The cause is unknown; if not successfully treated, the condition can progress to eclampsia. Eclampsia is the third most common cause of maternal death in the United States after hemorrhage and infection.

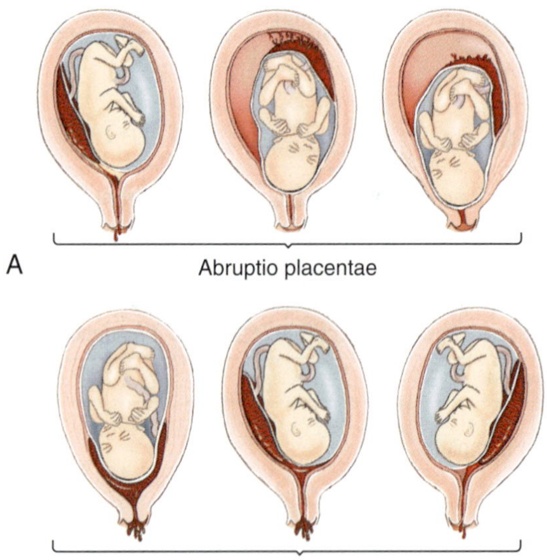

FIG. 9.5 Various presentations of abruptio placentae **(A)** and placenta previa **(B)**.

EXERCISE 15

Practice saying aloud each of the Obstetric Disease and Disorder Terms NOT Built from Word Parts.

> To hear the terms, go to Evolve Resources at evolve.elsevier.com and select:
> Practice Student Resources > Student Resources > Chapter 9 > **Pronounce and Spell**
>
> See Appendix B for instructions.

❑ Check the box when complete.

EXERCISE 16

Write the definitions of the following terms.

1. abruptio placentae ______________________________
2. abortion ______________________________
3. placenta previa ______________________________
4. eclampsia ______________________________
5. ectopic pregnancy ______________________________
6. preeclampsia ______________________________

EXERCISE 17

Write the term for each of the following definitions.

1. premature separation of the placenta from the uterine wall ______________
2. severe complication and progression of preeclampsia ______________
3. termination of pregnancy by the expulsion from the uterus of an embryo or fetus ______________
4. pregnancy occurring outside the uterus ______________
5. abnormally low implantation of the placenta on the uterine wall ______________
6. characterized by high blood pressure and proteinuria, but with no convulsions ______________

EXERCISE 18

Spell each of the Obstetric Disease and Disorder Terms NOT Built from Word Parts by having someone dictate them to you. Use a separate sheet of paper.

> To hear and spell the terms, go to Evolve Resources at evolve.elsevier.com and select:
> Practice Student Resources > Student Resources > Chapter 9 > **Pronounce and Spell**
>
> See Appendix B for instructions.

❑ Check the box when complete.

Neonatology Disease and Disorder Terms

BUILT FROM WORD PARTS

The following terms can be translated using definitions of word parts. Further explanation is provided within parentheses as needed.

EXERCISE FIGURE A

Fill in the blanks to label the diagram.

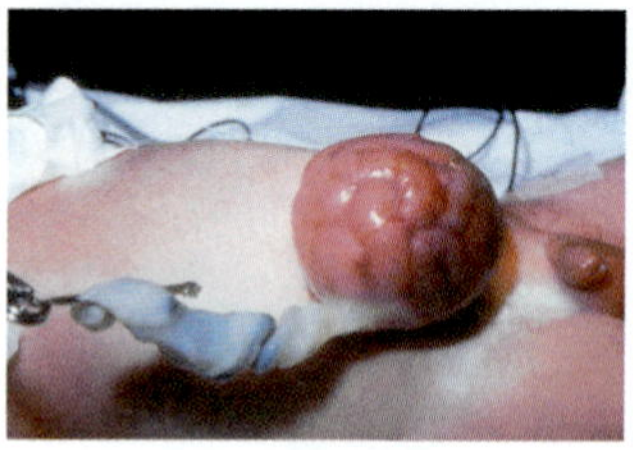

_____ / cv / _____
umbilicus herniation

TERM	DEFINITION
microcephalus (*mī*-krō-SEF-a-lus)	(fetus with a very) small head
omphalitis (*om*-fa-LĪ-tis)	inflammation of the umbilicus
omphalocele (OM-fal-ō-*sēl*)	herniation at the umbilicus (a part of the intestine protrudes through the abdominal wall at birth) (Exercise Figure A).
pyloric stenosis (pī-LOR-ik) (ste-NŌ-sis)	narrowing pertaining to the pyloric sphincter. (Congenital pyloric stenosis occurs in 1 of every 200 newborns.)
tracheoesophageal fistula (*trā*-kē-ō-ē-*sof*-a-JĒ-al) (FIS-tū-la)	abnormal passageway pertaining to the trachea and esophagus (between the trachea and esophagus)

EXERCISE 19

Practice saying aloud each of the Neonatology Disease and Disorder Terms Built from Word Parts.

To hear the terms, go to Evolve Resources at evolve.elsevier.com and select:
Practice Student Resources > Student Resources > Chapter 9 > **Pronounce and Spell**

See Appendix B for instructions.

❑ Check the box when complete.

EXERCISE 20

Analyze and define the following disease and disorder terms.

1. pyloric (stenosis)

_____

_____

2. omphalocele

_____

_____

3. omphalitis

_____

_____

4. microcephalus

_____

_____

5. tracheoesophageal (fistula)

_____

_____

EXERCISE 21

Build disease and disorder terms for the following definitions by using the word parts you have learned.

1. herniation at the umbilicus ______ WR / CV / S
2. (fetus with a very) small head ______ P / WR / S
3. (narrowing) pertaining to the pyloric sphincter ______ WR / S stenosis
4. abnormal passageway pertaining to the trachea and the esophagus (between the trachea and esophagus) ______ WR / CV / WR / S fistula
5. inflammation of the umbilicus ______ WR / S

EXERCISE 22

Spell each of the Neonatology Disease and Disorder Terms Built from Word Parts by having someone dictate them to you. Use a separate sheet of paper.

To hear and spell the terms, go to Evolve Resources at evolve.elsevier.com and select: Practice Student Resources > Student Resources > Chapter 9 > **Pronounce and Spell**

See Appendix B for instructions.

❑ Check the box when complete.

Neonatology Disease and Disorder Terms

NOT BUILT FROM WORD PARTS

Word parts may be present in the following terms; however, their full meanings cannot be translated using definitions of word parts alone.

TERM	DEFINITION
cleft lip or palate (kleft) (lip) (PAL-at)	congenital split of the lip or roof of the mouth, one or both deformities may be present (*cleft* indicates a fissure) (Fig. 9.6)
Down syndrome (down) (SIN-drōm)	genetic condition caused by a chromosomal abnormality characterized by varying degrees of intellectual, developmental, and physical disorders or defects (there is an extra 21st chromosome; hence, it is also called **trisomy 21**) (Fig. 9.7)
erythroblastosis fetalis (e-*rith*-rō-blas-TŌ-sis) (fē-TAL-is)	condition of the newborn characterized by hemolysis of the erythrocytes. The condition is usually caused by incompatibility of the infant's and mother's blood, occurring when the mother's blood is Rh negative and the infant's blood is Rh positive.

BIRTHMARKS

are benign discolorations in the neonate's skin. Common birthmarks include: **congenital dermal melanocytosis**, which are bluish-black areas of hyperpigmentation often found on the lower back or buttocks of darker-skinned neonates and **hemangiomas**, which are various benign vascular tumors or stains that cause reddish discoloration and/or malformations of the skin surface. **Nevus flammeus**, also called port-wine stain, is common, often temporary, and is caused by the dilation of certain blood vessels.

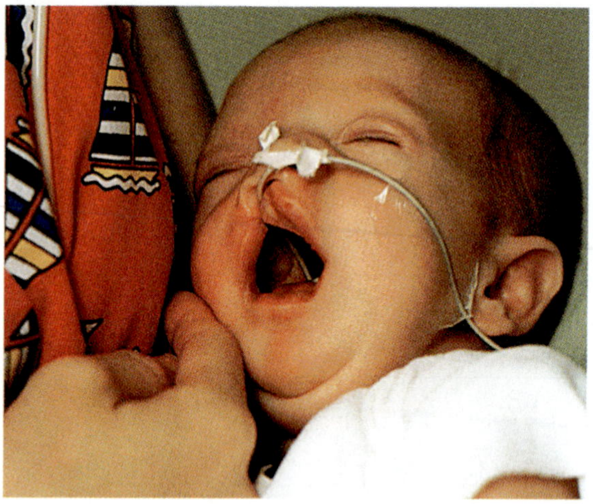

FIG. 9.6 Unilateral cleft lip. Note the nasogastric feeding tube in place. Neonates born with a cleft lip, palate, or both may require assistive feeding due to an impaired ability to suck.

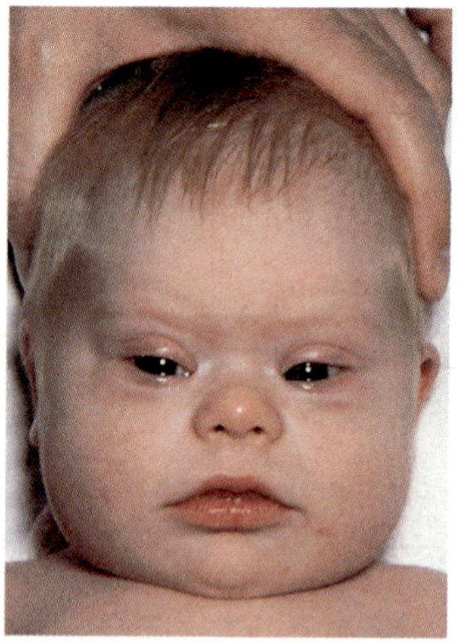

FIG. 9.7 Neonate with Down syndrome.

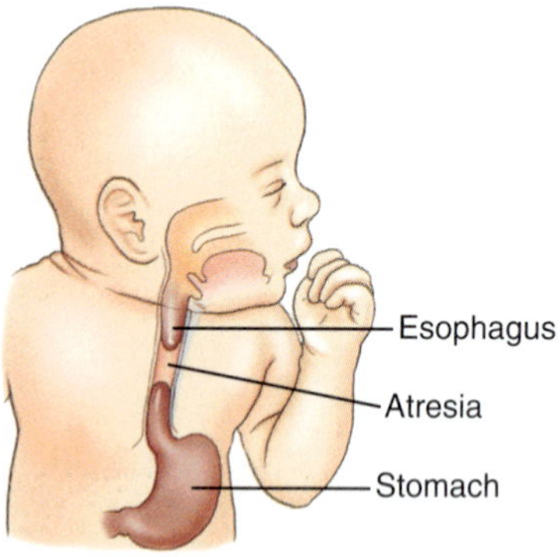

FIG. 9.8 Esophageal atresia.

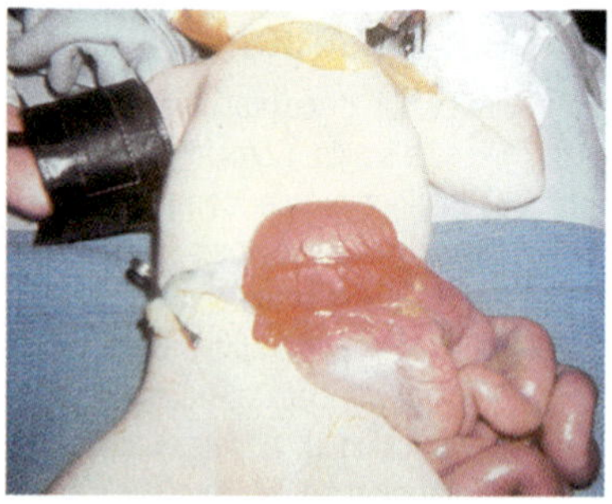

FIG. 9.9 Gastroschisis.

Neonatology Disease and Disorder Terms—cont'd

TERM	DEFINITION
esophageal atresia (e-*sof*-a-JĒ-al) (a-TRĒ-zha)	congenital absence of part of the esophagus. Food cannot pass from the baby's mouth to the stomach (Fig. 9.8).
fetal alcohol syndrome (FAS) (FĒ-tal) (AL-kō-hol) (SIN-drōm)	condition caused by excessive alcohol consumption by the mother during pregnancy. Various birth defects may be present, including central nervous system dysfunction and malformations of the skull and face.
gastroschisis (gas-TROS-ki-sis)	congenital fissure of the abdominal wall that is not at the umbilicus. Enterocele, protrusion of the intestine, is usually present (Fig. 9.9).
respiratory distress syndrome (RDS) (RES-pi-ra-*tōr*-ē) (di-STRESS) (SIN-drōm)	respiratory complication in the newborn, especially in premature infants. In premature infants RDS is caused by normal immaturity of the respiratory system resulting in compromised respiration (formerly called **hyaline membrane disease**).
spina bifida (SPĪ-na) (BIF-i-da)	congenital defect in the vertebral column caused by the failure of the vertebral arch to close. If the meninges protrude through the opening the condition is called meningocele. Protrusion of both the meninges and spinal cord is called meningomyelocele (Fig. 9.10).

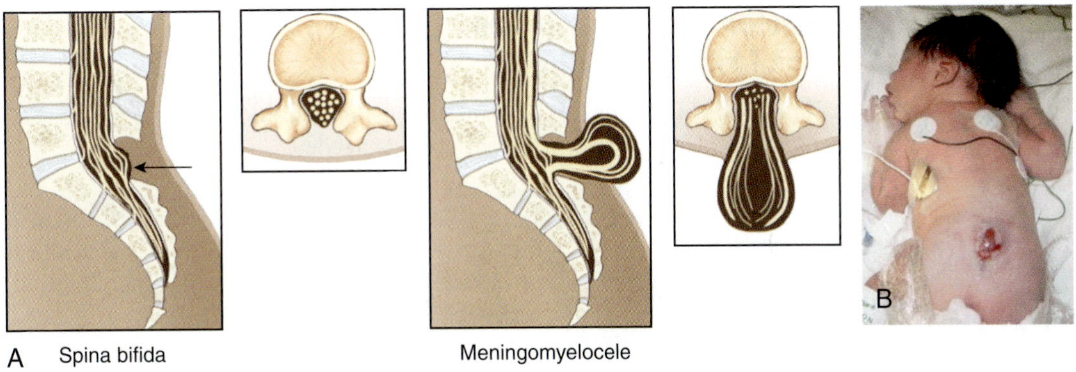

FIG. 9.10 A, Drawings of spina bifida and meningomyelocele. **B,** Photograph of meningomyelocele.

EXERCISE 23

Practice saying aloud each of the Neonatology Disease and Disorder Terms NOT Built from Word Parts.

> To hear the terms, go to Evolve Resources at evolve.elsevier.com and select:
> Practice Student Resources > Student Resources > Chapter 9 > **Pronounce and Spell**
>
> See Appendix B for instructions.

❑ Check the box when complete.

EXERCISE 24

Match the terms in the first column with their correct definitions in the second column.

_____ 1. Down syndrome	a. defect of the vertebral column
_____ 2. cleft lip or palate	b. respiratory complication of neonates
_____ 3. spina bifida	c. split of the lip or roof of the mouth
_____ 4. erythroblastosis fetalis	d. caused by incompatibility of the infant's and the mother's blood
_____ 5. fetal alcohol syndrome	e. congenital fissure of the abdominal wall
_____ 6. respiratory distress syndrome	f. genetic condition caused by chromosomal abnormality
_____ 7. esophageal atresia	g. congenital absence of part of the esophagus
_____ 8. gastroschisis	h. causes various birth defects, including central nervous system dysfunction

EXERCISE 25

Spell each of the Neonatology Disease and Disorder Terms NOT Built from Word Parts by having someone dictate them to you. Use a separate sheet of paper.

> To hear and spell the terms, go to Evolve Resources at evolve.elsevier.com and select:
> Practice Student Resources > Student Resources > Chapter 9 > **Pronounce and Spell**
>
> See Appendix B for instructions.

❑ Check the box when complete.

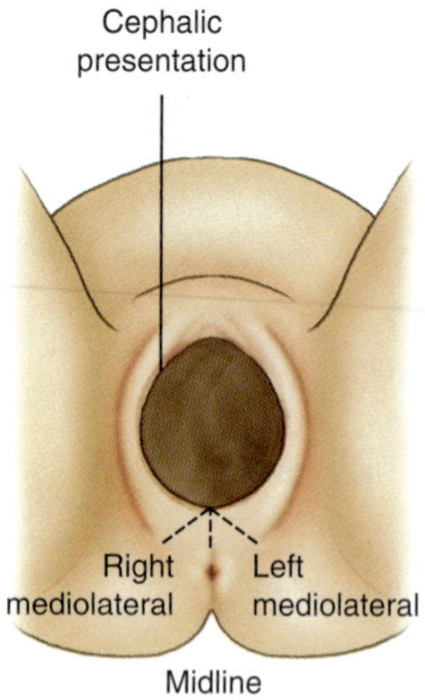

FIG. 9.11 Episiotomies.

CHORIONIC VILLUS SAMPLING (CVS)

is a prenatal test performed on a sample of chorionic villa removed from the placenta between 10 and 13 weeks of pregnancy. The sample is taken through the abdominal wall or the cervix. **Amniocentesis** is also a prenatal test performed after 15 weeks of pregnancy and the sample is taken by inserting a needle into the uterus through the abdominal wall. Both tests are used to diagnose genetic disorders such as cystic fibrosis and to assess fetal health.

Obstetric Surgical Terms

BUILT FROM WORD PARTS

The following terms can be translated using definitions of word parts. Further explanation is provided within parentheses as needed.

TERM	DEFINITION
amniotomy (*am*-nē-OT-o-mē)	incision into the amnion (rupture of the fetal membrane to induce labor; a special hook is generally used to make the incision)
episiotomy (e-*piz*-ē-OT-o-mē)	incision into the vulva (perineum) (sometimes performed during delivery to prevent a traumatic tear of the vulva) (also called **perineotomy**) (Fig. 9.11)

Obstetric Diagnostic Terms

BUILT FROM WORD PARTS

TERM	DEFINITION
DIAGNOSTIC IMAGING	
pelvic sonography (PEL-vik) (so-NOG-ra-fē)	pertaining to the pelvis, process of recording sound (pelvic ultrasound is used extensively to evaluate the fetus and pregnancy) (also called **pelvic ultrasonography, pelvic ultrasound,** and **obstetric ultrasonography**) (Fig. 9.12)
OTHER	
amniocentesis (*am*-nē-ō-sen-TĒ-sis)	surgical puncture to aspirate amniotic fluid (the needle is inserted through the abdominal and uterine walls, using ultrasound to guide the needle. It is a prenatal test in which the fluid is used for the assessment of fetal health and maturity to aid in diagnosing fetal abnormalities.) (Fig. 9.13).

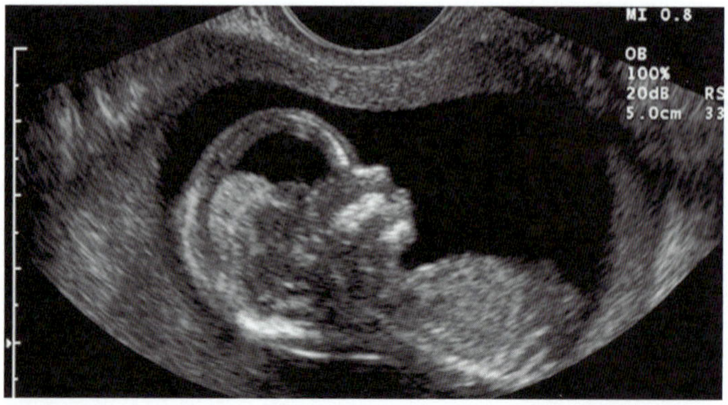

FIG. 9.12 Pelvic sonography image showing a fetal profile. Some specific uses are to: (1) diagnose early abnormal pregnancy, (2) determine the age of the fetus, (3) measure fetal growth, and (4) determine fetal position.

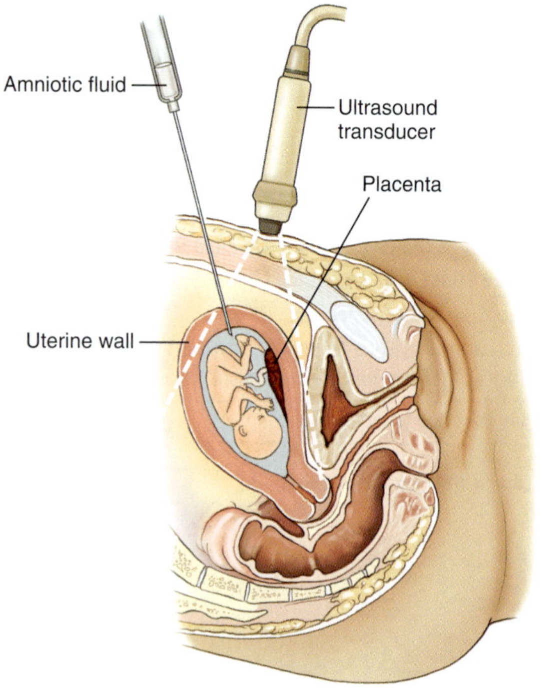

FIG. 9.13 Amniocentesis. Ultrasound is used to guide the needle through the abdominal and uterine walls.

EXERCISE 26

Practice saying aloud each of the Obstetric Surgical and Diagnostic Terms Built from Word Parts.

To hear the terms, go to Evolve Resources at evolve.elsevier.com and select:
Practice Student Resources > Student Resources > Chapter 9 > **Pronounce and Spell**

See Appendix B for instructions.

❑ Check the box when complete.

EXERCISE 27

Analyze and define the following obstetric surgical and diagnostic terms.

1. episiotomy

____

____

2. amniotomy

____

____

3. pelvic sonography

____

____

4. amniocentesis

____

____

EXERCISE 28

Build obstetric surgical and diagnostic terms for the following definitions by using the word parts you have learned.

1. incision into the amnion ______ / ______ / ______
   WR / CV / S

2. incision into the vulva ______ / ______ / ______
   WR / CV / S

3. surgical puncture to aspirate amniotic fluid ______ / ______ / ______
   WR / CV / S

4. pertaining to the pelvis, process of recording sound ______ / ______
   WR / S

   ______ / ______ / ______
   WR / CV / S

EXERCISE 29

Spell each of the Obstetric Surgical and Diagnostic Terms Built from Word Parts by having someone dictate them to you. Use a separate sheet of paper.

To hear and spell the terms, go to Evolve Resources at evolve.elsevier.com and select:
Practice Student Resources > Student Resources > Chapter 9 > **Pronounce and Spell**

See Appendix B for instructions.

❑ Check the box when complete.

Obstetric and Neonatal Complementary Terms
BUILT FROM WORD PARTS

The following terms can be translated using definitions of word parts. Further explanation is provided within parentheses as needed.

TERM	DEFINITION
amniochorial (*am*-nē-ō-KOR-ē-al)	pertaining to the amnion and chorion
amniorrhea (*am*-nē-ō-RĒ-a)	discharge (escape) of amniotic fluid
amniorrhexis (*am*-nē-ō-REK-sis)	rupture of the amnion
antepartum (*an*-tē-PAR-tum)	before childbirth (reference to the mother)
embryogenic (*em*-brē-ō-JEN-ik)	producing an embryo
embryoid (EM-brē-oyd)	resembling an embryo
fetal (FĒ-tal)	pertaining to the fetus
gravida (GRAV-i-da)	pregnant (woman); (a woman who is or has been pregnant, regardless of pregnancy outcome)
gravidopuerperal (*grav*-i-dō-pū-ER-per-al)	pertaining to pregnancy and childbirth (from delivery until reproductive organs return to normal)
intrapartum (*in*-tra-PAR-tum)	within (during) labor and childbirth
lactic (LAK-tik)	pertaining to milk
lactogenic (*lak*-tō-JEN-ik)	producing milk (by stimulation)
lactorrhea (*lak*-tō-RĒ-a)	(spontaneous) discharge of milk
multigravida (*mul*-ti-GRAV-i-da)	many pregnancies (a woman who has been pregnant two or more times)
multipara (multip) (mul-TIP-a-ra)	many births (a woman who has given birth to two or more viable offspring)
natal (NĀ-tal)	pertaining to birth
neonate (NĒ-ō-nāt)	new birth (an infant from birth to 4 weeks of age) (synonymous with **newborn [NB]**) (Exercise Figure B)

AN EXAMPLE OF USING GRAVIDA AND PARA IN MEDICAL SHORTHAND IN A CLINICAL SETTING

A 27 y/o **G4P2113** is a woman who has had **four** pregnancies, **two** term births, **one** preterm birth, **one** abortion, and has **three** living children.

TERM	DEFINITION
neonatologist (*nē*-ō-nā-TOL-o-jist)	physician who studies and treats disorders of the newborn
neonatology (*nē*-ō-nā-TOL-o-jē)	study of the newborn (branch of medicine that deals with diagnosis and treatment of disorders in newborns)
nulligravida (*nul*-li-GRAV-i-da)	no pregnancies (a woman who has never been pregnant)
nullipara (nu-LIP-a-ra)	no births (a woman who has not given birth to a viable offspring)
para (PAR-a)	birth (a woman who has given birth to an offspring after the point of viability—20 weeks, whether the fetus is alive or stillborn)
postnatal (pōst-NĀ-tal)	pertaining to after birth (reference to the newborn)
postpartum (pōst-PAR-tum)	after childbirth (reference to the mother)
prenatal (prē-NĀ-tal)	pertaining to before birth (reference to the newborn)
primigravida (prī-mi-GRAV-i-da)	first pregnancy (a woman in her first pregnancy)
primipara (primip) (*prī*-MIP-a-ra)	first birth (a woman who has given birth to an offspring after the point of viability—20 weeks)
pseudocyesis (*sū*-dō-sī-Ē-sis)	false pregnancy (a woman who believes she is pregnant—this may be a psychological condition or related to underlying pathology, such as a uterine tumor)
puerpera (pū-ER-per-a)	childbirth (a woman who has just given birth)
puerperal (pū-ER-per-al)	pertaining to (immediately after) childbirth
teratogen (TER-a-tō-jen)	(any agent) producing malformations (in the developing embryo). Teratogens include chemical agents such as drugs, alcohol, viruses, x-rays, and environmental factors.
teratogenic (*ter*-a-tō-JEN-ik)	producing malformations (in the developing embryo)
teratology (*ter*-a-TOL-o-jē)	study of malformations (usually in regard to malformations caused by teratogens on the developing embryo)

EXERCISE FIGURE B

Fill in the blanks to label the diagram.

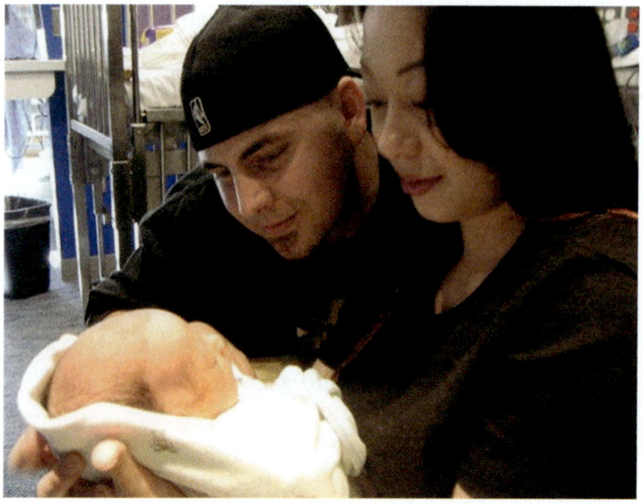

_____ / _____ / e
new / birth /

TABLE 9.1 Terms Relating to Mother and Newborn

	BEFORE BIRTH	AFTER BIRTH
Mother	antepartum	postpartum
Newborn	prenatal	postnatal

TABLE 9.2 Comparing Terms: Gravid/o and Par/o

GRAVID/O (PREGNANCY)	PAR/O (BIRTH)
nulli/gravid/a – no pregnancies	nulli/par/a – no births
primi/gravid/a – first pregnancy	primi/par/a – first birth
multi/gravid/a – many pregnancies	multi/par/a – many births

EXERCISE 30

Practice saying aloud each of the Complementary Terms Built from Word Parts.

> To hear the terms, go to Evolve Resources at evolve.elsevier.com and select:
> Practice Student Resources > Student Resources > Chapter 9 > **Pronounce and Spell**
>
> See Appendix B for instructions.

❑ Check the box when complete.

EXERCISE 31

Analyze and define the following obstetric and neonatal complementary terms.

1. puerpera

____

____

2. amniorrhexis

____

____

3. antepartum

4. pseudocyesis

5. prenatal

6. lactic

7. lactorrhea

8. amniorrhea

9. multipara

10. embryogenic

11. embryoid

12. fetal

13. gravida

14. amniochorial

15. multigravida

16. lactogenic

17. natal

18. gravidopuerperal

19. neonatology

20. nullipara

21. para

____

____

22. primigravida

____

____

23. postpartum

____

____

24. neonate

____

____

25. primipara

____

____

26. puerperal

____

____

27. nulligravida

____

____

28. intrapartum

____

____

29. teratogen

____

____

30. postnatal

____

____

31. teratology

____

____

32. neonatologist

____

____

33. teratogenic

____

____

EXERCISE 32

Build the complementary terms for the following definitions by using the word parts you have learned.

1. pertaining to the amnion and chorion ______ / ______ / ______ / ______
   WR / CV / WR / S

2. before childbirth (reference to the mother) ______ / ______ / ______
   P / WR / S

3. producing an embryo ______ / ______ / ______
   WR / CV / S

4. pertaining to the fetus ______ / ______
   WR / S

5. pertaining to before birth (reference to the newborn) ______ / ______ / ______ (P / WR / S)

6. pertaining to milk ______ / ______ (WR / S)

7. (spontaneous) discharge of milk ______ / ______ / ______ (WR / CV / S)

8. discharge (escape) of amniotic fluid ______ / ______ / ______ (WR / CV / S)

9. false pregnancy ______ / ______ / ______ (WR / CV / S)

10. producing milk (by stimulation) ______ / ______ / ______ (WR / CV / S)

11. rupture of the amnion ______ / ______ / ______ (WR / CV / S)

12. resembling an embryo ______ / ______ (WR / S)

13. pregnant (woman) ______ / ______ (WR / S)

14. pertaining to pregnancy and childbirth ______ / ______ / ______ / ______ (WR / CV / WR / S)

15. many births ______ / ______ / ______ (P / WR / S)

16. pertaining to birth ______ / ______ (WR / S)

17. new birth (an infant from birth to 4 weeks of age) ______ / ______ / ______ (P / WR / S)

18. study of the newborn ______ / ______ / ______ / ______ (P / WR / CV / S)

19. no births ______ / ______ / ______ (P / WR / S)

20. birth ______ / ______ (WR / S)

21. first pregnancy ______ / ______ / ______ / ______ (WR / CV / WR / S)

22. after childbirth (reference to the mother) ______ / ______ / ______ (P / WR / S)

23. first birth ________ / ____ / ________ / ________
WR / CV / WR / S

24. many pregnancies ________ / ________ / ________
P / WR / S

25. pertaining to (immediately after) childbirth ________ / ________
WR / S

26. no pregnancies ________ / ________ / ________
P / WR / S

27. (any agent) producing malformations ________ / ____ / ________
WR / CV / S

28. childbirth ________ / ________
WR / S

29. within (during) labor and childbirth ________ / ________ / ________
P / WR / S

30. producing malformations ________ / ____ / ________
WR / CV / S

31. physician who studies and treats disorders of the newborn ________ / ________ / ____ / ________
P / WR / CV / S

32. pertaining to after birth (reference to the newborn) ________ / ________ / ________
P / WR / S

33. study of malformations ________ / ____ / ________
WR / CV / S

EXERCISE 33

Spell each of the Complementary Terms Built from Word Parts by having someone dictate them to you. Use a separate sheet of paper.

> To hear and spell the terms, go to Evolve Resources at evolve.elsevier.com and select:
> Practice Student Resources > Student Resources > Chapter 9 > **Pronounce and Spell**
>
> See Appendix B for instructions.

❑ Check the box when complete.

Obstetric and Neonatal Complementary Terms

NOT BUILT FROM WORD PARTS

Word parts may be present in the following terms; however, their full meanings cannot be translated using definitions of word parts alone.

TERM	DEFINITION
Apgar score (AP-gar) (skor)	system for rapid neonatal assessment at 1 minute and 5 minutes after birth (Fig. 9.14)
breech presentation (brēch) (prē-zen-TĀ-shun)	birth position in which the buttocks, feet, or knees emerge first (Fig. 9.15A)
cephalic presentation (se-FAL-ik) (prē-zen-TĀ-shun)	birth position in which any part of the head emerges first. It is the most common presentation (Fig. 9.15B).
cesarean section (CS, C-section) (se-ZĀR-ē-an) (SEK-shun)	birth of a fetus through an incision in the mother's abdomen and uterus (may also be spelled **caesarean**)
colostrum (ke-LOS-trem)	thin, milky fluid secreted by the breast during pregnancy and during the first days after birth before lactation begins
congenital anomaly (kon-JEN-i-tal) (a-NOM-a-lē)	abnormality present at birth; often discovered before birth by sonography and/or amniocentesis
in vitro fertilization (IVF) (in) (VĒ-trō) (*fer*-ti-li-ZĀ-shun)	method of fertilizing human ova outside the body and placing the zygote into the uterus; used when infertility is present. Infertility management techniques that artificially combine both the ova and the sperm are called **assisted reproductive technology (ART).** (Fig. 9.16)
lactation (lak-TĀ-shun)	secretion of milk
lochia (LŌ-kē-a)	vaginal discharge after childbirth

CESAREAN SECTION (C-SECTION)

The origin of this term has no relation to the birth of Julius Caesar, as is commonly believed. One suggested etymology is that from 715 to 672 BC it was Roman law that the operation be performed on dying women in the last few months of pregnancy in the hope of saving the child. At that time the operation was called a **caeso matris utero**, which means **the cutting of the mother's uterus**.

SIGN	SCORE 0	SCORE 1	SCORE 2
Heart rate	Absent	Below 100	Over 100
Respiratory effort	Absent	Slow, irregular	Good, crying
Muscle tone	Limp	Some flexion of extremities	Active motion
Response to catheter in nostril (tested after oropharynx is clear)	No response	Grimace	Cough or sneeze
Color	Blue, pale	Body pink, extremities blue	Completely pink

FIG. 9.14 Apgar score. Developed in 1952 by Virginia Apgar, MD, the Apgar score provides a basic framework for rapid neonatal assessment by health care providers at 1 minute and 5 minutes after birth. Five vital criteria (**heartrate, respiration, muscle tone, response to stimulation**, and **color**) are assessed and scored on a 0-2 scale. The score is totaled, with a 5-minute Apgar score of 7 to 10 considered normal. The Apgar score is used only for quickly reporting a neonate's status and does not predict future health outcomes.

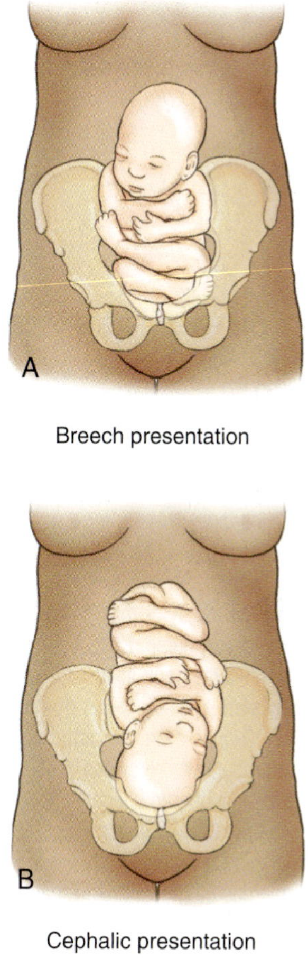

FIG. 9.15 A, Breech presentation. **B,** Cephalic presentation.

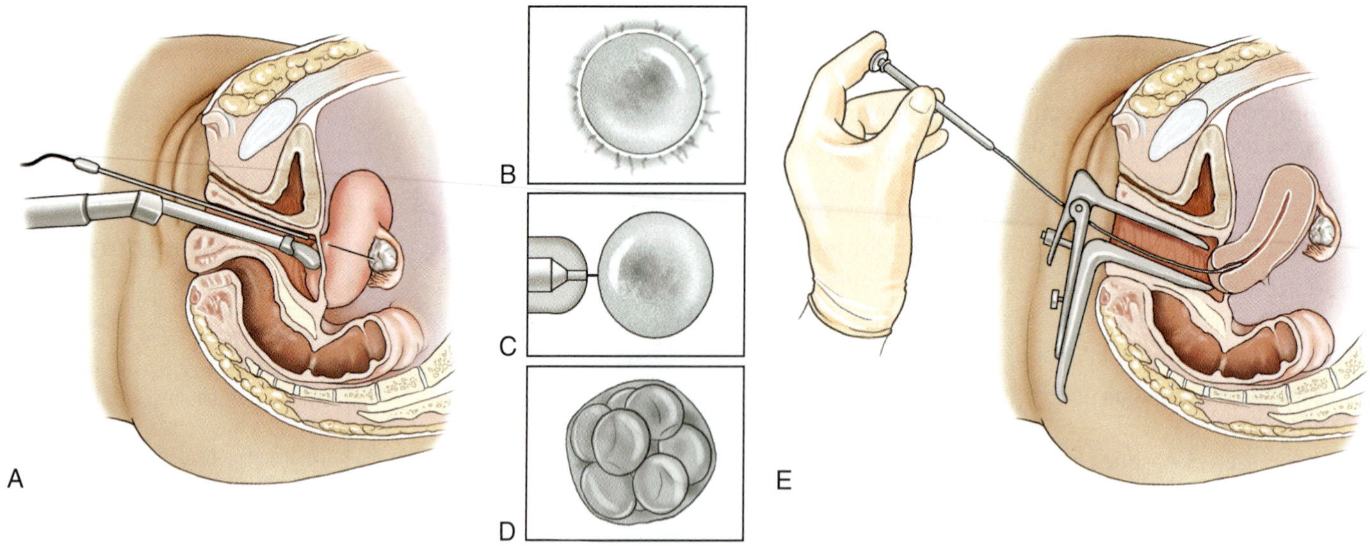

FIG. 9.16 In vitro fertilization (IVF). After ovarian stimulation, ova are retrieved from the ovary by ultrasound-guided transvaginal needle aspiration **(A).** The ova are fertilized outside the body in a dish with spermatozoa obtained from semen **(B).** A technique using a single sperm called intracytoplasmic sperm injection may also be used **(C).** After 48 hours the fertilized ova (zygotes) **(D)** are injected into the uterus for implantation **(E).** The first pregnancy after in vitro fertilization was reported more than 3 decades ago. Since then **assisted reproductive technology (ART)** has achieved hundreds of thousands of pregnancies worldwide.

Obstetric and Neonatal Complementary Terms—cont'd

TERM	DEFINITION
meconium (me-KŌ-nē-um)	first stool of the newborn (greenish-black)
midwife (MID-wīf)	individual who practices midwifery
midwifery (MID-wif-rē)	practice of assisting in childbirth
obstetrician (*ob*-ste-TRISH-an)	physician who specializes in obstetrics
obstetrics (OB) (ob-STET-riks)	medical specialty dealing with pregnancy, childbirth, and puerperium
parturition (*par*-tū-RISH-un)	act of giving birth
premature infant (PRĒ-ma-tur) (IN-fent)	infant born before completing 37 weeks of gestation (also called **preterm infant**)
puerperium (*pū*-er-PĒ-rē-um)	period from delivery until the reproductive organs return to normal (approximately 6 weeks)
quickening (KWIK-en-ing)	first feeling of movement of the fetus in utero by the pregnant woman. It usually occurs between 16 and 20 weeks of gestation.
stillborn (STIL-born)	born dead (death of fetus after 20 weeks of pregnancy)

COMPARE MIDWIFE & DOULA

Midwives practice midwifery, supervise pregnancy, labor, delivery, and puerperium. They assist with delivery independently, care for the newborn, and obtain medical assistance as necessary. A **midwife** may or may not be a registered nurse. Education, certification, and licensure vary by state and country. A **doula** (DOO-la) is a trained birth attendant who provides continual physical and emotional support to the laboring woman. **Doulas** provide a complementary role to the obstetric health care team.

Refer to **Appendix F** for pharmacology terms related to obstetrics and neonatology.

EXERCISE 34

Practice saying aloud each of the Complementary Terms NOT Built from Word Parts.

To hear the terms, go to Evolve Resources at evolve.elsevier.com and select:
Practice Student Resources > Student Resources > Chapter 9 > **Pronounce and Spell**

See Appendix B for instructions.

❑ Check the box when complete.

EXERCISE 35

Match the definitions in the first column with the correct terms in the second column.

______	1. vaginal discharge after childbirth	a. lochia
______	2. medical specialty dealing with pregnancy and childbirth	b. obstetrician
______	3. abnormality present at birth	c. premature infant
______	4. period after delivery, lasts approximately 6 weeks	d. meconium
______	5. giving birth	e. obstetrics
______	6. physician specializing in obstetrics	f. parturition
______	7. birth position with buttocks, feet, or knees first	g. puerperium
______	8. first stool	h. cesarean section
______	9. born before completing 37 weeks of gestation	i. congenital anomaly
______	10. birth through an abdominal and uterine incision	j. breech presentation

EXERCISE 36

Match the definitions in the first column with the correct terms in the second column

______	1. assisting in childbirth	a. quickening
______	2. one who assists in childbirth	b. lactation
______	3. secretion of milk	c. cephalic presentation
______	4. birth position with the head first	d. colostrum
______	5. neonatal assessment	e. midwife
______	6. born dead	f. stillborn
______	7. first feeling of movement of the fetus	g. in vitro fertilization
______	8. secreted before lactation	h. midwifery
______	9. method of fertilizing ova outside the body	i. Apgar score

EXERCISE 37

Write the definitions of the following terms.

1. meconium ______________________________
2. obstetrics ______________________________
3. premature infant ______________________________
4. lochia ______________________________
5. puerperium ______________________________
6. parturition ______________________________
7. obstetrician ______________________________

8. congenital anomaly ______________________________
9. breech presentation ______________________________
10. cesarean section ______________________________
11. quickening ______________________________
12. lactation ______________________________
13. cephalic presentation ______________________________
14. colostrum ______________________________
15. midwife ______________________________
16. stillborn ______________________________
17. midwifery ______________________________
18. in vitro fertilization ______________________________
19. Apgar score ______________________________

EXERCISE 38

Spell each of the Complementary Terms NOT Built from Word Parts by having someone dictate them to you. Use a separate sheet of paper.

To hear and spell the terms, go to Evolve Resources at evolve.elsevier.com and select:
Practice Student Resources > Student Resources > Chapter 9 > **Pronounce and Spell**

See Appendix B for instructions.

❑ Check the box when complete.

WEB LINK

For more information about obstetrics, visit The American College of Obstetricians and Gynecologists at ***www.acog.org***. Additional information regarding assistive reproductive technology (ART) can be found at the *Centers for Disease Control and Prevention* website at ***www.cdc.gov/ART***.

Abbreviations

ABBREVIATION	TERM
AB	abortion
CS, C-section	cesarean section
CVS	chorionic villus sampling
DOB	date of birth
EDD	expected (estimated) date of delivery
FAS	fetal alcohol syndrome
IVF	in vitro fertilization
LMP	last menstrual period
multip	multipara
NB	newborn
OB	obstetrics
primip	primipara
RDS	respiratory distress syndrome
VBAC	vaginal birth after cesarean section

Refer to **Appendix E** for a complete list of abbreviations.

EXERCISE 39

Write the medical term abbreviated.

1. OB ____________________
2. EDD ____________________
3. LMP ____________________
4. DOB ____________________
5. NB ____________________
6. multip ____________________
7. CS, C-section ____________________
8. VBAC ____________________
9. RDS ____________________
10. primip ____________________
11. FAS ____________________
12. IVF ____________________
13. AB ____________________
14. CVS ____________________

For additional practice with Abbreviations, go to Evolve Resources at evolve.elsevier.com and select: Practice Student Resources > Student Resources > Chapter 9 > **Flashcards:** Abbreviations

See Appendix B for instructions.

PRACTICAL APPLICATION

EXERCISE 40 *Case Study: Translate Between Everyday Language and Medical Language*

CASE STUDY: Charlene Birch

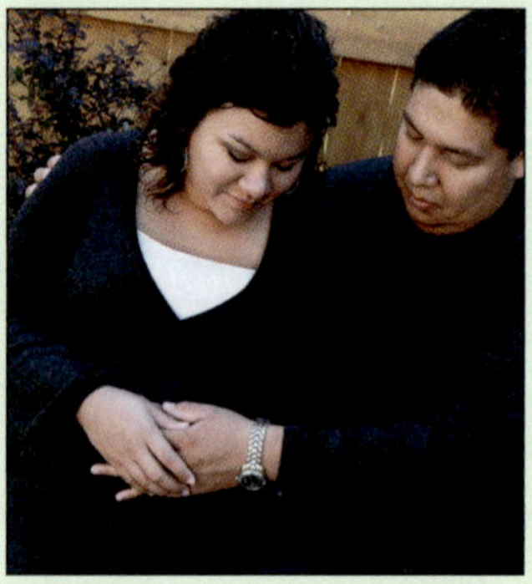

Charlene Birch is pregnant for the third time. She gave birth to one healthy baby about 4 years ago. The other baby was born dead when she was about 7 months into her pregnancy. Now she is about 3 months pregnant. She had an ultrasound test done when she first found out she was pregnant. This week she had some blood tests done and the doctor told her that the results suggest that her developing baby may have a genetic condition that causes physical and mental problems. He is suggesting a test where they use a needle to take fluid out of her womb and look at it under a microscope. She and her husband are very concerned and are not sure what to do.

Now that you have worked through Chapter 9 on obstetrics and neonatology, consider the medical terms that might be used to describe Charlene's experience. See the Review of Terms at the end of the chapter for a list of terms that might apply.

A. *Underline phrases in the case study that could be substituted with medical terms presented in Chapter 9 and previous chapters.*

B. *Write the medical term and its definition for three of the phrases you underlined.*

MEDICAL TERM	DEFINITION
1. ______________	______________
2. ______________	______________
3. ______________	______________

DOCUMENTATION: Excerpt From the Obstetrics Clinic Visit

Charlene is a 37-year-old gravida 3 para 2 female with an EDD of January 15, 20xx. Her prenatal history has been unremarkable up to this point. Recently, however, her prenatal screening tests came back suspicious for Down syndrome. I have recommended an amniocentesis to confirm this diagnosis. She is aware of the risks of the procedure, including the small possibility of spontaneous abortion. I have recommended that she have a very close follow up. We will attempt to detect any conditions including cardiac congenital anomalies or gastrointestinal malformation such as tracheoesophageal fistula. We will plan to have a neonatologist present at the time of birth.

C. *Underline medical terms presented in Chapter 9 used in the previous excerpt from Charlene's medical record. See the Review of Terms at the end of the chapter for a complete list.*

D. *Select and define three of the medical terms you underlined. To check your answers, go to Appendix A.*

MEDICAL TERM	DEFINITION
1. ______________	______________
2. ______________	______________
______________	______________

EXERCISE 41 *Interact With Medical Documents and Electronic Health Records*

A. Read the report and complete it by writing medical terms on answer lines within the document. Definitions of terms to be written appear after the document.

17432-OBN CISNEROS, Gloria

File Patient Navigate Custom Fields Help

Chart Review | Encounters | Notes | Labs | Imaging | Procedures | Rx | Documents | Referrals | Scheduling | Billing

Name: **CISNEROS, Gloria** MR#: 17432-OBN DOB: 08/26/19XX Gender: F Age: 24 **Allergies:** Penicillin **PCP:** Cynthia Bracken MD

History: Gloria Cisneros is a 24-year-old married 1. ____________________ 2 and 2. ____________________ 1 (abbreviated as G2P1) who is here today with her husband. Her 3. ____________________ is 1 week from today. She has received 4. ____________________ care here at the Medical Center Obstetrics Clinic since her second month of pregnancy. This pregnancy has been uncomplicated with no spotting, albuminuria, hypertension, edema, or glycosuria. Patient has attended Lamaze classes with her husband.

Physical exam: Her breasts are enlarged. She has gained 2 pounds since her last visit and she has gained 25 pounds throughout her pregnancy. Her current weight is 164 pounds. Her cervix is 1 cm dilated. Routine 5. ________________________ reveals a single fetus low in the pelvis in the 6. __________________.

Plan: Patient will return to clinic once a week until delivery.

Electronically signed: Heather Strom, MD 9/23/20XX 11:53

Start | Log On/Off | Print | Edit

LAMAZE

is a method of psychophysical preparation for childbirth started in the 1950s by a French obstetrician, Fernand Lamaze. The method requires classes and practice before and coaching during labor and delivery.

Definitions of Medical Terms to Complete the Document

Write the medical terms defined on corresponding answer lines in the document.

1. pregnant (woman)
2. birth
3. abbreviation for expected delivery date
4. pertaining to before birth (reference to the newborn)
5. pertaining to the pelvis, process of recording sound
6. birth position in which any part of the head emerges first

EXERCISE 41 *Interact With Medical Documents and Electronic Health Records—cont'd*

B. Read the medical report and answer the questions below it.

053447 SMITH, EMMALINE

File Patient Navigate Custom Fields Help

Patient Chart | Lab | Rad | Notes | Documents | Rx | Scheduling | Images | Billing

Name: **SMITH, EMMALINE** MR#: **053447** Gender: **F** Allergies: **ASA, Phenergan**

DOB: **3/17/XX** Age: **32** PCP: **Joseph Plains, MD**

RADIOLOGY REPORT

DATE: 04/17/20XX

INDICATION: Lower abdominal pain

EXAMINATION: Pelvic sonography

HISTORY: Thirty-two-year-old primip with menstrual irregularity and abdominal pain. History of pelvic inflammatory disease and spontaneous abortion x1.

FINDINGS: Sagittal and transverse images reveal an extrauterine sac containing a fetus in the left uterine tube. Cystic mass (hematoma) is evident in the rectouterine pouch. No fetal heart activity is noted.

OPINION: Ectopic pregnancy, left uterine tube.

Electronically signed by: A.W. Tyat, MD 4/17/20XX 21:07

Start | Log On/Off | Print | Edit

Use the medical report above to answer the questions.

1. The patient has:
    a. been pregnant two or more times
    b. given birth to two or more viable offspring
    c. borne one viable offspring
    d. never been pregnant

2. **True** or **False** The patient has experienced one abortion.

3. **True** or **False** Radiographic images were used to determine the findings.

C. Complete the **three medical documents** within the electronic health record (EHR) on Evolve.

Topic: Cesarean Section
Documents: Operative Report, Ultrasound Report, Obstetrics Delivery Note

To complete the three medical records, go to Evolve Resources at evolve.elsevier.com and select:
Practice Student Resources > Student Resources > Chapter 9 > **Electronic Heath Records**

See Appendix B for instructions.

EXERCISE 42 *Pronounce Medical Terms in Use*

Practice pronunciation of terms by reading aloud the following paragraph. Use the phonetic spellings following medical terms from the chapter to assist with pronunciation. The script also contains medical terms not presented in the chapter. Treat them as information only or look for their meanings in a medical dictionary or a reliable online source.

Josephine Alcotts is a 34-year-old **gravida** (GRAV-i-da) 2 **para** (PAR-a) 1 woman. Her LMP was April 20, 20XX. The EDD is January 25, 20XX. The **obstetrician** (*ob*-ste-TRISH-an) prescribed folic acid to prevent **spina bifida** (SPĪ-na) (BIF-i-da). The patient's first pregnancy was complicated by **preeclampsia** (prē-ē-KLAMP-sē-a) and a **breech presentation** (brēch) (prē-zen-TĀ-shun), which required a **cesarean section** (se-ZĀR-ē-an) (SEK-shun). **Pelvic sonography** (PEL-vik) (so-NOG-ra-fē) showed a single female fetus with normal development. She went on to deliver a healthy baby by VBAC 3 days before her expected delivery date.

EXERCISE 43 *Chapter Content Quiz*

Test your understanding of terms and abbreviations introduced in this chapter. Circle the letter for the medical term, definition, or abbreviation related to the words in italics.

1. During the second trimester the patient had a pelvic sonogram, which revealed *less than expected amniotic fluid*. Etiology may be related to disorders of fetal urinary system.
   a. chorioamnionitis
   b. oligohydramnios
   c. polyhydramnios
2. Because of inadequate uterine contractions, the patient was experiencing *difficult labor*.
   a. dysphasia
   b. dystocia
   c. dysuria
3. Down syndrome can be diagnosed by two prenatal tests: chorionic villus sampling done at 10-13 weeks of pregnancy, or a *surgical puncture to aspirate amniotic fluid* after 15 weeks of pregnancy.
   a. amniocentesis
   b. CVS
   c. amniorrhea
4. Infection of the Zika virus during pregnancy is linked to an increase in premature births, blindness, neurological disorders, and *small heads* in newborns.
   a. microcephalus
   b. omphalocele
   c. gastroschisis
5. *Antepartum* hemorrhage is considered an emergency.
   a. during labor
   b. after childbirth
   c. before childbirth
6. In the EHR, the medical assistant recorded that the patient *has never been pregnant*.
   a. nullipara
   b. nulligravida
   c. prenatal

7. At 20 weeks of gestation the patient was diagnosed with preeclampsia. The *disease progressed and she began having convulsions.* She was then diagnosed as having:
   a. eclampsia
   b. abruptio placentae
   c. placenta previa
8. The premature newborn was diagnosed with *RDS.*
   a. respiratory distress symptom
   b. right dominate syndrome
   c. respiratory distress syndrome
9. The mother was experiencing *vaginal discharge* throughout her postpartum period.
   a. lactation
   b. lochia
   c. meconium
10. The drug thalidomide taken by the mother was a *producing malformation* risk for the fetus.
    a. lactogenic
    b. teratogenic
    c. embryogenic
11. After a complete infertility evaluation, the physician recommended *IVF* for the couple.
    a. in vivo fertilization
    b. in vitro fertilization
    c. in vitro fetus
12. The patient was *pregnant with her third child.* She was referred to as:
    a. multigravida
    b. multipara
    c. nullipara

CHAPTER REVIEW

REVIEW OF CHAPTER CONTENT ON EVOLVE RESOURCES

Go to evolve.elsevier.com and click on Gradable Student Resources and Practice Student Resources. Online learning activities found there can be used to review chapter content and to assess your learning of word parts, medical terms, and abbreviations. Place check marks in the boxes next to activities used for review and assessment.

GRADABLE STUDENT RESOURCES

Chapter 09 >	Exercises >	☐ Word Parts ☐ Terms Built from Word Parts ☐ Terms Not Built from Word Parts ☐ Abbreviations
	Quizzes >	☐ Quiz 1: Disease and Disorder Terms ☐ Quiz 2: Complementary Terms

PRACTICE STUDENT RESOURCES > STUDENT RESOURCES

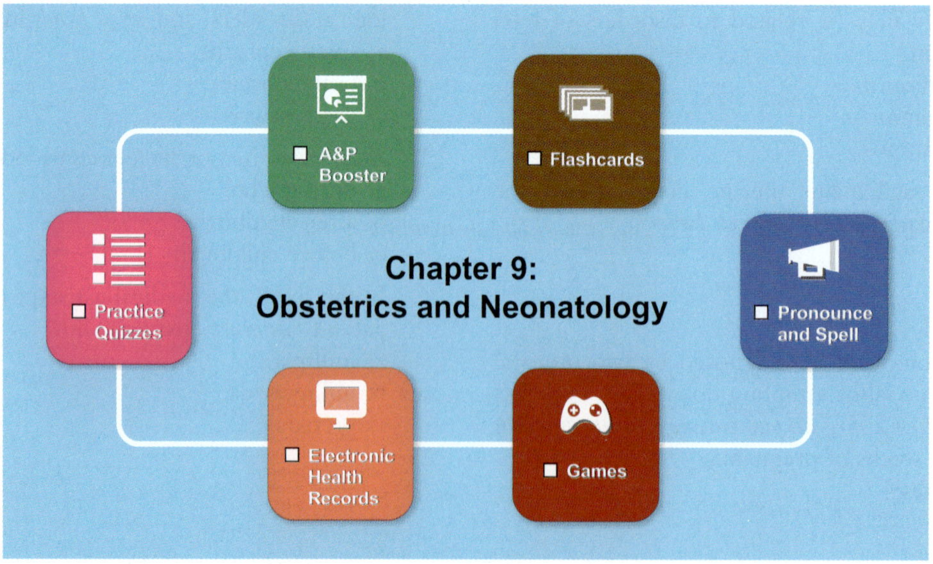

REVIEW OF WORD PARTS

Can you define and spell the following word parts?

COMBINING FORMS			PREFIXES	SUFFIXES
amni/o	fet/o	prim/i	ante-	-amnios
amnion/o	gravid/o	pseud/o	micro-	-cyesis
cephal/o	lact/o	puerper/o	multi-	-e
chori/o	nat/o	pylor/o	nulli-	-is
embry/o	omphal/o	terat/o	post-	-rrhexis
esophag/o	par/o		pre-	-tocia
fet/i	part/o			-um
				-us

REVIEW OF TERMS

Can you build, analyze, define, pronounce, and spell the following terms *built from word parts*?

DISEASES AND DISORDERS (OBSTETRICS)	DISEASES AND DISORDERS (NEONATOLOGY)	SURGICAL (OBSTETRICS)	DIAGNOSTIC (OBSTETRICS)	COMPLEMENTARY (OBSTETRICS AND NEONATOLOGY)	
amnionitis	microcephalus	amniotomy	amniocentesis	amniochorial	multigravida
chorioamnionitis	omphalitis	episiotomy	pelvic sonography	amniorrhea	multipara (multip)
choriocarcinoma	omphalocele			amniorrhexis	natal
dystocia	pyloric stenosis			antepartum	neonate
hysterorrhexis	tracheoesophageal fistula			embryogenic	neonatologist
oligohydramnios				embryoid	neonatology
polyhydramnios				fetal	nulligravida
				gravida	nullipara
				gravidopuerperal	para
				intrapartum	postnatal
				lactic	postpartum
				lactogenic	prenatal
				lactorrhea	primigravida
					primipara (primip)
					pseudocyesis
					puerpera
					puerperal
					teratogen
					teratogenic
					teratology

Can you define, pronounce, and spell the following terms *NOT built from word parts?*

DISEASES AND DISORDERS (OBSTETRICS)	DISEASES AND DISORDERS (NEONATOLOGY)	COMPLEMENTARY (OBSTETRICS AND NEONATOLOGY)	
abortion (AB)	cleft lip or palate	Apgar score	midwife
abruptio placentae	Down syndrome	breech presentation	midwifery
eclampsia	erythroblastosis fetalis	cephalic presentation	obstetrician
ectopic pregnancy	esophageal atresia	cesarean section (CS, C-section)	obstetrics (OB)
placenta previa	fetal alcohol syndrome (FAS)	colostrum	parturition
preeclampsia	gastroschisis	congenital anomaly	premature infant
	respiratory distress syndrome (RDS)	in vitro fertilization (IVF)	puerperium
	spina bifida	lactation	quickening
		lochia	stillborn
		meconium	

Chapter 10

Cardiovascular, Immune, Lymphatic Systems and Blood

Objectives

Upon completion of this chapter you will be able to:

1. Pronounce organs and anatomic structures.
2. Define and spell word parts.
3. Define, pronounce, and spell disease and disorder terms related to the cardiovascular and lymphatic systems and blood.
4. Define, pronounce, and spell surgical terms related to the cardiovascular and lymphatic systems and blood.
5. Define, pronounce, and spell diagnostic terms related to the cardiovascular system and blood.
6. Define, pronounce, and spell complementary terms related to the cardiovascular and immune systems and blood.
7. Interpret the meaning of abbreviations presented in the chapter.
8. Apply medical language in clinical contexts.

Outline

ANATOMY

At first glance this may seem like an overabundance of material in one chapter. It is a lot to cover, but as you will see **the systems have interactive functions**. The lymphatic and immune systems support each other by providing an immune response to invading microorganisms and foreign substances. The lymphatic system and blood share macrophages and lymphocytes. Lymph is drained into large veins of the cardiovascular system, and the cardiovascular system is responsible for circulating blood throughout the body.

Cardiovascular System

The cardiovascular system consists of the heart and a closed network of blood vessels composed of arteries, capillaries, and veins (Fig. 10.1).

FUNCTION

The heart functions as two pumps operating simultaneously. The right side of the heart pumps blood to the lungs while the left side pumps blood to the rest of the body. The exchange of gases, nutrients, and waste between the blood and body tissue takes place in the capillaries. The blood with carbon dioxide and waste is carried from the tissues through veins to organs of excretion. The cardiovascular system also serves a critical role in the body's ability to regulate temperature.

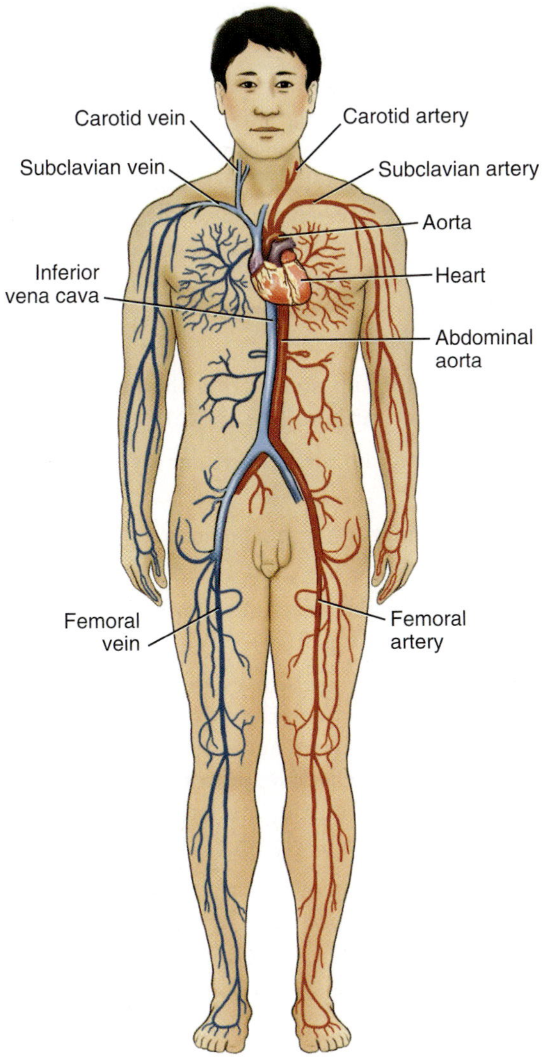

FIG. 10.1 Cardiovascular system.

Organs and Anatomic Structures of the Cardiovascular System

TERM	DEFINITION
heart (hart)	muscular cone-shaped organ the size of a fist, located behind the sternum (breast bone) and between the lungs. The pumping action of the heart circulates blood throughout the body (Fig. 10.2). The heart consists of two smaller upper chambers, the **right atrium** and the **left atrium** (pl. **atria**), and two larger lower chambers, the **right ventricle** and the **left ventricle** (pl. **ventricles**). The right atrium receives blood returning from the body through the veins and contracts to fill the right ventricle, which then pumps blood to the lungs. The left atrium receives blood from the lungs and contracts to fill the left ventricle, which then contracts to pump blood from the heart through the arteries to body tissues. The **atrial septum** separates the atria and the **ventricular septum** separates the ventricles.
atrioventricular valves (*ā*-trē-ō-ven-TRIK-ū-ler) (valvz)	consist of the **tricuspid** and **mitral** valves, which lie between the right atrium and the right ventricle and the left atrium and left ventricle, respectively. Valves of the heart keep blood flowing in one direction.
semilunar valves (*sem*-ē-LOO-ner) (valvz)	**pulmonary** and **aortic** valves located between the right ventricle and the pulmonary artery and between the left ventricle and the aorta, respectively.
pericardium (*per*-i-KAR-dē-um)	two-layer sac surrounding the heart, consisting of an external fibrous and an internal serous layer. The internal serous layer is then divided into two parts: the outer layer, called the parietal pericardium, and the inner layer, called the epicardium. Between these is the pericardial space, which contains fluid produced by the serous layer that facilitates movement of the heart.
epicardium (*ep*-i-KAR-dē-um)	outer lining covering the heart; also part of the pericardium (see above)
myocardium (*my*-ō-KAR-dē-um)	middle, thick, muscular layer of the heart
endocardium (*en*-dō-KAR-dē-um)	inner lining of the heart
blood vessels (blud) (VES-els)	tubelike structures that carry blood throughout the body (Fig. 10.3)
arteries (AR-ter-ēz)	blood vessels that carry blood away from the heart. All arteries, with the exception of the pulmonary artery, carry oxygen and other nutrients from the heart to the body cells. The **pulmonary artery**, in contrast, carries carbon dioxide and other waste products from the heart to the lungs.

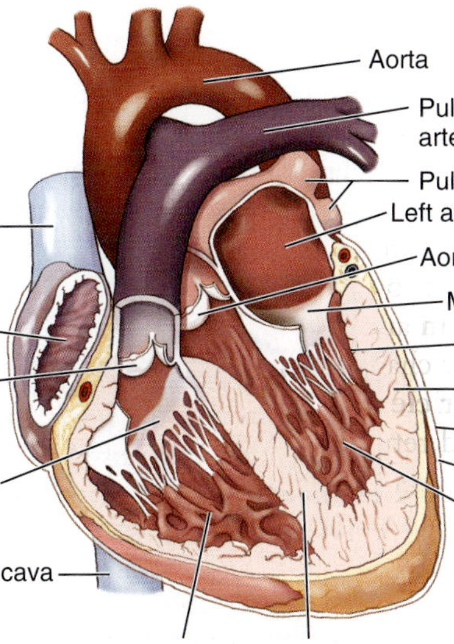

FIG. 10.2 Interior of the heart.

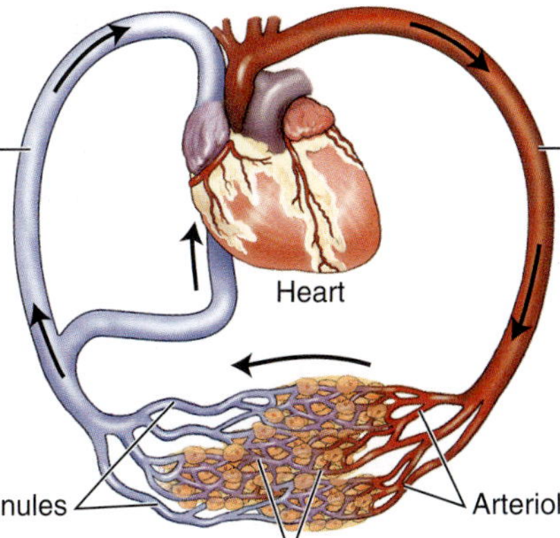

FIG. 10.3 Types of blood vessels.

TERM	DEFINITION
arterioles (ar-TĒR-ē-ōlz)	smallest arteries
aorta (ā-OR-ta)	largest artery in the body, which originates at the left ventricle, briefly ascends as the arch of the aorta, then descends through the thorax and abdomen
veins (vānz)	blood vessels that carry blood back to the heart. All veins, with the exception of the pulmonary veins, carry blood containing carbon dioxide and other waste products. The **pulmonary veins** carry oxygenated blood from the lungs to the heart.
venules (VEN-ūlz)	smallest veins
venae cavae (VĒ-nā) (KĀ-vā)	largest veins in the body. The **inferior vena cava** carries blood to the heart from body parts below the diaphragm, and the **superior vena cava** returns the blood to the heart from the upper part of the body.
capillaries (KAP-i-*lār*-ēz)	microscopic blood vessels that connect arterioles with venules. Materials are passed between the blood and tissue through the capillary walls.

Blood

FUNCTION

Activities of the blood include transportation of nutrients, waste, oxygen, carbon dioxide, and hormones; protection of the body against microorganisms; and regulation by controlling body temperature and maintaining fluid and electrolyte balance (Fig. 10.4 and Fig. 10.5).

Composition of Blood

TERM	DEFINITION
blood (blud)	fluid circulated through the heart, arteries, capillaries, and veins; composed of **plasma** and **formed elements**, such as erythrocytes, leukocytes, and thrombocytes (platelets)
plasma (PLAZ-ma)	clear, straw-colored, liquid portion of blood in which cells are suspended. Plasma is approximately 90% water. The other 10% is composed of solutes (dissolved substances), which include proteins, electrolytes, and vitamins. Plasma comprises approximately 55% of the total blood volume.
serum (SĒR-um)	clear, watery fluid portion of the blood that remains after a clot has formed
cells (formed elements)	
erythrocytes (e-RITH-rō-sītes)	red blood cells that carry oxygen. Erythrocytes develop in bone marrow.
leukocytes (LOO-kō-sītes)	white blood cells that combat infection and respond to inflammation. There are five types of white blood cells.
thrombocytes (THROM-bō-sītes)	one of the formed elements in the blood that is responsible for aiding in the clotting process (also called **platelets**)

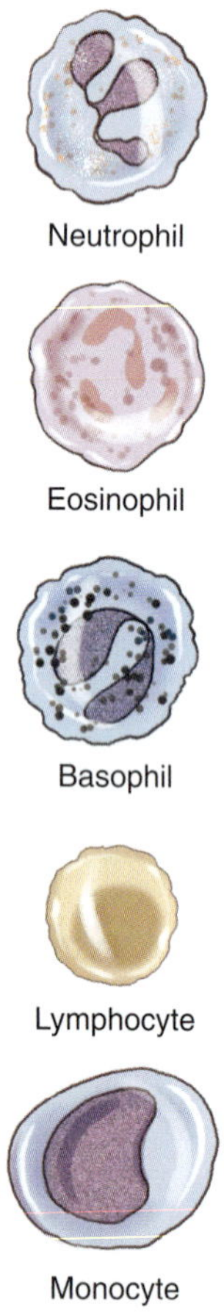

FIG. 10.4 Types of leukocytes. Each leukocyte plays a different role in providing immune responses to pathogens, foreign agents, allergies, and abnormal body cells.

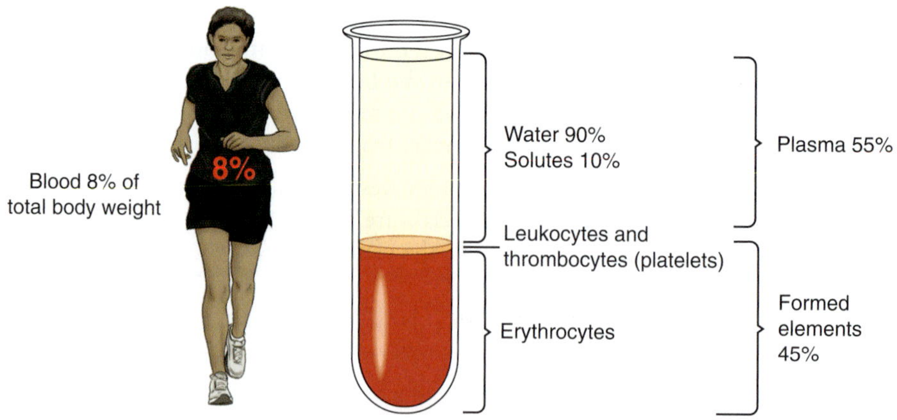

FIG. 10.5 Composition of blood.

Lymphatic System

The lymphatic system consists of lymph transported through lymphatic vessels, lymph nodes, the spleen, and thymus gland (Fig. 10.6).

FUNCTION

Three functions of the lymphatic system are to return excessive tissue fluid to the blood, absorb fats and fat-soluble vitamins from the small intestine and transport them to the blood, and provide defense against infections and other diseases. Collected extracellular fluid called lymph travels away from body tissue toward the heart and is drained into the cardiovascular system through ducts in the upper chest. Breathing and muscle action help propel lymph through the vessels.

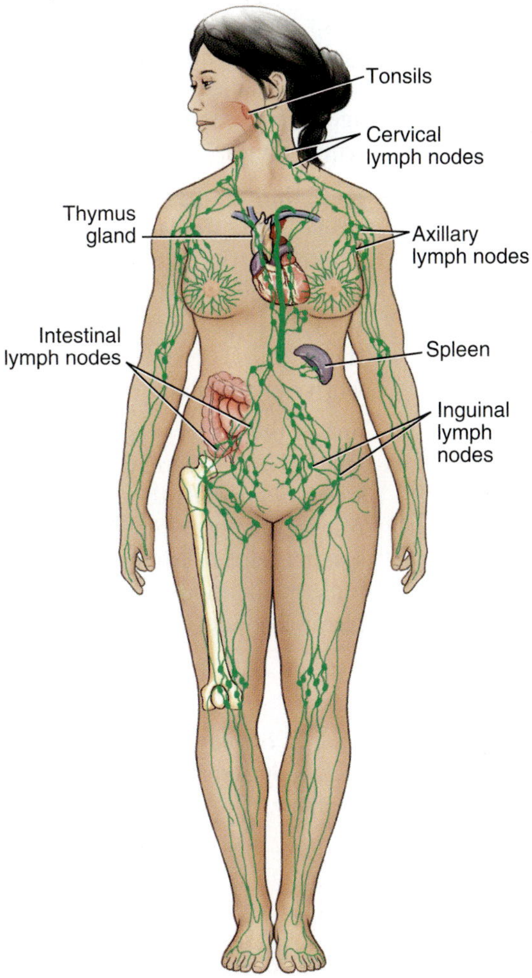

FIG. 10.6 Lymphatic system.

Organs and Anatomic Structures of the Lymphatic System

TERM	DEFINITION
lymph (limf)	transparent, colorless, tissue fluid; contains **lymphocytes** and **monocytes** and flows in a one-way direction to the heart
lymphatic vessels (lim-FAT-ik) (VES-els)	transport lymph from body tissues into the right and left subclavian veins, which then empty into the superior vena cava. The lymphatic vessels begin as capillaries spread throughout the body then merge into larger tubes that eventually become ducts in the chest. They provide a one-way flow for lymph, which enters through veins into the circulatory system.
lymph nodes (limf) (nōdz)	small, spherical bodies composed of lymphoid tissue. They may be singular or grouped together along the path of the lymph vessels. The nodes filter lymph to keep substances such as bacteria and other foreign agents from entering the blood. They also produce lymphocytes.
spleen (splēn)	located in the left side of the abdominal cavity between the stomach and the diaphragm. In adulthood, the spleen is the largest lymphatic organ in the body. Blood, rather than lymph, flows through the spleen. Blood is cleansed of microorganisms in the spleen. The spleen stores blood and destroys worn out red blood cells.
thymus gland (THĪ-mus) (gland)	one of the primary lymphatic organs, it is located anterior to the ascending aorta and posterior to the sternum between the lungs. It plays an important role in the development of the body's immune system, particularly from infancy to puberty. Around puberty the thymus gland shrinks so that most of the gland is connective tissue.

Immune System

The immune system does not have its own organs and structures. Its function depends on organs and structures of other body systems, including the spleen, liver, intestinal tract, lymph nodes, and bone marrow.

FUNCTION

The immune system protects the body against pathogens (disease-causing organisms such as bacteria, fungi, and viruses), foreign agents that cause allergic reactions (e.g., peanuts) or toxins (e.g., insect bites), and abnormal body cells (e.g., cancer). Immune function depends on three layers of protection, often referred to as lines of defense. (Fig. 10.7)

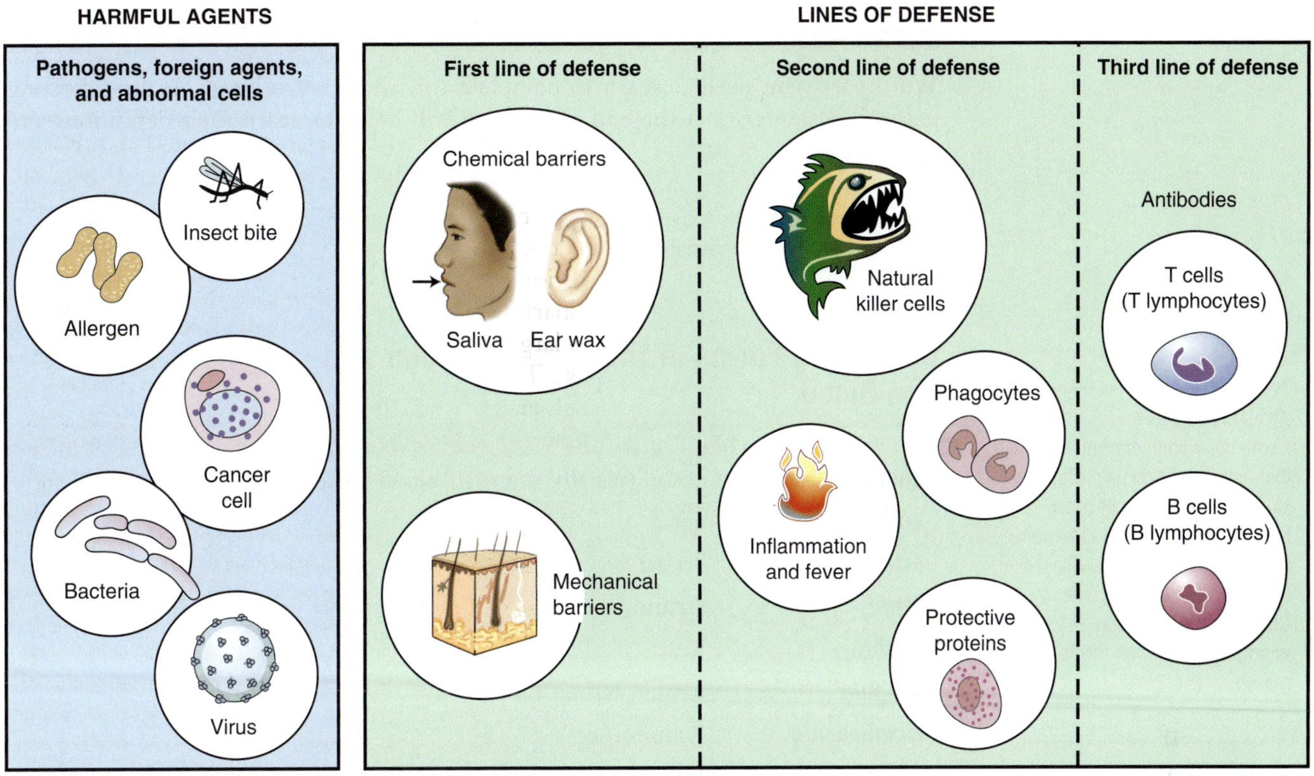

FIG. 10.7 Three lines of defense provided by the immune system to protect the body against pathogens, foreign agents, and cancer.

The first line of defense is the prevention of foreign substances from entering the body. Unbroken skin and mucous membranes act as mechanical barriers. Ear wax and saliva act as chemical barriers. If the first line of defense is penetrated by pathogens, a second line of defense continues to battle disease. Second-line defenses include inflammation and fever plus phagocytosis, a process in which some of the white blood cells destroy the invading microorganisms. Also activated are protective proteins such as interferons, which fight viruses, and natural killer (NK) cells, which are effective against microorganisms and cancer cells. Specific immunity, the third line of defense, provides protection against specific pathogens, such as the polio virus, by forming specific antibodies to fight against the infectious agent.

A&P Booster

For more anatomy and physiology, go to Evolve Resources at evolve.elsevier.com and select:
Practice Student Resources > Student Resources > Chapter 10 > **A&P Booster**

See Appendix B for instructions.

EXERCISE 1

Practice saying aloud each of the Organs and Anatomic Structures.

To hear the terms, go to Evolve Resources at evolve.elsevier.com and select:
Practice Student Resources > Student Resources > Chapter 10 > **Pronounce and Spell**

See Appendix B for instructions.

❑ Check the box when complete.

WORD PARTS

Word parts you need to learn to complete this chapter are listed on the following pages. The exercises at the end of each list will help you learn their definitions and spellings.

Use the flashcards accompanying this text or electronic flashcards to assist you in memorizing the word parts for this chapter.

VITAL AIR

It was believed in ancient times that **arteries** carried air. Vital air, or pneuma, did not allow blood in the arteries. A cut in an artery allowed vital air to escape and blood to replace it. The Greek **arteria**, meaning **windpipe**, was given for this reason.

VENTRICLE

is derived from the Latin **venter**, meaning **"little belly."** It was first applied to the belly and then to the stomach. Later it was extended to mean any small cavity in an organ or body. Modern clinical usage refers to the ventricles located in the heart or brain.

Combining Forms of the Cardiovascular and Lymphatic Systems and Blood

COMBINING FORM	DEFINITION
angi/o	vessel (usually refers to blood vessel)
aort/o	aorta
arteri/o	artery
atri/o	atrium
cardi/o	heart
lymph/o	lymph, lymph tissue
lymphaden/o	lymph node
myel/o	bone marrow *(Note: myel/o also means spinal cord; see Chapter 15)*
phleb/o, ven/o	vein
plasm/o	plasma
splen/o	spleen *(Note: Only one e in the word root for spleen)*
thym/o	thymus gland
valv/o, valvul/o	valve
ventricul/o	ventricle

lymphaden/o
When used in reference to the lymphatic system, the combining form lymphaden/o refers to a collection of lymphatic tissue and is called a lymph **node** rather than the literal translation of lymph gland.

EXERCISE 2

Fill in the blanks with combining forms in this diagram of a cutaway section of the heart. *To check your answers, go to Appendix A.*

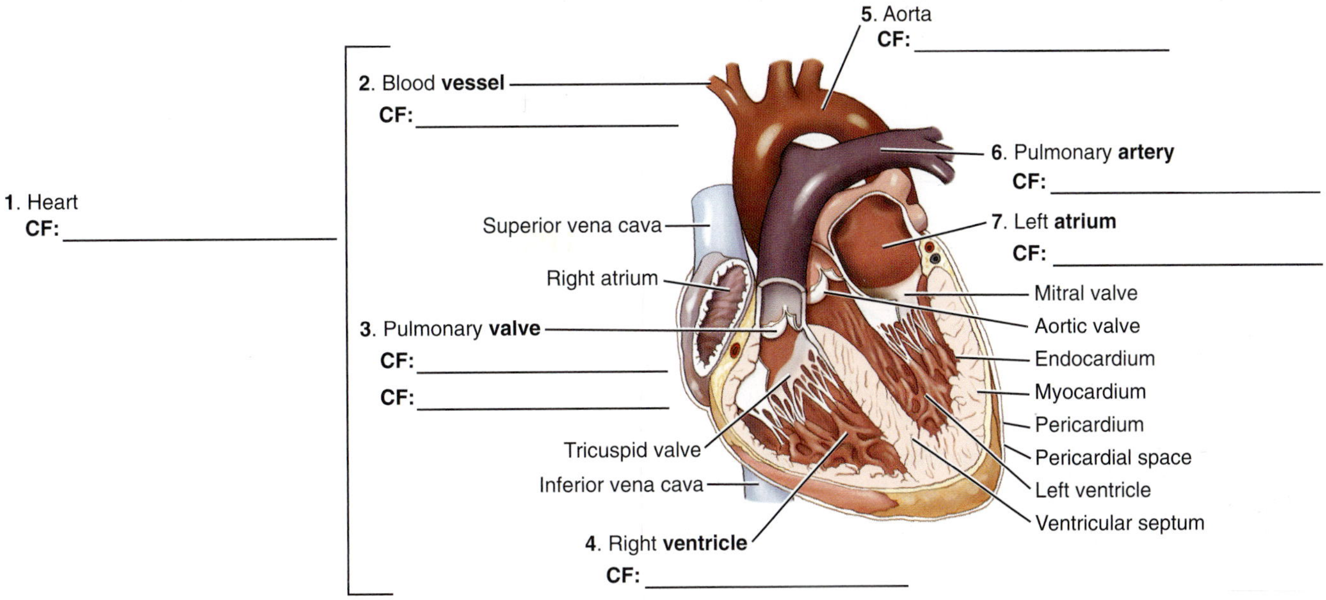

EXERCISE 3

Fill in the blanks with combining forms for the lymphatic system.

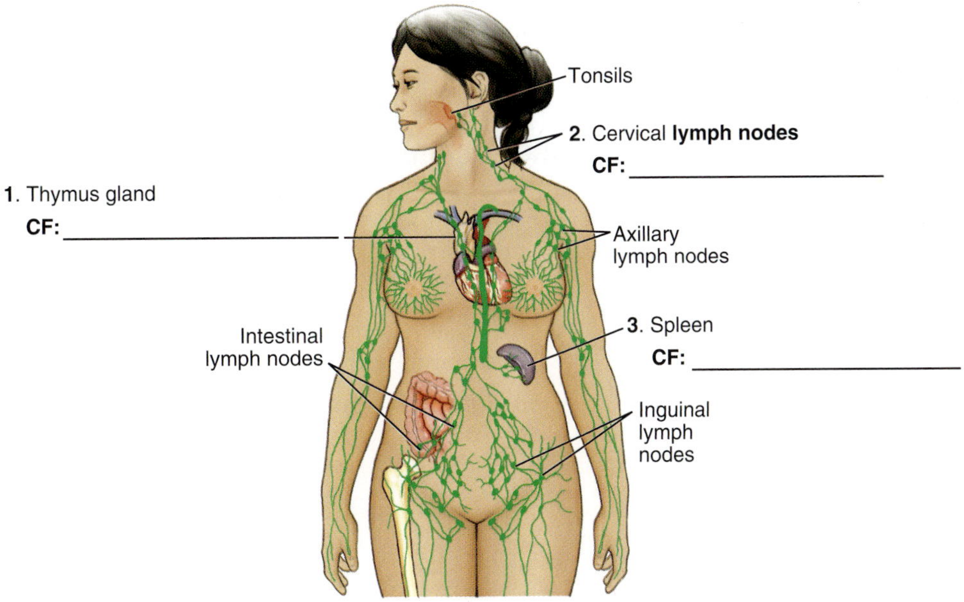

EXERCISE 4

Write the combining form(s) for each of the following terms.

1. vein a. ____________
   b. ____________
2. lymph, lymph tissue ____________
3. vessel (usually blood vessel) ____________
4. plasma ____________
5. bone marrow ____________

EXERCISE 5

Step 1: Write the definitions after the following combining forms.
Step 2: Match the descriptions on the right with the combining forms and definitions.

_____ 1. cardi/o, ______________________________
_____ 2. myel/o, ______________________________
_____ 3. valv/o, ______________________________
_____ 4. arteri/o, ______________________________
_____ 5. lymph/o, ______________________________
_____ 6. thym/o, ______________________________
_____ 7. ven/o, ______________________________

a. structures that keep blood flowing in one direction
b. transparent, colorless, tissue fluid
c. blood vessels that carry blood away from the heart
d. blood vessels that carry blood back to the heart
e. lymphatic organ important in the development of immunity
f. where erythrocytes develop
g. pumping action circulates blood throughout the body

EXERCISE 6

Step 1: Write the definitions after the following combining forms.
Step 2: Match the descriptions on the right with the combining forms and definitions.

_____ 1. lymphaden/o, ______________________________
_____ 2. aort/o, ______________________________
_____ 3. ventricul/o, ______________________________
_____ 4. phleb/o, ______________________________
_____ 5. angi/o, ______________________________
_____ 6. valvul/o, ______________________________
_____ 7. plasm/o, ______________________________
_____ 8. atri/o, ______________________________

a. small upper chamber in the heart
b. clear, straw-colored, liquid portion of blood
c. larger lower chamber in the heart
d. small, spherical bodies composed of lymphoid tissue
e. largest artery in the body
f. tubelike structures that carry blood or other fluids
g. blood vessels that carry blood back to the heart
h. structures that keep blood flowing in one direction

Combining Forms Commonly Used With the Cardiovascular System and Blood

COMBINING FORM	DEFINITION
ather/o	yellowish, fatty plaque
ech/o	sound
electr/o	electricity, electrical activity
isch/o	deficiency, blockage
therm/o	heat
thromb/o	clot

EXERCISE 7

Write the definition of the following combining forms.

1. ech/o ______________________________
2. thromb/o ______________________________
3. isch/o ______________________________
4. therm/o ______________________________
5. ather/o ______________________________
6. electr/o ______________________________

EXERCISE 8

Write the combining form for each of the following.

1. clot ______________________
2. sound ______________________
3. deficiency, blockage ______________________
4. yellowish, fatty plaque ______________________
5. heat ______________________
6. electricity, electrical activity ______________________

Prefixes

PREFIX	DEFINITION
brady-	slow
pan-	all, total

Suffixes

SUFFIX	DEFINITION
-ac	pertaining to
-apheresis	removal
-penia	abnormal reduction in number
-poiesis	formation
-sclerosis	hardening

Refer to **Appendix C** and **Appendix D** for alphabetical lists of word parts and their meanings.

EXERCISE 9

Write the definitions of the following prefixes and suffixes.

1. brady- ______________________
2. pan- ______________________
3. -penia ______________________
____
4. -sclerosis ______________________
5. -apheresis ______________________
6. -poiesis ______________________
7. -ac ______________________

EXERCISE 10

Write the suffix or prefix for each of the following.

1. formation ______________________
2. pertaining to ______________________
3. hardening ______________________
4. all, total ______________________
5. abnormal reduction in number ______________________
6. slow ______________________
7. removal ______________________

For additional practice with Word Parts, go to Evolve Resources at evolve.elsevier.com and select:
Practice Student Resources > Student Resources > Chapter 10 > **Flashcards**

See Appendix B for instructions.

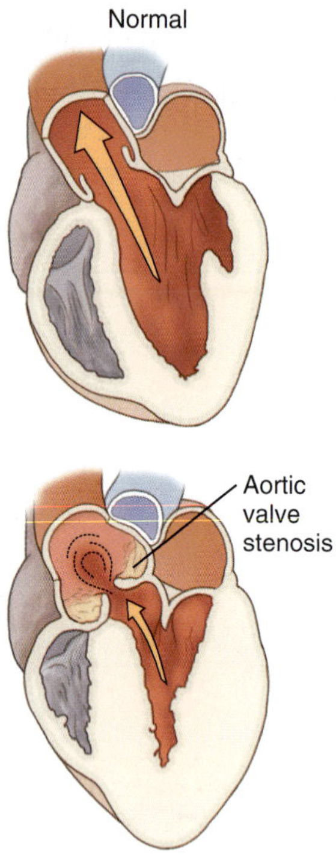

FIG. 10.8 Aortic stenosis.

EXERCISE FIGURE A

Fill in the blanks with word parts defined to label the diagram.

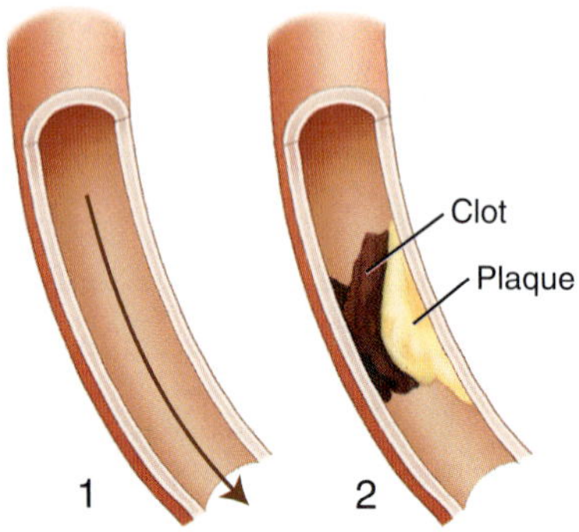

1. Healthy artery with smooth blood flow.
2. Blocked artery due to:

________ / ________
(blood) clot / abnormal condition

and ________ / ________ / ________
fatty plaque / CV / hardening

MEDICAL TERMS

The terms you need to learn to complete this chapter are listed below. The exercises following each list will help you learn the definition and the spelling of each word.

Disease and Disorder Terms
BUILT FROM WORD PARTS

The following terms can be translated using definitions of word parts. Further explanation is provided within parentheses as needed.

TERM	DEFINITION
CARDIOVASCULAR SYSTEM	
angioma (an-jē-Ō-ma)	tumor composed of blood vessels
angiostenosis (*an*-jē-ō-ste-NŌ-sis)	narrowing of a blood vessel
aortic stenosis (ā-OR-tik) (ste-NŌ-sis)	narrowing, pertaining to aorta (narrowing of the aortic valve) (Fig. 10.8)
arteriosclerosis (ar-*tēr*-ē-ō-skle-RŌ-sis)	hardening of the arteries
atherosclerosis (*ath*-er-ō-skle-RŌ-sis)	hardening of fatty plaque (deposited on the arterial wall) (Exercise Figure A)
bradycardia (*brad*-ē-KAR-dē-a)	condition of a slow heart (rate less than 60 beats per minute) *(Note: The i in cardi/o has been dropped)*
cardiomegaly (*kar*-dē-ō-MEG-a-lē)	enlargement of the heart
cardiomyopathy (*kar*-dē-ō-mī-OP-a-thē)	disease of the heart muscle
endocarditis (*en*-dō-kar-DĪ-tis)	inflammation of the inner (lining) of the heart (particularly heart valves)
ischemia (is-KĒ-mē-a)	deficiency in blood (flow); (caused by constriction or obstruction of a blood vessel. For example, in myocardial ischemia a deficient flow of blood to the heart muscle through the coronary arteries is caused by vessel constriction commonly due to atherosclerosis and can lead to myocardial infarction.)
myocarditis (*mī*-ō-kar-DĪ-tis)	inflammation of the muscle of the heart
pericarditis (*per*-i-kar-DĪ-tis)	inflammation of the sac surrounding the heart (Fig. 10.13)
phlebitis (fle-BĪ-tis)	inflammation of a vein
polyarteritis (*pol*-ē-*ar*-te-RĪ-tis)	inflammation of many (sites in the) arteries *(Note: The i in arteri/o has been dropped)*
tachycardia (*tak*-i-KAR-dē-a)	condition of a rapid heart (rate of more than 100 beats per min) *(Note: The i in cardi/o has been dropped)*
thrombophlebitis (*throm*-bō-fle-BĪ-tis)	inflammation of a vein associated with a (blood) clot

TERM	DEFINITION
valvulitis (*val*-vū-LĪ-tis)	inflammation of a valve (of the heart)
BLOOD	
erythrocytopenia (e-rith-rō-sī-tō-PĒ-nē-a)	abnormal reduction of red (blood) cells (this term is synonymous with **anemia**)
hematoma (*hē*-ma-TŌ-ma)	tumor of blood (collection that has leaked out of a broken vessel into the surrounding tissue) (Exercise Figure B)
leukocytopenia (lū-kō-sī-tō-PĒ-nē-a)	abnormal reduction of white (blood) cells (also called **leukopenia**)
multiple myeloma (MUL-te-pl) (*mī*-e-LŌ-ma)	tumors of the bone marrow (a blood malignancy that most often occurs after age 65. Signs and symptoms may include bone pain, infections, weight loss, anemia, and fatigue.)
pancytopenia (*pan*-sī-tō-PĒ-nē-a)	abnormal reduction of all (blood) cells
thrombocytopenia (throm-bō-sī-tō-PĒ-nē-a)	abnormal reduction of (blood) clotting cells (platelets)
thrombosis (throm-BŌ-sis)	abnormal condition of a (blood) clot (Exercise Figure A)
thrombus (THROM-bus)	(blood) clot (attached to the interior wall of an artery or vein)
LYMPHATIC SYSTEM	
lymphadenitis (*lim*-fad-e-NĪ-tis)	inflammation of lymph nodes
lymphadenopathy (lim-*fad*-e-NOP-a-thē)	disease of lymph nodes (characterized by abnormal enlargement of the lymph nodes associated with an infection or malignancy)
lymphoma (lim-FŌ-ma)	tumor of lymphatic tissue (malignant)
splenomegaly (*splē*-nō-MEG-a-lē)	enlargement of the spleen
thymoma (thī-MŌ-ma)	tumor of the thymus gland

EXERCISE FIGURE B

Fill in the blanks with word parts defined to complete labeling of the image.

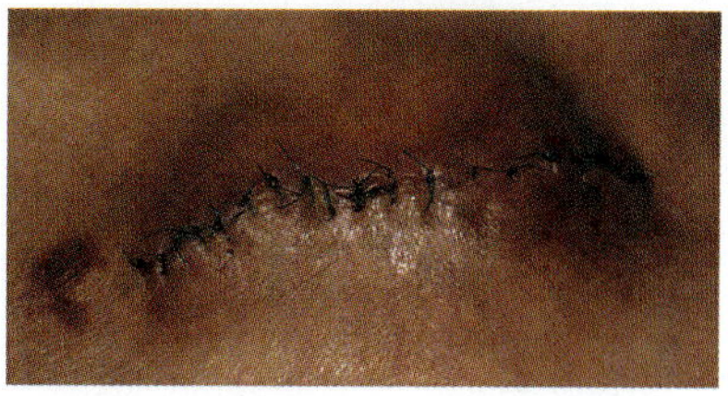

Post-surgical site displaying swelling and formation of a ______ / ______
blood / tumor

INTEGRATIVE MEDICINE TERM

Mindfulness-based stress reduction (MBSR) developed by Dr. Jon Kabat-Zinn, incorporates the techniques of meditation and yoga to effectively address health issues and promote physiologic and psychologic health and well-being. Research has demonstrated the efficacy of utilizing MBSR to improve quality of life and reduce elevated levels of blood pressure, heart rate, and depression associated with cardiovascular disease.

EMBOLUS/THROMBUS

An **embolus** circulates in the bloodstream until it becomes lodged in a vessel, whereas a **thrombus** is attached to the interior wall of a vessel. When any part of a **thrombus** breaks away and circulates in the bloodstream, it becomes known as an **embolus**.

EXERCISE 11

Practice saying aloud each of the Disease and Disorder Terms Built from Word Parts.

To hear the terms, go to Evolve Resources at evolve.elsevier.com and select:
Practice Student Resources > Student Resources > Chapter 10 > **Pronounce and Spell**

See Appendix B for instructions.

❑ Check the box when complete.

EXERCISE 12

Analyze and define the following terms.

1. endocarditis
2. bradycardia
3. cardiomegaly
4. arteriosclerosis
5. valvulitis
6. (multiple) myeloma
7. tachycardia
8. angiostenosis
9. thrombus
10. pericarditis
11. aortic (stenosis)
12. thrombosis
13. atherosclerosis
14. myocarditis
15. angioma
16. thymoma
17. lymphoma
18. lymphadenitis

19. splenomegaly

____
____

20. hematoma

____
____

21. polyarteritis

____
____

22. cardiomyopathy

____
____

23. lymphadenopathy

____
____

24. thrombophlebitis

____
____

25. phlebitis

____
____

26. pancytopenia

____
____

27. erythrocytopenia

____
____

28. leukocytopenia

____
____

29. thrombocytopenia

____
____

30. ischemia

____
____

EXERCISE 13

Build disease and disorder terms for the following definitions by using the word parts you have learned.

1. tumors of the bone marrow — multiple _______ WR / _______ S
2. enlargement of the heart — _______ WR / CV / _______ S
3. inflammation of the inner (layer) of the heart — _______ P / _______ WR / _______ S
4. condition of slow heart rate — _______ P / _______ WR / _______ S
5. hardening of the arteries — _______ WR / CV / _______ S
6. abnormal condition of a (blood) clot — _______ WR / _______ S

7. inflammation of the muscle of the heart ______ / ______ / ______ / ______
WR / CV / WR / S

8. narrowing of a blood vessel ______ / ______ / ______
WR / CV / S

9. condition of a rapid heart (rate) ______ / ______ / ______
P / WR / S

10. hardening of fatty plaque (deposited on the arterial wall) ______ / ______ / ______
WR / CV / S

11. tumor composed of blood vessels ______ / ______
WR / S

12. inflammation of a valve (of the heart) ______ / ______
WR / S

13. narrowing, pertaining to the aorta (narrowing of the aortic valve) ______ / ______ stenosis
WR / S

14. inflammation of the sac surrounding the heart ______ / ______ / ______
P / WR / S

15. tumor of lymphatic tissue ______ / ______
WR / S

16. deficiency in blood (flow) ______ / ______
WR / S

17. tumor of the thymus gland ______ / ______
WR / S

18. enlargement of the spleen ______ / ______ / ______
WR / CV / S

19. tumor (collection) of blood ______ / ______
WR / S

20. inflammation of lymph nodes ______ / ______
WR / S

21. disease of the heart muscle ______ / ______ / ______ / ______ / ______
WR / CV / WR / CV / S

22. inflammation of many (sites in the) arteries ______ / ______ / ______
P / WR / S

23. disease of lymph nodes ______ / ______ / ______
WR / CV / S

24. inflammation of a vein associated with a clot ______ / ______ / ______ / ______
WR / CV / WR / S

25. inflammation of a vein ______ / ______
WR / S

26. (blood) clot ________ WR / ________ S

27. abnormal reduction of all (blood) cells ________ P / ________ WR / CV / ________ S

28. abnormal reduction of red (blood) cells ________ WR / CV / ________ WR / CV / ________ S

29. abnormal reduction of white (blood) cells ________ WR / CV / ________ WR / CV / ________ S

30. abnormal reduction of (blood) clotting cells ________ WR / CV / ________ WR / CV / ________ S

EXERCISE 14

Spell each of the Disease and Disorder Terms Built from Word Parts by having someone dictate them to you. Use a separate sheet of paper.

To hear and spell the terms, go to Evolve Resources at evolve.elsevier.com and select:
Practice Student Resources > Student Resources > Chapter 10 > **Pronounce and Spell**

See Appendix B for instructions.

❑ Check the box when complete.

Disease and Disorder Terms
NOT BUILT FROM WORD PARTS

Word parts may be present in the following terms; however, their full meanings cannot be translated using definitions of word parts alone.

TERM	DEFINITION
CARDIOVASCULAR SYSTEM	
acute coronary syndrome (ACS) (a-KŪT) (KOR-o-*nar*-ē) (SIN-drōm)	sudden symptoms of insufficient blood supply to the heart indicating unstable angina or acute myocardial infarction. Rapid assessment is necessary to determine the diagnosis and treatment and to minimize heart damage.
aneurysm (AN-ū-riz-em)	ballooning of a weakened portion of an arterial wall (Fig. 10.9)
angina pectoris (an-JĪ-na) (PEK-to-ris)	chest pain, which may radiate to the left arm and jaw, that occurs when there is an insufficient supply of blood to the heart muscle
arrhythmia (ā-RITH-mē-a)	any disturbance or abnormality in the heart's normal rhythmic pattern

ANGINA PECTORIS was believed by the ancients to be a disorder of the breast. The Latin **angere**, meaning to throttle, was used to represent the sudden pain and was added to pectus, meaning breast.

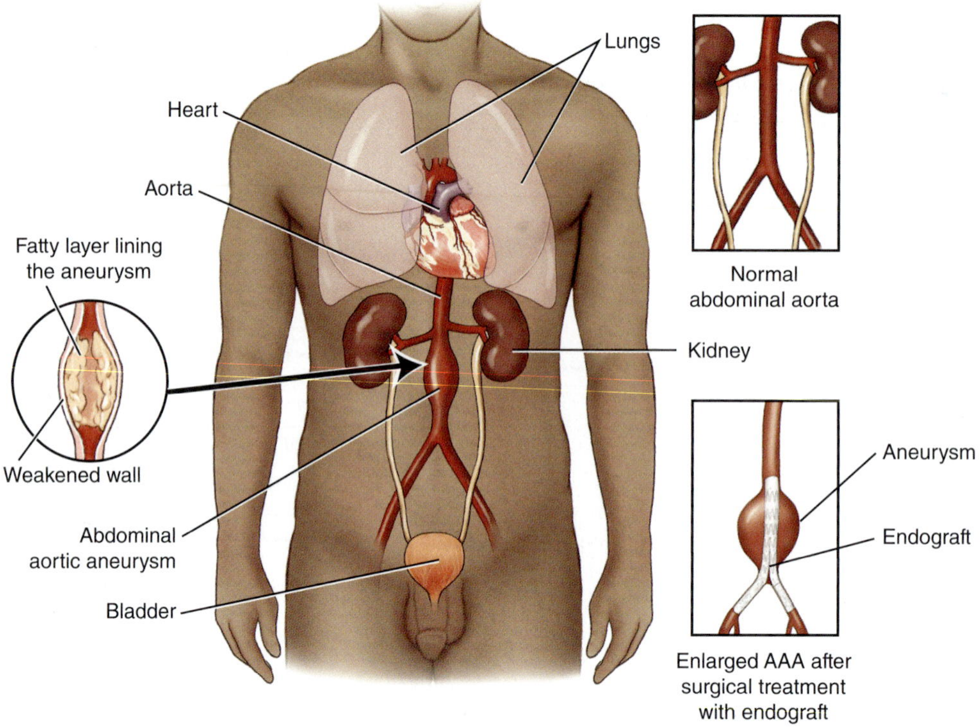

FIG. 10.9 Abdominal aortic aneurysm. An abdominal aortic aneurysm (AAA) is located in the abdominal area of the aorta, the main blood vessel that transports blood away from the heart. Because the success rate of surgery is much lower once an aneurysm has ruptured, more emphasis is being placed on diagnosis. AAA's can be detected by physical examination but are more frequently detected by abdominal ultrasound or computerized tomography (CT). Smaller AAAs have a very low risk of rupture and are usually followed closely to make sure they don't enlarge. Larger AAAs are usually repaired surgically. The preferred surgical intervention, called **endovascular stenting,** is performed through a puncture in the femoral artery, using a radiographic procedure called fluoroscopy. With this technique, an **endograft** can be placed within an aneurysm.

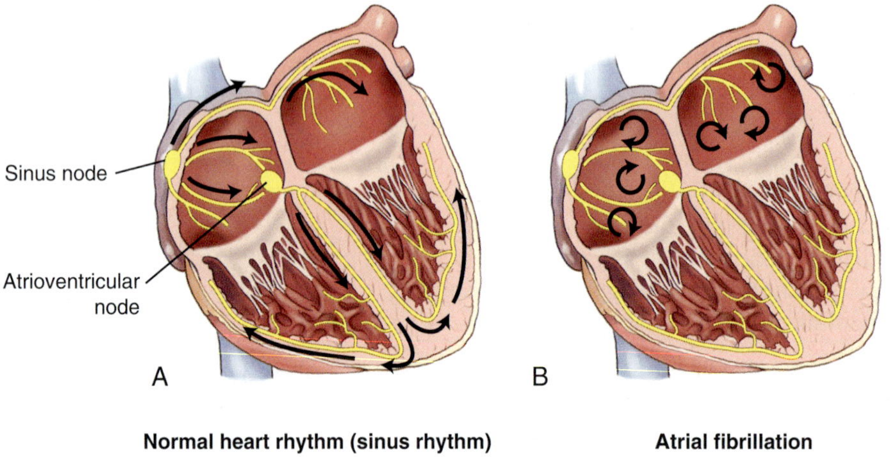

FIG. 10.10 Atrial fibrillation (AFib). **A,** Normal heart rhythm. Arrows indicate the normal travel of electrical impulses though the heart, stimulating coordinated contraction of chambers. **B,** Atrial fibrillation showing chaotic, rapid electrical impulses.

Disease and Disorder Terms—cont'd

TERM	DEFINITION
atrial fibrillation (AFib) (Ā-trē-al) (fi-bri-LĀ-shun)	cardiac arrhythmia characterized by chaotic, rapid electrical impulses in the atria. The atria quiver instead of contracting, causing an irregular ventricular response. Not all of the blood is ejected with each contraction, and the remaining blood flow becomes turbulent. This increases the risk of clot formation. Two types of AFib are **paroxysmal atrial fibrillation (PAF),** which is intermittent, and **chronic atrial fibrillation,** which is sustained (Fig. 10.10).

TERM	DEFINITION
cardiac arrest (KAR-dē-ak) (a-REST)	sudden cessation of cardiac output and effective circulation, which requires cardiopulmonary resuscitation (CPR)
cardiac tamponade (KAR-dē-ak) (tam-po-NĀD)	acute compression of the heart caused by fluid accumulation in the pericardial cavity
coarctation of the aorta (*kō*-ark-TĀ-shun) (ā-OR-ta)	congenital stenosis (narrowing) which occurs in the arch of the aorta (Fig. 10.11)
congenital heart disease (kon-JEN-i-tal) (hart) (di-ZĒZ)	heart abnormality present at birth
coronary artery disease (CAD) (KOR-o-*nar*-ē) (AR-te-rē) (di-ZĒZ)	condition that reduces the flow of blood through the coronary arteries to the myocardium that may progress to depriving the heart tissue of sufficient oxygen and nutrients to function normally; most often caused by coronary atherosclerosis. CAD is a common cause of **heart failure** and **myocardial infarction.**
cor pulmonale (kor) (pul-mō-NAL-ē)	enlargement of the heart's right ventricle due to pulmonary disease
deep vein thrombosis (DVT) (dēp) (vān) (throm-BŌ-sis)	condition of thrombus (clot) in a deep vein of the body. Most often occurs in the lower extremities. A clot, or part of a clot, can break off and travel to the lungs, causing a pulmonary embolism.
heart failure (HF) (hart) (fāl-ŪR)	condition in which there is an inability of the heart to pump enough blood through the body to supply the tissues and organs with nutrients and oxygen (also called **congestive heart failure** [CHF])
hypertensive heart disease (HHD) (*hī*-per-TEN-siv) (hart) (di-ZĒZ)	disorder of the heart caused by persistent high blood pressure; it may be associated with hypertrophy (abnormal thickening of the heart muscle) or dilation of the chambers of the heart (due to thinning and stretching of the heart muscle)
intermittent claudication (*in*-ter-MIT-ent) (*klaw*-di-KĀ-shun)	condition of pain, tension and weakness in a limb that starts when walking is begun, increases until walking is no longer possible, and then completely resolves when the patient is at rest. It is caused by reversible muscle ischemia that occurs with peripheral artery disease.
mitral valve stenosis (MĪ-tral) (ste-NŌ-sis)	narrowing of the mitral valve from scarring, usually caused by episodes of **rheumatic fever**
myocardial infarction (MI) (*mī*-ō-KAR-dē-al) (in-FARK-shun)	death (necrosis) of a portion of the myocardium caused by lack of oxygen resulting from an interrupted blood supply (also called **heart attack**)

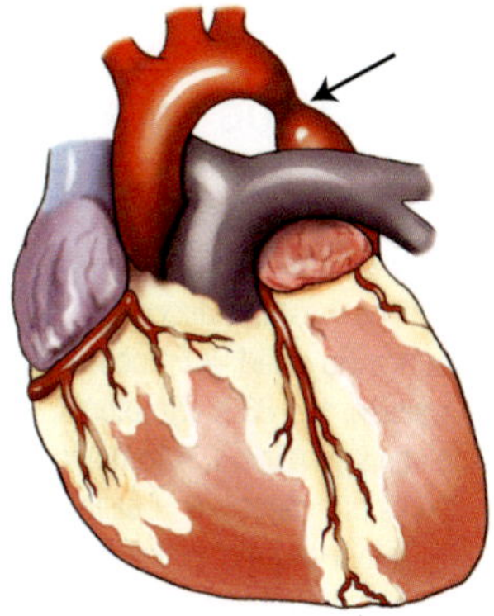

FIG. 10.11 Coarctation of the aorta (*arrow*).

CORONARY
is derived from the Latin coronalis, meaning crown or wreath. It describes the arteries encircling the heart.

Disease and Disorder Terms—cont'd

TERM	DEFINITION
peripheral artery disease (PAD) (pe-RIF-er-al) (AR-ter-ē) (di-ZĒZ)	disease of the arteries in the arms and legs, resulting in narrowing or complete obstruction of the artery. This is caused most commonly by atherosclerosis, but occasionally by inflammatory diseases, emboli, or thrombus formation. The most common symptom of peripheral artery disease is intermittent claudication. (also called **peripheral vascular disease [PVD]**)
rheumatic heart disease (rū-MAT-ik) (hart) (di-ZĒZ)	damage to the heart muscle or heart valves caused by one or more episodes of **rheumatic fever**
varicose veins (VAR-i-kōs) (vānz)	distended or tortuous veins usually found in the lower extremities (Fig. 10.12)
BLOOD	
anemia (a-NĒ-mē-a)	condition in which there is a reduction in the number of erythrocytes (RBCs). Anemia may be caused by blood loss, by decreased production of RBCs, or by increased destruction of RBCs. (Table 10.1)
embolus (pl. emboli) (EM-bō-lus) (EM-bo-lī)	blood clot or foreign material, such as air or fat, that enters the bloodstream and moves until it lodges at another point in the circulation
hemophilia (hē-mō-FIL-ē-a)	inherited bleeding disease most commonly caused by a deficiency of the coagulation factor VIII
leukemia (lū-KĒ-mē-a)	malignant disease characterized by excessive increase in abnormal leukocytes (white blood cells) formed in the bone marrow (Table 10.2)
sepsis (SEP-sis)	systemic inflammatory response caused by pathogenic microorganisms, usually bacteria, entering the bloodstream and multiplying; life-threatening condition, which may lead to tissue damage, organ failure, and death. The overwhelming presence of pathogens in the blood is called septicemia.

RAYNAUD (RĀ-NŌ) PHENOMENON

is classified as a **peripheral artery disease (PAD)**. The condition was first described by Maurice Raynaud, a French physician, in 1862. Symptoms include intermittent, symmetric attacks of cyanosis and pallor of the distal ends of the fingers and toes often caused by exposure to cold temperature.

RHEUMATIC FEVER

is an inflammatory disease, usually occurring in children and young adults after an upper respiratory tract streptococcal infection. One of the most serious symptoms is valvulitis (inflammation of a cardiac valve). While antibiotics have greatly decreased the incidence of this disease in developed nations, it is still a significant threat in developing nations.

VARICOSE VEINS AND CURRENT TREATMENT

Varicose veins usually occur in the superficial veins of the legs. One-way valves in the veins help move the blood upward. When these valves fail, or the veins lose their elasticity, the blood flows backward, pools, and forms varicose veins. Causes are heredity, obesity, pregnancy, illness, or injury. Current therapies include laser ablation, ambulatory phlebectomy, and sclerotherapy.

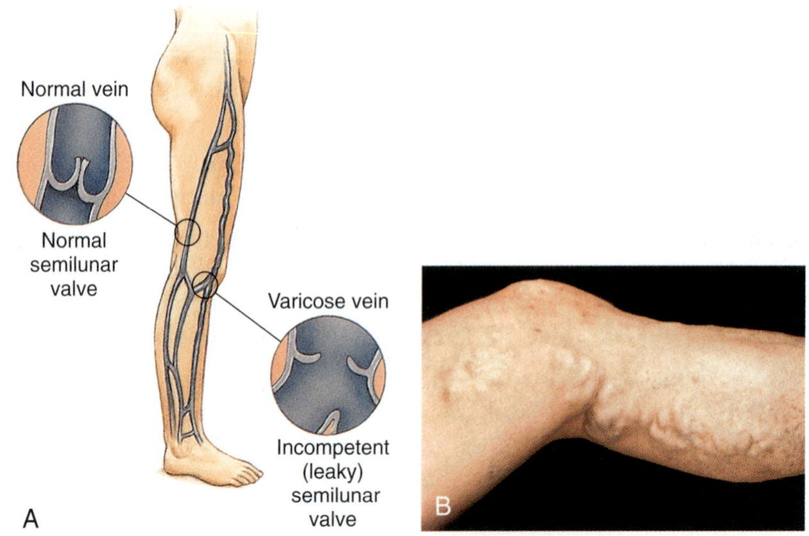

FIG. 10.12 **A,** Normal and varicose veins. **B,** Appearance of varicose veins.

TABLE 10.1 Common Types of Anemia

TYPE	DESCRIPTION
Anemia due to blood loss	• acute blood loss anemia as a result of hemorrhage
Anemia due to decreased production of red blood cells	• iron deficiency anemia: not enough iron in the body to produce hemoglobin • pernicious anemia: ineffective production of red blood cells due to vitamin B-12 deficiency • aplastic anemia: resulting from bone marrow failure
Anemia due to increased destruction of red blood cells	• hemolytic anemia: reduced life of blood cells (such as in sickle cell anemia)

TABLE 10.2 Leukemia

Leukemia is differentiated by the type of leukocyte that is affected and how quickly the disease develops and progresses.

Acute Leukemia develops quickly with rapid progression of the disease. Both adults and children may develop acute leukemia. Acute leukemia is the most common form of cancer in children and adolescents.

Chronic Leukemia develops slowly with gradual disease progression and most often occurs in adults.

Lymphocytic Leukemia affects the lymphoid cells (lymphocytes), which form lymph tissue (part of the immune system).

Myelogenous Leukemia affects the myeloid cells, which form red blood cells, white blood cells, and platelets.

MAJOR TYPES OF LEUKEMIA

- **acute lymphocytic leukemia (ALL):** the most common type in young children, can affect adults (also called acute lymphoblastic leukemia)
- **acute myelogenous leukemia (AML):** most common acute leukemia in adults, can also affect children
- **chronic lymphocytic leukemia (CLL):** most common chronic adult leukemia; patient may feel well for years without needing treatment
- **chronic myelogenous leukemia (CML):** occurs mostly in older adults

Rare Types of Leukemia include hairy cell leukemia **(HCL)**, myelodysplastic syndromes, and myeloproliferative disorders

TERM	DEFINITION
LYMPHATIC SYSTEM	
Hodgkin disease (HOJ-kin) (di-ZĒZ)	malignant disorder of the lymphatic tissue characterized by progressive enlargement of the lymph nodes, usually beginning in the cervical nodes (also called **Hodgkin lymphoma**)
infectious mononucleosis (in-FEK-shus) (*mon*-ō-*nū*-klē-Ō-sis)	acute infection caused by the Epstein-Barr virus characterized by swollen lymph nodes, sore throat, fatigue, and fever. The disease affects mostly young people and is often transmitted by saliva.

HODGKIN DISEASE was first described in 1832 by Thomas Hodgkin, a pathologist at Guy's Hospital in London. In 1865 the name Hodgkin's disease was given to the condition by another English physician, Sir Samuel Wilks.

EXERCISE 15

Practice saying aloud each of the Disease and Disorder Terms NOT Built from Word Parts.

To hear the terms, go to Evolve Resources at evolve.elsevier.com and select:
Practice Student Resources > Student Resources > Chapter 10 > **Pronounce and Spell**

See Appendix B for instructions.

❑ Check the box when complete.

EXERCISE 16

Fill in the blanks with the correct terms.

1. A congenital narrowing (stenosis) of the arch of the aorta is called ____________________ of the aorta.
2. A blood clot or foreign material that enters the bloodstream and moves until it lodges at another point in the circulation is called a(n) ____________________.
3. Sudden cessation of cardiac output and effective circulation is referred to as a(n) ____________________ ____________________.
4. ____________________ heart disease is the name given to a heart abnormality present at birth.
5. Veins that are distended or tortuous are called ____________________ ____________________.
6. ____________________ is the name given to the ballooning of a weakened portion of an artery wall.
7. ____________________ ____________________ is the name given to a malignant disorder of lymphatic tissue characterized by enlarged lymph nodes.
8. ____________________ ____________________ ____________________ is a condition most often caused by coronary atherosclerosis, which deprives the heart tissue of sufficient oxygen and nutrients to function normally.
9. ____________________ ____________________ is a cardiac condition characterized by chest pain caused by an insufficient blood supply to the cardiac muscle.
10. Death of a portion of myocardial muscle caused by lack of oxygen resulting from an interrupted blood supply is called a(n) ____________________ ____________________.
11. ____________________ ____________________ is a cardiac arrhythmia characterized by chaotic, rapid electrical impulses.
12. Any disturbance or abnormality in the heart's normal rhythmic pattern is called a(n) ____________________.
13. A disorder of the heart caused by a persistently high blood pressure is called ____________________ heart disease.
14. ____________________ ____________________ is the inability of the heart to pump enough blood through the body to supply tissues and organs.
15. ____________________ ____________________ ____________________ is a disease of the arteries in the arms and legs resulting in narrowing or complete obstruction of an artery.
16. ____________________ is an inherited bleeding disease most commonly caused by a deficiency of the coagulation factor VIII.
17. ____________________ is a malignant disease in which the number of abnormal white blood cells formed in the bone marrow is excessively increased.
18. A reduction in the number of erythrocytes results in a condition known as ____________________.

19. ____________________ ____________________ is an infection caused by the Epstein-Barr virus.

20. ____________________ ____________________ is a condition in which a patient has pain and discomfort in calf muscles while walking.

21. Acute compression of the heart caused by fluid accumulation in the pericardial cavity is known as ______________ ____________________.

22. Episodes of rheumatic fever can cause ____________________ ____________________ ____________________ and ____________________ heart ____________________.

23. ____________________ ____________________ ____________________ is the condition of a thrombus, most often occurring in the lower extremities.

24. ____________________ ____________________ ____________________ is a sudden insufficient blood supply to the heart, indicating unstable angina or myocardial infarction.

25. ____________________ is a systemic inflammatory response caused by pathogenic microorganisms.

26. Enlargement of the heart's right ventricle due to pulmonary disease is called __________ ______________.

EXERCISE 17

Match the terms in the first column with the correct definitions in the second column.

______	1. anemia	a. sudden cessation of cardiac output and effective circulation
______	2. aneurysm	b. ballooning of a weak portion of an arterial wall
______	3. angina pectoris	c. reduction in the number of erythrocytes in the blood
______	4. arrhythmia	d. any disturbance or abnormality in the heart's normal rhythmic pattern
______	5. cardiac arrest	e. chest pain occurring because of insufficient blood supply to the heart muscle
______	6. cardiac tamponade	f. inability of the heart to pump enough blood through the body to supply tissues or organs
______	7. coarctation of the aorta	g. pain in calf muscles while walking
______	8. congenital heart disease	h. congenital stenosis (narrowing), which occurs in the arch of the aorta
______	9. heart failure	i. acute compression of the heart caused by fluid in the pericardial cavity
______	10. intermittent claudication	j. heart abnormality present at birth
______	11. deep vein thrombosis	k. clot in a deep vein
______	12. coronary artery disease	l. disease of the arteries in the arms and legs resulting in narrowing or complete obstruction of the artery
______	13. peripheral artery disease	m. condition that reduces the flow of blood through the coronary arteries

EXERCISE 18

Match the terms in the first column with the correct definitions in the second column.

_____ 1. embolus
_____ 2. atrial fibrillation
_____ 3. hemophilia
_____ 4. infectious mononucleosis
_____ 5. Hodgkin disease
_____ 6. hypertensive heart disease
_____ 7. leukemia
_____ 8. myocardial infarction
_____ 9. mitral valve stenosis
_____ 10. acute coronary syndrome
_____ 11. varicose veins
_____ 12. rheumatic heart disease
_____ 13. sepsis
_____ 14. cor pulmonale

a. inherited bleeding disease most commonly caused by a deficiency of the coagulation factor VIII
b. heart disorder brought on by persistent high blood pressure
c. distended or tortuous veins
d. malignant disease, characterized by excessive increase of abnormal white blood cells formed in the bone marrow
e. characterized by chaotic, rapid electrical impulses of the atria
f. systemic inflammatory response caused by pathogenic microorganisms
g. symptoms indicating unstable angina or myocardial infarction
h. infectious disease that affects mostly young people; characterized by swollen lymph glands
i. blood clot or foreign material that enters the bloodstream and moves until it lodges at another point
j. malignant disorder of lymphatic tissue with enlargement of lymph nodes
k. death of a portion of myocardium caused by lack of oxygen resulting from an interrupted blood supply
l. narrowing of the valve between the left atrium and left ventricle
m. damage to the heart caused by episodes of rheumatic fever
n. enlargement of the heart's right ventricle due to pulmonary disease

EXERCISE 19

Spell each of the Disease and Disorder Terms NOT Built from Word Parts by having someone dictate them to you. Use a separate sheet of paper.

To hear and spell the terms, go to Evolve Resources at evolve.elsevier.com and select:
Practice Student Resources > Student Resources > Chapter 10 > **Pronounce and Spell**

See Appendix B for instructions.

❑ Check the box when complete.

Surgical Terms
BUILT FROM WORD PARTS

The following terms can be translated using definitions of word parts. Further explanation is provided within parentheses as needed.

TERM	DEFINITION
CARDIOVASCULAR SYSTEM	
angioplasty (AN-jē-ō-*plas*-tē)	surgical repair of a blood vessel
atherectomy (ath-er-EK-to-mē)	excision of fatty plaque (from a blocked artery using a specialized catheter and a rotary cutter)

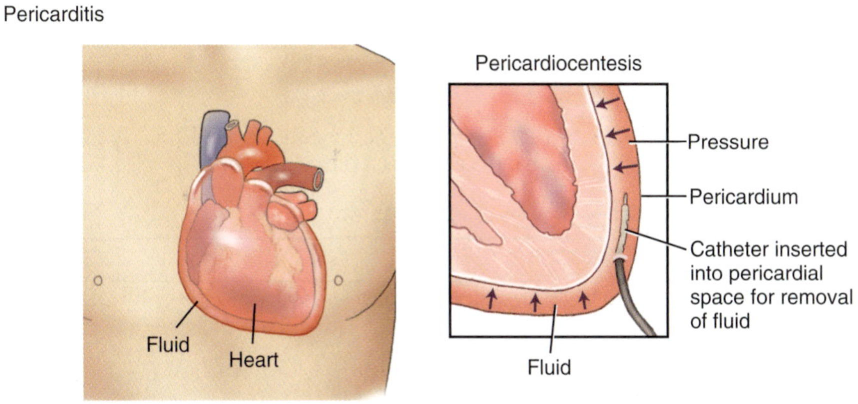

FIG. 10.13 Pericarditis may produce excess fluid in the pericardium. If the fluid seriously affects the heart's ability to pump blood, pericardiocentesis may be performed to remove the fluid.

TERM	DEFINITION
endarterectomy (*end*-ar-ter-EK-to-mē)	excision within the artery (excision of plaque from the arterial wall). This procedure is usually named for the artery to be cleaned out, such as carotid endarterectomy, which means removal of plaque from the wall of the carotid artery (Exercise Figure C). *(Note: the o from endo- is dropped for easier pronunciation)*
pericardiocentesis (*per*-i-kar-dē-ō-sen-TĒ-sis)	surgical puncture to aspirate fluid from the sac surrounding the heart (usually to relieve cardiac tamponade and/or for diagnostic investigation) (Fig. 10.13)
phlebectomy (fle-BEK-to-mē)	excision of a vein
phlebotomy (fle-BOT-o-mē)	incision into a vein (with a needle to remove blood or to give blood or intravenous fluids) (also called **venipuncture**)
valvuloplasty (VAL-vū-lō-*plas*-tē)	surgical repair of a valve (cardiac or venous)
LYMPHATIC SYSTEM	
splenectomy (splē-NEK-to-mē)	excision of the spleen
splenorrhaphy (sple-NOR-a-fē)	suturing, repairing of the spleen
thymectomy (thī-MEK-to-mē)	excision of the thymus gland

EXERCISE FIGURE C

Fill in the blanks with word parts defined to label the diagram.

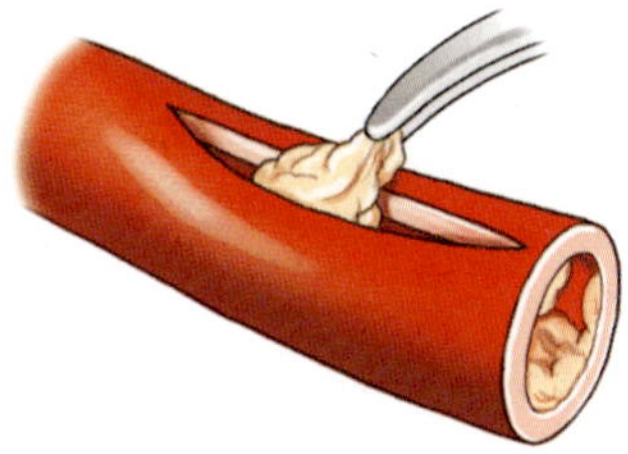

_____ / _____ / _____
within / artery / excision

EXERCISE 20

Practice saying aloud each of the Surgical Terms Built from Word Parts.

To hear the terms, go to Evolve Resources at evolve.elsevier.com and select:
Practice Student Resources > Student Resources > Chapter 10 > **Pronounce and Spell**

See Appendix B for instructions.

❑ Check the box when complete.

EXERCISE 21

Analyze and define the following surgical terms.

1. pericardiocentesis
____
____

2. thymectomy
____
____

3. angioplasty
____
____

4. splenorrhaphy
____
____

5. valvuloplasty
____
____

6. endarterectomy
____
____

7. phlebotomy
____
____

8. splenectomy
____
____

9. phlebectomy
____
____

10. atherectomy
____
____

EXERCISE 22

Build surgical terms for the following definitions by using the word parts you have learned.

1. excision within the artery ______ / ______ / ______ (P / WR / S)
2. suturing, repairing of the spleen ______ / ______ / ______ (WR / CV / S)
3. surgical repair of a valve ______ / ______ / ______ (WR / CV / S)
4. incision into a vein ______ / ______ / ______ (WR / CV / S)
5. excision of the thymus gland ______ / ______ (WR / S)
6. surgical puncture to aspirate fluid from the sac surrounding the heart ______ / ______ / ______ / ______ (P / WR / CV / S)

7. surgical repair of a blood vessel ______ WR / CV / ______ S

8. excision of the spleen ______ WR / ______ S

9. excision of a vein ______ WR / ______ S

10. excision of fatty plaque ______ WR / ______ S

EXERCISE 23

Spell each of the Surgical Terms Built from Word Parts by having someone dictate them to you. Use a separate sheet of paper.

To hear and spell the terms, go to Evolve Resources at evolve.elsevier.com and select:
Practice Student Resources > Student Resources > Chapter 10 > **Pronounce and Spell**

See Appendix B for instructions.

❑ Check the box when complete.

Surgical Terms
NOT BUILT FROM WORD PARTS

Word parts may be present in the following terms; however, their full meanings cannot be translated using definitions of word parts alone.

TERM	DEFINITION
CARDIOVASCULAR SYSTEM	
aneurysmectomy (*an*-ū-riz-MEK-to-mē)	surgical excision of an aneurysm
artificial cardiac pacemaker (*ar*-ti-FISH-el) (KAR-dē-ak) (PĀS-mā-kr)	battery-powered apparatus implanted under the skin with leads placed on the heart or in the chamber of the heart used to treat an abnormal heart rhythm, usually one that is too slow, secondary to an abnormal sinus node
automatic implantable cardiac defibrillator (AICD) (aw-to-MAT-ik) (im-PLANT-a-bl) (KAR-dē-ak) (dē-FIB-ri-lā-tor)	device implanted in the body that continuously monitors the heart rhythm. If life-threatening arrhythmias occur, the device delivers an electric shock to convert the arrhythmia back to a normal rhythm.
catheter ablation (KATH-e-ter) (ab-LĀ-shun)	procedure in which abnormal cells that trigger abnormal heart rhythms (arrhythmias) are destroyed by using a device that heats or freezes the cells (Fig. 10.14)
coronary artery bypass graft (CABG) (KOR-o-*nar*-ē) (AR-te-rē) (BĪ-pas) (graft)	surgical technique to bring a new blood supply to heart muscle by detouring around blocked arteries

SINUS NODE of the heart is the body's natural pacemaker. Also called the sinoatrial or SA node, it consists of specialized fibers that are responsible for initiating nerve impulses that tell the heart muscles when to contract. When the SA node is working properly, the pumping motion of the heart chambers is coordinated and well-timed. If the SA node (or other parts of the heart's conduction system) doesn't work properly, arrhythmias may occur.

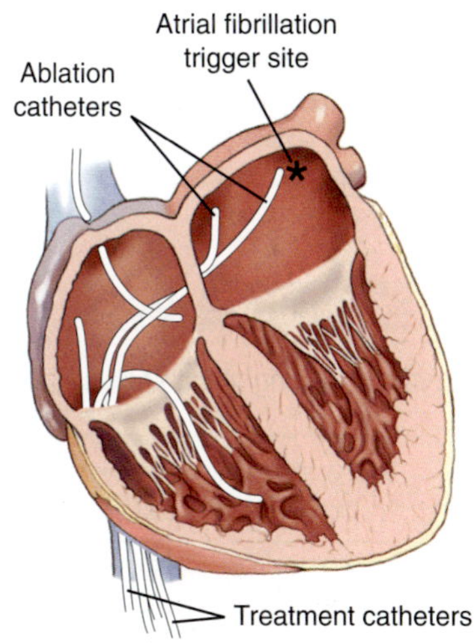

FIG. 10.14 Catheter ablation is used to treat atrial fibrillation if drug therapy is not effective.

Surgical Terms—cont'd

TERM	DEFINITION
coronary stent (KOR-o-*nar*-ē) (stent)	supportive scaffold device placed in the coronary artery; used to prevent closure of the artery after angioplasty or atherectomy; used to treat an artery occluded by plaque
embolectomy (*em*-bo-LEK-to-mē)	surgical removal of an embolus or clot, usually with a balloon catheter, inflating the balloon beyond the clot, then pulling the balloon back to the incision and bringing the clot with it
femoropopliteal bypass (*fem*-o-rō-pop-LIT-ē-al) (BĪ-pass)	surgery to establish an alternate route from femoral artery to popliteal artery to bypass an obstruction
percutaneous transluminal coronary angioplasty (PTCA) (*per*-kū-TĀ-nē-us) (trans-LŪ-min-al) (KOR-o-*nar*-ē) (AN-jē-ō-*plas*-tē)	procedure in which a balloon is advanced into a coronary artery to the area where plaque has formed. When the balloon is inflated, the vessel wall expands, allowing blood to flow more freely. (also called **balloon angioplasty**)
thrombolytic therapy (*throm*-bō-LIT-ik) (THER-a-pē)	injection of a medication either intravenously or intra-arterially to dissolve blood clots. It is often used in emergency departments for acute myocardial infarction.
BLOOD	
bone marrow aspiration (bōn) (MAR-ō) (*as*-pi-RĀ-shun)	procedure to obtain a sample of the **liquid** portion of the bone marrow, usually from the ilium (upper hip bone) for study; used to diagnose leukemia, infections, some types of anemia, and other blood disorders
bone marrow biopsy (bōn) (MAR-ō) (BĪ-op-sē)	procedure to obtain a sample of the **solid** portion of bone marrow, usually from the ilium, for study; used to diagnose leukemia, infections, some types of anemia, and other blood disorders. May be performed at the same time as bone marrow aspiration.
bone marrow transplant (bōn) (MAR-ō) (TRANS-plant)	infusion of healthy bone marrow cells from a matched donor into a patient with severely diseased or damaged bone marrow; the donor cells may establish a colony of new, healthy tissue in the recipient's bone marrow

BONE MARROW

is contained within spongy bone, which is located primarily at the ends of long bones and in the center of other bones. Stem cells within the bone marrow turn into thrombocytes, red blood cells, and white blood cells.

PERIPHERAL BLOOD STEM CELL TRANSPLANT (PBSCT)

is similar to bone marrow transplant. Stem cells are collected by apheresis, a process in which blood is removed from the patient or a matched donor and spun through a machine to harvest stem cells. The concentrated stem cells are given to the recipient by infusion. Both types of transplant are used to treat certain blood-related cancers and disorders, such as leukemia or anemia.

EXERCISE 24

Practice saying aloud each of the Surgical Terms NOT Built from Word Parts.

To hear the terms, go to Evolve Resources at evolve.elsevier.com and select:
Practice Student Resources > Student Resources > Chapter 10 > **Pronounce and Spell**

See Appendix B for instructions.

❑ Check the box when complete.

EXERCISE 25

Match the terms in the first column with their correct definitions in the second column.

______ 1. embolectomy
______ 2. bone marrow transplant
______ 3. aneurysmectomy
______ 4. thrombolytic therapy
______ 5. artificial cardiac pacemaker

a. battery powered apparatus used to treat an abnormal heart rhythm
b. injection of a medication to treat blood clots
c. surgical removal of an embolus or clot, usually with a balloon catheter
d. infusion of healthy bone marrow cells into a patient with diseased or damaged bone marrow
e. surgical excision of an aneurysm

EXERCISE 26

Write the medical term pictured and defined.

1. ______________________________

____

procedure to obtain a sample of the **liquid** portion of the bone marrow

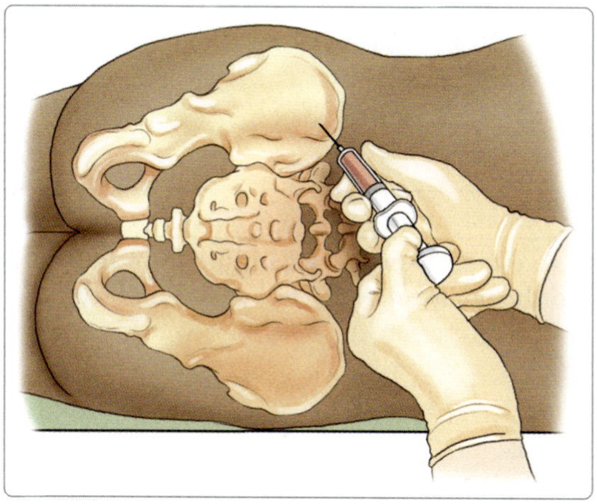

2. ______________________________

____

procedure to obtain a sample of the **solid** portion of bone marrow

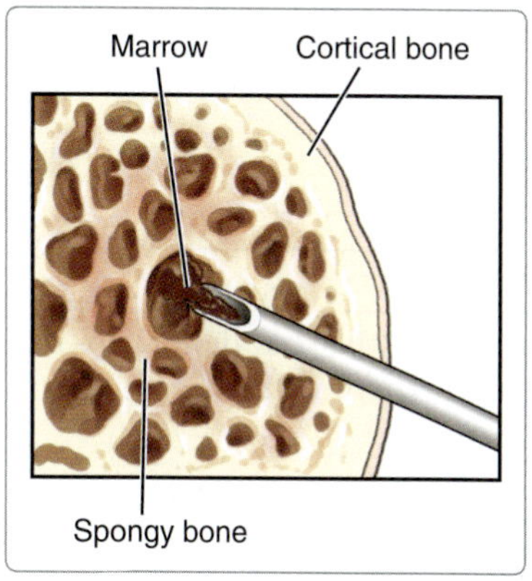

3. ______________________________

____

surgical technique to bring a new blood supply to heart muscle by detouring around blocked arteries

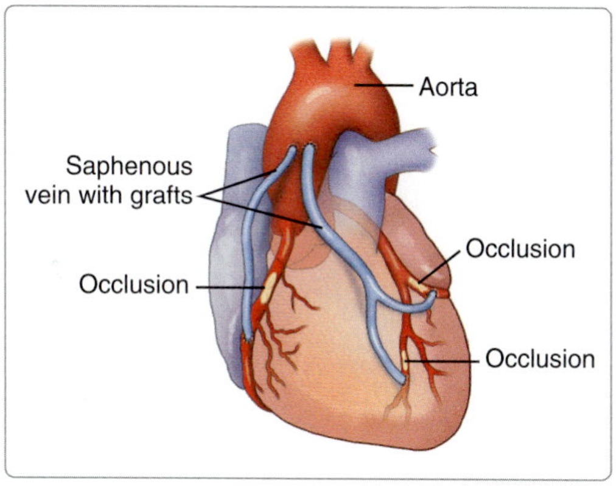

4. ______________________________

____

procedure in which abnormal cells that trigger abnormal heart rhythms (arrhythmias) are destroyed by using a device that heats or freezes the cells

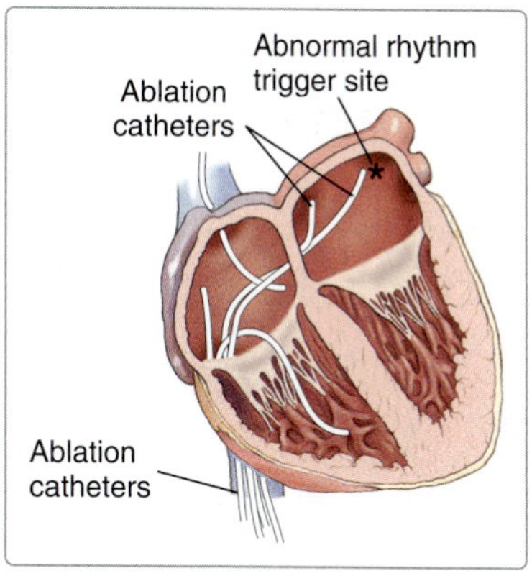

EXERCISE 26 *Pictured and Defined—cont'd*

5. ______________________________

____

supportive scaffold device placed in the coronary artery; used to prevent closure of the artery after angioplasty or atherectomy

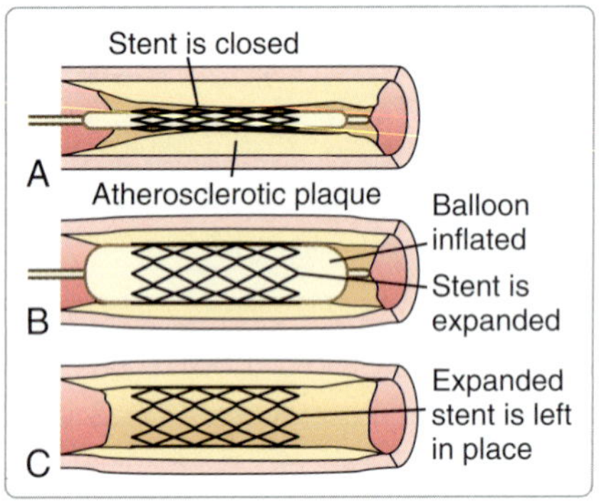

6. ______________________________

____

procedure in which a balloon is advanced into the coronary artery, to where plaque has formed. The balloon is inflated, the vessel wall expands, allowing blood to flow more freely

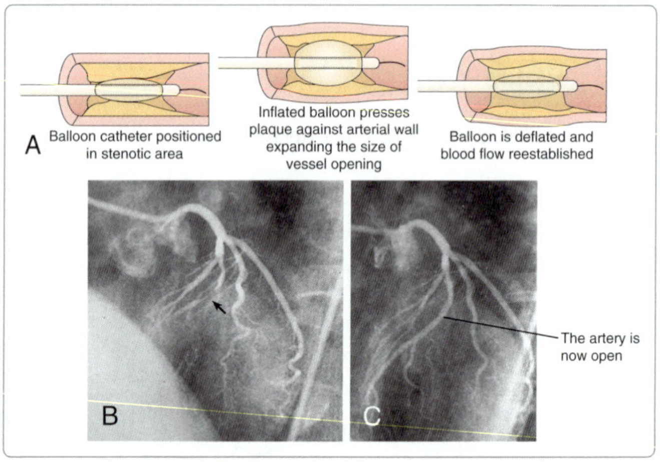

7. ______________________________

____

device implanted in the body that can deliver an electric shock to convert arrhythmia back to a normal rhythm

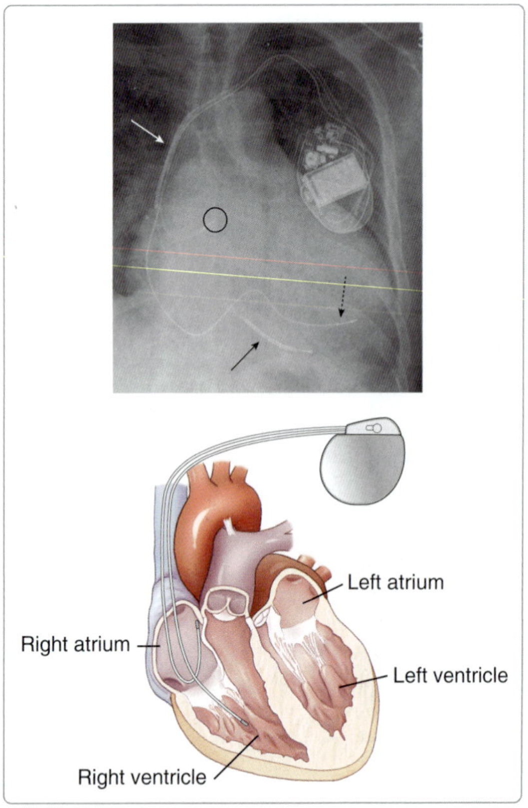

8. ______________________________

____

surgery to establish an alternate route from the femoral artery to the popliteal artery to bypass an obstruction

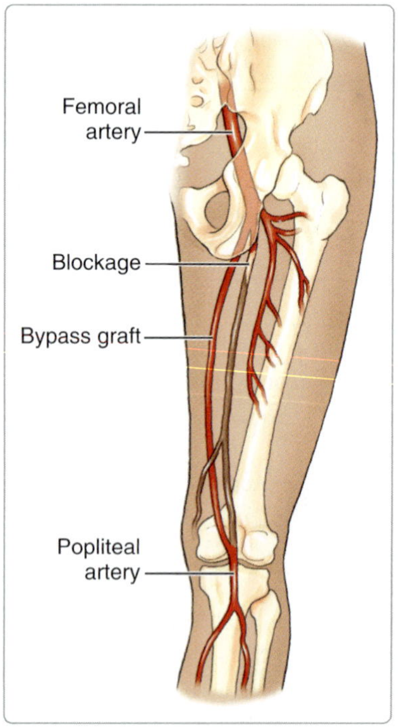

EXERCISE 27

Spell each of the Surgical Terms NOT Built from Word Parts by having someone dictate them to you. Use a separate sheet of paper.

To hear and spell the terms, go to Evolve Resources at evolve.elsevier.com and select:
Practice Student Resources > Student Resources > Chapter 10 > **Pronounce and Spell**

See Appendix B for instructions.

❑ Check the box when complete.

Diagnostic Terms
BUILT FROM WORD PARTS

The following terms can be translated using definitions of word parts. Further explanation is provided within parentheses as needed.

TERM	DEFINITION
CARDIOVASCULAR SYSTEM	
DIAGNOSTIC IMAGING	
angiography (*an*-jē-OG-ra-fē)	radiographic imaging of blood vessels (the procedure is named for the vessel to be studied, e.g., **femoral angiography** or **coronary angiography**) (Table 10-3)
angioscope (AN-jē-ō-skōp)	instrument used for visual examination (of the inside) of a blood vessel

TABLE 10.3 Types of Angiography

CORONARY ARTERY VISUALIZATION

Coronary angiography is an **invasive procedure** in which a catheter is inserted into an artery in the groin, arm or neck, then advanced into the coronary vessels. Next, contrast media are injected, and images are recorded. It is considered the best technique for determining the percentage of blockage in the coronary arteries.

OTHER VASCULAR VISUALIZATION

Magnetic resonance angiography (MRA) is a **noninvasive procedure** that does not require catheterization and uses specialized MR imaging to study vascular structures of the body. MRA may be chosen over computed tomography angiography because there is no exposure to ionizing radiation.

Computed tomography angiography (CTA) is a **noninvasive procedure** that uses a high-resolution CT system to study vascular structures of the body after the injection of intravenous contrast media.

Digital subtraction angiography (DSA) is an **invasive procedure** in which an image is taken and stored in the computer, then contrast medium is injected. A second image is taken and stored in the computer. The computer compares the two images and subtracts the first image from the second, removing structures not being studied. DSA enables better visualization of the arteries than regular angiography.

Diagnostic Terms—cont'd

TERM	DEFINITION
angioscopy (*an*-jē-OS-ko-pē)	visual examination (of the inside) of a blood vessel
aortogram (ā-ŌR-to-gram)	radiographic image of the aorta (after an injection of contrast media)
arteriogram (ar-TĒR-ē-ō-gram)	radiographic image of an artery (after an injection of contrast media) (Exercise Figure D)
venogram (VĒ-nō-gram)	radiographic image of a vein (after an injection of contrast media) (Exercise Figure E)
CARDIOVASCULAR PROCEDURES	
echocardiogram (ECHO) (*ek*-ō-KAR-dē-ō-gram)	record of the heart (structure and motion) using sound (waves); (used to detect valvular disease and evaluate heart function)
electrocardiogram (ECG, EKG) (ē-*lek*-trō-KAR-dē-ō-gram)	record of the electrical activity of the heart (Exercise Figure F)
electrocardiograph (ē-*lek*-trō-KAR-dē-ō-graf)	instrument used to record the electrical activity of the heart
electrocardiography (ē-*lek*-trō-*kar*-dē-OG-ra-fē)	process of recording the electrical activity of the heart

EXERCISE FIGURE D

Fill in the blanks with word parts defined to complete labeling of the diagram.

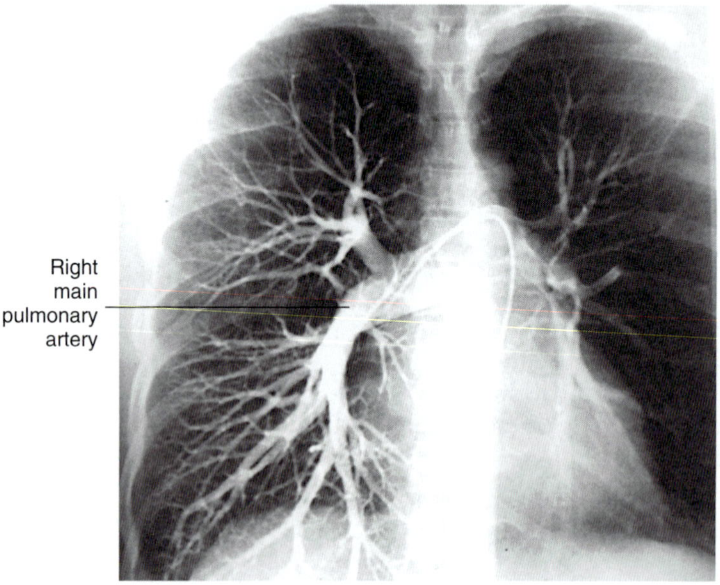

_______ / _______ / _______
artery / CV / radiographic image

showing the right main pulmonary artery. This procedure was performed after injection of contrast media.

EXERCISE FIGURE E

Fill in the blanks with word parts defined to complete labeling of the diagram.

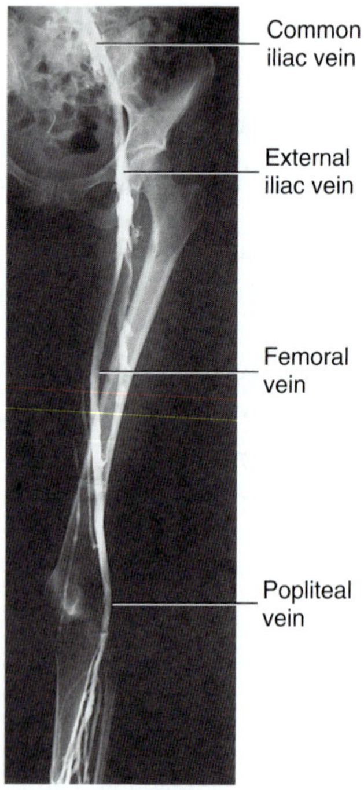

Normal _______ / _______ / _______, left lower limb
vein / CV / radiographic image

EXERCISE FIGURE F

Fill in the blanks with word parts defined to complete labeling of the diagram.

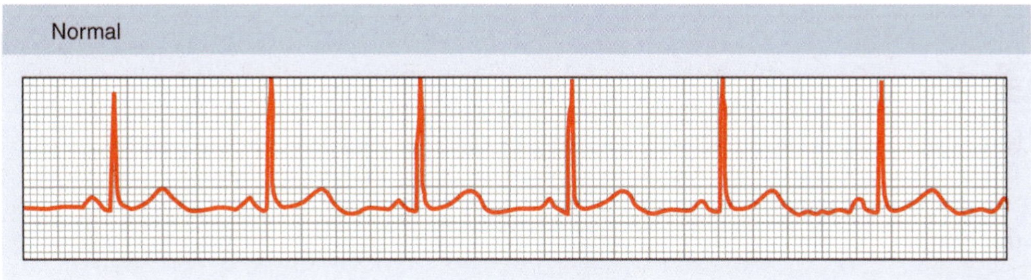

_______ / ___ / _______ / ___ / _______ showing a normal sinus rhythm.

electrical activity / CV / heart / CV / record

EXERCISE 28

Practice saying aloud each of the Diagnostic Terms Built from Word Parts.

> To hear the terms, go to Evolve Resources at evolve.elsevier.com and select:
> Practice Student Resources > Student Resources > Chapter 10 > **Pronounce and Spell**
>
> See Appendix B for instructions.

❑ Check the box when complete.

EXERCISE 29

Analyze and define the following diagnostic terms.

1. electrocardiograph
   ____
   ____
2. venogram
   ____
   ____
3. angiography
   ____
   ____
4. echocardiogram
   ____
   ____
5. aortogram
   ____
   ____
6. electrocardiogram
   ____
   ____
7. arteriogram
   ____
   ____
8. electrocardiography
   ____
   ____

9. angioscopy

____

____

10. angioscope

____

____

EXERCISE 30

Build diagnostic terms that correspond to the following definitions by using the word parts you have learned.

1. instrument used to record the electrical activity of the heart
   ____ / ____ / ____ / ____ / ____
   WR / CV / WR / CV / S
2. radiographic image of an artery (after an injection of contrast media)
   ____ / ____ / ____
   WR / CV / S
3. radiographic image of a vein (after an injection of contrast media)
   ____ / ____ / ____
   WR / CV / S
4. radiographic imaging of blood vessels
   ____ / ____ / ____
   WR / CV / S
5. record of the electrical activity of the heart
   ____ / ____ / ____ / ____ / ____
   WR / CV / WR / CV / S
6. record of the heart (structure and motion) using sound (waves)
   ____ / ____ / ____ / ____ / ____
   WR / CV / WR / CV / S
7. radiographic image of the aorta (after an injection of contrast media)
   ____ / ____ / ____
   WR / CV / S
8. process of recording the electrical activity of the heart
   ____ / ____ / ____ / ____ / ____
   WR / CV / WR / CV / S
9. visual examination (of the inside) of a blood vessel
   ____ / ____ / ____
   WR / CV / S
10. instrument used for visual examination (of the inside) of a blood vessel
   ____ / ____ / ____
   WR / CV / S

EXERCISE 31

Spell each of the Diagnostic Terms Built from Word Parts by having someone dictate them to you. Use a separate sheet of paper.

> To hear and spell the terms, go to Evolve Resources at evolve.elsevier.com and select:
> Practice Student Resources > Student Resources > Chapter 10 > **Pronounce and Spell**
>
> See Appendix B for instructions.

❑ Check the box when complete.

Diagnostic Terms

NOT BUILT FROM WORD PARTS

Word parts may be present in the following terms; however, their full meanings cannot be translated using definitions of word parts alone.

TERM	DEFINITION
CARDIOVASCULAR SYSTEM	
DIAGNOSTIC IMAGING	
digital subtraction angiography (DSA) (DIJ-i-tal) (sub-TRAK-shun) (*an*-jē-OG-ra-fē)	process of digital radiographic imaging of the blood vessels that "subtracts" or removes structures not being studied (Table 10.3)
Doppler ultrasound (DOP-ler) (UL-tra-sound)	study that uses high-frequency sound waves for detection of blood flow within the vessels; used to assess intermittent claudication, deep vein thrombosis, and other blood flow abnormalities
sestamibi test (*ses*-ta-MIB-ē) (test)	nuclear medicine test used to diagnose coronary artery disease and assess revascularization after coronary artery bypass surgery. Sestamibi, a radioactive isotope, is taken up by normal myocardial cells, but not in ischemia or infarction. These areas are identified as "cold" spots on the images produced.
single-photon emission computed tomography (SPECT) (SING-el-fō-ton) (ē-MISH-on) (com-PŪ-ted) (tō-MOG-ra-fē)	nuclear medicine scan that visualizes the heart from several different angles, producing three-dimensional images; used to assess damage to cardiac tissue
transesophageal echocardiogram (TEE) (*trans*-e-*sof*-a-JĒ-al) (*ek*-ō-KAR-dē-ō-*gram*)	ultrasound test that examines cardiac function and structure by using an ultrasound probe placed in the esophagus, which provides more direct views of the heart structures
DIAGNOSTIC PROCEDURES	
cardiac catheterization (KAR-dē-ak) (*kath*-e-ter-i-ZĀ-shun)	diagnostic procedure performed by passing a catheter into the heart from a blood vessel in the groin or arm to examine the condition of the heart and surrounding blood vessels; used to diagnose and treat cardiovascular conditions such as coronary artery disease
exercise stress test (EK-ser-sīz) (stres) (test)	study that evaluates cardiac function during physical stress by riding a bike or walking on a treadmill. **Electrocardiography** is the most common method, but **echocardiography,** and **nuclear medicine scanning** (diagnostic imaging tests) can also be used to measure cardiac function while exercising.

CHEMICAL STRESS TESTING

is the **use of drugs to simulate the stress of physical exercise** on the body. It is used to study cardiac function in patients who are unable to exercise.

Diagnostic Terms—cont'd

TERM	DEFINITION
OTHER	
blood pressure (BP) (blud) (PRES-ūr)	pressure exerted by the blood against the blood vessel walls. A blood pressure measurement written as **systolic** pressure (120) and **diastolic** pressure (80) is commonly recorded as 120/80 (blood pressure is measured in millimeters of mercury [mm Hg]).
pulse (puls)	contraction of the heart, which can be felt with a fingertip. The pulse is most commonly felt over the radial artery (in the wrist); however, the pulsations can be felt over a number of sites, including the femoral (groin) and carotid (neck) arteries.
sphygmomanometer (*sfig*-mō-ma-NOM-e-ter)	device used for measuring blood pressure
LABORATORY	
C-reactive protein (CRP) (C)-(rē-AK-tiv) (PRŌ-tēn)	blood test to measure the amount of C-reactive protein in the blood, which when elevated, indicates inflammation in the body. It is sometimes used in assessing the risk of cardiovascular disease.
creatine phosphokinase (CPK) (KRĒ-a-tin) (*fos*-fō-KĪ-nās)	blood test used to measure the level of creatine phosphokinase, an enzyme of heart and skeletal muscle released into the blood after muscle injury or necrosis. The test is useful in evaluating patients with acute myocardial infarction.
lipid profile (LIP-id) (PRŌ-fīl)	blood test used to measure the amount and type of lipids (fat-like substances) in a sample of blood. This test is used to evaluate one of the risks of cardiovascular disease, and to monitor therapy for patients taking lipid-lowering medications (Table 10-4).
troponin (TRŌ-pō-nin)	blood test that measures troponin, a heart muscle enzyme. Troponins are released into the blood approximately 3 hours after necrosis of the heart muscle and may remain elevated from 7 to 10 days. The test is useful in the diagnosis of a myocardial infarction.
BLOOD	
LABORATORY	
activated partial thromboplastin time (aPTT) (AK-ti-*vāt*-ed) (PAR-shel) (*throm*-bō-PLAS-tin) (tīm)	blood test used to monitor anticoagulation therapy for patients taking heparin, an intravenous anticoagulant medication
coagulation time (kō-*ag*-ū-LĀ-shun) (tīm)	blood test to determine the time it takes for blood to form a clot
complete blood count (CBC) and differential (Diff) (com-PLĒT) (blud) (kownt) (and) (*dif*-er-EN-shal)	laboratory test for basic blood screening that measures various aspects of erythrocytes, leukocytes, and thrombocytes (platelets); this automated test quickly provides a tremendous amount of information about the blood

BIOMARKER

is a naturally occurring substance of certain body cells that can be measured in the blood and used to aid in the diagnosis of various disorders. **Troponin, creatinine phosphokinase**, and **C-reactive protein** are biomarkers, and elevated levels are used in diagnosing various disorders occurring in the body.

TABLE 10.4 Understanding a Lipid Profile

Cholesterol—a compound important in the production of sex hormones, steroids, cell membranes, and bile acids. Cholesterol is produced by the body and is also contained in foods such as animal fats. Cholesterol is transported by lipoproteins.
High-density lipoprotein (HDL)—a type of lipoprotein that removes cholesterol from the tissues and transports it to the liver to be excreted in the bile. Elevated levels of HDL are considered protective against development of atherosclerosis, which may lead to coronary artery disease. HDL is often referred to as the "good" cholesterol.
Low-density lipoprotein (LDL)—a type of lipoprotein that transports cholesterol to the tissue and deposits it on the walls of the arteries. High levels of LDL are associated with the presence of atherosclerosis, which may lead to coronary artery disease. LDL is often referred to as the "bad" cholesterol.
Total cholesterol—a measurement of the cholesterol components LDL, HDL, and VLDL (triglyceride carriers) in the blood.
Triglycerides (TGs)—a form of fat in the blood. Triglycerides are synthesized in the liver and used to store energy. Test results are used to assess the risk of coronary artery disease.
Very-low-density lipoprotein (VLDL)—a type of lipoprotein that transports most of the triglycerides in the blood. Elevated levels of VLDL, to a lesser degree than LDL, indicate a risk for developing coronary artery disease.

TERM	DEFINITION
hematocrit (Hct) (hē-MAT-o-crit)	percentage of a blood sample that is composed of erythrocytes. It is used in the diagnosis and evaluation of anemic patients.
hemoglobin (Hgb) (HĒ-mō-*glō*-bin)	blood test that measures the amount of hemoglobin (the protein in red blood cells that carries oxygen) in the blood
prothrombin time (PT) (prō-THROM-bin) (tīm)	blood test used to determine certain coagulation activity defects and to monitor anticoagulation therapy for patients taking warfarin, an oral anticoagulant medication

PT/INR

stands for **prothrombin time/ international normalized ratio**. Most institutions, on the recommendation of the World Health Organization, report both absolute numbers and INR numbers, which provide uniform PT results to physicians worldwide.

EXERCISE 32

Practice saying aloud each of the Diagnostic Terms NOT Built from Word Parts.

To hear the terms, go to Evolve Resources at evolve.elsevier.com and select:
Practice Student Resources > Student Resources > Chapter 10 > **Pronounce and Spell**

See Appendix B for instructions.

❑ Check the box when complete.

EXERCISE 33

A. Fill in the blanks with the correct terms.

1. A device for measuring blood pressure is called a(n) ______________________.
2. ______________ ______________ is a blood test that determines the time it takes for blood to form a clot.
3. A blood test used to determine certain coagulation activity defects and to monitor oral anticoagulation therapy for patients taking warfarin is called ______________ ______________.
4. A blood test used to determine the oxygen-carrying protein in the blood is called ______________.
5. ______________ ______________ is a test in which an ultrasound probe provides views of the heart structures from the esophagus.
6. A blood test used to monitor anticoagulation therapy for patients taking heparin is called a(n) ______________ ______________ ______________ ______________.
7. A nuclear medicine test that visualizes the heart from several different angles, producing three dimensional images, is called a(n) ______________ ______________ ______________ ______________.
8. A blood test to measure an enzyme of the heart released into the bloodstream after muscle injury is called ______________ ______________.
9. An elevated ______________ ______________ indicates inflammation in the body.
10. ______________ is the rhythmic expansion of an artery created by contraction of the heart that can be felt with a fingertip.
11. ______________ is a heart muscle enzyme released into the bloodstream approximately 3 hours after heart muscle necrosis.
12. ______________ ______________ is the name of the blood test that measures the amount and type of lipids in the blood.
13. A test that determines the percentage of a blood sample that is composed of erythrocytes, and is used in the diagnosis and evaluation of anemic patients is called ______________.

B. Write the medical term pictured and defined.

1. ______________________
study that uses high-frequency sound waves for detection of blood flow within the vessels

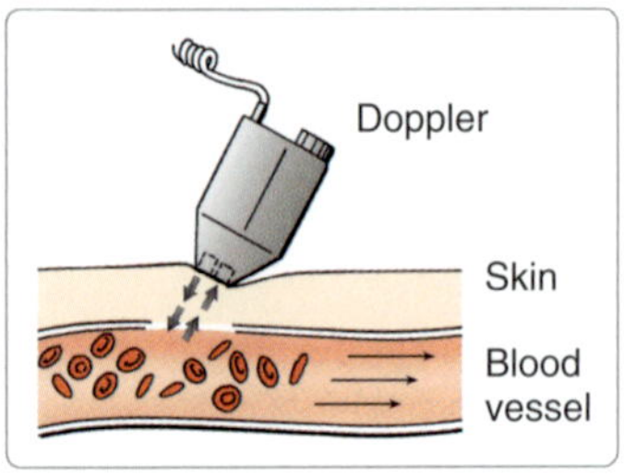

2. ______________________
____
laboratory test for basic blood screening that measures various aspects of erythrocytes, leukocytes, and thrombocytes (platelets)

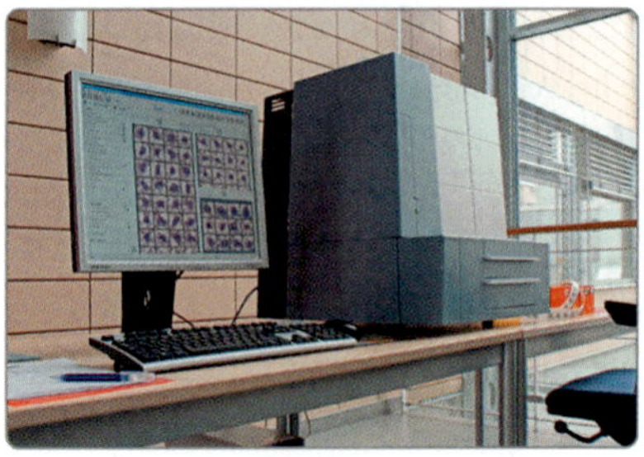

3. ______________________________

study that elevates cardiac function during physical stress by riding a bike or walking on a treadmill

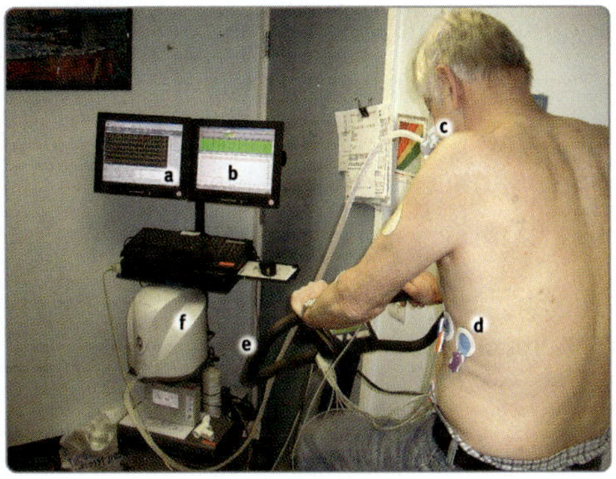

4. ______________________________

nuclear medicine test used to diagnose coronary artery disease and assess revascularization after CABG surgery

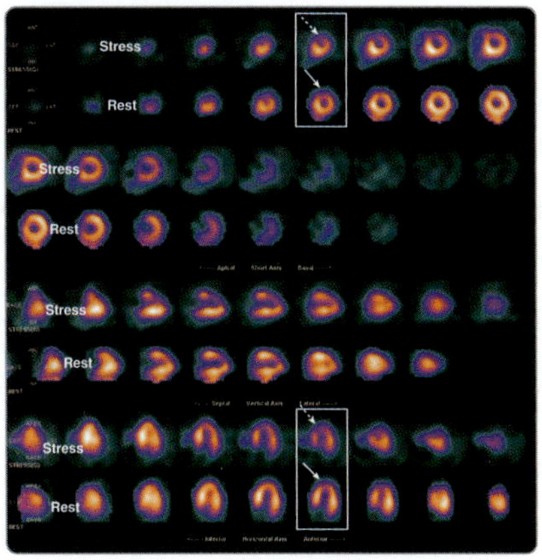

5. ______________________________

____

process of digital radiographic imaging of the blood vessels that "subtracts" or removes structures not being studied

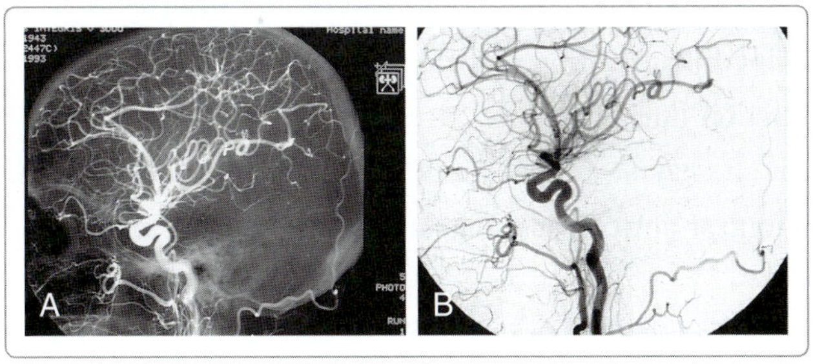

6. ______________________________

pressure exerted by the blood against the blood vessel walls

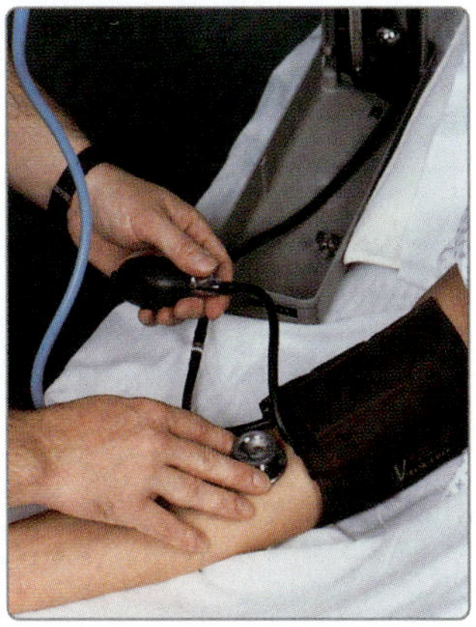

7. ______________________________

diagnostic procedure performed by passing a catheter into the heart from a vessel in the groin or arm to examine the condition of the heart and surrounding blood vessels

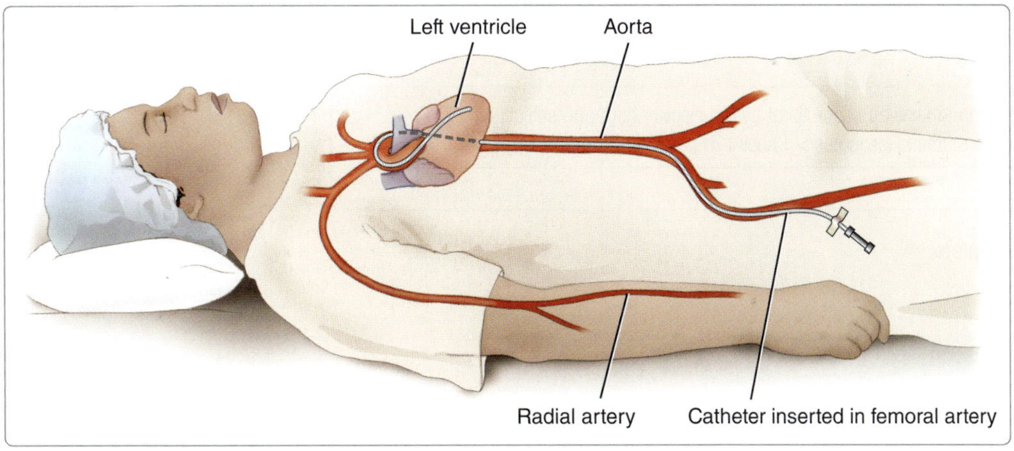

EXERCISE 34

Match the terms in the first column with their correct definitions in the second column.

_____ 1. cardiac catheterization
_____ 2. complete blood count and differential
_____ 3. coagulation time
_____ 4. hemoglobin
_____ 5. Doppler ultrasound
_____ 6. prothrombin time
_____ 7. sphygmomanometer
_____ 8. single-photon emission computed tomography
_____ 9. digital subtraction angiography
_____ 10. sestamibi test
_____ 11. transesophageal echocardiogram

a. device used for measuring blood pressure
b. digital radiographic imaging of blood vessels
c. test to determine certain coagulation activity defects
d. passage of a catheter into the heart to examine the condition of the heart and surrounding blood vessels
e. visualizes the heart from several different angles
f. used to assess revascularization after CABG
g. blood test used to determine the amount of oxygen-carrying proteins in the blood
h. basic blood-screening test
i. an ultrasound test that provides views of the heart from the esophagus
j. study in which high-frequency sound waves are used to determine the flow of blood within the vessels
k. determines the time it takes for blood to form a clot

EXERCISE 35

Match the terms in the first column with the correct definitions in the second column.

_____ 1. exercise stress test
_____ 2. activated partial thromboplastin time
_____ 3. C-reactive protein
_____ 4. blood pressure
_____ 5. creatine phosphokinase
_____ 6. hematocrit
_____ 7. pulse
_____ 8. lipid profile
_____ 9. troponin

a. the percentage of a blood sample that is composed of erythrocytes
b. blood test to determine inflammation or risk of cardiovascular disease
c. measures cardiac function during physical stress
d. measures the level of an enzyme released into the blood after muscle injury
e. blood test used to monitor anticoagulation therapy for patients taking heparin
f. pressure exerted by blood against the blood vessel walls
g. measured most often over the radial artery
h. blood test used to measure the amount and type of lipids in a sample of blood
i. measures an enzyme released within hours after damage to the heart muscle

EXERCISE 36

Spell each of the Diagnostic Terms NOT Built from Word Parts by having someone dictate them to you. Use a separate sheet of paper.

To hear and spell the terms, go to Evolve Resources at evolve.elsevier.com and select:
Practice Student Resources > Student Resources > Chapter10 > **Pronounce and Spell**

See Appendix B for instructions.

❑ Check the box when complete.

Complementary Terms
BUILT FROM WORD PARTS

The following terms can be translated using definitions of word parts. Further explanation is provided within parentheses as needed.

TERM	DEFINITION
CARDIOVASCULAR SYSTEM	
atrioventricular (AV) (*ā*-trē-ō-ven-TRIK-ū-ler)	pertaining to the atrium and ventricle
cardiac (KAR-dē-ak)	pertaining to the heart
cardiogenic (*kar*-dē-ō-JEN-ik)	originating in the heart
cardiologist (*kar*-dē-OL-o-jist)	physician who studies and treats diseases of the heart
cardiology (*kar*-dē-OL-o-jē)	study of the heart (a branch of medicine that deals with diseases of the heart)
hypothermia (*hī*-pō-THER-mē-a)	condition of (body) temperature that is below (normal) (sometimes induced for various surgical procedures, such as bypass surgery)
intravenous (IV) (*in*-tra-VĒ-nus)	pertaining to within the vein (Exercise Figure G)
BLOOD	
hematologist (*hē*-ma-TOL-o-jist)	physician who studies and treats diseases of the blood
hematology (*hē*-ma-TOL-o-jē)	study of the blood (branch of medicine that deals with diseases of the blood)
hematopoiesis (*hē*-ma-tō-poy-Ē-sis)	formation of blood (cells)
hemolysis (*hē*-MOL-i-sis)	dissolution of (red) blood (cells)
hemostasis (*hē*-mō-STĀ-sis)	stoppage of bleeding
myelopoiesis (*mī*-e-lō-poy-Ē-sis)	formation of bone marrow
plasmapheresis (*plaz*-ma-fe-RĒ-sis)	removal of plasma (from withdrawn blood); (the cells [formed elements] are then reinfused into the donor or into another patient who needs blood cells rather than whole blood)
thrombolysis (throm-BOL-i-sis)	dissolution of a clot

ELECTROPHYSIOLOGIST

is a **cardiologist** who specializes in the diagnosis and treatment of patients with arrhythmias.

INTRAVENOUS (IV) THERAPY

is **the infusion of a substance directly into a vein** for therapeutic purposes. **IV therapy** is a very common and essential component of medical care, serving as a direct, efficient route for the administration of fluids, medications, and blood products.

EXERCISE FIGURE G

Fill in the blanks with word parts defined to complete labeling of the diagram.

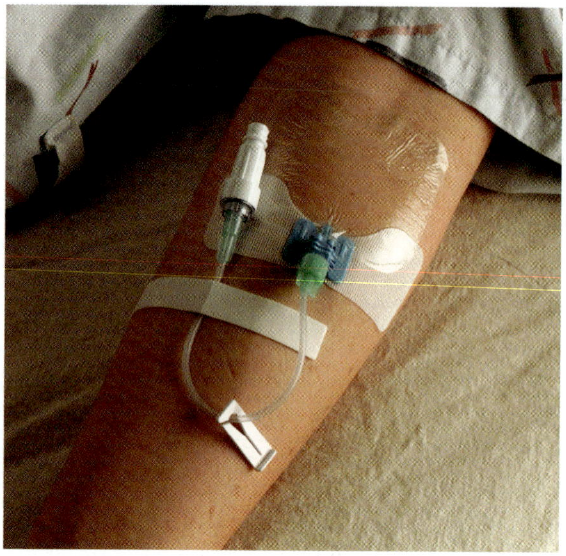

Patient's arm with an ________ / ________ / ________ (IV) catheter.
within / vein / pertaining to

EXERCISE 37

Practice saying aloud each of the Complementary Terms Built from Word Parts.

To hear the terms, go to Evolve Resources at evolve.elsevier.com and select:
Practice Student Resources > Student Resources > Chapter 10 > **Pronounce and Spell**

See Appendix B for instructions.

❑ Check the box when complete.

EXERCISE 38

Analyze and define the following complementary terms.

1. hypothermia
____
____

2. hematopoiesis
____
____

3. cardiology
____
____

4. cardiologist
____
____

5. hemolysis
____
____

6. hematologist
____
____

7. cardiac

____

____

8. hematology

____

____

9. plasmapheresis

____

____

10. hemostasis

____

____

11. cardiogenic

____

____

12. myelopoiesis

____

____

13. thrombolysis

____

____

14. atrioventricular

____

____

15. intravenous

____

____

EXERCISE 39

Build the complementary terms for the following definitions by using the word parts you have learned.

1. study of the heart ______ WR / CV / S
2. formation of blood (cells) ______ WR / CV / S
3. condition of (body) temperature that is below (normal) ______ P / WR / S
4. dissolution of (red) blood (cells) ______ WR / CV / S
5. removal of plasma (from withdrawn blood) ______ WR / S
6. physician who studies and treats diseases of the blood ______ WR / CV / S
7. pertaining to the heart ______ WR / S
8. physician who studies and treats diseases of the heart ______ WR / CV / S

9. study of the blood ______ WR / CV / S

10. stoppage of bleeding ______ WR / CV / S

11. formation of bone marrow ______ WR / CV / S

12. originating in the heart ______ WR / CV / S

13. dissolution of a clot ______ WR / CV / S

14. pertaining to the atrium and ventricle ______ WR / CV / WR / S

15. pertaining to within the vein ______ P / WR / S

EXERCISE 40

Spell each of the Complementary Terms Built from Word Parts by having someone dictate them to you. Use a separate sheet of paper.

> To hear and spell the terms, go to Evolve Resources at evolve.elsevier.com and select:
> Practice Student Resources > Student Resources > Chapter 10 > **Pronounce and Spell**
>
> See Appendix B for instructions.

❑ Check the box when complete.

Cardiovascular System and Blood Complementary Terms

NOT BUILT FROM WORD PARTS

Word parts may be present in the following terms; however, their full meanings cannot be translated using definitions of word parts alone.

TERM	DEFINITION
CARDIOVASCULAR SYSTEM	
bruit (broo-Ē)	abnormal vascular sound heard through auscultation, caused by turbulent blood flow through arteries or veins. Cardiovascular system abnormalities, such as **aneurysm**, create a distinctive bruit. Bruits may occur in numerous sites throughout the body where blood flow or body system functioning is abnormal.
cardiopulmonary resuscitation (CPR) (*kar*-dē-ō-PUL-mo-nar-ē) (rē-*sus*-i-TĀ-shun)	emergency procedure consisting of external cardiac compressions; may be accompanied by artificial ventilation

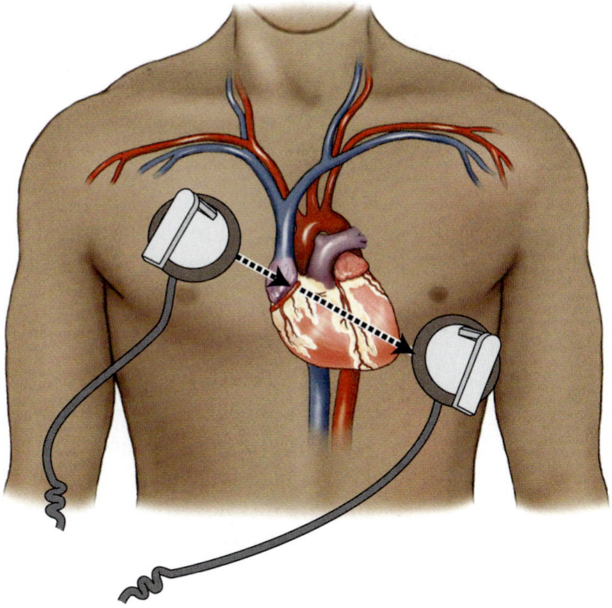

FIG. 10.15 Placement of defibrillator paddles on the chest.

TERM	DEFINITION
defibrillation (dē-*fib*-ri-LĀ-shun)	application of an electric shock to the myocardium through the chest wall to restore normal cardiac rhythm (Fig. 10.15)
diastole (dī-AS-tō-lē)	phase in the cardiac cycle in which the ventricles relax and fill with blood between contractions (diastolic is the lower number of a blood pressure reading)
extracorporeal (*ek*-stra-kōr-POR-ē-al)	occurring outside the body. During open-heart surgery, extracorporeal circulation occurs when blood is diverted outside the body to a heart-lung machine.
extravasation (ek-*strav*-a-SĀ-shun)	escape of blood or other fluid from a vessel into the tissue
fibrillation (fi-bri-LĀ-shun)	rapid, quivering, uncoordinated contractions of the atria or ventricles
hypercholesterolemia (*hī*-per-k-*les*-ter-ol-Ē-mē-a)	excessive amount of cholesterol in the blood; associated with an increased risk of cardiovascular disease
hyperlipidemia (*hī*-per-*lip*-i-DĒ-mē-a)	excessive amount of any type of fats (lipoproteins, triglycerides, and cholesterol) in the blood; associated with an increased risk of cardiovascular disease
hypertension (HTN) (*hī*-per-TEN-shun)	blood pressure that is above normal (greater than 140/90 mm Hg in an adult under the age of 60)
hypertriglyceridemia (*hī*-per-trī-*glis*-er-rī-DĒ-mē-a)	excessive amount of triglycerides in the blood; associated with an increased risk of cardiovascular disease

Cardiovascular System and Blood Complementary Terms—cont'd

TERM	DEFINITION
hypotension (*hī*-pō-TEN-shun)	blood pressure that is below normal (less than 90/60 mm Hg in an adult under the age of 60)
lipids (LIP-ids)	fats and fatlike substances that serve as a source of fuel in the body and are an important constituent of cell structure
lumen (LŪ-men)	the cavity or channel within a tube or tubular organ
murmur (MER-mer)	abnormal cardiac sound heard through auscultation; caused by turbulent blood flow through the heart. Murmurs are short-duration sounds heard in the cardiac region that are distinct from normal heart sounds. Heart valve defects, such as **mitral valve stenosis**, create a distinctive murmur.
occlude (o-KLŪD)	to close tightly, to block
phlebotomist (fle-BOT-ō-mist)	person who performs phlebotomy (incision into a vein) for the purpose of drawing blood or injecting IV fluids
systole (SIS-tō-lē)	phase in the cardiac cycle in which the ventricles contract and eject blood (systolic is the upper number of a blood pressure reading)
vasoconstrictor (*vās*-ō-kon-STRIK-tor)	agent or nerve that narrows the diameter of the blood vessels
vasodilator (*vās*-ō-DĪ-lā-tor)	agent or nerve that expands the diameter of the blood vessels
venipuncture (VEN-i-*punk*-chur)	procedure used to puncture a vein with a needle to remove blood, instill a medication, or start an intravenous infusion
BLOOD	
anticoagulant (*an*-tī-kō-AG-ū-lant)	agent that slows the blood clotting process
blood dyscrasia (blud) (dis-KRĀ-zha)	abnormal or pathologic condition of the blood
hemorrhage (HEM-o-rij)	rapid loss of blood, as in bleeding

DYSCRASIA
is made up of the Greek word parts **dys-**, meaning difficult, painful or abnormal, and **-crasia**, meaning mixture. Blood disease in ancient Greek times was thought to be an abnormal mixture of the four humors: blood, black bile, yellow bile, and phlegm. Today the term remains, but its full meaning can no longer be directly translated from its word parts.

EXERCISE 41

Practice saying aloud each of the Cardiovascular System and Blood Complementary Terms NOT Built from Word Parts.

To hear the terms, go to Evolve Resources at evolve.elsevier.com and select:
Practice Student Resources > Student Resources > Chapter 10 > **Pronounce and Spell**

See Appendix B for instructions.

❑ Check the box when complete.

EXERCISE 42

Write the term for each of the following definitions.

1. agent that narrows the blood vessels ____________________
2. cavity or channel within a tube or tubular organ ____________________
3. emergency procedure consisting of external cardiac compressions, which may be accompanied by artificial ventilation ____________________
4. phase in the cardiac cycle in which the ventricles relax ____________________
5. noncoordinated contractions of the atria or ventricles ____________________
6. blood pressure that is below normal ____________________
7. escape of blood or other fluid from the vessel into the tissue ____________________
8. puncture of a vein to remove blood ____________________
9. phase in the cardiac cycle in which the ventricles contract ____________________
10. agent that enlarges the diameter of blood vessels ____________________
11. blood pressure that is above normal ____________________
12. to close tightly ____________________
13. excessive amount of triglycerides in the blood ____________________
14. excessive amount of any type of fats in the blood ____________________
15. rapid loss of blood ____________________
16. excessive amount of cholesterol in the blood ____________________
17. pathologic condition of the blood ____________________
18. abnormal cardiac sound heard through auscultation ____________________
19. occurring outside the body ____________________
20. fats and fatlike substances ____________________
21. used to restore normal cardiac rhythm ____________________
22. agent that slows the clotting process ____________________
23. abnormal vascular sound heard through auscultation ____________________
24. person who performs phlebotomy for the purpose of drawing blood or injecting IV fluids ____________________

EXERCISE 43

Spell each of the Cardiovascular System and Blood Complementary Terms NOT Built from Word Parts by having someone dictate them to you. Use a separate sheet of paper.

> To hear and spell the terms, go to Evolve Resources at evolve.elsevier.com and select:
> Practice Student Resources > Student Resources > Chapter 10 > **Pronounce and Spell**
>
> See Appendix B for instructions.

❑ Check the box when complete.

Immune System Complementary Terms

NOT BUILT FROM WORD PARTS

Word parts may be present in the following terms; however, their full meanings cannot be translated using definitions of word parts alone.

HYPERSENSITIVITY

refers to a condition in which the body "overreacts" to something which it perceives to be a foreign substance, such as an **allergen**.

TERM	DEFINITION
allergen (AL-er-jen)	environmental substance capable of producing a hypersensitivity reaction (allergy) in the body. Common allergens are house dust, pollen, animal dander, and various foods.
allergist (AL-er-jist)	physician who studies and treats allergic conditions
allergy (AL-er-jē)	hypersensitivity to a substance, resulting in an inflammatory immune response
anaphylaxis (*an*-a-fe-LAK-sis)	exaggerated reaction to a previously encountered antigen such as bee venom, peanuts, or latex. While symptoms may initially be mild, such as hives or sneezing, anaphylaxis can quickly become severe. When it leads to a drop in blood pressure and blockage of the airway (which can lead to death within minutes), it is called **anaphylactic shock**.
antibody (AN-ti-*bod*-ē)	substance produced by lymphocytes that inactivates or destroys antigens (also called **immunoglobulins**)
antigen (AN-ti-jen)	substance that triggers an immune response when introduced into the body. Examples of antigens are transplant tissue, toxins, and infectious organisms.
autoimmune disease (*aw*-tō-i-MŪN) (di-ZĒZ)	disease caused by the body's inability to distinguish its own cells from foreign bodies, thus producing antibodies that attack its own tissue. **Rheumatoid arthritis** and **systemic lupus erythematosus** are examples of autoimmune diseases.
immune (i-MŪN)	being resistant to specific invading pathogens
immunodeficiency (*im*-ū-nō-de-FISH-en-sē)	deficient immune response caused by immune system dysfunction brought on by disease (such as HIV infection) or immunosuppressive drugs (such as prednisone or cancer chemotherapy)
immunologist (*im*-ū-NOL-o-jist)	physician who studies and treats immune system disorders
immunology (*im*-ū-NOL-o-jē)	branch of medicine dealing with immune system disorders
phagocytosis (*fā*-gō-sī-TŌ-sis)	process in which some of the white blood cells destroy the invading microorganism and old cells
vaccine (vak-SĒN)	suspension of weakened or killed microorganisms administered by injection, mouth, or nasal spray, which induces immunity to prevent an infectious disease

TYPES OF IMMUNITY

Inherited immunity: immunity to certain diseases develops before birth; also called inborn immunity

Acquired immunity: develops after birth; can be *natural* (exposure to the cause is not deliberate) or *artificial* (exposure to the cause is deliberate)

Refer to **Appendix F** for pharmacology terms related to the cardiovascular system and blood.

EXERCISE 44

Practice saying aloud each of the Immune System Complementary Terms NOT Built from Word Parts.

To hear the terms, go to Evolve Resources at evolve.elsevier.com and select:
Practice Student Resources > Student Resources > Chapter 10 > **Pronounce and Spell**

See Appendix B for instructions.

❑ Check the box when complete.

EXERCISE 45

Match the immune system terms in the first column with the phrases in the second column.

_____	1. allergen	a. deficient immune response
_____	2. autoimmune disease	b. branch of medicine dealing with immune system disorders
_____	3. immunologist	c. administered by injection, nasal spray, or orally to prevent an infectious disease
_____	4. antigen	d. inactivate or destroy antigens
_____	5. immune	e. house dust, pollen, animal dander
_____	6. allergist	f. transplant tissue, toxin, infectious organisms
_____	7. antibodies	g. physician who treats allergic conditions
_____	8. immunodeficiency	h. white blood cells destroy invading microorganisms
_____	9. phagocytosis	i. hypersensitivity to a substance
_____	10. vaccine	j. rheumatoid arthritis is an example
_____	11. allergy	k. exaggerated reaction to a previously encountered antigen
_____	12. immunology	l. resistant to specific invading pathogens
_____	13. anaphylaxis	m. physician who treats immune system disorders

EXERCISE 46

Spell each of the Immune System Complementary Terms NOT Built from Word Parts by having someone dictate them to you. Use a separate sheet of paper.

To hear and spell the terms, go to Evolve Resources at evolve.elsevier.com and select:
Practice Student Resources > Student Resources > Chapter 10 > **Pronounce and Spell**

See Appendix B for instructions.

❑ Check the box when complete.

Abbreviations

ABBREVIATION	TERM
ACS	acute coronary syndrome
AFib	atrial fibrillation
AICD	automatic implantable cardiac defibrillator
aPTT	activated partial thromboplastin time
AV	atrioventricular
BP	blood pressure
CABG	coronary artery bypass graft
CAD	coronary artery disease

WEB LINK

For additional information on the cardiovascular system, visit the **American Heart Association at** ***www.heart.org.***

WEB LINK

For additional information on the lymphatic system and blood, visit the **Leukemia and Lymphoma Society at** ***www.lls.org.***

Abbreviations—cont'd

ABBREVIATION	TERM
CBC and Diff	complete blood count and differential
CCU	coronary care unit
CPK	creatine phosphokinase
CPR	cardiopulmonary resuscitation
CRP	C-reactive protein
DSA	digital subtraction angiography
DVT	deep vein thrombosis
ECG, EKG	electrocardiogram
ECHO	echocardiogram
Hct	hematocrit
HF	heart failure
Hgb	hemoglobin
HHD	hypertensive heart disease
HTN	hypertension
IV	intravenous
MI	myocardial infarction
PAD	peripheral artery disease
PT	prothrombin time
PTCA	percutaneous transluminal coronary angioplasty
RBC	red blood cell (erythrocyte)
SPECT	single-photon emission computed tomography
TEE	transesophageal echocardiogram
WBC	white blood cell (leukocyte)

Refer to **Appendix E** for a complete list of abbreviations.

EXERCISE 47

Write the terms abbreviated.

1. **CAD** __________ __________ __________ has received growing interest over the past several years. Diagnostic procedures for new patients usually begin with an exercise **ECG** __________ __________. Patients whose stress tests are borderline usually proceed to noninvasive imaging such as **SPECT** __________ __________ __________ __________ and stress **ECHO** __________.
2. **DVT** __________ __________ __________ is common in hospitalized patients. Early detection is important because DVT can result in death from a pulmonary embolism. Doppler ultrasound is a noninvasive diagnostic procedure used to diagnose DVT. MRI and venography may be used as well.
3. The **CBC** __________ __________ __________ and **Diff** __________ are a series of automated laboratory tests of the peripheral blood that provide a great deal of information about the blood and other body organs. Tests performed as part of the CBC are **RBC** __________ __________ __________ count, **WBC** __________ __________ __________ count and differential, **Hgb** __________, and **Hct** __________.

4. Standard surgical treatment for CAD includes **CABG** _______________ _______________ _______________ _______________. There is a growth in the use of minimally invasive techniques to treat CAD, which include transmyocardial laser revascularization and **PTCA** _______________ _______________ _______________ _______________, atherectomy, and stent placement.
5. Hospitalized patients diagnosed with **MI** _______________ _______________ are cared for in the **CCU** _______________ _______________ _______________.
6. A sphygmomanometer is used to measure **BP** _______________ _______________.
7. Diagnosis used to indicate that a patient's heart is unable to pump enough blood through the body to supply tissues is **HF** _______________ _______________.
8. If the patient's heart and/or lungs have ceased to function, the medical team must begin **CPR** _______________ _______________.
9. A patient with persistently elevated blood pressure is likely to be diagnosed with **HHD** _______________ _______________ _______________.
10. When scheduling blood tests for a patient on oral anticoagulant medication, the doctor is likely to include a **PT** _______________ _______________.
11. Any interruption of the conduction of electrical impulses from the atria to the ventricles is called **AV** _______________ block.
12. The treatment of **ACS** _______________ _______________ _______________ is aimed at preventing thrombus formation and restoring blood flow to the occluded coronary artery.
13. Stopping smoking, exercising, and proper diet are important in the medical management of **PAD** _______________ _______________ _______________.
14. **DSA** _______________ _______________ _______________ is especially valuable in cardiac diagnostic applications.
15. The physician ordered a **TEE** _______________ _______________ to examine the patient's heart structure and function.
16. Two blood tests used in assessing and evaluating cardiovascular diseases are **CRP** _______________ _______________ and **CPK** _______________ _______________.
17. A patient experiencing **AFib** _______________ _______________ may be referred to an electrophysiologist, a cardiology subspecialist.
18. An **AICD** _______________ _______________ _______________ _______________ delivers an electric shock to convert an arrhythmia back to normal rhythm.
19. The patient with dehydration was ordered **IV** _______________ fluids by her physician.
20. **HTN** _______________ is usually diagnosed when a patient has elevated blood pressure on two separate occasions.

For additional practice with Abbreviations, go to Evolve Resources at evolve.elsevier.com and select: Practice Student Resources > Student Resources > Chapter 10 **Flashcards:** Abbreviations

See Appendix B for instructions.

PRACTICAL APPLICATION

EXERCISE 48 *Case Study: Translate Between Everyday Language and Medical Language*

CASE STUDY: Natalia Krouse

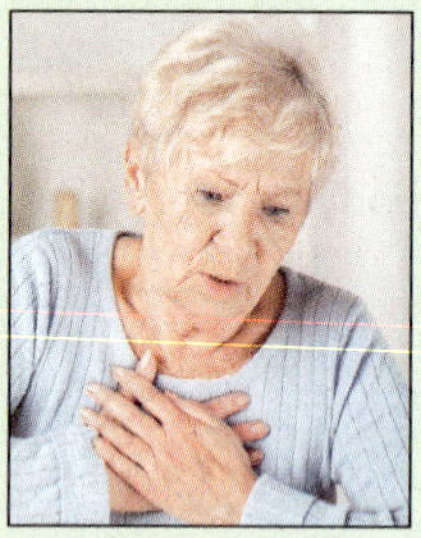

Natalia has not been feeling well lately. She seems to feel "wiped out" most of the time. She wonders if maybe her medicine for high blood pressure isn't working as well as it used to. Tonight she went for her usual walk after dinner with her dogs. She had barely made it down the driveway when she started feeling pain in her chest. It felt like something pushing down on her and squeezing her. She noticed pain in her left arm and even in her jaw. She noticed her heart was racing, and she was breathing faster than usual. She was also feeling dizzy at the same time and was afraid she might pass out. She stopped to sit down and after about 5 minutes she started feeling a little better. Her neighbor saw her and called 911. An ambulance came and took her to the Emergency Department.

Now that you have worked through Chapter 10 on the cardiovascular system, consider the medical terms that might be used to describe Natalia's experience. See the Review of Terms at the end of the chapter for a list of terms that might apply.

A. *Underline phrases in the case study that could be substituted with medical terms.*

B. *Write the medical term and its definition for three of the phrases you underlined.*

MEDICAL TERM	DEFINITION
1. ______________________	______________________________________
2. ______________________	______________________________________
3. ______________________	______________________________________

DOCUMENTATION: Excerpt From Hospital Admission Report

Natalia was brought to the emergency department and was admitted to the cardiology floor of the hospital. A portion of her history from the electronic medical record is noted below.

History of Present Illness: The patient has an extensive history of chronic cardiovascular issues. Coronary artery disease risk factors include hypertension and hypercholesterolemia. She also has extensive varicose veins of the lower extremities bilaterally. Her family physician referred her to a cardiologist in 2003 for medical management of these complications. She smokes one pack of cigarettes a day and has previously declined participation in a smoking cessation program. She is not diabetic. Family history reveals a brother who had coronary artery bypass grafts and a mother deceased from abdominal aortic aneurysm rupture.

C. *Underline medical terms presented in Chapter 10 in the previous excerpt from Natalia's medical record. See the Review of Terms at the end of the chapter for a complete list.*

D. *Select and define three of the medical terms you underlined. To check your answers, go to Appendix A.*

MEDICAL TERM	DEFINITION
1. ______________________	______________________________________
2. ______________________	______________________________________
3. ______________________	______________________________________

EXERCISE 49 *Interact With Medical Documents and Electronic Health Records*

A. Read the report and complete it by writing medical terms on answer lines within the document. Definitions of terms to be written appear after the document.

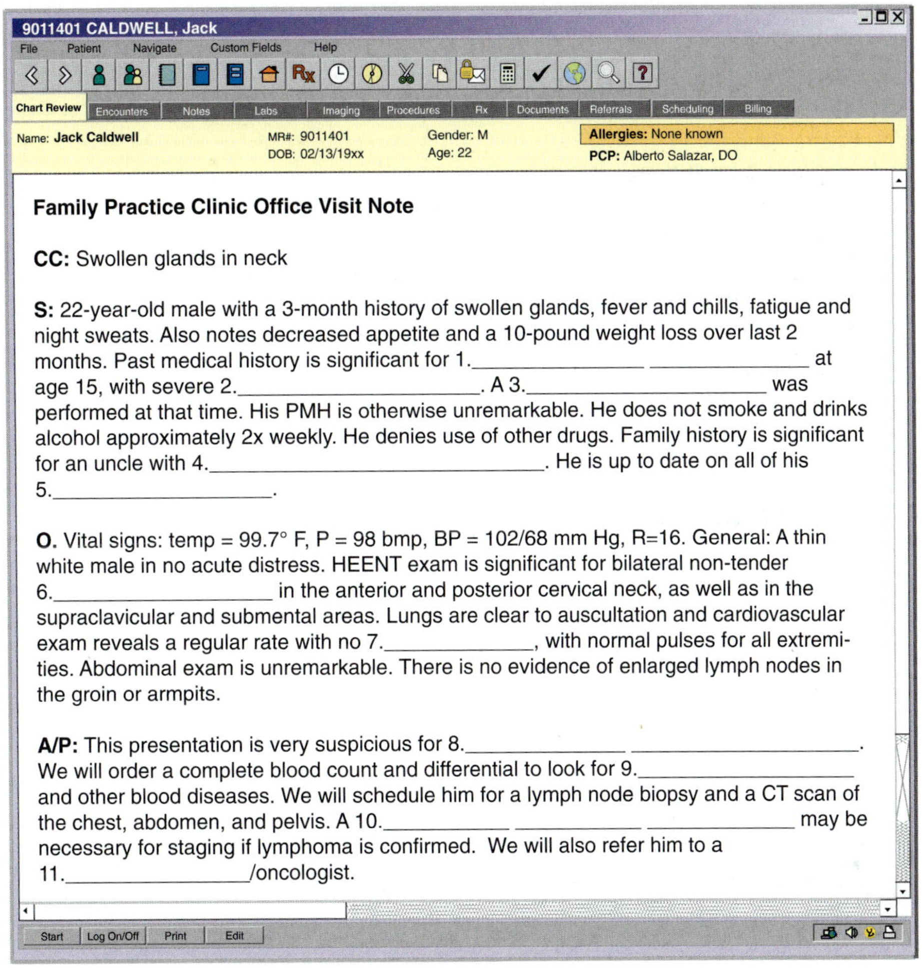
9011401 CALDWELL, Jack

File Patient Navigate Custom Fields Help

Chart Review | Encounters | Notes | Labs | Imaging | Procedures | Rx | Documents | Referrals | Scheduling | Billing

Name: **Jack Caldwell** MR#: 9011401 DOB: 02/13/19xx Gender: M Age: 22 **Allergies:** None known **PCP:** Alberto Salazar, DO

Family Practice Clinic Office Visit Note

CC: Swollen glands in neck

S: 22-year-old male with a 3-month history of swollen glands, fever and chills, fatigue and night sweats. Also notes decreased appetite and a 10-pound weight loss over last 2 months. Past medical history is significant for 1.______________ ______________ at age 15, with severe 2.____________________. A 3.____________________ was performed at that time. His PMH is otherwise unremarkable. He does not smoke and drinks alcohol approximately 2x weekly. He denies use of other drugs. Family history is significant for an uncle with 4.____________________________. He is up to date on all of his 5.__________________.

O. Vital signs: temp = 99.7° F, P = 98 bmp, BP = 102/68 mm Hg, R=16. General: A thin white male in no acute distress. HEENT exam is significant for bilateral non-tender 6.__________________ in the anterior and posterior cervical neck, as well as in the supraclavicular and submental areas. Lungs are clear to auscultation and cardiovascular exam reveals a regular rate with no 7.____________, with normal pulses for all extremities. Abdominal exam is unremarkable. There is no evidence of enlarged lymph nodes in the groin or armpits.

A/P: This presentation is very suspicious for 8.______________ ____________________. We will order a complete blood count and differential to look for 9.__________________ and other blood diseases. We will schedule him for a lymph node biopsy and a CT scan of the chest, abdomen, and pelvis. A 10.______________ ____________ ____________ may be necessary for staging if lymphoma is confirmed. We will also refer him to a 11.______________/oncologist.

Start | Log On/Off | Print | Edit

Definitions of Medical Terms to Complete the Document

Write the medical terms defined on corresponding answer lines in the document.

1. acute infection caused by the Epstein-Barr virus characterized by swollen lymph nodes, sore throat, fatigue, and fever
2. enlargement of the spleen
3. excision of the spleen
4. tumor of lymphatic tissue (malignant)
5. suspension of weakened or killed microorganisms administered by injection, mouth, or nasal spray
6. disease of lymph nodes
7. any disturbance or abnormality in the heart's normal rhythmic pattern
8. malignant disorder of the lymphatic tissue characterized by progressive enlargement of the lymph nodes, usually beginning in the cervical nodes
9. malignant disease characterized by excessive increase in abnormal leukocytes formed in the bone marrow
10. procedure to obtain a sample of the solid portion of bone marrow, usually from the ilium, for study
11. physician who studies and treats diseases of the blood

EXERCISE 49 *Interact With Medical Documents and Electronic Health Records—cont'd*

B. Read the medical report and answer the questions below it.

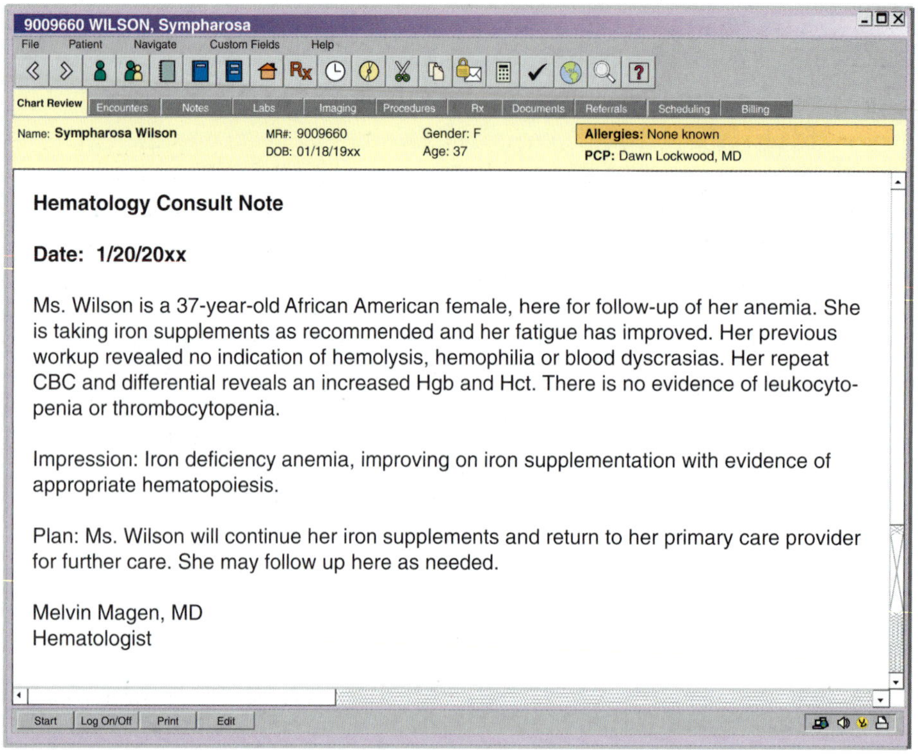

Hematology Consult Note

Date: 1/20/20xx

Ms. Wilson is a 37-year-old African American female, here for follow-up of her anemia. She is taking iron supplements as recommended and her fatigue has improved. Her previous workup revealed no indication of hemolysis, hemophilia or blood dyscrasias. Her repeat CBC and differential reveals an increased Hgb and Hct. There is no evidence of leukocytopenia or thrombocytopenia.

Impression: Iron deficiency anemia, improving on iron supplementation with evidence of appropriate hematopoiesis.

Plan: Ms. Wilson will continue her iron supplements and return to her primary care provider for further care. She may follow up here as needed.

Melvin Magen, MD
Hematologist

Use the medical report above to answer the questions.

1. Ms. Wilson was seen in the hematology clinic for:
   a. a low platelet count
   b. a low erythrocyte count
   c. a low white blood cell count
2. Her repeat CBC and differential revealed an improved:
   a. hemoglobin and C-reactive protein
   b. hematocrit and troponin
   c. hemoglobin and hematocrit
3. The consulting doctor was a physician who studies and treats:
   a. immune system disorders
   b. diseases of the blood
   c. diseases of the heart
4. **True** or **False**: the patient had evidence of dissolution of red blood cells.
5. **True** or **False**: the reason for the hematology consult was erythrocytopenia.

C. Complete the **three medical documents** within the electronic health record (EHR) on Evolve.

Topic: CAD
Documents: Echocardiogram Report, Cardiovascular Operative Report, Discharge Summary

To complete the three medical records, go to Evolve Resources at evolve.elsevier.com and select:
Practice Student Resources > Student Resources > Chapter 10 > **Electronic Heath Records**

See Appendix B for instructions.

EXERCISE 50 *Pronounce Medical Terms in Use*

Practice pronunciation of terms by reading aloud the following paragraph. Use the phonetic spellings following medical terms from the chapter to assist with pronunciation. The script also contains medical terms not presented in the chapter. Treat them as information only or look for their meanings in a medical dictionary or a reliable online source.

A 55-year-old man presented to his doctor with pain in the calf and swelling in the left foot and ankle. Three days prior, the patient had completed trans-Pacific airline travel, spending several hours in a sitting position. He has a history of **varicose veins** (VAR-i-kōs) (vānz). No previous history of **hypertension** (*hī*-per-TEN-shun) or **thrombophlebitis** (*throm*-bō-fle-BĪ-tis) existed. Physical examination revealed an edematous left lower extremity and a tender calf. The pedal **pulse** (puls) was intact. A **Doppler ultrasound** (DOP-ler) (UL-tra-sound) was obtained, which revealed **deep vein thrombosis** (dēp) (vān) (throm-BŌ-sis). The patient was hospitalized and subcutaneous low molecular weight heparin was begun. Concurrently, Coumadin was started and will continue for 6 months. The oral **anticoagulant** (*an*-tī-cō-AG-ū-lant) therapy will be monitored monthly by **prothrombin time** (prō-THROM-bin) (tīm).

EXERCISE 51 *Chapter Content Quiz*

Test your understanding of terms and abbreviations introduced in this chapter. Circle the letter for the medical term or abbreviation related to the words in italics.

1. Ms. Tompkins was diagnosed with sickle cell disease and was sent to a *physician who studies and treats diseases of the blood* for further evaluation.
   a. cardiologist
   b. immunologist
   c. hematologist
2. Following a trans-Pacific flight, Kenji Makoto developed *inflammation of the vein associated with a (blood) clot*, which was probably due to sitting for a long period of time.
   a. thrombophlebitis
   b. lymphadenitis
   c. atherosclerosis
3. Ted Lauer had a *record of the electrical activity of the heart* to follow up on his atrial fibrillation.
   a. CPR
   b. ECG
   c. ECHO
4. Mr. Schonfeld was diagnosed with a 6-centimeter abdominal aortic *ballooning of a weakened portion of a vessel wall*, which required surgical repair with an endograft.
   a. coarctation
   b. thrombosis
   c. aneurysm
5. On physical examination of the neck, Samantha Winslow was noted to have *disease of lymph nodes (abnormal enlargement of the lymph nodes)*.
   a. lymphoma
   b. lymphadenopathy
   c. lymphadenitis
6. After finishing a course of immunosuppressive medication for cancer treatment, a CBC revealed that the patient had *abnormal reduction of white blood cells*.
   a. leukocytopenia
   b. anemia
   c. thrombocytopenia
7. Mr. Matthews has an allergy to peanuts; he carries an EpiPen to prevent *episodes of exaggerated reaction to a previously encountered antigen which can lead to death within minutes*.
   a. immunodeficiency
   b. anaphylaxis
   c. autoimmune disease
8. Mrs. Patel was experiencing *episodes of chest pain that occurs when there is an insufficient amount of blood to the heart muscle* and was scheduled for an exercise stress test.
   a. acute coronary syndrome
   b. atrial fibrillation
   c. angina pectoris

9. Because Mr. Jiang is taking warfarin, he needs to have his *blood test used to determine certain coagulation activity defects and to monitor anticoagulation therapy* tested regularly.
   a. prothrombin time
   b. coagulation time
   c. troponin
10. Mr. MacDougal was brought to the emergency department after suffering chest trauma in a motor vehicle accident. His symptoms and chest x-ray were suspicious for aortic rupture, so a(n) *radiographic image of the aorta* was obtained.
   a. arteriogram
   b. aortogram
   c. venogram
11. After her myocardial infarction, Mrs. Alvarez was found to have 95% blockage in three sections of her coronary arteries. Thus, a *surgical technique to bring a new blood supply to heart muscle by detouring around blocked arteries* was performed.
   a. coronary stent
   b. angiography
   c. coronary artery bypass graft
12. Mr. Williams suffered from pancytopenia after his chemotherapy, so the hematologist ordered a(n) *infusion of healthy bone marrow cells from a matched donor into a patient with severely diseased or damaged bone marrow*.
   a. bone marrow aspiration
   b. bone marrow biopsy
   c. bone marrow transplant
13. Kelly Anastopoulis was recently diagnosed with rheumatoid arthritis, a(n) *disease caused by the body's inability to distinguish its own cells from foreign bodies*, when she had symptoms of joint pain and swelling in her hands.
   a. immunodeficiency
   b. blood dyscrasia
   c. autoimmune disease
14. Mrs. Rosenberg was admitted to the hospital to rule out a myocardial infarction. A phlebotomist performed a venipuncture to obtain labs, including a *blood test to measure the level of an enzyme of heart and skeletal muscle released into the blood after muscle injury or necrosis*.
   a. CPK
   b. CRP
   c. CBC
15. Ryan Lee developed *inflammation of the sac surrounding the heart* after a viral upper respiratory infection.
   a. myocarditis
   b. pericarditis
   c. endocarditis
16. Mr. O'Leary presented with symptoms of a stroke. *Process of digital radiographic imaging of the blood vessels that "subtracts" or removes structures not being studied* was performed to see if thrombolytic therapy was appropriate.
   a. digital subtraction angiography
   b. transesophageal echocardiogram
   c. single-photon emission computed tomography
17. During his high school sports physical, Habib El-Amin was found to have a(n) *abnormal cardiac sound heard through auscultation, caused by turbulent blood flow through the heart*.
   a. extravasation
   b. murmur
   c. bruit
18. The surgeon performed an emergency *suturing, repairing of the spleen* after Theresa Pangilinan ruptured it playing lacrosse.
   a. splenectomy
   b. thymectomy
   c. splenorrhaphy
19. The cardiologist recommended a *battery-powered apparatus implanted under the skin to treat an abnormal heart rhythm* for Mr. Jones, who had episodes of severe bradycardia.
   a. artificial cardiac pacemaker
   b. automatic implantable cardiac defibrillator
   c. percutaneous transluminal coronary angioplasty
20. Because she was over the age of 65, the physician recommended a pneumonia *suspension of weakened or killed microorganisms administered by injection, mouth, or nasal spray* for Mrs. Kurtz.
   a. venipuncture
   b. vaccine
   c. vasoconstrictor

C CHAPTER REVIEW

REVIEW OF CHAPTER CONTENT ON EVOLVE RESOURCES

Go to evolve.elsevier.com and click on Gradable Student Resources and Practice Student Resources. Online learning activities found there can be used to review chapter content and to assess your learning of word parts, medical terms, and abbreviations. Place check marks in the boxes next to activities used for review and assessment.

GRADABLE STUDENT RESOURCES

Chapter 10 >	Exercises >	☐ Word Parts ☐ Terms Built from Word Parts ☐ Terms Not Built from Word Parts ☐ Abbreviations
	Quizzes >	☐ Quiz 1: Disease and Disorder Terms ☐ Quiz 2: Surgical Terms ☐ Quiz 3: Diagnostic Terms ☐ Quiz 4: Complementary Terms

PRACTICE STUDENT RESOURCES > STUDENT RESOURCES

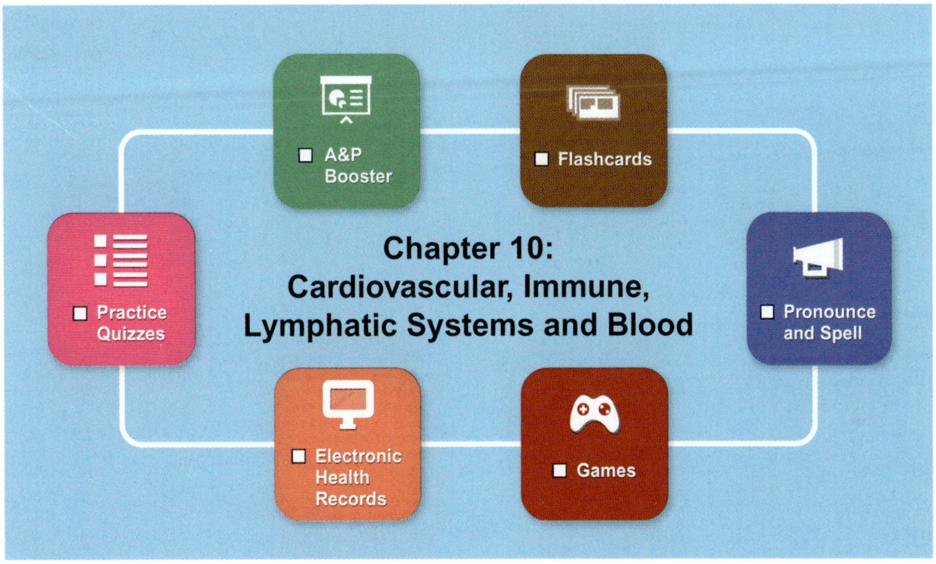

REVIEW OF WORD PARTS

Can you define and spell the following word parts?

COMBINING FORMS		PREFIXES	SUFFIXES
angi/o	myel/o	brady-	-ac
aort/o	phleb/o	pan-	-apheresis
arteri/o	plasm/o		-penia
ather/o	splen/o		-poiesis
atri/o	therm/o		-sclerosis
cardi/o	thromb/o		
ech/o	thym/o		
electr/o	valv/o		
isch/o	valvul/o		
lymph/o	ven/o		
lymphaden/o	ventricul/o		

REVIEW OF TERMS

Can you define, pronounce, and spell the following terms *built from word parts*?

DISEASES AND DISORDERS	SURGICAL	DIAGNOSTIC	COMPLEMENTARY
Cardiovascular System	***Cardiovascular System***	***Cardiovascular System***	***Cardiovascular System***
angioma	angioplasty	angiography	atrioventricular (AV)
angiostenosis	atherectomy	angioscope	cardiac
aortic stenosis	endarterectomy	angioscopy	cardiogenic
arteriosclerosis	pericardiocentesis	aortogram	cardiologist
atherosclerosis	phlebectomy	arteriogram	cardiology
bradycardia	phlebotomy	echocardiogram (ECHO)	hypothermia
cardiomegaly	valvuloplasty	electrocardiogram (ECG, EKG)	intravenous (IV)
cardiomyopathy	***Lymphatic System***	electrocardiograph	***Blood***
endocarditis	splenectomy	electrocardiography	hematologist
ischemia	splenorrhaphy	venogram	hematology
myocarditis	thymectomy		hematopoiesis
pericarditis			hemolysis
phlebitis			hemostasis
polyarteritis			myelopoiesis
tachycardia			plasmapheresis
thrombophlebitis			thrombolysis
valvulitis			
Blood			
erythrocytopenia			
hematoma			
leukocytopenia			
multiple myeloma			
pancytopenia			
thrombocytopenia			
thrombosis			
thrombus			
Lymphatic System			
lymphadenitis			
lymphadenopathy			
lymphoma			
splenomegaly			
thymoma			

Can you define, pronounce, and spell the following terms *NOT built from word parts?*

DISEASES AND DISORDERS

Cardiovascular System

acute coronary syndrome (ACS)
aneurysm
angina pectoris
arrhythmia
atrial fibrillation (AFib)
cardiac arrest
cardiac tamponade
coarctation of the aorta
congenital heart disease
coronary artery disease (CAD)
cor pulmonale
deep vein thrombosis (DVT)
heart failure (HF)
hypertensive heart disease (HHD)
intermittent claudication
mitral valve stenosis
myocardial infarction (MI)
peripheral artery disease (PAD)
rheumatic heart disease
varicose veins

Blood

anemia
embolus, pl. emboli
hemophilia
leukemia
sepsis

Lymphatic System

Hodgkin disease
infectious mononucleosis

SURGICAL

Cardiovascular System

aneurysmectomy
artificial cardiac pacemaker
automatic implantable cardiac defibrillator (AICD)
catheter ablation
coronary artery bypass graft (CABG)
coronary stent
embolectomy
femoropopliteal bypass
percutaneous transluminal coronary angioplasty (PTCA)
thrombolytic therapy

Blood

bone marrow aspiration
bone marrow biopsy
bone marrow transplant

DIAGNOSTIC

Cardiovascular System

blood pressure (BP)
cardiac catheterization
C-reactive protein (CRP)
creatine phosphokinase (CPK)
digital subtraction angiography (DSA)
Doppler ultrasound
exercise stress test
lipid profile
pulse
sestamibi test
single-photon emission computed tomography (SPECT)
sphygmomanometer
transesophageal echocardiogram (TEE)
troponin

Blood

activated partial thromboplastin time (aPTT)
coagulation time
complete blood count and differential (CBC and Diff)
hematocrit (Hct)
hemoglobin (Hgb)
prothrombin time (PT)

COMPLEMENTARY

Cardiovascular System

bruit
cardiopulmonary resuscitation (CPR)
defibrillation
diastole
extracorporeal
extravasation
fibrillation
heart murmur
hypercholesterolemia
hyperlipidemia
hypertension (HTN)
hypertriglyceridemia
hypotension
lipids
lumen
murmur
occlude
phlebotomist
systole
vasoconstrictor
vasodilator
venipuncture

Blood

anticoagulant
blood dyscrasia
hemorrhage

Immune System

allergen
allergist
allergy
anaphylaxis
antibody
antigen
autoimmune disease
immune
immunodeficiency
immunologist
immunology
phagocytosis
vaccine

Chapter 11

Digestive System

Objectives

Upon completion of this chapter you will be able to:

1. Pronounce organs and anatomic structures of the digestive system.
2. Define and spell word parts related to the digestive system.
3. Define, pronounce, and spell disease and disorder terms related to the digestive system.
4. Define, pronounce, and spell surgical terms related to the digestive system.
5. Define, pronounce, and spell diagnostic terms related to the digestive system.
6. Define, pronounce, and spell complementary terms related to the digestive system.
7. Interpret the meaning of abbreviations related to the digestive system.
8. Apply medical language in clinical contexts.

Outline

ANATOMY

The digestive system, also known as the alimentary canal or the gastrointestinal tract and abbreviated as GI tract, is a long continuous tube comprising the mouth, pharynx, esophagus, stomach, small intestine, large intestine, rectum, and anus. Accessory organs of the digestive system are the salivary glands, liver, bile ducts, gallbladder, and pancreas. (Figs. 11.1 through 11.5)

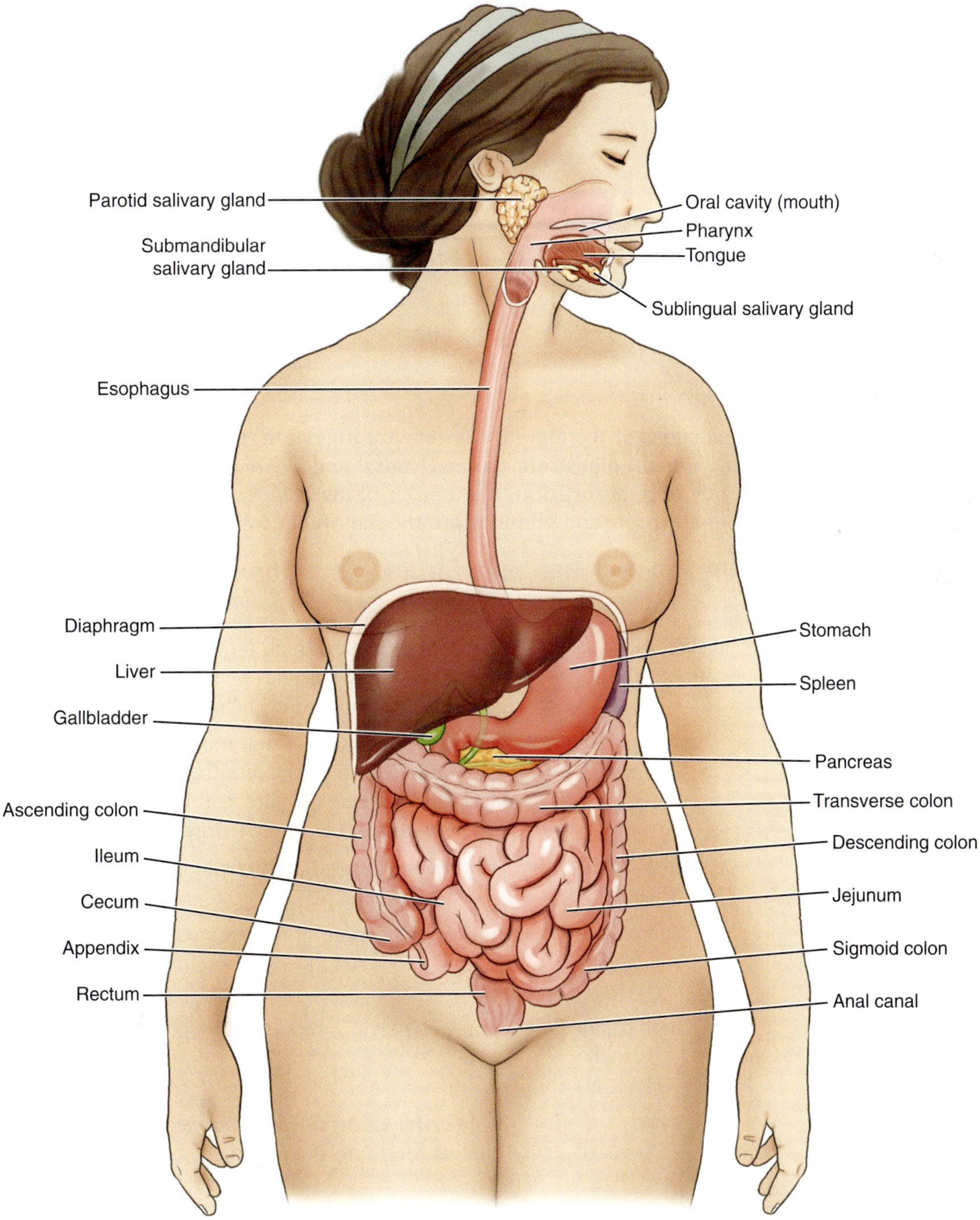

FIG. 11.1 Organs of the digestive system.

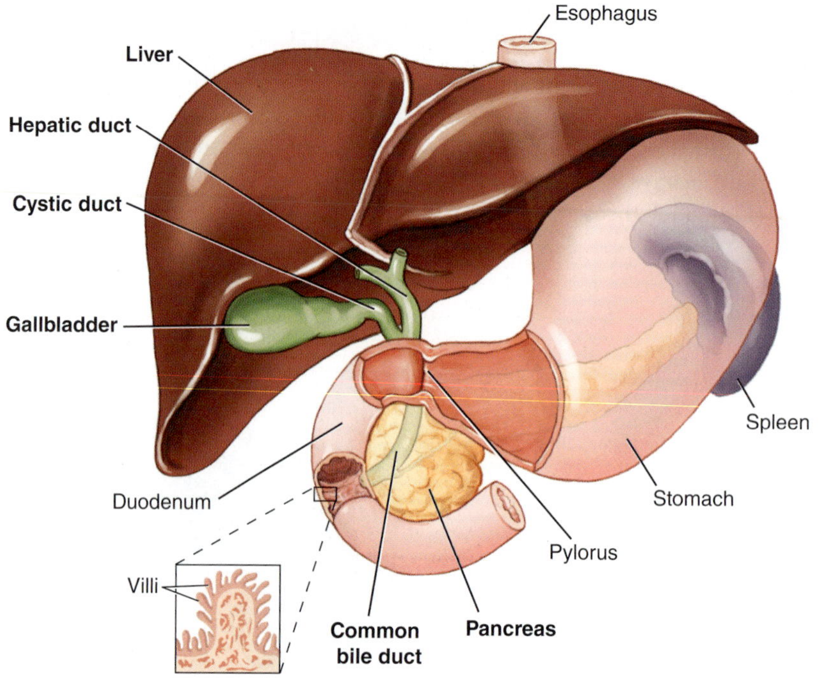

FIG. 11.2 Accessory organs: liver, hepatic duct, cystic duct, gallbladder, common bile duct, and pancreas.

Function

Functions of the digestive system are **ingestion**, the taking in of nutrients through the mouth; **digestion**, the mechanical and chemical breakdown of food for use by body cells; **absorption**, the transfer of digested food from the small intestine to the blood stream; and **elimination**, the removal of solid waste from the body.

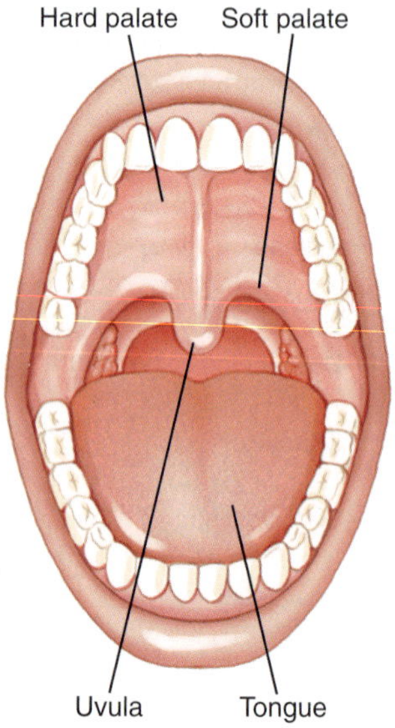

FIG. 11.3 The oral cavity.

Organs and Anatomic Structures of the Digestive System

TERM	DEFINITION
mouth (mouth)	opening through which food passes into the body; breaks food into small particles by mastication (chewing) and mixing with saliva (Fig. 11.3)
tongue (tung)	consists mostly of skeletal muscle; attached in the posterior region of the mouth. It provides movement of food for mastication, directs food to the pharynx for swallowing, and is a major organ for taste and speech.
palate (PAL-et)	separates the nasal cavity from the oral cavity
soft palate (sawft) (PAL-et)	posterior portion, not supported by bone
hard palate (hawrd) (PAL-et)	anterior portion, supported by bone
uvula (Ū-vū-la)	soft V-shaped structure that extends from the soft palate; directs food into the throat

TERM	DEFINITION
pharynx (FAR-inks)	performs the swallowing action that passes food from the mouth into the esophagus (also called **throat**)
esophagus (e-SOF-a-gus)	10-inch (25 cm) tube that is a passageway for food extending from the pharynx to the stomach. **Peristalsis**, involuntary wavelike movements that propel food along the gastrointestinal tract, begins in the esophagus.
stomach (STUM-ek)	J-shaped sac that mixes and stores food. It secretes chemicals for digestion and hormones for local communication control.
cardia (KAR-dē-a)	area around the opening of the esophagus
fundus (FUN-dus)	proximal domed portion of the stomach
body (BOD-ē)	central portion of the stomach, distal to the fundus
antrum (AN-trum)	distal portion of the stomach
pylorus (pī-LOR-us)	portion of the stomach that connects to the small intestine
pyloric sphincter (pī-LOR-ik) (SFINK-ter)	ring of muscle that guards the opening between the stomach and the duodenum
small intestine (smal) (in-TES-tin)	20-foot (6 m) tube extending from the pyloric sphincter to the large intestine. **Digestion** is completed in the small intestine. **Absorption**, the passage of the nutrients (end products of digestion) from the small intestine to the bloodstream, takes place through the **villi**, tiny fingerlike projections that line the walls of the small intestine.
duodenum (dū-OD-e-num)	first 10 to 12 inches (25 cm) of the small intestine
jejunum (je-JŪ-num)	second portion of the small intestine, approximately 8 feet (2.4 m) long
ileum (IL-ē-um)	third portion of the small intestine, approximately 11 feet (3.3 m) long, which connects with the large intestine
large intestine (larj) (in-TES-tin)	approximately 5 feet (1.5 m) long tube that extends from the ileum to the anus (Fig. 11.4). **Absorption** of water and transit of the solid waste products of digestion take place in the large intestine.
cecum (SĒ-kum)	U-shaped pouch that is the first portion of the large intestine
colon (KŌ-lun)	main portion of the large intestine. The colon is divided into four parts: ascending colon, transverse colon, descending colon, and sigmoid colon.
rectum (REK-tum)	distal portion of the large intestine, approximately 8 to 10 inches (20 cm) long, extending from the sigmoid colon to the anus

DUODENUM

is derived from the Latin **duodeni**, meaning **12 each**, a reference to its length. It was named in 240 BC by a Greek physician.

Jejunum is derived from the Latin **jejunus**, meaning **empty**; it was so named because the early anatomists always found it empty.

Ileum is derived from the Greek **eilein**, meaning to **roll**, a reference to the peristaltic waves that move food along the gastrointestinal tract. This term was first used in the early part of the seventeenth century.

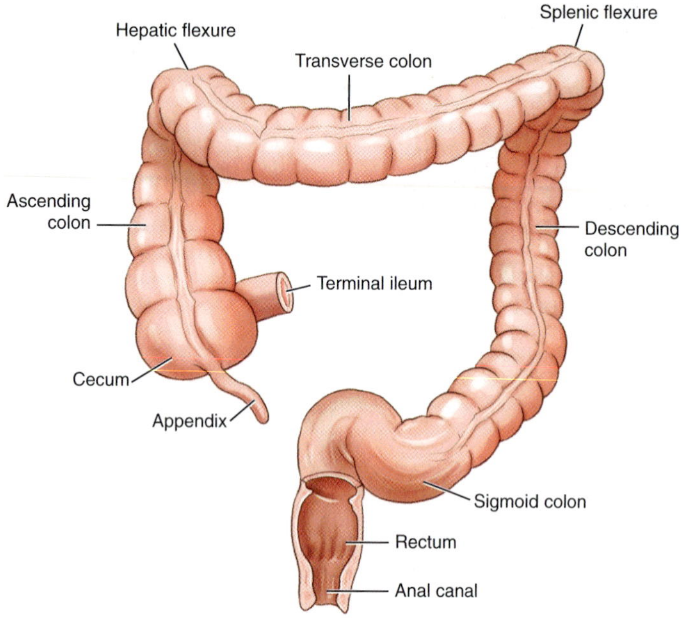

FIG. 11.4 Anatomy of the large intestine.

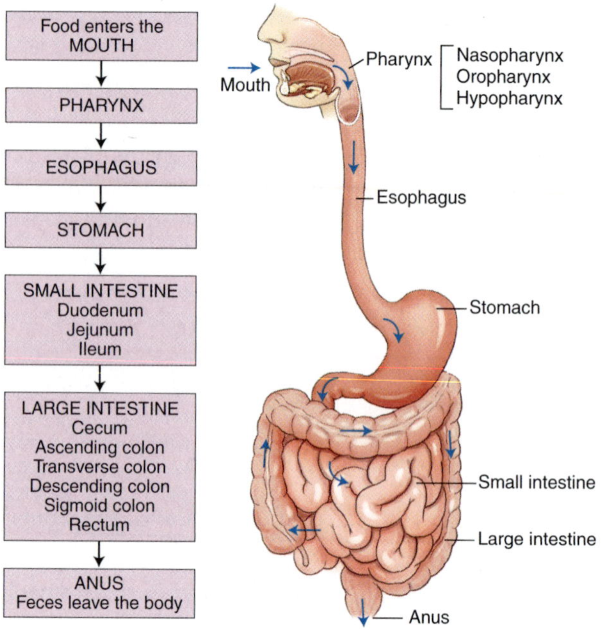

FIG. 11.5 Pathway of food.

Organs and Anatomic Structures of the Digestive System—cont'd

TERM	DEFINITION
anus (Ā-nus)	sphincter muscle (ringlike band of muscle fiber that keeps an opening tight) at the end of the gastrointestinal tract. Provides for **elimination** of solid waste products of digestion.
ACCESSORY ORGANS (Fig. 11.2)	
salivary glands (SAL-i-*ver*-ē) (glans)	produce saliva, which flows into the mouth (Fig. 11.1)
liver (LIV-er)	produces bile, which is necessary for the digestion of fats. The liver performs many other functions concerned with digestion and metabolism.
bile ducts (bīl) (dukts)	passageways that carry bile: the **hepatic duct** is a passageway for bile from the liver, and the **cystic duct** carries bile to and from the gallbladder. They join to form the **common bile duct**, which conveys bile to the duodenum. Collectively, these passageways are referred to as the **biliary tract**.
gallbladder (GAWL-blad-er)	small, saclike structure that stores bile produced by the liver
pancreas (PAN-krē-us)	produces pancreatic juice, which helps digest all types of food; secretes insulin for carbohydrate metabolism

BILIARY SYSTEM

The liver, bile ducts, and gallbladder comprise the biliary system, which creates, transports, stores, and releases bile into the small intestine to facilitate the absorption of fat.

PANCREAS

is derived from the Greek **pan**, meaning **all**, and **krea**, meaning **flesh**. The pancreas was first described in 300 BC. It was so named because of its fleshy appearance.

TERM	DEFINITION
OTHER STRUCTURES	
peritoneum (*per*-i-tō-NĒ-um)	serous saclike lining of the abdominal and pelvic cavities
appendix (a-PEN-diks)	small pouch, which has no known function in digestion; attached to the cecum (also called **vermiform appendix**)
abdomen (AB-duh-men)	portion of the body between the thorax and the pelvis

A&P Booster
For more anatomy and physiology, go to Evolve Resources at evolve.elsevier.com and select:
Practice Student Resources > Student Resources > Chapter 11 > **A&P Booster**

See Appendix B for instructions.

EXERCISE 1

Practice saying aloud each of the Organs and Anatomic Structures of the Digestive System.

To hear the terms, go to Evolve Resources at evolve.elsevier.com and select:
Practice Student Resources > Student Resources > Chapter 11 > **Pronounce and Spell**

See Appendix B for instructions.

❑ Check the box when complete.

WORD PARTS

Word parts you need to learn to complete this chapter are listed on the following pages. The exercises at the end of each list will help you learn their definitions and spellings.

Use the flashcards accompanying this text or electronic flashcards to assist you in memorizing the word parts for this chapter.

Combining Forms of the Digestive System

COMBINING FORM	DEFINITION
an/o	anus
antr/o	antrum
cec/o	cecum
col/o, colon/o	colon (large intestine)
duoden/o	duodenum
enter/o	intestine(s) (small intestine)
esophag/o	esophagus *(Note: esophag/o was covered in Chapter 9.)*
gastr/o	stomach
ile/o	ileum
jejun/o	jejunum
or/o, stomat/o	mouth
proct/o, rect/o	rectum
sigmoid/o	sigmoid colon

EXERCISE 2

Fill in the blanks with combining forms in this diagram of the digestive system. *To check your answers, go to Appendix A at the back of the textbook.*

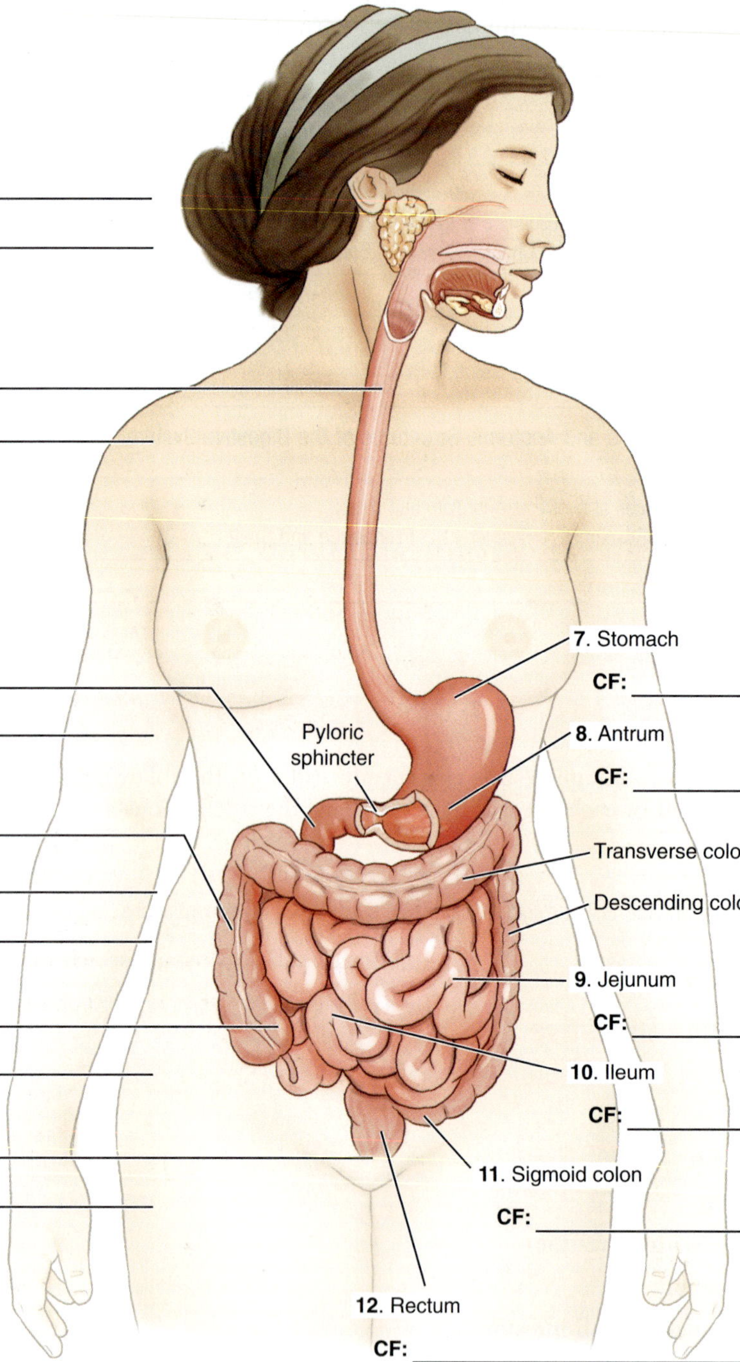

EXERCISE 3

Step 1: Write the definitions after the following combining forms.

Step 2: Match the descriptions on the right with the combining forms and definitions.

_____ 1. jejun/o, ______________________________

_____ 2. an/o, ______________________________

_____ 3. gastr/o, ______________________________

_____ 4. rect/o, ______________________________

_____ 5. or/o, ______________________________

_____ 6. col/o, ______________________________

_____ 7. sigmoid/o, ______________________________

_____ 8. enter/o, ______________________________

a. opening through which food passes into the body
b. distal portion of the large intestine
c. main portion of the large intestine
d. 20-foot (6 m) tube extending from the pyloric sphincter to the large intestine
e. second portion of the small intestine
f. portion of large intestine between descending colon and rectum
g. sphincter muscle at the end of the gastrointestinal tract
h. J-shaped sac that mixes and stores food

EXERCISE 4

Step 1: Write the definitions after the following combining forms.

Step 2: Match the descriptions on the right with the combining forms and definitions.

_____ 1. ile/o, ______________________________

_____ 2. stomat/o, ______________________________

_____ 3. proct/o, ______________________________

_____ 4. esophag/o, ______________________________

_____ 5. antr/o, ______________________________

_____ 6. colon/o, ______________________________

_____ 7. duoden/o, ______________________________

_____ 8. cec/o, ______________________________

a. distal portion of the stomach
b. first 10 to 12 inches (25 cm) of the small intestine
c. U-shaped pouch that is the first portion of the large intestine
d. third portion of the small intestine, approximately 11 feet (3.3 m) long
e. 10-inch (25 cm) tube that is a passageway for food extending from the pharynx to the stomach
f. main portion of the large intestine
g. opening through which food passes into the body
h. distal portion of the large intestine

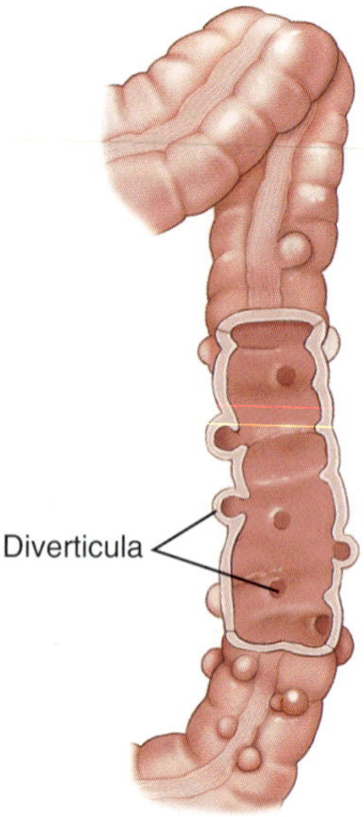

FIG. 11.6 Diverticula of the large intestine.

HERNIA

Types in the digestive system include abdominal, hiatal or diaphragmatic, inguinal, and umbilical hernia.

Combining Forms of the Accessory Organs/Combining Forms Commonly Used With Digestive System Terms

COMBINING FORM	DEFINITION
abdomin/o, celi/o, lapar/o	abdomen, abdominal cavity
append/o, appendic/o	appendix
cheil/o	lip(s)
cholangi/o	bile duct(s)
chol/e	gall, bile *(Note: the combining vowel is* e.*)*
choledoch/o	common bile duct
diverticul/o	diverticulum, pl. diverticula (pouch extending from a hollow organ) (Fig. 11.6)
gingiv/o	gum(s)
gloss/o, lingu/o	tongue
hepat/o	liver
herni/o	hernia (protrusion of an organ through a membrane or cavity wall) (Fig. 11.7)
palat/o	palate
pancreat/o	pancreas
peritone/o	peritoneum
polyp/o	polyp, small growth
pylor/o	pylorus, pyloric sphincter *(NOTE:* pylor/o *was covered in Chapter 9.)*
sial/o	saliva, salivary gland
steat/o	fat
uvul/o	uvula

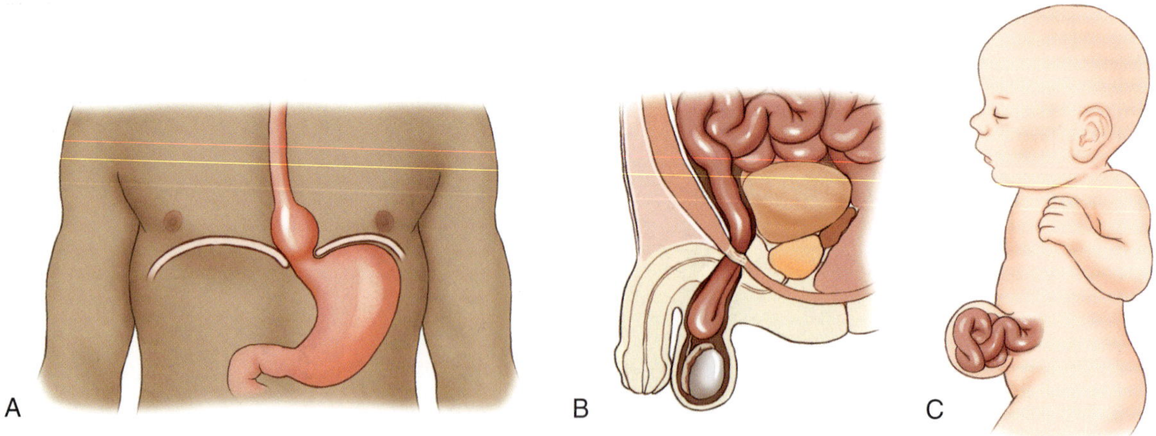

FIG. 11.7 Digestive hernias. **A**, Hiatal. **B**, Inguinal. **C**, Umbilical.

EXERCISE 5

Fill in the blanks with combining forms in this diagram of the digestive system and associated structures.

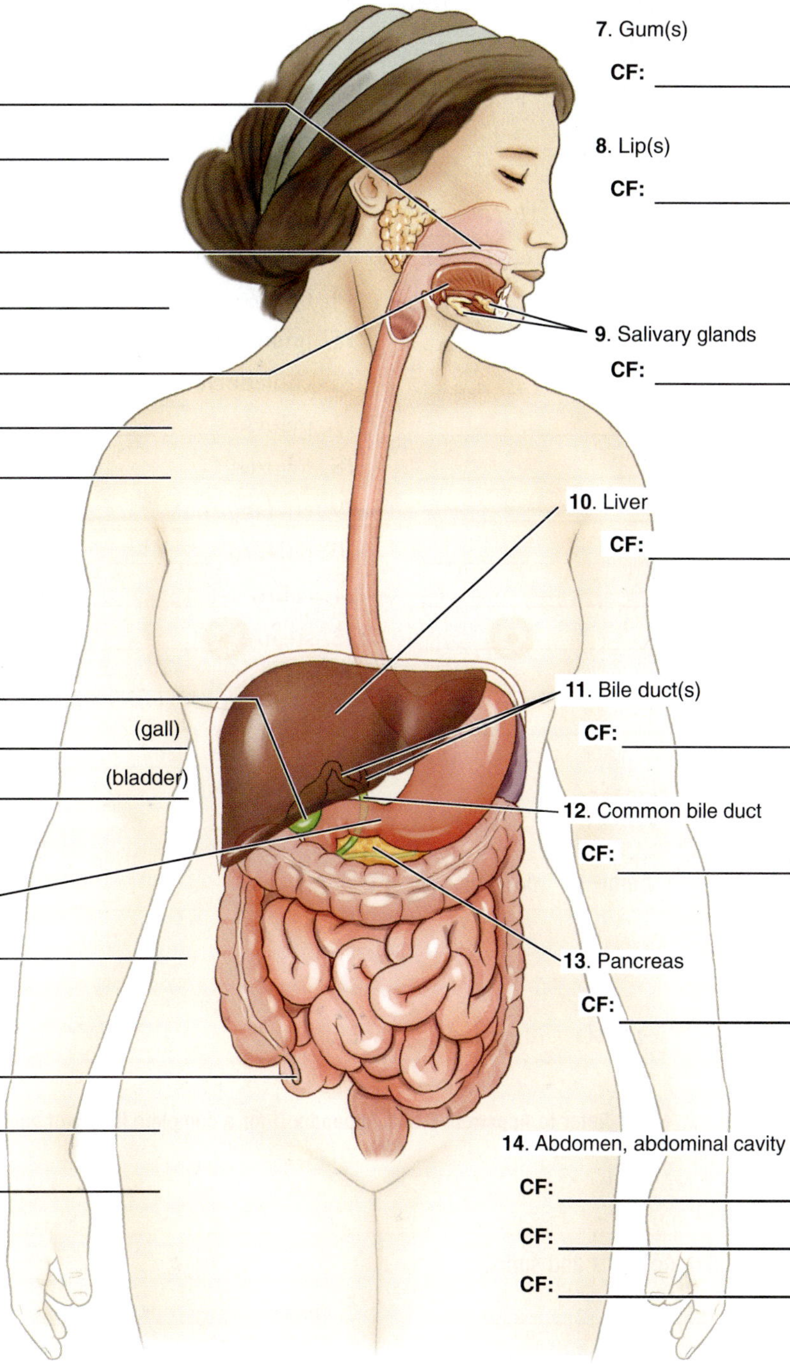

EXERCISE 6

Write the combining form for each of the following.

1. peritoneum ______
2. gall, bile ______
3. hernia ______
4. diverticulum ______
5. polyp, small growth ______
6. fat ______

EXERCISE 7

Write the definitions of the following combining forms.

1. herni/o ______
2. abdomin/o ______
3. sial/o ______
4. chol/e ______
5. diverticul/o ______
6. gingiv/o ______
7. appendic/o ______
8. gloss/o ______
9. hepat/o ______
10. cheil/o ______
11. peritone/o ______
12. palat/o ______
13. pancreat/o ______
14. lapar/o ______
15. lingu/o ______
16. choledoch/o ______
17. pylor/o ______
18. uvul/o ______
19. cholangi/o ______
20. polyp/o ______
21. celi/o ______
22. steat/o ______
23. append/o ______

Prefix

PREFIX	DEFINITION
hemi-	half

Suffix

SUFFIX	DEFINITION
-pepsia	digestion

Refer to **Appendix C** and **Appendix D** for a complete listing of word parts.

EXERCISE 8

A. Write the definitions for the following prefix and suffix.

1. -pepsia ______
2. hemi- ______

B. Write the prefix and suffix for the following definitions.

1. digestion ______
2. half ______

For additional practice with Word Parts, go to Evolve Resources at evolve.elsevier.com and select:
Practice Student Resources > Student Resources > Chapter 11 > **Flashcards**

See Appendix B for instructions.

MEDICAL TERMS

The terms you need to learn to complete this chapter are presented on the following pages. The exercises following each list will help you learn the definition and the spelling of each word.

Disease and Disorder Terms
BUILT FROM WORD PARTS

The following terms can be translated using definitions of word parts. Further explanation is provided within parentheses as needed.

TERM	DEFINITION
appendicitis (a-*pen*-di-SĪ-tis)	inflammation of the appendix (Exercise Figure A)
cholangioma (kō-*lan*-jē-Ō-ma)	tumor of the bile duct
cholecystitis (*kō*-lē-sis-TĪ-tis)	inflammation of the gallbladder
choledocholithiasis (kō-*led*-o-kō-li-THĪ-a-sis)	condition of stones in the common bile duct (Exercise Figure B)
cholelithiasis (*kō*-le-li-THĪ-a-sis)	condition of gallstones (Exercise Figure B)

EXERCISE FIGURE A

Fill in the blanks with word parts defined to complete labeling of the diagram.

1
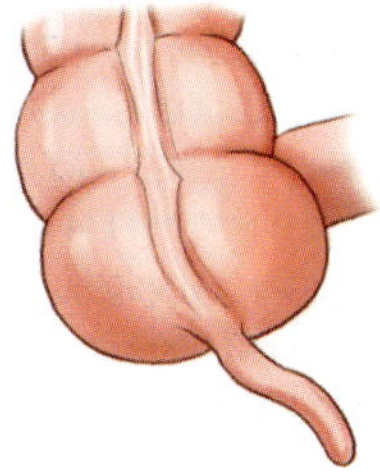

1. Normal appendix.

2
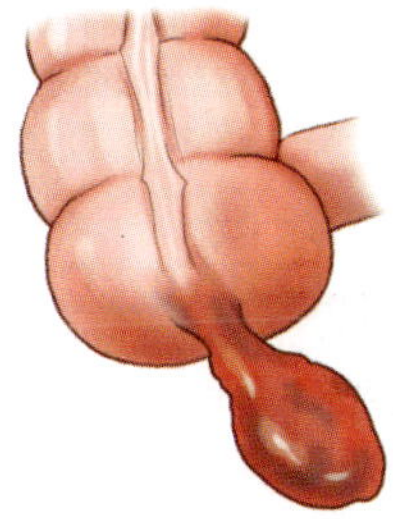

2. ______ / ______.
appendix / inflammation

EXERCISE FIGURE B

Fill in the blanks to complete labeling of the diagram.

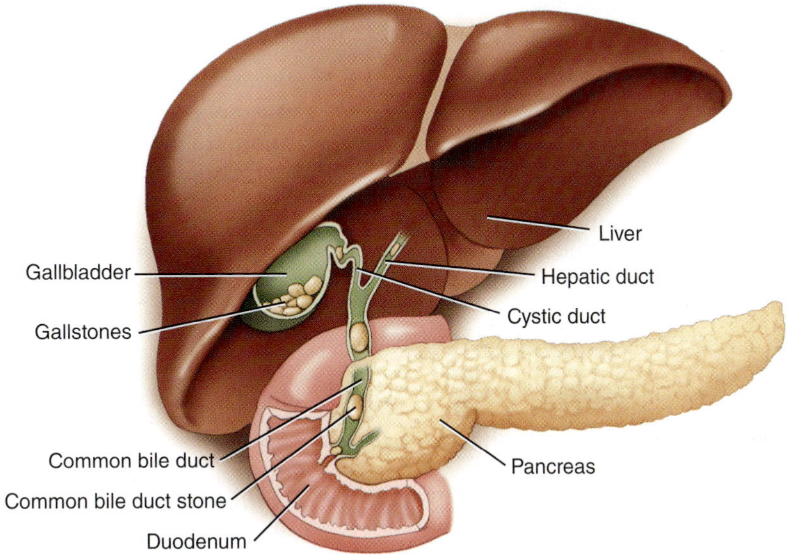

Common sites of

______ / ______ / ______ / ______ and ______ / ______ / ______ / ______.
gall / cv / stone / condition of — common bile duct / cv / stone / condition of

ANTIBIOTIC-ASSOCIATED COLITIS

Antibiotic-associated colitis is caused by a bacterium called ***Clostridium difficile*** (***C. difficile***). It was traditionally found in hospitalized patients; however, it is also now occurring more frequently in the general community. Symptoms include diarrhea and abdominal pain. Treatment includes using a different antibiotic or **fecal microbiota transplantation** (FMT), a fecal transplant, which is the infusion (usually via colonoscopy) of purified fecal bacteria from a healthy donor.

CAREER VIDEOS

To see interviews with a **Dental Hygienist** and a **Dietitian**, go to evolve.elsevier.com and select **Career Videos** located under the **Extra Content** tab.

See Appendix B for instructions.

Disease and Disorder Terms—cont'd

TERM	DEFINITION
colitis (ko-LĪ-tis)	inflammation of the colon
diverticulitis (*dī*-ver-*tik*-ū-LĪ-tis)	inflammation of a diverticulum
diverticulosis (*dī*-ver-*tik*-ū-LŌ-sis)	abnormal condition of having diverticula (Figs. 11.6 and 11.14B)
enteritis (*en*-ter-Ī-tis)	inflammation of the intestines
esophagitis (e-*sof*-a-JĪ-tis)	inflammation of the esophagus
gastritis (gas-TRĪ-tis)	inflammation of the stomach
gastroenteritis (*gas*-trō-*en*-te-RĪ-tis)	inflammation of the stomach and intestines
gingivitis (*jin*-ji-VĪ-tis)	inflammation of the gums
glossitis (glos-Ī-tis)	inflammation of the tongue
hepatitis (*hep*-a-TĪ-tis)	inflammation of the liver
hepatoma (*hep*-a-TŌ-ma)	tumor of the liver
palatitis (*pal*-a-TĪ-tis)	inflammation of the palate
pancreatitis (*pan*-krē-a-TĪ-tis)	inflammation of the pancreas
peritonitis (*per*-i-tō-NĪ-tis)	inflammation of the peritoneum *(Note: the* e *is dropped from the combining form* peritone/o.*)*
polyposis (*pol*-i-PŌ-sis)	abnormal condition of (multiple) polyps (in the mucous membrane of the intestine, especially the colon.) (Familial polyposis is a syndrome with a high potential for malignancy if polyps are not removed when they are small.) (Fig. 11.8)
proctitis (prok-TĪ-tis)	inflammation of the rectum
rectocele (REK-tō-sēl)	hernia of the rectum
sialolith (sī-AL-ō-lith)	stone in the salivary gland
steatohepatitis (*stē*-a-tō-*hep*-a-TĪ-tis)	inflammation of the liver associated with (excess) fat; (often caused by alcohol abuse and obesity; over time may cause cirrhosis)
uvulitis (*ū*-vū-LĪ-tis)	inflammation of the uvula

NASH SYNDROME

or **nonalcoholic steatohepatitis** may occur in nonalcoholic patients who are obese and/or suffer from type 2 diabetes mellitus.

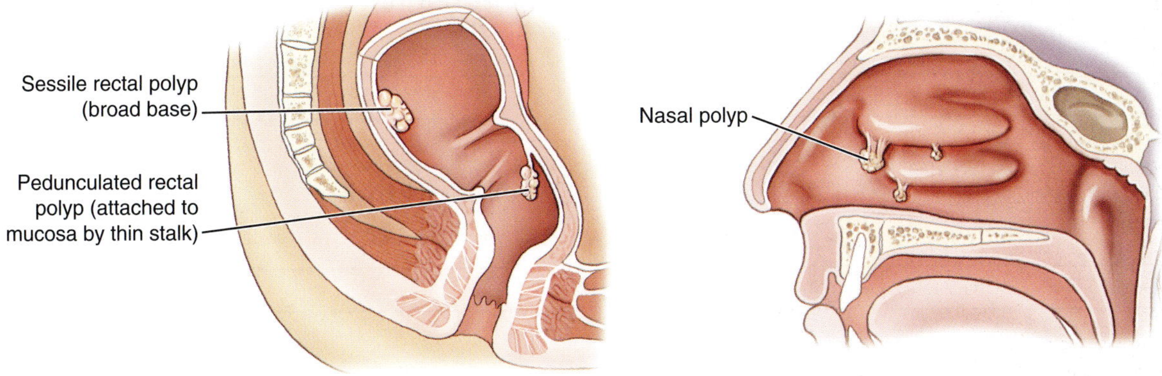

FIG. 11.8 Polyp is a general term used to describe a protruding growth from a mucous membrane. Polyps are commonly found in the nose, throat, intestines, uterus, and urinary bladder.

EXERCISE 9

Practice saying aloud each of the Disease and Disorder Terms Built from Word Parts.

To hear the terms, go to Evolve Resources at evolve.elsevier.com and select:
Practice Student Resources > Student Resources > Chapter 11 > **Pronounce and Spell**

See Appendix B for instructions.

❑ Check the box when complete.

EXERCISE 10

Analyze and define the following terms.

1. cholelithiasis

____

____

2. diverticulosis

____

____

3. sialolith

____

____

4. hepatoma

____

____

5. uvulitis

____

____

6. pancreatitis

____

____

7. proctitis

____

____

8. gingivitis

____

____

9. gastritis

____
____

10. rectocele

____
____

11. palatitis

____
____

12. hepatitis

____
____

13. appendicitis

____
____

14. cholecystitis

____
____

15. diverticulitis

____
____

16. gastroenteritis

____
____

17. enteritis

____
____

18. choledocholithiasis

____
____

19. cholangioma

____
____

20. polyposis

____
____

21. esophagitis

____
____

22. peritonitis

____
____

23. steatohepatitis

____
____

24. glossitis

____
____

25. colitis

____
____

EXERCISE 11

Build disease and disorder terms for the following definitions by using the word parts you have learned.

1. tumor of the liver ______ WR / ______ S
2. inflammation of the stomach ______ WR / ______ S
3. stone in the salivary gland ______ WR / CV / ______ WR
4. inflammation of the appendix ______ WR / ______ S
5. inflammation of a diverticulum ______ WR / ______ S
6. inflammation of the gallbladder ______ WR / CV / ______ WR / ______ S
7. abnormal condition of having diverticula ______ WR / ______ S
8. inflammation of the stomach and intestines ______ WR / CV / ______ WR / ______ S
9. inflammation of the rectum ______ WR / ______ S
10. hernia of the rectum ______ WR / CV / ______ S
11. inflammation of the uvula ______ WR / ______ S
12. inflammation of the gums ______ WR / ______ S
13. inflammation of the liver ______ WR / ______ S
14. inflammation of the palate ______ WR / ______ S
15. condition of gallstones ______ WR / CV / ______ WR / ______ S
16. inflammation of the liver associated with (excess) fat ______ WR / CV / ______ WR / ______ S
17. inflammation of the intestines ______ WR / ______ S

18. inflammation of the pancreas ______ / ______
WR / S

19. tumor of the bile duct ______ / ______
WR / S

20. inflammation of the esophagus ______ / ______
WR / S

21. condition of stones in the common bile duct ______ / ______ / ______ / ______
WR / CV / WR / S

22. abnormal condition of (multiple) polyps ______ / ______
WR / S

23. inflammation of the peritoneum ______ / ______
WR / S

24. inflammation of the tongue ______ / ______
WR / S

25. inflammation of the colon ______ / ______
WR / S

EXERCISE 12

Spell each of the Disease and Disorder Terms Built from Word Parts by having someone dictate them to you. Use a separate sheet of paper.

> To hear and spell the terms, go to Evolve Resources at evolve.elsevier.com and select:
> Practice Student Resources > Student Resources > Chapter 11 > **Pronounce and Spell**
>
> See Appendix B for instructions.

❑ Check the box when complete.

Disease and Disorder Terms
NOT BUILT FROM WORD PARTS

Word parts may be present in the following terms; however, their full meanings cannot be translated using definitions of word parts alone.

TERM	DEFINITION
adhesion (ad-HĒ-zhun)	abnormal growing together of two peritoneal surfaces that normally are separated. This may occur after abdominal surgery. Surgical treatment is called **adhesiolysis** or **adhesiotomy.**

TERM	DEFINITION
celiac disease (SĒ-lē-ak) (di-ZĒZ)	malabsorption syndrome caused by an immune reaction to gluten (a protein in wheat, rye, and barley), which may damage the lining of the small intestine that is responsible for absorption of food into the bloodstream. Celiac disease is considered a multisystem disorder with varying signs and symptoms, including abdominal bloating and pain, chronic diarrhea or constipation, steatorrhea (excessive fat in the stool), vomiting, weight loss, fatigue, and iron deficiency anemia. A pruritic skin rash known as dermatitis herpetiformis may be associated with celiac disease (also called **gluten enteropathy**).
cirrhosis (sir-RŌ-sis)	chronic disease of the liver with gradual destruction of cells and formation of scar tissue; commonly caused by alcoholism and certain types of viral hepatitis
Crohn disease (krōn) (di-ZĒZ)	chronic inflammation of the intestinal tract usually affecting the ileum and colon; characterized by cobblestone ulcerations and the formation of scar tissue that may lead to intestinal obstruction (also called **regional ileitis** or **regional enteritis**)
gastroesophageal reflux disease (GERD) (gas-trō-e-sof-a-JĒ-al) (RĒ-fluks) (di-ZĒZ)	abnormal backward flow of the gastrointestinal contents into the esophagus, causing heartburn and the gradual breakdown of the mucous barrier of the esophagus
hemochromatosis (hē-mō-krō-ma-TŌ-sis)	iron metabolism disorder that occurs when too much iron is absorbed from food, resulting in excessive deposits of iron in the tissue; can cause heart failure, diabetes, cirrhosis, or cancer of the liver
hemorrhoids (HEM-o-roydz)	swollen or distended veins in the rectum or anus, which are called internal or external, respectively, and can be a source of rectal bleeding and pain
ileus (IL-ē-us)	non-mechanical obstruction of the intestine, caused by a lack of effective peristalsis
intussusception (*in*-tu-sus-SEP-shun)	telescoping of a segment of the intestine
irritable bowel syndrome (IBS) (IR-i-ta-bl) (BOW-el) (SIN-drōm)	periodic disturbances of bowel function, such as diarrhea and/or constipation, usually associated with abdominal pain
obesity (ō-BĒS-i-tē)	excess of body fat, which increases body weight; a condition in which body mass index (BMI) is greater than 30 kg/m^2. **Overweight** is defined as BMI between 25 and 29.9 kg/m^2. **Morbid obesity** is defined as a BMI over 40 kg/m^2.

GASTROESOPHAGEAL REFLUX DISEASE (GERD)

is a common gastrointestinal disorder. The acidity of the regurgitated stomach contents causes inflammation of the esophagus (reflux esophagitis). In addition to heartburn, GERD may also cause chronic cough and excessive throat clearing. **Chronic GERD** may cause cellular changes in the lower esophagus called **Barrett esophagus**, which increases the risk of cancer.

INTEGRATIVE MEDICINE TERM

Hypnotherapy is the use of the power of suggestion and a state of altered consciousness involving focused attention to promote wellness. Studies have demonstrated that hypnosis has provided relief of symptoms and improvement in quality of life for patients with **irritable bowel syndrome**.

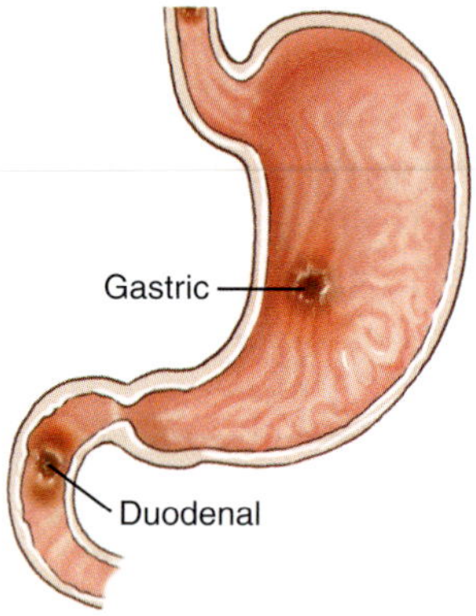

FIG. 11.9 Sites of peptic ulcers.

Disease and Disorder Terms—cont'd

TERM	DEFINITION
peptic ulcer (PEP-tik) (UL-ser)	erosion of the mucous membrane of the stomach or duodenum associated with increased secretion of acid from the stomach, bacterial infection (*H. pylori*), or medications such as nonsteroidal anti-inflammatory drugs (often referred to as **gastric** or **duodenal ulcer**, depending on its location) (Fig. 11.9)
polyp (POL-ip)	tumorlike growth extending outward from a mucous membrane; usually benign; common sites are in the nose, throat, and intestines (Figs. 11.8 and 11.11)
ulcerative colitis (UC) (UL-ser-a-tiv) (kō-LĪ-tis)	disease characterized by inflammation of the colon with the formation of ulcers, which can cause bloody diarrhea. A proctocolectomy with permanent ileostomy may become necessary if the patient doesn't respond to medical therapy.
volvulus (VOL-vū-lus)	twisting or kinking of the intestine, causing intestinal obstruction

EXERCISE 13

Practice saying aloud each of the Disease and Disorder Terms NOT Built from Word Parts.

To hear the terms, go to Evolve Resources at evolve.elsevier.com and select:
Practice Student Resources > Student Resources > Chapter 11 > **Pronounce and Spell**

See Appendix B for instructions.

EXERCISE 14A

Match the terms in the first column with the definitions in the second column.

_____ 1. hemochromatosis
_____ 2. cirrhosis
_____ 3. ulcerative colitis
_____ 4. ileus
_____ 5. celiac disease
_____ 6. irritable bowel syndrome
_____ 7. Crohn disease
_____ 8. obesity

a. excess of body fat, which increases body weight
b. non-mechanical obstruction of the intestine
c. disease characterized by inflammation of the colon with the formation of ulcers, which can cause bloody diarrhea
d. chronic inflammation of the intestinal tract usually affecting the ileum and colon with cobblestone ulcerations
e. iron metabolism disorder resulting in excessive deposits of iron in the tissue; can cause cirrhosis or liver cancer
f. malabsorption syndrome caused by an immune reaction to gluten
g. chronic disease of the liver with gradual destruction of cells and formation of scar tissue
h. periodic disturbances of bowel function, such as diarrhea and/or constipation, usually associated with abdominal pain

EXERCISE 14B

Write the medical term pictured and defined.

1. ______________________________
erosion of the mucous membrane of the stomach or duodenum associated with increased secretion of acid from the stomach

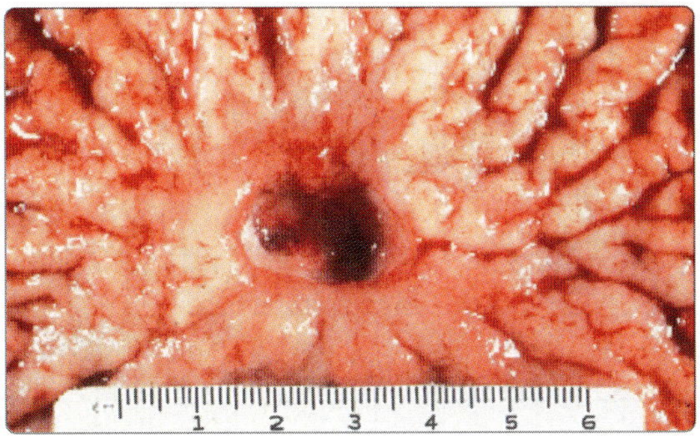

2. ______________________________
twisting or kinking of the intestine, causing intestinal obstruction

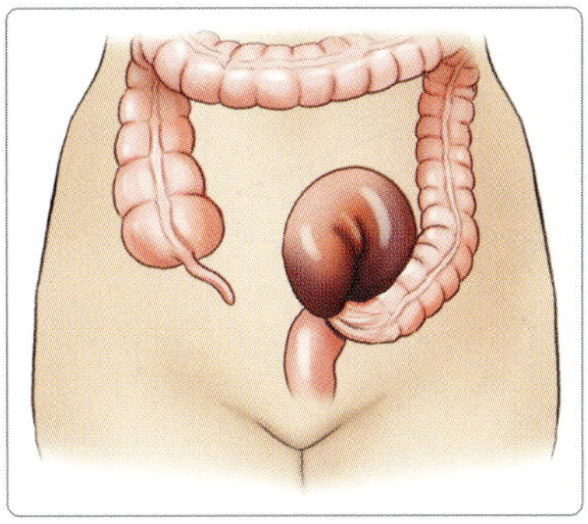

3. ______________________________
tumor-like growth extending outward from a mucous membrane; usually benign

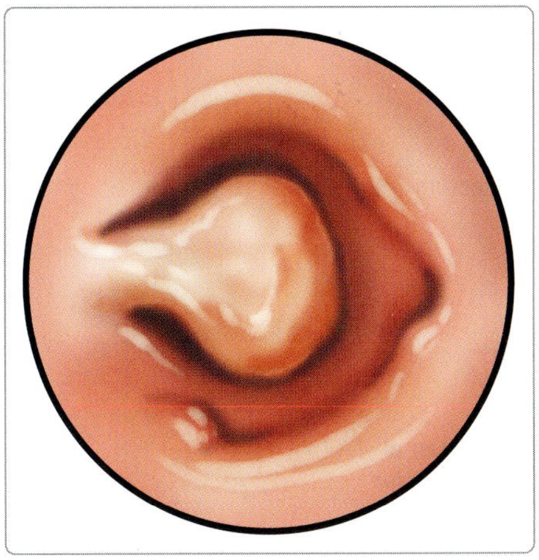

4. ______________________________
abnormal backward flow of the gastrointestinal contents into the esophagus

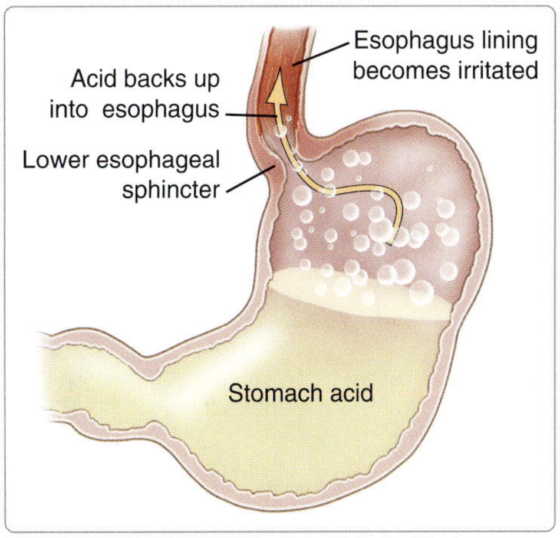

EXERCISE 14B *Pictured and Defined—cont'd*

5. ______________________________
abnormal growing together of two peritoneal surfaces that normally are separated

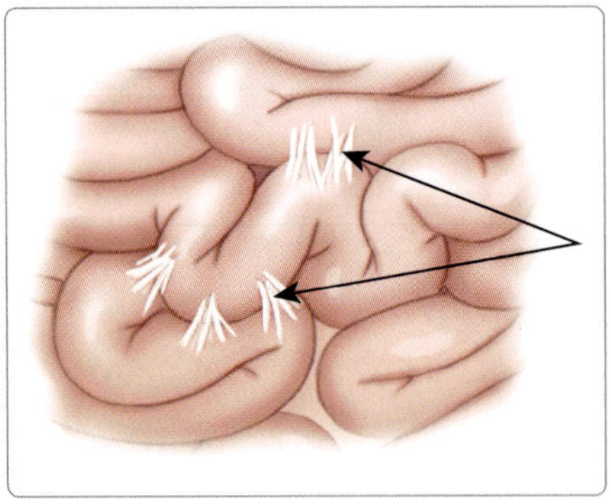

6. ______________________________
telescoping of a segment of the intestine

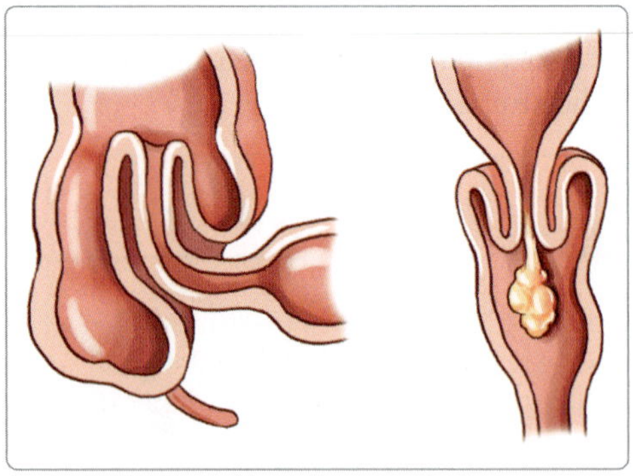

7. ______________________________
swollen or distended veins in the rectum or anus, which can be a source of rectal bleeding and pain

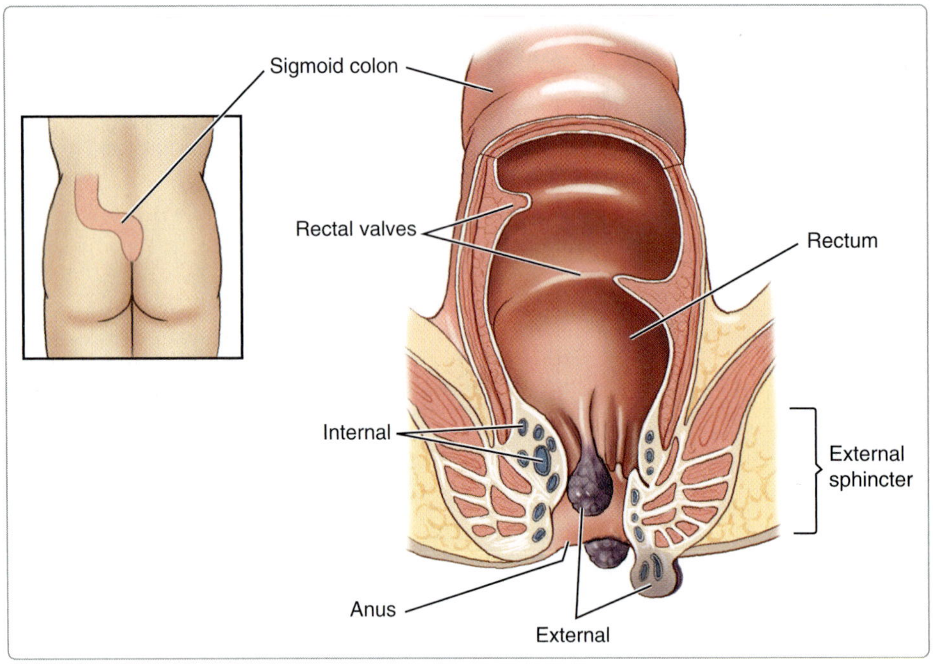

EXERCISE 15

Spell each of the Disease and Disorder Terms NOT Built from Word Parts by having someone dictate them to you. Use a separate sheet of paper.

To hear and spell the terms, go to Evolve Resources at evolve.elsevier.com and select:
Practice Student Resources > Student Resources > Chapter 11 > **Pronounce and Spell**

See Appendix B for instructions.

❑ Check the box when complete.

Surgical Terms

BUILT FROM WORD PARTS

The following terms can be translated using definitions of word parts. Further explanation is provided within parentheses as needed.

TERM	DEFINITION
abdominocentesis (ab-*dom*-i-nō-sen-TĒ-sis)	surgical puncture to aspirate fluid from the abdominal cavity (also called **paracentesis**)
abdominoplasty (ab-DOM-i-nō-*plas*-tē)	surgical repair of the abdomen
anoplasty (Ā-nō-*plas*-tē)	surgical repair of the anus
antrectomy (an-TREK-to-mē)	excision of the antrum (of the stomach)
appendectomy (*ap*-en-DEK-to-mē)	excision of the appendix
cheiloplasty (KĪ-lō-*plas*-tē)	surgical repair of the lip
cholecystectomy (*kō*-le-sis-TEK-to-mē)	excision of the gallbladder (Fig. 11.10)
choledocholithotomy (kō-*led*-o-kō-li-THOT-o-mē)	incision into the common bile duct to remove a stone

CHOLECYSTECTOMY was first performed in 1882 by a German surgeon. **Laparoscopic cholecystectomy** was first performed in 1987 in France.

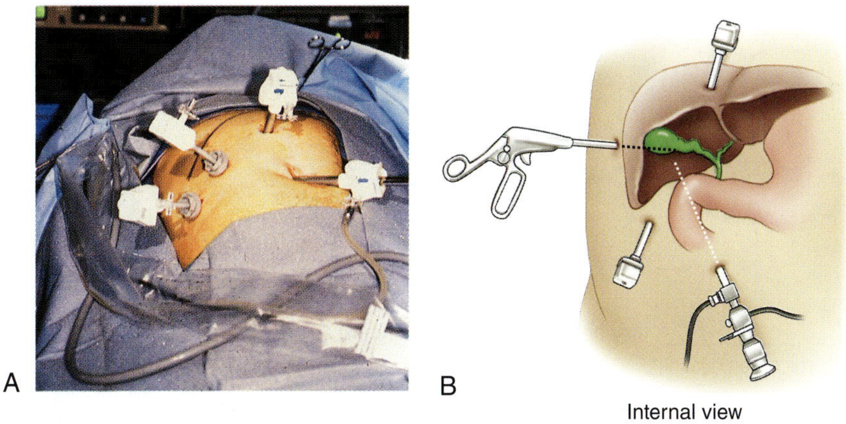

FIG. 11.10 In **laparoscopic cholecystectomy**, a type of endoscopic surgery, carbon dioxide (CO_2) is introduced into the abdominal cavity for better visualization. A tiny camera and surgical instruments, including a laparoscope, are passed through small incisions. **A,** External view. **B,** Internal view.

Surgical Terms—cont'd

TERM	DEFINITION
colectomy (kō-LEK-to-mē)	excision of the colon
colostomy (ko-LOS-to-mē)	creation of an artificial opening into the colon (through the abdominal wall). (Used for the passage of stool. A colostomy, which creates a mouthlike opening on the abdominal wall called a **stoma**, may be permanent or temporary; performed as treatment for bowel obstruction, cancer, or diverticulitis.) (Exercise Figure E)
diverticulectomy (*dī*-ver-*tik*-ū-LEK-to-mē)	excision of a diverticulum
enterorrhaphy (*en*-ter-OR-a-fē)	suturing of the intestine
esophagogastroplasty (e-*sof*-a-gō-GAS-trō-*plas*-tē)	surgical repair of the esophagus and the stomach
gastrectomy (gas-TREK-to-mē)	excision of the stomach (or part of the stomach) (Exercise Figure C)
gastrojejunostomy (*gas*-trō-je-jū-NOS-to-mē)	creation of an artificial opening between the stomach and jejunum
gastroplasty (GAS-trō-*plas*-tē)	surgical repair of the stomach
gastrostomy (gas-TROS-to-mē)	creation of an artificial opening into the stomach (through the abdominal wall). (A tube is inserted through the opening for administration of food when swallowing is impossible.) (Exercise Figure D)

EXERCISE FIGURE C

Fill in the blanks with word parts defined to label the diagram.

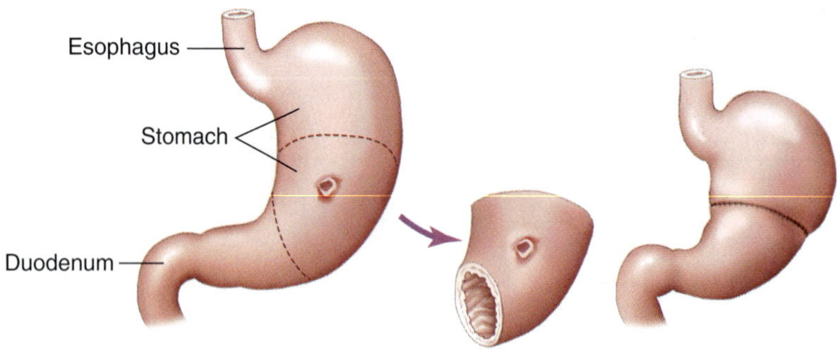

Partial ______ / ______ may be performed to treat chronic gastric ulcers.
stomach / surgical removal

EXERCISE FIGURE D

Fill in the blanks with word parts defined to label the diagram.

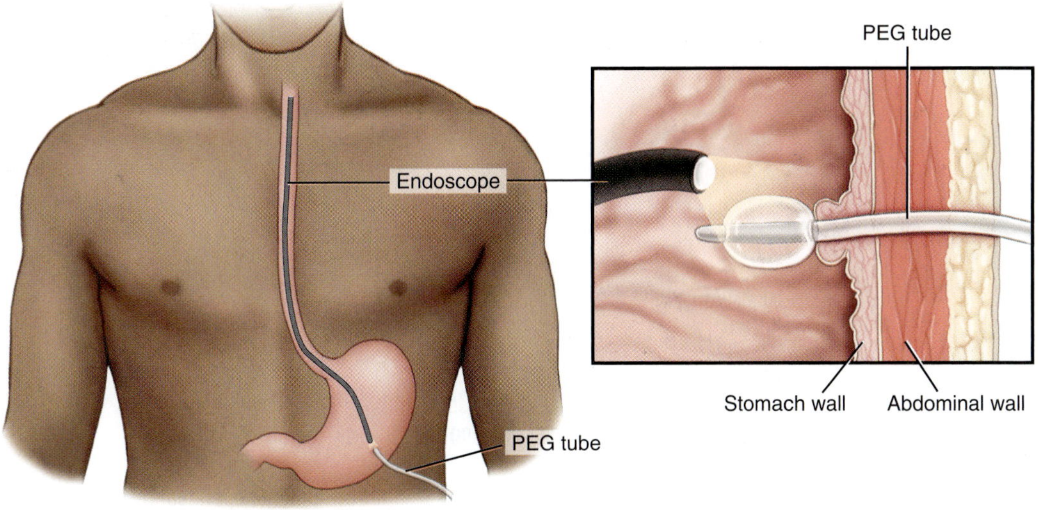

_____ / _____ / _____
through / skin / pertaining to

_____ / _____
within / pertaining to visual examination

_____ / _____ / _____
stomach / cv / creation of an artificial opening

is a procedure used to place a tube into the stomach through the abdominal wall to administer liquids for nutrition and hydration.

TERM	DEFINITION
gingivectomy (*jin*-ji-VEK-to-mē)	surgical removal of gum (tissue)
glossorrhaphy (glo-SOR-a-fē)	suturing of the tongue
hemicolectomy (*hem*-ē-kō-LEK-to-mē)	excision of half of the colon
herniorrhaphy (*her*-nē-OR-a-fē)	suturing of a hernia (for repair)
ileostomy (*il*-ē-OS-to-mē)	creation of an artificial opening into the ileum (through the abdominal wall creating a stoma, a mouthlike opening on the abdominal wall). (Used for the passage of stool. It is performed following total proctocolectomy for ulcerative colitis, Crohn disease, or cancer.) (Exercise Figure E)

EXERCISE FIGURE E

Fill in the blanks with word parts defined to complete labeling of the diagram.

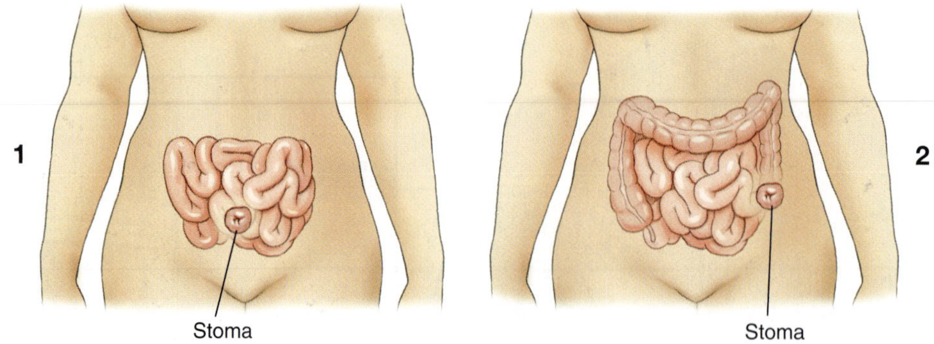

1. ______ / ______ / ______ after a total colectomy.
   ileum / cv / creation of an artificial opening

2. ______ / ______ / ______ after an abdominoperineal resection.
   colon / cv / creation of an artificial opening

Surgical Terms—cont'd

TERM	DEFINITION
laparotomy (*lap*-a-ROT-o-mē)	incision into the abdominal cavity (also called **celiotomy**)
palatoplasty (PAL-a-tō-*plas*-tē)	surgical repair of the palate
polypectomy (*pol*-i-PEK-to-mē)	excision of a polyp (Fig. 11.11)
pyloromyotomy (pī-*lor*-ō-mī-OT-o-mē)	incision into the pyloric muscle (performed to correct pyloric stenosis)
pyloroplasty (pī-LOR-ō-*plas*-tē)	surgical repair of the pylorus
uvulectomy (*ū*-vū-LEK-to-mē)	excision of the uvula
uvulopalatopharyngoplasty (UPPP) (*ū*-vū-lō-*pal*-a-*tō*-fa-RING-gō-*plas*-tē)	surgical repair of the uvula, palate, and pharynx (performed to correct obstructive sleep apnea) (see Fig. 5.7)

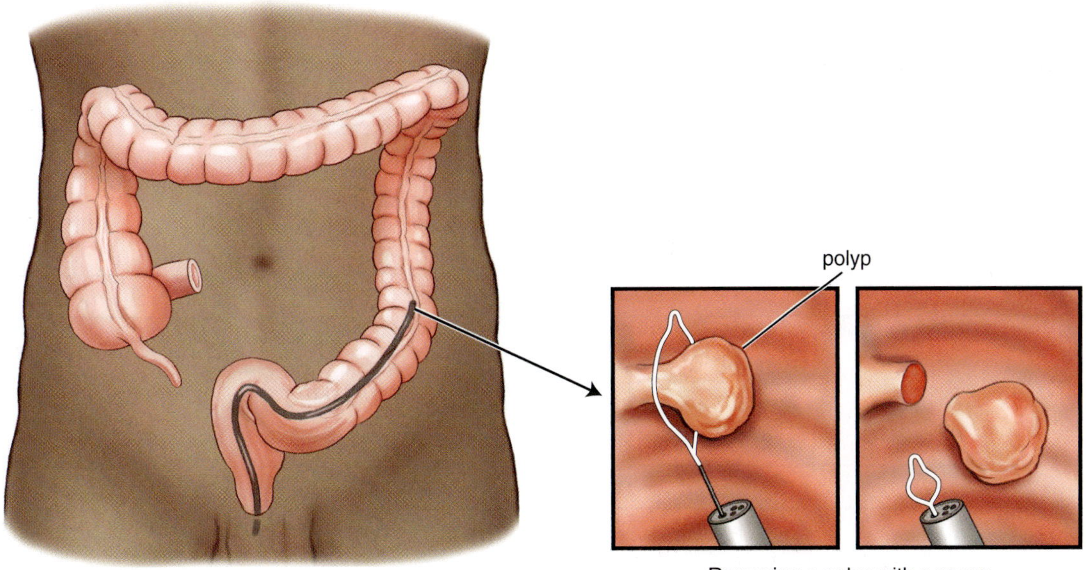

FIG. 11.11 Polypectomy performed using a colonoscope.

EXERCISE 16

Practice saying aloud each of the Surgical Terms Built from Word Parts.

To hear the terms, go to Evolve Resources at evolve.elsevier.com and select:
Practice Student Resources > Student Resources > Chapter 11 > **Pronounce and Spell**

See Appendix B for instructions.

❑ Check the box when complete.

EXERCISE 17

Analyze and define the following terms.

1. gastrectomy

____

____

2. esophagogastroplasty

____

____

3. diverticulectomy

____

____

4. antrectomy

____

____

5. palatoplasty

____

____

6. uvulectomy

____

____

7. gastrojejunostomy

____

____

8. cholecystectomy

____

____

9. colectomy

____

____

10. colostomy

____

____

11. pyloroplasty

____

____

12. anoplasty

____

____

13. appendectomy

____

____

14. cheiloplasty

____

____

15. gingivectomy

____

____

16. laparotomy

____

____

17. ileostomy

____

____

18. gastrostomy

____

____

19. herniorrhaphy

____

____

20. glossorrhaphy

____

____

21. choledocholithotomy

____

____

22. hemicolectomy

____

____

23. polypectomy

____

____

24. enterorrhaphy

____

____

25. abdominoplasty

____

____

26. pyloromyotomy

____

____

27. uvulopalatopharyngoplasty

____

____

28. gastroplasty

____

____

29. abdominocentesis

____

____

EXERCISE 18

Build surgical terms for the following definitions by using the word parts you have learned.

1. excision of the appendix ______ WR / ______ S
2. suturing of the tongue ______ WR / CV / ______ S
3. surgical repair of the esophagus and stomach ______ WR / CV / ______ WR / CV / ______ S
4. excision of a diverticulum ______ WR / ______ S
5. creation of an artificial opening into the ileum ______ WR / CV / ______ S
6. surgical removal of gum (tissue) ______ WR / ______ S
7. incision into the abdominal cavity ______ WR / CV / ______ S
8. surgical repair of the anus ______ WR / CV / ______ S
9. excision of the antrum ______ WR / ______ S
10. excision of the gallbladder ______ WR / CV / ______ WR / ______ S
11. excision of the colon ______ WR / ______ S

12. creation of an artificial opening into the colon
    ______ WR / CV / S
13. excision of the stomach
    ______ WR / S
14. creation of an artificial opening into the stomach
    ______ WR / CV / S
15. creation of an artificial opening between the stomach and jejunum
    ______ WR / CV / WR / CV / S
16. excision of the uvula
    ______ WR / S
17. surgical repair of the palate
    ______ WR / CV / S
18. surgical repair of the pylorus
    ______ WR / CV / S
19. suturing of a hernia
    ______ WR / CV / S
20. surgical repair of the lip
    ______ WR / CV / S
21. excision of half of the colon
    ______ P / WR / S
22. incision into the common bile duct to remove a stone
    ______ WR / CV / WR / CV / S
23. excision of a polyp
    ______ WR / S
24. suturing of the intestine
    ______ WR / CV / S
25. surgical repair of the abdomen
    ______ WR / CV / S
26. incision into the pylorus muscle
    ______ WR / CV / WR / CV / S
27. surgical repair of the uvula, palate, and pharynx
    ______ WR / CV / WR / CV / WR / CV / S
28. surgical repair of the stomach
    ______ WR / CV / S
29. surgical puncture to aspirate fluid from the abdominal cavity
    ______ WR / CV / S

EXERCISE 19

Spell each of the Surgical Terms Built from Word Parts by having someone dictate them to you. Use a separate sheet of paper.

To hear and spell the terms, go to Evolve Resources at evolve.elsevier.com and select:
Practice Student Resources > Student Resources > Chapter 11 > **Pronounce and Spell**

See Appendix B for instructions.

❑ Check the box when complete.

Surgical Terms
NOT BUILT FROM WORD PARTS

Word parts may be present in the following terms; however, their full meanings cannot be translated using definitions of word parts alone.

TERM	DEFINITION
abdominoperineal resection (APR) (ab-*dom*-i-nō-per-i-NĒ-el) (rē-SEK-shun)	removal of the distal colon, rectum, and anal sphincter through both abdominal and perineal approaches; performed to treat some colorectal cancers and inflammatory diseases of the lower large intestine. The patient will have a colostomy (see Exercise Figure E2).
anastomosis (pl. anastomoses) (a-*nas*-to-MŌ-sis) (a-*nas*-to-MŌ-sēz)	connection created by surgically joining two structures, such as blood vessels or bowel segments (Fig. 11.12)
bariatric surgery (*bar*-ē-AT-rik) (SUR-jer-ē)	surgical reduction of gastric capacity to treat morbid obesity, a condition which can cause serious illness (Table 11.1)
hemorrhoidectomy (*hem*-o-royd-EK-to-mē)	excision of hemorrhoids, the swollen or distended veins in the lower rectum and anus
vagotomy (vā-GOT-o-mē)	cutting of certain branches of the vagus nerve, performed with gastric surgery to reduce the amount of gastric acid produced and thus reduce the recurrence of ulcers

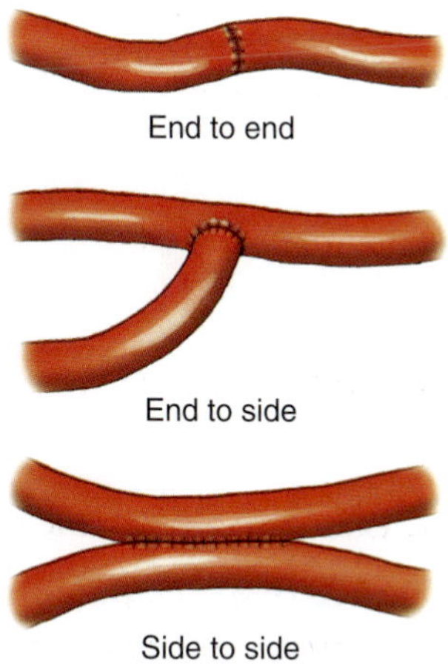

FIG. 11.12 Types of anastomoses.

BARIATRIC

contains the word roots **bar**, meaning **weight**, and **iatr**, meaning **treatment**.

EXERCISE 20

Practice saying aloud each of the Surgical Terms NOT Built from Word Parts.

To hear the terms, go to Evolve Resources at evolve.elsevier.com and select:
Practice Student Resources > Student Resources > Chapter 11 > **Pronounce and Spell**

See Appendix B for instructions.

❑ Check the box when complete.

TABLE 11.1 Bariatric Surgery

Bariatric surgery may be used to treat morbid obesity for patients with a BMI greater than 40 or those with a BMI greater than 35 associated with a serious medical condition. During surgery, a small stomach pouch is created for the purpose of restricting the amount of food an individual can eat. The following are three types of surgeries performed.

ROUX-EN-Y GASTRIC BYPASS (RYGB)

Creation of a small gastric pouch with drainage of food to the rest of the gastrointestinal tract through a restricted stoma; the duodenum and part of the jejunum are bypassed. RYGB, the most common form of bariatric surgery performed in the United States, restricts food intake and calorie absorption rate.

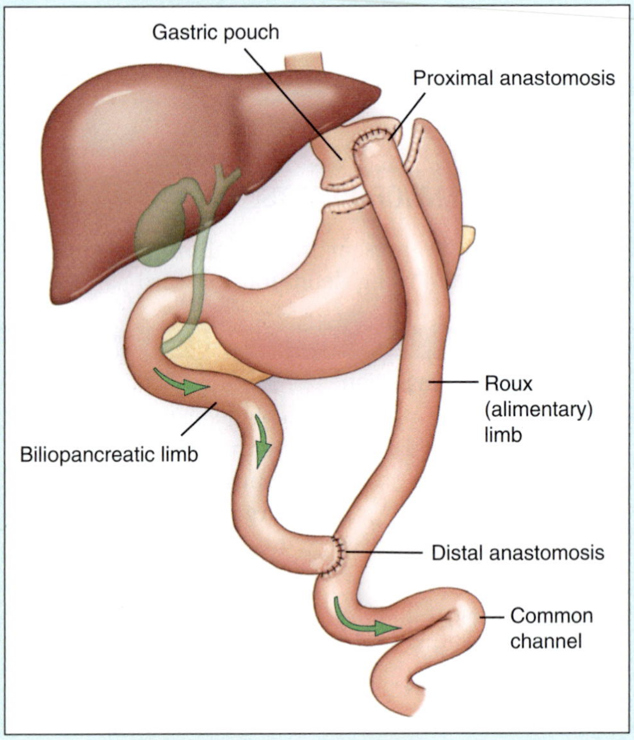

SLEEVE GASTRECOMY

The majority of the stomach is removed and a smaller tubular stomach is created. The capacity of the stomach is therefore significantly reduced.

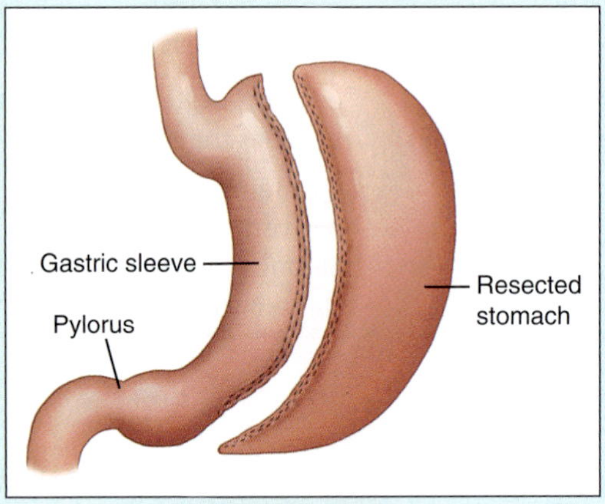

LAPAROSCOPIC ADJUSTABLE GASTRIC BANDING (LAGB)

Creation of a small gastric pouch by the placement of a band around the upper portion of the stomach; the band can be adjusted to change the size of the stomach through a subcutaneous port.

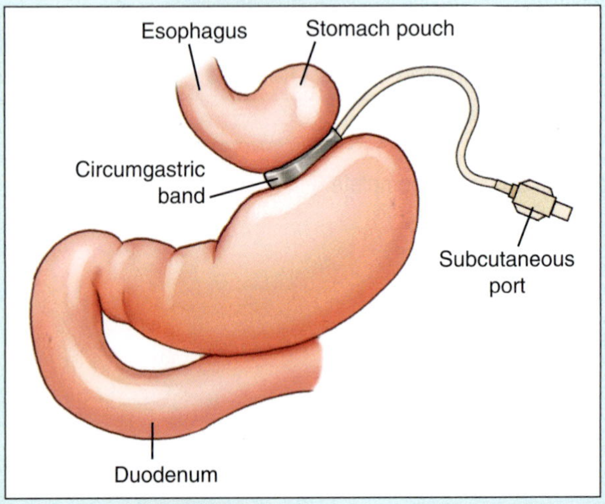

EXERCISE 21

Write the term for each of the following definitions.

1. cutting certain branches of the vagus nerve ______________________
2. connection created by surgically joining two structures ______________________
3. removal of the distal colon, rectum, and anal sphincter ______________________
4. surgical reduction of gastric capacity to treat morbid obesity ______________________
5. excision of swollen or distended veins in the lower rectum and anus ______________________

EXERCISE 22

Spell each of the Surgical Terms NOT Built from Word Parts by having someone dictate them to you. Use a separate sheet of paper.

To hear and spell the terms, go to Evolve Resources at evolve.elsevier.com and select:
Practice Student Resources > Student Resources > Chapter 11 > **Pronounce and Spell**

See Appendix B for instructions.

❑ Check the box when complete.

Diagnostic Terms
BUILT FROM WORD PARTS

The following terms can be translated using definitions of word parts. Further explanation is provided within parentheses as needed.

TERM	DEFINITION
DIAGNOSTIC IMAGING	
cholangiogram (kō-LAN-jē-ō-gram)	radiographic image of the bile ducts
cholangiography (kō-*lan*-jē-OG-ra-fē)	radiographic imaging of the bile ducts (after administration of contrast media to outline the ducts)
CT colonography (C-T) (*kō*-lon-OG-ra-fē)	radiographic imaging of the colon (using computed tomography) (Exercise Figure F)
esophagogram (e-SOF-a-gō-gram)	radiographic image of the esophagus (and pharynx). (A contrast medium, such as barium, is used to study function and form of swallowing related to the pharynx and esophagus.) (also called **esophagram** and **barium swallow**)

OPERATIVE CHOLANGIOGRAPHY

is performed during surgery to check for residual stones after the removal of the gallbladder. Postoperative cholangiography, also called T-tube cholangiography, is performed in the radiology department after a cholecystectomy, also to check for residual stones. Both use the injection of contrast media into the common bile duct.

EXERCISE FIGURE F

Fill in the blanks with word parts defined to complete labeling of the diagram.

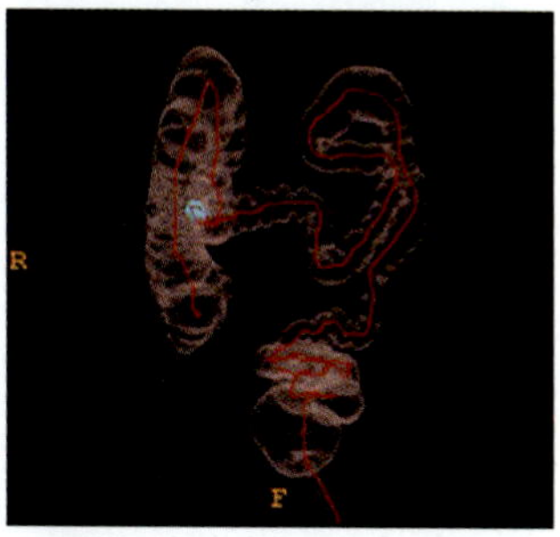

Image obtained using CT ______ / ______ / ______
colon / cv / radiographic imaging

also called virtual colonoscopy. It is less invasive than conventional colonoscopy but still requires a thorough emptying of the bowels (bowel prep) prior to the procedure.

Diagnostic Terms—cont'd

TERM	DEFINITION
ENDOSCOPY	
capsule endoscopy (KAP-sel) (en-DOS-ko-pē)	(capsule) visual examination within (a hollow organ); (procedure that uses a tiny wireless camera to take pictures of the gastrointestinal tract, especially the small intestine [which is not easily accessed by traditional endoscopy]; used to find obscure causes of gastrointestinal bleeding and to diagnose disorders such as Crohn disease, celiac disease, and cancer [also called **camera endoscopy**]) (Fig. 11.13)
colonoscope (kō-LON-ō-skōp)	instrument used for visual examination of the colon (Fig. 11.11)
colonoscopy (*kō*-lon-OS-ko-pē)	visual examination of the colon (Figs. 11.14 and 11.15)
esophagogastroduodenoscopy (EGD) (*e-sof*-a-gō-*gas*-trō-*dū*-od-e-NOS-ko-pē)	visual examination of the esophagus, stomach, and duodenum
esophagoscopy (e-*sof*-a-GOS-ko-pē)	visual examination of the esophagus
gastroscope (GAS-trō-skōp)	instrument used for visual examination of the stomach (Exercise Figure G2)

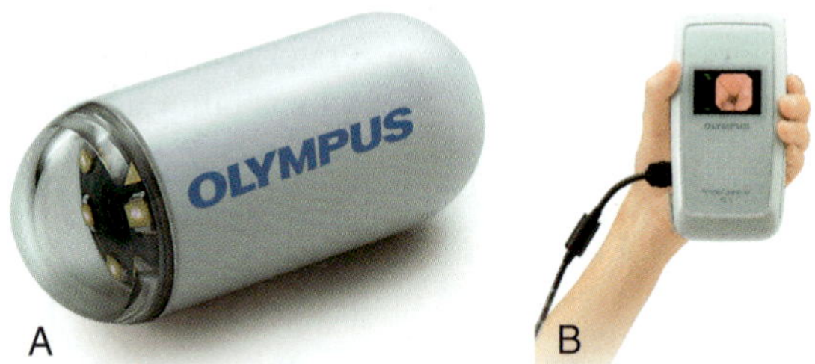

FIG. 11.13 Capsule endoscopy, also known as **camera endoscopy**. **A,** Patients swallow a capsule containing a camera, about the size of a vitamin pill. The camera takes pictures as it moves naturally through the gastrointestinal tract, and records thousands of images on a small device worn around the patient's waist. **B,** The recording device is then returned to the physician and the images are transferred to a computer for examination. The video capsule is expelled in the bowel movement and not retrieved.

TERM	DEFINITION
gastroscopy (gas-TROS-ko-pē)	visual examination of the stomach (Exercise Figure G1)
laparoscope (LAP-a-rō-skōp)	instrument used for visual examination of the abdominal cavity. (Also used to perform laparoscopic surgery, a method that sometimes replaces **laparotomy**, open abdominal incisional surgery.) (Fig. 11.10)
laparoscopy (*lap*-a-ROS-ko-pē)	visual examination of the abdominal cavity
proctoscope (PROK-tō-skōp)	instrument used for visual examination of the rectum
proctoscopy (prok-TOS-ko-pē)	visual examination of the rectum
sigmoidoscopy (*sig*-moy-DOS-ko-pē)	visual examination of the sigmoid colon (Fig. 11.15)

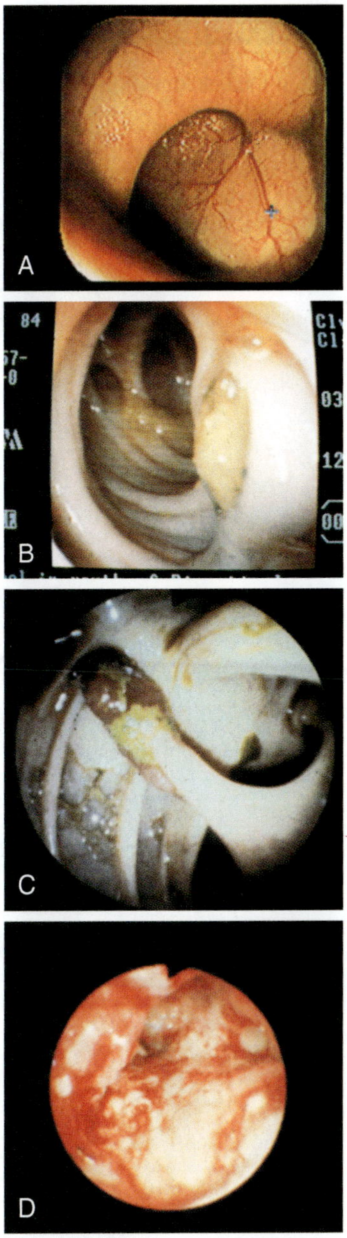

FIG. 11.14 Images obtained during colonoscopy reveal a normal colon **(A),** diverticulosis **(B),** a colon polyp **(C),** and colon cancer **(D).**

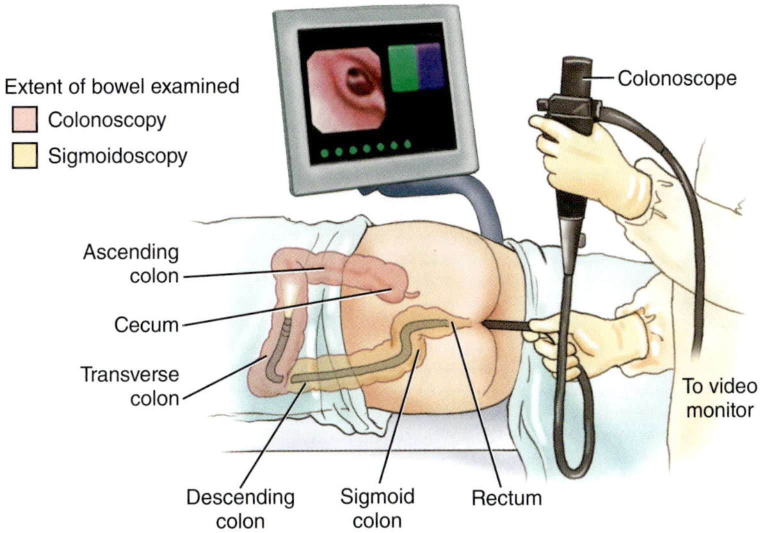

FIG. 11.15 Sigmoidoscopy, colonoscopy.

EXERCISE FIGURE G

Fill in the blanks with word parts defined to complete labeling of the diagram.

1
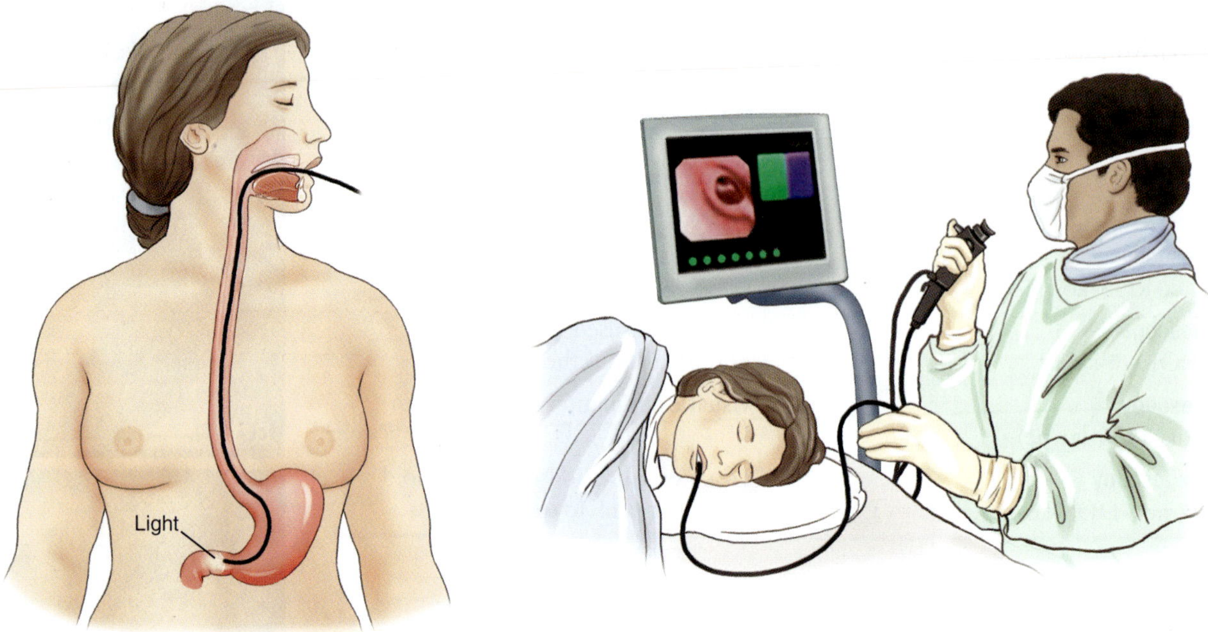

1, ________ / ________ / ________
stomach / cv / visual examination

2
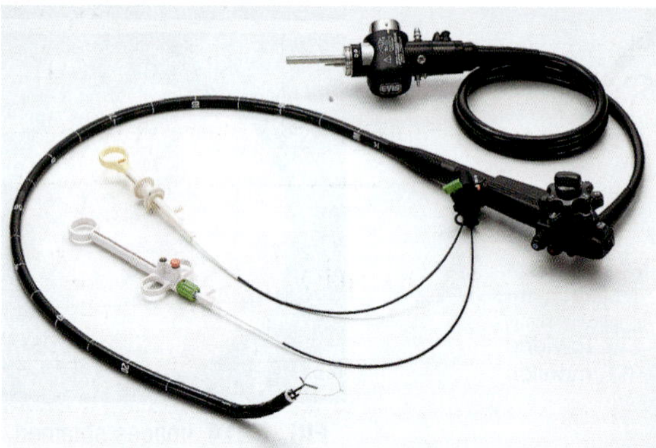

2, Fiberscope, a type of ________ / ________ / ________ that
stomach / cv / instrument used for visual examination
has glass fibers in a flexible tube, allows for light to be transmitted back to the examiner.

EXERCISE 23

Practice saying aloud each of the Diagnostic Terms Built from Word Parts.

> To hear the terms, go to Evolve Resources at evolve.elsevier.com and select:
> Practice Student Resources > Student Resources > Chapter 11 > **Pronounce and Spell**
>
> See Appendix B for instructions.

❑ Check the box when complete.

EXERCISE 24

Analyze and define the following terms.

1. esophagoscopy
2. gastroscope
3. gastroscopy
4. proctoscope
5. proctoscopy
6. (capsule) endoscopy
7. sigmoidoscopy
8. cholangiogram
9. esophagogastroduodenoscopy
10. colonoscope
11. laparoscope
12. colonoscopy
13. laparoscopy
14. (CT) colonography
15. esophagogram
16. cholangiography

EXERCISE 25

Build diagnostic terms for the following definitions by using the word parts you have learned.

1. (capsule) visual examination within (a hollow organ)	capsule ______ / ______ P / S(WR)
2. instrument used for visual examination of the stomach	WR / CV / S
3. instrument used for visual examination of the rectum	WR / CV / S
4. visual examination of the rectum	WR / CV / S
5. visual examination of the esophagus	WR / CV / S
6. visual examination of the sigmoid colon	WR / CV / S
7. radiographic image of the bile ducts	WR / CV / S
8. visual examination of the stomach	WR / CV / S
9. instrument used for visual examination of the abdominal cavity	WR / CV / S
10. visual examination of the esophagus, stomach, and duodenum	WR / CV / WR / CV / WR / CV / S
11. visual examination of the colon	WR / CV / S
12. visual examination of the abdominal cavity	WR / CV / S
13. instrument used for visual examination of the colon	WR / CV / S
14. radiographic imaging of the colon (using computed tomography)	CT ______ WR / CV / S
15. radiographic imaging of the bile ducts	WR / CV / S
16. radiographic image of the esophagus	WR / CV / S

EXERCISE 26

Spell each of the Diagnostic Terms Built from Word Parts by having someone dictate them to you. Use a separate sheet of paper.

To hear and spell the terms, go to Evolve Resources at evolve.elsevier.com and select:
Practice Student Resources > Student Resources > Chapter 11 > **Pronounce and Spell**

See Appendix B for instructions.

❑ Check the box when complete.

Diagnostic Terms
NOT BUILT FROM WORD PARTS

Word parts may be present in the following terms; however, their full meanings cannot be translated using definitions of word parts alone.

TERM	DEFINITION
DIAGNOSTIC IMAGING	
abdominal sonography (ab-DOM-i-nal) (so-NOG-ra-fē)	ultrasound scan of the abdominal cavity in which the size and structure of organs such as the aorta, liver, gallbladder, bile ducts, and pancreas can be visualized. Liver cysts, abscesses, tumors, cholelithiasis, pancreatitis, and pancreatic tumors may be detected. May also be used to evaluate the kidneys and the portion of the aorta extending through the abdominal cavity (Table 11.2).
barium enema (BE) (BAR-ē-um) (EN-e-ma)	series of radiographic images taken of the large intestine after the contrast agent barium has been administered rectally (also called **lower GI series**) (Fig. 11.16)
endoscopic retrograde cholangiopancreatography (ERCP) (*en*-dō-SKOP-ic) (RET-rō-grād) (kō-*lan*-jē-ō-*pan*-krē-a-TOG-rah-fē)	procedure in which contrast media is introduced (through an endoscope in the duodenum) into the biliary and pancreatic ducts; used to evaluate obstructions, strictures, stone diseases, pancreatitis, and pancreatic cancer (Fig. 11.17)
endoscopic ultrasound (EUS) (*en*-dō-SKOP-ic) (UL-tra-sound)	procedure using an endoscope fitted with an ultrasound probe that provides images of the esophageal and stomach linings, as well as the walls of the small and large intestines; used to detect tumors and cystic growths and for staging of malignant tumors
upper GI series (up-PER) (G-Ī) (SE-rēz)	series of radiographic images taken of the pharynx, esophagus, stomach, and duodenum after the contrast agent barium has been administered orally (also called **upper gastrointestinal series**)

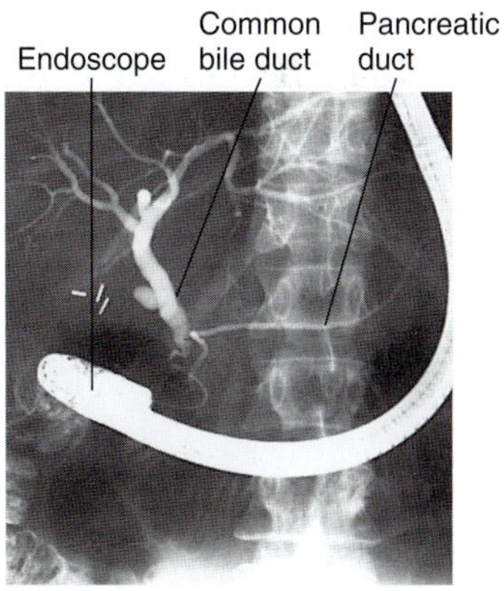

FIG. 11.17 Endoscopic retrograde cholangiopancreatography (ERCP).

TABLE 11.2 Abdominal Sonography

AREAS VISUALIZED AND POSSIBLE FINDINGS

- **Liver**—cysts, abscess, tumors, hepatitis, fatty infiltration, cirrhosis, hepatomegaly
- **Gallbladder and Bile Ducts**—cholelithiasis, choledocholithiasis, inflammation, obstruction, tumors (including polyps)
- **Pancreas**—inflammation, tumors, abscess, pseudocysts, obstruction
- **Kidney**—calculi, cysts, tumors, hydronephrosis, malformations, abscess, inflammation, scarring, atrophy
- **Aorta**—aneurysm, dissection, atherosclerosis

IMAGE

Abdominal ultrasound showing cholelithiasis. *GB*, Gallbladder; *St*, stone

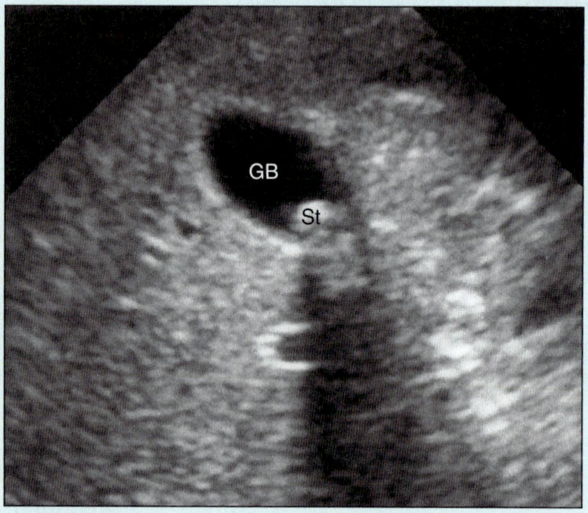

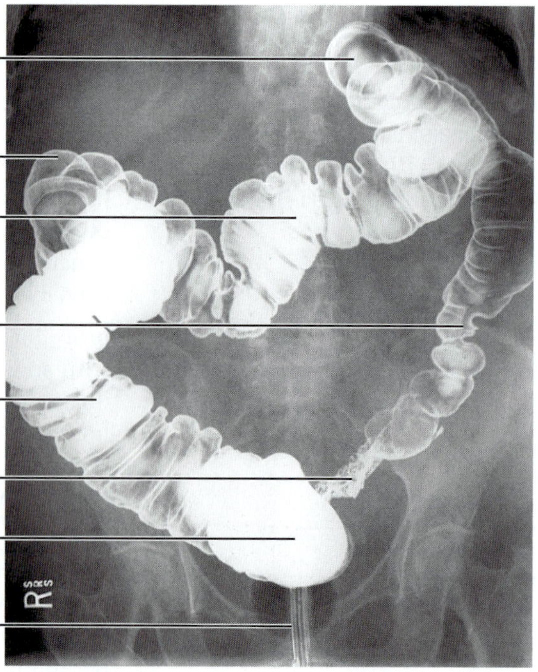

FIG. 11.16 Barium enema (BE); also called a **lower GI series.**

Diagnostic Terms—cont'd

TERM	DEFINITION
LABORATORY	
fecal occult blood test (FOBT) (FĒ-kl) (o-KULT) (blud) (test)	test to detect occult blood in feces. It is used to screen for colon cancer or polyps. Occult blood refers to blood that is present but can only be detected by chemical testing or by microscope.
***Helicobacter pylori* (*H. pylori*) antibodies test** (*hel*-i-kō-BAK-ter) (pī-LŌ-rē) (AN-ti-bod-ēs) (test)	blood test to determine the presence of *H. pylori* bacteria. The bacteria can be found in the lining of the stomach and can cause peptic ulcers. Tests for *H. pylori* are also performed on biopsy specimens and by breath test.

FECAL IMMUNOCHEMICAL TEST (FIT) FOR OCCULT BLOOD

is currently the standard stool test for screening for colorectal cancer and large polyps that may become cancerous. The FIT test requires only one stool specimen and is specific for occult blood in the lower gastrointestinal tract.

EXERCISE 27

Practice saying aloud each of the Diagnostic Terms NOT Built from Word Parts.

To hear the terms, go to Evolve Resources at evolve.elsevier.com and select:
Practice Student Resources > Student Resources > Chapter 11 > **Pronounce and Spell**

See Appendix B for instructions.

❑ Check the box when complete.

EXERCISE 28

Match the procedures in the first column with their correct definitions in the second column.

_____ 1. fecal occult blood test
_____ 2. barium enema
_____ 3. *Helicobacter pylori* antibodies test
_____ 4. upper GI series
_____ 5. endoscopic retrograde cholangiopancreatography
_____ 6. abdominal sonography
_____ 7. endoscopic ultrasound

a. used to diagnose peptic ulcers
b. radiographic images of the pharynx, esophagus, stomach, and duodenum
c. provides images of esophageal and stomach linings, and also walls of the intestines
d. detects blood in feces
e. radiographic imaging of biliary and pancreatic ducts
f. radiographic images of the large intestine
g. ultrasound scan of the abdominal cavity

EXERCISE 29

Spell each of the Diagnostic Terms NOT Built from Word Parts by having someone dictate them to you. Use a separate sheet of paper.

To hear and spell the terms, go to Evolve Resources at evolve.elsevier.com and select:
Practice Student Resources > Student Resources > Chapter 11 > **Pronounce and Spell**

See Appendix B for instructions.

❑ Check the box when complete.

Complementary Terms
BUILT FROM WORD PARTS

The following terms can be translated using definitions of word parts. Further explanation is provided within parentheses as needed.

TERM	DEFINITION
abdominal (ab-DOM-i-nal)	pertaining to the abdomen
anal (Ā-nal)	pertaining to the anus
aphagia (a-FĀ-ja)	without swallowing (the inability to)
celiac (SĒ-lē-ak)	pertaining to the abdomen
colorectal (*kō*-lō-REK-tal)	pertaining to the colon and rectum
duodenal (dū-OD-e-nal)	pertaining to the duodenum
dyspepsia (dis-PEP-sē-a)	difficult digestion (often used to describe GI symptoms, such as abdominal pain and bloating)
dysphagia (dis-FĀ-ja)	difficult swallowing
enteropathy (*en*-ter-OP-a-thē)	disease of the intestine
esophageal (e-*sof*-a-JĒ-al)	pertaining to the esophagus
gastric (GAS-trik)	pertaining to the stomach
gastroenterologist (*gas*-trō-*en*-ter-OL-o-jist)	physician who studies and treats diseases of the stomach and intestines (GI tract and accessory organs)
gastroenterology (*gas*-trō-*en*-ter-OL-o-jē)	study of the stomach and intestines (branch of medicine that deals with treating diseases of the GI tract and accessory organs)
gastromalacia (*gas*-trō-ma-LĀ-sha)	softening of the stomach
hepatomegaly (*hep*-a-tō-MEG-a-lē)	enlargement of the liver
ileocecal (*il*-ē-ō-SĒ-kal)	pertaining to the ileum and cecum
nasogastric (*nā*-zō-GAS-trik)	pertaining to the nose and stomach
oral (OR-al)	pertaining to the mouth
orogastric (*or*-ō-GAS-trik)	pertaining to the mouth and stomach
pancreatic (*pan*-krē-AT-ik)	pertaining to the pancreas

TERM	DEFINITION
peritoneal (*per*-i-tō-NĒ-al)	pertaining to the peritoneum
proctology (prok-TOL-o-jē)	study of the rectum (branch of medicine that deals with disorders of the rectum and anus)
rectal (REK-tal)	pertaining to the rectum
steatorrhea (*stē*-a-tō-RĒ-a)	discharge of fat (excessive amount of fat in the stool, causing frothy, foul-smelling fecal matter usually associated with the malabsorption of fat in conditions such as chronic pancreatitis and celiac disease)
steatosis (*stē*-a-TŌ-sis)	abnormal condition of fat (increased fat at the cellular level often affecting the liver)
stomatitis (*stō*-ma-TĪ-tis)	inflammation of the mouth (mucous membrane)
sublingual (sub-LING-gwal)	pertaining to under the tongue

EXERCISE 30

Practice saying aloud each of the Complementary Terms Built from Word Parts.

To hear the terms, go to Evolve Resources at evolve.elsevier.com and select:
Practice Student Resources > Student Resources > Chapter 11 > **Pronounce and Spell**

See Appendix B for instructions.

❑ Check the box when complete.

EXERCISE 31

Analyze and define the following complementary terms.

1. aphagia
____
____

2. dyspepsia
____
____

3. anal
____
____

4. dysphagia
____
____

5. hepatomegaly
____
____

6. ileocecal
____
____

7. oral

8. orogastric

9. gastromalacia

10. pancreatic

11. peritoneal

12. steatosis

13. sublingual

14. proctology

15. nasogastric

16. abdominal

17. gastroenterology

18. gastroenterologist

19. colorectal

20. rectal

21. steatorrhea

22. stomatitis

23. enteropathy

24. gastric

25. duodenal

____

____

26. esophageal

____

____

27. celiac

____

____

EXERCISE 32

Build the complementary terms for the following definitions by using the word parts you have learned.

1. enlargement of the liver ______ / ______ / ______ (WR / CV / S)
2. without swallowing (the inability to) ______ / ______ (P / S(WR))
3. pertaining to under the tongue ______ / ______ / ______ (P / WR / S)
4. pertaining to the nose and the stomach ______ / ______ / ______ / ______ (WR / CV / WR / S)
5. pertaining to the mouth and the stomach ______ / ______ / ______ / ______ (WR / CV / WR / S)
6. pertaining to the anus ______ / ______ (WR / S)
7. pertaining to the peritoneum ______ / ______ (WR / S)
8. pertaining to the abdomen
   a. ______ / ______ (WR / S)
   b. ______ / ______ (WR / S)
9. difficult swallowing ______ / ______ (P / S(WR))
10. pertaining to the ileum and cecum ______ / ______ / ______ / ______ (WR / CV / WR / S)
11. softening of the stomach ______ / ______ / ______ (WR / CV / S)

12. difficult digestion ______ P / ______ S(WR)

13. pertaining to the pancreas ______ WR / ______ S

14. study of the rectum ______ WR / CV / ______ S

15. discharge of fat (in the stool) ______ WR / CV / ______ S

16. pertaining to the mouth ______ WR / ______ S

17. physician who studies and treats diseases of the stomach and intestines ______ WR / CV / ______ WR / CV / ______ S

18. study of the stomach and intestines ______ WR / CV / ______ WR / CV / ______ S

19. pertaining to the colon and rectum ______ WR / CV / ______ WR / ______ S

20. pertaining to the rectum ______ WR / ______ S

21. abnormal condition of fat (such as in the liver) ______ WR / ______ S

22. pertaining to the esophagus ______ WR / ______ S

23. pertaining to the stomach ______ WR / ______ S

24. pertaining to the duodenum ______ WR / ______ S

25. disease of the intestine ______ WR / CV / ______ S

26. inflammation of the mouth (mucous membrane) ______ WR / ______ S

EXERCISE 33

Spell each of the Complementary Terms Built from Word Parts by having someone dictate them to you. Use a separate sheet of paper.

To hear and spell the terms, go to Evolve Resources at evolve.elsevier.com and select:
Practice Student Resources > Student Resources > Chapter 11 > **Pronounce and Spell**

See Appendix B for instructions.

❑ Check the box when complete.

Complementary Terms

NOT BUILT FROM WORD PARTS

Word parts may be present in the following terms; however, their full meanings cannot be translated using definitions of word parts alone.

TERM	DEFINITION
ascites (a-SĪ-tēz)	abnormal collection of fluid in the peritoneal cavity (Fig. 11.18)
diarrhea (dī-a-RĒ-a)	frequent discharge of liquid stool *(Note:* diarrhea *is composed of* dia-, *meaning through, and* -rrhea, *meaning flow.)*
dysentery (DIS-en-*ter*-ē)	disorder that involves inflammation of the intestine (usually the large intestine) associated with abdominal pain and diarrhea that is often bloody
emesis (EM-e-sis)	expelling matter from the stomach through the mouth (also called **vomiting**)
feces (FĒ-sēz)	waste from the gastrointestinal tract expelled through the rectum (also called **stool** or **fecal matter**)
flatus (FLĀ-tus)	gas in the gastrointestinal tract or expelled through the anus
gastric lavage (GAS-trik) (la-VOZH)	washing out of the stomach
gavage (ga-VOZH)	process of feeding a person through a tube
hematemesis (*hē*-ma-TEM-e-sis)	vomiting of blood
hematochezia (*hē*-ma-tō-KĒ-zha)	passage of visibly bloody feces
malabsorption (*mal*-ab-SORP-shun)	impaired digestion or intestinal absorption of nutrients
melena (me-LĒ-na)	black, tarry stool that contains digested blood; usually a result of bleeding in the upper GI tract
nausea (NAW-zē-a)	urge to vomit
palpate (PAL-pāt)	to examine by hand; to feel
peristalsis (*per*-i-STAL-sis)	involuntary wavelike contractions that propel food along the gastrointestinal tract

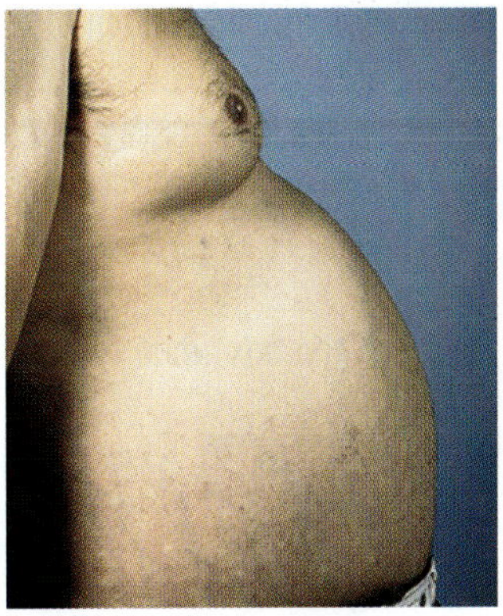

FIG. 11.18 Ascites.

Complementary Terms—cont'd

TERM	DEFINITION
reflux (RĒ-fluks)	abnormal backward flow. In esophageal reflux, the stomach contents flow back into the esophagus.
stoma (STŌ-ma)	surgical opening between an organ and the surface of the body, such as the opening established in the abdominal wall by colostomy, ileostomy, or a similar operation (see Exercise Figure E). Stoma may also refer to an opening created between body structures or between portions of the intestines.

Refer to **Appendix F** for pharmacology terms related to the digestive system.

EXERCISE 34

Practice saying aloud each of the Complementary Terms NOT Built from Word Parts.

To hear the terms, go to Evolve Resources at evolve.elsevier.com and select:
Practice Student Resources > Student Resources > Chapter 11 > **Pronounce and Spell**

See Appendix B for instructions.

❑ Check the box when complete.

EXERCISE 35

Match the definitions in the first column with the correct terms in the second column.

_____ 1. abnormal collection of fluid
_____ 2. expelling matter from the stomach
_____ 3. feeding a person through a tube
_____ 4. washing out of the stomach
_____ 5. urge to vomit
_____ 6. frequent discharge of liquid stool
_____ 7. waste expelled from the rectum
_____ 8. vomiting of blood
_____ 9. abnormal backward flow
_____ 10. inflammation of the intestine associated with abdominal pain and diarrhea that is often bloody
_____ 11. gas expelled through the anus
_____ 12. involuntary wavelike contractions
_____ 13. black, tarry stools
_____ 14. surgical opening between an organ and the surface of the body
_____ 15. to examine by hand
_____ 16. passage of visibly bloody feces
_____ 17. impaired digestion or intestinal absorption

a. hematemesis
b. flatus
c. gastric lavage
d. reflux
e. emesis
f. gavage
g. melena
h. dysentery
i. diarrhea
j. peristalsis
k. feces
l. nausea
m. ascites
n. hematochezia
o. stoma
p. malabsorption
q. palpate

EXERCISE 36

Write definitions for each of the following terms.

1. ascites ____
2. gavage ____
3. gastric lavage ____
4. feces ____
5. nausea ____
6. dysentery ____
7. diarrhea ____
8. flatus ____
9. reflux ____
10. hematemesis ____
11. peristalsis ____
12. melena ____
13. stoma ____
14. hematochezia ____
15. emesis ____
16. malabsorption ____
17. palpate ____

EXERCISE 37

Spell each of the Complementary Terms NOT Built from Word Parts by having someone dictate them to you. Use a separate sheet of paper.

To hear and spell the terms, go to Evolve Resources at evolve.elsevier.com and select:
Practice Student Resources > Student Resources > Chapter 11 > **Pronounce and Spell**

See Appendix B for instructions.

❑ Check the box when complete.

Abbreviations

ABBREVIATION	TERM
APR	abdominoperineal resection
BE	barium enema
EGD	esophagogastroduodenoscopy
ERCP	endoscopic retrograde cholangiopancreatography
EUS	endoscopic ultrasound
FOBT	fecal occult blood test
GERD	gastroesophageal reflux disease
GI	gastrointestinal
H. pylori	*Helicobacter pylori*
IBS	irritable bowel syndrome
N&V	nausea and vomiting

WEB LINK

For more information about diseases and disorders of the digestive system and the latest treatments available, please visit the National Digestive Diseases Information Clearing House at *digestive .niddk.nih.gov.*

Abbreviations—cont'd

ABBREVIATION	TERM
PEG	percutaneous endoscopic gastrostomy
UC	ulcerative colitis
UGI	upper gastrointestinal
UPPP	uvulopalatopharyngoplasty

Refer to **Appendix E** for a complete list of abbreviations.

EXERCISE 38

Write the abbreviations for the terms listed below.

1. upper gastrointestinal ______________________
2. *Helicobacter pylori* ______________________
3. nausea and vomiting ______________________
4. endoscopic retrograde cholangiopancreatography ______________________
5. gastrointestinal ______________________
6. uvulopalatopharyngoplasty ______________________
7. gastroesophageal reflux disease ______________________
8. ulcerative colitis ______________________
9. barium enema ______________________
10. irritable bowel syndrome ______________________
11. esophagogastroduodenoscopy ______________________
12. percutaneous endoscopic gastrostomy ______________________
13. endoscopic ultrasound ______________________
14. abdominoperineal resection ______________________
15. fecal occult blood test ______________________

For additional practice with Abbreviations, go to Evolve Resources at evolve.elsevier.com and select:
Practice Student Resources > Student Resources > Chapter 11 > **Flashcards:** Abbreviations

See Appendix B for instructions.

For nutrition terms and dental terms, go to Evolve Resources at evolve.elsevier.com and select:
Practice Student Resources > Student Resources > Extra Content > **Appendix L:** Nutrition Terms
Appendix M: Dental Terms

See Appendix B for instructions.

PRACTICAL APPLICATION

EXERCISE 39 *Case Study: Translate Between Everyday Language and Medical Language*

CASE STUDY: Ruth Clifton

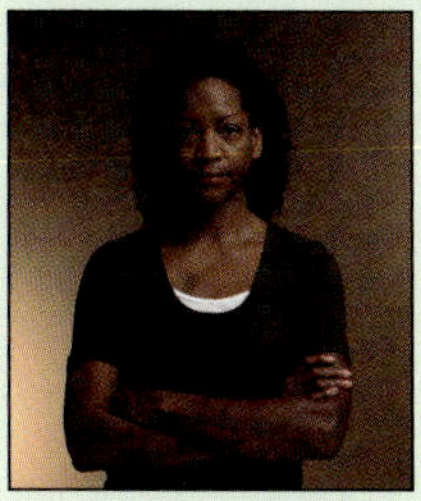

Ruth is worried about her stomach. She has been having pain on and off for about 3 months. At first it was just once in a while but now it seems to be every day. Her pain seems to be worse when she hasn't eaten for a while and after she eats something bland it usually gets a bit better. She bought some antacids at the pharmacy and chewing those also seems to help. Lately the pain in her stomach has been waking her up at night. A glass of milk usually helps with that. The last few days, though, she has felt sick to her stomach, has been throwing up, and is finding it difficult to eat. Her friend recommends that she see a stomach doctor, who helped her when she had similar problems.

Now that you have worked through Chapter 11 on the digestive system, consider the medical terms that might be used to describe Ruth Clifton's experience. See the Review of Terms at the end of this chapter for a list of terms that might apply.

A. *Underline phrases in the case study that could be substituted with medical terms.*

B. *Write the medical term and its definition for three of the phrases you underlined.*

MEDICAL TERM	DEFINITION
1. ____________	____________
2. ____________	____________
3. ____________	____________

DOCUMENTATION: Excerpt From Endoscopic Procedure Report

Ms. Clifton made an appointment with a gastroenterologist. He recommended an endoscopic procedure; a portion of the report is documented below.

ENDOSCOPY REPORT: Procedure: Esophagogastroduodenoscopy

The patient was given 2 mg of intravenous midazolam along with lidocaine spray to the pharynx. After she was placed in the left lateral decubitus position, the gastroscope was passed into the pharynx without difficulty. No abnormalities were noted in the esophagus, or in the cardia and the body of the stomach. A biopsy of the gastric mucosa was obtained for *Helicobacter pylori* antibodies test. In the distal antrum, some mild erythematous changes were noted. The pylorus appeared normal, but a single 1 cm ulceration of the proximal duodenum, a peptic ulcer, was observed.

C. *Underline medical terms presented in Chapter 11 in the previous excerpt from Ms. Clifton's medical record. See the Review of Terms at the end of the chapter for a complete list.*

D. *Select and define three of the medical terms you underlined. To check your answers, go to Appendix A.*

MEDICAL TERM	DEFINITION
1. ____________	____________
2. ____________	____________
3. ____________	____________

EXERCISE 40 *Interact With Medical Documents and Electronic Health Records*

A. Read the report and complete it by writing medical terms on answer lines within the document. Definitions of terms to be written appear after the document.

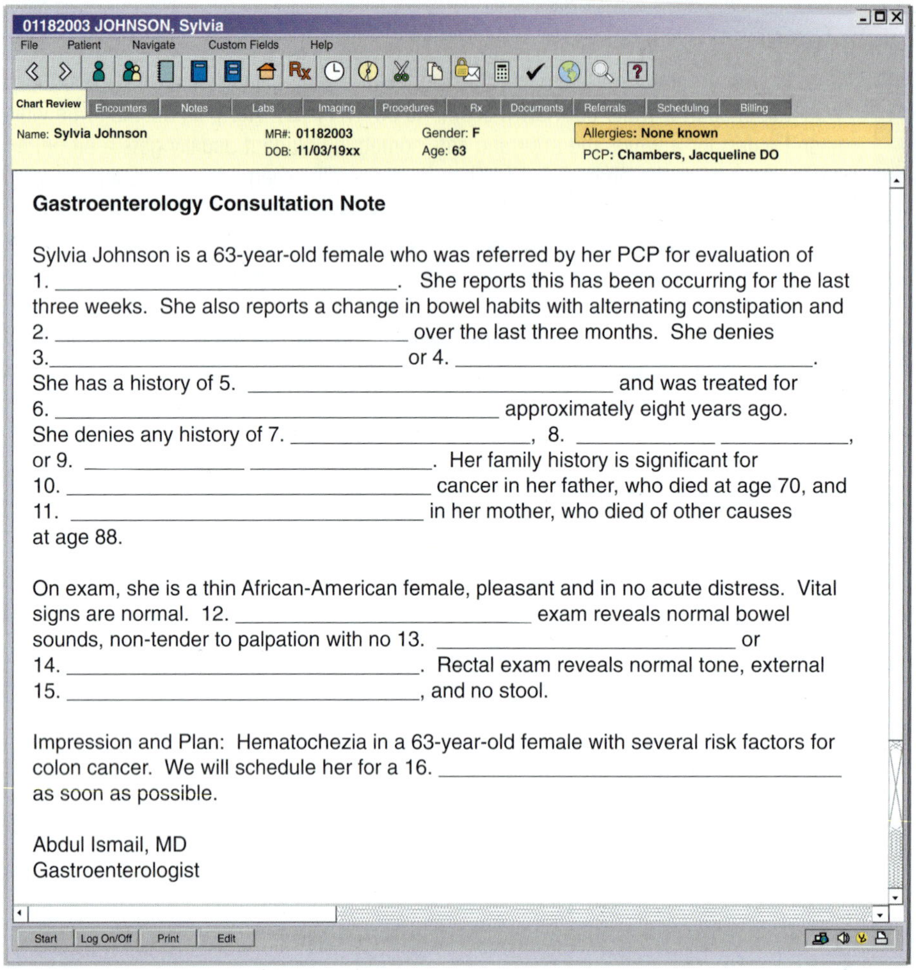

Gastroenterology Consultation Note

Sylvia Johnson is a 63-year-old female who was referred by her PCP for evaluation of 1. ______________________. She reports this has been occurring for the last three weeks. She also reports a change in bowel habits with alternating constipation and 2. ______________________ over the last three months. She denies 3. ______________________ or 4. ______________________. She has a history of 5. ______________________ and was treated for 6. ______________________ approximately eight years ago. She denies any history of 7. ______________________, 8. __________ __________, or 9. __________ __________. Her family history is significant for 10. ______________________ cancer in her father, who died at age 70, and 11. ______________________ in her mother, who died of other causes at age 88.

On exam, she is a thin African-American female, pleasant and in no acute distress. Vital signs are normal. 12. ______________________ exam reveals normal bowel sounds, non-tender to palpation with no 13. ______________________ or 14. ______________________. Rectal exam reveals normal tone, external 15. ______________________, and no stool.

Impression and Plan: Hematochezia in a 63-year-old female with several risk factors for colon cancer. We will schedule her for a 16. ______________________ as soon as possible.

Abdul Ismail, MD
Gastroenterologist

Definitions of Medical Terms to Complete the Document

Write the medical terms defined on corresponding answer lines in the document.

1. discharge of visibly bloody feces
2. frequent discharge of liquid stool
3. urge to vomit
4. expelling matter from the stomach through the mouth
5. abnormal backward flow of the gastrointestinal contents into the esophagus
6. blood test to determine the presence of *a bacteria found in the lining* of the stomach that can cause peptic ulcers
7. erosion of the mucous membrane of the stomach or duodenum
8. chronic inflammation of the intestinal tract characterized by cobblestone ulcerations and the formation of scar tissue that may lead to intestinal obstruction
9. disease characterized by inflammation of the colon with the formation of ulcers, which can cause bloody diarrhea
10. pertaining to the colon and rectum
11. inflammation of the esophagus
12. pertaining to the abdomen
13. abnormal collection of fluid in the peritoneal cavity
14. enlargement of the liver
15. swollen or distended veins in the rectum or anus
16. visual examination of the colon

B. Read the medical report and answer the questions below it.

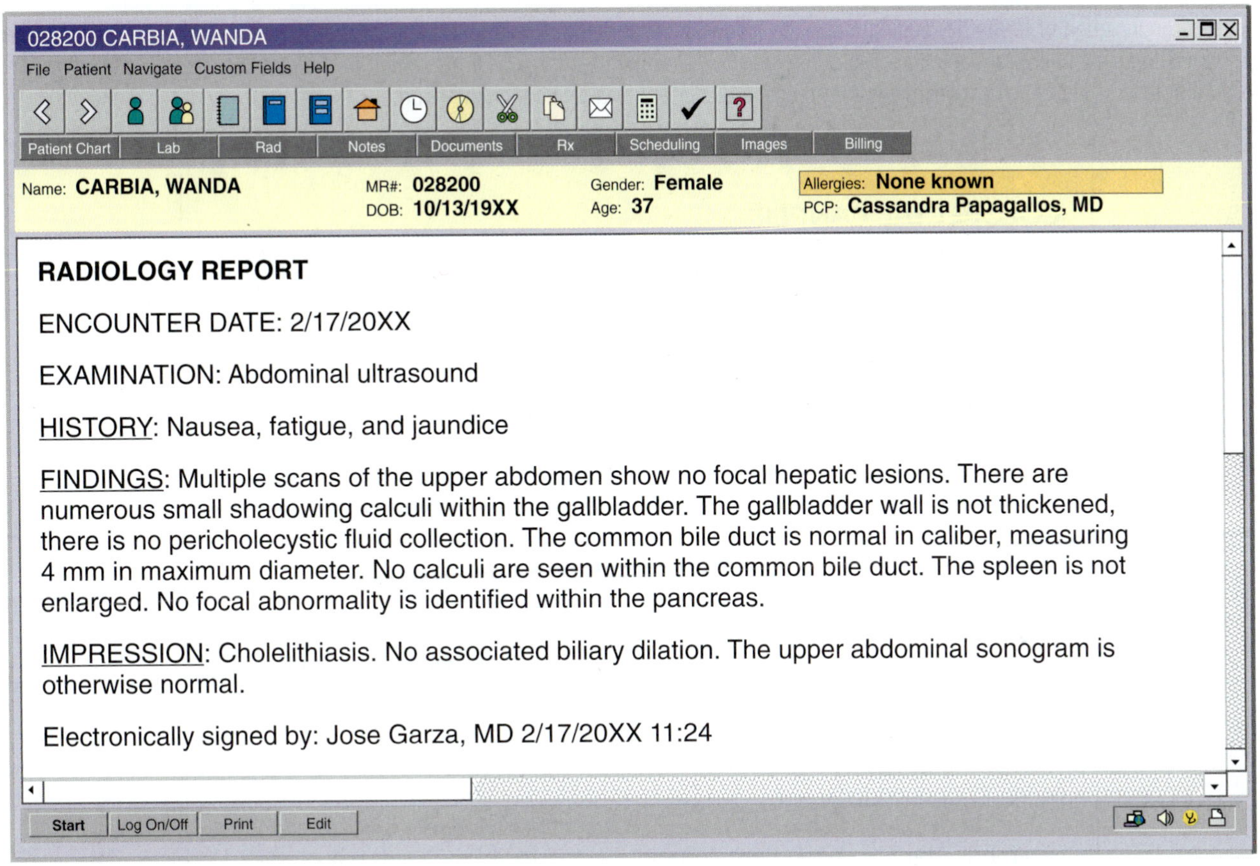

028200 CARBIA, WANDA

File Patient Navigate Custom Fields Help

Patient Chart | Lab | Rad | Notes | Documents | Rx | Scheduling | Images | Billing

Name: **CARBIA, WANDA** MR#: **028200** DOB: **10/13/19XX** Gender: **Female** Age: **37** Allergies: **None known** PCP: **Cassandra Papagallos, MD**

RADIOLOGY REPORT

ENCOUNTER DATE: 2/17/20XX

EXAMINATION: Abdominal ultrasound

HISTORY: Nausea, fatigue, and jaundice

FINDINGS: Multiple scans of the upper abdomen show no focal hepatic lesions. There are numerous small shadowing calculi within the gallbladder. The gallbladder wall is not thickened, there is no pericholecystic fluid collection. The common bile duct is normal in caliber, measuring 4 mm in maximum diameter. No calculi are seen within the common bile duct. The spleen is not enlarged. No focal abnormality is identified within the pancreas.

IMPRESSION: Cholelithiasis. No associated biliary dilation. The upper abdominal sonogram is otherwise normal.

Electronically signed by: Jose Garza, MD 2/17/20XX 11:24

Start | Log On/Off | Print | Edit

Use the medical report above to answer the questions.

1. The exam included which diagnostic procedure:
   a. radiographic imaging of the colon with computerized tomography
   b. radiographic imaging of the bile ducts after administration of contrast media
   c. use of an endoscope fitted with an ultrasound probe to obtain images of layers of the intestinal wall
   d. recording images of organs with sound waves produced by a transducer placed directly on the skin
2. The patient's symptoms included:
   a. expelling matter from the stomach through the mouth
   b. condition characterized by a yellow tinge to the skin
   c. bluish discoloration of the skin
   d. erythroderma
3. The examination revealed the presence of:
   a. stones within the gallbladder
   b. stones within the common bile duct
   c. lesions in the liver
   d. inflammation of the pancreas
4. "Biliary dilation" would most likely refer to:
   a. inflammation of the pancreas
   b. the presence of fluid in the upper abdomen
   c. choledocholithiasis
   d. widening of the bile ducts or gallbladder

C. Complete the **three medical documents** within the electronic health record (EHR) on Evolve.

Topic: Bowel Obstruction
Documents: Office Visit, Radiology Report, Colonoscopy Report

To complete the three medical records, go to Evolve Resources at evolve.elsevier.com and select:
Practice Student Resources > Student Resources > Chapter 11 > **Electronic Heath Records**

See Appendix B for instructions.

EXERCISE 41 *Pronounce Medical Terms in Use*

Practice pronunciation of terms by reading aloud the following paragraphs. Use the phonetic spellings following medical terms from the chapter to assist with pronunciation. The script also contains medical terms not presented in the chapter. Treat them as information only or look for their meanings in a medical dictionary or a reliable online source.

COLORECTAL CANCER

Colorectal (kō-lō-REK-tal) cancer begins in the colon or rectum and is the second leading cause of cancer deaths in the United States. Most are adenocarcinomas that originate as a benign, adenomatous **polyp** (POL-ip).

Many people have no symptoms until the tumor is quite advanced, and symptoms vary depending on the location of the tumor. Warning signs are altered bowel habits, **rectal** (REK-tal) bleeding, **abdominal** (ab-DOM-i-nal) cramps, **flatus** (FLĀ-tus) and bloating, iron deficiency anemia, and weight loss.

Screening and diagnostic tests for colorectal cancer include digital rectal examination, **fecal occult blood test** (FĒ-kl) (o-KULT) (blud) (test), **sigmoidoscopy** (*sig*-moy-DOS-ko-pē), **colonoscopy** (kō-lon-OS-ko-pē), and **barium enema** (BAR-ē-um) (EN-e-ma). As well as being an important diagnostic tool, colonos-copy may be used for biopsy and for the removal of pedunculated **polyps** (POL-ips). To perform a **polypectomy** (*pol*-i-PEK-to-mē), a braided wire snare is inserted into the **colonoscope** (kō-LON-ō-skōp). A snare loop, like a noose, is placed around the stem of the polyp. With electrosurgical power attached to the snare, the polyp is detached. The polyp is removed from the colon for histologic examination.

For cancer beyond the early stage, conventional surgery is the main treatment. The type of surgery depends on the location and stage of the tumor. Types of surgeries performed are left or right-sided **hemicolectomy** (*hem*-ē-kō-LEK-to-mē) with **anastomosis** (a-*nas*-to-MŌ-sis), sigmoid **colectomy** (kō-LEK-to-mē), and **abdominoperineal resection** (ab-*dom*-i-nō-per-i-NĒ-el) (rē-SEK-shun) with **colostomy** (ko-LOS-to-mē). Currently, colorectal surgeons can sometimes perform low anterior resection (LAR), which preserves the anal sphincter and prevents the need for a colostomy.

EXERCISE 42 *Chapter Content Quiz*

Test your understanding of terms and abbreviations introduced in this chapter. Circle the letter for the medical term or abbreviation related to the words in italics.

1. Mr. Gomez was tentatively diagnosed with *gallstones*, or
   a. cholelithiasis
   b. cholecystitis
   c. choledocholithiasis
2. An abdominal ultrasound confirmed the diagnosis, and Mr. Gomez is now scheduled for a laparoscopic *excision of the gallbladder*, or
   a. cholecystostomy
   b. cholecystectomy
   c. colectomy
3. After prior surgeries to remove portions of his intestines due to Crohn disease, Mr. Kipling was able to have *connections created by surgically joining two structures* when his disease went into remission. (hint: plural form)
   a. anastomoses
   b. anastomosis
   c. anastomosices

4. Mrs. Marshall was having symptoms of bloody diarrhea, abdominal pain and cramping, and fatigue. She was eventually diagnosed with *disease characterized by inflammation of the colon with the formation of ulcers, which can cause bloody diarrhea.*
   a. UC
   b. UPPP
   c. UGI

5. As an infant, Cameron Liu had an episode of *telescoping of a segment of the intestine*, which was diagnosed and treated by a barium enema.
   a. irritable bowel syndrome
   b. ileum
   c. intussusception

6. Because of her frequent heartburn, Mrs. Patel had a(n) *series of radiographic images taken of the pharynx, esophagus, stomach, and duodenum after the contrast agent barium has been administered orally*.
   a. upper GI series
   b. endoscopic ultrasound
   c. barium enema

7. After years of taking medication for peptic ulcers with no relief, it was recommended that Mr. Ezaki have *cutting of certain branches of the vagus nerve* to help treat his symptoms.
   a. gastrectomy
   b. pyloroplasty
   c. vagotomy

8. Mrs. Schwartz found that she *experienced difficult digestion, (such as abdominal pain and bloating)*, shortly after taking her osteoporosis medication.
   a. dyspepsia
   b. diarrhea
   c. dysphagia

9. During the colonoscopy, Dr. Mostafa found it difficult to visualize the colon all the way to the *pertaining to the ileum and cecum* valve.
   a. esophageal
   b. ileocecal
   c. peritoneal

10. After multiple surgeries for various gynecologic and gastrointestinal problems, Ms. Harding developed *abnormal growing together of two peritoneal surfaces that normally are separated.*
    a. hemorrhoids
    b. celiac disease
    c. adhesions

11. Mrs. Palmeri had an abdominal ultrasound that revealed *enlargement of the liver*, which was thought to be due to steatosis.
    a. hepatitis
    b. hepatoma
    c. hepatomegaly

12. A percutaneous endoscopic *creation of an artificial opening into the stomach (PEG)* tube was used for Mrs. McKee after her stroke.
    a. gastrostomy
    b. gastrectomy
    c. gastrotomy

13. John Begay saw his doctor because of right upper quadrant pain after eating fatty foods. An abdominal ultrasound revealed a stone in the common bile duct. A(n) *procedure in which contrast media is introduced into the biliary and pancreatic ducts* was performed and the stone was removed.
    a. ERCP
    b. EUS
    c. EGD

14. Mrs. Martinez, who was morbidly obese, was struggling with diabetes and hypertension. Her physician referred her for *a surgical reduction of gastric capacity to treat morbid obesity, a condition which can cause serious illness.*
    a. abdominocentesis
    b. bariatric surgery
    c. abdominoperineal resection

15. After his last episode of diverticulitis, Mr. Small developed *inflammation of the peritoneum*.
    a. peristalsis
    b. pancreatitis
    c. peritonitis

16. As a result of her Parkinson disease, Mrs. Borders developed *difficult swallowing*.
    a. dysphagia
    b. aphagia
    c. dysentery

17. Laura Schmidt complained of *discharge of fat (excessive amount of fat in the stool, causing frothy, foul-smelling fecal matter)* which later led to her diagnosis of celiac disease.
    a. steatohepatitis
    b. steatosis
    c. steatorrhea

18. Many years ago, Jaime Garza had *excision of the uvula* for treatment of his sleep apnea.
    a. gingivectomy
    b. uvulectomy
    c. uvulopalatopharyngoplasty

19. Indu Deshmukh was born with cleft palate and cleft lip. She had palatoplasty and *surgical repair of the lip* during her childhood.
    a. pyloroplasty
    b. cheiloplasty
    c. gastroplasty

20. After eating very spicy Vietnamese food, Johan Johanssen developed *inflammation of the tongue*.
    a. gingivitis
    b. palatitis
    c. glossitis

CHAPTER REVIEW

REVIEW OF CHAPTER CONTENT ON EVOLVE RESOURCES

Go to evolve.elsevier.com and click on Gradable Student Resources and Practice Student Resources. Online learning activities found there can be used to review chapter content and to assess your learning of word parts, medical terms, and abbreviations. Place check marks in the boxes next to activities used for review and assessment.

GRADABLE STUDENT RESOURCES

Chapter 11 >	Exercises >	☐ Word Parts ☐ Terms Built from Word Parts ☐ Terms Not Built from Word Parts ☐ Abbreviations
	Quizzes >	☐ Quiz 1: Disease and Disorder Terms ☐ Quiz 2: Surgical Terms ☐ Quiz 3: Diagnostic Terms ☐ Quiz 4: Complementary Terms

PRACTICE STUDENT RESOURCES > STUDENT RESOURCES

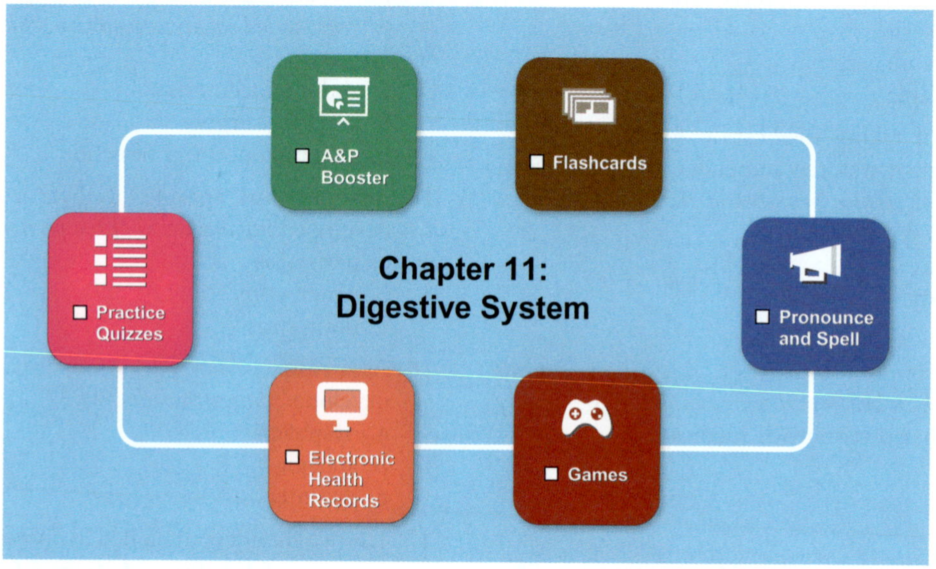

REVIEW OF WORD PARTS

Can you define and spell the following word parts?

COMBINING FORMS			PREFIX	SUFFIX
abdomin/o	duoden/o	palat/o	hemi-	-pepsia
an/o	enter/o	pancreat/o		
antr/o	esophag/o	peritone/o		
append/o	gastr/o	polyp/o		
appendic/o	gingiv/o	proct/o		
cec/o	gloss/o	pylor/o		
celi/o	hepat/o	rect/o		
cheil/o	herni/o	sial/o		
cholangi/o	ile/o	sigmoid/o		
chol/e	jejun/o	steat/o		
choledoch/o	lapar/o	stomat/o		
col/o	lingu/o	uvul/o		
colon/o	or/o			
diverticul/o				

REVIEW OF TERMS

Can you define, pronounce, and spell the following terms *built from word parts*?

DISEASES AND DISORDERS	SURGICAL	DIAGNOSTIC	COMPLEMENTARY
appendicitis	abdominocentesis	capsule endoscopy	abdominal
cholangioma	abdominoplasty	cholangiogram	anal
cholecystitis	anoplasty	cholangiography	aphagia
choledocholithiasis	antrectomy	colonoscope	celiac
cholelithiasis	appendectomy	colonoscopy	colorectal
colitis	cheiloplasty	CT colonography	duodenal
diverticulitis	cholecystectomy	esophagogastroduodenoscopy (EGD)	dyspepsia
diverticulosis	choledocholithotomy	esophagogram	dysphagia
enteritis	colectomy	esophagoscopy	enteropathy
esophagitis	colostomy	gastroscope	esophageal
gastritis	diverticulectomy	gastroscopy	gastric
gastroenteritis	enterorrhaphy	laparoscope	gastroenterologist
gastroenterocolitis	esophagogastroplasty	laparoscopy	gastroenterology
gingivitis	gastrectomy	proctoscope	gastromalacia
glossitis	gastrojejunostomy	proctoscopy	hepatomegaly
hepatitis	gastroplasty	sigmoidoscopy	ileocecal
hepatoma	gastrostomy		nasogastric
palatitis	gingivectomy		oral
pancreatitis	glossorrhaphy		orogastric
peritonitis	hemicolectomy		pancreatic
polyposis	herniorrhaphy		peritoneal
proctitis	ileostomy		proctology
rectocele	laparotomy		rectal
sialolith	palatoplasty		steatorrhea
steatohepatitis	polypectomy		steatosis
uvulitis	pyloromyotomy		stomatitis
	pyloroplasty		sublingual
	uvulectomy		
	uvulopalatopharyngoplasty (UPPP)		

Can you build, analyze, define, pronounce, and spell the following terms *NOT built from word parts?*

DISEASES AND DISORDERS	SURGICAL	DIAGNOSTIC	COMPLEMENTARY
adhesion	abdominoperineal resection (APR)	abdominal sonography	ascites
celiac disease	anastomosis (pl. anastomoses)	barium enema (BE)	diarrhea
cirrhosis	bariatric surgery	endoscopic retrograde cholangiopancreatography (ERCP)	dysentery
Crohn disease	hemorrhoidectomy	endoscopic ultrasound (EUS)	emesis
gastroesophageal reflux disease (GERD)	vagotomy	fecal occult blood test (FOBT)	feces
hemochromatosis		*Helicobacter pylori* (*H. pylori*) antibodies test	flatus
hemorrhoids		upper GI series	gastric lavage
ileus			gavage
intussusception			hematemesis
irritable bowel syndrome (IBS)			hematochezia
obesity			malabsorption
peptic ulcer			melena
polyp			nausea
ulcerative colitis (UC)			palpate
volvulus			peristalsis
			reflux
			stoma

Chapter 12

Eye

Objectives

Upon completion of this chapter you will be able to:

1. Pronounce organs and anatomic structures of the eye.
2. Define and spell word parts related to the eye.
3. Define, pronounce, and spell disease and disorder terms related to the eye.
4. Define, pronounce, and spell surgical terms related to the eye.
5. Define, pronounce, and spell diagnostic terms related to the eye.
6. Define, pronounce, and spell complementary terms related to the eye.
7. Interpret the meaning of abbreviations related to the eye.
8. Apply medical language in clinical contexts.

Outline

ANATOMY

Function

The eyes are organs of vision and are located in a bony protective cavity of the skull called the orbit. Only a small portion of the eye is visible from the exterior (Figs. 12.1 and 12.2).

Organs and Anatomic Structures of the Eye

TERM	DEFINITION
eye (ī)	organ of vision
sclera (SKLER-ah)	outer protective layer of the eye; the portion seen on the anterior portion of the eyeball is referred to as the **white of the eye**
cornea (KŌR-nē-a)	transparent anterior part of the sclera, which is anterior to the aqueous humor and lies over the iris. It allows the light rays to enter the eye.
choroid (KŌR-oid)	middle layer of the eye, which is interlaced with many blood vessels that supply nutrients to the eye
iris (Ī-ris)	pigmented muscular structure that regulates the amount of light entering the eye by controlling the size of the pupil
pupil (PŪ-pil)	opening in the center of the iris
lens (lenz)	lies directly behind the pupil; its function is to focus and bend light
retina (RET-i-nah)	innermost layer of the eye, which contains the vision receptors (Fig. 12.3)
aqueous humor (Ā-kwē-us) (HŪ-mor)	watery liquid found in the anterior cavity of the eye. It provides nourishment to nearby structures and maintains shape in the anterior part of the eye.
vitreous humor (VIT-rē-us) (HŪ-mor)	jellylike substance found behind the lens in the posterior cavity of the eye that maintains its shape
meibomian glands (mī-BŌ-mē-an) (glans)	oil glands found in the upper and lower edges of the eyelids that help lubricate the eye
lacrimal apparatus (LAK-ri-mal) (*ap*-ah-RAT-us)	network of glands, ducts, canals, and sacs that produce and drain tears; the lacrimal gland produces tears, which then flow through the lacrimal ducts to cover the surface of the eye. Tears drain into lacrimal canals, flow into the lacrimal sac (tear sac) and then into the nasolacrimal duct, which opens into the nasal cavity. (Fig. 12.1C)
optic nerve (OP-tik) (nurv)	carries visual impulses from the retina to the brain
conjunctiva (kon-JUNK-ti-vah)	mucous membrane lining the eyelids and covering the anterior portion of the sclera

IRIS
was the special messenger of the Queen of Heaven according to Greek mythology. In this role she passed from heaven to earth over the rainbow while dressed in rainbow hues. Her name was applied to the **circular eye muscle** because of its varied colors.

A&P Booster
For more anatomy and physiology, go to Evolve Resources at evolve.elsevier.com and select: Practice Student Resources > Student Resources > Chapter 12 > **A&P Booster**

See Appendix B for instructions.

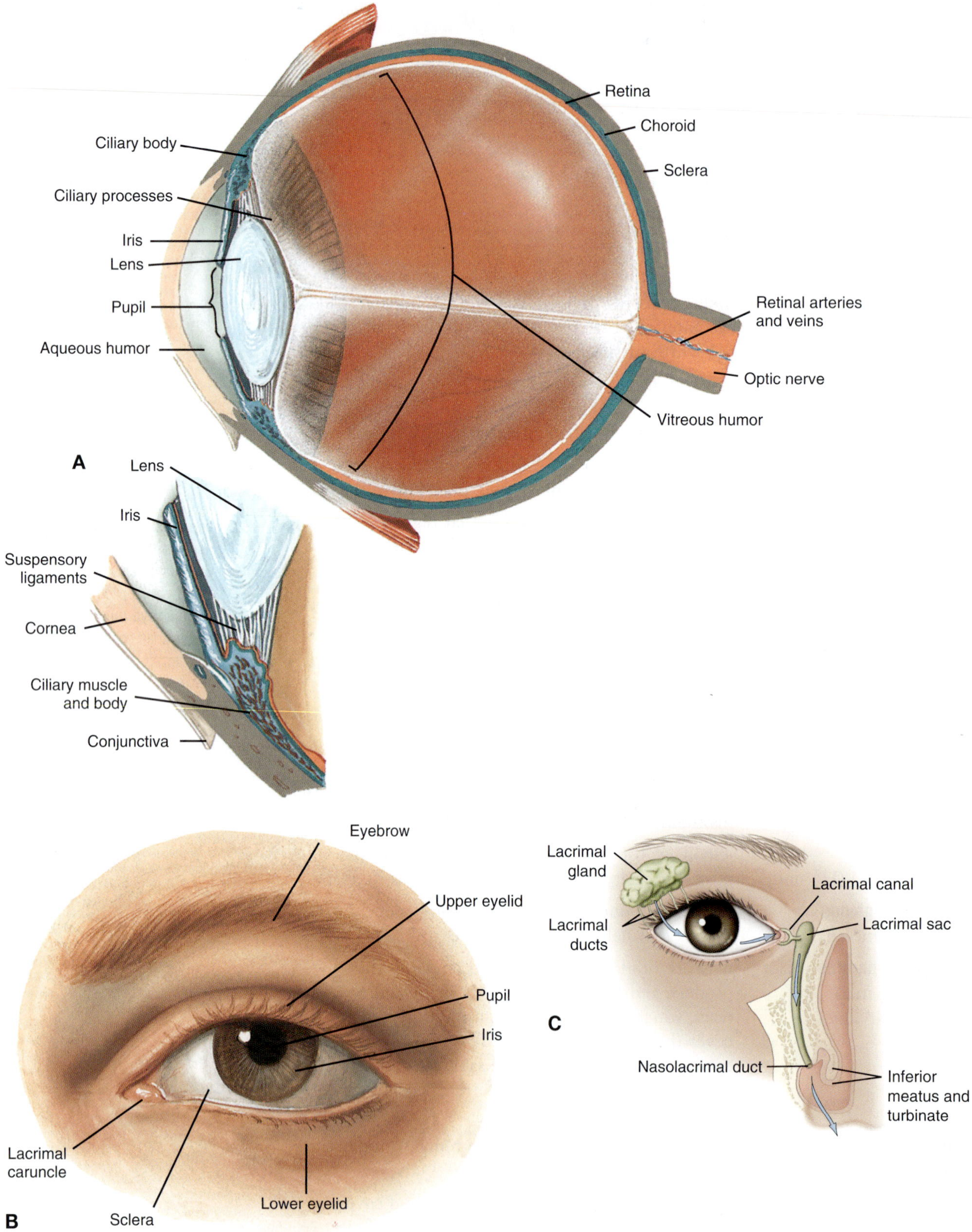

FIG. 12.1 **A,** Anatomy of the eye. **B,** Visible surface of the eye. **C,** Lacrimal apparatus.

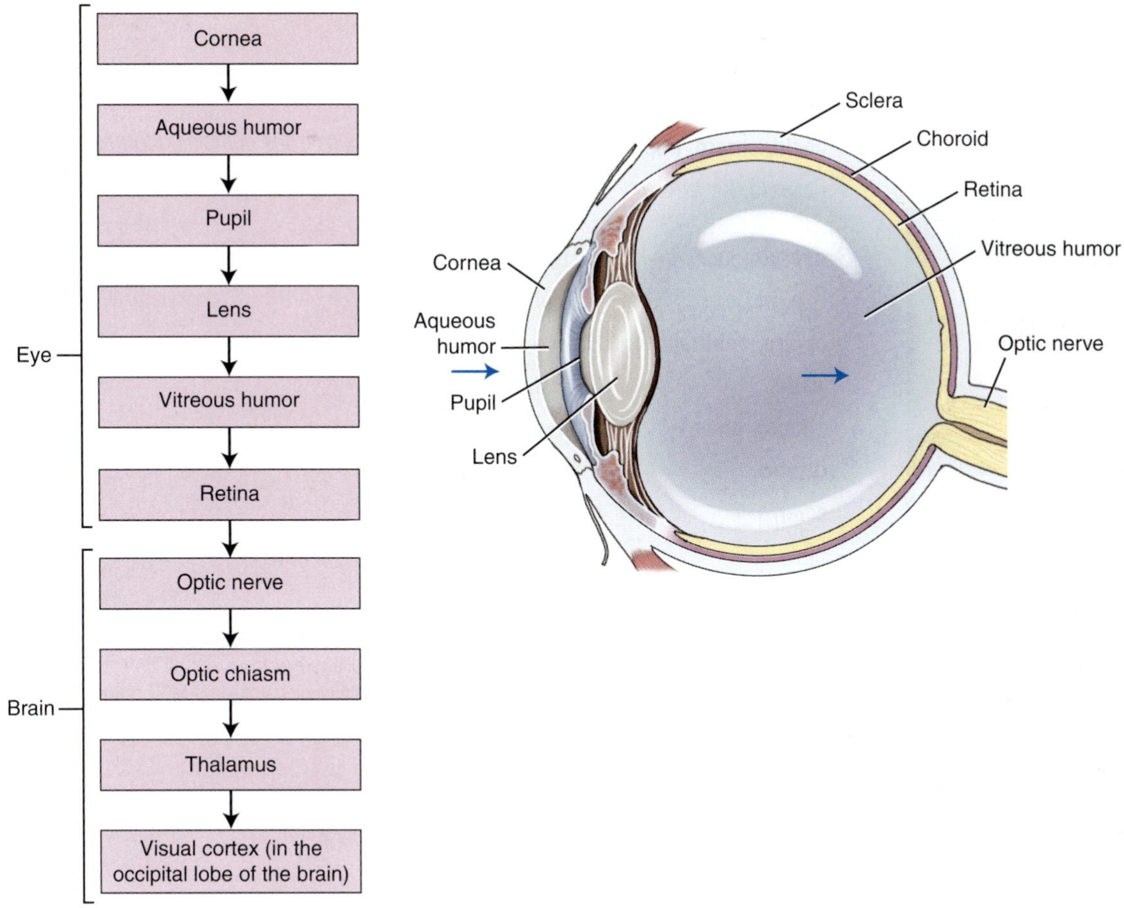

FIG. 12.2 Pathway of light.

EXERCISE 1

Practice saying aloud each of the Organs and Anatomic Structures of the Eye.

To hear the terms, go to Evolve Resources at evolve.elsevier.com and select:
Practice Student Resources > Student Resources > Chapter 12 > **Pronounce and Spell**

See Appendix B for instructions.

❑ Check the box when complete.

WORD PARTS

Combining Forms of the Eye

Word parts you need to learn to complete this chapter are listed on the following pages. The exercises at the end of each list will help you learn their definitions and spellings.

Use the flashcards accompanying this text or electronic flashcards to assist you in memorizing the word parts for this chapter.

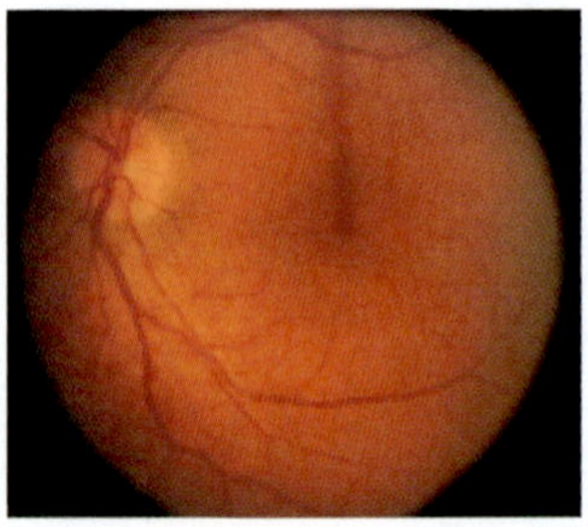

FIG. 12.3 Ophthalmoscopic view of the retina.

COMBINING FORM	DEFINITION
blephar/o	eyelid
conjunctiv/o	conjunctiva
cor/o, core/o, pupill/o	pupil *(Note: pupil has one* l; *the combining form has two* ls.*)*
corne/o, kerat/o	cornea *(Note: kerat/o also means* hard *or* horny tissue; *see Chapter 4.)*
dacry/o, lacrim/o	tear(s)
ir/o, irid/o	iris
ocul/o, ophthalm/o	eye
opt/o	vision
phac/o, phak/o	lens
retin/o	retina (Fig. 12.3)
scler/o	sclera

SPELLING *OPHTHALM*

Look closely at the spelling of the word root **ophthalm**. Medical terms containing **ophthalm** are often misspelled by omitting the first h; **ph** gives the **f** sound followed by the sound of **thal**. Think pronunciation when spelling terms that contain **ophthalm**, as in ophthalmology (of[ph]-thal-MOL-o-jē).

EXERCISE 2

Fill in the blanks with combining forms of the eye. *To check your answers, go to Appendix A.*

1. Eye

   CF: ______________________

   CF: ______________________

2. Eyelid

   CF: ______________________

3. Lacrimal (tear) sac

   CF: ______________________

   CF: ______________________

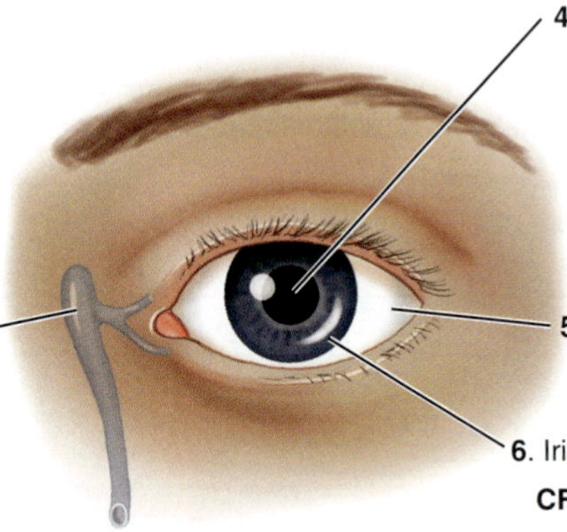

4. Pupil

   CF: ______________________

   CF: ______________________

   CF: ______________________

5. Sclera

   CF: ______________________

6. Iris

   CF: ______________________

   CF: ______________________

7. Vision

   CF: ______________________

8. Conjunctiva

CF: ______________________

9. Cornea

CF: ______________________

CF: ______________________

10. Lens

CF: ______________________

CF: ______________________

11. Retina

CF: ______________________

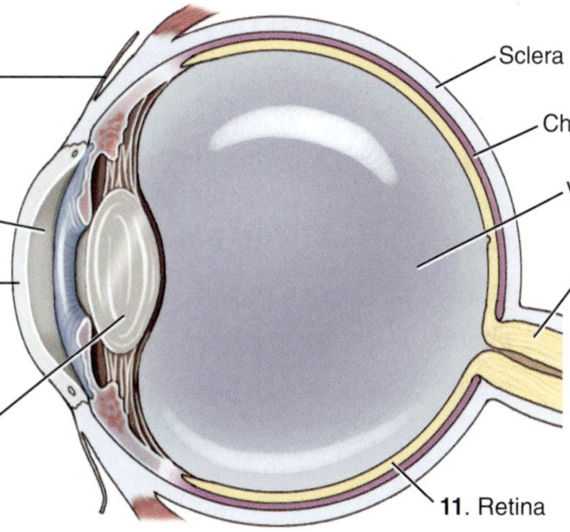

EXERCISE 3

Step 1: Write the definitions after the following combining forms.

Step 2: Match the descriptions on the right with the combining forms and definitions. Answers may be used more than once; no answer line appears for those not described in a lettered item.

_____ 1. scler/o, ______________________

_____ 2. cor/o, core/o, ______________________

_____ 3. corne/o, ______________________

_____ 4. conjunctiv/o, ______________________

_____ 5. lacrim/o, ______________________

_____ 6. retin/o, ______________________

_____ 7. phac/o, phak/o, ______________________

_____ 8. ocul/o, ______________________

_____ 9. ir/o, irid/o, ______________________

_____ 10. pupill/o, ______________________

_____ 11. kerat/o, ______________________

_____ 12. ophthalm/o, ______________________

_____ 13. dacry/o, ______________________

14. blephar/o, ______________________

15. opt/o, ______________________

a. opening in the center of the iris

b. lies directly behind the pupil; focuses and bends light

c. organ of vision

d. pigmented muscular structure regulating the amount of light entering the eye

e. outer protective layer of the eye

f. produced by and drained by the lacrimal apparatus

g. innermost layer of the eye containing vision receptors

h. mucous membrane lining the eyelids and the anterior portion of the sclera

i. transparent anterior part of the sclera

DACR/O + CYST/O

When the combining forms **dacr/o** and **cyst/o** appear together, the medical term refers to the lacrimal sac (directly translated as the "tear sac").

Combining Forms Commonly Used With the Eye

COMBINING FORM	DEFINITION
cry/o	cold
cyst/o	bladder, sac *(Note: In terms describing the eye, the definition "sac" is used when cyst/o appears within a term.)*
dipl/o	two, double
is/o	equal
phot/o	light
ton/o	tension, pressure

EXERCISE 4

Write the definitions of the following combining forms.

1. ton/o ______________________
2. phot/o ______________________
3. cry/o ______________________
4. dipl/o ______________________
5. is/o ______________________
6. cyst/o ______________________

EXERCISE 5

Write the combining form for each of the following.

1. cold ______________________
2. tension, pressure ______________________
3. bladder, sac ______________________
4. two, double ______________________
5. light ______________________
6. equal ______________________

Prefixes and Suffixes

PREFIXES	DEFINITION
bi-, bin-	two
SUFFIXES	**DEFINITIONS**
-opia	vision (condition)
-phobia	abnormal fear of or aversion to specific things
-plegia	paralysis

Refer to **Appendix C** and **Appendix D** for a complete listing of word parts.

EXERCISE 6

A. Write the definition of the following prefixes and suffixes.

1. -opia ______________________
2. bi- ______________________
3. -plegia ______________________
4. -phobia ______________________
5. bin- ______________________

B. Write the prefixes or suffixes for each of the following definitions.

1. paralysis ____________________
2. two a. ____________________
   b. ____________________
3. abnormal fear of or aversion to specific things ____________________
4. vision (condition) ____________________

For additional practice with Word Parts, go to Evolve Resources at evolve.elsevier.com and select: Practice Student Resources > Student Resources > Chapter 12 > **Flashcards**

See Appendix B for instructions.

MEDICAL TERMS

The terms you need to learn to complete this chapter are listed on the following pages. The exercises following each list will help you learn the definition and the spelling of each word.

Disease and Disorder Terms
BUILT FROM WORD PARTS

The following terms can be translated using definitions of word parts. Further explanation is provided within parentheses as needed.

TERM	DEFINITION
aphakia (a-FĀ-kē-a)	condition of without a lens (may be congenital, though often is the result of extraction of a cataract without the placement of an intraocular lens)
blepharitis (*blef*-a-RĪ-tis)	inflammation of the eyelid (Exercise Figure A)
blepharoptosis (*blef*-ar-op-TŌ-sis)	drooping of the eyelid (Exercise Figure B) (commonly called **ptosis**)
conjunctivitis (kon-*junk*-ti-VĪ-tis)	inflammation of the conjunctiva (commonly called **pinkeye**)
dacryocystitis (*dak*-rē-ō-sis-TĪ-tis)	inflammation of the tear (lacrimal) sac (Exercise Figure C)
diplopia (di-PLŌ-pē-a)	double vision
endophthalmitis (*en*-dof-thal-MĪ-tis)	inflammation within the eye *(Note: the* o *in* endo *is dropped.)*
iridoplegia (*īr*-i-dō-PLĒ-ja)	paralysis of the iris
iritis (*ī*-RĪ-tis)	inflammation of the iris
keratitis (*ker*-a-TĪ-tis)	inflammation of the cornea
keratomalacia (*ker*-a-tō-ma-LĀ-sha)	softening of the cornea (usually a bilateral condition associated with vitamin A deficiency)
leukocoria (*lū*-kō-KŌ-rē-a)	condition of white pupil
oculomycosis (*ok*-ū-lō-mī-KŌ-sis)	abnormal condition of the eye caused by a fungus

EXERCISE FIGURE A

Fill in the blanks with word parts defined to label the diagram.

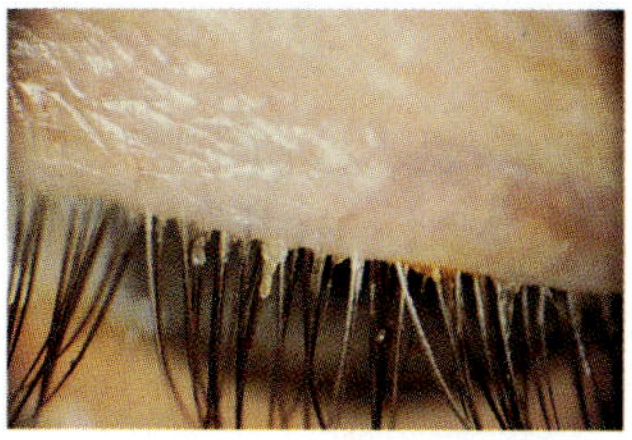

________ / ________
eyelid / inflammation
with thickened lids and crusts around the lashes.

EXERCISE FIGURE B

Fill in the blanks with word parts defined to label the diagram.

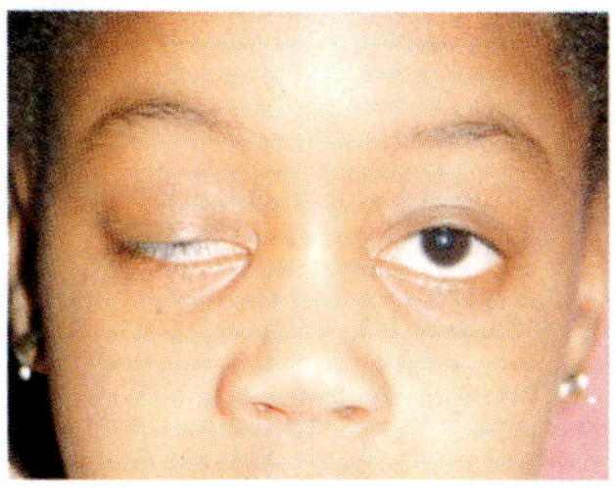

________ / ________ / ________
eyelid / cv / drooping

Disease and Disorder Terms—cont'd

TERM	DEFINITION
ophthalmalgia (*of-thal*-MAL-ja)	pain in the eye
ophthalmoplegia (of-thal-mō-PLĒ-ja)	paralysis of the eye (muscle)
phacomalacia (*făk*-ō-ma-LĀ-sha)	softening of the lens
photophobia (*fō*-tō-FŌ-bē-a)	abnormal fear of (sensitivity to) light
retinoblastoma (*ret*-i-nō-blas-TŌ-ma)	tumor arising from a developing retinal cell (malignant, may be congenital; occurs mainly in children)
retinopathy (*ret*-i-NOP-a-thē)	(any noninflammatory) disease of the retina (such as **diabetic retinopathy**)
scleritis (skle-RĪ-tis)	inflammation of the sclera
scleromalacia (*sklĕr*-ō-ma-LĀ-sha)	softening of the sclera
xerophthalmia (*zēr*-of-THAL-mē-a)	condition of dry eye (conjunctiva and cornea)

EXERCISE FIGURE C

Fill in the blanks with word parts defined to label the diagram.

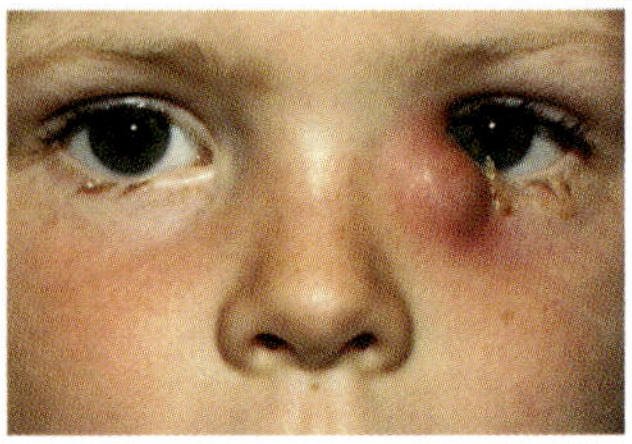

_____ / _____ / _____ / _____
tear / cv / sac / inflammation

EXERCISE 7

Practice saying aloud each of the Disease and Disorder Terms Built from Word Parts.

To hear the terms, go to Evolve Resources at evolve.elsevier.com and select:
Practice Student Resources > Student Resources > Chapter 12 > **Pronounce and Spell**

See Appendix B for instructions.

❑ Check the box when complete.

EXERCISE 8

Analyze and define the following terms.

1. scleritis
____
____

2. ophthalmalgia
____
____

3. blepharoptosis
____
____

4. diplopia
____
____

5. conjunctivitis

6. leukocoria

7. iridoplegia

8. scleromalacia

9. photophobia

10. blepharitis

11. oculomycosis

12. dacryocystitis

13. endophthalmitis

14. iritis

15. retinoblastoma

16. keratitis

17. ophthalmoplegia

18. retinopathy

19. xerophthalmia

20. keratomalacia

21. phacomalacia

22. aphakia

EXERCISE 9

Build disease and disorder terms for the following definitions by using the word parts you have learned.

1. inflammation of the conjunctiva ______ WR / ______ S
2. abnormal condition of the eye caused by a fungus ______ WR / CV / ______ WR / ______ S
3. pain in the eye ______ WR / ______ S
4. double vision ______ WR / ______ S
5. inflammation of the eyelid ______ WR / ______ S
6. condition of white pupil ______ WR / CV / ______ WR / ______ S
7. paralysis of the iris ______ WR / CV / ______ S
8. drooping of the eyelid ______ WR / CV / ______ S
9. inflammation of the iris ______ WR / ______ S
10. tumor arising from a developing retinal cell ______ WR / CV / ______ WR / ______ S
11. softening of the sclera ______ WR / CV / ______ S
12. inflammation of a tear (lacrimal) sac ______ WR / CV / ______ WR / ______ S
13. inflammation of the sclera ______ WR / ______ S
14. abnormal fear of (sensitivity to) light ______ WR / CV / ______ S
15. inflammation of the cornea ______ WR / ______ S
16. disease of the retina ______ WR / CV / ______ S
17. inflammation within the eye ______ P / ______ WR / ______ S

18. paralysis of the eye (muscle) ________ WR / CV / ________ S

19. condition of dry eye ________ WR / ________ WR / ________ S

20. softening of the cornea ________ WR / CV / ________ S

21. condition of without a lens ________ P / ________ WR / ________ S

22. softening of the lens ________ WR / CV / ________ S

EXERCISE 10

Spell each of the Disease and Disorder Terms Built from Word Parts by having someone dictate them to you. Use a separate sheet of paper.

> To hear and spell the terms, go to Evolve Resources at evolve.elsevier.com and select:
> Practice Student Resources > Student Resources > Chapter 12 > **Pronounce and Spell**
>
> See Appendix B for instructions.

❑ Check the box when complete.

Disease and Disorder Terms
NOT BUILT FROM WORD PARTS

Word parts may be present in the following terms; however, their full meanings cannot be translated using definitions of word parts alone.

TERM	DEFINITION
amblyopia (*am*-blē-Ō-pē-a)	reduced vision in one eye caused by disuse or misuse associated with strabismus, unequal refractive errors, or otherwise impaired vision. The brain suppresses images from the impaired eye to avoid double vision (commonly called **lazy eye**).
anisometropia (an-*i*-sō-ma-TRŌ-pē-a)	significant unequal refractive error between two eyes
astigmatism (Ast) (a-STIG-ma-tizm)	blurred vision caused by irregular curvature of the cornea or lens. Light refracts improperly, resulting in diffused, rather than points of light focusing on the retina. (Fig. 12.5C)
cataract (KAT-a-rakt)	clouding of the lens of the eye (Fig. 12.4)
chalazion (ka-LĀ-zē-on)	non-infected obstruction of an oil gland of the eyelid (also called **meibomian cyst)**
drusen (DRŪ-zen)	yellowish deposits located under the retina; commonly associated with aging and macular degeneration

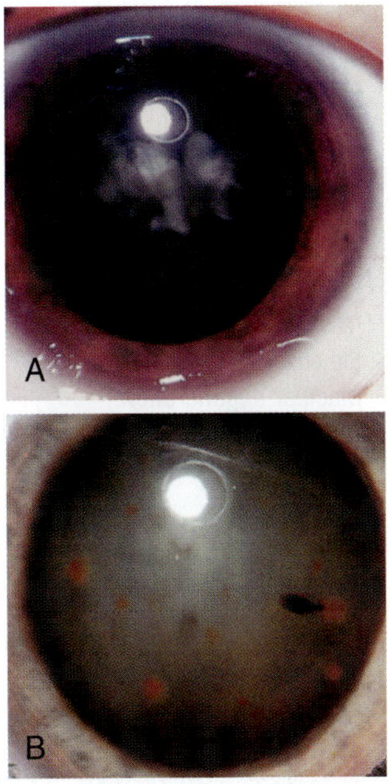

FIG. 12.4 A, Snowflake cataract. **B,** Senile cataract.

CATARACT
is derived from the Greek **kato**, meaning **down**, and **raktos**, meaning **precipice**. Together, the words were interpreted as **waterfall**. The individual with a cataract sees things as through a watery veil of mist or waterfall.

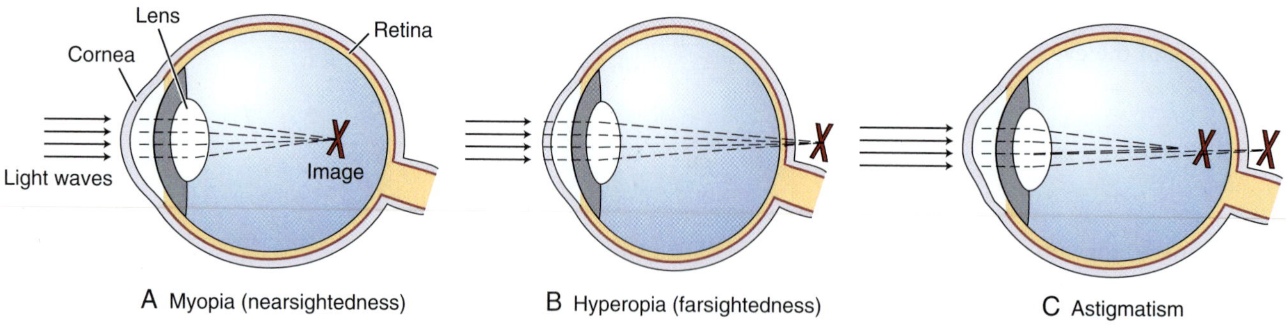

FIG. 12.5 Refraction errors. **A,** Myopia, nearsightedness. **B,** Hyperopia, farsightedness. **C,** Astigmatism.

GLAUCOMA
is composed of the Greek **glaukos**, meaning **blue-gray** or **sea green**, and **oma**, meaning a morbid condition. The term was given to any condition in which gray or green replaced the black in the pupil.

INTEGRATIVE MEDICINE TERM
Vitamin therapy is the use of nutrition, through diet and supplements, to promote optimal health and as preventive support, reduce the incidence and progression of disease and symptoms. Current research has yielded suggestive evidence that dietary supplementation with specific vitamins and minerals may serve to prevent or delay the onset of age-related **macular degeneration**.

Disease and Disorder Terms—cont'd

TERM	DEFINITION
glaucoma (glaw-KŌ-ma)	eye disorder characterized by increase of intraocular pressure (IOP). If left untreated may progress to optic nerve damage and visual impairment or loss.
hyperopia (*hī*-per-Ō-pē-a)	farsightedness (Fig. 12.5B)
hyphema (hī-FĒ-ma)	hemorrhage within the anterior chamber of the eye; most often caused by blunt trauma (also called **hyphemia**)
macular degeneration (MAC-ū-lar) (dē-*gen*-e-RĀ-shun)	progressive deterioration of the portion of the retina called the **macula**, resulting in loss of central vision (Fig. 12.6). Age-related macular degeneration (ARMD) is the leading cause of legal blindness in persons older than 65 years; onset occurs between the ages of 50 and 60.
myopia (mī-Ō-pē-a)	nearsightedness (Fig. 12.5A)

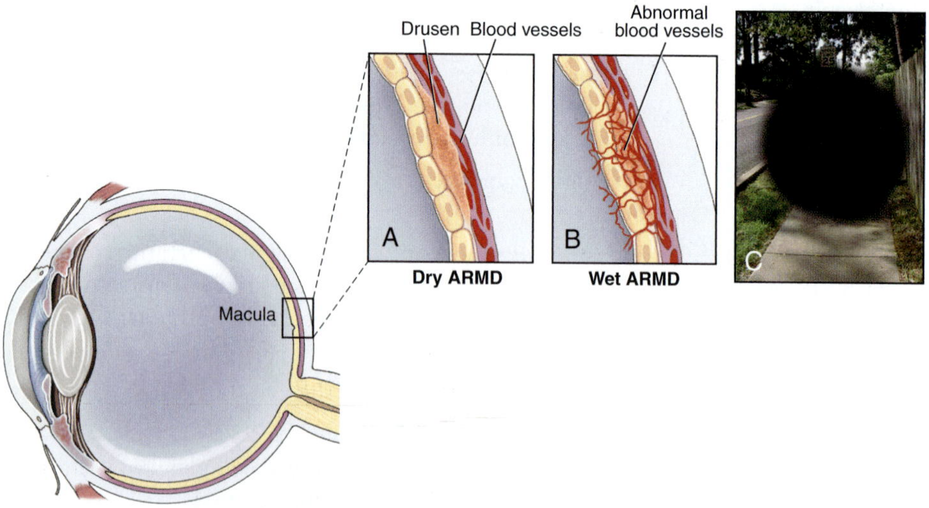

FIG. 12.6 Atrophic macular degeneration (AMD). **A, Dry macular degeneration,** where blood vessels under the macula become brittle and yellow deposits called drusen form, is the most common form of age-related macular degeneration (ARMD). **B, Wet macular degeneration,** where new abnormal blood vessels form under the macula, is less common though more likely to cause legal blindness. **C, Central vision loss** as may be experienced in ARMD.

TERM	DEFINITION
nyctalopia (*nik*-ta-LŌ-pē-a)	poor vision at night or in faint light (commonly called **night blindness**)
nystagmus (nis-TAG-mus)	involuntary, jerking movements of the eyes
pinguecula (ping-GWEH-kū-la)	yellowish mass on the conjunctiva that may be related to long-term exposure to ultraviolet light, dry climates, and dust. A pinguecula that spreads onto the cornea becomes a **pterygium.**
presbyopia (*pres*-bē-Ō-pē-a)	impaired vision as a result of aging
pterygium (te-RIJ-ē-um)	thin tissue growing onto the cornea from the conjunctiva, usually caused by sun exposure
retinal detachment (RET-in-al) (dē-TACH-ment)	separation of the retina from the choroid in back of the eye (Fig. 12.7)
retinitis pigmentosa (*ret*-i-NĪ-tis) (*pig*-men-TŌ-sa)	hereditary, progressive disease marked by night blindness with atrophy and retinal pigment changes
strabismus (stra-BIZ-mus)	condition in which the eyes look in different directions; caused by dysfunction of the external eye muscles or an uncorrected refractive error (called **cross-eyed** when one eye turns in)
sty (stī)	infection of an oil gland of the eyelid (also spelled **stye** and also called **hordeolum**)

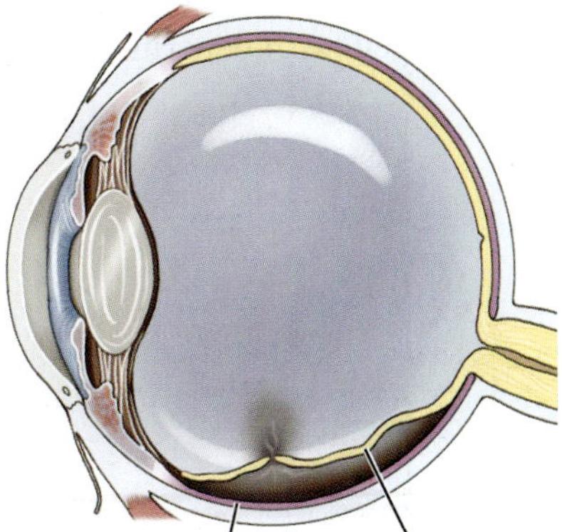

FIG. 12.7 Retinal detachment. Vitreous fluid has seeped through a tear in the retina, causing the retina to separate from the choroid.

EXERCISE 11

Practice saying aloud each of the Disease and Disorder Terms NOT Built from Word Parts.

To hear the terms, go to Evolve Resources at evolve.elsevier.com and select:
Practice Student Resources > Student Resources > Chapter 12 > **Pronounce and Spell**

See Appendix B for instructions.

❑ Check the box when complete.

EXERCISE 12

Fill in the blanks with the correct terms.

1. Another name for nearsightedness is ______________________.
2. Impaired vision as a result of aging is ______________________.
3. Significant unequal refractive error between two eyes is ______________________.
4. Irregular curvature of the cornea or lens causes a condition known as ______________________.
5. ______________________ is the name given to involuntary, jerking movements of the eye.
6. Eye disorder characterized by the increase of intraocular pressure is ______________________.
7. Another name for farsightedness is ______________________.
8. ______________________ is a hereditary, progressive disease causing night blindness with retinal pigment changes and atrophy.

9. Another name for night blindness is ________________________________.
10. Another name for lazy eye is ________________________________.

EXERCISE 13

Write the medical term pictured and defined.

1. ________________________________
yellowish deposits located under the retina

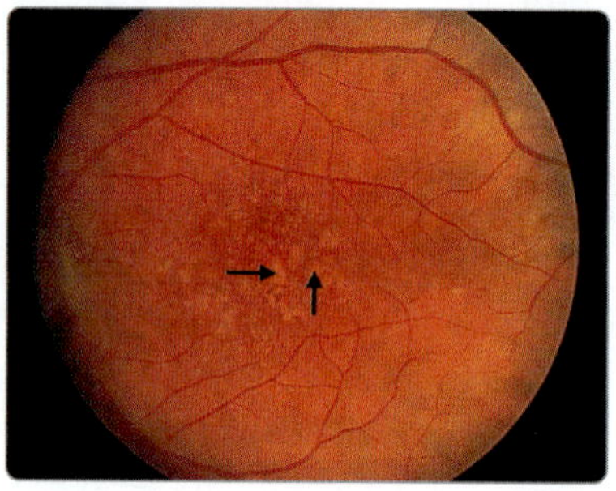

2. ________________________________
progressive deterioration of the portion of the retina called the macula, resulting in loss of central vision

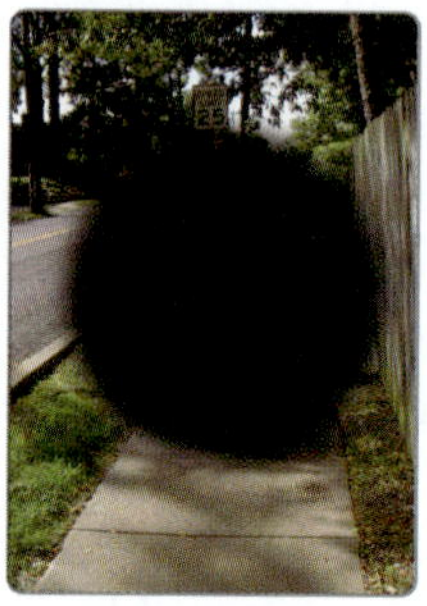

3. ________________________________
thin tissue growing onto the cornea from the conjunctiva, usually caused by sun exposure

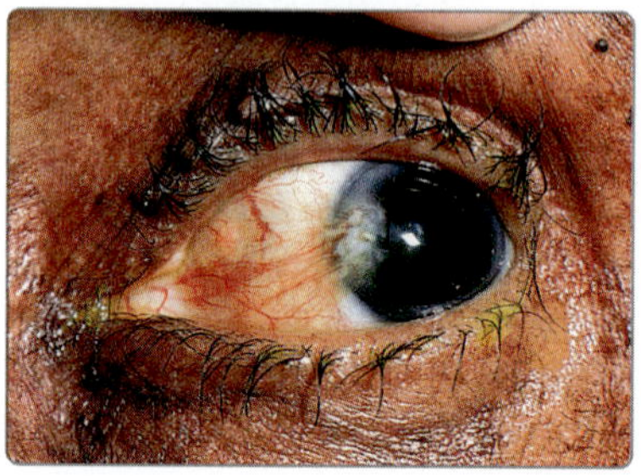

4. ________________________________
yellowish mass on the conjunctiva that may be related to long-term exposure to ultraviolet light, dry climates, and dust

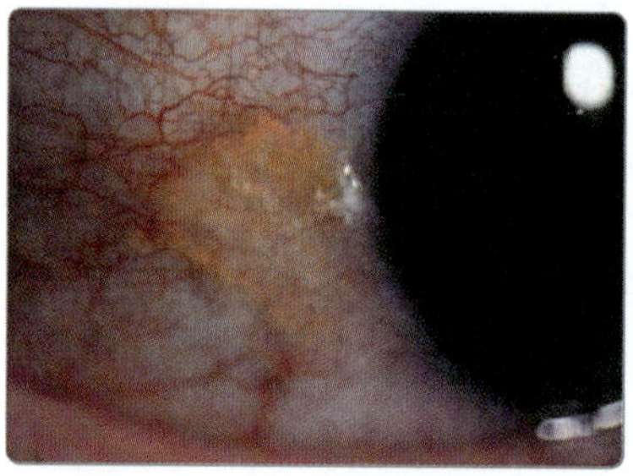

5. ________________________________
non-infected obstruction of an oil gland of the eyelid

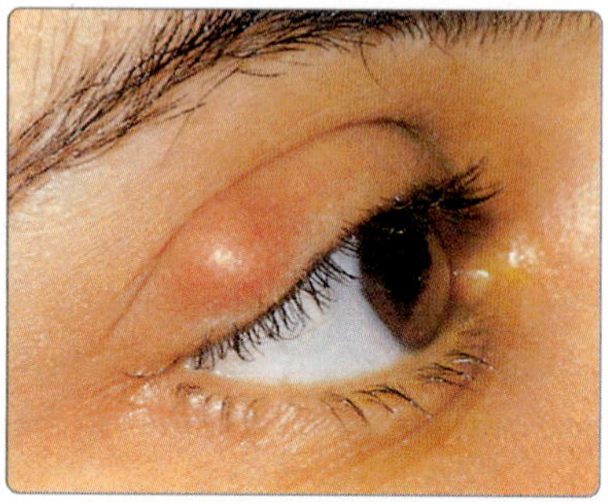

6. ________________________________
infection of an oil gland of the eyelid

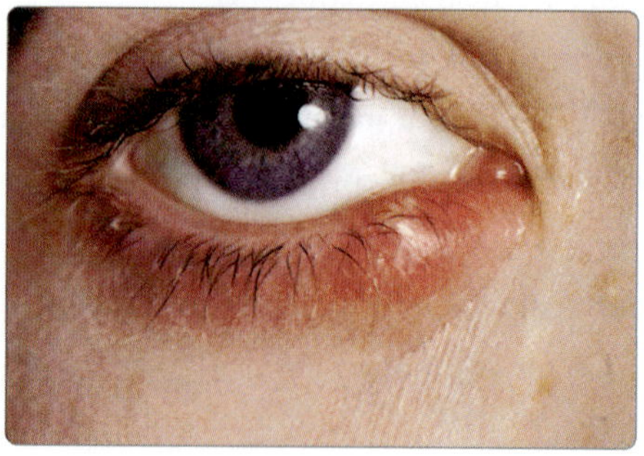

7. ______________________________
clouding of the lens of the eye

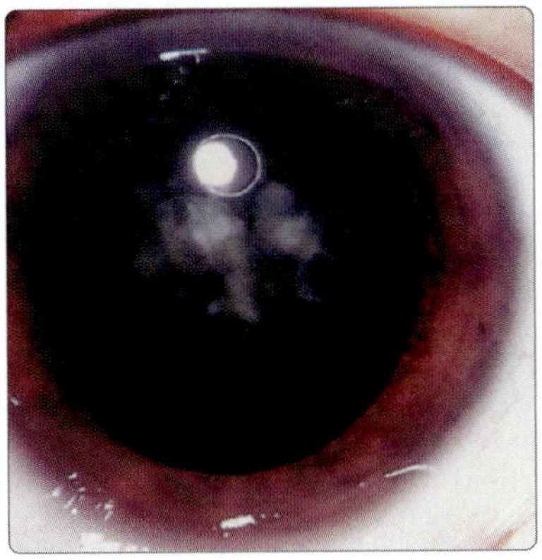

8. ______________________________
hemorrhage within the anterior chamber of the eye; most often caused by blunt trauma

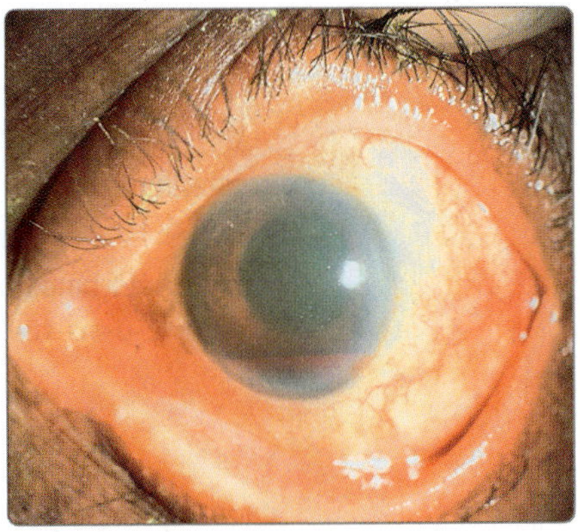

9. ______________________________
condition in which the eyes look in different directions

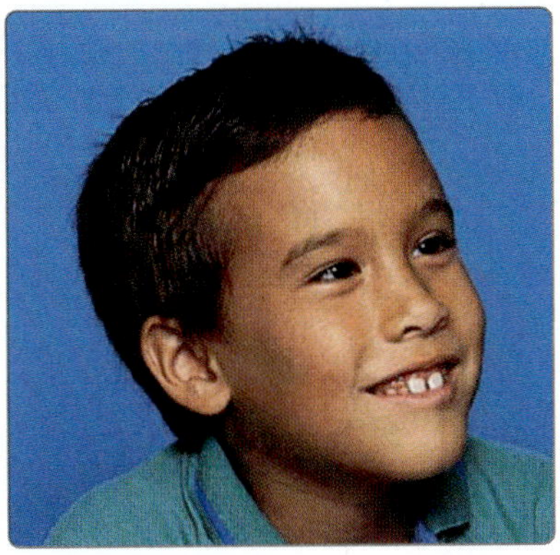

10. ______________________________
separation of the retina from the choroid in back of the eye

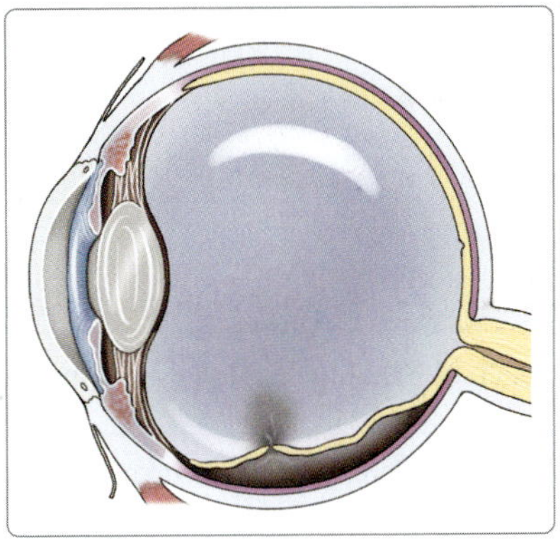

EXERCISE 14

Spell each of the Disease and Disorder Terms NOT Built from Word Parts by having someone dictate them to you. Use a separate sheet of paper.

To hear and spell the terms, go to Evolve Resources at evolve.elsevier.com and select:
Practice Student Resources > Student Resources > Chapter 12 > **Pronounce and Spell**

See Appendix B for instructions.

❑ Check the box when complete.

Surgical Terms
BUILT FROM WORD PARTS

The following terms can be translated using definitions of word parts. Further explanation is provided within parentheses as needed.

TERM	DEFINITION
blepharoplasty (BLEF-a-rō-*plas*-tē)	surgical repair of the eyelid
cryoretinopexy (*krī*-ō-RE-tin-ō-*pek*-sē)	surgical fixation of the retina by using extreme cold (carbon dioxide)
dacryocystorhinostomy (*dak*-rē-ō-sis-tō-rī-NOS-to-mē)	creation of an artificial opening between the tear (lacrimal) sac and the nose (to restore drainage into the nose when the nasolacrimal duct is obstructed or obliterated)
dacryocystotomy *dak*-rē-ō-sis-TOT-o-mē)	incision into the tear (lacrimal) sac
iridectomy (*ir*-i-DEK-to-mē)	excision (of part) of the iris
iridotomy (*ir*-i-DOT-o-mē)	incision into the iris
keratoplasty (KER-a-tō-*plas*-tē)	surgical repair of the cornea (corneal transplant) (Fig. 12.8)
sclerotomy (skle-ROT-o-mē)	incision into the sclera

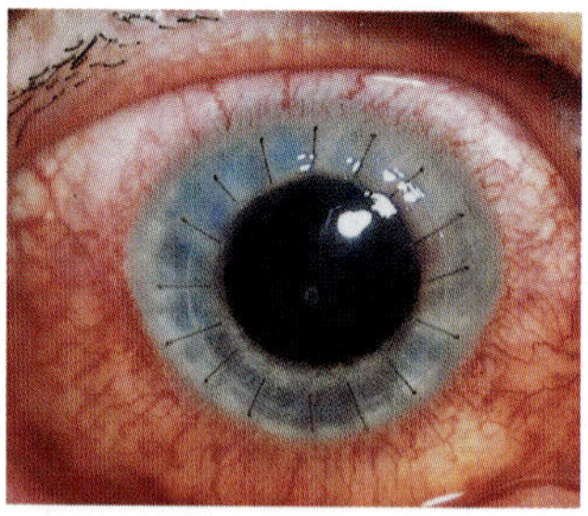
FIG. 12.8 Appearance of eye after keratoplasty.

EXERCISE 15

Practice saying aloud each of the Surgical Terms Built from Word Parts.

To hear the terms, go to Evolve Resources at evolve.elsevier.com and select:
Practice Student Resources > Student Resources > Chapter 12 > **Pronounce and Spell**

See Appendix B for instructions.

❑ Check the box when complete.

EXERCISE 16

Analyze and define the following surgical terms.

1. keratoplasty

____

____

2. sclerotomy

____

____

3. dacryocystotomy

____

____

4. cryoretinopexy

____

____

5. blepharoplasty

____

____

6. iridectomy

____

____

7. dacryocystorhinostomy

____

____

8. iridotomy

____

____

EXERCISE 17

Build surgical terms for the following definitions by using the word parts you have learned.

1. creation of an artificial opening between the tear (lacrimal) sac and the nose ______ WR / CV / WR / CV / WR / CV / S
2. excision (of part) of the iris ______ WR / S
3. surgical repair of the cornea ______ WR / CV / S
4. incision into the sclera ______ WR / CV / S
5. incision into the iris ______ WR / CV / S
6. surgical repair of the eyelid ______ WR / CV / S
7. surgical fixation of the retina using extreme cold ______ WR / CV / WR / CV / S
8. incision into the (lacrimal) tear sac ______ WR / CV / WR / CV / S

EXERCISE 18

Spell each of the Surgical Terms Built from Word Parts by having someone dictate them to you. Use a separate sheet of paper.

To hear and spell the terms, go to Evolve Resources at evolve.elsevier.com and select:
Practice Student Resources > Student Resources > Chapter 12 > **Pronounce and Spell**

See Appendix B for instructions.

❑ Check the box when complete.

Surgical Terms
NOT BUILT FROM WORD PARTS

Word parts may be present in the following terms; however, their full meanings cannot be translated using definitions of word parts alone.

TERM	DEFINITION
enucleation (ē-*nū*-klē-Ā-shun)	surgical removal of the eyeball (also, the removal of any organ that comes out clean and whole)
LASIK (laser-assisted in situ keratomileusis) (LĀ-sik) (*ker*-a-tō-mi-LOO-sis)	laser procedure that reshapes the corneal tissue beneath the surface of the cornea to correct astigmatism, hyperopia, and myopia. LASIK is a combination of excimer laser and lamellar keratoplasty. It differs from photorefractive keratectomy (PRK) in that it reshapes corneal tissue beneath the surface rather than on the surface (Fig. 12.9B).
phacoemulsification (PHACO) (*fa*-kō-ē-*mul*-si-fi-KĀ-shun)	method to remove cataracts in which an ultrasonic needle probe breaks up the lens, which is then aspirated
photorefractive keratectomy (PRK) (*fō*-tō-rē-FRAK-tiv) (*ker*-a-TEK-to-mē)	procedure for the treatment of astigmatism, hyperopia, and myopia in which an excimer laser is used to reshape (flatten) the corneal surface by removing a portion of the cornea (Fig. 12.9A)
retinal photocoagulation (RET-in-al) (*fō*-tō-kō-*ag*-ū-LĀ-shun)	intense beam of light from a laser condenses retinal tissue to seal leaking blood vessels, to destroy abnormal tissue or lesions, or to bond the retina to the back of the eye. Used to treat retinal tears, diabetic retinopathy, wet macular degeneration, glaucoma, and intraocular tumors.
scleral buckling (SKLER-al) (BUK-ling)	procedure to repair retinal detachment. A strip of sclera is resected, or a fold is made in the sclera. An exoplant is used to hold and buckle the sclera (Fig. 12.10).

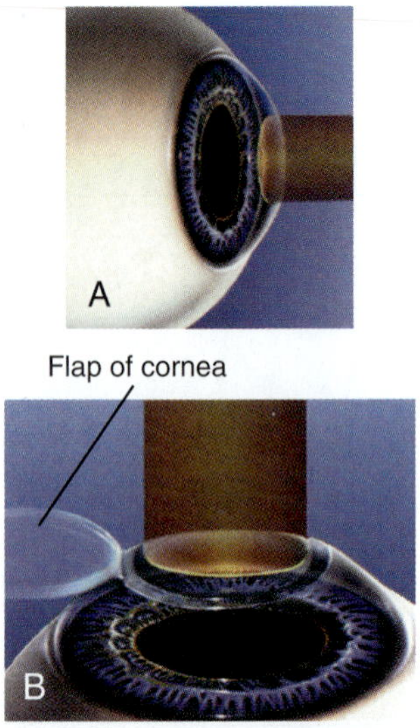

FIG. 12.9 Excimer laser treatments for near-sightedness. **A, Photorefractive keratectomy** (PRK) removes tissue from the surface of the cornea. **B, LASIK** (laser-assisted in situ keratomileusis): reshapes corneal tissue below the surface of the cornea. The excimer laser was invented in the early 1980s. It is a computer-controlled ultraviolet beam of light that reshapes the cornea. It has replaced **RK** (radial keratotomy), a surgery in which spokelike incisions are made to reshape the cornea.

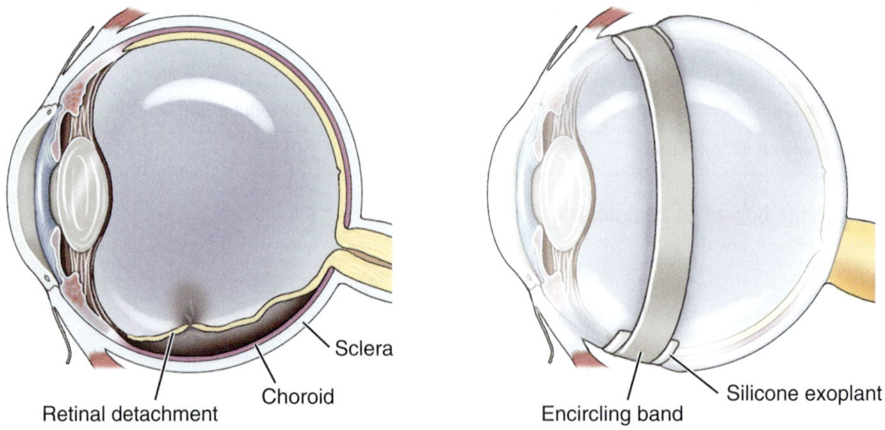

FIG. 12.10 Scleral buckling. A surgical procedure to repair a detached retina.

TERM	DEFINITION
trabeculectomy (tra-*bek*-ū-LEK-to-mē)	surgical creation of an opening that allows aqueous humor to drain out of the eye to underneath the conjunctiva where it is absorbed; used to treat glaucoma by reducing intraocular pressure. (Laser trabeculoplasty may also be used.)
vitrectomy (vi-TREK-to-mē)	surgical removal of all or part of the vitreous humor (used to treat diabetic retinopathy)

EXERCISE 19

Practice saying aloud each of the Surgical Terms NOT Built from Word Parts.

To hear the terms, go to Evolve Resources at evolve.elsevier.com and select:
Practice Student Resources > Student Resources > Chapter 12 > **Pronounce and Spell**

See Appendix B for instructions.

❑ Check the box when complete.

EXERCISE 20

Fill in the blank with the correct terms.

1. ________________ ________________ is the use of a laser beam to condense retinal tissue to seal leaking blood vessels, destroy abnormal tissue, or bond the retina to the back of the eye.
2. Surgical removal of an eyeball is called a(n) ________________.
3. ________________ is the name given to the procedure that breaks up the lens with ultrasound and then aspirates it.
4. Procedure using the excimer laser and lamellar keratoplasty to correct hyperopia, myopia, and astigmatism is called ________________.
5. ________________ is the surgical creation of an opening that allows aqueous humor to drain out of the eye to reduce intraocular pressure.
6. Operation to repair retinal detachment in which the sclera is folded or resected and an exoplant is used to buckle and hold the sclera is called ________________ ________________.
7. Surgery to remove vitreous humor from the eye is called ________________.
8. ________________ ________________ is a procedure for the treatment of astigmatism, hyperopia, and myopia in which an excimer laser is used to reshape the corneal surface by removing the outer most layer of the cornea.

EXERCISE 21

Match the terms in the first column with their correct definitions in the second column.

____ 1. LASIK
____ 2. enucleation
____ 3. trabeculectomy
____ 4. retinal photocoagulation
____ 5. phacoemulsification
____ 6. scleral buckling
____ 7. vitrectomy
____ 8. photorefractive keratectomy

a. use of a laser beam to repair retinal tears and detachment, as well as other retinopathies
b. surgical creation of an opening to reduce intraocular pressure
c. procedure for the treatment of astigmatism, hyperopia, and myopia in which an excimer laser is used to reshape the corneal surface by removing the outermost layer of the cornea
d. procedure in which the lens is broken up by ultrasound and aspirated
e. procedure used to correct astigmatism, nearsightedness, and farsightedness by reshaping tissue beneath the corneal surface
f. surgical removal of an eyeball
g. surgical removal of vitreous humor
h. detached retina surgery in which the sclera is folded and an exoplant is used to buckle and hold the sclera

EXERCISE 22

Spell each of the Surgical Terms NOT Built from Word Parts by having someone dictate them to you. Use a separate sheet of paper.

To hear and spell the terms, go to Evolve Resources at evolve.elsevier.com and select:
Practice Student Resources > Student Resources > Chapter 12 > **Pronounce and Spell**

See Appendix B for instructions.

❑ Check the box when complete.

Diagnostic Terms
BUILT FROM WORD PARTS

The following terms can be translated using definitions of word parts. Further explanation is provided within parentheses as needed.

TERM	DEFINITION
DIAGNOSTIC IMAGING	
fluorescein angiography (flō-RES-ēn) (*an*-jē-OG-ra-fē)	radiographic imaging of blood vessels (of the eye with fluorescing dye)
OPHTHALMIC EVALUATION	
keratometer (*ker*-a-TOM-e-ter)	instrument used to measure (the curvature of) the cornea (used for fitting contact lenses)
ophthalmoscope (of-THAL-mō-skōp)	instrument used for visual examination (of the interior) of the eye (Exercise Figure D)
ophthalmoscopy (*of*-thal-MOS-ko-pē)	visual examination of the eye (Exercise Figure D)

TERM	DEFINITION
optometry (op-TOM-e-trē)	measurement of vision (also measurement of the eye and visual processing system)
pupillometer (*pū*-pil-OM-e-ter)	instrument used to measure (the diameter of) the pupil
pupilloscope (pū-PIL-ō-skōp)	instrument used for visual examination of the pupil
retinoscopy (*ret*-i-NOS-ko-pē)	visual examination of the retina
tonometer (tō-NOM-e-ter)	instrument used to measure pressure (within the eye, used to diagnose glaucoma)
tonometry (tō-NOM-e-trē)	measurement of pressure (within the eye)

EXERCISE FIGURE D

Fill in the blanks with word parts defined to label the diagram.

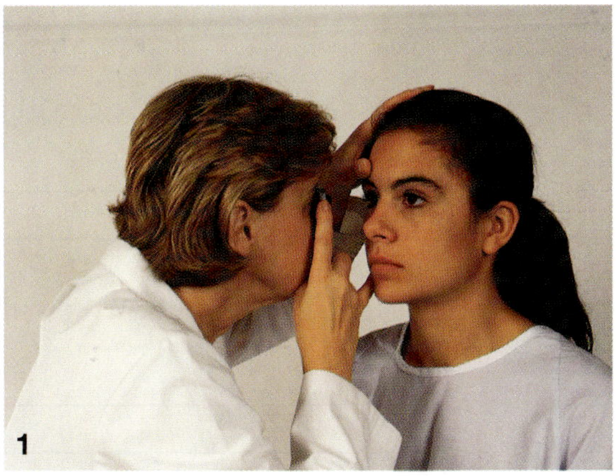

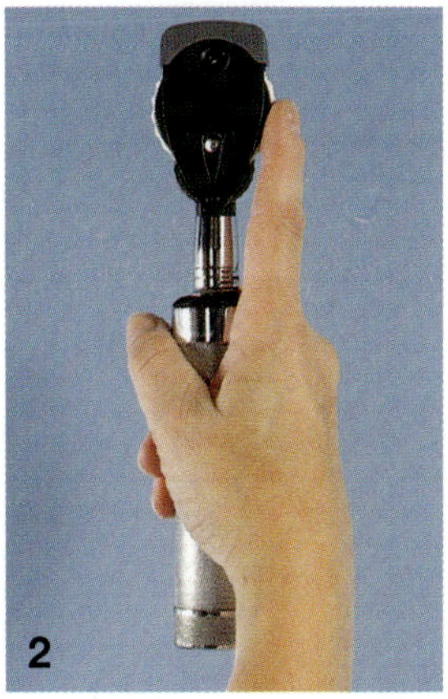

1) _____ / _____ / _____
eye / cv / visual examination

2) _____ / _____ / _____
eye / cv / instrument used for visual examination

EXERCISE 23

Practice saying aloud each of the Diagnostic Terms Built from Word Parts.

To hear the terms, go to Evolve Resources at evolve.elsevier.com and select:
Practice Student Resources > Student Resources > Chapter 12 > **Pronounce and Spell**

See Appendix B for instructions.

❑ Check the box when complete.

EXERCISE 24

Analyze and define the following diagnostic terms.

1. pupilloscope

____

____

2. optometry

____

____

3. ophthalmoscope

____

____

4. tonometry

____

____

5. pupillometer

____

____

6. tonometer

____

____

7. keratometer

____

____

8. ophthalmoscopy

____

____

9. (fluorescein) angiography

____

____

10. retinoscopy

____

____

EXERCISE 25

Build diagnostic terms that correspond to the following definitions by using the word parts you have learned.

1. measurement of pressure (within the eye) ______ WR / CV / ______ S

2. instrument used to measure (the diameter of) the pupil ______ WR / CV / ______ S

3. instrument used to measure (the curvature of) the cornea ______ WR / CV / ______ S

4. measurement of vision ______ WR / CV / ______ S

5. instrument used for visual examination of the eye ______ WR / CV / ______ S

6. instrument used to measure pressure (within the eye) ______ WR / CV / ______ S

7. instrument used for visual examination of the pupil

_______ / _______ / _______
WR / CV / S

8. visual examination of the eye

_______ / _______ / _______
WR / CV / S

9. radiographic imaging of blood vessels (of the eye with fluorescing dye)

fluorescein _______ / _______ / _______
WR / CV / S

10. visual examination of the retina

_______ / _______ / _______
WR / CV / S

EXERCISE 26

Spell each of the Diagnostic Terms Built from Word Parts by having someone dictate them to you. Use a separate sheet of paper.

To hear and spell the terms, go to Evolve Resources at evolve.elsevier.com and select:
Practice Student Resources > Student Resources > Chapter 12 > **Pronounce and Spell**

See Appendix B for instructions.

❑ Check the box when complete.

Complementary Terms
BUILT FROM WORD PARTS

The following terms can be translated using definitions of word parts. Further explanation is provided within parentheses as needed.

TERM	DEFINITION
anisocoria (an-ī-sō-KŌR-ē-a)	condition of absence of equal pupil (size) (unequal size of pupils)
binocular (bin-OK-ū-lar)	pertaining to two or both eyes
corneal (KOR-nē-al)	pertaining to the cornea
intraocular (*in*-tra-OK-ū-lar)	pertaining to within the eye
isocoria (ī-sō-KŌR-ē-a)	condition of equal pupil (size)
lacrimal (LAK-ri-mal)	pertaining to tear(s)
nasolacrimal (*nā*-zō-LAK-ri-mal)	pertaining to the nose and tear (ducts)
ophthalmic (of-THAL-mik)	pertaining to the eye
ophthalmologist (*of*-thal-MOL-o-jist)	physician (surgeon) who studies and treats diseases of the eye
ophthalmology (Ophth) (*of*-thal-MOL-o-jē)	study of the eye (branch of medicine that treats diseases of the eye)

Complementary Terms—cont'd

TERM	DEFINITION
ophthalmopathy (*of*-thal-MOP-a-thē)	(any) disease of the eye
optic (OP-tik)	pertaining to vision
pseudophakia (*soo*-dō-FĀ-ke-a)	condition of false lens (placement of an intraocular lens during surgery to treat cataracts)
pupillary (PŪ-pi-lar-ē)	pertaining to the pupil
retinal (RET-i-nal)	pertaining to the retina

EXERCISE 27

Practice saying aloud each of the Complementary Terms Built from Word Parts.

To hear the terms, go to Evolve Resources at evolve.elsevier.com and select:
Practice Student Resources > Student Resources > Chapter 12 > **Pronounce and Spell**

See Appendix B for instructions.

❑ Check the box when complete.

EXERCISE 28

Analyze and define the following complementary terms.

1. ophthalmology

____
____

2. binocular

____
____

3. lacrimal

____
____

4. pupillary

____
____

5. ophthalmologist

____
____

6. corneal

____
____

7. ophthalmic

____
____

8. nasolacrimal

____
____

9. optic

____

____

10. intraocular

____

____

11. retinal

____

____

12. ophthalmopathy

____

____

13. isocoria

____

____

14. anisocoria

____

____

15. pseudophakia

____

____

EXERCISE 29

Build the complementary terms for the following definitions by using the word parts you have learned.

1. study of the eye ________ WR / CV / S
2. pertaining to two or both eyes ________ P / WR / S
3. pertaining to the retina ________ WR / S
4. pertaining to within the eye ________ P / WR / S
5. physician who studies and treats diseases of the eye ________ WR / CV / S
6. pertaining to tear(s) ________ WR / S
7. pertaining to vision ________ WR / S
8. pertaining to the eye ________ WR / S
9. pertaining to the cornea ________ WR / S

10. pertaining to the nose and tear (ducts) ____ WR / CV / WR / S

11. disease of the eye ____ WR / CV / S

12. pertaining to the pupil ____ WR / S

13. condition of false lens ____ WR / CV / WR / S

14. condition of equal pupil (size) ____ WR / CV / WR / S

15. condition of absence of equal pupil (size) ____ P / WR / CV / WR / S

EXERCISE 30

Spell each of the Complementary Terms Built from Word Parts by having someone dictate them to you. Use a separate sheet of paper.

> To hear and spell the terms, go to Evolve Resources at evolve.elsevier.com and select:
> Practice Student Resources > Student Resources > Chapter 12 > **Pronounce and Spell**
>
> See Appendix B for instructions.

❑ Check the box when complete.

Complementary Terms
NOT BUILT FROM WORD PARTS

Word parts may be present in the following terms; however, their full meanings cannot be translated using definitions of word parts alone.

TERM	DEFINITION
emmetropia (Em) (*em*-e-TRŌ-pē-a)	normal refractive condition of the eye
intraocular lens (IOL) (*in*-tra-OK-ū-lar) (lenz)	artificial lens implanted within the eye during cataract surgery
miotic (mī-OT-ik)	agent that constricts the pupil
mydriatic (*mid*-rē-AT-ik)	agent that dilates the pupil
optician (op-TISH-in)	specialist who fills prescriptions for lenses (cannot prescribe lenses)
optometrist (op-TOM-e-trist)	health professional who diagnoses, treats, and manages diseases and disorders of the eyes and visual processing system; doctor of optometry (OD)
visual acuity (VA) (VIZH-ū-al) (a-KŪ-i-tē)	sharpness of vision for either distance or near

> **OPTOMETRIST**
> is derived from the Greek **optikos**, meaning **sight**, and **metron**, meaning **measure**. Literally, an optometrist is a person who measures sight.

Refer to **Appendix F** for pharmacology terms related to the eye.

EXERCISE 31

Practice saying aloud each of the Complementary Terms NOT Built from Word Parts.

To hear the terms, go to Evolve Resources at evolve.elsevier.com and select:
Practice Student Resources > Student Resources > Chapter 12 > **Pronounce and Spell**

See Appendix B for instructions.

❑ Check the box when complete.

EXERCISE 32

Write the definitions for the following complementary terms.

1. optometrist ____________________
2. mydriatic ____________________
3. visual acuity ____________________
4. miotic ____________________
5. optician ____________________
6. emmetropia ____________________
7. intraocular lens ____________________

EXERCISE 33

Fill in the blanks with the correct terms.

1. Agent that dilates the pupil is a(n) ________________.
2. Agent that constricts the pupil is a(n) ________________.
3. Health professional who diagnoses, treats, and manages diseases and disorders of the eyes and visual processing system is a(n) ________________.
4. Another term for sharpness of vision is ________________ ________________.
5. Specialist who fills prescriptions for lenses but who cannot prescribe lenses is a(n) ________________.
6. Normal refractive condition of the eye is called ________________.
7. After the removal of the lens by phacoemulsification to treat cataracts, often an artificial lens, or ________________ ________________, is implanted within the eye.

EXERCISE 34

Spell each of the Complementary Terms NOT Built from Word Parts by having someone dictate them to you. Use a separate sheet of paper.

To hear and spell the terms, go to Evolve Resources at evolve.elsevier.com and select:
Practice Student Resources > Student Resources > Chapter 12 > **Pronounce and Spell**

See Appendix B for instructions.

❑ Check the box when complete.

Abbreviations

WEB LINK

To learn more about conditions of the eye and vision, visit the American Optometric Association's website at *www.aoa.org*.

ABBREVIATION	TERM
ARMD	age-related macular degeneration
Ast	astigmatism
Em	emmetropia
IOL	intraocular lens
IOP	intraocular pressure
LASIK	laser-assisted in situ keratomileusis
Ophth	ophthalmology
PHACO	phacoemulsification
PRK	photorefractive keratectomy
VA	visual acuity

EXERCISE 35

Write the term abbreviated.

1. VA ______________________________
2. Ast ______________________________
3. IOP ______________________________
4. Em ______________________________
5. Ophth ______________________________
6. ARMD ______________________________
7. PHACO ______________________________
8. IOL ______________________________
9. PRK ______________________________
10. LASIK ______________________________

For additional practice with Abbreviations, go to Evolve Resources at evolve.elsevier.com and select: Practice Student Resources > Student Resources > Chapter 12 > **Flashcards:** Abbreviations

See Appendix B for instructions.

PRACTICAL APPLICATION

EXERCISE 36 *Case Study: Translate Between Everyday Language and Medical Language*

CASE STUDY: Anjit Singh

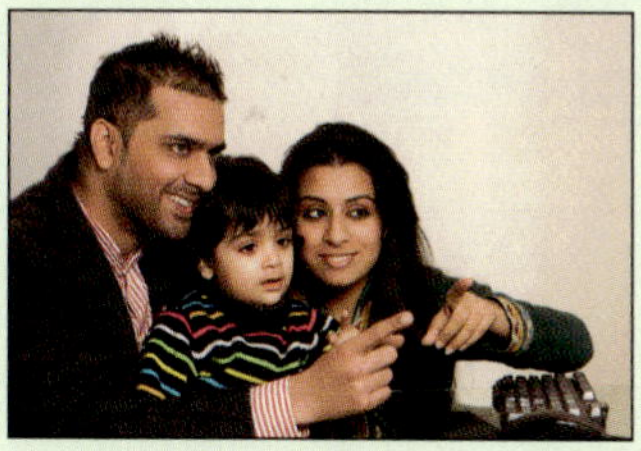

Anjit Singh, a 2-year-old boy, was brought by his parents to the pediatrician for his well-child examination. His mother noted that lately he seemed to be having trouble seeing things that he could identify previously, and that one of his eyes seemed to move more slowly and to look in a different direction. Also, the white part of the same eye seemed to be irritated and looked red and inflamed. She also noticed that on a recent flash photograph that she took of her son, one pupil had a typical "red eye" look, but the other pupil looked white. The pediatrician agreed that there was a problem and sent Anjit to an eye physician for further work-up.

Now that you have worked through Chapter 12, consider the medical terms that might be used to describe Anjit's experience. See the Review of Terms at the end of the chapter for a list of terms that might apply.

A. *Underline phrases in the case study that could be substituted with medical terms.*

B. *Write the medical term and its definition for three of the phrases you underlined.*

MEDICAL TERM	DEFINITION
1. ____________	____________
2. ____________	____________
3. ____________	____________

DOCUMENTATION: Excerpt From Ophthalmology Visit

Anjit was examined by an ophthalmologist; an excerpt from the medical record is documented below.

Anjit Singh is a 2-year-old male referred by his pediatrician for issues related to his left eye. He is accompanied by his mother and father. History is significant for leukocoria, strabismus with resultant amblyopia, and scleritis. There is no family history of eye disease. Ophthalmoscopy reveals the absence of a red reflex on the left, with confirmation of leukocoria in that eye. The left eye also deviates outward on extraocular motor testing, and visual acuity is markedly decreased on the left. Retinal exam reveals a normal right eye and a mass suspicious for retinoblastoma in the left.

C. *Underline medical terms presented in Chapter 12 used in the previous excerpt from Anjit's medical record. See the Review of Terms at the end of the chapter for a complete list.*

D. *Select and define three of the medical terms you underlined. To check your answers, go to Appendix A.*

MEDICAL TERM	DEFINITION
1. ____________	____________
2. ____________	____________
3. ____________	____________

EXERCISE 37 *Interact With Medical Documents and Electronic Health Records*

A. Read the report and complete it by writing medical terms on answer lines within the document. Definitions of terms to be written appear after the document.

763217 GRAVES, William

File Patient Navigate Custom Fields Help

Chart Review | Encounters | Notes | Labs | Imaging | Procedures | Rx | Documents | Referrals | Scheduling | Billing

Name: **GRAVES, William** MR#: 763217 DOB: 6/27/19XX Sex: M Age: 66 **Allergies:** None known **PCP:** Murphy, Clara MD

Ophthalmology Clinic Visit
Date: 03 April 20XX 10:15

Subjective: Mr. Graves is a 66-year-old male here today for his annual 1.______________________ exam. He has no current complaint. He has a family history of 2.______________________ in his brother. He has a history of hypertension and type 2 diabetes mellitus. A 3.___________________ was removed from his right eye 5 years ago.

Medications: Glyburide 5 mg bid and metoprolol 50 mg bid.

Objective:
Visual Acuities: Aided: right eye 20/25 left eye 20/30-1 both eyes 20/25
Unaided: right eye 20/100 left eye 20/80-1 both eyes 20/80

Externals: 2 mm 4.____right eye.
PERLA (pupils equal and reactive to light and accommodation).
EOMI (extraocular movements intact).

Ophthalmoscopic:
Lens: left eye showed early cortical spokes
Disk: margins normal
Cup-to-disk ratio: 0.2 both eyes
Fundus: scattered microaneurysms bilaterally, with dot and blot hemorrhages noted in all four quadrants of both eyes
Refraction: right eye 1.00-0.50 x 90 20/20, left eye 1.25-0.25 x 90 20/20
Tonometry: 14 mm Hg/right eye, 13 mm Hg/left eye

Visual Field: Full

Assessment: Patient has compound myopic 5.______________________________ and 6.________________________________ with diabetic 7.___________________ and grade 2 hypertension. He also shows an early 8.______________________________________ in the left eye.

Plan: Provide prescription for corrective lenses. See patient for follow-up visit in 6 months to reevaluate diabetic retinopathy and cataract. Counseled patient to report any sudden changes in vision.

Electronically signed: Rwabunihi, Anella MD on 05 April 20XX 14:00

Start | Log On/Off | Print | Edit

Definitions of Medical Terms to Complete the Document

Write the medical terms defined on corresponding answer lines in the document.

1. study of the eye
2. eye disorder characterized by the increase of intraocular pressure
3. thin tissue growing into the cornea from the conjunctiva
4. drooping of eyelid
5. irregular curvature of the cornea or lens
6. impaired vision as a result of aging
7. (any noninflammatory) disease of the retina
8. clouding of the lens of the eye

B. Read the patient profile and answer the questions below it.

Patient Profile

This 70-year-old woman was admitted for surgical treatment of chronic, poorly controlled **glaucoma** and for **cataract** extraction.

Subjective: The patient reported a progressive loss of **visual acuity** in her right eye; she complained of headaches and problems with glare (particularly at night) and said she perceives halos around lights.

Objective: Vision testing and physical examination (i.e., **ophthalmoscopy,** slit lamp microscopy, and **tonometry**) revealed acuity (unaided) of 10/100 for the right eye and 20/60 for the left eye. Opacification of right lens was evident, as was moderate **corneal** edema.

Therapeutic Management: After a **mydriatic** agent was applied to the right pupil, a combined procedure **phacoemulsification** of the cataract and **trabeculectomy** with releasable sutures (to minimize **IOP**) was performed with the patient under local anesthesia. The patient tolerated the procedure well and returned to her room wearing a 12-hour collagen shield on the treated eye.

Use the patient profile above to answer the questions.

1. Vision testing and physical examination of the patient revealed opacification of the right lens, confirming the need for:
   a. PRK
   b. phacoemulsification
   c. scleral buckling
   d. enucleation
2. Application of a mydriatic agent would:
   a. reduce tears
   b. produce tears
   c. constrict the pupil
   d. dilate the pupil
3. A trabeculectomy was performed because the patient had a history of:
   a. condition of crossed eyes
   b. disorder characterized by increased intraocular pressure
   c. nearsightedness
   d. progressive deterioration of a portion of the retina
4. The abbreviation IOP stands for:
   a. both eyes
   b. normal vision
   c. intraocular pressure
   d. iris outer pupil

C. Complete the **three medical documents** within the electronic health record (EHR) on Evolve.

Topic: Glaucoma
Documents: New Patient Evaluation, Consultation Letter to PCP, Operative Note

To complete the three medical records, go to Evolve Resources at evolve.elsevier.com and select:
Practice Student Resources > Student Resources > Chapter 12 > **Electronic Heath Records**

See Appendix B for instructions.

EXERCISE 38 *Pronounce Medical Terms in Use*

Practice pronunciation of terms by reading aloud the following paragraphs. Use the phonetic spellings following medical terms from the chapter to assist with pronunciation. The script also contains medical terms not presented in the chapter. Treat them as information only or look for their meanings in a medical dictionary or a reliable online source.

An elderly gentleman visited his **ophthalmologist** (*of*-thal-MOL-o-jist) because of decreased vision. A **tonometry** (tō-NOM-e-trē) examination showed borderline readings. **Visual acuity** (VIZH-ū-al) (a-KŪ-i-tē) measurement indicated a mild degree of **myopia** (mī-Ō-pē–a) and **presbyopia** (*pres*-bē-Ō-pē-a). A diagnosis of **glaucoma** (glaw-KŌ-ma) is suspected in this case and timolol eye drops were prescribed, one drop daily.

A **cataract** (KAT-a-rakt) of the right eye was found. Lens implant surgery, which places an **intraocular lens** (in-tra-OK-ū-lar) (lenz), will be performed when the cataract matures sufficiently. Approximately 5 years ago the patient had a **retinal detachment** (RET-in-al) (dē-TACH-ment) of the left eye. A **scleral buckling** (SKLER-al) (BUK-ling) procedure was performed and was successful in halting the progression of retinal detachment.

EXERCISE 39 *Chapter Content Quiz*

Test your understanding of terms and abbreviations introduced in this chapter. Circle the letter for the medical term or abbreviation related to the words in italics.

1. Before the exam, a medication to *dilate the pupils* was placed in the patient's eyes using a dropper.
   a. miotic
   b. mydriatic
   c. myopia
2. A person with an *irregular curvature of the cornea or lens* of the eye has:
   a. astigmatism
   b. glaucoma
   c. strabismus
3. To *measure the pressure within the patient's eye*, the optometrist used a:
   a. pupillometer
   b. tonometer
   c. keratometer
4. A patient with an *involuntary jerking movement of the eyes* has a condition known as:
   a. astigmatism
   b. anisometropia
   c. nystagmus
5. The ophthalmologist ordered a *radiographic imaging of the blood vessels of the eye with a dye* to assess the progression of the patient's diabetic retinopathy.
   a. fluorescein angiography
   b. tonometry
   c. ophthalmoscopy
6. A person who is *farsighted* has:
   a. hyperopia
   b. myopia
   c. diplopia
7. *Health professionals who diagnose, treat, and manage diseases and disorders of the eyes and visual processing system* are licensed by the state and have earned doctorate degrees abbreviated as OD.
   a. optician
   b. optometrist
   c. ophthalmologist
8. *Inflammation of the white of the eye* can be very painful and may be associated with an underlying autoimmune disorder, such as rheumatoid arthritis and systemic lupus erythematosus.
   a. scleritis
   b. scleromalacia
   c. conjunctivitis
9. The surgery schedule indicated the patient being treated for cataracts would undergo right eye *PHACO* with IOL.
   a. photorefractive keratectomy
   b. photocoagulation
   c. phacoemulsification

10. After *surgical placement of the intraocular lens*, the patient's right eye would be described as:
    a. anisocoria
    b. aphakia
    c. pseudophakia
11. *Progressive deterioration of the retina, resulting in loss of central vision* may be described as dry, where the blood vessels become thin and brittle, or wet, where new abnormal vessels develop under the macula.
    a. retinitis pigmentosa
    b. macular degeneration
    c. presbyopia
12. The patient explained that she experienced an *abnormal sensitivity to light* before her migraine.
    a. photophobia
    b. nyctalopia
    c. isocoria
13. In hopes of giving up her glasses, the patient elected to have *a laser procedure to reshape her corneal tissue beneath the surface of the cornea* to treat nearsightedness.
    a. PRK
    b. LASIK
    c. IOP
14. In a surgical procedure, *retinal tissue was condensed using an intense beam of light* to repair retinal tears in the patient's left eye and prevent retinal detachment.
    a. retinal photocoagulation
    b. phacoemulsification
    c. scleral buckling
15. *Inflammation of the tear sac* is an infection of the lacrimal sac, which may be acute or chronic.
    a. blepharitis
    b. endophthalmitis
    c. dacryocystitis
16. The *instrument used to measure the diameter of the pupil* may be used as a part of a neurological examination to provide an objective measure of pupillary response.
    a. tonometer
    b. pupillometer
    c. keratometer

CHAPTER REVIEW

REVIEW OF CHAPTER CONTENT ON EVOLVE RESOURCES

Go to evolve.elsevier.com and click on Gradable Student Resources and Practice Student Resources. Online learning activities found there can be used to review chapter content and to assess your learning of word parts, medical terms, and abbreviations. Place check marks in the boxes next to activities used for review and assessment.

GRADABLE STUDENT RESOURCES

Chapter 12 >	Exercises >	□ Word Parts □ Terms Built from Word Parts □ Terms Not Built from Word Parts □ Abbreviations
	Quizzes >	□ Quiz 1: Disease and Disorder Terms □ Quiz 2: Surgical Terms □ Quiz 3: Diagnostic Terms □ Quiz 4: Complementary Terms

PRACTICE STUDENT RESOURCES > STUDENT RESOURCES

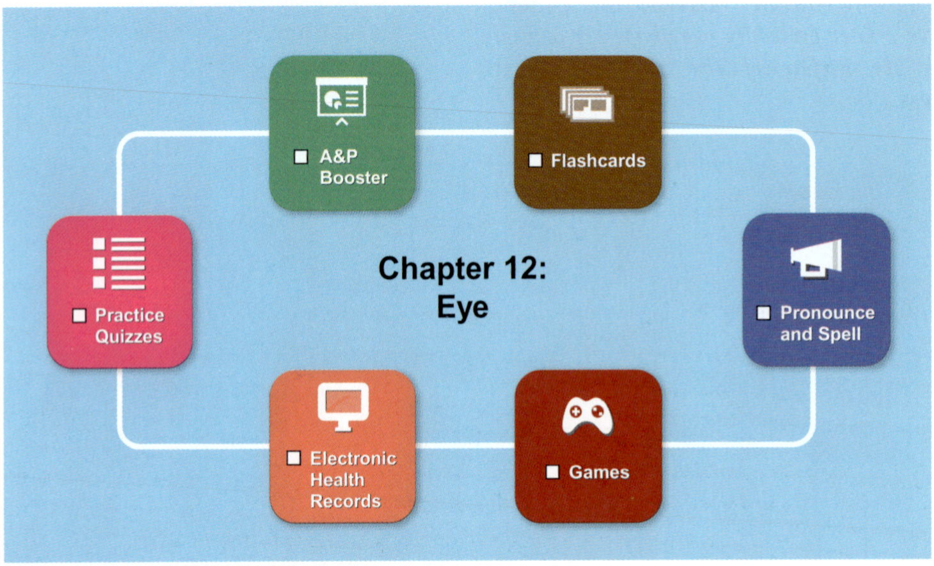

REVIEW OF WORD PARTS

Can you define and spell the following word parts?

COMBINING FORMS			PREFIXES	SUFFIXES
blephar/o	dipl/o	opt/o	bi-	-opia
conjunctiv/o	ir/o	phac/o	bin-	-phobia
cor/o	irid/o	phak/o		-plegia
core/o	is/o	phot/o		
corne/o	kerat/o	pupill/o		
cry/o	lacrim/o	retin/o		
cyst/o	ocul/o	scler/o		
dacry/o	ophthalm/o	ton/o		

REVIEW OF TERMS

Can you define, pronounce, and spell the following terms *built from word parts?*

DISEASES AND DISORDERS	SURGICAL	DIAGNOSTIC	COMPLEMENTARY
aphakia	blepharoplasty	fluorescein angiography	anisocoria
blepharitis	cryoretinopexy	keratometer	binocular
blepharoptosis	dacryocystorhinostomy	ophthalmoscope	corneal
conjunctivitis	dacryocystotomy	ophthalmoscopy	intraocular
dacryocystitis	iridectomy	optometry	isocoria
diplopia	iridotomy	pupillometer	lacrimal
endophthalmitis	keratoplasty	pupilloscope	nasolacrimal
iridoplegia	sclerotomy	retinoscopy	ophthalmic
iritis		tonometer	ophthalmologist
keratitis		tonometry	ophthalmology (Ophth)
keratomalacia			ophthalmopathy
leukocoria			optic
oculomycosis			pseudophakia
ophthalmalgia			pupillary
ophthalmoplegia			retinal
phacomalacia			
photophobia			
retinoblastoma			
retinopathy			
scleritis			
scleromalacia			
xerophthalmia			

Can you define, pronounce, and spell the following terms *NOT built from word parts*?

DISEASES AND DISORDERS		SURGICAL	COMPLEMENTARY
amblyopia	myopia	enucleation	emmetropia (Em)
anisometropia	nyctalopia	LASIK (laser-assisted in situ keratomileusis)	intraocular lens (IOL)
astigmatism (Ast)	nystagmus	phacoemulsification (PHACO)	miotic
cataract	pinguecula	photorefractive keratectomy (PRK)	mydriatic
chalazion	presbyopia	retinal photocoagulation	optician
drusen	pterygium	scleral buckling	optometrist
glaucoma	retinal detachment	trabeculectomy	visual acuity (VA)
hyperopia	retinitis pigmentosa	vitrectomy	
hyphema	strabismus		
macular degeneration	sty		

Chapter 13 Ear

Objectives

Upon completion of this chapter you will be able to:

1. Pronounce organs and anatomic structures of the ear.
2. Define and spell word parts related to the ear.
3. Define, pronounce, and spell disease and disorder terms related to the ear.
4. Define, pronounce, and spell surgical terms related to the ear.
5. Define, pronounce, and spell diagnostic terms related to the ear.
6. Define, pronounce, and spell complementary terms related to the ear.
7. Interpret the meaning of abbreviations related to the ear.
8. Apply medical language in clinical contexts.

Outline

ANATOMY

Function

The two functions of the ear are to hear and to provide the sense of balance. The ear is made up of three parts: the **external ear**, the **middle ear**, and the **inner ear** (Figs. 13.1 and 13.2). The process of hearing begins with the **auricles** directing sound waves into the **external auditory canal.** As the sound waves ripple through the external ear, the **tympanic membrane** vibrates. The **ossicles** in the middle ear carry the vibration to the inner ear, where the stimulus is transmitted by the cochlear nerve to the brain and is interpreted as sound.

Balance is a function of the **inner ear** and is maintained through a series of complex processes. The vestibular nerve transmits information about motion and body position from the semicircular canals and the vestibule to the brain for interpretation.

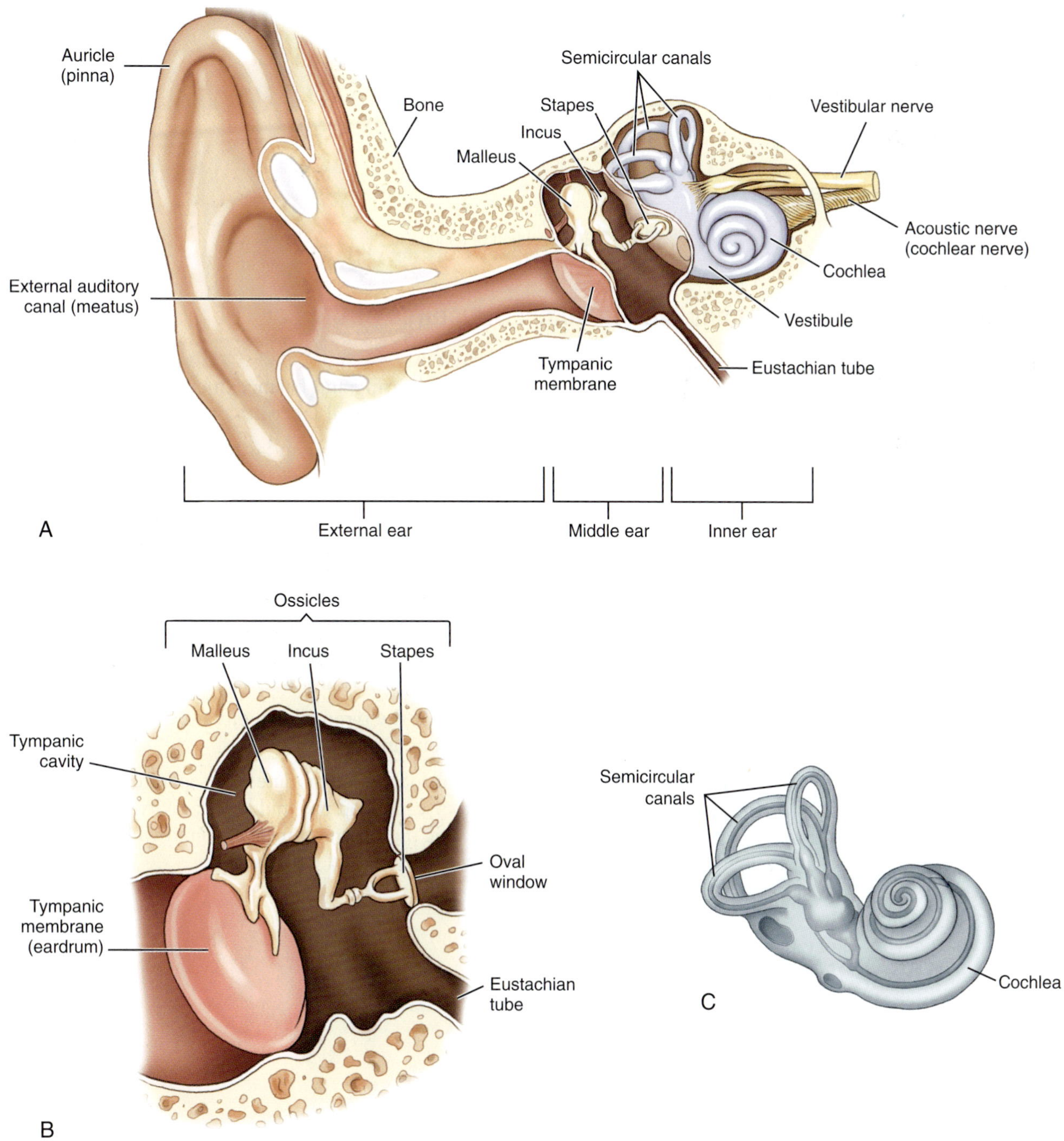

FIG. 13.1 A, Gross anatomy of the ear. **B,** The middle ear. **C,** Labyrinth.

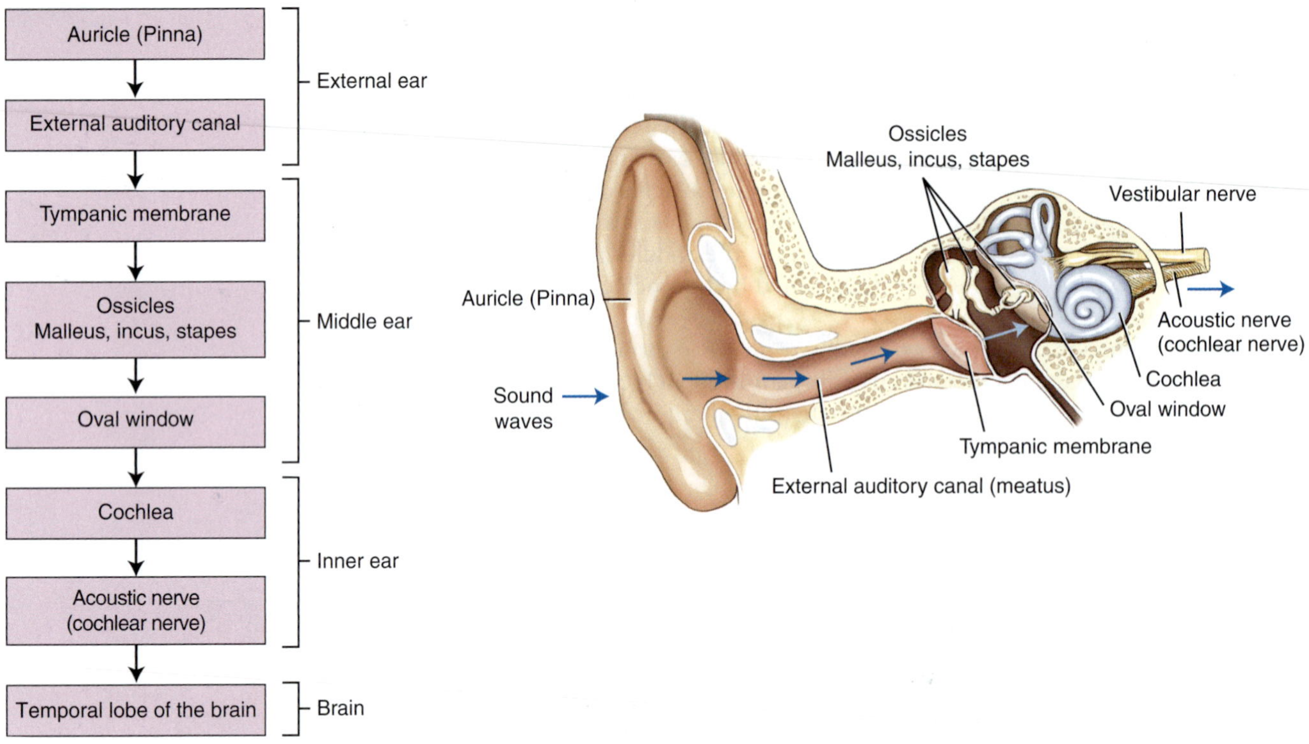

FIG. 13.2 Perception of sound.

Organs and Anatomic Structures of the Ear

TERM	DEFINITION
ear (ēr)	organ of hearing and balance; includes the external ear, middle ear, and labyrinth or inner ear
external ear (ek-STER-nal) (ēr)	consists of the auricle and external auditory canal (meatus)
auricle (AW-ri-kl)	external, visible part of the ear located on both sides of the head; directs sound waves into the external auditory canal. (also called **pinna**)
external auditory canal (ek-STER-nal) (AW-di-tor-ē) (kah-NAL)	short tube that ends at the tympanic membrane. The inner part lies within the temporal bone of the skull and contains the glands that secrete earwax (cerumen). (also called **external auditory meatus**)
middle ear (MID-l) (ēr)	consists of the tympanic membrane and the tympanic cavity containing the ossicles
tympanic membrane (tim-PAN-ik) (MEM-brān)	semitransparent membrane that separates the external auditory canal and the middle ear cavity. The tympanic membrane transmits sound vibrations to the ossicles. (also called **eardrum**)

TYMPANIC MEMBRANE
is derived from the Greek **tympanon**, meaning **drum**, because of its resemblance to a drum or tambourine.

TERM	DEFINITION
ossicles (OS-i-kalz)	bones of the middle ear that carry sound vibrations. The ossicles are composed of the **malleus** (hammer), **incus** (anvil), and **stapes** (stirrup). The stapes connects to the **oval window**, which transmits the sound vibrations to the cochlea of the inner ear.
eustachian tube (yū-STĀ-shan) (toob)	passage between the middle ear and the pharynx; equalizes air pressure on both sides of the tympanic membrane
inner ear (IN-ar) (ēr)	consists of the labyrinth and connectors of the vestibular and the cochlear nerves
labyrinth (LAB-e-rinth)	bony spaces within the temporal bone of the skull made up of three distinct parts, the cochlea, the semicircular canals, and the vestibule. The cochlea facilitates hearing. The semicircular canals and the vestibule facilitate equilibrium and balance.
cochlea (KŌK-lē-ah)	coiled portion of the inner ear containing the sensory organ for hearing; connects to the oval window in the middle ear
semicircular canals and vestibule (*sem*-ī-SUR-kū-lar) (kah-NALS), (VES-ti-būl)	sensory organs of balance; contain receptors and endolymph that provide sensory information about the body's position to maintain equilibrium
mastoid bone (MAS-toid) (bōn)	portion of the temporal bone of the skull posterior and inferior to each auditory canal; contains mastoid air cells that drain into the middle ear cavity behind the external auditory canal. (also called **mastoid process**)

STAPES
is Latin for **stirrup**. The anatomic stapes was so named for its stirrup-like shape.

A&P Booster
For more anatomy and physiology, go to Evolve Resources at evolve.elsevier.com and select:
Practice Student Resources > Student Resources > Chapter 13 > **A&P Booster**

See Appendix B for instructions.

EXERCISE 1

Practice saying aloud each of the Organs and Anatomic Structures of the Ear.

To hear the terms, go to Evolve Resources at evolve.elsevier.com and select:
Practice Student Resources > Student Resources > Chapter 13 > **Pronounce and Spell**

See Appendix B for instructions.

❑ Check the box when complete.

Use the flashcards accompanying this text or electronic flashcards to assist you in memorizing the word parts for this chapter.

WORD PARTS

Word parts you need to learn to complete this chapter are as follows. The exercises at the end of each list will help you learn their definitions and spellings.

Combining Forms of the Ear

COMBINING FORM	DEFINITION
audi/o	hearing
aur/i, ot/o	ear
cochle/o	cochlea
labyrinth/o	labyrinth
mastoid/o	mastoid bone
myring/o	tympanic membrane (eardrum)
staped/o	stapes
tympan/o	middle ear
vestibul/o	vestibule

Refer to **Appendix C** and **Appendix D** for a complete list of word parts.

EXERCISE 2

A. Fill in the blanks with combining forms of the ear. To check your answers, go to Appendix A.

1. Ear

CF: ____________________

CF: ____________________

2. Hearing

CF: ____________________

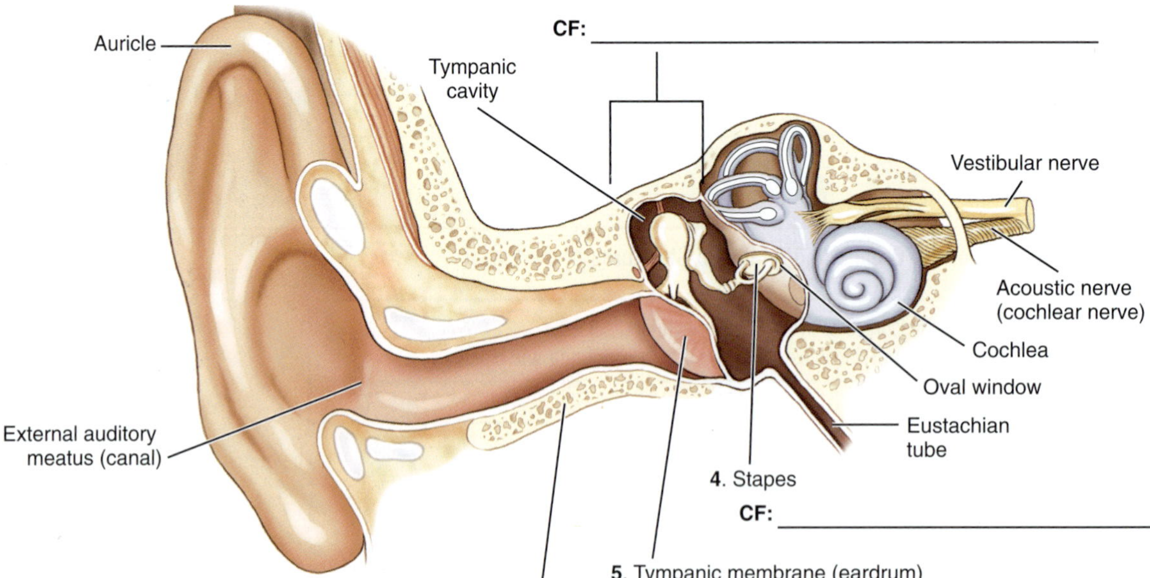

3. Middle ear

CF: ____________________

4. Stapes

CF: ____________________

5. Tympanic membrane (eardrum)

CF: ____________________

6. Mastoid bone

CF: ____________________

B. Fill in the blanks with combining forms of the ear.

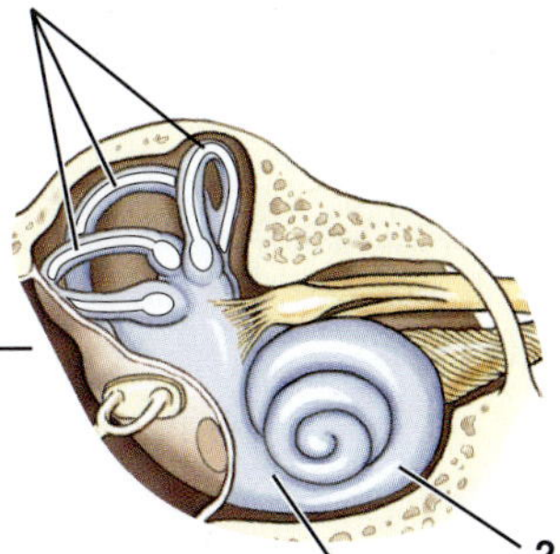

EXERCISE 3

Step 1: Write the definitions after the following combining forms.

Step 2: Match the descriptions on the right with the combining forms and definitions. Answers may be used more than once; no answer line appears for those not described in a lettered item.

_____ 1. staped/o, ______________________

_____ 2. vestibul/o, ______________________

_____ 3. aur/i, ______________________

_____ 4. cochle/o, ______________________

_____ 5. labyrinth/o, ______________________

_____ 6. myring/o, ______________________

_____ 7. tympan/o, ______________________

_____ 8. ot/o, ______________________

_____ 9. mastoid/o, ______________________

10. audi/o, ______________________

a. organ of hearing and balance

b. semitransparent membrane that separates the external auditory canal and the middle ear cavity

c. portion of the temporal bone of the skull posterior and inferior to each auditory canal

d. sensory organ of balance containing receptors and endolymph

e. bony spaces within the temporal bone of the skull made up of three distinct parts, the cochlea, the semicircular canals, and the vestibule

f. coiled portion of the inner ear containing the sensory organ for hearing

g. one of three bones of the middle ear; shaped like a stirrup and connected to the oval window

h. portion of the ear containing the tympanic membrane and the tympanic cavity

For additional practice with Word Parts, go to Evolve Resources at evolve.elsevier.com and select:
Practice Student Resources > Student Resources > Chapter 13 > **Flashcards**

See Appendix B for instructions.

MEDICAL TERMS

The terms you need to learn to complete this chapter are listed on the following pages. The exercises following each list will help you learn the definition and spelling of each word.

Disease and Disorder Terms

BUILT FROM WORD PARTS

The following terms can be translated using definitions of word parts. Further explanation is provided within parentheses as needed.

TERM	DEFINITION
labyrinthitis (*lab*-i-rin-THĪ-tis)	inflammation of the labyrinth
mastoiditis (*mas*-toyd-Ī-tis)	inflammation of the mastoid bone
myringitis (*mir*-in-JĪ-tis)	inflammation of the tympanic membrane (eardrum)
otalgia (ō-TAL-ja)	pain in the ear
otomastoiditis (*ō*-tō-*mas*-toyd-Ī-tis)	inflammation of the ear and the mastoid bone
otomycosis (*ō*-tō-mī-KŌ-sis)	abnormal condition of fungus in the ear (usually affects the external auditory canal)
otopyorrhea (*ō*-tō-*pī*-ō-RĒ-a)	discharge of pus from the ear
otorrhea (*ō*-tō-RĒ-a)	discharge from the ear (may be serous, bloody, consisting of pus, or containing cerebrospinal fluid)
otosclerosis (*ō*-tō-skle-RŌ-sis)	hardening of the ear (stapes) (caused by irregular bone development and resulting in hearing loss)

EXERCISE 4

Practice saying aloud each of the Disease and Disorder Terms Built from Word Parts.

To hear the terms, go to Evolve Resources at evolve.elsevier.com and select:
Practice Student Resources > Student Resources > Chapter 13 > **Pronounce and Spell**

See Appendix B for instructions.

❑ Check the box when complete.

EXERCISE 5

Analyze and define the following terms.

1. otomycosis

____

____

2. otomastoiditis

____

____

3. otalgia

____

____

4. labyrinthitis

____

____

5. myringitis

____

____

6. otosclerosis

____

____

7. mastoiditis

____

____

8. otopyorrhea

____

____

9. otorrhea

____

____

EXERCISE 6

Build disease and disorder terms for the following definitions with the word parts you have learned.

1. inflammation of the tympanic membrane ______ / ______ (WR / S)
2. discharge of pus from the ear ______ / ______ / ______ / ______ / ______ (WR / CV / WR / CV / S)
3. inflammation of the mastoid bone ______ / ______ (WR / S)
4. pain in the ear ______ / ______ (WR / S)
5. hardening of the ear (stapes) ______ / ______ / ______ (WR / CV / S)
6. abnormal condition of fungus in the ear ______ / ______ / ______ / ______ (WR / CV / WR / S)
7. inflammation of the ear and the mastoid bone ______ / ______ / ______ / ______ (WR / CV / WR / S)
8. inflammation of the labyrinth ______ / ______ (WR / S)
9. discharge from the ear ______ / ______ / ______ (WR / CV / S)

EXERCISE 7

Spell each of the Disease and Disorder Terms Built from Word Parts by having someone dictate them to you. Use a separate sheet of paper.

To hear and spell the terms, go to Evolve Resources at evolve.elsevier.com and select:
Practice Student Resources > Student Resources > Chapter 13 > **Pronounce and Spell**

See Appendix B for instructions.

❑ Check the box when complete.

Disease and Disorder Terms
NOT BUILT FROM WORD PARTS

Word parts may be present in the following terms; however, their full meanings cannot be translated using definitions of word parts alone.

INTEGRATIVE MEDICINE TERM

Music and sound therapy is the use of music or sounds within a therapeutic relationship to address physical, emotional, cognitive, and social needs of individuals. Music and sound therapy studies have shown promising clinical efficacy in the treatment of **tinnitus** and the rehabilitation of post-cochlear implant patients.

TERM	DEFINITION
acoustic neuroma (a-KOOS-tik) (nū-RŌ-ma)	benign tumor within the internal auditory canal growing from the acoustic nerve (cochlear branch of the vestibulocochlear nerve); may cause hearing loss and may damage structures of the cerebellum as it grows
cholesteatoma (*ko*-le-stē-a-TŌ-ma)	cystlike mass composed of epithelial cells and cholesterol occurring in the middle ear; may be associated with chronic otitis media
Ménière disease (me-NYĀR) (di-ZĒZ)	chronic disease of the inner ear characterized by a sensation of spinning motion (vertigo), ringing in the ear (tinnitus), aural fullness, and fluctuating hearing loss; symptoms are related to a change in volume or composition of fluid within the labyrinth
otitis externa (ō-TĪ-tis) (eks-TER-na)	inflammation of the outer ear
otitis media (OM) (ō-TĪ-tis) (MĒ-dē-a)	inflammation of the middle ear (Fig. 13.3A)

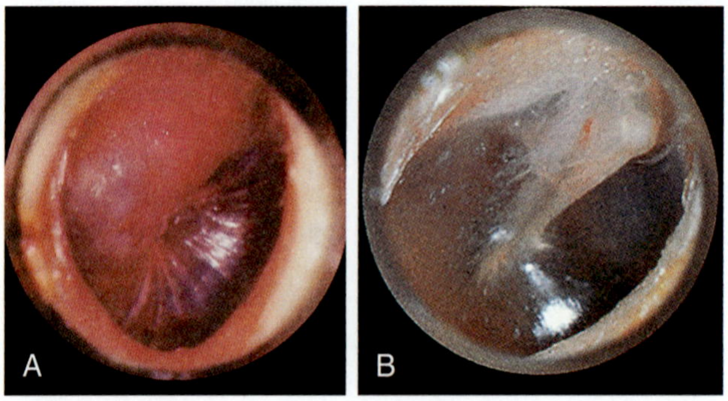

FIG. 13.3 Otitis media. Signs include bulging, perforated, reddened, or retracted tympanic membrane. **A,** Tympanic membrane demonstrating **acute otitis media (AOM)**. **B,** Normal tympanic membrane.

TERM	DEFINITION
presbycusis (*prez*-bi-KŪ-sis)	hearing impairment occurring with age
tinnitus (tin-NĪ-tus)	ringing in the ears
vertigo (VER-ti-gō)	sense that either one's own body (subjective vertigo) or the environment (objective vertigo) is revolving; may indicate inner ear disease

TINNITUS

Note the spelling of **tinnitus**. The ending is **itus** and not **itis**, the ending most familiar to you, meaning inflammation.

BENIGN PAROXYSMAL POSITIONAL VERTIGO (BPPV)

is characterized by brief episodes of vertigo associated with a change in the position of the head, such as turning over in bed or sitting up in the morning. In BPPV, normal calcium carbonate crystals called otoconia break loose and shift within the labyrinth, triggering an episode of vertigo.

EXERCISE 8

Practice saying aloud each of the Disease and Disorder Terms NOT Built from Word Parts.

To hear the terms, go to Evolve Resources at evolve.elsevier.com and select:
Practice Student Resources > Student Resources > Chapter 13 > **Pronounce and Spell**

See Appendix B for instructions.

❑ Check the box when complete.

EXERCISE 9

A. Fill in the blanks with the correct terms.

1. The patient reported that her body seemed to be revolving, or ____________________, and ringing in the ears, or ____________________.
2. A chronic ear disease characterized by vertigo, tinnitus, aural fullness, and fluctuating hearing loss is called ____________________ disease.
3. ____________________ is hearing impairment occurring with age.

EXERCISE 9—*cont'd*

B. Write the medical term pictured and defined.

1. ______________________________

inflammation of the outer ear

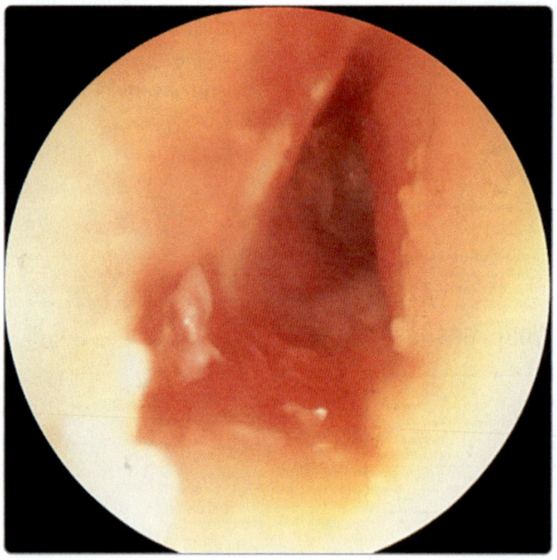

2. ______________________________

inflammation of the middle ear

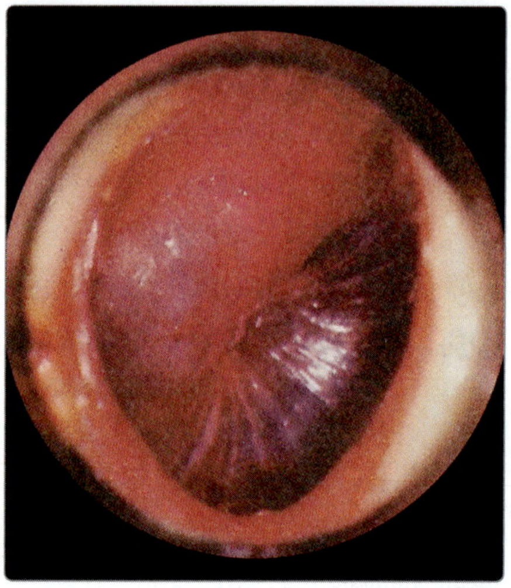

3. ______________________________

cystlike mass composed of epithelial cells and cholesterol occurring in the middle ear

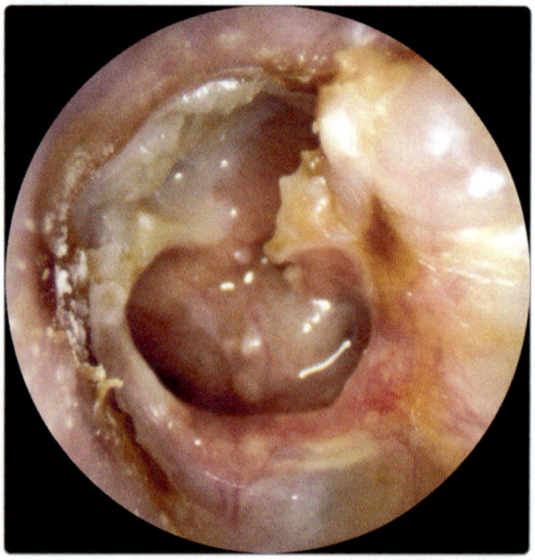

4. ______________________________

benign tumor within the internal auditory canal growing from the acoustic nerve

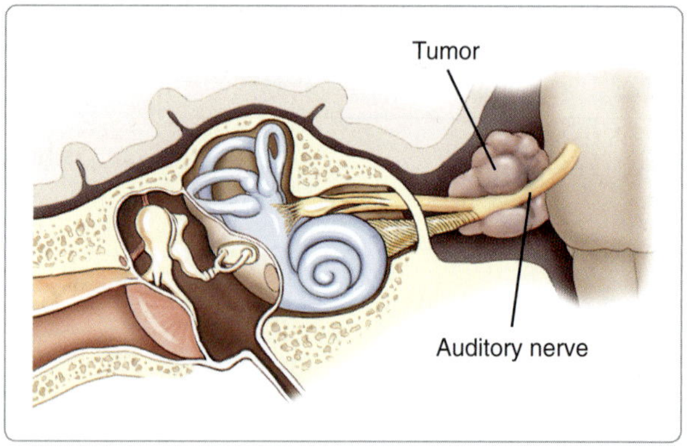

EXERCISE 10

Match the terms in the first column with the correct definitions in the second column.

______ 1. vertigo	a. inflammation of the middle ear
______ 2. tinnitus	b. chronic ear problem characterized by vertigo, tinnitus, and fluctuating hearing loss
______ 3. Ménière disease	c. benign tumor arising from the acoustic nerve
______ 4. otitis externa	d. sense of revolving of one's own body or the environment
______ 5. acoustic neuroma	e. ringing in the ears
______ 6. otitis media	f. inflammation of the outer ear
______ 7. presbycusis	g. hearing impairment occurring with age
______ 8. cholesteatoma	h. mass composed of epithelial cells and cholesterol

EXERCISE 11

Spell each of the Disease and Disorder Terms NOT Built from Word Parts by having someone dictate them to you. Use a separate sheet of paper.

To hear and spell the terms, go to Evolve Resources at evolve.elsevier.com and select:
Practice Student Resources > Student Resources > Chapter 13 > **Pronounce and Spell**

See Appendix B for instructions.

❑ Check the box when complete.

Surgical Terms

BUILT FROM WORD PARTS

The following terms can be translated using definitions of word parts. Further explanation is provided within parentheses as needed.

TERM	DEFINITION
cochlear implant (KŌK-lē-ar) (IM-plant)	pertaining to the cochlea implant (surgically inserted electronic device that converts sound into electrical impulses. The impulses stimulate the auditory nerve to carry the signal to the brain which learns to interpret the signal as sound. The damaged part of the ear is bypassed.) (Fig. 13.4)
labyrinthectomy (*lab*-i-rin-THEK-to-mē)	excision of the labyrinth
mastoidectomy (*mas*-toy-DEK-to-mē)	excision of the mastoid bone
mastoidotomy (*mas*-toy-DOT-o-mē)	incision into the mastoid bone
myringoplasty (mi-RING-gō-*plas*-tē)	surgical repair of the tympanic membrane
myringotomy (*mir*-ing-GOT-o-mē)	incision into the tympanic membrane (performed to relieve pressure in the middle ear by releasing pus or fluid and for the placement of tubes) (Exercise Figure A)

EXERCISE FIGURE A

Fill in the blanks with word parts defined to label the diagram.

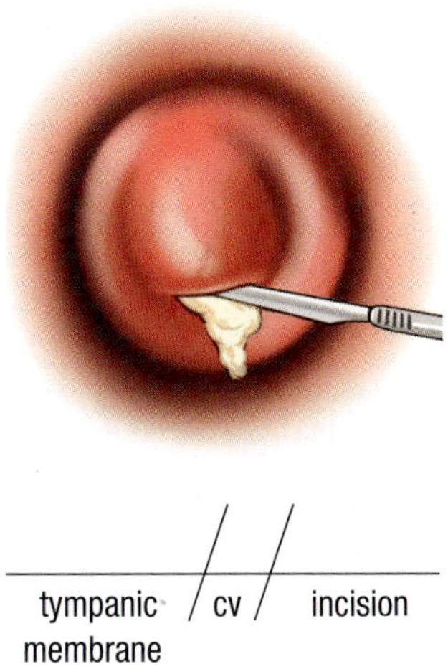

is performed to release pus from the middle ear through the tympanic membrane to treat acute otitis media.

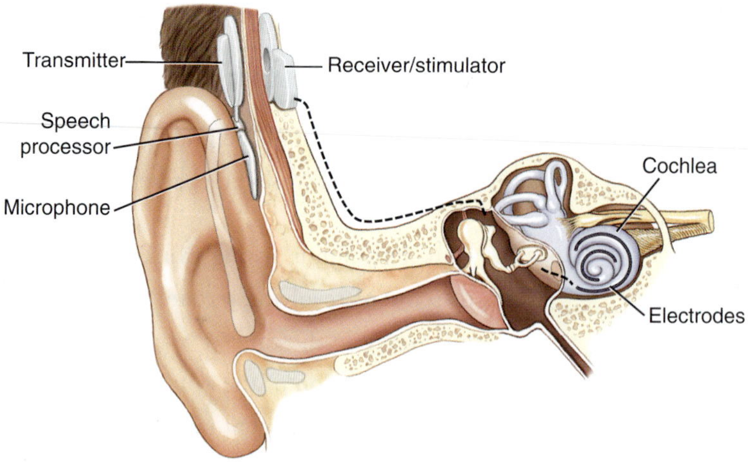

FIG. 13.4 Cochlear implants are fitted in adults and children who are deaf or severely hard of hearing.

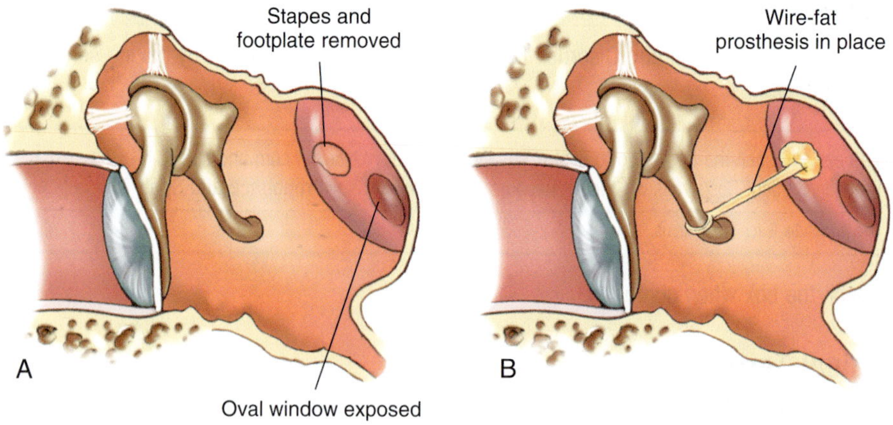

FIG. 13.5 Stapedectomy. **A,** Stapes is removed. **B,** Prosthesis is in place.

Surgical Terms—cont'd

TERM	DEFINITION
stapedectomy (*stā*-pe-DEK-to-mē)	excision of the stapes (performed to restore hearing in cases of otosclerosis; the stapes is replaced by a prosthesis) (Fig. 13.5)
tympanoplasty (TIM-pa-nō-*plas*-tē)	surgical repair (of the hearing mechanism) of the middle ear (including the tympanic membrane and the ossicles)

EXERCISE 12

Practice saying aloud each of the Surgical Terms Built from Word Parts.

To hear the terms, go to Evolve Resources at evolve.elsevier.com and select:
Practice Student Resources > Student Resources > Chapter 13 > **Pronounce and Spell**

See Appendix B for instructions.

❑ Check the box when complete.

EXERCISE 13

Analyze and define the following surgical terms.

1. mastoidectomy
____
____

2. myringotomy
____
____

3. labyrinthectomy
____
____

4. mastoidotomy
____
____

5. tympanoplasty
____
____

6. myringoplasty
____
____

7. stapedectomy
____
____

8. cochlear (implant)
____
____

EXERCISE 14

Build surgical terms for the following definitions by using the word parts you have learned.

1. incision into the mastoid bone ______ / ______ / ______
WR / CV / S

2. excision of the labyrinth ______ / ______
WR / S

3. surgical repair (of the hearing mechanism) of the middle ear ______ / ______ / ______
WR / CV / S

4. excision of the mastoid bone ______ / ______
WR / S

5. incision into the tympanic membrane ______ / ______ / ______
WR / CV / S

6. surgical repair of the tympanic membrane ______ / ______ / ______
WR / CV / S

7. excision of the stapes ______ / ______
WR / S

8. pertaining to the cochlea ______ / ______ implant
WR / S

EXERCISE 15

Spell each of the Surgical Terms Built from Word Parts by having someone dictate them to you. Use a separate sheet of paper.

To hear and spell the terms, go to Evolve Resources at evolve.elsevier.com and select:
Practice Student Resources > Student Resources > Chapter 13 > **Pronounce and Spell**

See Appendix B for instructions.

❑ Check the box when complete.

Diagnostic Terms
BUILT FROM WORD PARTS

The following terms can be translated using definitions of word parts. Further explanation is provided within parentheses as needed.

TERM	DEFINITION
audiogram (AW-dē-ō-*gram*)	(graphic) record of hearing (Fig. 13.6B)
audiometer (*aw*-dē-OM-e-ter)	instrument used to measure hearing (Fig. 13.6A)
audiometry (*aw*-dē-OM-e-trē)	measurement of hearing
electrocochleography (ē-*lek*-trō-*kok*-lē-OG-ra-fē)	process of recording the electrical activity in the cochlea (in response to sound)
otoscope (Ō-tō-skōp)	instrument used for visual examination of the ear (Exercise Figure B)
otoscopy (ō-TOS-ko-pē)	visual examination of the ear (Exercise Figure B)
tympanometer (*tim*-pa-NOM-e-ter)	instrument used to measure middle ear (function) (Exercise Figure C)
tympanometry (*tim*-pa-NOM-e-trē)	measurement of middle ear (function)

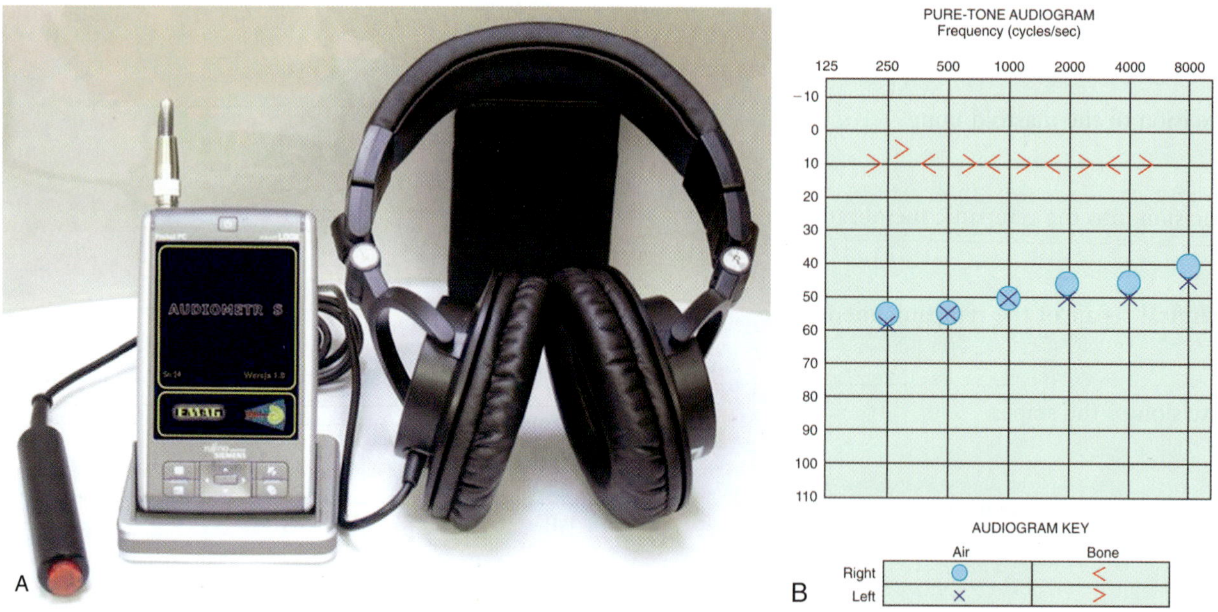

FIG. 13.6 A, Audiometer. **B,** Audiogram.

EXERCISE FIGURE B

Fill in the blanks with word parts defined to label the diagram.

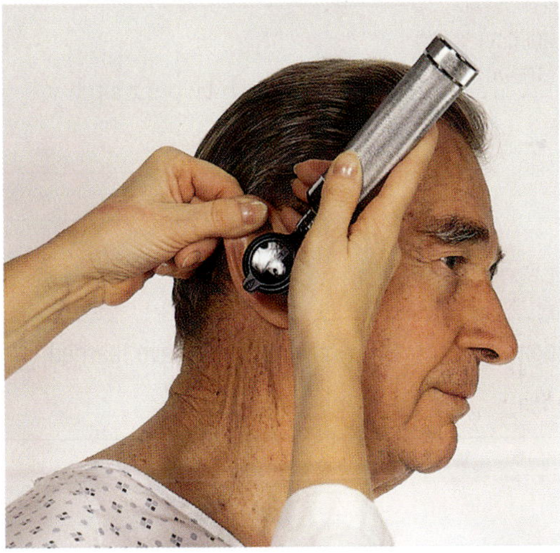

______ / ______ / ______ performed with an ______ / ______ / ______.
ear / cv / visual examination ... ear / cv / instrument used for visual examination

EXERCISE FIGURE C

Fill in the blanks with word parts defined to label the diagram.

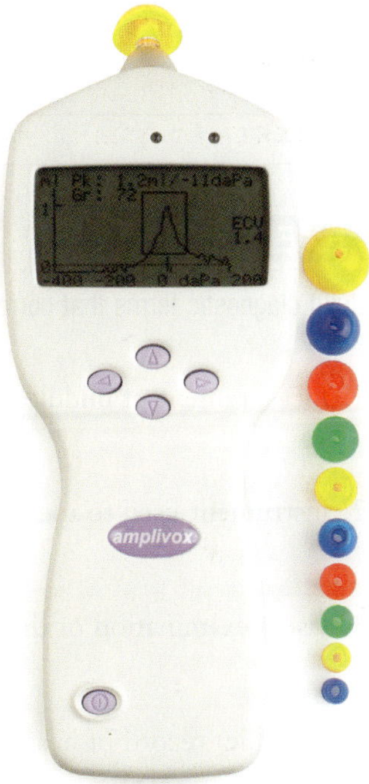

______ / ______ / ______
middle ear / cv / instrument used to measure

EXERCISE 16

Practice saying aloud each of the Diagnostic Terms Built from Word Parts.

To hear the terms, go to Evolve Resources at evolve.elsevier.com and select:
Practice Student Resources > Student Resources > Chapter 13 > **Pronounce and Spell**

See Appendix B for instructions.

❑ Check the box when complete.

EXERCISE 17

Analyze and define the following diagnostic terms.

1. otoscope

____

____

2. audiometry

____

____

3. audiogram

____

____

4. otoscopy

____

____

5. audiometer

____

____

6. tympanometry

____

____

7. tympanometer

____

____

8. electrocochleography

____

____

EXERCISE 18

Build diagnostic terms that correspond to the following definitions by using the word parts you have learned.

1. measurement of middle ear (function) ____ / ____ / ____ (WR / CV / S)
2. instrument used to measure hearing ____ / ____ / ____ (WR / CV / S)
3. visual examination of the ear ____ / ____ / ____ (WR / CV / S)
4. (graphic) record of hearing ____ / ____ / ____ (WR / CV / S)
5. instrument used for visual examination of the ear ____ / ____ / ____ (WR / CV / S)
6. measurement of hearing ____ / ____ / ____ (WR / CV / S)
7. instrument used to measure middle ear (function) ____ / ____ / ____ (WR / CV / S)
8. process of recording the electrical activity in the cochlea ____ / ____ / ____ / ____ / ____ (WR / CV / WR / CV / S)

EXERCISE 19

Spell each of the Diagnostic Terms Built from Word Parts by having someone dictate them to you. Use a separate sheet of paper.

> To hear and spell the terms, go to Evolve Resources at evolve.elsevier.com and select:
> Practice Student Resources > Student Resources > Chapter 13 > **Pronounce and Spell**
>
> See Appendix B for instructions.

❑ Check the box when complete.

Complementary Terms
BUILT FROM WORD PARTS

The following terms can be translated using definitions of word parts. Further explanation is provided within parentheses as needed.

TERM	DEFINITION
audiologist (*aw*-dē-OL-o-jist)	one who studies and specializes in hearing
audiology (*aw*-dē-OL-o-jē)	study of hearing
aural (AW-rul)	pertaining to the ear
cochlear (KOK-lē-ar)	pertaining to the cochlea
otolaryngologist (ENT) (*ō*-tō-*lar*-ing-GOL-o-jist)	physician who studies and treats diseases of the ear, (nose), and larynx (throat)
otologist (ō-TOL-o-jist)	physician who studies and treats diseases of the ear
otology (ō-TOL-o-jē)	study of the ear (a branch of medicine that deals with diseases of the ear)
vestibular (ves-TIB-ū-lar)	pertaining to the vestibule
vestibulocochlear (ves-*tib*-ū-lō-KOK-lē-ar)	pertaining to the vestibule and the cochlea

AUDIOLOGIST

To see an interview with an **audiologist**, go to Evolve Resources at evolve.elsevier.com and select: Practice Student Resources > Extra Content > **Career Videos**

See Appendix B for instructions.

Refer to **Appendix F** for pharmacology terms related to the ear.

EXERCISE 20

Practice saying aloud each of the Complementary Terms Built from Word Parts.

To hear the terms, go to Evolve Resources at evolve.elsevier.com and select: Practice Student Resources > Student Resources > Chapter 13 > **Pronounce and Spell**

See Appendix B for instructions.

❑ Check the box when complete.

EXERCISE 21

Analyze and define the following complementary terms.

1. otology
____
____

2. audiologist
____
____

3. otolaryngologist
____
____

4. audiology
____
____

5. otologist
____
____

6. aural
____
____

7. cochlear
____
____

8. vestibular
____
____

9. vestibulocochlear
____
____

EXERCISE 22

Build the complementary terms for the following definitions by using the word parts you have learned.

1. study of hearing ______ / ___ / ______
WR / CV / S

2. physician who studies and treats diseases of the ear, (nose), and larynx (throat) ______ / ___ / ______ / ___ / ______
WR / CV / WR / CV / S

3. study of the ear ______ / ___ / ______
WR / CV / S

4. one who studies and specializes in hearing ______ / ___ / ______
WR / CV / S

5. physician who studies and treats diseases of the ear ______ / ___ / ______
WR / CV / S

6. pertaining to the ear ______ / ______
WR / S

7. pertaining to the vestibule and the cochlea ________ / ____ / ________ / ________
WR / CV / WR / S

8. pertaining to the vestibule ________ / ________
WR / S

9. pertaining to the cochlea ________ / ________
WR / S

EXERCISE 23

Spell each of the Complementary Terms Built from Word Parts by having someone dictate them to you. Use a separate sheet of paper.

> To hear and spell the terms, go to Evolve Resources at evolve.elsevier.com and select:
> Practice Student Resources > Student Resources > Chapter 13 > **Pronounce and Spell**
>
> See Appendix B for instructions.

❑ Check the box when complete.

Abbreviations

ABBREVIATION	TERM
AOM	acute otitis media
ENT	ears, nose, throat; otolaryngologist
HOH	hard of hearing
OM	otitis media

EXERCISE 24

Write the meaning of the following abbreviations.

1. ENT ________ ________ ________ and ________
2. HOH ________ ________ ________
3. OM ________ ________
4. AOM ________ ________ ________

> For additional practice with Abbreviations, go to Evolve Resources at evolve.elsevier.com and select:
> Practice Student Resources > Student Resources > Chapter 13 > **Flashcards:** Abbreviations
>
> See Appendix B for instructions.

PRACTICAL APPLICATION

EXERCISE 25 *Case Study: Translate Between Everyday Language and Medical Language*

CASE STUDY: Marisol Montoya

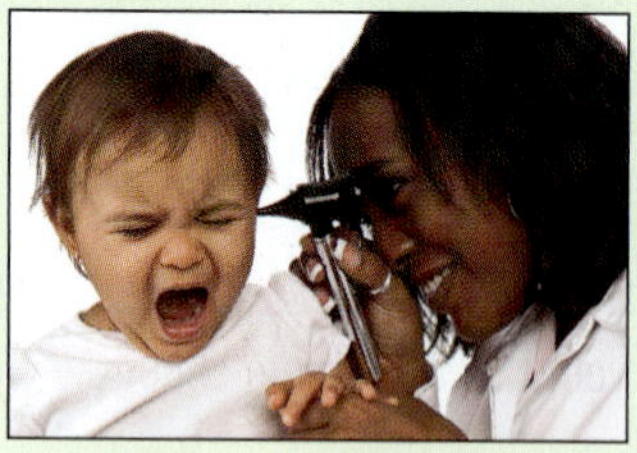

Marisol Montoya is only 13 months old and she has already had five episodes of middle ear infections (inflammation). For the last few days she has had a fever and she keeps pulling on her ear as if it is painful. Today her mother noticed a pus-like liquid coming out of her left ear. Now her mother is seeing redness and swelling on her skull behind Marisol's earlobe. She calls her pediatrician, who arranges an immediate referral to an ear, nose, and throat physician.

Now that you have worked through Chapter 13, consider the medical terms that might be used to describe Marisol's experience. See the Review of Terms at the end of the chapter for a list of terms that might apply.

A. *Underline phrases in the case study that could be substituted with medical terms.*

B. *Write the medical term and its definition for three of the phrases you underlined.*

MEDICAL TERM	DEFINITION
1. ______________	______________________________
2. ______________	______________________________
3. ______________	______________________________

DOCUMENTATION: Excerpt from Otolaryngology Visit

Marisol was examined by an otolaryngologist; an excerpt from the medical record is documented below.

Marisol Montoya is a thirteen-month-old female referred by her pediatrician for possible mastoiditis. Her mother reports a history of frequent episodes of otitis media, and she currently has symptoms of fever, otalgia, and otopyorrhea. Today her mother noted inflammation in the left mastoid region. Physical exam reveals an unhappy child with a temperature of 101.7 degrees Fahrenheit. Otoscopy is difficult due to pain but shows both otitis externa in the left ear and otitis media bilaterally. Tympanometry shows evidence of poor mobility and suggests a collection of fluid and pressure in the middle ear. Examination of the left mastoid region reveals erythema, edema, and severe tenderness. My impression is that this child has acute mastoiditis. We will perform bilateral myringotomies and send the fluid for cultures. In the meantime, we will start antibiotics and obtain a CT scan of the affected area. If she worsens or does not improve, mastoidectomy will be considered.

C. *Underline medical terms presented in Chapter 13 used in the previous excerpt from Marisol's medical record. See the Review of Terms at the end of the chapter for a complete list.*

D. *Select and define three of the medical terms you underlined. To check your answers, go to Appendix A.*

MEDICAL TERM	DEFINITION
1. ______________	______________________________
2. ______________	______________________________
3. ______________	______________________________

EXERCISE 26 *Interact with Medical Documents and Electronic Health Records*

A. Read the report and complete it by writing medical terms on answer lines within the document. Definitions of terms to be written appear after the document.

99665-AUD TOHE, Jimmy

File Patient Navigate Custom Fields Help

Chart Review | Encounters | Notes | Labs | Imaging | Procedures | Rx | Documents | Referrals | Scheduling | Billing

Name: **TOHE, Jimmy** MR#: **99665-AUD** DOB: 03/09/19XX Gender: M Age: 62 **Allergies: Demerol** **PCP: Unknown**

ENT Clinic Visit
Date: 04 September 20XX 10:00

Subjective: Jimmy Tohe is a 62-year-old male, appearing younger than his stated age. He was brought into the 1. ________________ clinic by his daughter, who states that he is unable to hear what is being said to him by family members. She states that this problem has existed for at least 30 years but that it appears to be getting markedly worse. The patient states he had several episodes of ear infections as a child and young adult. He denies any 2. ________________ or 3.________________.

Objective: Temperature, 99.4. Pulse, 72. Respirations, 20. Blood pressure, 136/76 mm Hg. Weight, 162 pounds. Patient ambulates without difficulty. Alert and oriented x3. 4. ________________ reveals scarring of the tympanic membranes bilaterally. Auditory canals appear normal bilaterally.

Assessment:
1. Mild loss of hearing bilaterally, probably caused by 5.________________ as a child.
2. Recent exacerbation of hearing loss most likely attributable to 6. ________________.

Plan:
1. Patient referred to 7. ________________ for complete 8. ________________ workup.

Electronically signed: McKeegan, Bridey MD, 09/04/20XX 10:30

Start | Log On/Off | Print | Edit

Definitions of Medical Terms to Complete the Document

Write the medical terms defined on corresponding answer lines in the document.

1. abbreviation for ears, nose, and throat
2. ringing in the ears
3. sense of one's own body or the environment revolving
4. visual examination of the ear
5. inflammation of the middle ear
6. hearing impairment occurring with age
7. one who studies and specializes in hearing
8. measurement of hearing

EXERCISE 26 *Interact with Medical Documents and Electronic Health Records—cont'd*

B. Read the medical report and answer the questions below it.

028464 MARIEB, PAULINA

File Patient Navigate Custom Fields Help

Patient Chart | Lab | Rad | Notes | Documents | Rx | Scheduling | Images | Billing

Name: **MARIEB, PAULINA** MR#: **028464** DOB: **3/24/19XX** Gender: **Female** Age: **65** Allergies: **None known** PCP: **Tamika Jefferson, MD**

CLINICAL NOTES REPORT

ENCOUNTER DATE: 1/7/20XX
PURPOSE OF VISIT: Referred by Dr. Tamika Jefferson for itching ears.

HISTORY: The patient is a 65-year-old female who has had about six months difficulty with itching in her outer ears. She was seen by an internist who has given her Cortaid cream to use in this area. She denies otorrhea or otalgia or aural fullness, congestion, vertigo, or hearing changes. She denies any ear surgeries or previous ear infections.

PHYSICAL EXAMINATION: Under the operating microscope, the left ear was examined. The external ear shows no edema, no involvement of cartilage. No chondritis noted, but along the conchal bowl there is some dry scaling of the skin. There was some cerumen which was removed with suction. Inspection of the right ear revealed more of the same. There are no fissures forming. There was no postauricular dermatitis noted on either ear. There was no lymphadenopathy or adenopathy.

IMPRESSION: Chronic otitis externa.

PLAN: Continue with the cream twice a day until itching symptoms resolve and then to use the cream once a day. The patient has been educated as to the importance of keeping her ears dry. We would be happy to see her back as needed if her symptoms worsen or persist.

Electronically signed by: David Lee, MD 1/7/20XX 16:24

Start | Log On/Off | Print | Edit

Use the medical report above to answer the questions.

1. The patient has been experiencing:
   a. itchiness
   b. hearing loss
   c. otalgia
   d. vertigo
2. In the patient's left ear, suction removed:
   a. scaling
   b. cerumen
   c. chondritis
   d. otorrhea
3. The patient's condition has been diagnosed as chronic:
   a. abnormal condition of fungus in the ear
   b. inflammation of the tympanic membrane
   c. hardening of the stapes
   d. inflammation of the outer ear

C. Complete the **three medical documents** within the electronic health record (EHR) on Evolve.

Topic: Acoustic Neuroma
Documents: Audiology Assessment, Urgent Care Clinic Note, Office Visit

To complete the three medical records, go to Evolve Resources at evolve.elsevier.com and select: Practice Student Resources > Student Resources > Chapter 13 > **Electronic Heath Records**

See Appendix B for instructions.

EXERCISE 27 *Pronounce Medical Terms in Use*

Practice pronunciation of terms by reading aloud the following paragraph. Use the phonetic spellings following medical terms from the chapter to assist with pronunciation. The script also contains medical terms not presented in the chapter. Treat them as information only or look for their meanings in a medical dictionary or a reliable online source.

ACUTE OTITIS MEDIA

Acute **otitis media** (ō-TĪ-tis) (MĒ-dē-a) is one of the most common pediatric infections. Most middle ear infections are caused by bacteria, and some by viruses. Symptoms include **otalgia** (ō-TAL-ja), **otorrhea** (ō-tō-RĒ-a), ear pulling, and irritability. The tympanic membrane will be bulging, red in color, with a thickened appearance and reduced translucency. Antibiotics may be ordered if the infection does not resolve on its own. If unresponsive to antibiotic treatment, a **myringotomy** (*mir*-ing-GOT-o-mē) may be performed to identify the causative pathogen, allowing for the appropriate antibiotic treatment to be prescribed.

EXERCISE 28 *Chapter Content Quiz*

Test your understanding of terms and abbreviations introduced in this chapter. Circle the letter for the medical term or abbreviation related to the words in italics.

1. The vestibular nerve and the auditory nerve are branches of the *pertaining to the vestibule and the cochlea* nerve.
   a. aural
   b. cochlear
   c. vestibulocochlear
2. The abbreviation *ENT*, meaning "ears, nose, and throat," can also refer to the following:
   a. otolaryngologist
   b. audiologist
   c. otoscopy
3. A(n) *physician who studies and treats diseases of the ear* is an ENT with one to three years of additional training in specific areas and functions of the ear.
   a. otolaryngology
   b. otologist
   c. audiologist
4. The patient reported being bothered by *ringing in the ears* for the last three weeks.
   a. tinnitus
   b. vertigo
   c. presbycusis
5. Vertigo, tinnitus, and fluctuating hearing loss in *chronic disease of the inner ear* usually occur in episodes that can last for several days.
   a. mastoiditis
   b. presbycusis
   c. Ménière disease
6. *Process of recording electrical activity in the cochlea in response to sound*, may be used in the diagnosis of Ménière disease.
   a. electrocochleography
   b. tympanometry
   c. audiometry
7. Thought to be caused by a viral infection, labyrinthitis may cause sudden intense *sensation of revolving*, nausea, vomiting, and imbalance.
   a. tinnitus
   b. vertigo
   c. aural fullness
8. A *cystlike mass composed of epithelial cells and cholesterol* may destroy adjacent bones, including the ossicles.
   a. cholesteatoma
   b. otosclerosis
   c. otitis media

9. Manifestations of *benign tumor within the auditory canal growing from the cochlear branch of the vestibulocochlear nerve* often begin with tinnitus and gradual hearing loss.
   a. otitis externa
   b. mastoiditis
   c. acoustic neuroma
10. Typical presentation of *abnormal condition of fungus in the ear* is with inflammation, pruritus, scaling, and extreme discomfort.
   a. otomycosis
   b. otalgia
   c. otopyorrhea
11. Mild *hardening of the ear* may be treated with a hearing aid.
   a. otalgia
   b. otomycosis
   c. otosclerosis
12. A(n) *instrument used to measure middle ear function* changes the air pressure in the ear causing the eardrum to move back and forth.
   a. tympanometer
   b. audiometer
   c. otoscope
13. *Surgical repair of the middle ear* may include placement of a graft to close perforation of the eardrum and improve hearing.
   a. myringotomy
   b. myringoplasty
   c. tympanoplasty
14. A *surgically implanted electronic device that converts sound into electrical impulses* has internal and external components.
   a. cochlear implant
   b. audiogram
   c. electrocochleography

C CHAPTER REVIEW

e REVIEW OF CHAPTER CONTENT ON EVOLVE RESOURCES

Go to evolve.elsevier.com and click on Gradable Student Resources and Practice Student Resources. Online learning activities found there can be used to review chapter content and to assess your learning of word parts, medical terms, and abbreviations. Place check marks in the boxes next to activities used for review and assessment.

GRADABLE STUDENT RESOURCES

Chapter 13 >	Exercises >	☐ Word Parts ☐ Terms Built from Word Parts ☐ Terms Not Built from Word Parts
	Quizzes >	☐ Quiz 1: Disease and Disorder and Complementary Terms ☐ Quiz 2: Surgical and Diagnostic Terms

PRACTICE STUDENT RESOURCES > STUDENT RESOURCES

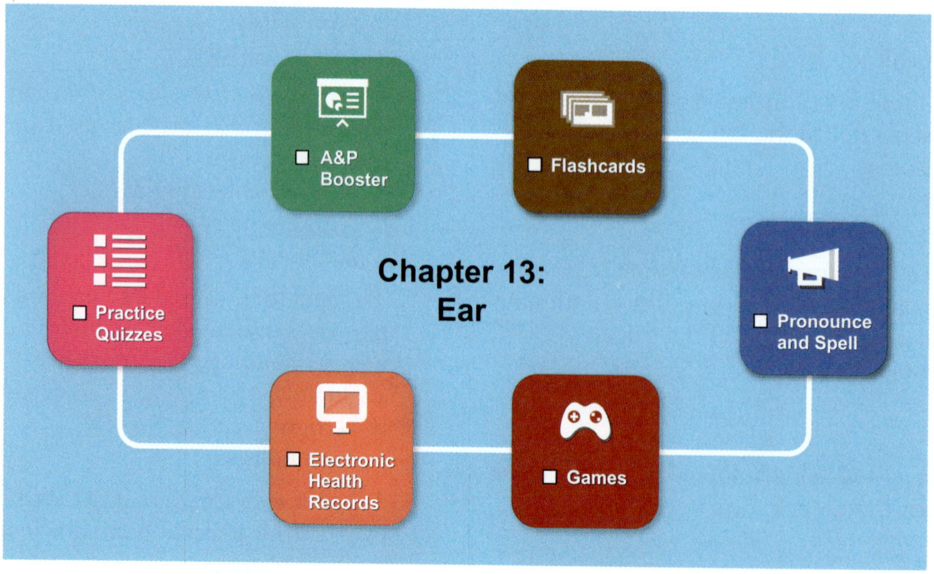

REVIEW OF WORD PARTS

Can you define and spell the following word parts?

COMBINING FORMS	
audi/o	myring/o
aur/i	ot/o
cochle/o	staped/o
labyrinth/o	tympan/o
mastoid/o	vestibul/o

REVIEW OF TERMS

Can you build, analyze, define, pronounce, and spell the following terms *built from word parts*?

DISEASES AND DISORDERS	SURGICAL	DIAGNOSTIC	COMPLEMENTARY
labyrinthitis	cochlear implant	audiogram	audiologist
mastoiditis	labyrinthectomy	audiometer	audiology
myringitis	mastoidectomy	audiometry	aural
otalgia	mastoidotomy	electrocochleography	cochlear
otomastoiditis	myringoplasty	otoscope	otolaryngologist (ENT)
otomycosis	myringotomy	otoscopy	otologist
otopyorrhea	stapedectomy	tympanometer	otology
otorrhea	tympanoplasty	tympanometry	vestibular
otosclerosis			vestibulocochlear

Can you define, pronounce, and spell the following terms *NOT built from word parts?*

DISEASES AND DISORDERS
acoustic neuroma
cholesteatoma
Ménière disease
otitis externa
otitis media (OM)
presbycusis
tinnitus
vertigo

Chapter 14

Musculoskeletal System

Objectives

Upon completion of this chapter you will be able to:

1. Pronounce anatomic structures of the musculoskeletal system.
2. Define and spell word parts related to the musculoskeletal system.
3. Define, pronounce, and spell disease and disorder terms related to the musculoskeletal system.
4. Define, pronounce, and spell surgical terms related to the musculoskeletal system.
5. Define, pronounce, and spell diagnostic terms related to the musculoskeletal system.
6. Define, pronounce, and spell complementary terms related to the musculoskeletal system.
7. Identify and define types of body movement.
8. Interpret the meaning of abbreviations related to the musculoskeletal system.
9. Apply medical language in clinical contexts.

Outline

ANATOMY

The musculoskeletal system consists of muscles, bones (Fig. 14.1), bone marrow, joints, cartilage, tendons, ligaments, and bursae. The adult human skeleton contains 206 bones (Fig. 14.2A and B and Fig. 14.3A and B) and more than 600 muscles. Joints form the union between bones and often allow for movement, although some do not. Most of the joints in the skeleton are freely moving and contain cartilage and bursae.

Function

The functions of the muscular system are movement, posture, joint stability, and heat production. The functions of the skeletal system are to provide a framework for the body, protect the soft body parts such as the brain, store calcium, and support and protect bone marrow (where blood cells are produced). The organs and structures of the musculoskeletal system work together to protect, support, and move the body.

Bone Structure

TERM	DEFINITION
periosteum (*per*-ē-OS-tē-um)	outermost layer of the bone, made up of fibrous tissue
compact bone (KOM-pakt) (bōn)	dense, hard layers of bone tissue that lie underneath the periosteum
cancellous bone (kan-SEL-us) (bōn)	contains little spaces like a sponge and is encased in the layers of compact bone (also called **spongy bone**)
endosteum (en-DOS-tē-um)	membranous lining of the hollow cavity of the bone
diaphysis (dī-AF-i-sis)	shaft of the long bones (Fig. 14.1)

PERIOSTEUM

is composed of the prefix **peri-**, meaning **surrounding**, and the word root **oste**, meaning **bone**.

ENDOSTEUM

is composed of the prefix **endo-**, meaning **within**, and the word root **oste**, meaning **bone**.

DIAPHYSIS

comes from the Greek **diaphusis**, meaning state of growing between.

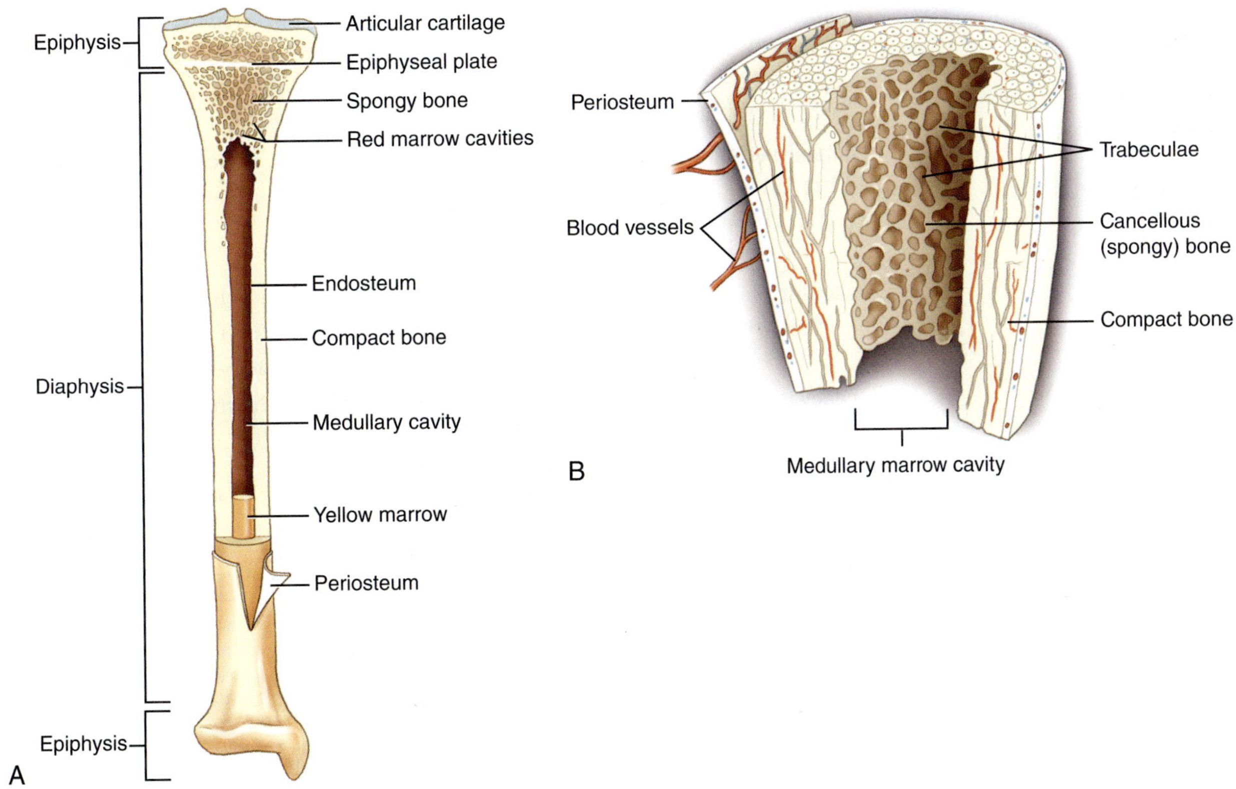

FIG. 14.1 **A,** Bone structure. **B,** Magnified view of bone structure.

> **EPIPHYSIS**
> has been used in the English language since the 1600s and retains the meaning given to it by a Greco-Roman physician. It means a **portion of bone attached for a time to another bone** by a cartilage, but that later combines with the principal bone. During the period of growth, the epiphysis is separated from the main portion of the bone by cartilage.

Bone Structure—cont'd

TERM	DEFINITION
epiphysis (pl. epiphyses) (e-PIF-i-sis), (e-PIF-i-sēz)	end of each long bone (Fig. 14.1)
bone marrow (bōn) (MAR-ō)	material found in the cavities of bones
red marrow (red) (MAR-ō)	thick, bloodlike material found in flat bones and the ends of long bones; location of blood cell formation
yellow marrow (YEL-ō) (MAR-ō)	soft, fatty material found in the medullary cavity of long bones

Skeletal Bones

TERM	DEFINITION
maxilla (mak-SIL-a)	upper jawbone
mandible (MAN-di-bul)	lower jawbone
vertebral column (ver-TĒ-brel) (KOL-em)	made up of bones called vertebrae (pl.) or vertebra (sing.) through which the spinal cord runs. The vertebral column protects the spinal cord, supports the head, and provides points of attachment for ribs and muscles. (Fig. 14.2)
cervical vertebrae (C1 to C7) (SUR-vi-kal) (VER-te-bray)	first set of seven bones, forming the neck
thoracic vertebrae (T1 to T12) (tha-RAS-ik) (VER-te-bray)	second set of 12 vertebrae. They articulate with the 12 pairs of ribs to form the outward curve of the spine.
lumbar vertebrae (L1 to L5) (LUM-bar) (VER-te-brāy)	third set of five larger vertebrae, which forms the inward curve of the spine
sacrum (SĀ-krum)	next five vertebrae, which fuse together to form a triangular bone positioned between the two hip bones, forming joints called the sacroiliac joints
coccyx (KOK-siks)	four vertebrae fused together to form the tailbone
lamina (pl. laminae) (LAM-i-na) (LAM-i-nā)	part of the vertebral arch
clavicle (KLAV-i-kul)	collarbone
scapula (SKAP-ū-la)	shoulder blade
acromion process (a-KRŌ-mē-on) (PRA-ses)	extension of the scapula, which forms the superior point of the shoulder

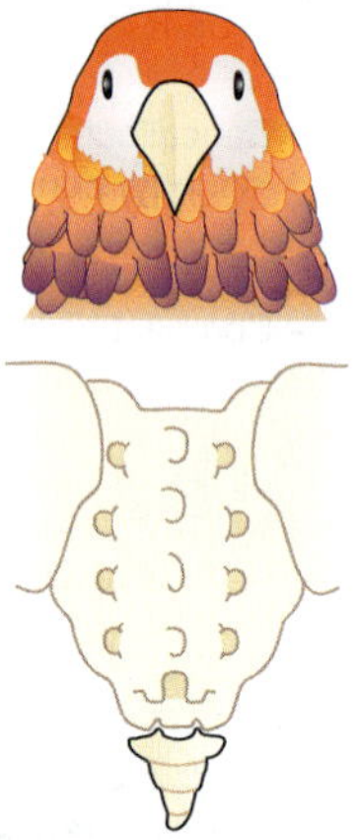

Coccyx is derived from the Greek word *cuckoo* because of its resemblance to a cuckoo's beak.

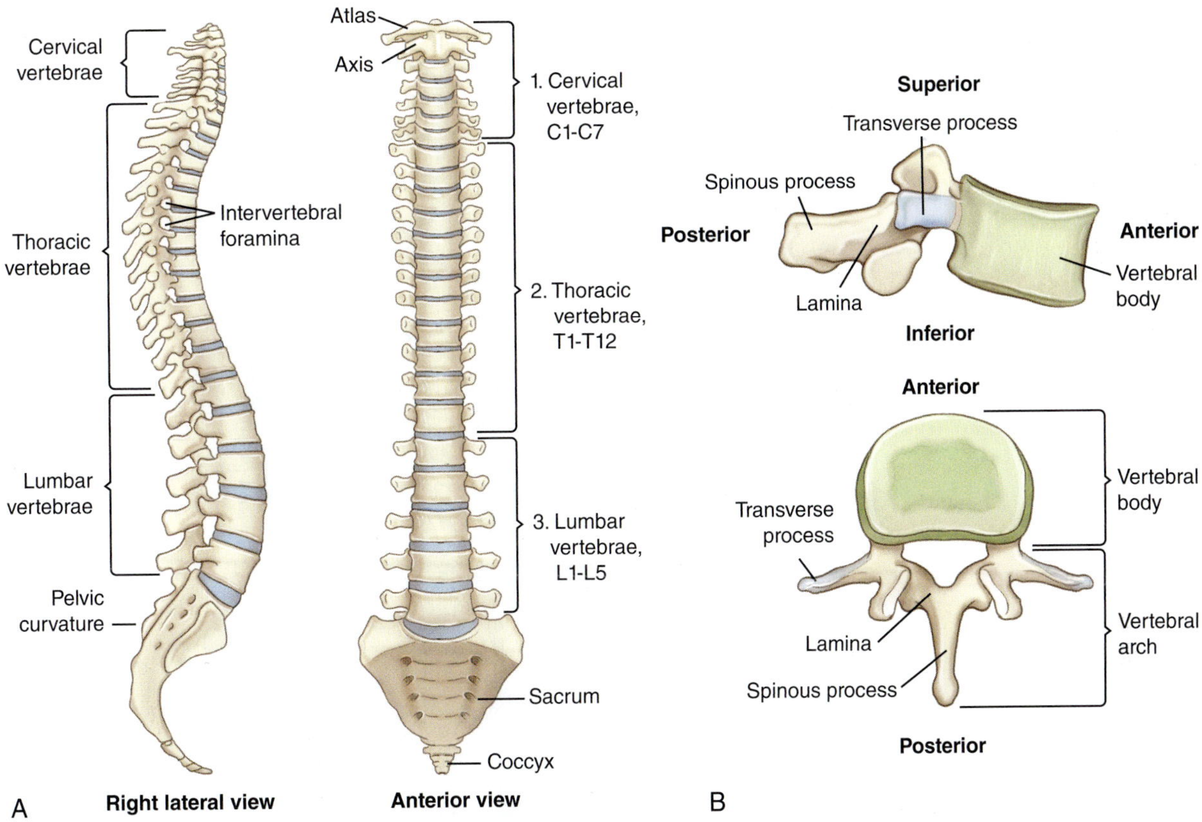

FIG. 14.2 A, Vertebral column, right lateral view and anterior view. **B,** A typical vertebra, lateral view and transverse view.

TERM	DEFINITION
sternum (STUR-num)	breastbone
xiphoid process (ZĪ-foid) (PRA-ses)	lower portion of the sternum
humerus (HŪ-mer-us)	upper arm bone
ulna and radius (UL-na), (RĀ-dē-us)	lower arm bones
olecranon process (ō-LEK-ra-non) (PRA-ses)	projection at the proximal end of the ulna that forms the bony point of the elbow
carpal bones (KAR-pal) (bōnz)	wrist bones
metacarpal bones (*met*-a-KAR-pal) (bōnz)	hand bones (also called **metacarpus**)
phalanx (pl. phalanges) (FĀ-lanks) (fa-LAN-jēz)	finger and toe bones

METACARPUS

literally means **beyond the wrist**. It is composed of the prefix **meta-**, meaning **beyond**, and **carpus**, meaning **wrist**.

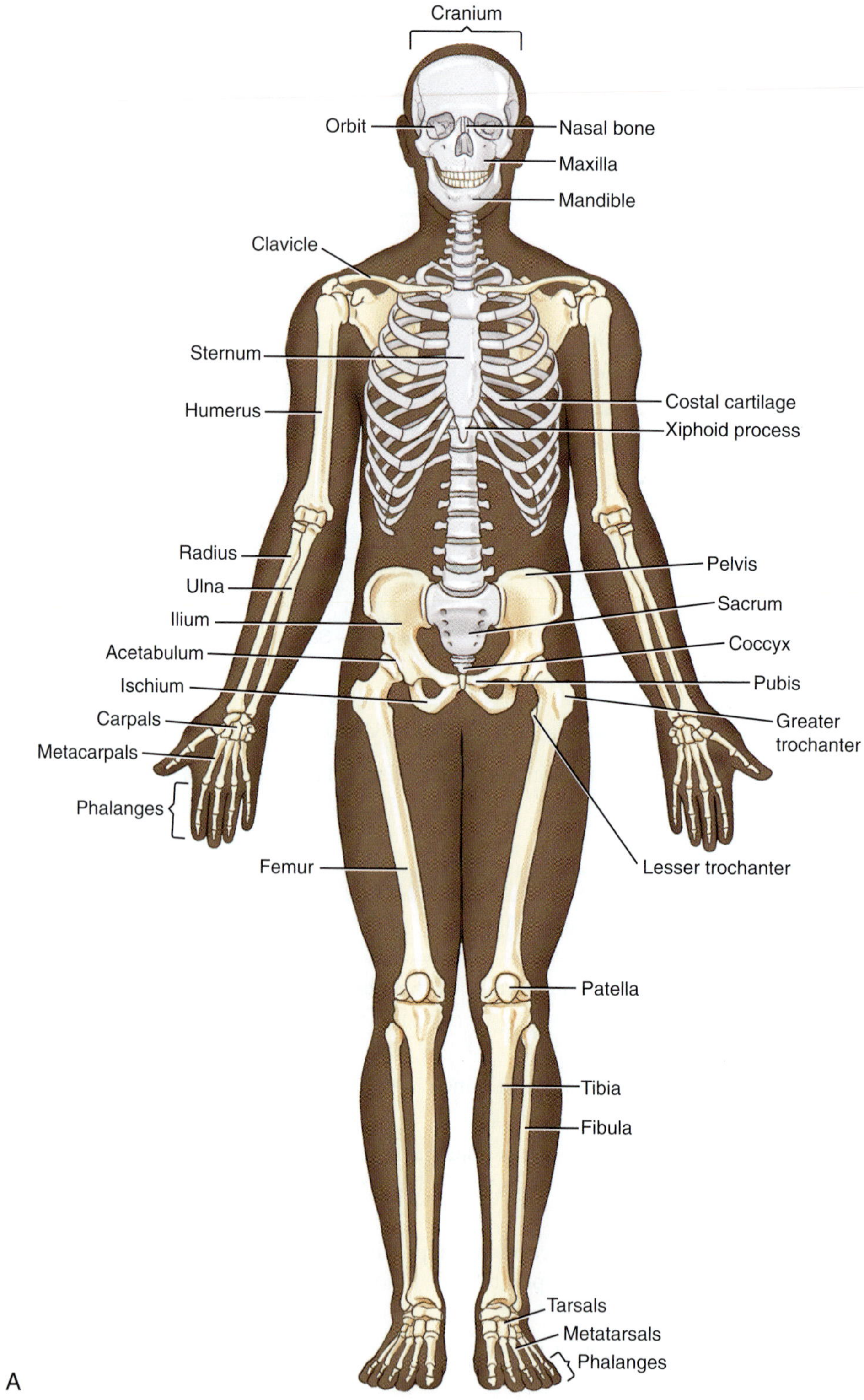

FIG. 14.3 **A,** Anterior view of the skeleton.

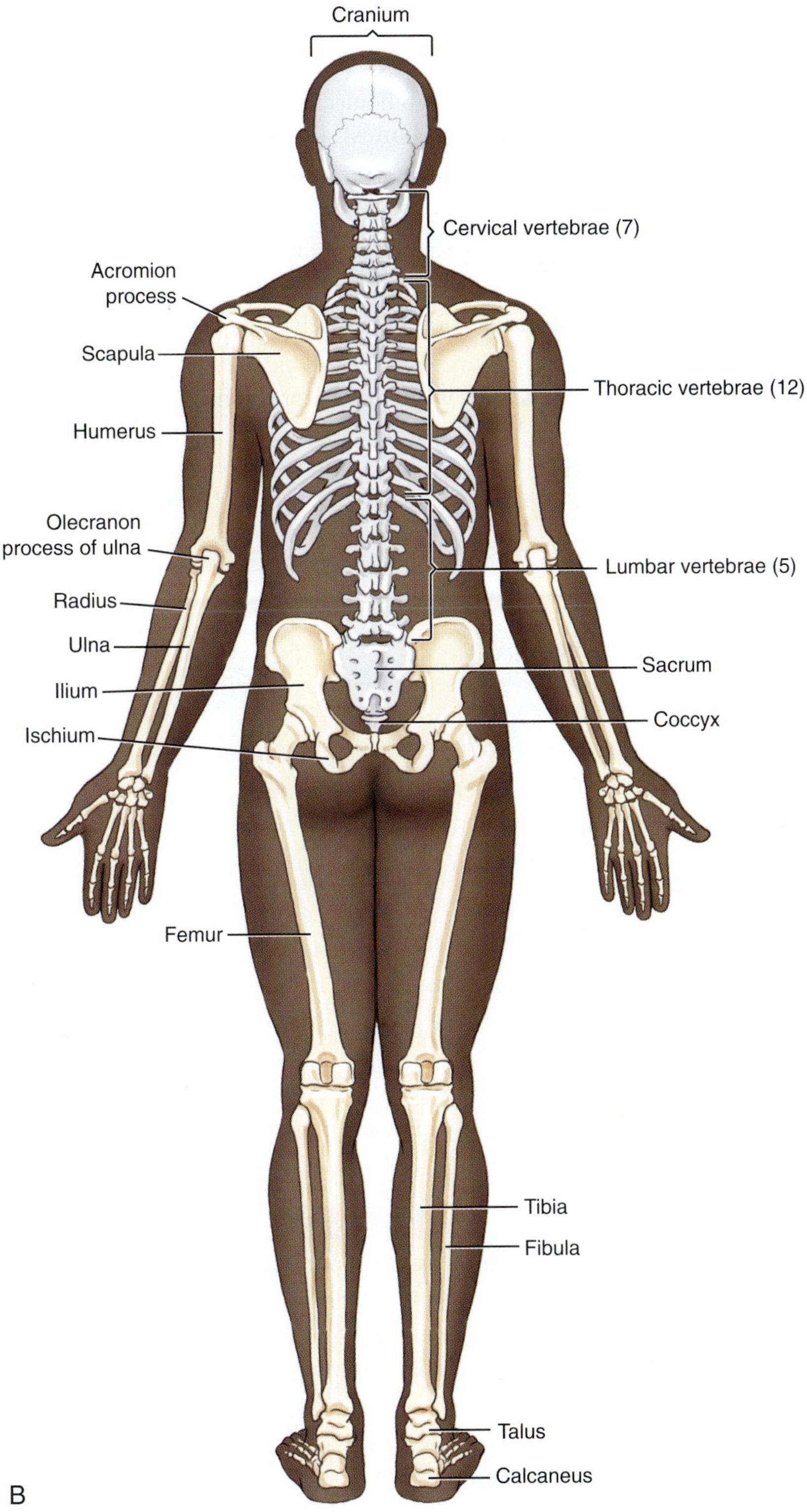

FIG. 14.3, cont'd B, Posterior view of the skeleton.

Skeletal Bones—cont'd

TERM	DEFINITION
pelvis (PEL-vis)	made up of three bones fused together (also called **pelvic bones** and **hip bones**)
ischium (is-KĒ-um)	lower, posterior portion of the pelvis on which one sits
ilium (IL-ē-um)	upper, wing-shaped part on each side of the pelvis
pubis (PŪ-bis)	anterior portion of the pelvis
acetabulum (*as*-a-TAB-ū-lum)	large socket in the pelvis for the head of the femur
femur (FĒ-mer)	upper leg bone
tibia and fibula (TIB-ē-a), (FIB-ū-la)	lower leg bones
patella (pl. patellae) (pa-TEL-a) (pa-TEL-ē)	kneecap
tarsal bones (TAR-sal) (bōnz)	ankle bones
calcaneus (kal-KĀ-nē-us)	heel bone
metatarsal bones (*met*-a-TAHR-sal) (bōnz)	foot bones

Joints

Joints, also called **articulations**, hold our bones together and make movement possible (in most joints) (Fig. 14.4).

TERM	DEFINITION
joint (joint)	junction of two or more bones, which often allows for movement of these bones
cartilage (KAR-ti-lej)	firm connective tissue primarily found in joints. Articular cartilage covers the contacting surfaces of bones.
meniscus (me-NIS-kus)	crescent-shaped cartilage found in some joints, including the knee
intervertebral disk (*in*-ter-VUR-tē-bral) (disk)	cartilaginous pad found between the vertebrae in the spine
pubic symphysis (PŪ-bik) (SIM-fi-sis)	cartilaginous joint at which two pubic bones come together anteriorly at the midline

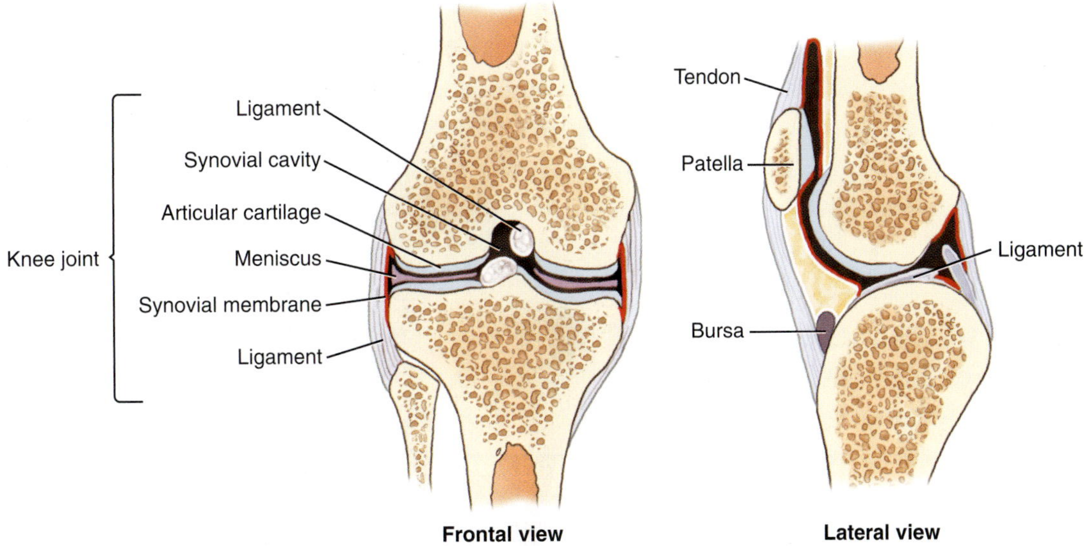

FIG. 14.4 Knee joint.

TERM	DEFINITION
synovia (si-NŌ-vē-a)	fluid secreted by the synovial membrane and found in joint cavities, bursae, and around tendons
bursa **(pl. bursae)** (BUR-sa) (BUR-sā)	fluid-filled sac that allows for easy movement of one part of a joint over another
ligament (LIG-a-ment)	flexible, tough band of fibrous connective tissue that attaches one bone to another at a joint
tendon (TEN-don)	band of fibrous connective tissue that attaches muscle to bone
aponeurosis (*ap*-ō-noo-RŌ-sis)	strong sheet of tissue that acts as a tendon to attach muscles to bone

Muscles

TERM	DEFINITION
skeletal muscles (SKEL-e-tal) (MUS-els)	attached to bones by tendons and make body movement possible. Skeletal muscles produce action by pulling and by working in pairs. They are also known as voluntary muscles because we have control over these muscles. Alternating dark and light bands create striations (stripes). (also called **striated muscles**) (Fig. 14.5A and B, Fig. 14.6A)
smooth muscles (smooth) (MUS-els)	located in internal organs such as the walls of blood vessels and the digestive tract. They are also known as involuntary muscles because they respond to impulses from the autonomic nerves and are not controlled voluntarily (also called **unstriated muscles**) (Fig. 14.6B).
cardiac muscle (KAR-dē-ak) (MUS-el)	forms most of the wall of the heart. Its involuntary contraction produces the heartbeat (also called **myocardium**) (Fig. 14.6C).

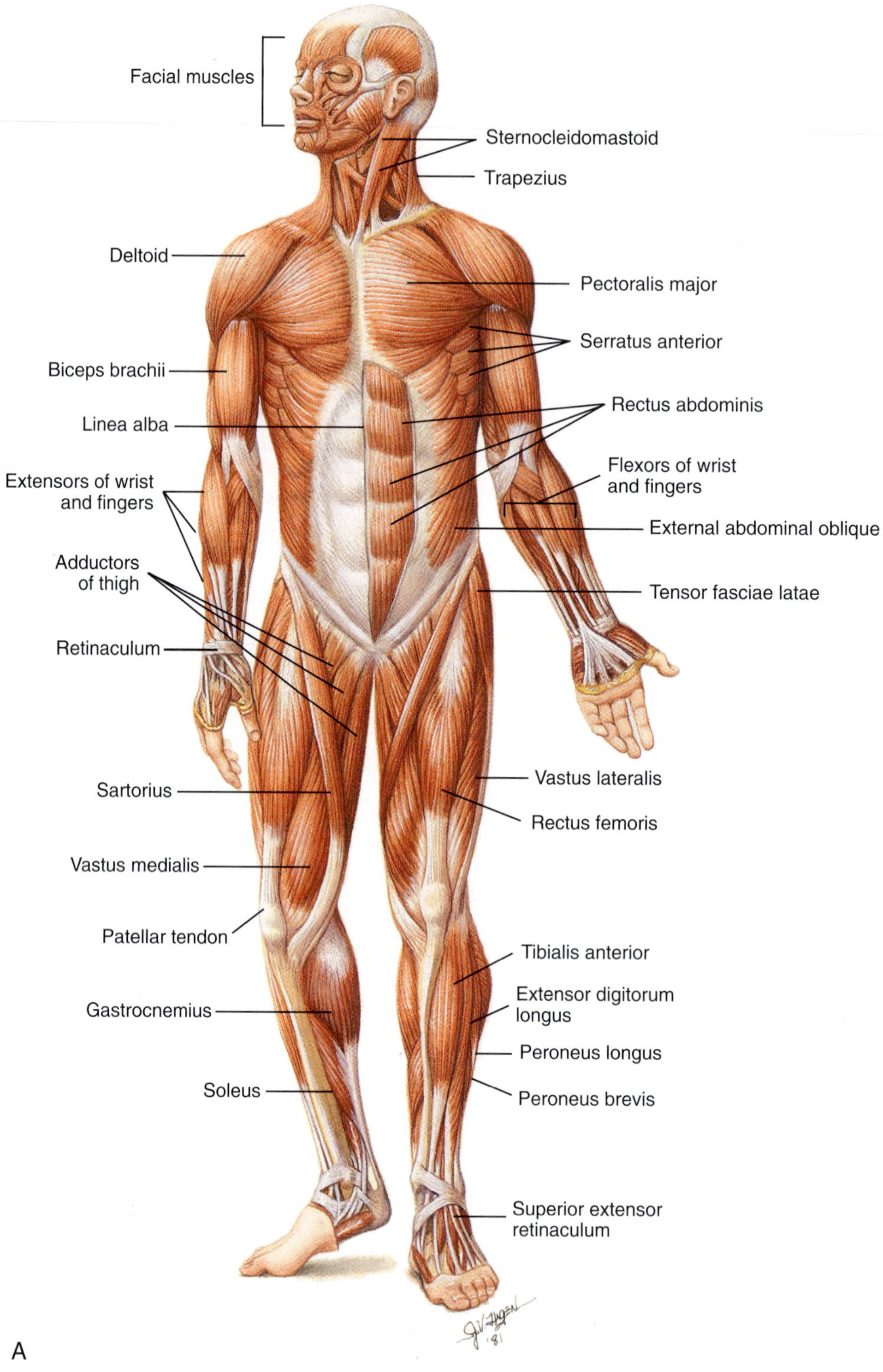

FIG. 14.5 A, Anterior view of the muscular system.

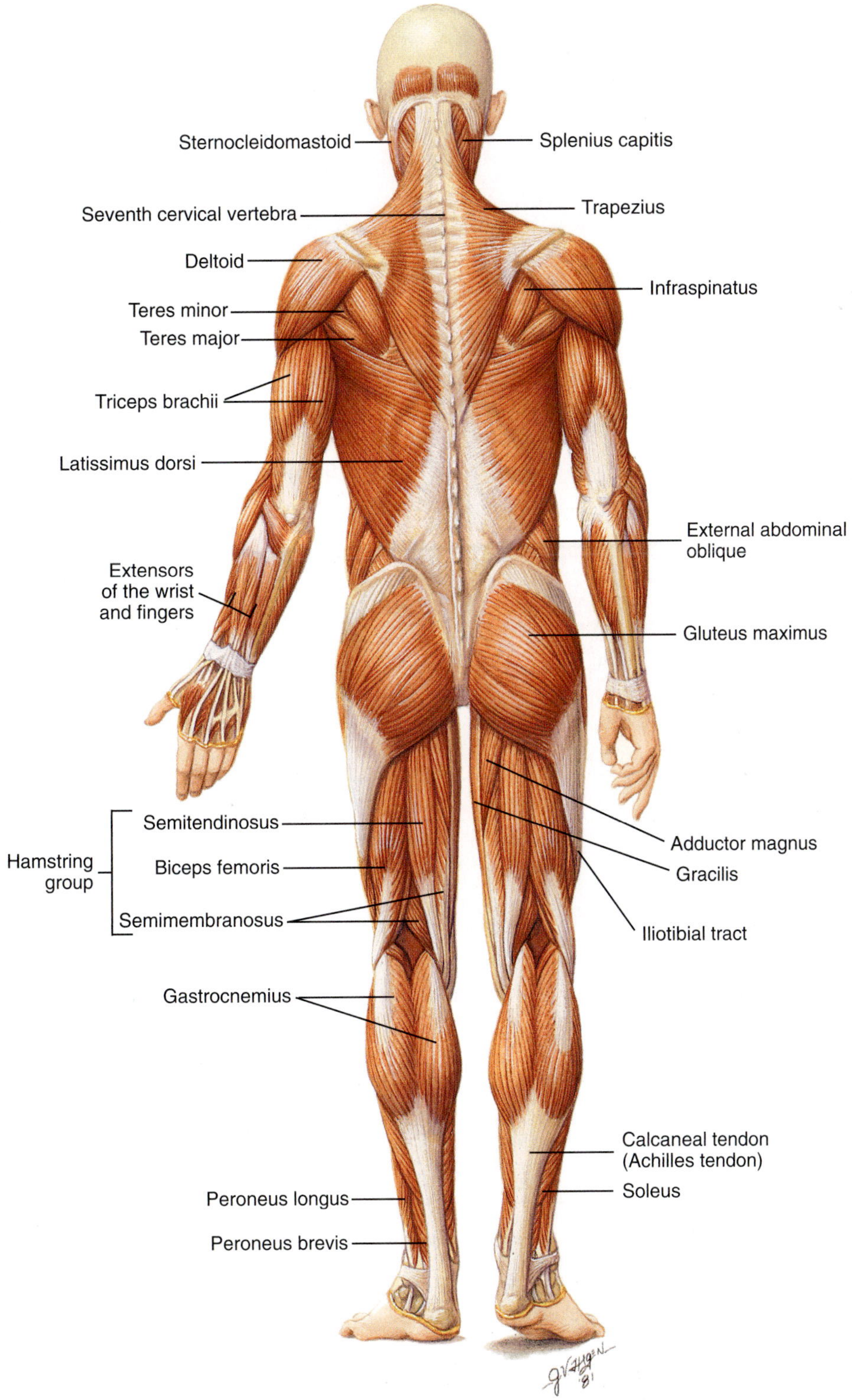

B

FIG. 14.5, cont'd B, Posterior view of the muscular system.

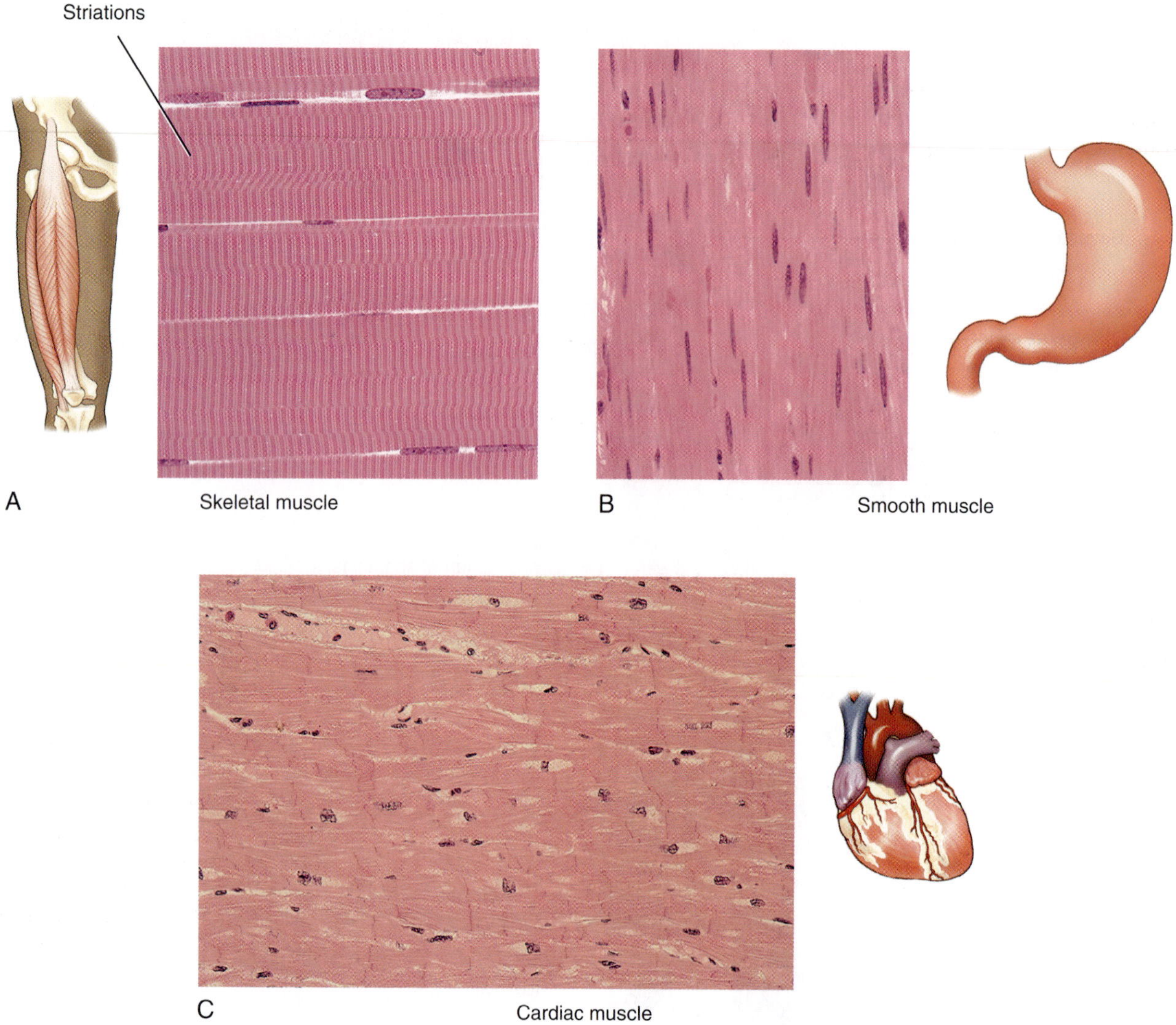

FIG. 14.6 Types of muscle tissue, with their related histology views.

A&P Booster

For more anatomy and physiology, go to Evolve Resources at evolve.elsevier.com and select:
Practice Student Resources > Student Resources > Chapter 14 > **A&P Booster**

See Appendix B for instructions.

EXERCISE 1

Practice saying aloud each of the Anatomic Structures of the Musculoskeletal System.

To hear the terms, go to Evolve Resources at evolve.elsevier.com and select:
Practice Student Resources > Student Resources > Chapter 14 > **Pronounce and Spell**

See Appendix B for instructions.

❑ Check the box when complete.

WORD PARTS

At first glance the number of word parts introduced in this chapter may seem overwhelming, but notice that many of them are names for bones already learned in the anatomic section. The definitions of the word parts include both anatomic terms and commonly used words. For example, both *carpals* and *wrist* are given as the definition of the combining form *carp/o*. Word parts you need to learn to complete this chapter are listed on the following pages. The exercises at the end of each list will help you learn their definitions and spellings.

Use the flashcards accompanying this text or electronic flashcards to assist you in memorizing the word parts for this chapter.

Combining Forms of the Musculoskeletal System

COMBINING FORM	DEFINITION
carp/o	carpals (wrist)
clavic/o, clavicul/o	clavicle (collarbone)
cost/o	rib
crani/o	cranium (skull)
femor/o	femur (upper leg bone) *(Note: The* u *in femur changes to an* o *in the word root femor/.)*
fibul/o	fibula (lower leg bone)
humer/o	humerus (upper arm bone)
ili/o	ilium
ischi/o	ischium
lumb/o	loin, lumbar region of the spine
mandibul/o	mandible (lower jawbone)
maxill/o	maxilla (upper jawbone)
patell/o	patella (kneecap)
pelv/i	pelvis, pelvic bones, pelvic cavity *(Note:* pelv/i *was introduced in Chapter 8.)*
phalang/o	phalanx (pl. phalanges) (any bone of the fingers or toes)
pub/o	pubis
rachi/o, spondyl/o, vertebr/o	vertebra, spine, vertebral column
radi/o	radius (lower arm bone)
sacr/o	sacrum
scapul/o	scapula (shoulder blade)
stern/o	sternum (breastbone)
tars/o	tarsals (ankle bones)
tibi/o	tibia (lower leg bone)
uln/o	ulna (lower arm bone)

ILIUM VS. ILEUM

Compare the combining form for ilium, **ili/o**, the portion of the pelvis, with the combining form for ileum, **ile/o**, the distal portion of the intestine. The pronunciation is the same. Think of **i**lium with an **i** and intestin**e** with an **e** to help distinguish the word roots.

EXERCISE 2

Fill in the blanks with combining forms in this diagram of the skeleton, anterior view. *To check your answers, go to Appendix A.*

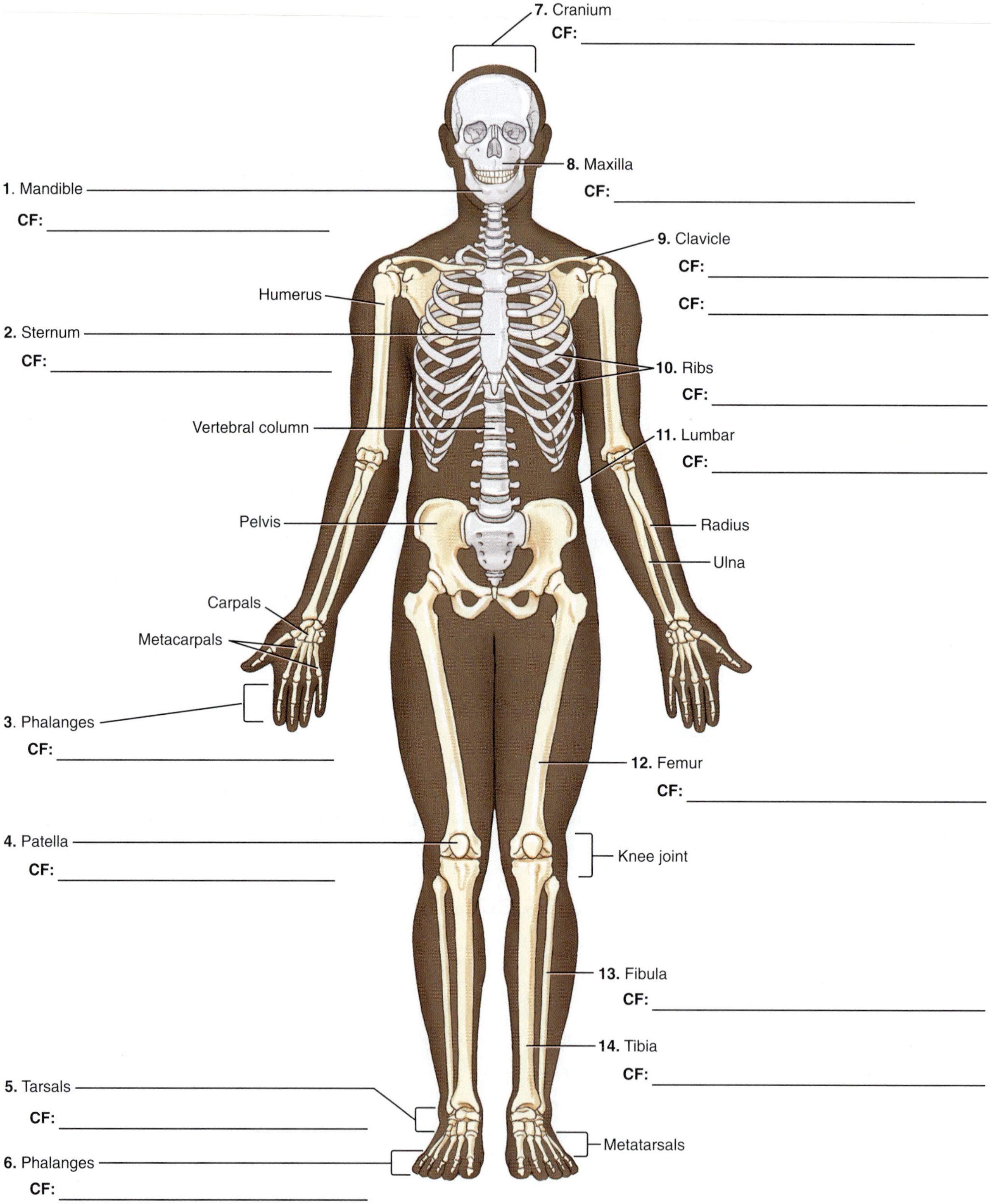

EXERCISE 3

Fill in the blanks with combining forms in this diagram of the skeleton, posterior view, and the pelvis.

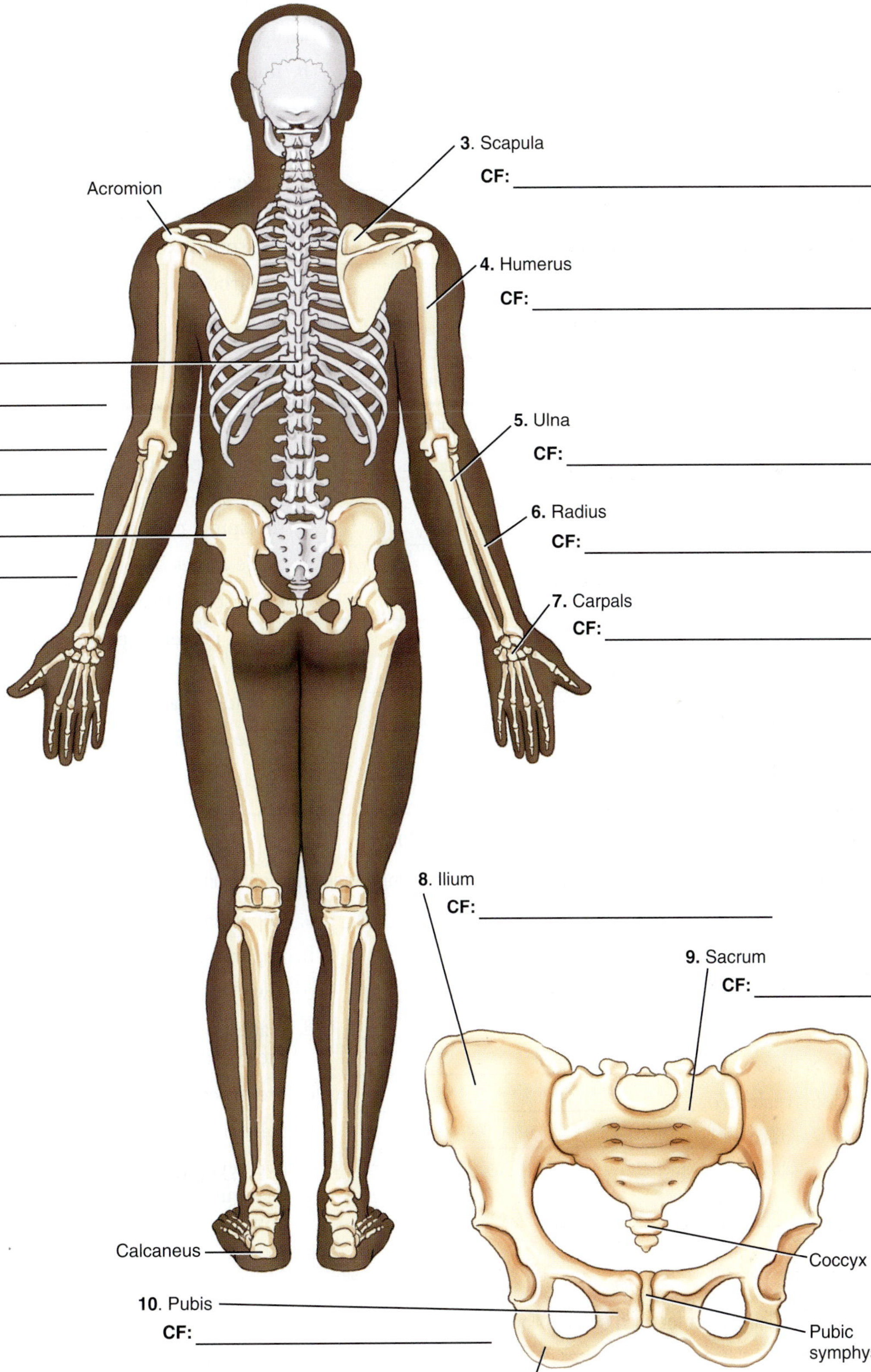

EXERCISE 4

Step 1: Write the definitions after the following combining forms.

Step 2: Match the descriptions on the right with the combining forms and definitions.

_____ 1. rachi/o, ______________________
_____ 2. patell/o, ______________________
_____ 3. maxill/o, ______________________
_____ 4. phalang/o, ______________________
_____ 5. carp/o, ______________________
_____ 6. clavic/o, ______________________
_____ 7. humer/o, ______________________

a. upper jawbone
b. finger and toe bones
c. wrist bones
d. kneecap
e. upper arm bone
f. made up of bones called vertebrae through which the spinal cord runs
g. collarbone

EXERCISE 5

Step 1: Write the definitions after the following combining forms.

Step 2: Match the descriptions on the right with the combining forms and definitions.

_____ 1. lumb/o, ______________________
_____ 2. ischi/o, ______________________
_____ 3. pub/o, ______________________
_____ 4. spondyl/o, ______________________
_____ 5. scapul/o, ______________________
_____ 6. tars/o, ______________________
_____ 7. pelv/i, ______________________

a. anterior portion of the pelvis
b. made up of bones called vertebrae through which the spinal cord runs
c. ankle bones
d. third set of five larger vertebrae
e. lower, posterior portion of the pelvis on which one sits
f. shoulder blade
g. made up of three bones fused together

EXERCISE 6

Step 1: Write the definitions after the following combining forms.

Step 2: Match the descriptions on the right with the combining forms and definitions.

_____ 1. mandibul/o, ______________________
_____ 2. sacr/o, ______________________
_____ 3. femor/o, ______________________
_____ 4. clavicul/o, ______________________
_____ 5. ili/o, ______________________
_____ 6. vertebr/o, ______________________
_____ 7. stern/o, ______________________

a. upper leg bone
b. upper, wing-shaped part on each side of the pelvis
c. lower jawbone
d. made up of bones called vertebrae through which the spinal cord runs
e. breastbone
f. collarbone
g. five vertebrae, which fuse together to form a triangular bone positioned between the two hip bones

EXERCISE 7

Write the combining form for each of the following terms.

1. rib ______________________
2. radius ______________________
3. tibia ______________________
4. fibula (lower leg bone) ______________________
5. ulna ______________________
6. cranium (skull) ______________________

Combining Forms of Joints

COMBINING FORM	DEFINITION
aponeur/o	aponeurosis
arthr/o	joint
burs/o	bursa (cavity)
chondr/o	cartilage
disk/o	intervertebral disk
menisc/o	meniscus (crescent)
synovi/o	synovia, synovial membrane
ten/o, tend/o, tendin/o	tendon

DISK
is from the Greek **diskos**, meaning **flat plate**. A variant spelling, *disc*, is also used, though chiefly in ophthalmology.

EXERCISE 8

Fill in the blanks with combining forms on these diagrams of the knee joint.

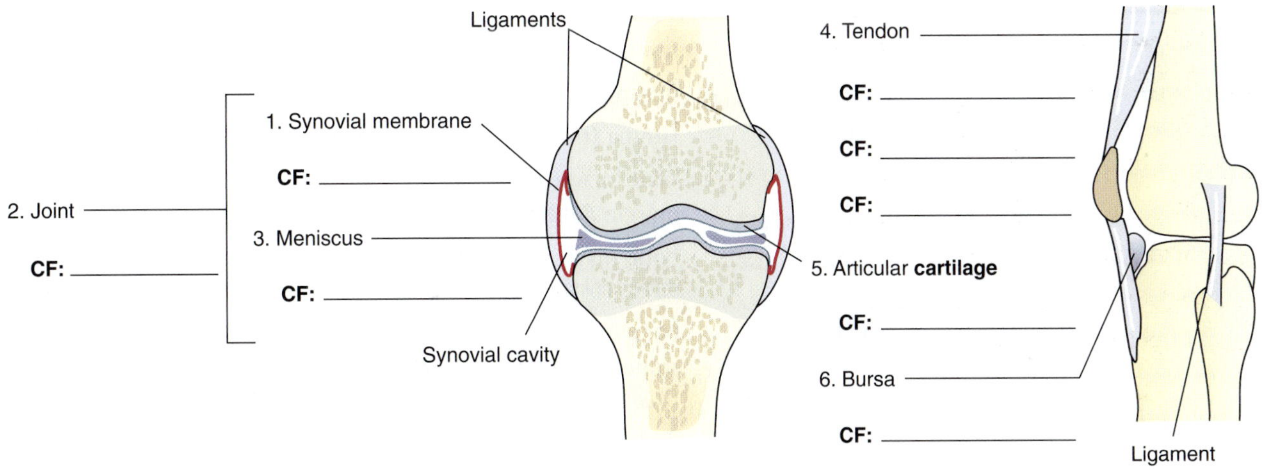

EXERCISE 9

Step 1: Write the definitions after the following combining forms.

Step 2: Match the descriptions on the right with the combining forms and definitions.

_____ 1. disk/o, ____________________

_____ 2. synovi/o, ____________________

_____ 3. aponeur/o, ____________________

_____ 4. ten/o, ____________________

_____ 5. arthr/o, ____________________

a. band of fibrous connective tissue that attaches muscle to bone

b. a junction of two or more bones, which often allows for movement of these bones

c. cartilaginous pad found between the vertebrae in the spine

d. fluid secreted by the synovial membrane

e. strong sheet of tissue that acts as a tendon to attach muscles to bone

EXERCISE 10

Step 1: Write the definitions after the following combining forms.

Step 2: Match the descriptions on the right with the combining forms and definitions. Answers may be used more than once.

_____ 1. tendin/o, ______________________________

_____ 2. burs/o, ______________________________

_____ 3. tend/o, ______________________________

_____ 4. menisc/o, ______________________________

_____ 5. chondr/o, ______________________________

a. firm connective tissue primarily found in joints

b. band of fibrous connective tissue that attaches muscle to bone

c. fluid-filled sac that allows for easy movement of one part of a joint over another

d. crescent-shaped cartilage found in some joints, including the knee

Combining Forms Commonly Used With Musculoskeletal System Terms

COMBINING FORM	DEFINITION
ankyl/o	stiff, bent
kinesi/o	movement, motion
kyph/o	hump (increased convexity of the spine)
lamin/o	lamina (thin, flat plate or layer)
lord/o	bent forward (increased concavity of the spine)
my/o, myos/o	muscle *(Note:* my/o *was introduced in Chapter 2.)*
myel/o	bone marrow (also covered in Chapter 10) *(Note:* myel/o *also means* spinal cord; *see Chapter 15.)*
oste/o	bone
petr/o	stone *(Note:* lith/o, *also a combining form for* stone, *was introduced in Chapter 6.)*
sarc/o	flesh, connective tissue *(Note: sarc/o was introduced in Chapter 2.)*
scoli/o	(lateral) curved (spine)

EXERCISE 11

Write the definitions of the following combining forms.

1. my/o ______________________________
2. petr/o ______________________________
3. kinesi/o ______________________________
4. oste/o ______________________________
5. lamin/o ______________________________
6. myel/o ______________________________
7. kyph/o ______________________________
8. ankyl/o ______________________________
9. scoli/o ______________________________
10. myos/o ______________________________
11. lord/o ______________________________
12. sarc/o ______________________________

EXERCISE 12

Write the combining form for each of the following.

1. muscle a. ______________________________
   b. ______________________________
2. stone ______________________________
3. movement, motion ______________________________
4. bone ______________________________
5. lamina ______________________________
6. bone marrow ______________________________
7. hump ______________________________
8. stiff, bent ______________________________
9. (lateral) curved (spine) ______________________________
10. bent forward ______________________________
11. flesh, connective tissue ______________________________

Prefixes

PREFIX	DEFINITION
inter-	between
supra-	above
sym-, syn-	together, joined

EXERCISE 13

Write the definition of the following prefixes.

1. supra- ______________________
2. sym-, syn- ______________________
3. inter- ______________________

EXERCISE 14

Write the prefix for each of the following definitions.

1. together, joined a. ______________________
   b. ______________________
2. between ______________________
3. above ______________________

Suffixes

SUFFIX	DEFINITION
-asthenia	weakness
-desis	surgical fixation, fusion
-physis	growth
-schisis	split, fissure
-trophy	nourishment, development

EXERCISE 15

Write the definitions of the following suffixes.

1. -physis ______________________
2. -desis ______________________
3. -schisis ______________________
4. -asthenia ______________________
5. -trophy ______________________

EXERCISE 16

Write the suffix for each of the following definitions.

1. growth ______________________
2. weakness ______________________
3. surgical fixation, fusion ______________________
4. split, fissure ______________________
5. nourishment, development ______________________

For additional practice with Word parts, go to Evolve Resources at evolve.elsevier.com and select: Practice Student Resources > Student Resources > Chapter 14 > **Flashcards**

See Appendix B for instructions.

MEDICAL TERMS

Disease and Disorder Terms
BUILT FROM WORD PARTS

The following terms can be translated using definitions of word parts. Further explanation is provided within parentheses as needed.

REPETITIVE MOTION DISORDERS (RMDs) are a group of musculoskeletal disorders caused by overuse and repetitive motions performed in the course of normal work or recreational activities. These disorders, which include **tendonitis, bursitis,** and **carpal tunnel syndrome,** are characterized by pain, swelling, numbness, and loss of strength or flexibility and most commonly affect the hands, wrists, elbows, and shoulders. Incorporating rest breaks, stretching, improved posture or ergonomics, antiinflammatory medications, and physical therapy provide the majority of treatment for RMDs. Surgery may be needed as treatment for permanent injuries. These disorders may also be referred to as **repetitive strain syndrome.**

TERM	DEFINITION
ankylosis (*ang*-ki-LŌ-sis)	abnormal condition of stiffness (often referring to fusion of a joint, such as the result of chronic rheumatoid arthritis)
arthritis (ar-THRĪ-tis)	inflammation of a joint. (The most common forms of arthritis are osteoarthritis and rheumatoid arthritis.) (Fig. 14.7)
bursitis (ber-SĪ-tis)	inflammation of a bursa
chondromalacia (*kon*-drō-ma-LĀ-sha)	softening of cartilage
cranioschisis (*krā*-nē-OS-ki-sis)	fissure (split) of the cranium (congenital)
diskitis (dis-KĪ-tis)	inflammation of an intervertebral disk (also spelled **discitis**)
fibromyalgia (*fī*-brō-mī-AL-ja)	pain in the fibrous tissues and muscles (a common condition characterized by widespread pain and stiffness of muscles, fatigue, and disturbed sleep)
kyphosis (kī-FŌ-sis)	abnormal condition of a hump (in the thoracic spine) (also called **hunchback** or **humpback**) (Exercise Figure A2)
lordosis (lōr-DŌ-sis)	abnormal condition of bending forward (in the lumbar spine) (also called **swayback**) (Exercise Figure A1)
maxillitis (*mak*-si-LĪ-tis)	inflammation of the maxilla
meniscitis (*men*-i-SĪ-tis)	inflammation of a meniscus
myasthenia (*mī*-as-THĒ-nē-a)	muscle weakness
myeloma (*mī*-e-LŌ-ma)	tumor of the bone marrow (malignant)
osteitis (*os*-tē-Ī-tis)	inflammation of the bone
osteoarthritis (OA) (*os*-tē-ō-ar-THRĪ-tis)	inflammation of the bone and joint (Fig. 14.7)
osteochondritis (*os*-tē-ō-kon-DRĪ-tis)	inflammation of the bone and cartilage
osteofibroma (*os*-tē-ō-fī-BRŌ-ma)	tumor of the bone and fibrous tissue (benign)
osteomalacia (*os*-tē-ō-ma-LĀ-sha)	softening of bone

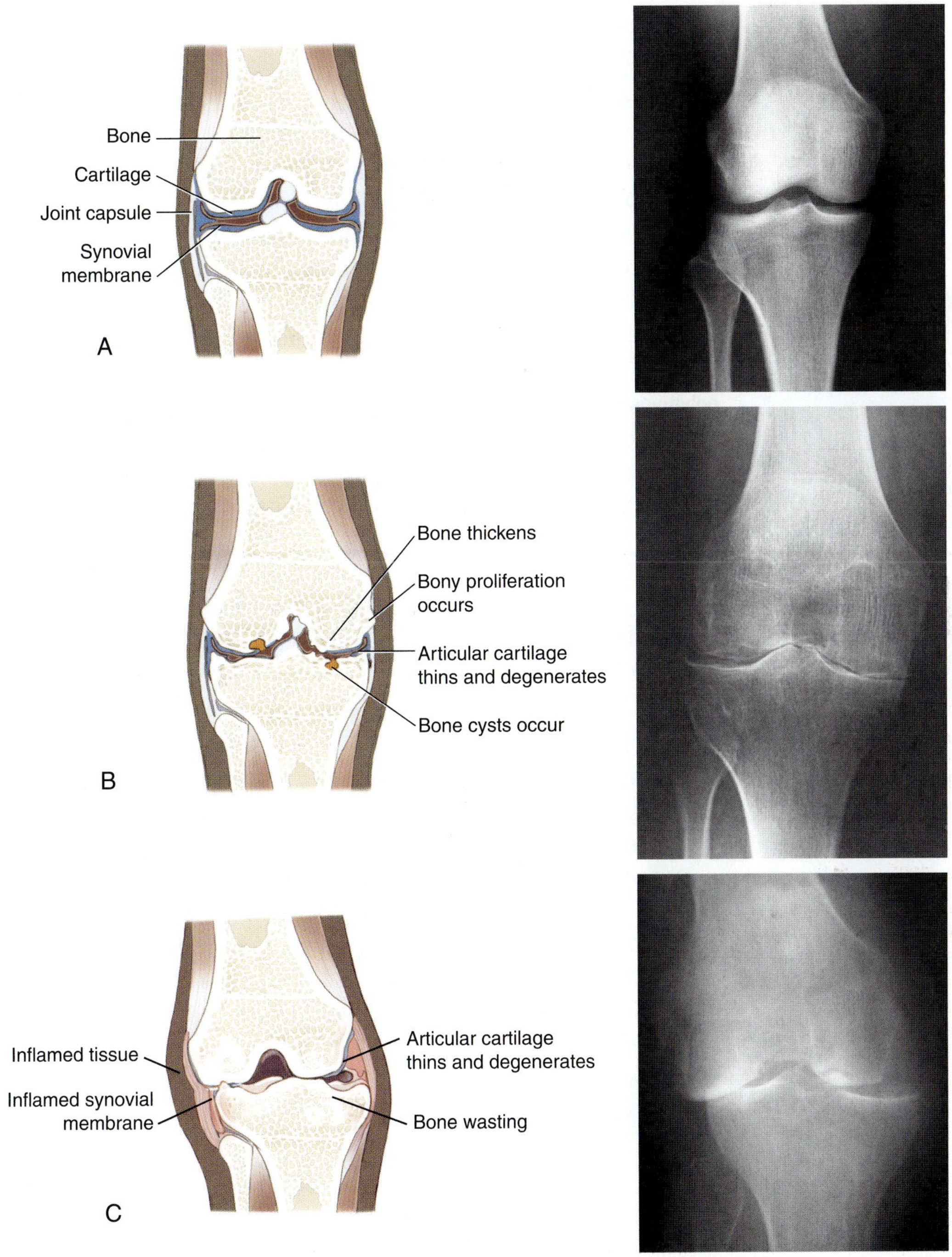

FIG. 14.7 Normal and arthritic knee joints. **A,** Normal knee joint, illustration and radiograph. **B,** Osteoarthritis of the knee joint, illustration and radiograph. **C,** Rheumatoid arthritis of the knee joint, illustration and radiograph.

Disease and Disorder Terms—cont'd

TERM	DEFINITION
osteomyelitis (*os*-tē-ō-*mī*-e-LĪ-tis)	inflammation of the bone and bone marrow (caused by bacterial infection)
osteopenia (*os*-tē-ō-PĒ-nē-a)	abnormal reduction of bone mass (caused by inadequate replacement of bone lost to normal bone lysis and can lead to osteoporosis)
osteopetrosis (*os*-tē-ō-pe-TRŌ-sis)	abnormal condition of stonelike bones (very dense bones caused by defective resorption of bone)
osteosarcoma (*os*-tē-ō-sar-KŌ-ma)	malignant tumor of the bone
polymyositis (*pol*-ē-*mī*-ō-SĪ-tis)	inflammation of many muscles
rachischisis (ra-KIS-ki-sis)	fissure (split) of the vertebral column (congenital) (also called **spina bifida**)
rhabdomyolysis (*rab*-dō-mī-OL-i-sis)	dissolution of striated muscle (caused by trauma, extreme exertion, or drug toxicity; in severe cases renal failure can result)
sarcopenia (*sar*-kō-PĒ-nē-a)	abnormal reduction of connective tissue (such as loss of skeletal muscle mass in the elderly)
scoliosis (*skō*-lē-Ō-sis)	abnormal condition of (lateral) curved (spine) (Fig. 14.8) (Exercise Figure A3)
spondylarthritis (*spon*-dil-ar-THRĪ-tis)	inflammation of the vertebral joints (also called **spondyloarthritis**)
spondylosis (*spon*-di-LŌ-sis)	abnormal condition of the vertebrae (a general term used to describe changes to the spine from osteoarthritis or ankylosis)
synoviosarcoma (si-*nō*-vē-ō-sar-KŌ-ma)	malignant tumor of the synovial membrane
tendinitis (*ten*-di-NĪ-tis)	inflammation of a tendon (also spelled **tendonitis**)
tenosynovitis (*ten*-ō-sin-ō-VĪ-tis)	inflammation of the tendon and synovial membrane *(Note: the* i *in* synovi *is dropped because the suffix begins with an* i.)

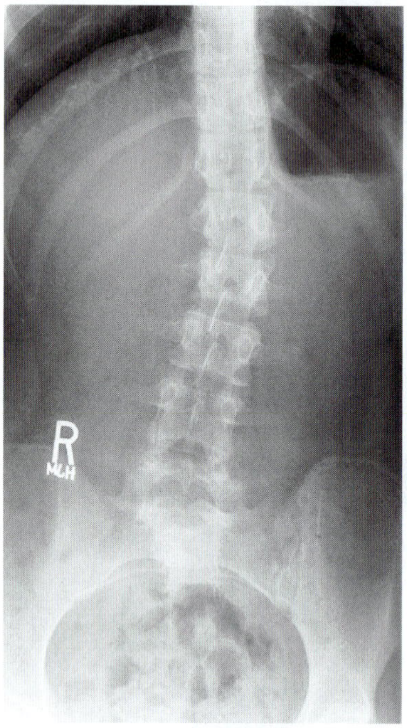

FIG. 14.8 AP lumbar spine radiograph demonstrating congenital scoliosis.

EXERCISE 17

Practice saying aloud each of the Disease and Disorder Terms Built from Word Parts.

To hear the terms, go to Evolve Resources at evolve.elsevier.com and select:
Practice Student Resources > Student Resources > Chapter 14 > **Pronounce and Spell**

See Appendix B for instructions.

❑ Check the box when complete.

EXERCISE FIGURE A

Fill in the blanks with word parts defined to label the diagram.

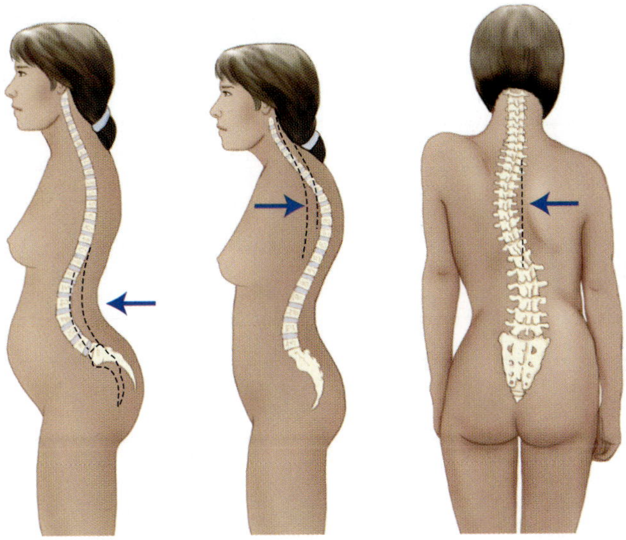

1. ______ / ______
bent forward / abnormal condition

2. ______ / ______
hump / abnormal condition

3. ______ / ______
(lateral) curved / abnormal condition

EXERCISE 18

Analyze and define the following disease and disorder terms.

1. osteitis

______

______

2. osteomyelitis

______

______

3. osteopetrosis

______

______

4. osteomalacia

______

______

5. osteochondritis

______

______

6. osteofibroma

______

______

7. arthritis

______

______

8. rhabdomyolysis

______

______

9. myeloma

10. tendinitis

11. osteopenia

12. spondylosis

13. bursitis

14. spondylarthritis

15. ankylosis

16. kyphosis

17. scoliosis

18. cranioschisis

19. maxillitis

20. meniscitis

21. rachischisis

22. myasthenia

23. osteosarcoma

24. chondromalacia

25. synoviosarcoma

26. tenosynovitis

27. polymyositis

____

____

28. diskitis

____

____

29. lordosis

____

____

30. osteoarthritis

____

____

31. fibromyalgia

____

____

32. sarcopenia

____

____

EXERCISE 19

Build disease and disorder terms for the following definitions with the word parts you have learned.

1. inflammation of the bone and cartilage ______ WR / CV / WR / S
2. tumor of the bone and fibrous tissue ______ WR / CV / WR / S
3. inflammation of a joint ______ WR / S
4. dissolution of striated muscle ______ WR / CV / WR / CV / S
5. tumor of the bone marrow ______ WR / S
6. inflammation of a tendon ______ WR / S
7. abnormal condition of the vertebrae ______ WR / S
8. abnormal reduction of bone mass ______ WR / CV / S
9. inflammation of the bursa ______ WR / S
10. inflammation of the vertebral joints ______ WR / WR / S
11. abnormal condition of stiffness ______ WR / S

12. abnormal condition of a hump (in the thoracic spine) ______ / ______
WR / S

13. abnormal condition of (lateral) curved (spine) ______ / ______
WR / S

14. fissure (split) of the cranium ______ / ___ / ______
WR / CV / S

15. inflammation of the maxilla ______ / ______
WR / S

16. inflammation of the meniscus ______ / ______
WR / S

17. fissure (split) of the vertebral column ______ / ______
WR / S

18. muscle weakness ______ / ______
WR / S

19. inflammation of the bone ______ / ______
WR / S

20. inflammation of the bone and bone marrow ______ / ___ / ______ / ______
WR / CV / WR / S

21. abnormal condition of stonelike bones (very dense bones) ______ / ___ / ______ / ______
WR / CV / WR / S

22. softening of bone ______ / ___ / ______
WR / CV / S

23. inflammation of the tendon and synovial membrane ______ / ___ / ______ / ______
WR / CV / WR / S

24. malignant tumor of the synovial membrane ______ / ___ / ______
WR / CV / S

25. malignant tumor of the bone ______ / ___ / ______
WR / CV / S

26. softening of cartilage ______ / ___ / ______
WR / CV / S

27. inflammation of an intervertebral disk ______ / ______
WR / S

28. inflammation of many muscles ______ / ______ / ______
P / WR / S

29. abnormal condition of bending forward (swayback) ______ / ______
WR / S

30. inflammation of the bone and joint ______ WR / CV / WR / S

31. pain in the fibrous tissues and muscles ______ WR / CV / WR / S

32. abnormal reduction of connective tissue ______ WR / CV / S

EXERCISE 20

Spell each of the Disease and Disorder Terms Built from Word Parts by having someone dictate them to you. Use a separate sheet of paper.

> To hear and spell the terms, go to Evolve Resources at evolve.elsevier.com and select:
> Practice Student Resources > Student Resources > Chapter 14 > **Pronounce and Spell**
>
> See Appendix B for instructions.

❑ Check the box when complete.

Disease and Disorder Terms

NOT BUILT FROM WORD PARTS

Word parts may be present in the following terms; however, their full meanings cannot be translated using definitions of word parts alone.

TERM	DEFINITION
ankylosing spondylitis (*ang*-ki-LŌ-sing) (*spon*-di-LĪ-tis)	form of arthritis that first affects the spine and adjacent structures and that, as it progresses, causes a forward bend of the spine (also called **Strümpell-Marie arthritis** or **disease,** or **rheumatoid spondylitis**)
bunion (BUN-yun)	abnormal prominence of the joint at the base of the great toe, the metatarsal-phalangeal joint. It is a common problem, often hereditary or caused by poorly fitted shoes (also called **hallux valgus**).
carpal tunnel syndrome (CTS) (KAR-pl) (TUN-el) (SIN-drōm)	common nerve entrapment disorder of the wrist caused by compression of the median nerve. Symptoms include pain and tingling in portions of the hand and fingers.
Colles fracture (KOL-ēz) (FRAK-chur)	type of wrist fracture. The fracture is at the distal end of the radius, the distal fragment being displaced backward.
exostosis (*ek*-sos-TŌ-sis)	abnormal benign growth on the surface of a bone (also called **spur**)
fracture (fx) (FRAK-chūr)	broken bone
gout (gowt)	disease in which an excessive amount of uric acid in the blood causes sodium urate crystals (**tophi**) to be deposited in the joints, producing arthritis. The great toe is frequently affected.

ANKYLOSING SPONDYLITIS was first described in 1884 by Adolf von Strümpell (1853–1925). It became known as **Strümpell-Marie disease** after von Strümpell and French physician Pierre Marie.

COLLES FRACTURE was first described in 1814 by Irish surgeon and anatomist **Abraham Colles** (1773–1843). In 1804 Colles was appointed Professor of Anatomy and Surgery at the Irish College of Surgeons.

Disease and Disorder Terms—cont'd

TERM	DEFINITION
herniated disk (HER-nē-*āt*-ed) (disk)	rupture of the intervertebral disk cartilage, which allows the contents to protrude through it, putting pressure on the spinal nerve roots (also called **slipped disk, ruptured disk, herniated intervertebral disk,** or **herniated nucleus pulposus [HNP]**)
Lyme disease (līm) (di-ZĒZ)	infection caused by a bite from a deer tick infected with *Borrelia burgdorferi.* This bacterium provokes an immune response in the body, the symptoms of which can mimic several musculoskeletal diseases. Patients may experience fever, headache, and joint pain. A rash (target lesion) may initially arise at the site of the tick bite. Lyme disease was first reported in Lyme, Connecticut, in 1975.
muscular dystrophy (MD) (MUS-kū-lar) (DIS-tro-fē)	group of hereditary diseases characterized by degeneration of muscle and weakness
myasthenia gravis (MG) (*mī*-as-THĒ-nē-a) (GRA-vis)	chronic disease characterized by muscle weakness and thought to be caused by a defect in the transmission of impulses from nerve to muscle cell. The face, larynx, and throat are frequently affected; no true paralysis of the muscles exists.
osteoporosis (*os*-tē-ō-po-RŌ-sis)	abnormal loss of bone density that may lead to an increase in fractures of the ribs, thoracic and lumbar vertebrae, hips, and wrists after slight trauma (occurs predominantly in postmenopausal women)
plantar fasciitis (PLAN-tar) (fas-ē-Ī-tis)	inflammation of plantar fascia, connective tissue of the sole of the foot, due to repetitive injury; common cause of heel pain
rheumatoid arthritis (RA) (RŪ-ma-toid) (ar-THRĪ-tis)	chronic systemic disease characterized by autoimmune inflammatory changes in the connective tissue throughout the body (Fig. 14.7C)
spinal stenosis (SPĪ-nal) (ste-NŌ-sis)	narrowing of the spinal canal with compression of nerve roots. The condition is either congenital or due to spinal degeneration. Symptoms are pain radiating to the thigh or lower legs and numbness or tingling in the lower extremities.
spondylolisthesis (*spon*-di-lō-lis-THĒ-sis)	forward slipping of one vertebra over another

INTEGRATIVE MEDICINE TERM

Tai Chi, often referred to as "meditation in motion," is an ancient Chinese art using slow movements and focused breathing to support mental and physical health. Studies suggest the measurable benefits of regular Tai Chi practice include improvement in cardiovascular health, muscle strength, mobility, and balance for a variety of populations including the elderly, and those who may have diabetes, **rheumatoid arthritis**, COPD, or Parkinson disease.

EXERCISE 21

Practice saying aloud each of the Disease and Disorder Terms NOT Built from Word Parts.

To hear the terms, go to Evolve Resources at evolve.elsevier.com and select:
Practice Student Resources > Student Resources > Chapter 14 > **Pronounce and Spell**

See Appendix B for instructions.

❑ Check the box when complete.

EXERCISE 22

Match the terms in the first column with their correct definition in the second column.

_____ 1. muscular dystrophy
_____ 2. exostosis
_____ 3. ankylosing spondylitis
_____ 4. myasthenia gravis

a. abnormal benign growth on the surface of a bone
b. form of arthritis that first affects the spine and adjacent structures and cause a forward bend of the spine
c. group of hereditary diseases characterized by degeneration of muscles and weakness
d. chronic disease characterized by muscle weakness and thought to be caused by a defect in the transmission of impulses from nerve to muscle cell

EXERCISE 23

Write the medical term pictured and defined.

1. ______________________
rupture of the intervertebral disk cartilage, which allows the contents to protrude through it, putting pressure on the spinal nerve roots

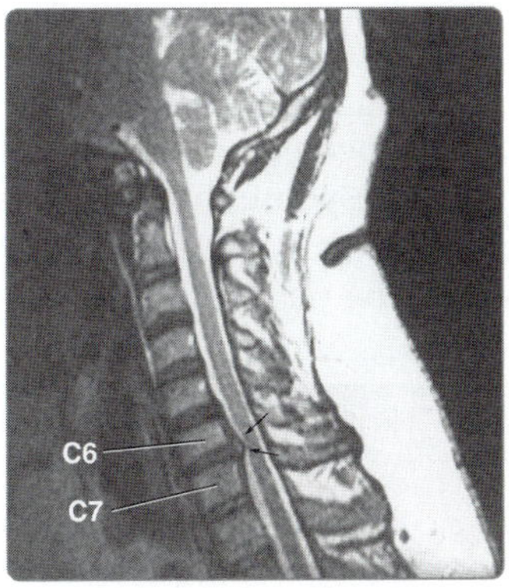

2. ______________________
chronic systemic disease characterized by autoimmune inflammatory changes in the connective tissue throughout the body

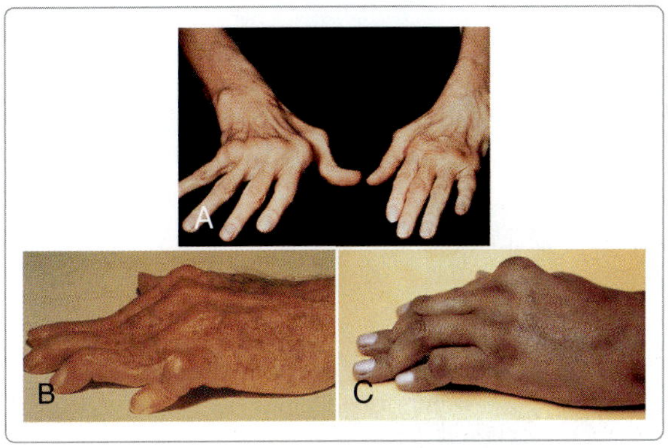

3. ______________________
common nerve entrapment disorder of the wrist caused by compression of the median nerve

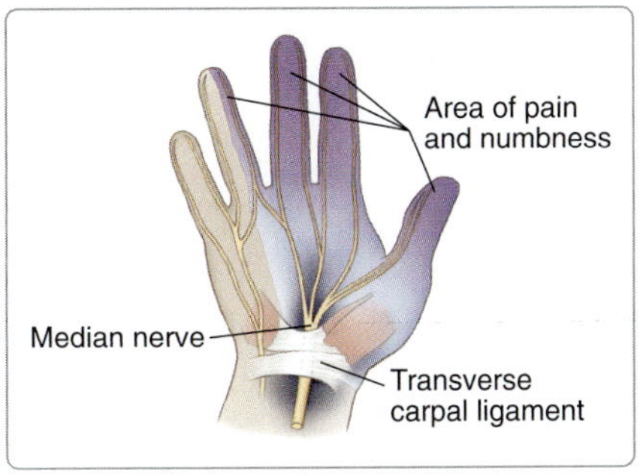

4. ______________________
forward slipping of one vertebra over the other

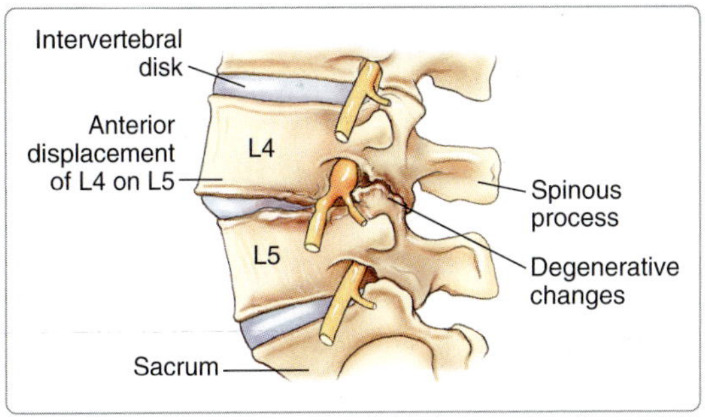

EXERCISE 23 *Pictured and Defined—cont'd*

5. ______________________________
disease in which an excessive amount of uric acid in the blood causes sodium urate crystals (tophi) to be deposited in the joints

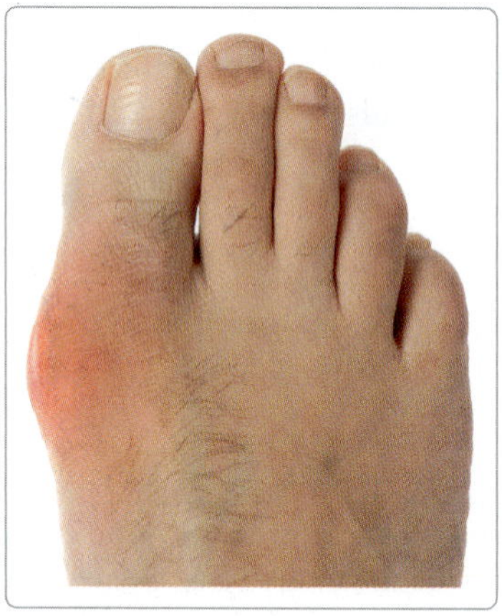

6. ______________________________
abnormal loss of density that may lead to an increase in fractures

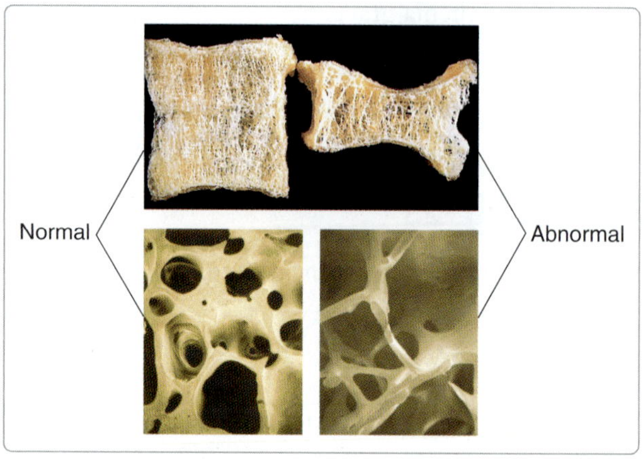

7. ______________________________
broken bone

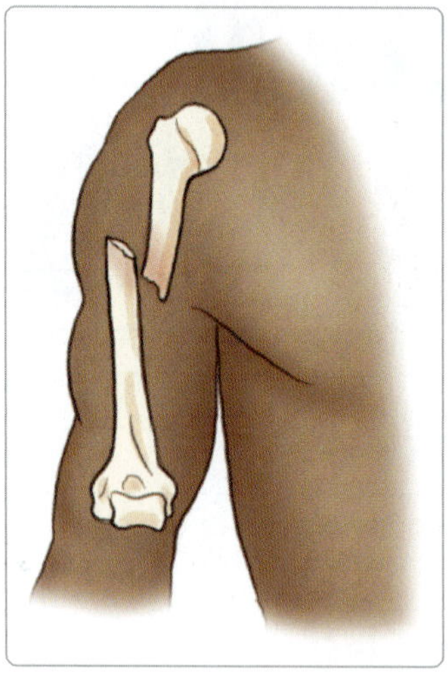

8. ______________________________
infecction caused by a bite from an infected deer tick, which provokes an immune response that can mimic several musculoskeletal diseases. A rash (target lesion) may be found at the site of the tick bite.

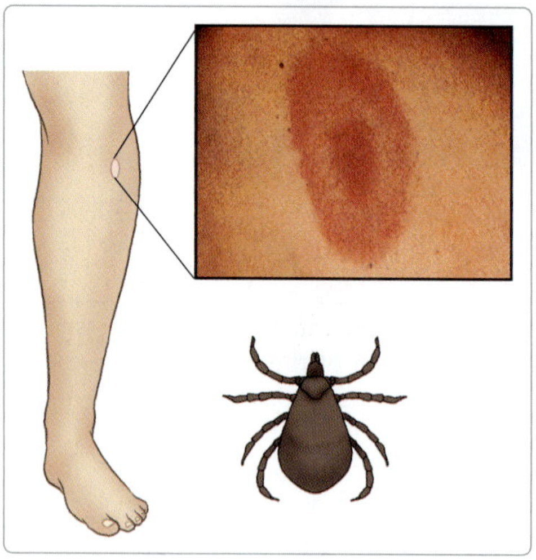

9. ____

abnormal prominence of the joint at the base of the great toe, the metatarsal-phalangeal joint

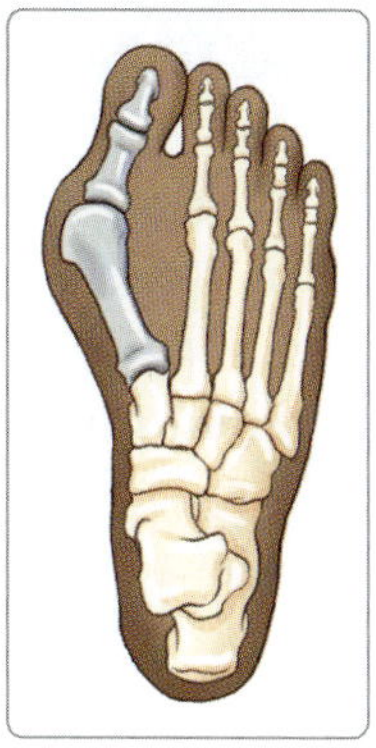

10. ____

narrowing of the spinal canal with compression of nerve roots

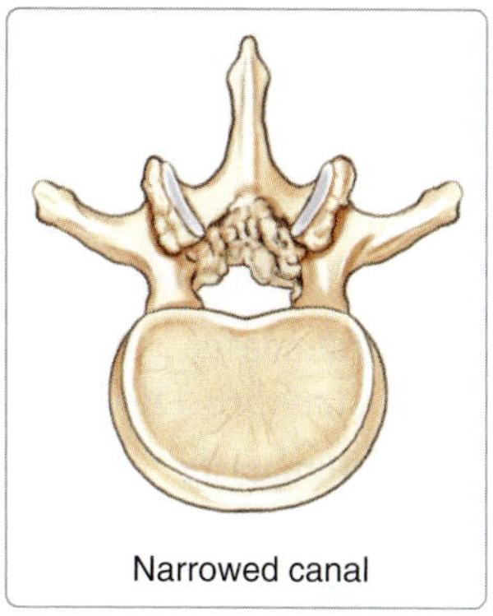

11. ____

inflammation of the connective tissue of the sole of the foot, common cause of heel pain

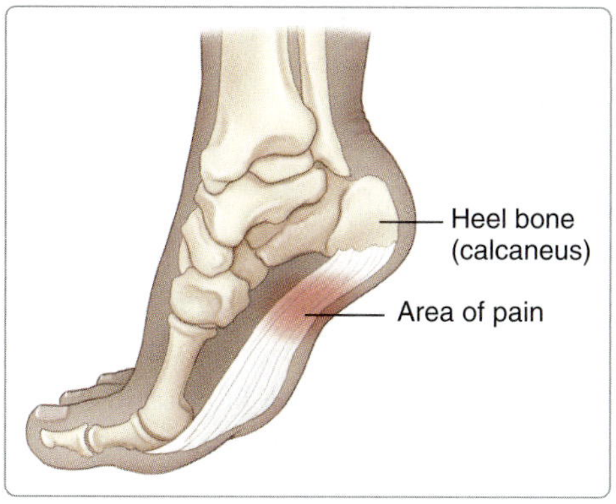

12. ____

type of wrist fracture, occurs at the distal end of the radius, the distal fragment being displaced backward

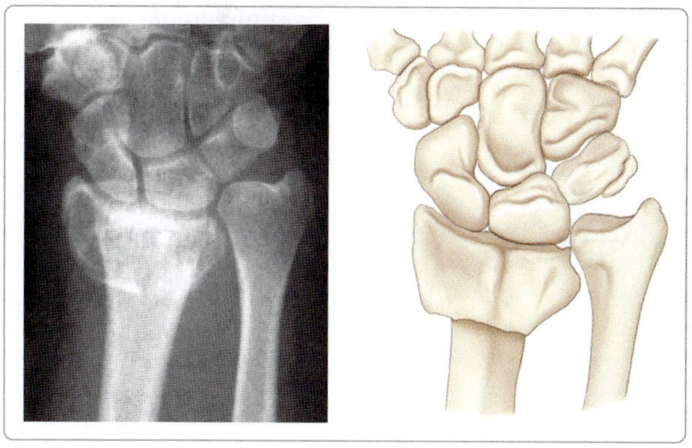

EXERCISE 24

Spell each of the Disease and Disorder Terms NOT Built from Word Parts by having someone dictate them to you. Use a separate sheet of paper.

To hear and spell the terms, go to Evolve Resources at evolve.elsevier.com and select:
Practice Student Resources > Student Resources > Chapter 14 > **Pronounce and Spell**

See Appendix B for instructions.

❑ Check the box when complete.

Surgical Terms
BUILT FROM WORD PARTS

The following terms can be translated using definitions of word parts. Further explanation is provided within parentheses as needed.

TERM	DEFINITION
aponeurorrhaphy (*ap*-ō-nū-ROR-a-fē)	suturing of an aponeurosis
arthrocentesis (*ar*-thrō-sen-TĒ-sis)	surgical puncture to aspirate fluid from a joint
arthrodesis (*ar*-thrō-DĒ-sis)	surgical fixation of a joint (also called **joint fusion**)
arthroplasty (AR-thrō-*plas*-tē)	surgical repair of a joint (Table 14.1)
bursectomy (bur-SEK-to-mē)	excision of a bursa
carpectomy (kar-PEK-to-mē)	excision of a carpal bone
chondrectomy (kon-DREK-to-mē)	excision of a cartilage
chondroplasty (KON-drō-*plas*-tē)	surgical repair of a cartilage
costectomy (kos-TEK-to-mē)	excision of a rib
cranioplasty (KRĀ-nē-ō-*plas*-tē)	surgical repair of the skull
craniotomy (*krā*-nē-OT-o-mē)	incision into the cranium (as for surgery of the brain)
diskectomy (dis-KEK-to-mē)	excision of an intervertebral disk (a portion of the disk is removed to relieve pressure on nerve roots) (also spelled **discectomy**) (Fig. 14.9)
laminectomy (*lam*-i-NEK-to-mē)	excision of a lamina (often performed to relieve pressure on the nerve roots in the lower spine caused by a herniated disk and other conditions)
maxillectomy (*mak*-si-LEK-to-mē)	excision of the maxilla
meniscectomy (*men*-i-SEK-to-mē)	excision of a meniscus (performed for a torn cartilage)
myorrhaphy (mī-OR-a-fē)	suturing of a muscle
ostectomy (os-TEK-to-mē)	excision of bone *(Note: the* e *is dropped from* oste.*)*
osteotomy (*os*-tē-OT-o-mē)	incision into a bone
patellectomy (*pat*-e-LEK-to-mē)	excision of a patella
phalangectomy (*fal*-an-JEK-to-mē)	excision of a finger or toe bone
rachiotomy (*rā*-kē-OT-o-mē)	incision into the vertebral column

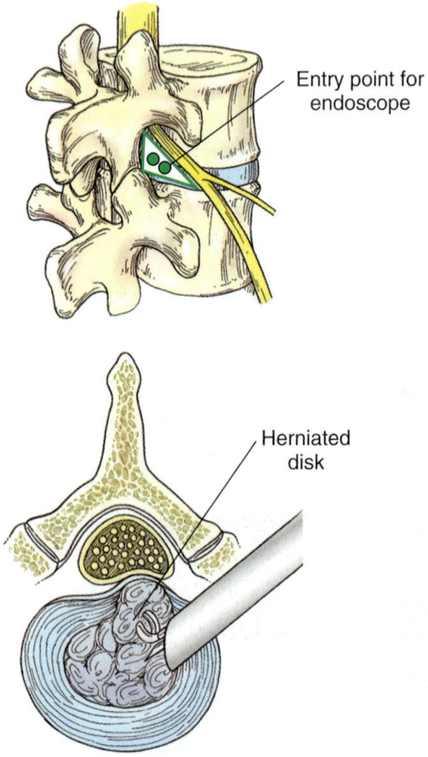

FIG. 14.9 Endoscopic discectomy.

MICROENDOSCOPIC DISKECTOMY (MED)
is a minimally-invasive procedure that uses a fluoroscope and special dilating instrumentation to create a small tunnel to the affected disk area. An endoscopic tool allows the surgeon to visualize and remove the thick, sticky nucleus of the herniated disk. The disk then softens and contracts, relieving severe low back and leg pain. Recovery time is significantly quicker than open diskectomy because of a small incision and less trauma to surrounding tissues.

TABLE 14.1 Types of Arthroplasty

Total hip arthroplasty (THA) is indicated for degenerative joint disease or rheumatoid arthritis. The operation originally involved replacement of the hip joint with a metallic femoral head and a plastic-coated acetabulum. More recently, however, many different materials have been used in an attempt to prevent the artificial joint from wearing out too quickly. These materials include joints composed of metal, ceramic, polyethylene (plastic), and combinations of each.

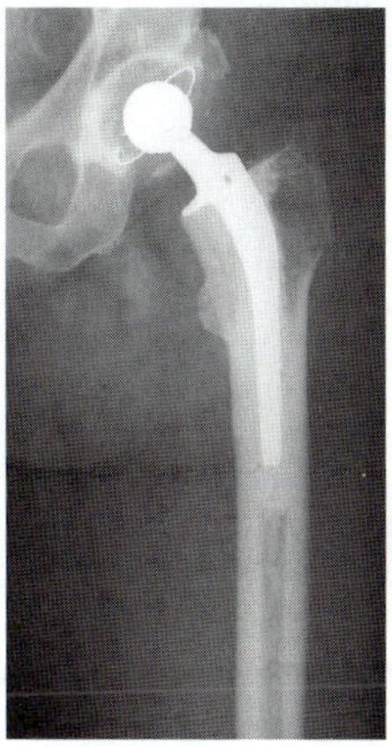

Total hip arthroplasty

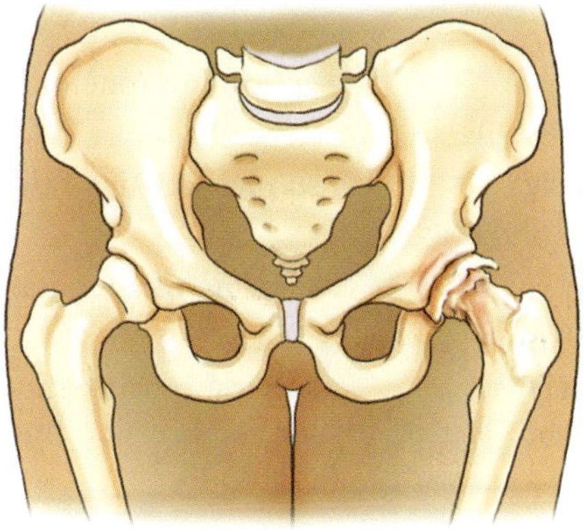

Normal hip joint

Hip joint damaged by osteoarthritis

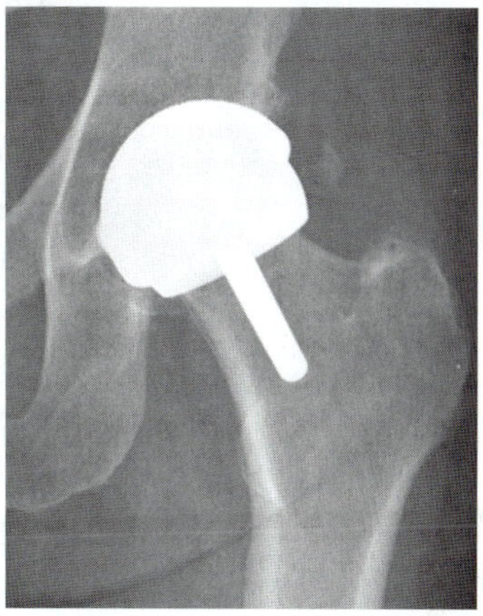

Hip resurfacing arthroplasty

Hip Resurfacing Arthroplasty (HRA) is a procedure that provides an option for younger, active patients needing a total hip arthroplasty. The procedure requires the removal of a few millimeters of bone from the femoral head instead of the removal of the entire femoral head required in total hip arthroplasty. A metal cap is then placed on top of the femur, and smooth metal is placed in the acetabulum. The risk of fracture of the neck of the femur is increased when smaller diameter components are used, making HRA less appropriate for women.

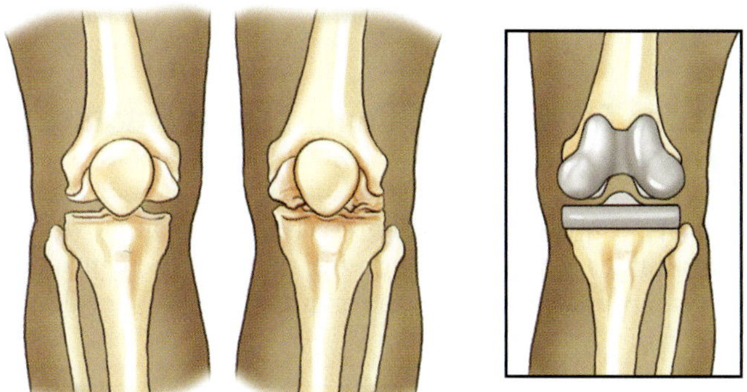

Normal knee joint

Knee joint damaged by osteoarthritis

Total knee replacement

Total Knee Arthroplasty (TKA) is designed to replace worn surfaces of the knee joint. Various prostheses (artificial parts) are used.

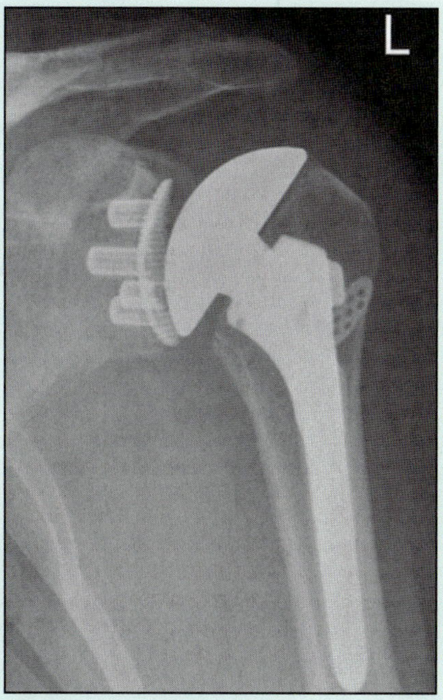

Shoulder Arthroplasty is a procedure that restores the major functions of this ball and socket joint: motion, stability, strength, and smoothness. Prostheses are applied to the head of the humerus and the glenoid cavity (part of the scapula). Osteoarthritis, rheumatoid arthritis, and severe rotator cuff tears are some of the most common reasons for this surgery.

Surgical Terms—cont'd

TERM	DEFINITION
spondylosyndesis (*spon*-di-lō-sin-DĒ-sis)	fusing together of the vertebrae (also called **spinal fusion**) *(Note: the prefix* syn- *appears in the middle of the term.)*
synovectomy (*sin*-ō-VEK-to-mē)	excision of the synovial membrane (of a joint) *(Note: the i in* synovi *is dropped because the suffix begins with a vowel.)*
tarsectomy (tar-SEK-to-mē)	excision of (one or more) tarsal bones
tenomyoplasty (*ten*-ō-MĪ-ō-*plas*-tē)	surgical repair of the tendon and muscle
tenorrhaphy (te-NOR-a-fē)	suturing of a tendon
vertebroplasty (VER-te-brō-*plas*-tē)	surgical repair of a vertebra (usually performed for compression fractures due to osteoporosis) (Table 14.2)

EXERCISE 25

Practice saying aloud each of the Surgical Terms Built from Word Parts.

To hear the terms, go to Evolve Resources at evolve.elsevier.com and select:
Practice Student Resources > Student Resources > Chapter 14 > **Pronounce and Spell**

See Appendix B for instructions.

❑ Check the box when complete.

TABLE 14.2 Procedures for Treatment of Compression Fractures Caused by Osteoporosis

Percutaneous vertebroplasty (PV) is a minimally invasive operation in which an interventional radiologist places a needle through the skin into the damaged vertebra. A special liquid cement is injected into the area through the needle to fill the holes left by osteoporosis.

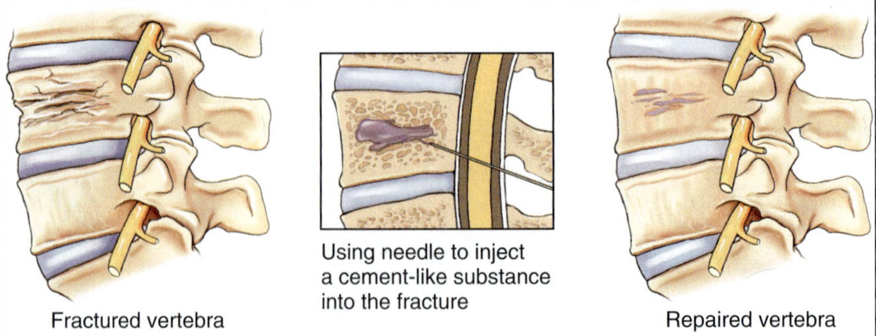

Percutaneous vertebroplasty

Kyphoplasty is similar to vertebroplasty except a balloonlike device is used to expand the compressed vertebra before the cement is injected. Recent studies have generated controversy as to whether these procedures are better than non-surgical management, such as pain medication and physical therapy. In either case, it is important to treat the underlying osteoporosis, to prevent future fractures.

EXERCISE 26

Analyze and define the following surgical terms.

1. osteotomy
2. ostectomy
3. arthrodesis
4. arthroplasty
5. chondrectomy
6. chondroplasty
7. myorrhaphy
8. tenomyoplasty
9. tenorrhaphy
10. costectomy
11. patellectomy
12. aponeurorrhaphy
13. carpectomy
14. phalangectomy
15. meniscectomy
16. spondylosyndesis
17. laminectomy
18. bursectomy

19. craniotomy

____

____

20. cranioplasty

____

____

21. maxillectomy

____

____

22. rachiotomy

____

____

23. tarsectomy

____

____

24. synovectomy

____

____

25. diskectomy

____

____

26. vertebroplasty

____

____

27. arthrocentesis

____

____

EXERCISE 27

Build surgical terms for the following definitions by using the word parts you have learned.

1. incision into a bone ______ / ______ / ______ (WR / CV / S)
2. excision of bone ______ / ______ (WR / S)
3. surgical fixation of a joint ______ / ______ / ______ (WR / CV / S)
4. surgical repair of a joint ______ / ______ / ______ (WR / CV / S)
5. excision of cartilage ______ / ______ (WR / S)
6. surgical repair of cartilage ______ / ______ / ______ (WR / CV / S)
7. suturing of a muscle ______ / ______ / ______ (WR / CV / S)

8. surgical repair of a tendon and muscle ______ / ______ / ______ / ______ / ______
WR / CV / WR / CV / S

9. suturing of a tendon ______ / ______ / ______
WR / CV / S

10. excision of a rib ______ / ______
WR / S

11. excision of a patella ______ / ______
WR / S

12. suturing of an aponeurosis ______ / ______ / ______
WR / CV / S

13. excision of a carpal bone ______ / ______
WR / S

14. excision of a finger or toe bone ______ / ______
WR / S

15. excision of a meniscus ______ / ______
WR / S

16. fusing together of the vertebrae ______ / ______ / ______ / ______
WR / CV / P / S

17. excision of a lamina ______ / ______
WR / S

18. excision of a bursa ______ / ______
WR / S

19. incision into the cranium ______ / ______ / ______
WR / CV / S

20. surgical repair of the skull ______ / ______ / ______
WR / CV / S

21. excision of the maxilla ______ / ______
WR / S

22. incision into the vertebral column ______ / ______ / ______
WR / CV / S

23. excision of (one or more) tarsal bones ______ / ______
WR / S

24. excision of the synovial membrane ______ / ______
WR / S

25. excision of an intervertebral disk ______ / ______
WR / S

26. surgical repair of a vertebra ________ / CV / ________
WR / CV / S

27. surgical puncture to aspirate fluid from a joint ________ / CV / ________
WR / CV / S

EXERCISE FIGURE B

Fill in the blanks with word parts defined to label the diagram.

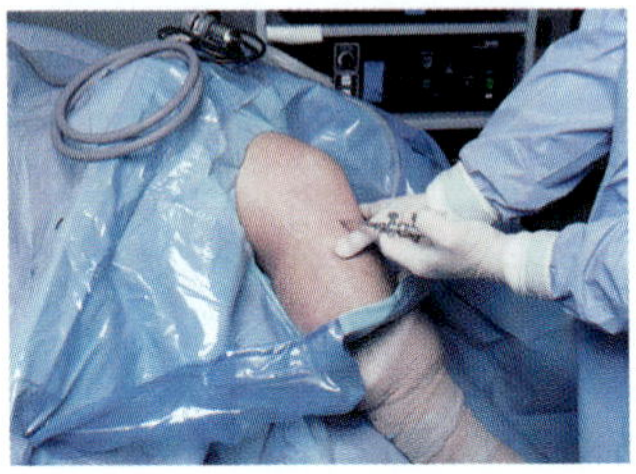

________ / ________ / ________
joint / cv / visual examination

EXERCISE FIGURE C

Fill in the blanks with word parts defined to label the diagram.

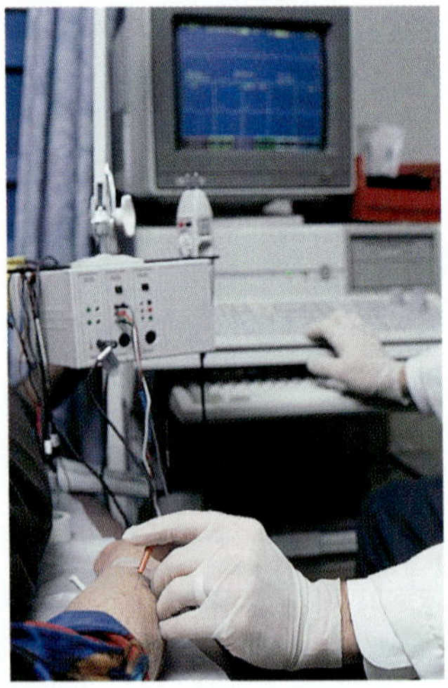

________ / ________ / ________ / ________ / ________
electrical activity / cv / muscle / cv / record

EXERCISE 28

Spell each of the Surgical Terms Built from Word Parts by having someone dictate them to you. Use a separate sheet of paper.

To hear and spell the terms, go to Evolve Resources at evolve.elsevier.com and select: Practice Student Resources > Student Resources > Chapter 14 > **Pronounce and Spell**

See Appendix B for instructions.

❑ Check the box when complete.

Diagnostic Terms

BUILT FROM WORD PARTS

The following terms can be translated using definitions of word parts. Further explanation is provided within parentheses as needed.

TERM	DEFINITION
DIAGNOSTIC IMAGING	
arthrography (ar-THROG-ra-fē)	radiographic imaging of a joint (with contrast media). (Magnetic resonance imaging [MRI] has mostly replaced conventional arthrography as the imaging technique for joints such as the knee, wrist, hip, and shoulder. Many of the remaining arthrograms are performed in conjunction with MRI. A conventional arthrogram might be used in situations in which a patient cannot have an MRI, such as a person with a cardiac pacemaker. See Table 14.3 for **diagnostic imaging procedures** used for the musculoskeletal system.)
ENDOSCOPY	
arthroscopy (ar-THROS-ko-pē)	visual examination of a joint (Exercise Figure B)
OTHER	
electromyogram (EMG) (ē-*lek*-trō-MĪ-ō-gram)	record of the (intrinsic) electrical activity in a (skeletal) muscle (Exercise Figure C)

TABLE 14.3 Diagnostic Imaging Procedures Used for the Musculoskeletal System

In addition to **arthrography**, listed previously, the following diagnostic imaging procedures are commonly used for diagnosing diseases, fractures, strains, and other conditions of the musculoskeletal system.

Bone densitometry is a method of determining the density of bone by radiographic techniques used to diagnose osteoporosis. **Dual-energy X-ray absorptiometry (DXA or DEXA)** is commonly used for this test (Fig. 14.10).

Bone scan (nuclear medicine test) is used to detect the presence of metastatic disease of the bone and to monitor degenerative bone disease (Fig. 14.12).

Magnetic resonance imaging (MRI) is used to evaluate the bones and soft tissue of the shoulders, hips, elbows, knees, ankles, feet, and spinal cord stenosis, spinal cord defects, and degenerative disk changes (Fig. 14.11).

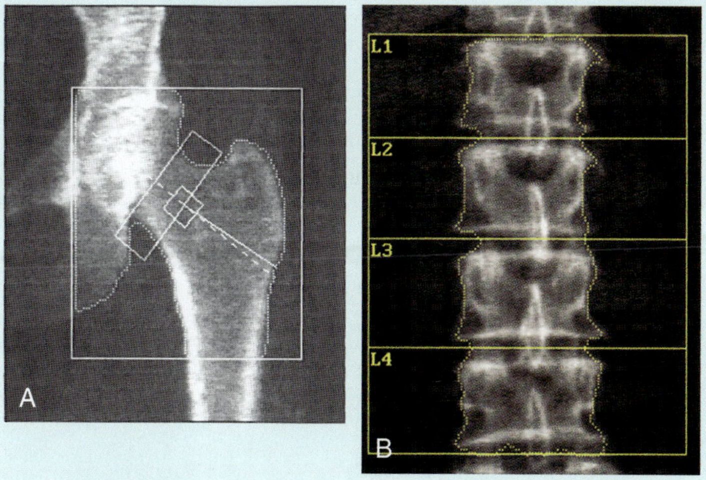

FIG. 14.10 DEXA images of the (A) left hip and (B) spine.

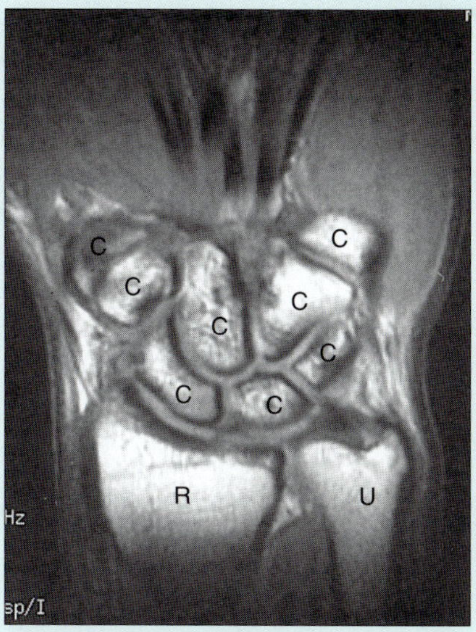

FIG. 14.11 Coronal MRI scan of the wrist. Marrow within the carpal bones (C), radius (R), and ulna (U).

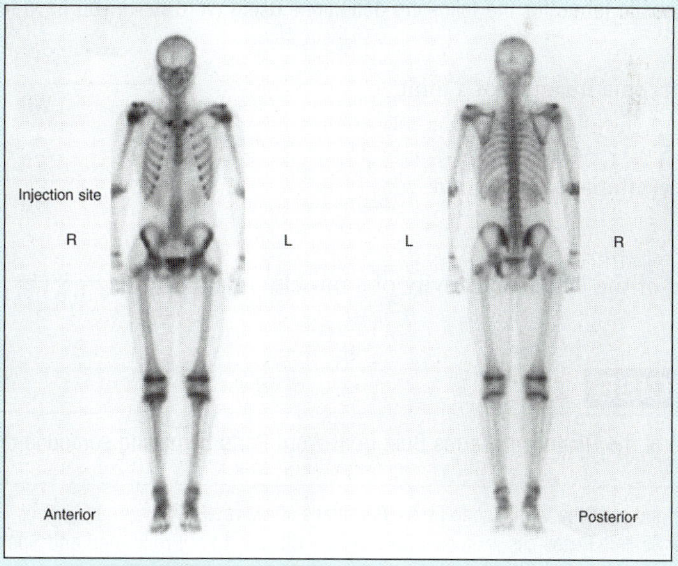

FIG. 14.12 Whole body nuclear medicine bone scan.

Radiography (radiographic imaging) of the bones and joints is used to identify fractures or tumors, monitor healing, or identify abnormal structures.

Single-photon emission computed tomography (SPECT) of the bone is an even more sensitive nuclear method for detecting bone abnormalities.

EXERCISE 29

Practice saying aloud each of the Diagnostic Terms Built from Word Parts.

To hear the terms, go to Evolve Resources at evolve.elsevier.com and select:
Practice Student Resources > Student Resources > Chapter 14 > **Pronounce and Spell**

See Appendix B for instructions.

❑ Check the box when complete.

EXERCISE 30

Analyze and define the following diagnostic terms.

1. electromyogram

____

____

2. arthrography

____

____

3. arthroscopy

____

____

EXERCISE 31

Build diagnostic terms for the following definitions using word parts you have learned.

1. radiographic imaging of a joint ________ WR / CV / S

2. visual examination of a joint ________ WR / CV / S

3. record of the electrical activity of a muscle ________ WR / CV / WR / CV / S

EXERCISE 32

Spell each of the Diagnostic Terms Built from Word Parts by having someone dictate them to you. Use a separate sheet of paper.

To hear and spell the terms, go to Evolve Resources at evolve.elsevier.com and select:
Practice Student Resources > Student Resources > Chapter 14 > **Pronounce and Spell**

See Appendix B for instructions.

❑ Check the box when complete.

Complementary Terms
BUILT FROM WORD PARTS

The following terms can be translated using definitions of word parts. Further explanation is provided within parentheses as needed.

TERM	DEFINITION
arthralgia (ar-THRAL-ja)	pain in the joint
atrophy (AT-ro-fē)	without development (process of wasting away)
bradykinesia (*brad*-ē-ki-NĒ-zha)	slow movement
carpal (CAR-pal)	pertaining to the wrist
clavicular (kla-VIK-ū-lar)	pertaining to the clavicle
costochondral (KOS-tō-kon-dral)	pertaining to the ribs and cartilage
cranial (KRĀ-nē-al)	pertaining to the cranium
dyskinesia (*dis*-ki-NĒ-zha)	difficult movement
dystrophy (DIS-tro-fē)	abnormal development
femoral (FEM-or-al)	pertaining to the femur
fibular (FIB-ū-lar)	pertaining to the fibula
humeral (HŪ-mer-al)	pertaining to the humerus
hyperkinesia (*hī*-per-ki-NĒ-zha)	excessive movement (hyperactive)
hypertrophy (hī-PER-tro-fē)	excessive development
iliofemoral (*il*-ē-ō-FEM-or-al)	pertaining to the ilium and femur
intercostal (*in*-ter-KOS-tal)	pertaining to between the ribs
intervertebral (*in*-ter-VER-te-bral)	pertaining to between the vertebrae
intracranial (*in*-tra-KRĀ-nē-al)	pertaining to within the cranium
ischiopubic (*is*-kē-ō-PŪ-bik)	pertaining to the ischium and pubis
lumbar (LUM-bar)	pertaining to the loins (the part of the back between the thorax and pelvis)
lumbocostal (*lum*-bō-KOS-tal)	pertaining to the loins and the ribs

Complementary Terms—cont'd

TERM	DEFINITION
lumbosacral (*lum*-bō-SĀ-kral)	pertaining to the lumbar regions (loin) and the sacrum
myalgia (mī-AL-ja)	pain in muscle
osteoblast (OS-tē-ō-*blast*)	developing bone cell
osteocyte (OS-tē-ō-*sīt*)	bone cell
osteonecrosis (*os*-tē-ō-ne-KRŌ-sis)	abnormal condition of bone death (due to lack of blood supply)
pelvic (PEL-vik)	pertaining to the pelvis
pubic (PŪ-bik)	pertaining to the pubis
radial (RĀ-dē-al)	pertaining to the radius
sacral (SĀ-kral)	pertaining to the sacrum
sternoclavicular (*ster*-nō-kla-VIK-ū-lar)	pertaining to the sternum and clavicle
sternoid (STER-noyd)	resembling the sternum
subcostal (sub-KOS-tal)	pertaining to below the rib
submandibular (*sub*-man-DIB-ū-lar)	pertaining to below the mandible
submaxillary (sub-MAK-si-*lar*-ē)	pertaining to below the maxilla
subscapular (sub-SKAP-ū-lar)	pertaining to below the scapula
substernal (sub-STER-nal)	pertaining to under the sternum
suprapatellar (*sū*-pra-pa-TEL-ar)	pertaining to above the patella
suprascapular (*sū*-pra-SKAP-ū-lar)	pertaining to above the scapula
symphysis (SIM-fi-sis)	growing together (as in symphysis pubis)
tibial (TIB-ē-al)	pertaining to the tibia
ulnoradial (ul-nō-RĀ-dē-al)	pertaining to the ulna and radius
vertebrocostal (*ver*-te-brō-KOS-tal)	pertaining to the vertebrae and ribs

MOVEMENT DISORDERS

are impairments in voluntary movement and are also known as **dyskinesias**. **Bradykinesia** is characterized by slowness of all voluntary movement and speech, while **hyperkinesia** describes excessive or involuntary movements. Parkinson disease and Tourette syndrome are some examples of movement disorders and will be addressed further in Chapter 15.

EXERCISE 33

Practice saying aloud each of the Complementary Terms Built from Word Parts.

To hear the terms, go to Evolve Resources at evolve.elsevier.com and select:
Practice Student Resources > Student Resources > Chapter 14 > **Pronounce and Spell**

See Appendix B for instructions.

❑ Check the box when complete.

EXERCISE 34

Analyze and define the following complementary terms.

1. symphysis
2. femoral
3. humeral
4. intervertebral
5. hyperkinesia
6. dyskinesia
7. bradykinesia
8. intracranial
9. sternoclavicular
10. iliofemoral
11. fibular
12. submaxillary
13. ischiopubic
14. submandibular

15. suprascapular

____
____

16. subcostal

____
____

17. vertebrocostal

____
____

18. subscapular

____
____

19. osteoblast

____
____

20. osteocyte

____
____

21. osteonecrosis

____
____

22. sternoid

____
____

23. arthralgia

____
____

24. carpal

____
____

25. lumbar

____
____

26. lumbocostal

____
____

27. lumbosacral

____
____

28. sacral

____
____

29. pubic

____
____

30. substernal

____
____

31. suprapatellar

____
____

32. dystrophy

____
____

33. atrophy

____

____

34. hypertrophy

____

____

35. intercostal

____

____

36. cranial

____

____

37. pelvic

____

____

38. clavicular

____

____

39. tibial

____

____

40. radial

____

____

41. ulnoradial

____

____

42. costochondral

____

____

43. myalgia

____

____

EXERCISE 35

Build the complementary terms for the following definitions by using the word parts you have learned.

1. growing together ______ P / ______ S(WR)

2. pertaining to the femur ______ WR / ______ S

3. pertaining to the humerus ______ WR / ______ S

4. pertaining to between the vertebrae ______ P / ______ WR / ______ S

5. excessive movement (hyperactive) ______ P / ______ WR / ______ S

6. difficult movement ______ P / ______ WR / ______ S

7. slow movement ______ P / ______ WR / ______ S

8. pertaining to within the cranium ______ P / ______ WR / ______ S

9. pertaining to the sternum and clavicle ______ WR / CV / ______ WR / ______ S

10. pertaining to the ilium and femur ______ WR / CV / ______ WR / ______ S

11. pertaining to the fibula ______ WR / ______ S

12. pertaining to below the maxilla ______ P / ______ WR / ______ S

13. pertaining to the ischium and pubis ______ WR / CV / ______ WR / ______ S

14. pertaining to below the mandible ______ P / ______ WR / ______ S

15. pertaining to above the scapula ______ P / ______ WR / ______ S

16. pertaining to below the rib ______ P / ______ WR / ______ S

17. pertaining to the vertebrae and ribs ______ WR / CV / ______ WR / ______ S

18. pertaining to below the scapula ______ P / ______ WR / ______ S

19. developing bone cell ______ WR / CV / ______ WR

20. bone cell ______ WR / CV / ______ S

21. abnormal condition of bone death ______ WR / CV / ______ WR / ______ S

22. resembling the sternum ______ WR / ______ S

23. pain in the joint ______ WR / ______ S

24. pertaining to the wrist
WR / S

25. pertaining to the sacrum
WR / S

26. pertaining to the loins
WR / S

27. pertaining to the pubis
WR / S

28. pertaining to the lumbar region (loin) and the sacrum
WR / CV / WR / S

29. pertaining to the loins and ribs
WR / CV / WR / S

30. pertaining to under the sternum
P / WR / S

31. pertaining to above the patella
P / WR / S

32. abnormal development
P / S(WR)

33. without development
P / S(WR)

34. excessive development
P / S(WR)

35. pertaining to the cranium
WR / S

36. pertaining to between the ribs
P / WR / S

37. pertaining to the pelvis
WR / S

38. pertaining to the clavicle
WR / S

39. pertaining to the tibia
WR / S

40. pertaining to the radius
WR / S

41. pertaining to the ulna and radius
WR / CV / WR / S

42. pertaining to the ribs and cartilage ______ WR / CV / ______ WR / ______ S

43. pain in muscle ______ WR / ______ S

EXERCISE 36

Spell each of the Complementary Terms Built from Word Parts by having someone dictate them to you. Use a separate sheet of paper.

> To hear and spell the terms, go to Evolve Resources at evolve.elsevier.com and select:
> Practice Student Resources > Student Resources > Chapter 14 > **Pronounce and Spell**
>
> See Appendix B for instructions.

❑ Check the box when complete.

Complementary Terms
NOT BUILT FROM WORD PARTS

Word parts may be present in the following terms; however, their full meanings cannot be translated using definitions of word parts alone.

> **CAREER VIDEOS**
> To see interviews with an **Occupational Therapist** and a **Physical Therapy Assistant**, go to Evolve resources at evolve.elsevier.com and select **Career Videos** located under the **Extra Content** Tab.

TERM	DEFINITION
chiropractic (*kī*-rō-PRAK-tik)	system of treatment that consists of manipulation of the vertebral column
chiropractor (DC) (KĪ-rō-*prak*-tor)	specialist in chiropractic
crepitus (KREP-i-tus)	crackling sensation heard or felt when two bones rub against each other or grating caused by the rubbing together of dry surfaces of a joint. (Crepitus is also used to describe the crackling sound heard with pneumonia.) (also called **crepitation**)
orthopedics (Ortho) (*or*-thō-PĒ-diks)	branch of medicine dealing with the study and treatment of diseases and abnormalities of the musculoskeletal system
orthopedist (*or*-thō-PĒ-dist)	physician who specializes in the study and treatment of diseases and abnormalities of the musculoskeletal system
orthotics (or-THOT-iks)	making and fitting of orthopedic appliances, such as arch supports, used to support, align, prevent, or correct deformities
orthotist (or-THOT-ist)	person who specializes in orthotics
osteoclast (OS-tē-ō-*klast*)	type of bone cell involved in absorption and removal of bone minerals. It works in balance with osteoblasts to maintain healthy bone tissue.
osteopath (DO) (OS-tē-ō-path)	physician who specializes in osteopathy

TERM	DEFINITION
osteopathy (*os*-tē-OP-a-thē)	system of medicine that uses the usual forms of diagnosis and treatment but places greater emphasis on the relation between body organs and the musculoskeletal system; manipulation may be used in addition to other treatments
podiatrist (pō-DĪ-a-trist)	specialist in treating and diagnosing diseases and disorders of the foot, including medical and surgical treatment
prosthesis (pl. prostheses) (pros-THĒ-sis), (pros-THĒ-sēz)	artificial substitute for a missing body part such as a leg, eye, or hip replacement
rheumatologist (roo-ma-TOL-ō-jist)	physician who specializes in the study and treatment of rheumatic diseases
rheumatology (roo-ma-TOL-ō-jē)	study and treatment of rheumatic diseases (musculoskeletal disorders characterized by inflammation and degeneration of structures)

RHEUMATOLOGY AND ORTHOPEDICS: WHAT IS THE DIFFERENCE?

While both medical specialties focus on the diagnosis and treatment of disease and disorders of the musculoskeletal system, **rheumatology** focuses on medical management for chronic conditions while **orthopedics** focuses on surgical treatment for acute or chronic conditions. For example, a patient with **rheumatoid arthritis** would see a **rheumatologist** for medications to manage symptoms of the disease and would be referred to an **orthopedist** if joint replacement surgery was warranted.

Refer to **Appendix F** for pharmacology terms related to the musculoskeletal system.

EXERCISE 37

Practice saying aloud each of the Complementary Terms NOT Built from Word Parts.

To hear the terms, go to Evolve Resources at evolve.elsevier.com and select:
Practice Student Resources > Student Resources > Chapter 14 > **Pronounce and Spell**

See Appendix B for instructions.

❑ Check the box when complete.

EXERCISE 38

Match the definitions in the first column with the correct terms in the second column.

_____ 1. specialist in manipulation of the vertebral column
_____ 2. study and treatment of diseases of the musculoskeletal system
_____ 3. physician who places emphasis on manipulation
_____ 4. foot specialist
_____ 5. substitute for a body part
_____ 6. system of treatment that consists of manipulation of the vertebral column
_____ 7. system of medicine that places greater emphasis on the relation between body organs and the musculoskeletal system
_____ 8. making of orthopedic appliances
_____ 9. skilled in orthotics
_____ 10. crackling or grating sensation
_____ 11. physician who specializes in treatment of diseases and abnormalities of the musculoskeletal system
_____ 12. maintains healthy bone tissue with osteoblasts
_____ 13. physician who specializes in the study and treatment of rheumatic diseases
_____ 14. study and treatment of rheumatic diseases

a. chiropractic
b. chiropractor
c. osteopath
d. osteopathy
e. orthopedics
f. orthopedist
g. podiatrist
h. orthotics
i. prosthesis
j. orthotist
k. crepitus
l. rheumatologist
m. osteoclast
n. rheumatology

EXERCISE 39

Write the definitions of the following.

1. chiropractor ____
2. chiropractic ____
3. orthopedics ____
4. orthopedist ____
5. podiatrist ____
6. osteopath ____
7. osteopathy ____
8. orthotics ____
9. prosthesis ____
10. orthotist ____
11. crepitus ____
12. osteoclast ____
13. rheumatologist ____
14. rheumatology ____

EXERCISE 40

Spell each of the Complementary Terms NOT Built from Word Parts by having someone dictate them to you. Use a separate sheet of paper.

> To hear and spell the terms, go to Evolve Resources at evolve.elsevier.com and select:
> Practice Student Resources > Student Resources > Chapter 14 > **Pronounce and Spell**
>
> See Appendix B for instructions.

❑ Check the box when complete.

Types of Body Movement

Bones and muscles work together to produce various types of body movement. Some are listed below (Fig. 14.13).

MIDLINE VS. MIDDLE

The two terms are synonyms, both describing an imaginary line that separates the body, or body part, into equal halves. In medical language, *midline* is the preferred term and is used as a common reference point.

TERM	DEFINITION
abduction (ab-DUK-shun)	moving away from the midline
adduction (ad-DUK-shun)	moving toward the midline
inversion (in-VER-zhun)	turning inward
eversion (ē-VER-zhun)	turning outward
extension (ek-STEN-shun)	movement in which a limb is placed in a straight position, increasing the angle between the bone and the joint
flexion (FLEK-shun)	movement in which a limb is bent, decreasing the angle between the bone and the joint

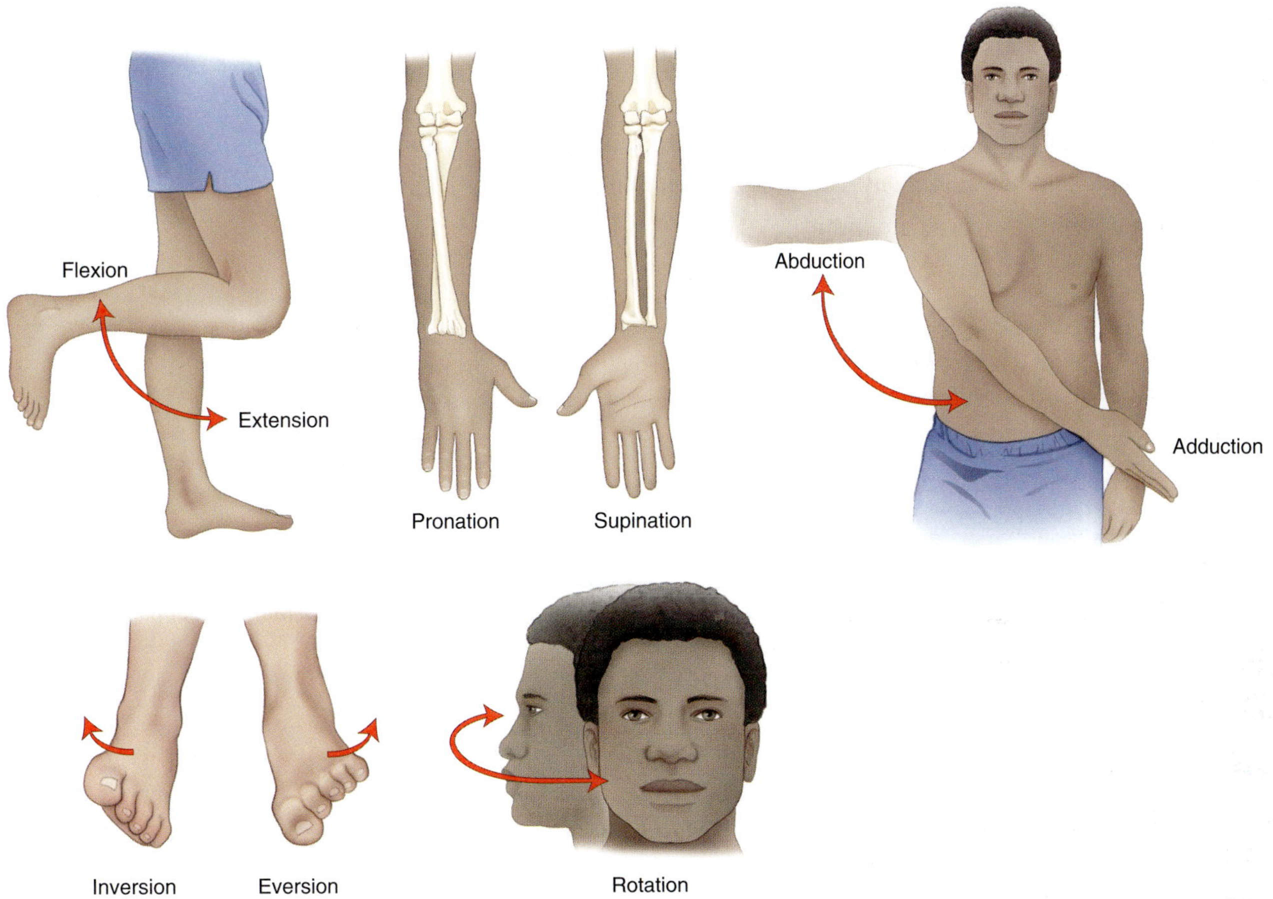

FIG. 14.13 Types of body movements.

TERM	DEFINITION
pronation (prō-NĀ-shun)	movement that turns the palm down
supination (sū-pi-NĀ-shun)	movement that turns the palm up
rotation (rō-TĀ-shun)	turning around its own axis

EXERCISE 41

Practice saying aloud each of the Types of Body Movement terms.

To hear the terms, go to Evolve Resources at evolve.elsevier.com and select:
Practice Student Resources > Student Resources > Chapter 14 > **Pronounce and Spell**

See Appendix B for instructions.

❑ Check the box when complete.

EXERCISE 42

Match the terms in the first column with the correct definitions in the second column.

______	1. abduction	a. movement in which a limb is placed in a straight position
______	2. adduction	b. movement that turns the palm up
______	3. pronation	c. turning outward
______	4. rotation	d. moving toward the midline
______	5. eversion	e. turning around its own axis
______	6. extension	f. turning inward
______	7. flexion	g. movement in which a limb is bent
______	8. inversion	h. moving away from the midline
______	9. supination	i. movement that turns the palm down

EXERCISE 43

Spell each of the Types of Body Movement terms by having someone dictate them to you. Use a separate sheet of paper.

To hear and spell the terms, go to Evolve Resources at evolve.elsevier.com and select:
Practice Student Resources > Student Resources > Chapter 14 > **Pronounce and Spell**

See Appendix B for instructions.

❑ Check the box when complete.

WEB LINK

For additional information on arthritis, visit the **Arthritis Foundation** at *www.arthritis.org.*

Abbreviations

ABBREVIATION	TERM
C1-C7	cervical vertebrae
CTS	carpal tunnel syndrome
DC	Doctor of Chiropractic
DO	Doctor of Osteopathy
EMG	electromyogram
fx	fracture
HNP	herniated nucleus pulposus
L1-L5	lumbar vertebrae
MD	muscular dystrophy
MG	myasthenia gravis
OA	osteoarthritis
Ortho	orthopedics
RA	rheumatoid arthritis
T1-T12	thoracic vertebrae
THA	total hip arthroplasty
TKA	total knee arthroplasty

Refer to **Appendix E** for a complete list of abbreviations.

EXERCISE 44

Write the terms abbreviated.

1. Vertebrae make up the bones of the spinal column. **C1 to C7** ____________ ____________ are the first set that form the neck. The second set **T1 to T12** ____________ ____________ articulate with the 12 pairs of ribs that form the outward curve of the spine. **L1 to L5** ____________ ____________, the third set, are larger and form the inward curve of the spine.
2. Patients with **RA** ______________ ______________ may experience muscle atrophy and weakness because of inactivity.
3. Water exercise or gentle movement, such as Tai Chi, is recommended for many patients with **OA** ____________ __________________, the most common joint disease.
4. **MG** ____________ ____________ most often affects women and the onset occurs at any age. It is an acquired autoimmune disorder.
5. **EMG** ________________________________ is used to evaluate patients with localized or diffuse muscle weakness, such as polymyositis.
6. **CTS** ____________ ____________ ____________ is a common condition in which, for various reasons, the median nerve in the wrist becomes compressed, causing numbness and pain.
7. Nine types of **MD** ____________ ____________ have been identified. Because symptoms of the disease are similar to other muscular disorders, diagnosis is often difficult.
8. **HNP** ____________ ____________ ____________ may also be referred to as slipped or ruptured disk or herniated intervertebral disk.
9. **THA** ____________ ____________ ____________ is used to treat severe osteoarthritis of the hip joints.
10. Taking a holistic view of medicine, the **DO** ____________ ______ ____________________ evaluates the patient's musculoskeletal system in relation to overall health.
11. Knee replacement surgery, also called **TKA** _______________ ______________ ____________________, is used in patients that have disabling pain due to arthritis.

For additional practice with Abbreviations, go to Evolve Resources at evolve.elsevier.com and select: Practice Student Resources > Student Resources > Chapter 14 > **Flashcards:** Abbreviations

See Appendix B for instructions.

PRACTICAL APPLICATION

EXERCISE 45 *Case Study: Translate Between Everyday Language and Medical Language*

CASE STUDY: Shanti Mehra

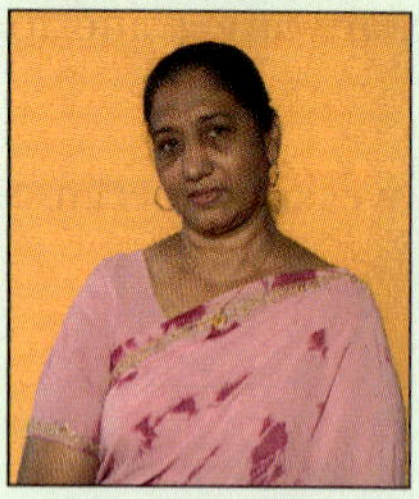

Shanti Mehra was walking to the store to buy more cigarettes. It was cold and icy and unfortunately, she slipped on some ice on the pavement. Her hand and wrist buckled under her when she fell. Now she is worried she may have broken some finger or wrist bones. She goes to the emergency department and an x-ray is done. She is told that she has broken both of her lower arm bones and is referred to a musculoskeletal specialist. She is also told that her bones are not dense enough and that she needs to have additional tests done.

Now that you have worked through Chapter 14, consider the medical terms that might be used to describe Mrs. Mehra's experience. See the Review of Terms at the end of the chapter for a list of terms that might apply.

A. *Underline phrases in the case study that could be substituted with medical terms.*

B. *Write the medical term and its definition for three of the phrases you underlined.*

MEDICAL TERM	DEFINITION
1. ______________	______________
2. ______________	______________
3. ______________	______________

DOCUMENTATION: Excerpt from Orthopedic Clinic Visit

Mrs. Mehra made an appointment with an orthopedist; a portion of the report is documented below.

Progress Note

Physical Examination: *She has prominent dorsal kyphosis in the thoracic vertebral column. AP and lateral radiographs of the right wrist reveal a Colles fracture and a distal ulnar fracture. Her bones show evidence of osteoporosis.*

Assessment and Plan: *A DEXA scan is recommended to assess bone mineral density. She was advised to continue immobilization of the radioulnar-carpal junction for 4 weeks.*

C. *Underline medical terms presented in Chapter 14 used in the previous excerpt from Mrs. Mehra's medical record. See the Review of Terms at the end of the chapter for a complete list.*

D. *Select and define three of the medical terms you underlined. To check your answers, go to Appendix A.*

MEDICAL TERM	DEFINITION
1. ______________	______________
2. ______________	______________
3. ______________	______________

EXERCISE 46 *Interact With Medical Documents and Electronic Health Records*

A. Read the report and complete it by writing medical terms on answer lines within the document. Definitions of terms to be written appear after the document.

10003-MKL McBRIDE, William

File Patient Navigate Custom Fields Help

Chart Review | Encounters | Notes | Labs | Imaging | Procedures | Rx | Documents | Referrals | Scheduling | Billing

Name: **McBRIDE, William** MR#: **10003-MKL** DOB: 12/04/19XX Gender: M Age: 55 **Allergies:** Penicillin, Promethazine **PCP:** Annie Morocco, MD

Operative Report:

History: William McBride is a 55-year-old male who reports pain in his left knee when walking and golfing. He states that his knees have "been painful" for many years since he quit playing semiprofessional hockey, but the pain has become much more severe in the last 6 months. He was admitted to the Medical Center's Outpatient 1.________________ Center for an 2.____________________ of his left knee.

Preoperative Diagnosis: Degenerative 3. __________________ of the left knee, with possible tear of the 4. _________________ meniscus.

Operative Report: After induction of spinal anesthetic, the patient was positioned on the operating table, and a tourniquet was applied over the upper left thigh. After positioning the leg in a circumferential holder, the end of the table was flexed to allow the leg to hang freely. The patient's left leg was prepped and draped in the usual manner. After exsanguination of the leg with an Esmarch bandage, the tourniquet was inflated to 300 mm Hg. The knee was inspected by anterolateral and anteromedial parapatellar portholes.

Findings: The synovium in the 5. _______________________ pouch showed moderate to severe inflammatory changes with villi formation and hyperemia. The undersurface of the patella showed loss of normal articular cartilage on the lateral patellar facet with exposed bone in that area and moderate to severe 6. ____________________________ of the medial facet. Similar changes were noted in the intercondylar groove. In the medial compartment, the patient had smooth articular cartilage on the femur and moderate chondromalacia of the tibial plateau. The medial meniscus appeared normal with no evidence of tears and a smooth articular surface on the femoral condyle. No additional 7. _______________________ being identified.

The tourniquet was then released and the knee flushed with lactated Ringer solution until the bleeding slowed. The wounds were Steri-Stripped closed, a sterile bandage with an external Ace wrap applied, and the patient returned to the postoperative recovery area in stable condition. The patient tolerated the procedure well.

Postoperative Diagnosis: Degenerative arthritis with mild chondromalacia of the left knee.

Electronically signed: Martin Spencer, DO 02/13/20XX 07:59

Start | Log On/Off | Print | Edit

Definitions of Medical Terms to Complete the Document

Write the medical terms defined on corresponding answer lines in the document.

1. branch of medicine dealing with the study and treatment of diseases and abnormalities of the musculoskeletal system
2. visual examination of a joint
3. inflammation of a joint
4. toward the middle or midline
5. pertaining to above the patella
6. softening of the cartilage
7. study of (body changes caused by) disease

EXERCISE 46 *Interact With Medical Documents and Electronic Health Records—cont'd*

B. Read the medical report and answer the questions below it.

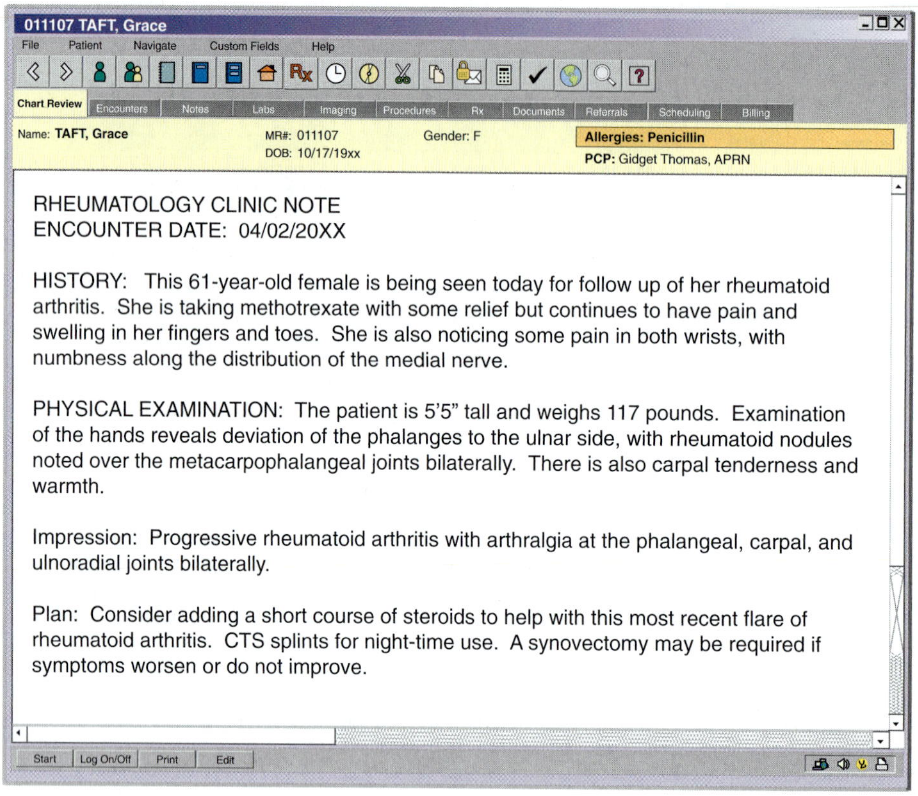
011107 TAFT, Grace

File Patient Navigate Custom Fields Help

Chart Review | Encounters | Notes | Labs | Imaging | Procedures | Rx | Documents | Referrals | Scheduling | Billing

Name: **TAFT, Grace** MR#: 011107 DOB: 10/17/19xx Gender: F **Allergies: Penicillin** **PCP:** Gidget Thomas, APRN

RHEUMATOLOGY CLINIC NOTE
ENCOUNTER DATE: 04/02/20XX

HISTORY: This 61-year-old female is being seen today for follow up of her rheumatoid arthritis. She is taking methotrexate with some relief but continues to have pain and swelling in her fingers and toes. She is also noticing some pain in both wrists, with numbness along the distribution of the medial nerve.

PHYSICAL EXAMINATION: The patient is 5'5" tall and weighs 117 pounds. Examination of the hands reveals deviation of the phalanges to the ulnar side, with rheumatoid nodules noted over the metacarpophalangeal joints bilaterally. There is also carpal tenderness and warmth.

Impression: Progressive rheumatoid arthritis with arthralgia at the phalangeal, carpal, and ulnoradial joints bilaterally.

Plan: Consider adding a short course of steroids to help with this most recent flare of rheumatoid arthritis. CTS splints for night-time use. A synovectomy may be required if symptoms worsen or do not improve.

Start | Log On/Off | Print | Edit

Use the medical report above to answer the questions.

1. Pain and numbness in the wrist with compression of the medial nerve could indicate
   a. ankylosing spondylitis
   b. gout
   c. carpal tunnel syndrome
   d. plantar fasciitis

2. The patient is exhibiting tenderness and warmth over the
   a. ankles
   b. wrists
   c. elbows
   d. knees

C. Complete the three medical documents within electronic health record (EHR) on Evolve.

Topic: Fracture, Parkinson Disease
Documents: Admission Note, Radiology Report, Neurology Consultation

To complete the three medical records, go to Evolve Resources at evolve.elsevier.com and select:
Practice Student Resources > Student Resources > Chapter 14 > **Electronic Heath Records**

See Appendix B for instructions.

EXERCISE 47 *Pronounce Medical Terms in Use*

Practice pronunciation of terms by reading aloud the following sentences. Use the phonetic spellings following medical terms from the chapter to assist with pronunciation. The script also contains medical terms not presented in the chapter. Treat them as information only or look for their meanings in a medical dictionary or a reliable online source.

1. The **orthopedist** (or-thō-PĒ-dist) recommended Mr. Shah have an **arthrodesis** (*ar*-thrō-DĒ-sis) to reduce pain caused from an ankle **fracture** (FRAK-chur) he sustained several years ago.
2. Mrs. Diaz severed a tendon by accidentally walking through a glass patio door. A **tenorrhaphy** (te-NOR-a-fē) was performed to repair the tendon.
3. An **electromyogram** (e-*lek*-trō-MĪ-ō-gram) can assist the physician in diagnosing **muscular dystrophy** (MUS-kū-lar) (DIS-trō-fē). **Atrophy** (AT-rō-fē) frequently occurs in patients with this disease.
4. Adjective forms of medical terms are used by health professionals to indicate areas of the body that describe anatomic locations, areas of pain, sites of injections, locations of lesions, and so forth. Below are some examples.
   a. **cranial** (KRĀ-nē-al) laceration
   b. **intercostal** (*in*-ter-KOS-tal) muscles
   c. pain in the **subcostal** (sub-KOS-tal) region
   d. herniation of an **intervertebral** (*in*-ter-VER-te-bral) disk
   e. **intracranial** (*in*-tra-KRĀ-nē-al) pressure
   f. **femoral** (FEM-or-al) artery
   g. strain of the **ischiopubic** (*is*-kē-ō-PŪ-bik) area
   h. degenerative disease of the **sternoclavicular** (*ster*-nō-kla-VIK-ū-lar) joint

EXERCISE 48 *Use Plural Endings*

Circle the correct singular or plural term to match the context of the sentence.

1. The (**epiphysis, epiphyses**) are the enlarged ends of the long bone.
2. The distal (**phalanx, phalanges**) of the ring finger was fractured.
3. Osteoporosis was present in four lumbar (**vertebrae, vertebra**).
4. A (**prosthesis, prostheses**) was implanted in the left hip.
5. Many synovial joints contain (**bursa, bursae**).

EXERCISE 49 *Chapter Content Quiz*

Test your understanding of terms and abbreviations introduced in this chapter. Circle the letter for the medical term or abbreviation related to the words in italics.

1. Jessie Steinbach was diagnosed with *an infection caused by a bite from a deer tick infected with Borrelia burgdorferi*, after noting symptoms of fever, headache and joint pain. Her symptoms started after a camping trip last summer.
   a. rheumatoid arthritis
   b. Lyme disease
   c. rhabdomyolysis
2. Tommy John surgery, named after the first professional baseball player to have it performed, involves *suturing of a tendon* of the ulnar collateral ligament, usually with a graft from a different tendon in the body.
   a. tenomyoplasty
   b. myorrhaphy
   c. tenorrhaphy

3. Orthopedists may perform *visual examination of a joint* to diagnose and sometimes treat problems in the knee, shoulder, or elbow.
   a. arthroscopy
   b. arthrography
   c. arthrocentesis
4. Ever since his initial diagnosis of ankylosing spondylitis, James Montoya has been seeing a *physician who specializes in the study and treatment of rheumatic diseases*.
   a. podiatrist
   b. rheumatologist
   c. chiropractor
5. Dr. Lu ordered an electromyogram (EMG) for Mr. Borunda when he suspected *chronic disease characterized by muscle weakness and thought to be caused by a defect in the transmission of impulses from nerve to muscle.*
   a. muscular dystrophy
   b. meniscitis
   c. myasthenia gravis
6. A total hip *surgical repair of a joint* was recommended for Mrs. Jiang, when she could no longer tolerate the pain from her osteoarthritis.
   a. arthrodesis
   b. arthroplasty
   c. chondroplasty
7. Ayaz Ismail noticed ulnoradial pain whenever he was asked to put his forearm into *movement that turns the palm up*.
   a. pronation
   b. eversion
   c. supination
8. The physician assistant explained to Mrs. Hayashi that the imbalance of *type of bone cell involved in absorption and removal of bone minerals* and osteoblasts was the cause of her osteoporosis.
   a. osteopaths
   b. osteoclasts
   c. osteocytes
9. A(n) *excision of a lamina* was performed on Mr. Lopez, who had been experiencing spinal stenosis for many years.
   a. laminectomy
   b. synovectomy
   c. vertebroplasty
10. Dawn Labenz had special *making and fitting of orthopedic appliances, such as arch supports* made for her shoes after experiencing plantar fasciitis for the second time.
    a. orthopedics
    b. prostheses
    c. orthotics
11. Mr. O'Rourke had a radiograph of his knee to determine how much *inflammation of the bone and joint* was present.
    a. OA
    b. RA
    c. DO
12. Mrs. Jerue developed *abnormal condition of bone death* of the jaw after a rather difficult tooth extraction.
    a. osteomalacia
    b. osteopetrosis
    c. osteonecrosis
13. Natalie Pageau experienced left *pertaining to below the rib* pain after she was in an automobile accident; luckily, her spleen was found to be intact.
    a. costochondral
    b. subcostal
    c. intercostal
14. Mr. Sadowsky's symptoms of *slow movement* worsened as his Parkinson disease progressed.
    a. bradykinesia
    b. hyperkinesia
    c. hypertrophy
15. After his fall from a ladder, Adam Murphy had an emergency *incision into the cranium* to relieve intracranial pressure.
    a. cranioplasty
    b. craniotomy
    c. rachiotomy
16. Tyler Williams complained of pain and numbness in the *pertaining to the lumbar regions and the sacrum* area when the doctor placed his right hip into flexion and his knee into extension.
    a. lumbar
    b. lumbocostal
    c. lumbosacral
17. Mr. Cohen complained of chronic wrist *pain in the joint*. A plain radiograph showed soft tissue swelling along with erosions in the carpal bones. Arthrocentesis revealed monosodium urate crystals and confirmed the diagnosis of gout.
    a. atrophy
    b. arthralgia
    c. myalgia
18. An osteotomy or partial phalangectomy may be required during *abnormal prominence of the joint at the base of the great toe* surgery to realign the metatarsal-phalangeal joint.
    a. carpal tunnel syndrome
    b. exostosis
    c. bunion

19. Lily Chakraborty developed severe *abnormal condition of (lateral) curved (spine)* as a teen; a partial costectomy and other corrective surgery was performed with good results.
    a. scoliosis
    b. kyphosis
    c. lordosis

20. Dr. Nair advised Melanie Chua to increase her calcium and vitamin D intake after radiographs showed *abnormal reduction of bone mass* at the distal radial portion of her wrist.
    a. osteosarcoma
    b. osteofibroma
    c. osteopenia

CHAPTER REVIEW

REVIEW OF CHAPTER CONTENT ON EVOLVE RESOURCES

Go to evolve.elsevier.com and click on Gradable Student Resources and Practice Student Resources. Online learning activities found there can be used to review chapter content and to assess your learning of word parts, medical terms, and abbreviations. Place check marks in the boxes next to activities used for review and assessment.

GRADABLE STUDENT RESOURCES

Chapter 14 >	Exercises >	□ Word Parts □ Terms Built from Word Parts □ Terms Not Built from Word Parts □ Abbreviations
	Quizzes >	□ Quiz 1: Disease and Disorder Terms □ Quiz 2: Surgical Terms □ Quiz 3: Complementary Terms

PRACTICE STUDENT RESOURCES > STUDENT RESOURCES

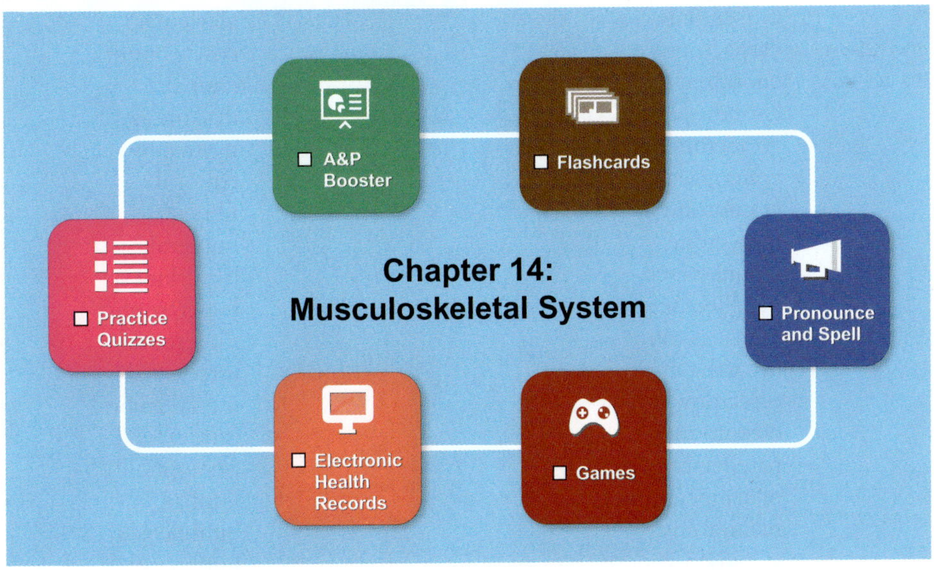

REVIEW OF WORD PARTS

Can you define and spell the following word parts?

COMBINING FORMS					PREFIXES	SUFFIXES
ankyl/o	disk/o	lumb/o	petr/o	synovi/o	inter-	-asthenia
aponeur/o	femor/o	mandibul/o	phalang/o	tars/o	supra-	-desis
arthr/o	fibul/o	maxill/o	pub/o	ten/o	sym-	-physis
burs/o	humer/o	menisc/o	rachi/o	tend/o	syn-	-schisis
carp/o	ili/o	my/o	radi/o	tendin/o		-trophy
chondr/o	ischi/o	myel/o	sacr/o	tibi/o		
clavic/o	kinesi/o	myos/o	sarc/o	uln/o		
clavicul/o	kyph/o	oste/o	scapul/o	vertebr/o		
cost/o	lamin/o	patell/o	scoli/o			
crani/o	lord/o	pelv/i	spondyl/o			
			stern/o			

REVIEW OF TERMS

Can you define, pronounce, and spell the following terms *built from word parts?*

DISEASES AND DISORDERS	SURGICAL	DIAGNOSTIC	COMPLEMENTARY	
ankylosis	aponeurorrhaphy	arthrography	arthralgia	osteoblast
arthritis	arthrocentesis	arthroscopy	atrophy	osteocyte
bursitis	arthrodesis	electromyogram (EMG)	bradykinesia	osteonecrosis
chondromalacia	arthroplasty		carpal	pelvic
cranioschisis	bursectomy		clavicular	pubic
diskitis	carpectomy		costochondral	radial
fibromyalgia	chondrectomy		cranial	sacral
kyphosis	chondroplasty		dyskinesia	sternoclavicular
lordosis	costectomy		dystrophy	sternoid
maxillitis	cranioplasty		femoral	subcostal
meniscitis	craniotomy		fibular	submandibular
myasthenia	diskectomy		humeral	submaxillary
myeloma	laminectomy		hyperkinesia	subscapular
osteitis	maxillectomy		hypertrophy	substernal
osteoarthritis (OA)	meniscectomy		iliofemoral	suprapatellar
osteochondritis	myorrhaphy		intercostal	suprascapular
osteofibroma	ostectomy		intervertebral	symphysis
osteomalacia	osteotomy		intracranial	tibial
osteomyelitis	patellectomy		ischiopubic	ulnoradial
osteopenia	phalangectomy		lumbar	vertebrocostal
osteopetrosis	rachiotomy		lumbocostal	
osteosarcoma	spondylosyndesis		lumbosacral	
polymyositis	synovectomy		myalgia	
rachischisis	tarsectomy			
rhabdomyolysis	tenomyoplasty			
sarcopenia	tenorrhaphy			
scoliosis	vertebroplasty			
spondylarthritis				
spondylosis				
synoviosarcoma				
tendinitis				
tenosynovitis				

Can you define, pronounce, and spell the following terms *NOT built from word parts?*

DISEASES AND DISORDERS	COMPLEMENTARY	TYPES OF BODY MOVEMENTS
ankylosing spondylitis	chiropractic	abduction
bunion	chiropractor (DC)	adduction
carpal tunnel syndrome (CTS)	crepitus	eversion
Colles fracture	orthopedics (Ortho)	extension
exostosis	orthopedist	flexion
fracture (fx)	orthotics	inversion
gout	orthotist	pronation
herniated disk	osteoclast	rotation
Lyme disease	osteopath (DO)	supination
muscular dystrophy (MD)	osteopathy	
myasthenia gravis (MG)	podiatrist	
osteoporosis	prosthesis (pl. prostheses)	
plantar fasciitis	rheumatologist	
rheumatoid arthritis (RA)	rheumatology	
spinal stenosis		
spondylolisthesis		

Chapter 15

Nervous System and Behavioral Health

Objectives

Upon completion of this chapter you will be able to:

1. Pronounce organs and anatomic structures of the nervous system.
2. Define and spell word parts related to the nervous system.
3. Define, pronounce, and spell disease and disorder terms related to the nervous system.
4. Define, pronounce, and spell surgical terms related to the nervous system.
5. Define, pronounce, and spell diagnostic terms related to the nervous system.
6. Define, pronounce, and spell complementary terms related to the nervous system.
7. Define, pronounce, and spell behavioral health terms.
8. Interpret the meaning of abbreviations related to the nervous system and behavioral health.
9. Apply medical language in clinical contexts.

Outline

ANATOMY

The nervous system consists of the brain, spinal cord, and nerves and may be divided into two parts: the **central nervous system** (CNS) and the **peripheral nervous system** (PNS). The central nervous system consists of the brain and spinal cord. The peripheral nervous system is the collection of spinal and cranial nerves, whose branches infiltrate virtually all parts of the body, conveying messages to and from the CNS (Figs. 15.1 and 15.2).

Function

The nervous system forms a complex communication system allowing for the coordination of body functions and activities. The nervous system can also be divided into two parts from a functional standpoint. The somatic nervous system is responsible for sending signals to the skeletal (voluntary) muscles and receives input from the senses. The autonomic nervous system generally operates on a "subconscious" level, meaning it governs itself without our conscious knowledge. It sends signals to the "involuntary" tissues, which include smooth muscles, cardiac muscles, glands, and fat. These tissues have receptors that send autonomic signals back to the brain and spinal cord. As a whole, the nervous system is designed to detect changes inside and outside the body, to evaluate this sensory information, and to send directions to muscles or glands in response. This system also provides for mental activities such as thought, memory, and emotions.

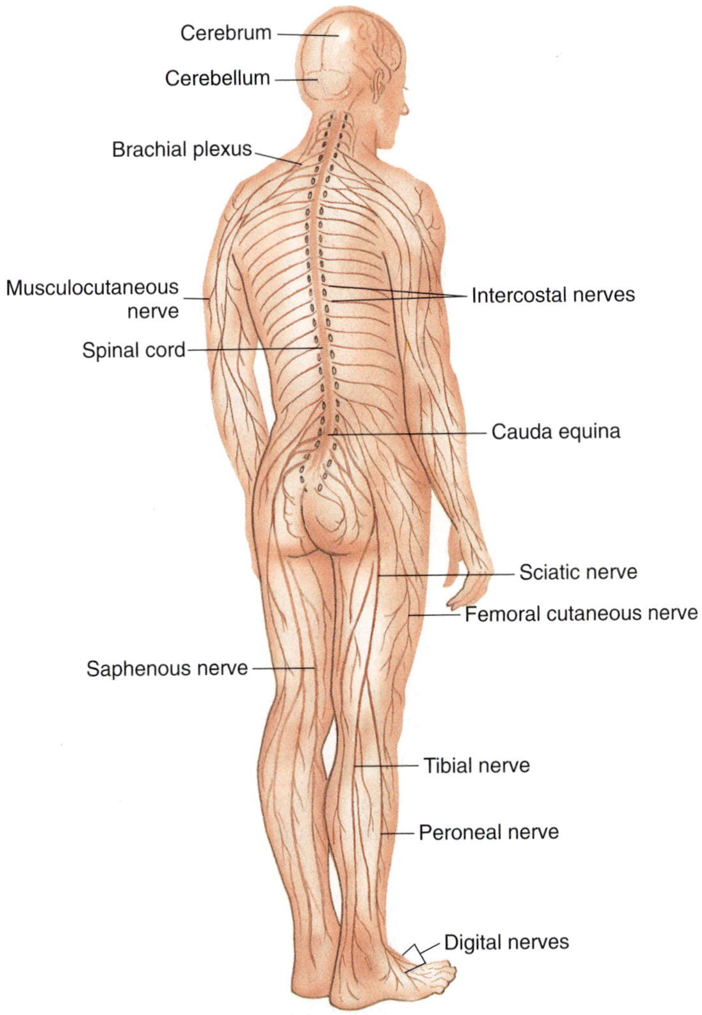

FIG. 15.1 Simplified view of the nervous system.

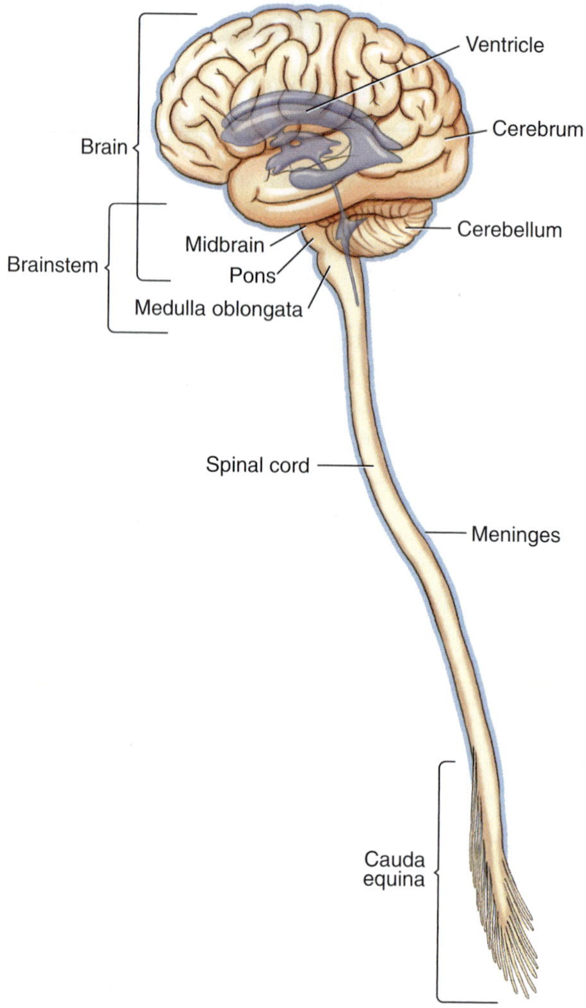

FIG. 15.2 Brain and spinal cord.

Organs and Anatomic Structures of the Nervous System

TERM	DEFINITION
brain (brān)	contained within the cranium, the center for coordinating body activities and comprises the cerebrum, cerebellum, and brainstem; the brainstem contains the pons, medulla oblongata, and midbrain (Fig. 15.2)
cerebrum (se-RĒ-brum)	largest portion of the brain, divided into left and right hemispheres. The cerebrum controls the skeletal muscles, interprets general senses (such as temperature, pain, and touch), and contains centers for sight and hearing. Intellect, memory, and emotional reactions also take place in the cerebrum.
ventricles (VEN-tri-kulz)	cavities (spaces) within the brain that contain **cerebrospinal fluid (CSF)**. The cerebrospinal fluid flows through the subarachnoid space around the brain and spinal cord.
cerebellum (*ser*-a-BEL-um)	located under the posterior portion of the cerebrum; assists in the coordination of skeletal muscles to maintain balance (also called **hindbrain**)

TERM	DEFINITION
brainstem (BRĀN-stem)	stemlike portion of the brain that connects with the spinal cord; contains centers that control respiration and heart rate. Three structures comprise the brainstem: pons, medulla oblongata, and midbrain.
pons (ponz)	literally means **bridge**. It connects the cerebrum with the cerebellum and brainstem.
medulla oblongata (ma-DŪL-a) (*ob*-long-GAH-ta)	located between the pons and spinal cord. It contains centers that control respiration, heart rate, and the muscles in the blood vessel walls, which assist in determining blood pressure.
midbrain (MID-brān)	most superior portion of the brainstem
cerebrospinal fluid (CSF) (*ser*-ē-brō-SPĪ-nal) (FLOO-id)	clear, colorless fluid contained in the ventricles that flows through the subarachnoid space around the brain and spinal cord. It cushions the brain and spinal cord from shock, transports nutrients, and clears metabolic waste.
spinal cord (SPĪ-nal) (kord)	passes through the vertebral canal extending from the medulla oblongata to the level of the second lumbar vertebra. The spinal cord conducts nerve impulses to and from the brain and initiates reflex action to sensory information without input from the brain.
meninges (me-NIN-jēz)	three layers of membrane that cover the brain and spinal cord (Fig. 15.3)
dura mater (DUR-a) (MĀ-ter)	tough outer layer of the meninges
arachnoid (a-RAK-noid)	delicate middle layer of the meninges. The arachnoid membrane is loosely attached to the pia mater by weblike fibers, which allow for the **subarachnoid space**.
pia mater (PĒ-a) (MĀ-ter)	thin inner layer of the meninges

CEREBELLUM

was named in the third century BC by Erasistratus, who also named the cerebrum. **Cerebellum** literally means **little brain** and is the diminutive of **cerebrum**, meaning **brain**. Although it was named long ago, its function was not understood until the nineteenth century.

MENINGES

were first named by a Persian physician in the tenth century. When translated into Latin, they became **dura mater**, meaning **hard mother** (because it is a tough membrane), and **pia mater**, meaning **soft mother** (because it is a delicate membrane). **Mater** was used because the Arabians believed that the meninges were the mother of all other body membranes.

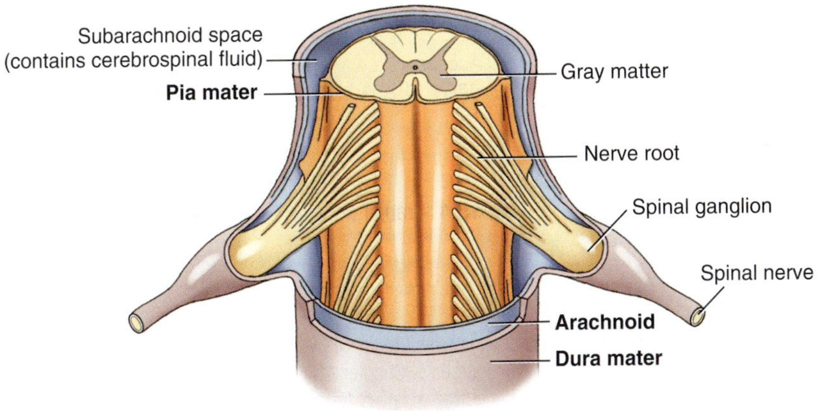

FIG. 15.3 Layers of meninges.

Organs and Anatomic Structures of the Nervous System—cont'd

TERM	DEFINITION
nerve (nurv)	cordlike structure made up of fibers that carries impulses from one part of the body to another. There are 12 pairs of cranial nerves and 31 pairs of spinal nerves (Figs. 15.1 and 15.4).
ganglion (pl. ganglia) (GANG-glē-on) (GANG-glē-a)	group of nerve cell bodies located outside the central nervous system
glia (GLĒ-a)	specialized cells that support and nourish nervous tissue. Some cells assist in the secretion of cerebrospinal fluid and others assist with phagocytosis. They do not conduct impulses. Schwann cells are glial cells in the peripheral nervous system. Types of glia in the central nervous system include **ependymal cells, astroglia, oligodendroglia,** and **microglia.** (also called **neuroglia**)
neuron (NŪR-on)	nerve cell that conducts nerve impulses to carry out the function of the nervous system. Destroyed neurons in the central nervous system cannot be replaced.

GLIA
the Greek word for **glue**, were named in 1856 by the pathologist Rudolph Virchow. These gelatinous cells were originally credited with holding the nerves together. Today we know that they perform many more tasks in the brain and spinal cord.

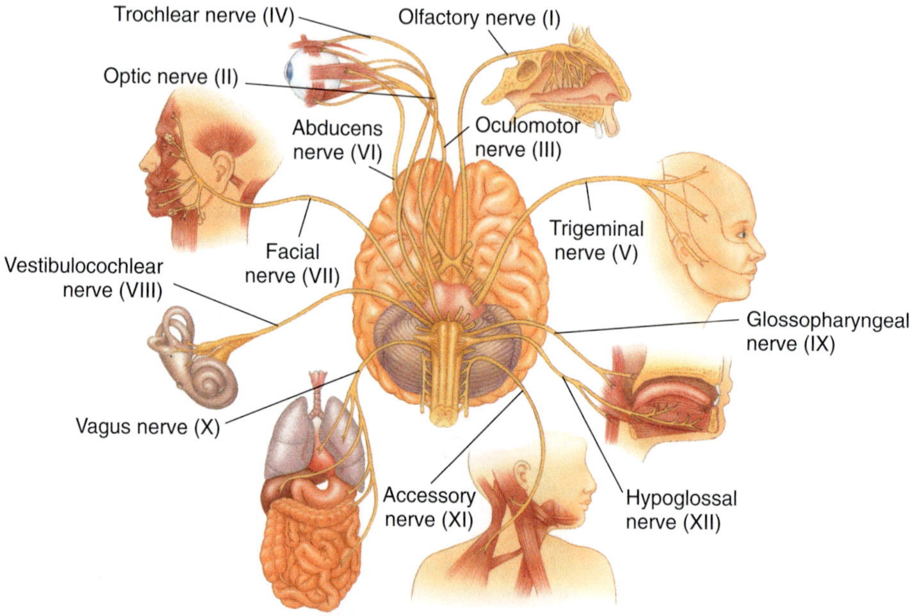

FIG. 15.4 Cranial nerves.

A&P Booster
For more anatomy and physiology, go to Evolve Resources at evolve.elsevier.com and select: Practice Student Resources > Student Resources > Chapter 15 > **A&P Booster**

See Appendix B for instructions.

EXERCISE 1

Practice saying aloud each of the Organs and Anatomic Structures of the Nervous System.

To hear the terms, go to Evolve Resources at evolve.elsevier.com and select:
Practice Student Resources > Student Resources > Chapter 15 > **Pronounce and Spell**

See Appendix B for instructions.

❑ Check the box when complete.

WORD PARTS

Word parts you need to learn to complete this chapter are listed on the following pages. The exercises at the end of each list will help you learn their definitions and spellings.

Use the flashcards accompanying this text or electronic flashcards to assist you in memorizing the word parts for this chapter.

Combining Forms of the Nervous System

COMBINING FORM	DEFINITION
cerebell/o	cerebellum
cerebr/o	cerebrum, brain
dur/o	hard, dura mater
encephal/o	brain
gangli/o, ganglion/o	ganglion
gli/o	glia
mening/o, meningi/o	meninges
myel/o	spinal cord *(Note: myel/o also means bone marrow; see Chapter 14.)*
neur/o	nerve *(Note: neur/o was introduced in Chapter 2.)*
radic/o, radicul/o, rhiz/o	nerve root (proximal end of a peripheral nerve, closest to the spinal cord)

EXERCISE 2

A. Fill in the blanks with combining forms in this diagram of the brain and spinal cord. *To check your answers, go to Appendix A.*

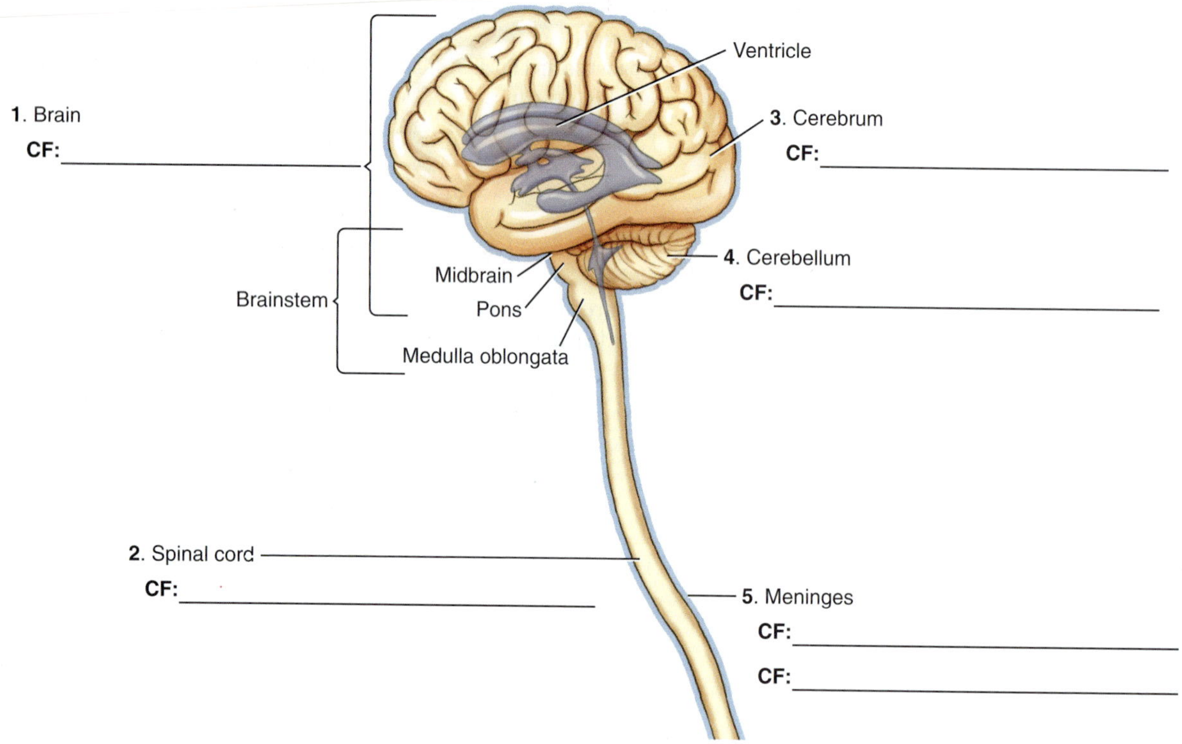

B. Fill in the blanks with combining forms in this diagram of the spinal cord and layers of meninges.

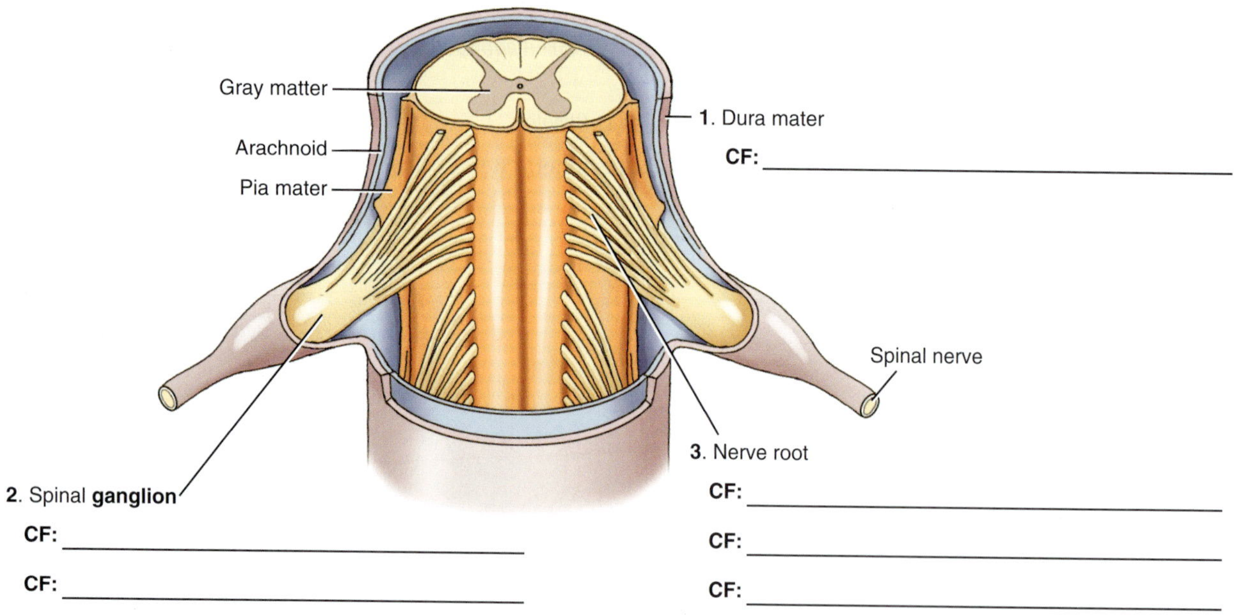

C. Write the combining form for the following definitions.

1. glia ______ 2. nerve ______

EXERCISE 3

Step 1: Write the definitions after the following combining forms.

Step 2: Match the descriptions on the right with the combining forms and definitions.

_____ 1. gangli/o, ______________________

_____ 2. dur/o, ______________________

_____ 3. encephal/o, ______________________

_____ 4. cerebell/o, ______________________

_____ 5. meningi/o, ______________________

_____ 6. neur/o, ______________________

a. assists in the coordination of skeletal muscles to maintain balance

b. cordlike structure made up of fibers that carries impulses from one part of the body to another

c. contained within the cranium, the center for coordinating body activities

d. tough outer layer of the meninges

e. group of nerve cell bodies located outside the central nervous system

f. three layers of membrane that cover the brain and spinal cord

EXERCISE 4

Step 1: Write the definitions after the following combining forms.

Step 2: Match the descriptions on the right with the combining forms and definitions.

_____ 1. gli/o, ______________________

_____ 2. ganglion/o, ______________________

_____ 3. mening/o, ______________________

_____ 4. cerebr/o, ______________________

_____ 5. myel/o, ______________________

a. conducts impulses to and from the brain and initiates reflex action to sensory information

b. specialized cells that support and nourish nervous tissue

c. largest portion of the brain, divided into left and right hemispheres

d. group of nerve cell bodies located outside the central nervous system

e. three layers of membrane that cover the brain and spinal cord

EXERCISE 5

Write the combining forms for the following term.

1. nerve root
   a. ______________________
   b. ______________________
   c. ______________________

Combining Forms Commonly Used With Nervous System Terms

COMBINING FORM	DEFINITION
esthesi/o	sensation, sensitivity, feeling
ment/o, psych/o	mind
mon/o	one, single
phas/o	speech
poli/o	gray matter
quadr/i	four *(Note: an i is the combining vowel in quadr/i.)*

EXERCISE 6

Write the definitions of the following combining forms.

1. mon/o ______________________
2. psych/o ______________________
3. quadr/i ______________________
4. ment/o ______________________
5. phas/o ______________________
6. esthesi/o ______________________
7. poli/o ______________________

EXERCISE 7

Write the combining form for each of the following.

1. four ______________________
2. one, single ______________________
3. mind a. ______________________
   b. ______________________
4. speech ______________________
5. gray matter ______________________
6. sensation, sensitivity, feeling ______________________

Suffixes

SUFFIX	DEFINITION
-iatrist	specialist, physician (*-logist* also means specialist, was covered in Chapter 2)
-iatry	treatment, specialty
-ictal	seizure, attack
-paresis	slight paralysis (*-plegia*, meaning *paralysis*, was covered in Chapter 12)

EXERCISE 8

Write the definitions of the following suffixes.

1. -paresis ______________________
2. -iatry ______________________
3. -ictal ______________________
4. -iatrist ______________________

EXERCISE 9

Write the suffix for each of the following.

1. slight paralysis ____________
2. treatment, specialty ____________
3. seizure, attack ____________
4. specialist, physician ____________

For additional practice with Word Parts, go to Evolve Resources at evolve.elsevier.com and select:
Practice Student Resources > Student Resources > Chapter 15 > **Flashcards**

See Appendix B for instructions.

MEDICAL TERMS

Disease and Disorder Terms

BUILT FROM WORD PARTS

The following terms can be translated using definitions of word parts. Further explanation is provided within parentheses as needed.

TERM	DEFINITION
cerebellitis (*ser*-e-bel-Ī-tis)	inflammation of the cerebellum
cerebral thrombosis (se-RĒ-bral) (throm-BŌ-sis)	pertaining to the cerebrum, abnormal condition of a clot (blood clot in a blood vessel of the brain. Onset of symptoms may appear from minutes to days after an obstruction occurs; a cause of **ischemic stroke**.)
duritis (dū-RĪ-tis)	inflammation of the dura mater
encephalitis (en-*sef*-a-LĪ-tis)	inflammation of the brain
encephalomalacia (en-*sef*-a-lō-ma-LĀ-sha)	softening of the brain
encephalomyeloradiculitis (en-*sef*-a-lō-*mī*-e-lō-ra-*dik*-ū-LĪ-tis)	inflammation of the brain, spinal cord, and nerve roots
gangliitis (*gang*-glē-Ī-tis)	inflammation of a ganglion
glioblastoma (*glī*-ō-blas-TŌ-ma)	tumor composed of developing glia (the most malignant primary tumor of the brain) (Fig. 15.5)
glioma (glī-Ō-ma)	tumor composed of glia. (Gliomas can develop from any of the four types of glial cells, or from their developing cells.)
meningioma (me-*nin*-jē-Ō-ma)	tumor of the meninges (usually benign and slow growing; most common tumor originating in the brain and surrounding tissues)

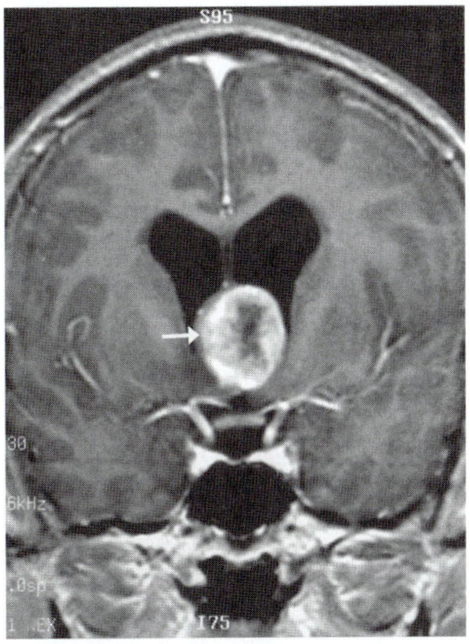

FIG. 15.5 MRI image of brain demonstrating glioblastoma *(arrow)*.

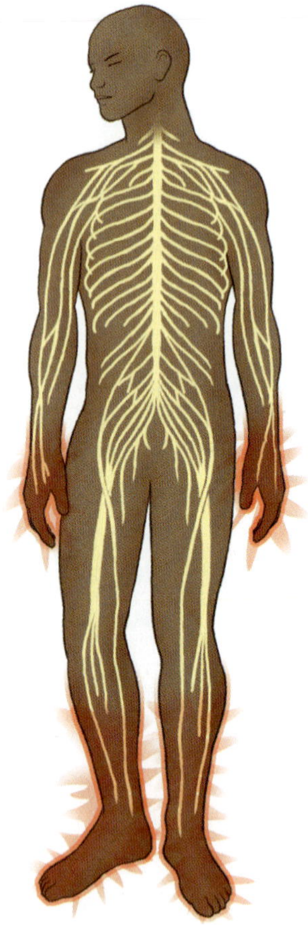
FIG. 15.6 Peripheral neuropathy.

PERIPHERAL NEUROPATHY

refers to disorders of the peripheral nervous system, including **radiculopathy**, **mononeuropathy**, and **polyneuropathy**.

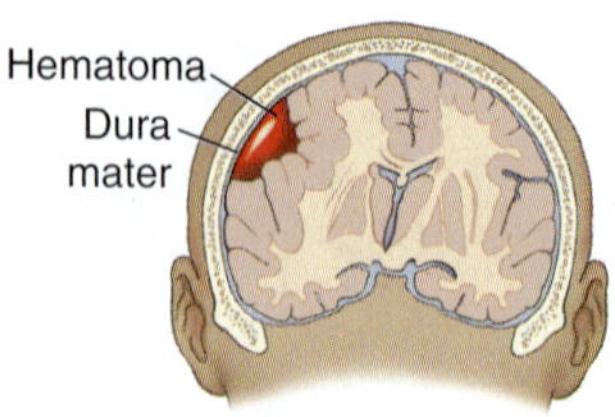

FIG. 15.7 Subdural hematoma.

Disease and Disorder Terms—cont'd

TERM	DEFINITION
meningitis (*men*-in-JĪ-tis)	inflammation of the meninges
meningocele (me-NING-gō-sēl)	protrusion of the meninges (through a defect in the skull or vertebral arch)
meningomyelocele (me-*ning*-gō-MĪ-e-lō-*sēl*)	protrusion of the meninges and spinal cord (through a neural arch defect in the vertebral column) (also called **myelomeningocele**) (see Fig. 9.10)
mononeuropathy (*mon*-ō-nū-ROP-a-thē)	disease affecting a single nerve (such as carpal tunnel syndrome)
neuralgia (nū-RAL-ja)	pain in a nerve
neuritis (nū-RĪ-tis)	inflammation of a nerve
neuroarthropathy (*nū*-rō-ar-THROP-a-thē)	disease of nerves and joints
neuropathy (nū-ROP-a-thē)	disease of the nerves (peripheral) (Fig. 15.6)
poliomyelitis (*pō*-lē-ō-*mī*-e-LĪ-tis)	inflammation of the gray matter of the spinal cord. (This infectious disease, commonly referred to as *polio*, is caused by one of three polio viruses.)
polyneuritis (*pol*-ē-nū-RĪ-tis)	inflammation of many nerves
polyneuropathy (*pol*-ē-nū-ROP-a-thē)	disease of many nerves (most often occurs as a complication of diabetes mellitus, but may also occur as a result of drug therapy, critical illness such as sepsis, or carcinoma; exhibiting symptoms of weakness, distal sensory loss, and burning)
radiculitis (ra-*dik*-ū-LĪ-tis)	inflammation of the nerve roots
radiculopathy (ra-*dik*-ū-LOP-a-thē)	disease of the nerve roots
rhizomeningomyelitis (*rī*-zō-me-*ning*-gō-*mī*-e-LĪ-tis)	inflammation of the nerve root, meninges, and spinal cord
subdural hematoma (sub-DŪ-ral) (*hē*-ma-TŌ-ma)	pertaining to below the dura mater, tumor of blood (*hematoma*, translated literally, means *blood tumor;* however, a hematoma is a collection of blood resulting from a broken blood vessel) (Fig. 15.7)

EXERCISE 10

Practice saying aloud each of the Disease and Disorder Terms Built from Word Parts

To hear the terms, go to Evolve Resources at evolve.elsevier.com and select:
Practice Student Resources > Student Resources > Chapter 15 > **Pronounce and Spell**

See Appendix B for instructions.

❑ Check the box when complete.

EXERCISE 11

Analyze and define the following terms.

1. neuritis
2. neuralgia
3. neuroarthropathy
4. meningioma
5. encephalomalacia
6. encephalitis
7. encephalomyeloradiculitis
8. meningitis
9. meningocele
10. meningomyelocele
11. radiculitis
12. cerebellitis
13. gangliitis
14. duritis

15. polyneuritis

____
____

16. poliomyelitis

____
____

17. cerebral thrombosis

____
____

18. subdural hematoma

____
____

19. rhizomeningomyelitis

____
____

20. mononeuropathy

____
____

21. neuropathy

____
____

22. radiculopathy

____
____

23. glioma

____
____

24. glioblastoma

____
____

25. polyneuropathy

____
____

EXERCISE 12

Build disease and disorder terms for the following definitions with the word parts you have learned.

1. inflammation of the nerve ______ / ______
WR / S

2. pain in a nerve ______ / ______
WR / S

3. disease of nerves and joints ______ / ____ / ______ / ____ / ______
WR / CV / WR / CV / S

4. disease of the nerve roots ______ / ____ / ______
WR / CV / S

5. softening of the brain ______ / ____ / ______
WR / CV / S

6. inflammation of the brain ______ / ______
WR / S

7. inflammation of the brain, spinal cord, and nerve roots

WR / CV / WR / CV / WR / S

8. inflammation of the meninges

WR / S

9. protrusion of the meninges (through a defect in the skull or vertebral column)

WR / CV / S

10. protrusion of the meninges and spinal cord (through the vertebral column)

WR / CV / WR / CV / S

11. inflammation of the nerve roots

WR / S

12. inflammation of the cerebellum

WR / S

13. inflammation of a ganglion

WR / S

14. inflammation of the dura mater

WR / S

15. inflammation of many nerves

P / WR / S

16. inflammation of the gray matter of the spinal cord

WR / CV / WR / S

17. pertaining to the cerebrum; abnormal condition of a clot

WR / S ; WR / S

18. pertaining to below the dura mater; tumor of blood

P / WR / S ; WR / S

19. inflammation of the nerve root, meninges, and spinal cord

WR / CV / WR / CV / WR / S

20. tumor of the meninges

WR / S

21. disease affecting a single nerve

WR / CV / WR / CV / S

22. disease of the nerves

WR / CV / S

23. tumor composed of glia

WR / S

24. tumor composed of developing glia

WR / CV / WR / S

25. disease of many nerves

P / WR / CV / S

EXERCISE 13

Spell each of the Disease and Disorder Terms Built from Word Parts by having someone dictate them to you. Use a separate sheet of paper.

To hear and spell the terms, go to Evolve Resources at evolve.elsevier.com and select:
Practice Student Resources > Student Resources > Chapter 15 > **Pronounce and Spell**

See Appendix B for instructions.

❑ Check the box when complete.

Disease and Disorder Terms
NOT BUILT FROM WORD PARTS

Word parts may be present in the following terms; however, their full meanings cannot be translated using definitions of word parts alone.

TERM	DEFINITION
Alzheimer disease (AD) (AWLTZ-hī-mer) (di-ZĒZ)	type of dementia that occurs more frequently after the age of 65, but can begin at any age. The brain shrinks dramatically as nerve cells die and tissues atrophy. The disease is slowly progressive and usually results in profound dementia in 5 to 10 years. A prominent feature of AD is the inability to remember the recent past, while memories of the distant past remain intact.
amyotrophic lateral sclerosis (ALS) (ā-mī-ō-TRŌ-fik) (LAT-er-al) (skle-RŌ-sis)	progressive muscle atrophy caused by degeneration and scarring of neurons along the lateral columns of the spinal cord that control muscles (also called **Lou Gehrig disease**)
Bell palsy (bel) (PAWL-zē)	paralysis of muscles on one side of the face caused by inflammation or compression of the facial nerve—cranial nerve VII. Signs include a sagging mouth on the affected side and nonclosure of the eyelid; paralysis is usually temporary.
cerebral aneurysm (se-RĒ-bral) (AN-ū-rizm)	aneurysm in the cerebrum. It is usually asymptomatic until it ruptures, which can be very serious and can result in death.
cerebral embolism (se-RĒ-bral) (EM-bō-lizm)	an embolus (usually a blood clot or a piece of atherosclerotic plaque arising from a distant site) lodges in a cerebral artery, causing sudden blockage of blood supply to the brain tissue. Atrial fibrillation is a common cause of cerebral embolism, which can lead to **ischemic stroke.**
cerebral palsy (CP) (se-RĒ-bral) (PAWL-zē)	condition characterized by lack of muscle control and partial paralysis, caused by a brain defect or lesion present at birth or shortly after
dementia (de-MEN-sha)	cognitive impairment characterized by loss of intellectual brain function. Patients have difficulty in various ways, including difficulty in performing complex tasks, reasoning, learning and retaining new information, orientation, word finding, and behavior. Dementia has several causes and is not considered part of normal aging (Table 15.1).

TERM	DEFINITION
epilepsy (EP-i-lep-sē)	condition characterized by recurrent seizures; a general term given to a group of neurologic disorders, all characterized by abnormal electrical activity in the brain
hydrocephalus (*hī*-drō-SEF-a-lus)	congenital or acquired disorder caused by obstructed circulation of cerebrospinal fluid, resulting in dilated cerebral ventricles and impaired brain function. For infants, hydrocephalus can cause enlargement of the cranium.
intracerebral hemorrhage (*in*-tra-SER-e-bral) (HEM-o-rij)	bleeding into the brain as a result of a ruptured blood vessel within the brain. Symptoms vary depending on the location of the hemorrhage; acute symptoms include dyspnea, dysphagia, aphasia, diminished level of consciousness, and hemiparesis. The symptoms often develop suddenly. Intracerebral hemorrhage, a cause of **hemorrhagic stroke,** is frequently associated with high blood pressure.
multiple sclerosis (MS) (MUL-ti-pl) (skle-RŌ-sis)	chronic degenerative disease characterized by sclerotic patches along the brain and spinal cord; signs and symptoms fluctuate over the course of the disease; more common symptoms include fatigue, balance and coordination impairments, numbness, and vision problems
Parkinson disease (PD) (PAR-kin-sun) (di-ZĒZ)	chronic degenerative disease of the central nervous system. Signs and symptoms include resting tremors of the hands and feet, rigidity, expressionless face, shuffling gait, and eventually dementia. It usually occurs after the age of 50 years. (also called **parkinsonism**)
sciatica (sī-AT-i-ka)	inflammation of the sciatic nerve, causing pain that travels from the thigh through the leg to the foot and toes; can be caused by injury, infection, arthritis, herniated disk, or from prolonged pressure on the nerve from sitting for long periods
shingles (SHING-gelz)	viral disease that affects the peripheral nerves and causes blisters on the skin that follow the course of the affected nerves (also called **herpes zoster**)
stroke (strōk)	interruption of blood supply to a region of the brain, depriving nerve cells in the affected area of oxygen and nutrients. The cells cannot perform and may be damaged or die within minutes. The parts of the body controlled by the involved cells will experience dysfunction. Speech, movement, memory, and other CNS functions may be affected in varying degrees. **Ischemic stroke** is a result of a blocked blood vessel. **Hemorrhagic stroke** is a result of bleeding. (also called **cerebrovascular accident [CVA],** or **brain attack**)

EPILEPSY

was written about by Hippocrates, in 400 BC, in a book titled **Sacred Disease**. It was believed at one time that epilepsy was a punishment for offending the gods. The Greek **epilepsia** meant **seizure** and is derived from **epi**, meaning upon, and **lambanein**, meaning **to seize**. The term literally means **seized upon** (by the gods).

HYDROCEPHALUS

literally means **water in the head** and is made of the word parts **hydro**, meaning **water**, and **cephal**, meaning **head**. The condition was first described around 30 AD in the book **De Medicina**.

PARKINSON DISEASE

was first described by James Parkinson, an English professor, in his **Essay on the Shaking Palsy** in 1817.

POSTHERPETIC NEURALGIA

is a complication of **shingles** (herpes zoster) and is caused by damage to the nerve fibers. Severe pain and hyperesthesia persist after the skin lesions disappear and may last months or even years.

Disease and Disorder Terms—cont'd

TERM	DEFINITION
subarachnoid hemorrhage (SAH) (*sub*-e-RAK-noid) (HEM-o-rij)	bleeding between the pia mater and arachnoid layers of the meninges (subarachnoid space), caused by a ruptured blood vessel (usually a cerebral aneurysm). The patient may experience an intense, sudden headache accompanied by nausea, vomiting, and neck pain. SAH is a critical condition which must be recognized and treated immediately to prevent permanent brain damage or death. (a cause of **hemorrhagic stroke**)
transient ischemic attack (TIA) (TRAN-sē-ent) (is-KĒ-mik) (a-TAK)	sudden deficient supply of blood to the brain lasting a short time. The symptoms may be similar to those of stroke, but with TIA the symptoms are temporary and the usual outcome is complete recovery. TIAs are often warning signs for eventual occurrence of a stroke.

TABLE 15.1 Types of Dementia

COMMON TYPES OF DEMENTIA	
Alzheimer disease	most common type of dementia, responsible for 60% to 80% of all cases. The disease, which appears to be due to a variety of causes, is a progressive neurodegenerative disorder characterized by diffuse brain atrophy and the presence of senile plaques and neurofibrillary tangles within the brain cortex. Women are affected more than men, possibly because women tend to live longer, and because the chances of having AD double with every 5 additional years of life after age 65.
Vascular or multiple infarct dementia	affects approximately 10% of patients with dementia. It is secondary to cerebrovascular disease and usually occurs in older patients. Dementia usually worsens in a step-wise fashion, and other neurological findings (like paralysis or cranial nerve abnormalities) are often present.
Lewy body dementia	usually a rapidly progressive form of dementia which is responsible for approximately 10% of all dementias. Lewy body dementia is characterized by hallucinations, fluctuations in severity, sleep disorders, and Parkinson symptoms, the latter of which occur less than one year before the dementia.
Parkinson dementia	generally does not develop until patients have advanced Parkinson disease; similar to Lewy body dementia
Frontotemporal dementia (Pick disease)	affects the anterior portions of the brain; most common symptoms are personality changes, disinhibition, and impulsiveness. Atrophy may be observed on brain CT or MRI.
LESS COMMON FORMS OF DEMENTIA	
Normal pressure hydrocephalus	imbalance of cerebrospinal fluid in the brain leads to a triad of dementia, urinary incontinence, and gait instability. Sometimes caused by trauma or subarachnoid hemorrhage; can be treated with a ventricular peritoneal shunt
Wernicke-Korsakoff syndrome	form of dementia found with chronic alcoholism; caused by thiamine deficiency and poor nutritional status
Infections	including Creutzfeldt-Jakob disease, HIV infection, syphilis, and tuberculosis
Tumors and chronic subdural hematomas	space-occupying lesions that prevent normal brain function

EXERCISE 14

Practice saying aloud each of the Disease and Disorder Terms NOT Built from Word Parts.

To hear the terms, go to Evolve Resources at evolve.elsevier.com and select:
Practice Student Resources > Student Resources > Chapter 15 > **Pronounce and Spell**

See Appendix B for instructions.

❑ Check the box when complete.

EXERCISE 15

A. Match the terms in the first column with the definitions in the second column.

_____ 1. multiple sclerosis
_____ 2. epilepsy
_____ 3. cerebral palsy
_____ 4. Parkinson disease
_____ 5. amyotrophic lateral sclerosis
_____ 6. dementia
_____ 7. hydrocephalus

a. condition characterized by lack of muscle control and partial paralysis, caused by a brain defect or a lesion present at birth or shortly after
b. progressive muscle atrophy caused by degeneration and scarring of neurons along the lateral columns of the spinal cord
c. cognitive impairment characterized by loss of intellectual brain function; not considered part of normal aging
d. chronic degenerative disease characterized by sclerotic patches along the brain and spinal cord
e. disorder caused by obstructed circulation of cerebrospinal fluid, resulting in dilated cerebral ventricles and impaired brain function
f. chronic degenerative disease of the central nervous system, characterized by resting tremors of the hands and feet, rigidity, expressionless face, shuffling gait, and dementia
g. condition characterized by recurrent seizures

B. Write the medical term pictured and defined.

1. ______________________________
sudden deficient supply of blood to the brain lasting a short time

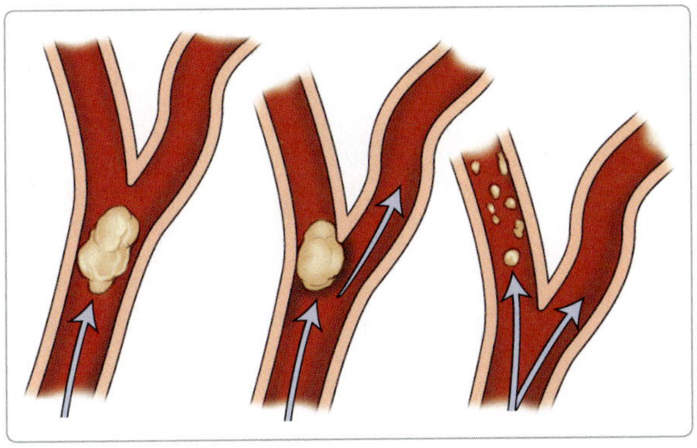

2. ______________________________
paralysis of muscles on one side of the face caused by inflammation or compression of the facial nerve

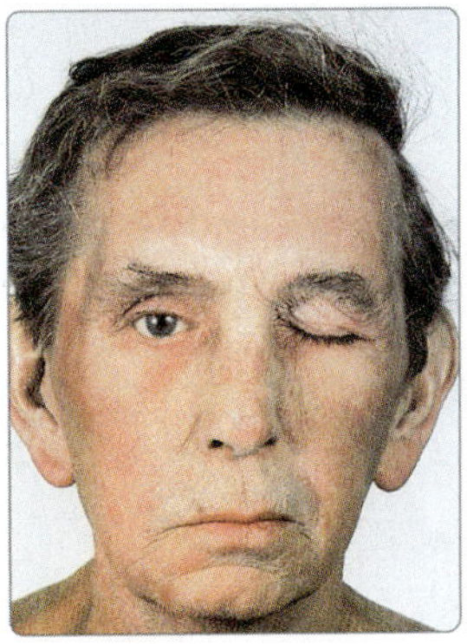

EXERCISE 15 *Pictured and Defined—cont'd*

3. ______________________________
inflammation of the sciatic nerve, causing pain that travels from the thigh through the leg to the foot and toes

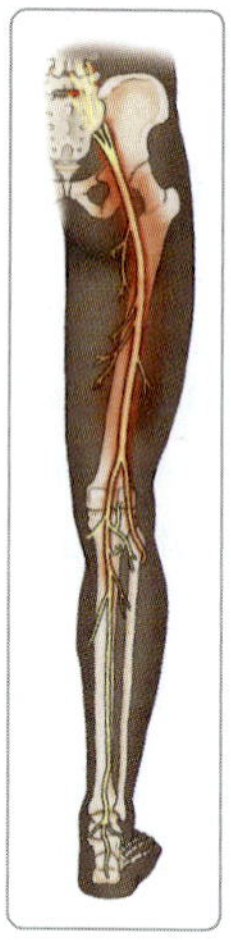

4. ______________________________
type of dementia that occurs more frequently after the age of 65; the brain shrinks dramatically

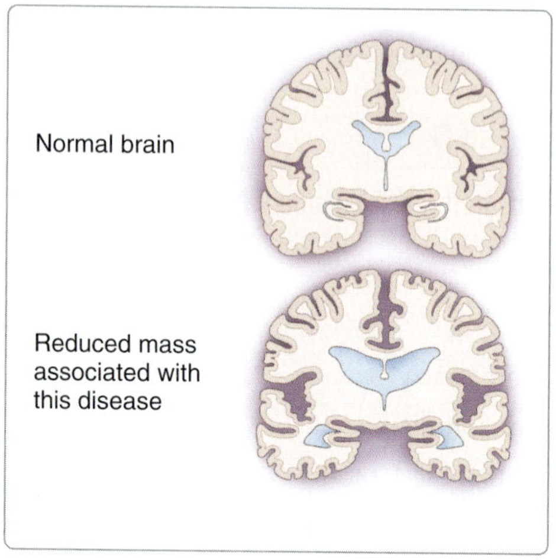

5. ______________________________
viral disease that affects the peripheral nerves and causes blisters on the skin that follow the course of the affected nerves

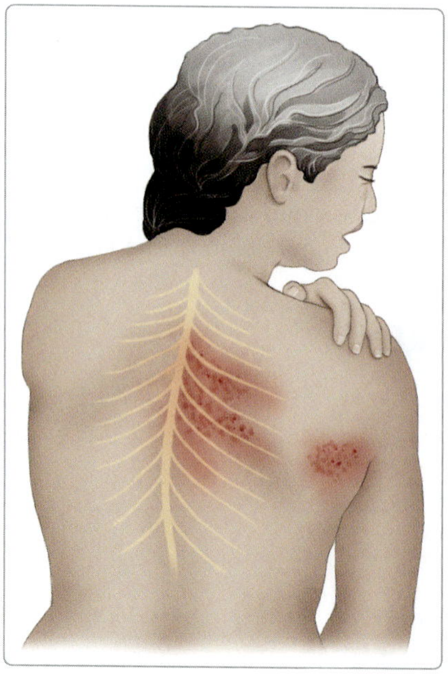

6. ______________________________
aneurysm in the cerebrum

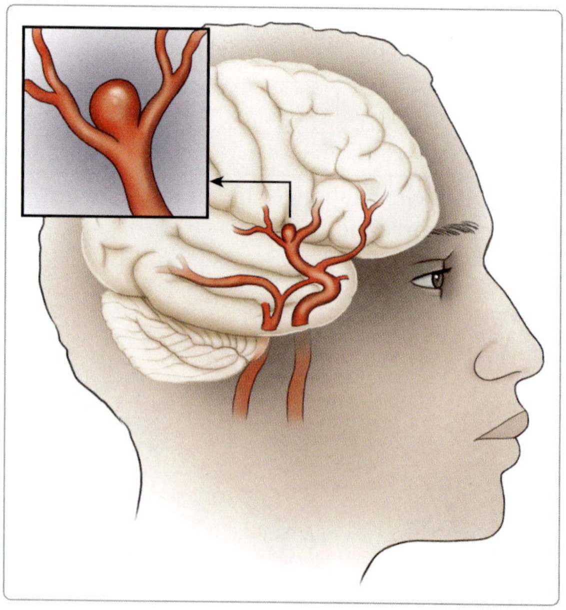

7. ______________________________
bleeding into the brain as a result of a ruptured blood vessel within the brain

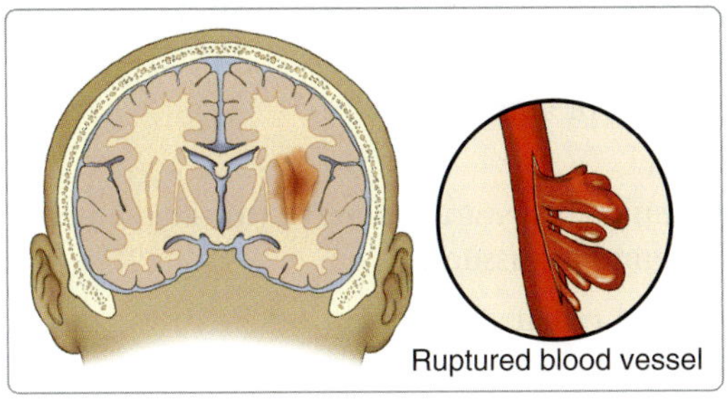

8. ______________________________
a blood clot or a piece of atherosclerotic plaque arising from a distant site lodges in a cerebral artery, causing sudden blockage of blood supply to the brain tissue

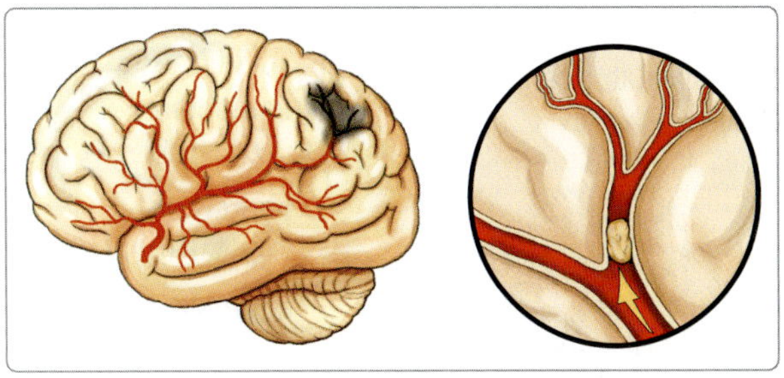

9. ______________________________
bleeding between the pia mater and arachnoid layers of the meninges caused by a ruptured blood vessel

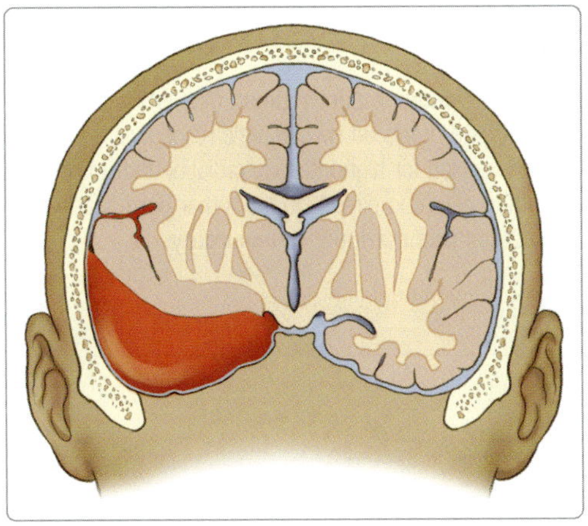

10. ______________________________
interruption of blood supply to a region of the brain, depriving nerve cells in the affected area of oxygen and nutrients

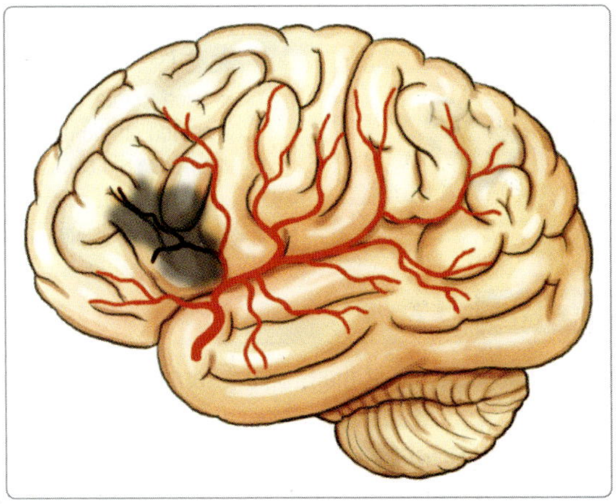

EXERCISE 16

Spell each of the Disease and Disorder Terms NOT Built from Word Parts by having someone dictate them to you. Use a separate sheet of paper.

> To hear and spell the terms, go to Evolve Resources at evolve.elsevier.com and select:
> Practice Student Resources > Student Resources > Chapter 15 > **Pronounce and Spell**
>
> See Appendix B for instructions.

❑ Check the box when complete.

Surgical Terms

BUILT FROM WORD PARTS

The following terms can be translated using definitions of word parts. Further explanation is provided within parentheses as needed.

EXERCISE FIGURE A

Fill in the blanks with word parts defined to label the diagram.

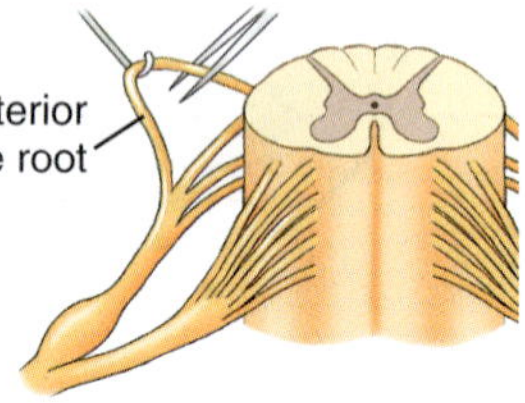

____ / ____ / ____
nerve root / cv / incision

OR

____ / ____ / ____
nerve root / cv / incision

TERM	DEFINITION
ganglionectomy (*gang*-glē-o-NEK-to-mē)	excision of a ganglion (also called **gangliectomy**)
neurectomy (nū-REK-to-mē)	excision of a nerve
neurolysis (nū-ROL-i-sis)	loosening, separating a nerve (to release it from surrounding tissues)
neuroplasty (NŪR-ō-*plas*-tē)	surgical repair of a nerve
neurorrhaphy (nū-ROR-a-fē)	suturing of a nerve
neurotomy (nū-ROT-o-mē)	incision into a nerve
radicotomy, rhizotomy (*rad*-i-KOT-o-mē), (rī-ZOT-o-mē)	incision into a nerve root (Exercise Figure A)

STEREOTACTIC RADIOSURGERY

is used to treat patients with **brain tumors** or **arteriovenous malformations (AVMs).** A special frame is mounted on the patient's head. Images of the brain are produced by magnetic resonance imaging (MRI). A high-powered computer uses the images to design a plan for high-intensity radiation that matches the exact size and shape of the tumor. Radiation is then delivered directly to the tumor only, sparing surrounding tissue. This procedure may also be called **Gamma-knife radiosurgery**.

EXERCISE 17

Practice saying aloud each of the Surgical Terms Built from Word Parts.

To hear the terms, go to Evolve Resources at evolve.elsevier.com and select:
Practice Student Resources > Student Resources > Chapter 15 > **Pronounce and Spell**

See Appendix B for instructions.

❑ Check the box when complete.

EXERCISE 18

Analyze and define the following surgical terms.

1. radicotomy

____

____

2. neurectomy

____

____

3. neurorrhaphy

____

____

4. ganglionectomy

____

____

5. neurotomy

____

____

6. neurolysis

____

____

7. neuroplasty

____

____

8. rhizotomy

____

____

EXERCISE 19

Build surgical terms for the following definitions by using the word parts you have learned.

1. incision into a nerve root

a. ________ / ____ / ________
WR / CV / S

b. ________ / ____ / ________
WR / CV / S

2. excision of a nerve ________ / ________
WR / S

3. suturing of a nerve ________ / ____ / ________
WR / CV / S

4. excision of a ganglion ________ / ________
WR / S

5. incision into a nerve ________ / ____ / ________
WR / CV / S

6. loosening, separating a nerve (to release it from surrounding tissue) ________ / ____ / ________
WR / CV / S

7. surgical repair of a nerve ________ / ____ / ________
WR / CV / S

EXERCISE 20

Spell each of the Surgical Terms Built from Word Parts by having someone dictate them to you. Use a separate sheet of paper.

> To hear and spell the terms, go to Evolve Resources at evolve.elsevier.com and select:
> Practice Student Resources > Student Resources > Chapter 15 > **Pronounce and Spell**
> See Appendix B for instructions.

❑ Check the box when complete.

EXERCISE FIGURE B

Fill in the blanks with word parts defined to label the diagram.

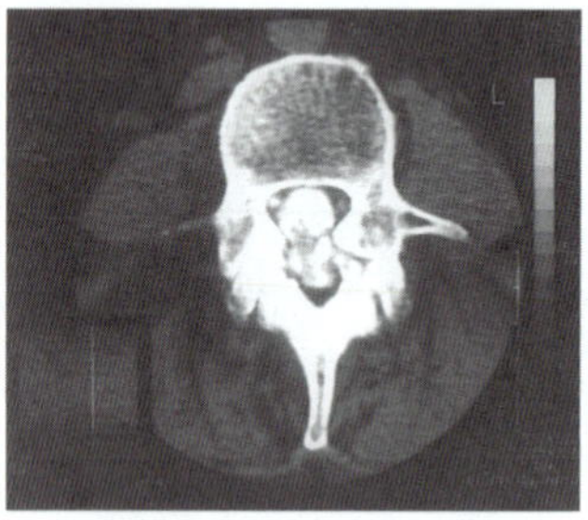

CT ______ / ______ / ______
spinal cord / cv / process of recording

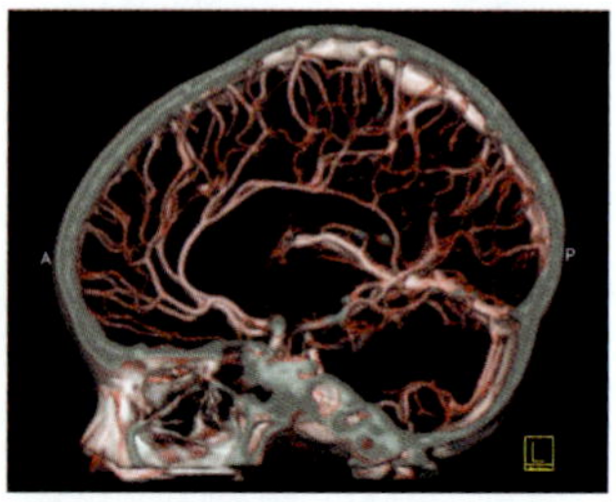

FIG. 15.8 Cerebral angiogram. CT imaging of cerebral venous circulation.

> ***Neurodiagnostic Technician***
> To see an interview with a **Neurodiagnostic Technician** who performs EEGs, go to Evolve Resources at evolve.elsevier.com and select **Career Videos** located under the **Extra Content** Tab.

Diagnostic Terms
BUILT FROM WORD PARTS

The following terms can be translated using definitions of word parts. Further explanation is provided within parentheses as needed.

TERM	DEFINITION
DIAGNOSTIC IMAGING	
cerebral angiography (se-RĒ-bral) (*an*-jē-OG-ra-fē)	process of recording (scan of) the (blood) vessels of the cerebrum (after an injection of contrast medium) (Fig. 15.8)
CT myelography (C-T) (*mī*-e-LOG-ra-fē)	process of recording (scan of) the spinal cord (after an injection of a contrast agent into the subarachnoid space by lumbar puncture. Size, shape, and position of the spinal cord and nerve roots are demonstrated.) (Exercise Figure B)
NEURODIAGNOSTIC PROCEDURES	
electroencephalogram (EEG) (ē-*lek*-trō-en-SEF-a-lō-gram)	record of electrical activity of the brain
electroencephalograph (ē-*lek*-trō-en-SEF-a-lō-graf)	instrument used to record electrical activity of the brain
electroencephalography (ē-*lek*-trō-en-*sef*-a-LOG-ra-fē)	process of recording the electrical activity of the brain

EXERCISE 21

Practice saying aloud each of the Diagnostic Terms Built from Word Parts.

> To hear the terms, go to Evolve Resources at evolve.elsevier.com and select:
> Practice Student Resources > Student Resources > Chapter 15 > **Pronounce and Spell**
> See Appendix B for instructions.

❑ Check the box when complete.

EXERCISE 22

Analyze and define the following diagnostic terms.

1. electroencephalogram

____

____

2. electroencephalograph

____

____

3. electroencephalography

____

____

4. CT myelography

____

____

5. cerebral angiography

____

____

EXERCISE 23

Build diagnostic terms that correspond to the following definitions by using the word parts you have learned.

1. record of electrical activity of the brain ______ WR / CV / WR / CV / S

2. instrument used to record electrical activity of the brain ______ WR / CV / WR / CV / S

3. process of recording the electrical activity of the brain ______ WR / CV / WR / CV / S

4. process of recording (scan of) the spinal cord CT ______ WR / CV / S

5. process of recording (scan of) the (blood) vessels of the cerebrum ______ WR / S ______ WR / CV / S

EXERCISE 24

Spell each of the Diagnostic Terms Built from Word Parts by having someone dictate them to you. Use a separate sheet of paper.

To hear and spell the terms, go to Evolve Resources at evolve.elsevier.com and select:
Practice Student Resources > Student Resources > Chapter 15 > **Pronounce and Spell**

See Appendix B for instructions.

❑ Check the box when complete.

Diagnostic Terms
NOT BUILT FROM WORD PARTS

Word parts may be present in the following terms; however, their full meanings cannot be translated using definitions of word parts alone.

TERM	DEFINITION
DIAGNOSTIC IMAGING	
computed tomography (CT) (com-PŪ-td) (tō-MOG-ra-fē)	computerized radiographic process producing a series of sectional images (slices) of tissue. CT imaging is commonly used in the brain, spine, neck, chest, abdomen, and pelvis.
magnetic resonance imaging (MRI) (mag-NET-ik) (REZ-ō-nans) (IM-a-jing)	high strength, computer-controlled magnetic fields producing a series of sectional images (slices) that visualize abnormalities such as swelling, infections, tumors, and herniated disks. In addition to the brain and spine, MR imaging is also commonly used in the abdomen, and throughout the musculoskeletal system.
positron emission tomography (PET) scan (POZ-i-tron) (ē-MISH-un) (tō-MOG-ra-fē) (skan)	nuclear medicine procedure combining CT and radioactive chemicals to produce sectional images of the brain or other organs to examine blood flow and metabolic activity
NEURODIAGNOSTIC PROCEDURES	
evoked potential studies (EP studies) (i-VŌKD) (pō-TEN-shal) (STUD-ēz)	group of diagnostic tests that measure changes and responses in brain waves elicited by visual, auditory, or somatosensory stimuli. Visual evoked response (VER) is a response to visual stimuli. Auditory evoked response (AER) is a response to auditory stimuli. Somatosensory evoked response (SSER) is a response to stimuli applied to the extremities.
OTHER	
lumbar puncture (LP) (LUM-bar) (PUNK-chur)	diagnostic procedure performed by insertion of a needle into the subarachnoid space usually between the third and fourth lumbar vertebrae; performed for many reasons, including the removal of cerebrospinal fluid (also called **spinal tap**)

EXERCISE 25

Practice saying aloud each of the Diagnostic Terms NOT Built from Word Parts.

> To hear the terms, go to Evolve Resources at evolve.elsevier.com and select:
> Practice Student Resources > Student Resources > Chapter 15 > **Pronounce and Spell**
>
> See Appendix B for instructions.

❑ Check the box when complete.

EXERCISE 26

Match the Diagnostic Terms NOT Built from Word Parts in the first column with the correct definitions in the second column.

_____ 1. evoked potential studies
_____ 2. positron emission tomography
_____ 3. lumbar puncture
_____ 4. magnetic resonance imaging
_____ 5. computed tomography

a. high strength, computer-controlled magnetic fields producing a series of sectional images (slices) that visualize abnormalities such as swelling, infections, tumors, and herniated disks
b. computerized radiographic process producing a series of sectional images (slices) of tissue
c. group of diagnostic tests that measure changes and responses in brain waves elicited by visual, auditory, or somatosensory stimuli
d. nuclear medicine procedure combining CT and radioactive chemicals to produce sectional images of the brain or other organs to examine blood flow and metabolic activity
e. diagnostic procedure performed by insertion of a needle into the subarachnoid space usually between the third and fourth lumbar vertebrae

EXERCISE 27

Write the medical term pictured and defined.

1. ______________________________

group of diagnostic tests that measure changes and responses in brain waves elicited by visual, auditory, or somatosensory stimuli

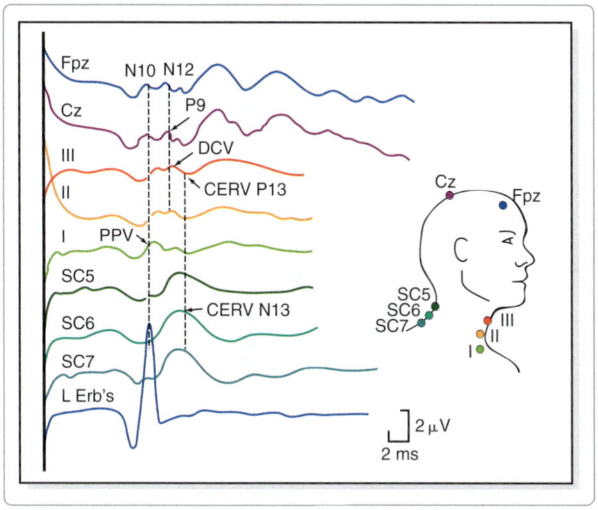

2. ______________________________

nuclear medicine procedure combining CT and radioactive chemicals to examine blood flow and metabolic activity

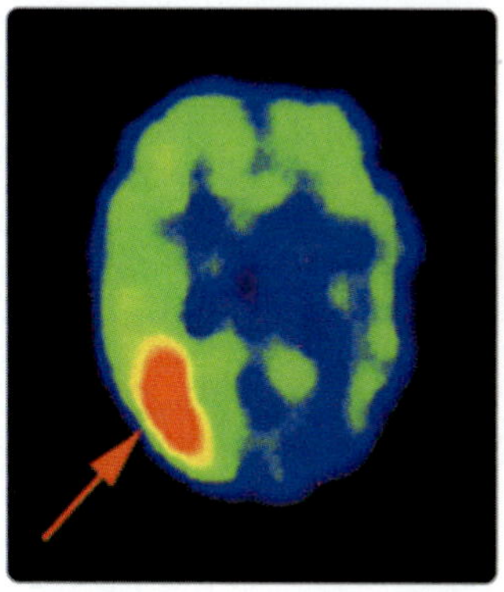

EXERCISE 27 *Pictured and Defined—cont'd*

3. ______________________________
computerized radiographic process producing a series of sectional images (slices) of tissue

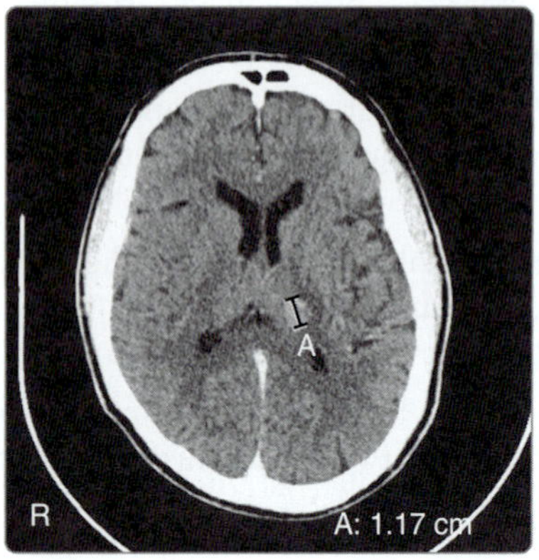

4. ______________________________
high strength, computer-controlled magnetic fields producing a series of sectional images

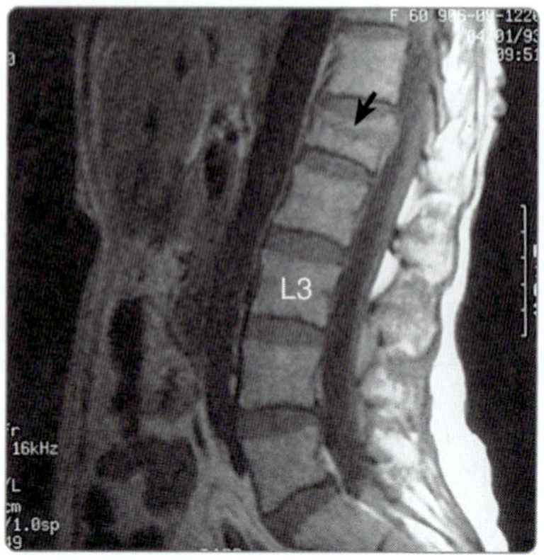

5. ______________________________
diagnostic procedure performed by insertion of a needle into the subarachnoid space

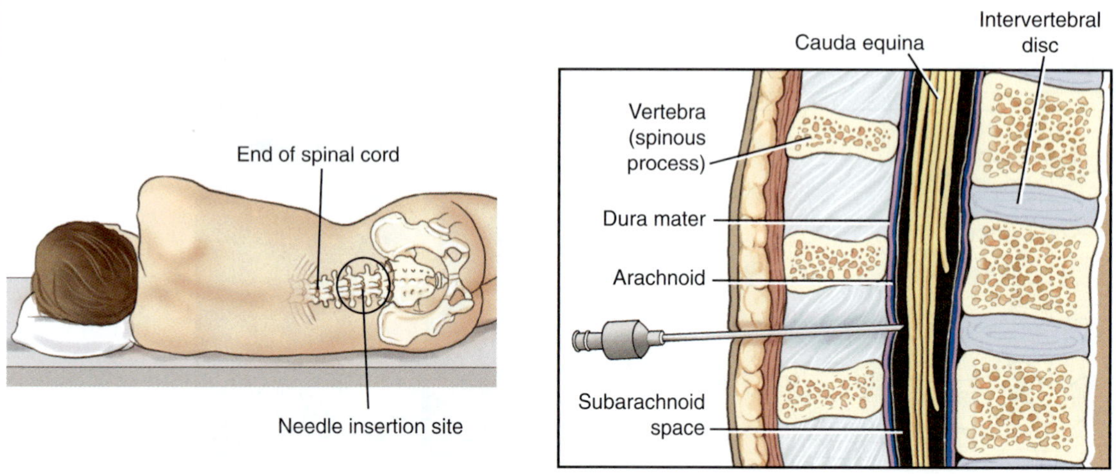

EXERCISE 28

Spell each of the Diagnostic Terms NOT Built from Word Parts by having someone dictate them to you. Use a separate sheet of paper.

To hear and spell the terms, go to Evolve Resources at evolve.elsevier.com and select:
Practice Student Resources > Student Resources > Chapter 15 > **Pronounce and Spell**

See Appendix B for instructions.

❑ Check the box when complete.

Complementary Terms
BUILT FROM WORD PARTS

The following terms can be translated using definitions of word parts. Further explanation is provided within parentheses as needed.

TERM	DEFINITION
anesthesia (*an*-es-THĒ-zha)	without (loss of) feeling or sensation
aphasia (a-FĀ-zha)	condition of without speaking (loss or impairment of the ability to speak)
cephalgia (sef-AL-ja)	pain in the head (headache) (Migraine, tension headache, and cluster headaches account for nearly 90% of all headaches.) *(NOTE: the* al *is dropped from the combining form cephal/o)*
cerebral (se-RĒ-bral)	pertaining to the cerebrum
craniocerebral (*krā*-nē-ō-su-RĒ-bral)	pertaining to the cranium and cerebrum
dysesthesia (dis-es-THĒ-zha)	painful sensation
dysphasia (dis-FĀ-zha)	condition of difficulty speaking
encephalopathy (en-*sef*-a-LOP-a-thē)	disease of the brain
gliocyte (GLĪ-ō-sīt)	glial cell
hemiparesis (*hem*-ē-pa-RĒ-sis)	slight paralysis of half (right or left side of the body)
hemiplegia (*hem*-ē-PLĒ-ja)	paralysis of half (right or left side of the body); (stroke is the most common cause of hemiplegia) (Exercise Figure C)
hyperesthesia (*hī*-per-es-THĒ-zha)	excessive sensitivity (to stimuli)
interictal (*in*-ter-IK-tal)	(occurring) between seizures or attacks
intracerebral (*in*-tra-SER-e-bral)	pertaining to within the cerebrum
mental (MEN-tel)	pertaining to the mind
monoparesis (*mon*-ō-pa-RĒ-sis)	slight paralysis of one (limb)
monoplegia (*mon*-ō-PLĒ-ja)	paralysis of one (limb)
myelomalacia (*mī*-e-lō-ma-LĀ-sha)	softening of the spinal cord

CHRONIC TRAUMATIC ENCEPHALOPATHY

(CTE) is a progressive disease of the brain which generally appears years or decades after head trauma. Originally diagnosed in boxers (dementia pugilistica), it has now been found in other professional athletes who experienced repeated head trauma, such as football, ice hockey, soccer, wrestling, and basketball players. Signs and symptoms include memory loss, aggression, confusion, attention deficits, poor judgment, aggression, anxiety, and depression. Currently, CTE can only be definitively diagnosed after death by brain autopsy, but in the future, diagnostic imaging, chemical biomarkers, and neuropsychological tests may be helpful.

Complementary Terms—cont'd

TERM	DEFINITION
neuroid (NŪ-royd)	resembling a nerve
neurologist (nū-ROL-o-jist)	physician who studies and treats diseases of the nervous system
neurology (nū-ROL-o-jē)	study of nerves (branch of medicine dealing with diseases of the nervous system)
paresthesia (*par*-es-THĒ-zha)	abnormal sensation (such as burning, prickling, or tingling sensation, often in the extremities; may be caused by nerve damage or peripheral neuropathy) *(Note: the a is dropped from the prefix para.)*
postictal (pōst-IK-tal)	(occurring) after a seizure or attack
preictal (prē-IK-tal)	(occurring) before a seizure or attack
quadriplegia (*kwod*-ri-PLĒ-ja)	paralysis of four (limbs) (Exercise Figure C)
subdural (sub-DŪ-ral)	pertaining to below the dura mater

EXERCISE 29

Practice saying aloud each of the Complementary Terms Built from Word Parts.

> To hear the terms, go to Evolve Resources at evolve.elsevier.com and select:
> Practice Student Resources > Student Resources > Chapter 15 > **Pronounce and Spell**
> See Appendix B for instructions.

❑ Check the box when complete.

EXERCISE FIGURE C

Fill in the blanks with word parts defined to label these diagrams of types of paralysis.

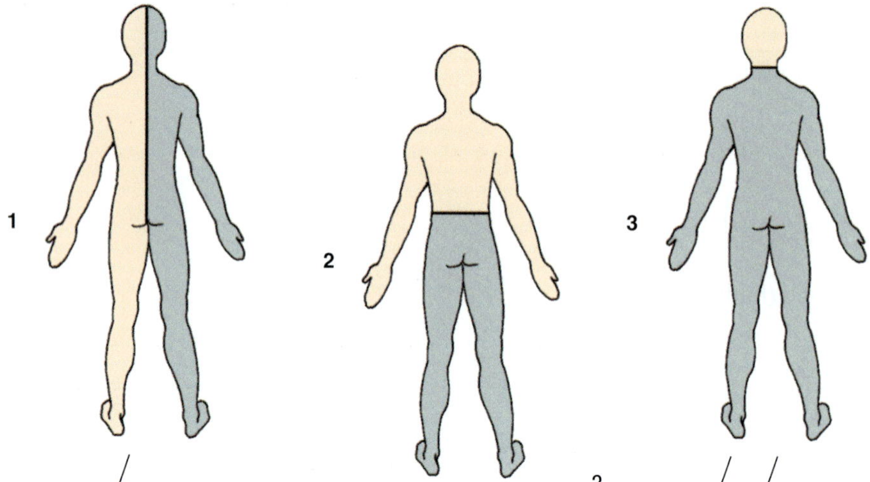

1. ________ / ________
half / paralysis

2. Paraplegia

3. ________ / ________ / ________
four / cv / paralysis

EXERCISE 30

Analyze and define the following complementary terms.

1. hemiplegia
2. paresthesia
3. neurologist
4. neurology
5. neuroid
6. quadriplegia
7. cerebral
8. monoplegia
9. aphasia
10. dysphasia
11. hemiparesis
12. anesthesia
13. hyperesthesia
14. subdural
15. cephalgia
16. craniocerebral
17. myelomalacia
18. encephalopathy

19. postictal

____

____

20. dysesthesia

____

____

21. interictal

____

____

22. monoparesis

____

____

23. preictal

____

____

24. intracerebral

____

____

25. gliocyte

____

____

26. mental

____

____

EXERCISE 31

Build the complementary terms for the following definitions by using the word parts you have learned.

1. slight paralysis of half (right or left side of the body) ______ / ______ P / S(WR)

2. without (loss of) feeling or sensation ______ / ______ / ______ P / WR / S

3. excessive sensitivity (to stimuli) ______ / ______ / ______ P / WR / S

4. pertaining to below the dura mater ______ / ______ / ______ P / WR / S

5. pain in the head (headache) ______ / ______ WR / S

6. pertaining to the cranium and cerebrum ______ / ______ / ______ / ______ WR / CV / WR / S

7. softening of the spinal cord ______ / ______ / ______ WR / CV / S

8. disease of the brain ______ / ______ / ______ WR / CV / S

9. paralysis of half (left or right side) of the body ______ / ______ P / S(WR)

10. physician who studies and treats diseases of the nervous system ______ / ______ / ______
WR / CV / S

11. study of nerves (branch of medicine dealing with diseases of the nervous system) ______ / ______ / ______
WR / CV / S

12. resembling a nerve ______ / ______
WR / S

13. paralysis of four (limbs) ______ / ______ / ______
WR / CV / S

14. pertaining to the cerebrum ______ / ______
WR / S

15. paralysis of one (limb) ______ / ______ / ______
WR / CV / S

16. condition of without speaking (loss or impairment of the ability to speak) ______ / ______ / ______
P / WR / S

17. condition of difficulty speaking ______ / ______ / ______
P / WR / S

18. (occurring) before a seizure or attack ______ / ______
P / S(WR)

19. slight paralysis of one (limb) ______ / ______ / ______
WR / CV / S

20. (occurring) after a seizure ______ / ______
P / S(WR)

21. painful sensation ______ / ______ / ______
P / WR / S

22. (occurring) between seizures or attacks ______ / ______
P / S(WR)

23. pertaining to within the cerebrum ______ / ______ / ______
P / WR / S

24. glial cell ______ / ______ / ______
WR / CV / S

25. abnormal sensation ______ / ______ / ______
P / WR / S

26. pertaining to the mind ______ / ______
WR / S

EXERCISE 32

Spell each of the Complementary Terms Built from Word Parts by having someone dictate them to you. Use a separate sheet of paper.

To hear and spell the terms, go to Evolve Resources at evolve.elsevier.com and select:
Practice Student Resources > Student Resources > Chapter 15 > **Pronounce and Spell**

See Appendix B for instructions.

❑ Check the box when complete.

Complementary Terms
NOT BUILT FROM WORD PARTS

Word parts may be present in the following terms; however, their full meanings cannot be translated using definitions of word parts alone.

TERM	DEFINITION
afferent (AF-er-ent)	conveying toward a center (for example, afferent nerves carry sensory impulses to the central nervous system)
ataxia (a-TAK-sē-a)	lack of muscle coordination
cognitive (COG-ni-tiv)	pertaining to the mental processes of comprehension, judgment, memory, and reason
coma (KŌ-ma)	state of profound unconsciousness
concussion (kon-KUSH-un)	injury to the brain caused by minor or major head trauma; symptoms include vertigo, headache, and possible loss of consciousness
conscious (KON-shus)	awake, alert, aware of one's surroundings
convulsion (kun-VUL-zhun)	sudden, involuntary contraction of a group of muscles; may be present during a seizure
disorientation (dis-*or*-ē-en-TĀ-shun)	state of mental confusion as to time, place, or identity
dysarthria (dis-AR-thrē-a)	inability to use speech that is distinct and connected because of a loss of muscle control after damage to the peripheral or central nervous system
efferent (EF-er-ent)	conveying away from the center (for example, efferent nerves carry impulses away from the central nervous system)
gait (gāt)	manner or style of walking
incoherent (*in*-kō-HĒR-ent)	unable to express one's thoughts or ideas in an orderly, intelligible manner
paraplegia (*par*-a-PLĒ-ja)	paralysis from the waist down caused by damage to the lower level of the spinal cord (Exercise Figure C)
seizure (SĒ-zher)	sudden, abnormal surge of electrical activity in the brain, resulting in involuntary body movements or behaviors

CONCUSSION
is a common type of **traumatic brain injury (TBI),** an umbrella term used to describe mild to severe damage to the brain sustained by a wide range of injuries. Falls, motor vehicle accidents, sports injuries, combat-related injuries or violence may all cause TBI.

PARAPLEGIA
is composed of the Greek **para**, meaning **beside**, and **plegia**, meaning **paralysis**. It has been used since Hippocrates' time and at first meant paralysis of any limb or side of the body. Since the nineteenth century, it has been used to mean paralysis from the waist down.

TERM	DEFINITION
shunt (shunt)	tube implanted in the body to redirect the flow of a fluid
syncope (SINK-o-pē)	fainting or sudden loss of consciousness caused by lack of blood supply to the cerebrum
unconsciousness (un-KON-shus-nes)	state of being unaware of surroundings and incapable of responding to stimuli as a result of injury, shock, illness, or drugs

TABLE 15.2 Types of Cognitive Impairment

Mild cognitive impairment (MCI)	presence of significant memory difficulty when adjusted for age-related norms. The patient usually has little difficulty performing activities of daily living. This condition may be an early manifestation of Alzheimer disease or other forms of dementia.
Age-associated memory impairment	refers to a normal aging process in which the speed of mental processing and the performance of tasks decreases, and recent memory and learning are more difficult. Verbal intelligence is preserved, and this condition is not a forerunner of dementia.
Delirium	potentially reversible acute disturbance of consciousness with impairment of cognition. A number of conditions can cause delirium by interfering with brain metabolism. Drugs, alcohol, systemic infections, head trauma, hypoglycemia, and electrolyte disturbances are common examples.
Pseudodementia	behavioral disorder resembling dementia but is not caused by brain tissue abnormalities. This can be found in mental illness, such as major depression, and can be reversible with treatment.

EXERCISE 33

Practice saying aloud each of the Complementary Terms NOT Built from Word Parts.

To hear the terms, go to Evolve Resources at evolve.elsevier.com and select:
Practice Student Resources > Student Resources > Chapter 15 > **Pronounce and Spell**

See Appendix B for instructions.

❑ Check the box when complete.

EXERCISE 34

Write the term for each of the following definitions.

1. injury to the brain caused by head trauma ______________________
2. state of being unaware of surroundings and incapable of responding to stimuli as a result of injury, shock, illness, or drugs ______________________
3. awake, alert, aware of one's surroundings ______________________
4. sudden, abnormal surge of electrical activity in the brain ______________________
5. sudden, involuntary contraction of a group of muscles ______________________
6. tube implanted in the body to redirect the flow of a fluid ______________________
7. paralysis from the waist down caused by damage to the lower level of the spinal cord ______________________
8. state of profound unconsciousness ______________________
9. fainting or sudden loss of consciousness ______________________

10. lack of muscle coordination ______________________________
11. manner or style of walking ______________________________
12. inability to use speech that is distinctive and connected ______________________________
13. unable to express one's thoughts or ideas in an orderly, intelligible manner ______________________________
14. state of mental confusion as to time, place, or identity ______________________________
15. pertaining to the mental processes of comprehension, judgment, memory, and reason ______________________________
16. conveying toward the center ______________________________
17. conveying away from the center ______________________________

EXERCISE 35

Match the definitions in the first column with the correct terms in the second column.

_____ 1. state of profound unconsciousness
_____ 2. fainting or sudden loss of consciousness
_____ 3. paralysis from the waist down caused by damage to the lower level of the spinal cord
_____ 4. lack of muscle coordination
_____ 5. tube implanted in the body to redirect the flow of a fluid
_____ 6. manner or style of walking
_____ 7. conveying away from the center
_____ 8. inability to use speech that is distinctive and connected
_____ 9. sudden, abnormal surge of electrical activity in the brain
_____ 10. unable to express one's thoughts or ideas in an orderly, intelligible manner
_____ 11. awake, alert, aware of one's surroundings
_____ 12. conveying toward the center
_____ 13. state of being unaware of surroundings and incapable of responding to stimuli as a result of injury, shock, illness, or drugs
_____ 14. pertaining to the mental processes of comprehension, judgment, memory, and reason
_____ 15. injury to the brain caused by head trauma
_____ 16. state of mental confusion as to time, place, or identity
_____ 17. sudden, involuntary contraction of a group of muscles

a. shunt
b. paraplegia
c. coma
d. concussion
e. unconsciousness
f. conscious
g. seizure
h. convulsion
i. syncope
j. ataxia
k. dysarthria
l. gait
m. cognitive
n. disorientation
o. incoherent
p. efferent
q. afferent

EXERCISE 36

Spell each of the Complementary Terms NOT Built from Word Parts by having someone dictate them to you. Use a separate sheet of paper.

To hear and spell the terms, go to Evolve Resources at evolve.elsevier.com and select:
Practice Student Resources > Student Resources > Chapter 15 > **Pronounce and Spell**

See Appendix B for instructions.

❑ Check the box when complete.

Behavioral Health Terms

Although the terms below are listed as behavioral health terms, medications, physical changes, substance abuse, and illness may contribute to these conditions.

BUILT FROM WORD PARTS

The following terms can be translated using definitions of word parts. Further explanation is provided within parentheses as needed.

TERM	DEFINITION
psychiatrist (sī-KĪ-a-trist)	physician who studies and treats disorders of the mind (Psychiatrists have additional training and experience in prevention, diagnosis, and treatment of mental, emotional, and behavioral disorders. Psychiatrists often prescribe medications for patients with these disorders.)
psychiatry (sī-KĪ-a-trē)	specialty of the mind (branch of medicine that deals with the treatment of mental disorders)
psychogenic (sī-*kō*-JEN-ik)	originating in the mind
psychologist (sī-KOL-o-jist)	specialist of the mind (Clinical psychologists have graduate training in clinical psychology, administer psychological tests, and treat individuals with disturbances of mental, emotional, and behavioral disorders by counseling therapy.)
psychology (sī-KOL-o-jē)	study of the mind (a profession that involves dealing with the mind and mental processes in relation to human behavior)
psychopathy (sī-KOP-a-thē)	(any) disease of the mind
psychosis (pl. psychoses) (sī-KO-sis), (sī-KO-sēz)	abnormal condition of the mind (major mental disorder characterized by extreme derangement, often with delusions and hallucinations)
psychosomatic (*sī*-kō-sō-MAT-ik)	pertaining to the mind and body (interrelations of)

Psychiatric Technician
To see an interview with a **Psychiatric Technician**, go to Evolve Resources at evolve.elsevier.com and select **Career Videos** located under the **Extra Content** Tab.

EXERCISE 37

Practice saying aloud each of the Behavioral Health Terms Built from Word Parts.

To hear the terms, go to Evolve Resources at evolve.elsevier.com and select:
Practice Student Resources > Student Resources > Chapter 15 > **Pronounce and Spell**

See Appendix B for instructions.

❑ Check the box when complete.

EXERCISE 38

Analyze and define the following terms.

1. psychosomatic

____
____

2. psychopathy

____
____

3. psychology

____
____

4. psychiatry

____
____

5. psychologist

____
____

6. psychogenic

____
____

7. psychiatrist

____
____

8. psychosis

____
____

EXERCISE 39

Build the behavioral health terms for the following definitions by using the word parts you have learned.

1. specialty of the mind (branch of medicine that deals with the treatment of mental disorders) ________ / ________ WR / S
2. abnormal condition of the mind ________ / ________ WR / S
3. study of the mind (a profession that involves dealing with the mind and mental processes in relation to human behavior) ________ / ___ / ________ WR / CV / S
4. originating in the mind ________ / ___ / ________ WR / CV / S
5. physician who studies and treats disorders of the mind ________ / ________ WR / S
6. specialist of the mind ________ / ___ / ________ WR / CV / S
7. pertaining to the mind and body ________ / ___ / ________ / ________ WR / CV / WR / S
8. disease of the mind ________ / ___ / ________ WR / CV / S

EXERCISE 40

Spell each of the Behavioral Health Terms Built from Word Parts by having someone dictate them to you. Use a separate sheet of paper.

> To hear and spell the terms, go to Evolve Resources at evolve.elsevier.com and select:
> Practice Student Resources > Student Resources > Chapter 15 > **Pronounce and Spell**
>
> See Appendix B for instructions.

❑ Check the box when complete.

Behavioral Health Terms
NOT BUILT FROM WORD PARTS

Word parts may be present in the following terms; however, their full meanings cannot be translated using definitions of word parts alone.

TERM	DEFINITION
anorexia nervosa (*an*-ō-REK-sē-a) (ner-VŌ-sa)	eating disorder characterized by a disturbed perception of body image resulting in failure to maintain body weight, intensive fear of gaining weight, pronounced desire for thinness, and, in females, amenorrhea
anxiety disorder (ang-ZĪ-e-tē) (dis-OR-der)	disorder characterized by feelings of apprehension, tension, or uneasiness arising typically from the anticipation of unreal or imagined danger
attention deficit/hyperactivity disorder (ADHD) (a-TEN-shun) (DEF-i-sit) (*hī*-per-ak-TIV-i-tē) (dis-OR-der)	disorder of learning and behavioral problems characterized by marked inattention, distractibility, impulsiveness, and hyperactivity
autism (AW-tizm)	spectrum of mental disorders, the features of which include onset during infancy or childhood, preoccupation with subjective mental activity, inability to interact socially, and impaired communication (also referred to as **autism spectrum disorders** [ASD])
bipolar disorder (bī-PŌ-lar) (dis-OR-der)	major psychological disorder typified by a disturbance in mood. The disorder is manifested by manic (elevated or irritated mood, excessive energy, impulsiveness) and depressive episodes that may alternate; or elements of both may occur simultaneously.
bulimia nervosa (bū-LĒ-mē-a) (ner-VŌ-sa)	eating disorder characterized by uncontrolled binge eating followed by purging (induced vomiting)

INTEGRATIVE MEDICINE TERM

Biofeedback, also referred to as neurofeedback, is learned self-control of physiologic responses utilizing electronic devices to provide monitoring information. Current research suggests that biofeedback is a viable alternative treatment for **attention deficit/hyperactivity disorder (ADHD)** and **autism spectrum disorders (ASD)**.

Behavioral Health Terms—cont'd

TERM	DEFINITION
major depression (MĀ-jor) (dē-PRESH-un)	mood disturbance characterized by feelings of sadness, despair, discouragement, hopelessness, lack of joy, altered sleep patterns, and difficulty with decision making and daily function. Depression ranges from normal feelings of sadness (resulting from and proportional to personal loss or tragedy), through dysthymia (chronic depressive neurosis), to major depression (also referred to as **clinical depression, mood disorder**).
obsessive-compulsive disorder (OCD) (ob-SES-iv-kom-PUL-siv) (dis-OR-der)	disorder characterized by intrusive, unwanted thoughts that result in the tendency to perform repetitive acts or rituals (compulsions), usually as a means of releasing tension or anxiety
panic attack (PAN-ik) (a-TAK)	episode of sudden onset of acute anxiety, occurring unpredictably, with feelings of acute apprehension, dyspnea, dizziness, sweating, and/or chest pain, depersonalization, paresthesia and fear of dying, loss of mind or control
phobia (FŌ-bē-a)	marked and persistent fear that is excessive or unreasonable cued by the presence or anticipation of a specific situation or object (such as claustrophobia, the abnormal fear of being in enclosed spaces)
pica (PĪ-ka)	compulsive eating of nonnutritive substances such as clay or ice. This condition may be a result of an iron deficiency. When iron deficiency is the cause of pica the condition will disappear in 1 or 2 weeks when treated with iron therapy.
posttraumatic stress disorder (PTSD) (*pōst*-tra-MAT-ik) (stres) (dis-OR-der)	significant behavioral health disorder in which some people exposed to a traumatic event go on to develop a series of symptoms related to it. These include mentally re-experiencing the event, increased autonomic arousal (the "fight or flight" response), avoidance of thoughts or activities that are reminders of the trauma, social withdrawal, and difficulty making emotional contacts with family and friends.
schizophrenia (*skit*-sō-FRĒ-nē-a)	any one of a large group of psychotic disorders characterized by gross distortions of reality, disturbance of language and communication, withdrawal from social interaction, and the disorganization and fragmentation of thought, perception, and emotional reaction
somatoform disorders (sō-MAT-ō-form) (dis-OR-derz)	disorders characterized by physical symptoms for which no known physical cause exists

Refer to **Appendix F** for pharmacology terms related to the nervous system and behavioral health.

For a list of behavioral health terms, go to Evolve Resources at evolve.elsevier.com and select: Practice Student Resources > Student Resources > **Extra Content** > Appendix J: Behavioral Health Terms

See Appendix B for instructions.

EXERCISE 41

Practice saying aloud each of the Behavioral Health Terms NOT Built from Word Parts.

To hear the terms, go to Evolve Resources at evolve.elsevier.com and select:
Practice Student Resources > Student Resources > Chapter 15 > **Pronounce and Spell**

See Appendix B for instructions.

❑ Check the box when complete.

EXERCISE 42

Match the definitions in the first column with the correct terms in the second column.

_____ 1. manifested by manic and depressive episodes
_____ 2. episode of acute anxiety, occurs unpredictably
_____ 3. characterized by feelings of apprehension and tension
_____ 4. disorder of learning and behavioral problems with distractibility
_____ 5. mood disturbance characterized by feelings of sadness, despair, and discouragement
_____ 6. marked and persistent fear that is excessive or unreasonable
_____ 7. binge eating followed by purging
_____ 8. physical symptoms for which no known physical cause exists
_____ 9. eating of nonnutritive substances, such as ice
_____ 10. disturbed perception of body image with failure to maintain body weight
_____ 11. characterized by gross distortions of reality and disturbance of language and communication
_____ 12. preoccupation with subjective mental activity, inability to interact socially, and impaired communication
_____ 13. mentally re-experiencing a traumatic event; avoidance of thoughts or activities that are reminders of the trauma
_____ 14. intrusive unwanted thoughts that result in rituals and/or repetitive acts

a. phobia
b. anxiety disorder
c. attention deficit/hyperactivity disorder
d. somatoform disorders
e. schizophrenia
f. anorexia nervosa
g. bulimia nervosa
h. pica
i. bipolar disorder
j. major depression
k. obsessive-compulsive disorder
l. posttraumatic stress disorder
m. panic attack
n. autism

EXERCISE 43

Spell each of the Behavioral Health Terms NOT Built from Word Parts by having someone dictate them to you. Use a separate sheet of paper.

To hear and spell the terms, go to Evolve Resources at evolve.elsevier.com and select:
Practice Student Resources > Student Resources > Chapter 15 > **Pronounce and Spell**

See Appendix B for instructions.

❑ Check the box when complete.

Abbreviations

ABBREVIATION	TERM
AD	Alzheimer disease
ADHD	attention deficit/hyperactivity disorder
ALS	amyotrophic lateral sclerosis
CNS	central nervous system
CP	cerebral palsy
CSF	cerebrospinal fluid
CT	computed tomography
CTE	chronic traumatic encephalopathy
CVA	cerebrovascular accident
EEG	electroencephalogram
EP studies	evoked potential studies
LP	lumbar puncture
MRI	magnetic resonance imaging
MS	multiple sclerosis
OCD	obsessive-compulsive disorder
PD	Parkinson disease
PET	positron emission tomography
PNS	peripheral nervous system
PTSD	posttraumatic stress disorder
SAH	subarachnoid hemorrhage
TIA	transient ischemic attack

Refer to **Appendix E** for a complete list of abbreviations.

EXERCISE 44

Write the terms abbreviated.

1. Diagnostic tests used to diagnose patients with diseases of the nervous system include **EEG** ____________ ____________, **CT** ____________ ____________, **MRI** ____________ ____________ ____________, **PET** ____________ ____________ ____________, **EP studies** ____________ ____________ ____________, and **LP** ____________ ____________.
2. Diseases that affect the nervous system are **AD** ____________ ____________, **ALS** ____________ ____________ ____________, **CP** ____________ ____________, **MS** ____________ ____________, and **PD** ____________ ____________.
3. Stroke is the disruption of normal blood supply to the brain; it often occurs suddenly. Because of this, Hippocrates used the term *apoplexy*, which literally means *struck down*, to describe the condition. The term *stroke* grew out of the term *apoplexy*. The term *brain attack* is used to signify that a stroke is in progress and an emergency situation exists. **CVA** ____________ ____________ is also used to describe a stroke. An ischemic stroke, which is caused by a thrombosis or embolus, is frequently preceded by a **TIA** ____________ ____________ ____________. A ruptured cerebral aneurysm is the most common cause of **SAH** ____________ ____________, a type of hemorrhagic stroke.

4. The examination of **CSF** ______________________ ______________ may assist in the diagnosis of cerebral hemorrhage, meningitis, encephalitis, and other diseases.
5. Two common psychiatric disorders are **OCD** ____________________ ____________________________, and **ADHD** ______________ ______________ / ___________________________ ______________.
6. The nervous system may be divided into the **CNS** ______________ ______________ ______________, and the **PNS** ______________ ______________ ______________.
7. Psychiatric disorders related to trauma include **PTSD** ______________ ______________ ______________ and **CTE** ______________ ______________ ______________.

For additional practice with Abbreviations, go to Evolve Resources at evolve.elsevier.com and select: Practice Student Resources > Student Resources > Chapter 15 > **Flashcards:** Abbreviations

See Appendix B for instructions.

PRACTICAL APPLICATION

EXERCISE 45 *Case Study: Translate Between Everyday Language and Medical Language*

CASE STUDY: Koji Kaneshiro

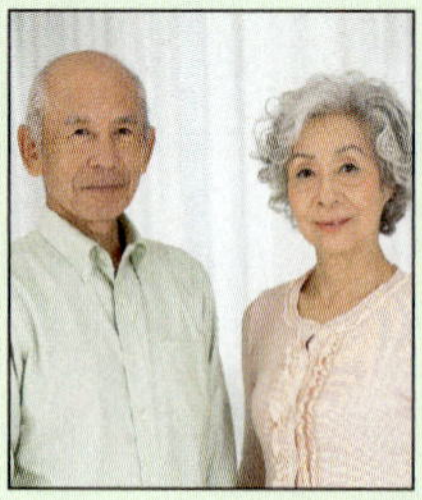

Kazuno Kaneshiro is worried about her husband, Koji. He was eating breakfast with her when he suddenly stopped speaking and dropped his spoon onto the table. "He never does that!" she thought. He seemed to be unable to speak. Also, his right arm was hanging limply by his side. She noticed that the left side of his face was also droopy. She had seen a billboard about strokes and was afraid he might be having one. She remembered the billboard saying that every minute counts so she called 911 immediately.

Now that you have worked through Chapter 15, consider the medical terms that might be used to describe Mr. Kaneshiro's experience. See the Review of Terms at the end of the chapter for a list of terms that might apply.

A. *Underline phrases in the case study that could be substituted with medical terms.*

B. *Write the medical term and its definition for three of the phrases you underlined.*

MEDICAL TERM	DEFINITION
1. ______________________	______________________________________
2. ______________________	______________________________________
3. ______________________	______________________________________

DOCUMENTATION: Excerpt from Emergency Department Visit

Mr. Kaneshiro was evaluated in the local emergency department; an excerpt from the medical record is documented below.

This 78-year-old male presented to the emergency department after the sudden onset of aphasia, right hemiplegia, and facial droop. Physical exam reveals an elderly male who is alert and oriented x 3, but shows evidence of dysphasia. Focused neurologic exam is significant for right-sided facial drooping with paralysis of the seventh cranial nerve. The rest of the cranial nerves appear normal. Motor exam reveals hemiparesis on the right. Paresthesias are also present on the right. Cerebellar exam is normal, though difficult to test on the right. Gait is not assessed due to the patient's weakness. A CT of the head without contrast indicates no evidence of cerebral or subarachnoid hemorrhage. The patient appears to be experiencing a CVA. We will start him on the stroke protocol.

C. *Underline medical terms presented in Chapter 15 used in the previous excerpt from Mr. Kaneshiro's medical record. See the Review of Terms at the end of the chapter for a complete list.*

D. *Select and define three of the medical terms you underlined. To check your answers, go to Appendix A.*

MEDICAL TERM	DEFINITION
1. ______________________	______________________________________
2. ______________________	______________________________________
3. ______________________	______________________________________

EXERCISE 46 *Interact With Medical Documents and Electronic Health Records*

A. Read the report and complete it by writing medical terms on answer lines within the document. Definitions of terms to be written appear after the document.

71086-NUR DRAKE, Eldon

File Patient Navigate Custom Fields Help

Chart Review | Encounters | Notes | Labs | Imaging | Procedures | Rx | Documents | Referrals | Scheduling | Billing

Name: **DRAKE, Eldon** MR#: 71086-NUR DOB: 08/12/19XX Gender: M Age: 85 **Allergies:** NKDA **PCP:** Maggie Alcott, APRN

History: Eldon Drake is an 85-year-old male who was admitted to the hospital on 01/02/20XX for fever and confusion. Mr. Drake was in his usual state of good health until 3 days before admission, when he began to show signs of confusion and 1. ______________________ accompanied by a fever of 38.5° C. His fever continued, and he showed a steady decline in 2. ______________ function. He developed expressive 3. ________________.

Objective Findings: On physical examination the patient was 4. ______________ and alert but disoriented to time and place. Blood pressure was 160/80 mm Hg. Pulse, 96. Respirations, 20. Temperature 38.8° C. There were no focal neurologic deficits. Chest radiograph, urinalysis, and blood cultures were negative. A 5. ______________ consultation was obtained. 6. ________________ ____________ ____________ of the brain was performed, which disclosed 7. ____________. An 8. ________________________ was markedly abnormal for his age.

Treatment Summary: The patient was given acyclovir by intravenous infusion. On the second hospital day, the patient developed a generalized 9. ________________. He was placed on intravenous phenytoin and lorazepam. He later lapsed into a semicomatose state. He responded to tactile and verbal stimuli but was completely 10. _________________________. A nasogastric tube was placed, and enteral feedings were begun. After 14 days of IV acyclovir, the patient slowly began to improve and by the third week of his illness, he was talking normally and taking nourishment.

Electronically signed: Rashid Maitryi MD 01/23/20XX 11:18

Start | Log On/Off | Print | Edit

Definitions of Medical Terms to Complete the Document

Write the medical terms defined on corresponding answer lines in the document.

1. a state of mental confusion as to time, place, or identity
2. pertaining to the mental processes of comprehension, judgment, memory, and reason
3. loss of the ability to speak
4. awake, alert, and aware of one's surroundings
5. study of nerves (branch of medicine dealing with diseases of the nervous system)
6. uses high-strength computer-controlled magnetic fields to produce sectional images
7. inflammation of the brain
8. record of electrical impulses of the brain
9. sudden, abnormal surge of electrical activity in the brain
10. unable to express one's thoughts or ideas in an orderly, intelligible manner

EXERCISE 46 *Interact With Medical Documents and Electronic Health Records—cont'd*

B. Read the medical report and answer the questions below it.

32463 CASTILLA, ALANZE

File Patient Navigate Custom Fields Help

Patient Chart | Lab | Rad | Notes | Documents | Rx | Scheduling | Images | Billing

Name: **CASTILLA, ALANZE** MR#: **32463** DOB: **04/11/19XX** Gender: **F** Allergies: **Sulfonamides** PCP: **Mei Shang, MD**

NEUROLOGY CONSULTATION

ENCOUNTER DATE: 06/04/20XX

HISTORY: The patient is a 63-year-old female referred to Neurology because of persistent low back and right leg pain and paresthesias of 6 months duration. The pain is described as dull and aching and is rated 6/10. The discomfort is worse when standing and intensifies after walking about a block. The pain improves when the patient is sitting or when bending over. Her general health is good and there has been no weight loss.

NEUROLOGIC EXAM: The gait is somewhat wide based. Balance is normal. No muscle atrophy is present. Muscle strength is normal for age. The right Achilles reflex is absent. Sensation to pinprick is diminished over the right S1 dermatome.

LAB AND IMAGING: CBC and sed rate are normal. Fasting blood sugar is 106 mg/dL. A lumbosacral spine radiograph shows spondylosis and spondylolisthesis of L5 over S1. A CT scan shows a moderate degree of facet joint arthropathy and bulging discs at L2-3 and L4-5 levels along with narrowing of the spinal canal at these levels.

IMPRESSION: Lumbar spinal stenosis with radiculopathy of the S1 nerve root.

RECOMMENDATION: Referral to Neuroanesthesia for a series of epidural steroid injections. Physical therapy is also advised. Surgical referral is not necessary at this time.

Electronically signed by: Susan Rand, MD 06/04/20XX 18:15

Start | Log On/Off | Print | Edit

Use the medical report above to answer the questions.

1. Spinal stenosis causes compression of nerve roots demonstrated by which of the following symptoms for the patient?
   a. total paralysis
   b. abnormal sensation of prickling and tingling
   c. paralysis of one limb
   d. slight paralysis

2. The patient's diagnosis is spinal stenosis with:
   a. disease of the nerve roots
   b. disease of peripheral nerves
   c. disease affecting a single nerve
   d. disease of many nerves

C. Complete the three medical documents within the electronic health record (EHR) on Evolve.

Topic: Migraine
Documents: Office Visit Report, Emergency Department Report, Diagnostic Imaging Report

To complete the three medical records, go to Evolve Resources at evolve.elsevier.com and select:
Practice Student Resources > Student Resources > Chapter 15 > **Electronic Health Records**

See Appendix B for instructions.

EXERCISE 47 *Pronounce Medical Terms in Use*

Practice pronunciation of terms by reading aloud the following paragraph. Use the phonetic spellings following medical terms from the chapter to assist with pronunciation. The script also contains medical terms not presented in the chapter. Treat them as information only or look for their meanings in a medical dictionary or a reliable online source.

A 36-year-old right-handed female presents to the emergency department for an episode of **monoparesis** (*mon*-ō-pa-RĒ-sis) of the right leg, which started earlier in the day. She has a history of **major depression** (MĀ-jor) (dē-PRESH-un), for which she sees a **psychiatrist** (sī-KĪ-a-trist), and is treated with medication. About 6 months ago she had an episode of optic **neuritis** (nū-RĪ-tis), which was treated with steroids. She denies any history of **seizures** (SĒ-zherz). On examination she was noted to have **gait** (gāt) difficulties due to the weakness of her right leg. There was no evidence of **paresthesia** (*par*-es-THĒ-zha) or **cognitive** (COG-ni-tiv) impairment. Because of her age, a diagnosis of **stroke** (strōk) or **TIA** (T-I-A) is unlikely. A **subdural hematoma** (sub-DŪ-ral) (*hē*-ma-TŌ-ma) or intracranial lesion, such as **meningioma** (me-*nin*-jē-Ō-ma) or **glioblastoma** (*glī*-ō-blas-TŌ-ma), must be ruled out. Her symptoms are suggestive of **multiple sclerosis** (MUL-ti-pl) (skle-RŌ-sis). We will order an **MRI** (M-R-I) of the brain with contrast to see if any characteristic lesions are present. If not, we will consider a **lumbar puncture** (LUM-bar) (PUNK-chur) and refer her to a **neurologist** (nū-ROL-o-jist) for **evoked potential studies** (i-VŌKD) (pō-TEN-shal) (STUD-ēz).

EXERCISE 48 *Chapter Content Quiz*

Test your understanding of terms and abbreviations introduced in this chapter. Circle the letter for the medical term or abbreviation related to the words in italics.

1. Jack Cheng was in a serious motorcycle accident that resulted in *paralysis of all four limbs.*
   a. quadriplegia
   b. monoplegia
   c. hemiplegia
2. During her stroke, Mrs. Delgado had *inability to speak.*
   a. dysarthria
   b. aphasia
   c. dysphasia
3. Jacob Mamula experienced a brief period of being *unaware of his or her surroundings and unable to respond to stimuli* after suffering a concussion from a hard hit during the football game.
   a. convulsion
   b. incoherent
   c. unconsciousness
4. The newborn had *meninges protruding through a defect in his skull.*
   a. myelomalacia
   b. myelomeningocele
   c. meningocele
5. Gabriella Moreno was advised to schedule an appointment with the *physician who studies and treats disorders of the mind* when she was diagnosed with bipolar disorder.
   a. neurologist
   b. psychologist
   c. psychiatrist
6. *Chronic degenerative disease characterized by sclerotic patches along the brain and spinal cord* is more common in women, and frequently presents in the fourth or fifth decade of life.
   a. multiple sclerosis
   b. schizophrenia
   c. amyotrophic lateral sclerosis
7. The *process of recording of electrical activity of the brain* was scheduled for Caleb Cook when he started experiencing seizures.
   a. electroencephalogram
   b. electroencephalography
   c. electroencephalograph

8. *Abnormal condition of a clot in the cerebrum* was the cause of the TIA that Mr. Hernandez experienced.
   a. cerebral thrombosis
   b. cerebral aneurysm
   c. cerebral embolism

9. Mrs. Patel was having headaches and blurred vision. Her doctor was concerned about a meningioma. She ordered a *diagnostic procedure to examine blood flow and metabolic activity.*
   a. computed tomography
   b. positron emission tomography
   c. magnetic resonance imaging

10. Misha Sanov was diagnosed with *viral disease that affects the peripheral nerves and causes blisters on the skin that follow the course of the affected nerves* over her upper abdomen.
    a. shingles
    b. sciatica
    c. epilepsy

11. Because of scarring from a burn injury to her right hand, Emma Sammani had *loosening, separating a nerve to release it from surrounding tissues* to provide pain relief.
    a. neurolysis
    b. neuralgia
    c. rhizotomy

12. Mr. Rosenthal was taking medication to try to prevent rapid progression of his *type of dementia that occurs more frequently after the age of 65, with dramatic brain shrinkage.*
    a. PD
    b. CP
    c. AD

13. After his military service ended, Brandon O'Rourke experienced *significant behavioral disorder in which some people exposed to a traumatic event go on to develop a series of symptoms related to it.*
    a. somatoform disorder
    b. panic attacks
    c. posttraumatic stress disorder

14. James Robbins had poliomyelitis as a child, and was left with *slight paralysis of one (limb)*, which made it difficult for him to walk without assistance.
    a. monoparesis
    b. monoplegia
    c. hemiparesis

15. The physician assistant thought that Mrs. Ng's complaints of headaches and abdominal pain, which started after she lost her job, might be *pertaining to the mind and body.*
    a. psychopathy
    b. psychogenic
    c. psychosomatic

16. Corrine Pageau was brought to the emergency department after experiencing a seizure. She was eventually diagnosed with herpes simplex *inflammation of the brain.*
    a. meningitis
    b. encephalitis
    c. radiculitis

17. Daniel Roth lost consciousness after complaining of severe cephalgia; a CT scan revealed *bleeding between the pia mater and arachnoid layers of the meninges caused by a ruptured blood vessel.*
    a. subarachnoid hemorrhage
    b. subdural hematoma
    c. hydrocephalus

18. Malia Williams has been receiving therapy in the psychology department for her *disorder characterized by intrusive, unwanted thoughts that result in the tendency to perform repetitive acts or rituals.*
    a. attention deficit/hyperactivity disorder
    b. bipolar disorder
    c. obsessive-compulsive disorder

CHAPTER REVIEW

REVIEW OF CHAPTER CONTENT ON EVOLVE RESOURCES

Go to evolve.elsevier.com and click on Gradable Student Resources and Practice Student Resources. Online learning activities found there can be used to review chapter content and to assess your learning of word parts, medical terms, and abbreviations. Place check marks in the boxes next to activities used for review and assessment.

GRADABLE STUDENT RESOURCES

Chapter 15 >	Exercises >	☐ Word Parts ☐ Terms Built from Word Parts ☐ Terms Not Built from Word Parts ☐ Abbreviations
	Quizzes >	☐ Quiz 1: Disease and Disorder Terms ☐ Quiz 2: Surgical and Diagnostic Terms ☐ Quiz 3: Complementary and Behavioral Health Terms

PRACTICE STUDENT RESOURCES > STUDENT RESOURCES

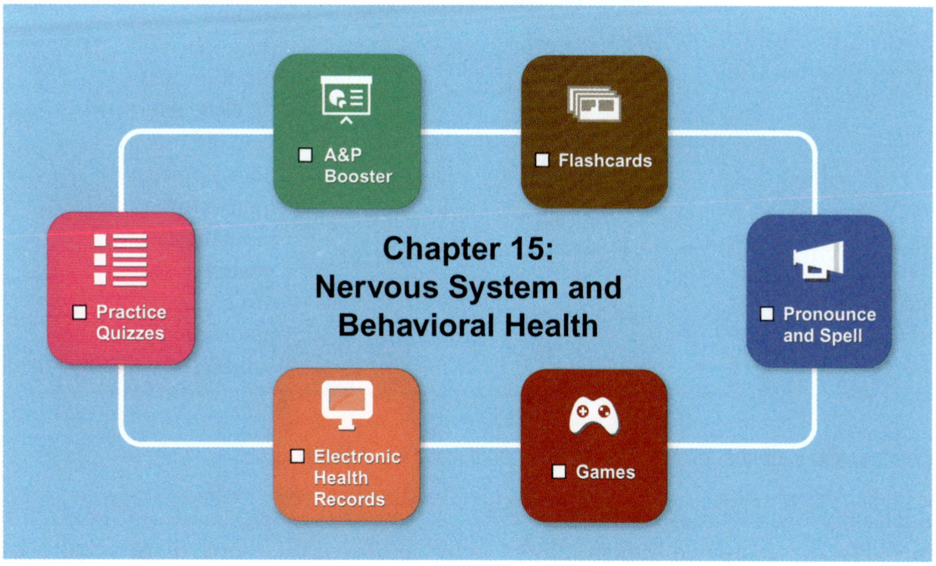

REVIEW OF WORD PARTS

Can you define and spell the following word parts?

COMBINING FORMS		SUFFIXES
cerebell/o	myel/o	-iatrist
cerebr/o	neur/o	-iatry
dur/o	phas/o	-ictal
encephal/o	poli/o	-paresis
esthesi/o	psych/o	
gangli/o	quadr/i	
ganglion/o	radic/o	
gli/o	radicul/o	
mening/i	rhiz/o	
meningi/o		
ment/o		
mon/o		

REVIEW OF TERMS

Can you build, analyze, define, pronounce, and spell the following terms *built from word parts?*

DISEASES AND DISORDERS

- cerebellitis
- cerebral thrombosis
- duritis
- encephalitis
- encephalomalacia
- encephalomyeloradiculitis
- gangliitis
- glioblastoma
- glioma
- meningioma
- meningitis
- meningocele
- meningomyelocele
- mononeuropathy
- neuralgia
- neuritis
- neuroarthropathy
- neuropathy
- poliomyelitis
- polyneuritis
- polyneuropathy
- radiculitis
- radiculopathy
- rhizomeningomyelitis
- subdural hematoma

SURGICAL

- ganglionectomy
- neurectomy
- neurolysis
- neuroplasty
- neurorrhaphy
- neurotomy
- radicotomy
- rhizotomy

DIAGNOSTIC

- cerebral angiography
- CT myelography
- electroencephalogram (EEG)
- electroencephalograph
- electroencephalography

COMPLEMENTARY

- anesthesia
- aphasia
- cephalgia
- cerebral
- craniocerebral
- dysesthesia
- dysphasia
- encephalopathy
- gliocyte
- hemiparesis
- hemiplegia
- hyperesthesia
- interictal
- intracerebral
- mental
- monoparesis
- monoplegia
- myelomalacia
- neuroid
- neurologist
- neurology
- paresthesia
- postictal
- preictal
- quadriplegia
- subdural

BEHAVIORAL HEALTH

- psychiatrist
- psychiatry
- psychogenic
- psychologist
- psychology
- psychopathy
- psychosis (pl. psychoses)
- psychosomatic

Can you define, pronounce, and spell the following terms *NOT built from word parts?*

DISEASES AND DISORDERS

- Alzheimer disease (AD)
- amyotrophic lateral sclerosis (ALS)
- Bell palsy
- cerebral aneurysm
- cerebral embolism
- cerebral palsy (CP)
- dementia
- epilepsy
- hydrocephalus
- intracerebral hemorrhage
- multiple sclerosis (MS)
- Parkinson disease (PD)
- sciatica
- shingles
- stroke
- subarachnoid hemorrhage (SAH)
- transient ischemic attack (TIA)

DIAGNOSTIC

- computed tomography (CT)
- evoked potential (EP) studies
- lumbar puncture (LP)
- magnetic resonance imaging (MRI)
- positron emission tomography (PET)

COMPLEMENTARY

- afferent
- ataxia
- cognitive
- coma
- concussion
- conscious
- convulsion
- disorientation
- dysarthria
- efferent
- gait
- incoherent
- paraplegia
- seizure
- shunt
- syncope
- unconsciousness

BEHAVIORAL HEALTH

- anorexia nervosa
- anxiety disorder
- attention deficit/hyperactivity disorder (ADHD)
- autism
- bipolar disorder
- bulimia nervosa
- major depression
- obsessive-compulsive disorder (OCD)
- panic attack
- phobia
- pica
- posttraumatic stress disorder (PTSD)
- schizophrenia
- somatoform disorders

Chapter 16

Endocrine System

Outline

Objectives

Upon completion of this chapter you will be able to:

1. Pronounce glands and hormones of the endocrine system.
2. Define and spell word parts related to the endocrine system.
3. Define, pronounce, and spell disease and disorder terms related to the endocrine system.
4. Define, pronounce, and spell surgical terms related to the endocrine system.
5. Define, pronounce, and spell diagnostic terms related to the endocrine system.
6. Define, pronounce, and spell complementary terms related to the endocrine system.
7. Interpret the meaning of abbreviations related to the endocrine system.
8. Apply medical language in clinical contexts.

ANATOMY

The endocrine system is composed of endocrine glands distributed throughout the body. The endocrine glands are: pituitary, thyroid, parathyroid, adrenal, pancreas, gonads (ovaries and testes), and thymus.

Function

The endocrine system regulates body activities through the use of chemical messengers called **hormones**, which when released into the bloodstream influence metabolic activities, growth, and development (Fig. 16.1). The nervous system also regulates body activities by receiving electrical impulses that convey information about the state of the body, and then activating glandular secretions in response. Hormones secreted by the **endocrine glands** that make up the endocrine system go directly into the bloodstream and are transported throughout the body. They are referred to as **ductless glands** because they do not have ducts to carry their secretions. In contrast, the **exocrine** or **duct glands** have ducts that carry their secretions from the producing gland to other parts of the body. An example is the parotid gland, which produces saliva that flows through the parotid duct into the mouth. Only those terms related to the major endocrine glands—pituitary, thyroid, parathyroids, adrenals, and the islets of Langerhans in the pancreas—are presented in this chapter. The thymus primarily functions as part of the lymphatic system and was presented in Chapter 10. The male and female sex glands were also presented in previous chapters.

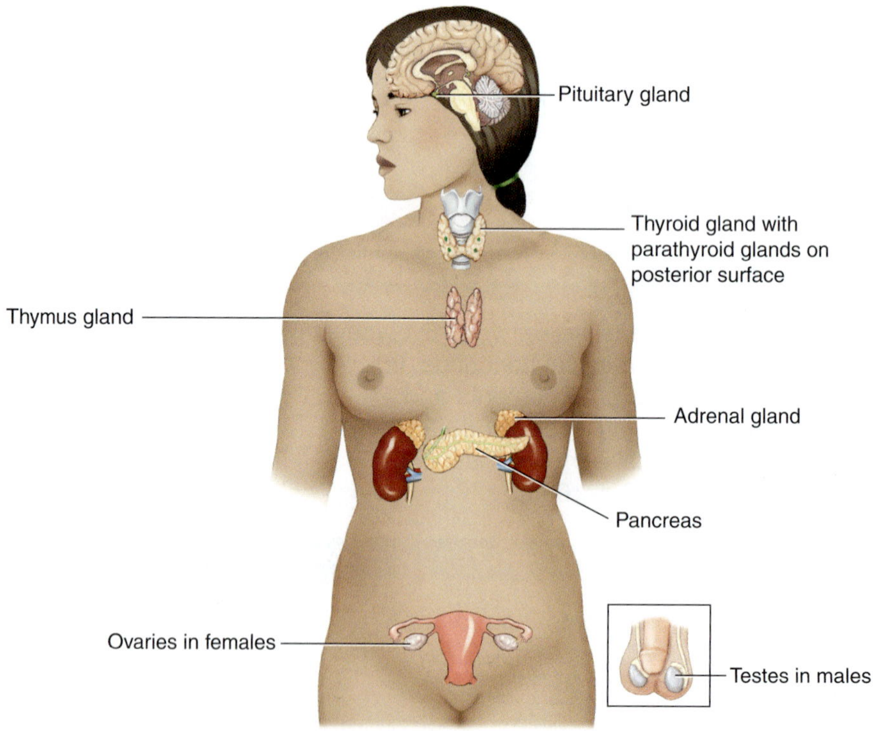

FIG. 16.1 The endocrine system.

Endocrine Glands and Hormones

TERM	DEFINITION
pituitary gland (pi-TOO-i-*tar*-ē) (gland)	approximately the size of a pea and located at the base of the brain. The pituitary is divided into two lobes. It is often referred to as the master gland because it produces hormones that stimulate the function of other endocrine glands (also called **hypophysis cerebri**) (Fig. 16.2).
anterior lobe (ān-TĒR-ē-er) (lōb)	produces and secretes the following hormones (also called **adenohypophysis**):
growth hormone (GH) (grohth) (HŌR-mōn)	regulates the growth of the body
adrenocorticotropic hormone (ACTH) (a-*drē*-nō-*kōr*-ti-kō-TRŌ-pik) (HŌR-mōn)	stimulates the adrenal cortex
thyroid-stimulating hormone (TSH) (*THĪ*-royd) (STIM-yuh-lāt-ing) (HŌR-mōn)	stimulates the thyroid gland
gonadotropic hormones (*gō-na*-dō-TRŌ-pik) (HŌR-mōns)	stimulate the gonads (the testes in males and ovaries in females). **Follicle-stimulating hormone** (FSH) and **luteinizing hormone** (LH) are the gonadotropic hormones released from the adenohypophysis.
prolactin (PRL) (prō-LAK-tin)	promotes development of glandular tissue during pregnancy and produces milk after birth of an infant

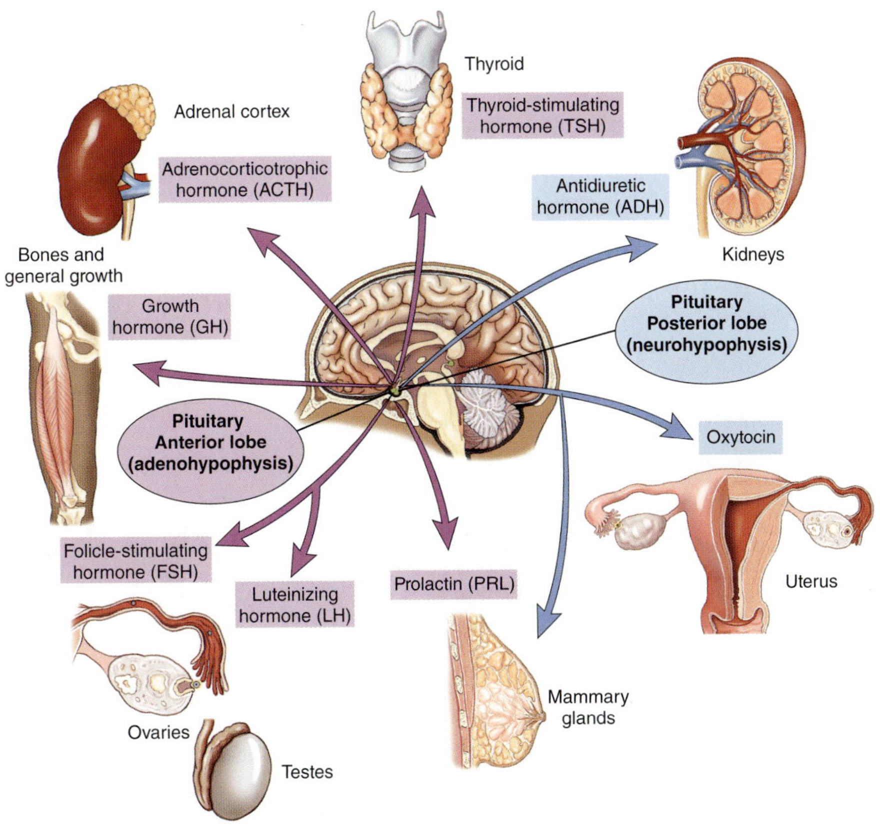

FIG. 16.2 Pituitary gland, hormones secreted, and target organs.

Endocrine Glands and Hormones—cont'd

TERM	DEFINITION
posterior lobe (po-STĒR-ē-er) (lōb)	stores and releases antidiuretic hormone and oxytocin (also called **neurohypophysis**)
antidiuretic hormone (ADH) (*an*-tē-*dī*-ū-*RET*-ik) (HŌR-mōn)	stimulates the kidney to reabsorb water and constricts blood vessels to help maintain blood pressure (also called **vasopressin**)
oxytocin (*ok*-sē-TŌ-sin)	stimulates uterine contractions during labor and postpartum, and milk let down by the breasts postpartum
hypothalamus (*hī*-pō-THAL-a-mus)	located superior to the pituitary gland in the brain. The hypothalamus secretes "releasing" hormones that function to stimulate or inhibit the release of pituitary gland hormones.
thyroid gland (THĪ-royd) (gland)	largest endocrine gland. It is located anteriorly in the neck below the larynx and comprises bilateral lobes connected by an isthmus (Fig. 16.3C). The thyroid gland secretes the hormones triiodothyronine (T_3) and thyroxine (T_4), which require iodine for their production. Thyroxine is necessary for body cell metabolism.
parathyroid glands (*par*-a-THĪ-royd) (glans)	four small bodies embedded in the posterior aspect of the lobes of the thyroid gland (Fig. 16.3D). Parathyroid hormone (PTH), the hormone produced by the glands, helps maintain the level of calcium in the blood by its effects on bone and kidneys.

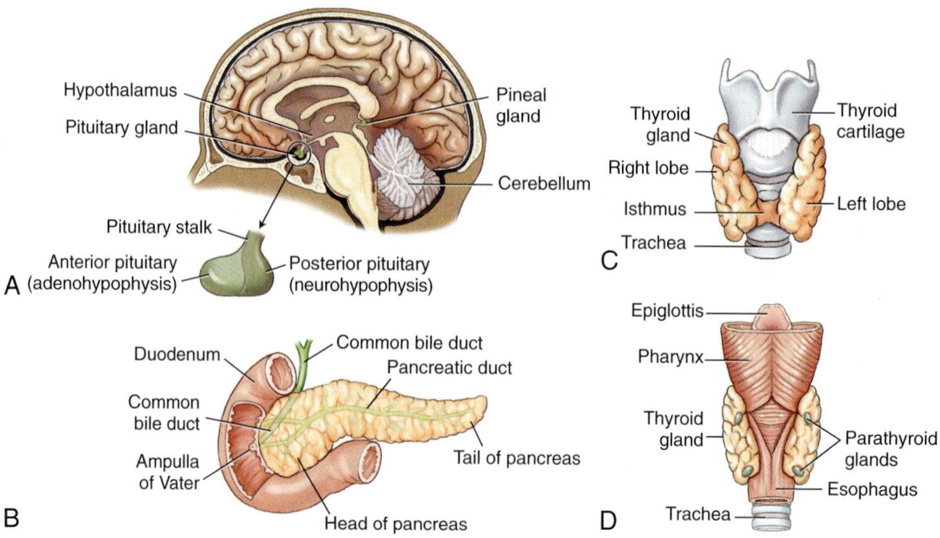

FIG. 16.3 A, Pituitary and pineal glands. **B,** Pancreas. **C,** Thyroid gland. **D,** Parathyroid glands, posterior view.

TERM	DEFINITION
islets of Langerhans (Ī-lets) (LAHNG-er-hahnz)	clusters of endocrine tissue found throughout the pancreas, made up of different cell types that secrete various hormones, including insulin and glucagon. Non-endocrine cells found throughout the pancreas produce enzymes that facilitate digestion (Fig. 16.4).
adrenal glands (a-DRĒ-nal) (glans)	paired glands, one of which is located superior to each kidney. The outer portion is called the **adrenal cortex,** and the inner portion is called the **adrenal medulla.** The following hormones are secreted by the adrenal glands:
cortisol (KOR-ti-sol)	secreted by the adrenal cortex. It aids the body during stress by increasing glucose levels to provide energy (also called **hydrocortisone**).
aldosterone (al-DOS-ter-ōn)	secreted by the adrenal cortex. Electrolytes (mineral salts) that are necessary for normal body function are regulated by this hormone.
epinephrine, norepinephrine (*ep*-i-NEF-rin), (*nor*-ep-i-NEF-rin)	secreted by the adrenal medulla. These hormones help the body to deal with stress by increasing the blood pressure, heartbeat, and respirations. (also called **adrenaline** and **noradrenaline**, respectively)

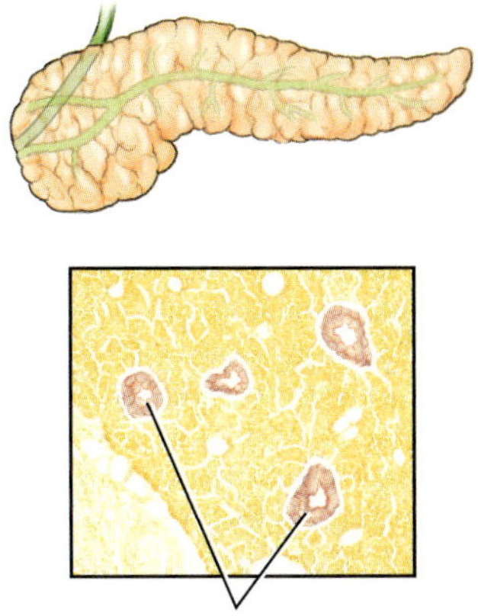

FIG. 16.4 Pancreas, with islets of Langerhans.

A&P Booster

For more anatomy and physiology, go to Evolve Resources at evolve.elsevier.com and select:
Practice Student Resources > Student Resources > Chapter 16 > **A&P Booster**

See Appendix B for instructions.

EXERCISE 1

Practice saying aloud each of the Glands and Hormones of the Endocrine System.

To hear the terms, go to Evolve Resources at evolve.elsevier.com and select:
Practice Student Resources > Student Resources > Chapter 16 > **Pronounce and Spell**

See Appendix B for instructions.

❑ Check the box when complete.

WORD PARTS

Word parts you need to learn to complete this chapter are listed on the following pages. The exercises at the end of each list will help you learn their definitions and spellings.

> Use the flashcards accompanying this text or electronic flashcards to assist you in memorizing the word parts for this chapter.

Combining Forms of the Endocrine System

COMBINING FORM	DEFINITION
adren/o, adrenal/o	adrenal glands
cortic/o	cortex (the outer layer of a body organ)
endocrin/o	endocrine
parathyroid/o	parathyroid glands
pituitar/o	pituitary gland
thyr/o, thyroid/o	thyroid gland

EXERCISE 2

Fill in the blanks with combining forms in this diagram of the endocrine glands. *To check your answers, go to Appendix A.*

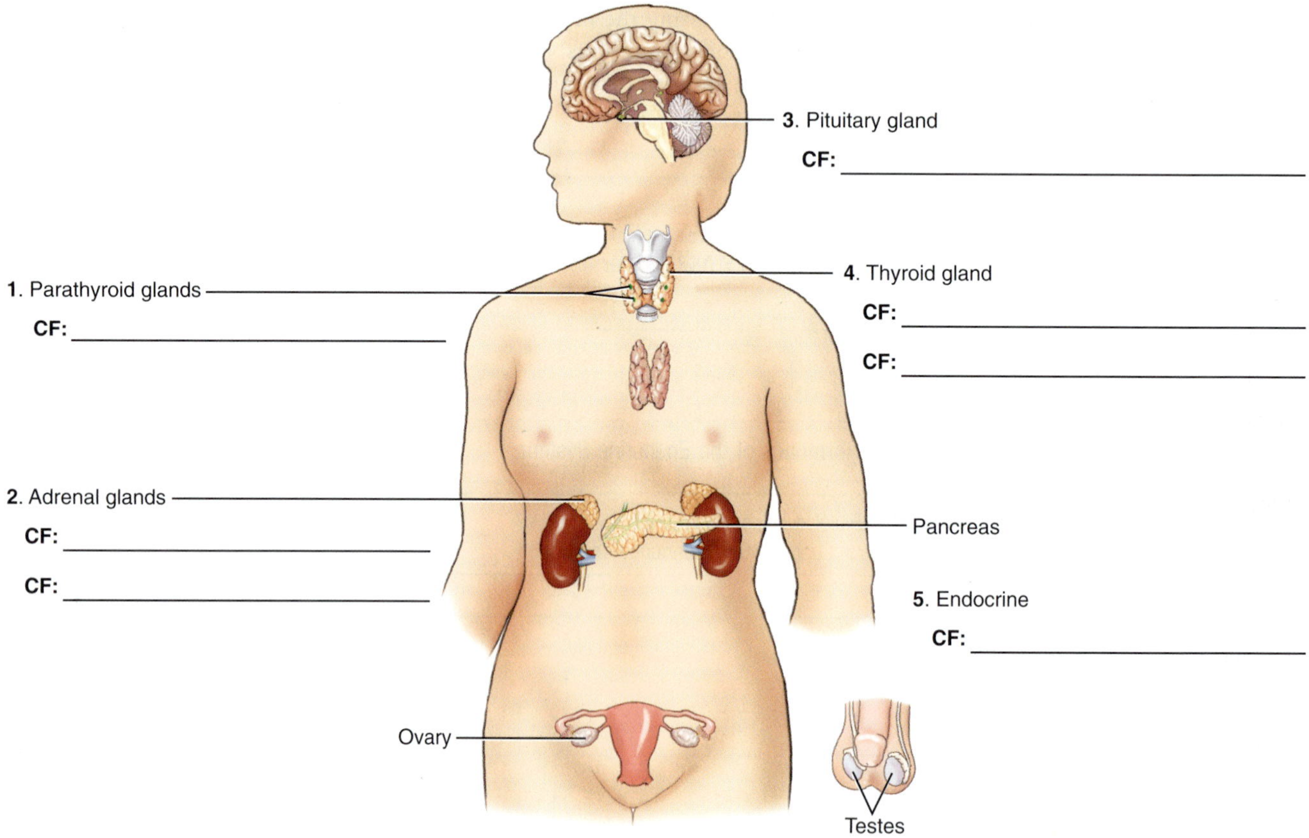

EXERCISE 3

Fill in the blank with the combining form in this diagram of adrenal glands (with transverse cross-sectional view).

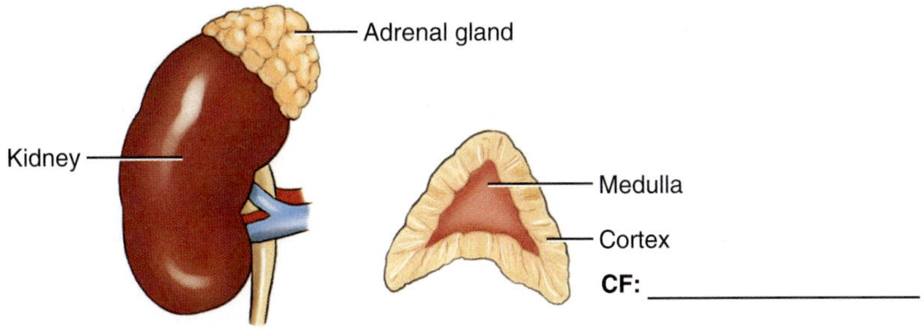

EXERCISE 4

Step 1: Write the definitions after the following combining forms.

Step 2: Match the descriptions on the right with the combining forms and definitions. Answers may be used more than once; no answer line appears for those not described in a lettered item.

_____ 1. thyr/o, ______________________________
_____ 2. adrenal/o, ______________________________
_____ 3. pituitar/o, ______________________________
_____ 4. cortic/o, ______________________________
_____ 5. parathyroid/o, ______________________________
_____ 6. adren/o, ______________________________
_____ 7. thyroid/o, ______________________________
8. endocrin/o, ______________________________

a. referred to as the master gland because it produces hormones that stimulate the function of other endocrine glands
b. four small bodies embedded in the posterior aspect of the lobes of the thyroid gland
c. largest endocrine gland, secretes triiodothyronine (T_3) and thyroxine (T_4)
d. paired glands, one of which is located above each kidney
e. outer portion of adrenal gland

Combining Forms Commonly Used with Endocrine System Terms

COMBINING FORM	DEFINITION
acr/o	extremities, height
calc/i	calcium *(Note: the combining vowel is* i.*)*
dips/o	thirst
kal/i	potassium *(Note: the combining vowel is* i.*)*
natr/o	sodium

EXERCISE 5

Write the definitions of the following combining forms.

1. dips/o ______________________________
2. kal/i ______________________________
3. calc/i ______________________________
4. acr/o ______________________________
5. natr/o ______________________________

EXERCISE 6

Write the combining form for each of the following.

1. extremities, height ______________________
2. calcium ______________________
3. thirst ______________________
4. potassium ______________________
5. sodium ______________________

Suffix

SUFFIX	DEFINITION
-drome	run, running

Refer to **Appendix C** and **Appendix D** for a complete list of word parts.

EXERCISE 7

Write the definition of the following word part.

1. -drome ______________________

EXERCISE 8

Write the suffix for the following.

1. run, running ______________________

For additional practice with Word Parts, go to Evolve Resources at evolve.elsevier.com and select: Practice Student Resources > Student Resources > Chapter 16 > **Flashcards**

See Appendix B for instructions.

EXERCISE FIGURE A

Fill in the blanks with word parts defined to label the photograph.

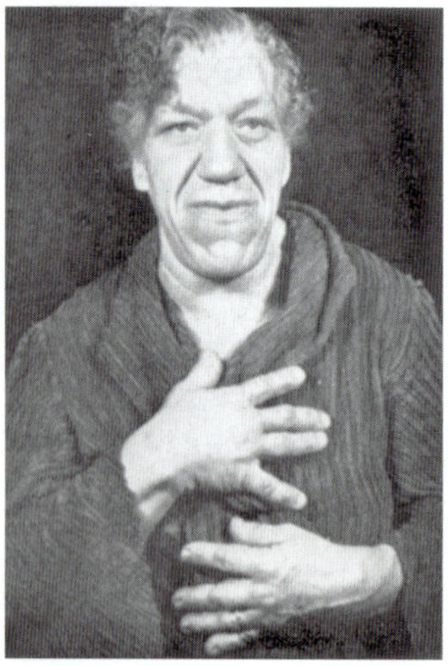

______ / ______ / ______
extremities / cv / enlargement

is a metabolic disorder characterized by marked enlargement of the face, jaw, and extremities.

MEDICAL TERMS

The terms you need to learn to complete this chapter are listed below. The exercises following each list will help you learn the definition and spelling of each word.

Disease and Disorder Terms

BUILT FROM WORD PARTS

The following terms can be translated using definitions of word parts. Further explanation is provided within parentheses as needed.

TERM	DEFINITION
acromegaly (*ak*-rō-MEG-a-lē)	enlargement of the extremities (and face due to increased soft tissue, bone, and cartilage; caused by excessive production of the growth hormone by the pituitary gland after puberty) (Exercise Figure A)
adrenalitis (a-*drē*-nal-Ī-tis)	inflammation of the adrenal glands
adrenomegaly (a-*drē*-nō-MEG-a-lē)	enlargement (of one or both) of the adrenal glands

TERM	DEFINITION
hypercalcemia (*hī*-per-kal-SĒ-mē-a)	excessive calcium in the blood
hyperglycemia (*hī*-per-glī-SĒ-mē-a)	excessive sugar in the blood
hyperkalemia (*hī*-per-ka-LĒ-mē-a)	excessive potassium in the blood
hyperparathyroidism (*hī*-per-*par*-a-THĪ-royd-izm)	state of excessive parathyroid gland activity (resulting in hypercalcemia and leading to osteoporosis, as well as symptoms of muscle weakness, abdominal pain, nausea, vomiting, and drowsiness)
hyperpituitarism (*hī*-per-pi-TOO-i-ta-*rizm*)	state of excessive pituitary gland activity (characterized by excessive secretion of pituitary hormones)
hyperthyroidism (*hī*-per-THĪ-royd-izm)	state of excessive thyroid gland activity (characterized by excessive secretion of thyroid hormones. Signs and symptoms include weight loss, irritability, and heat intolerance.)
hypocalcemia (*hī*-pō-kal-SĒ-mē-a)	deficient calcium in the blood
hypoglycemia (*hī*-pō-glī-SĒ-mē-a)	deficient sugar in the blood
hypokalemia (*hī*-pō-ka-LĒ-mē-a)	deficient potassium in the blood
hyponatremia (*hī*-pō-na-TRĒ-mē-a)	deficient sodium in the blood
hypopituitarism (*hī*-pō-pi-TŪ-i-ta-*rizm*)	state of deficient pituitary gland activity (characterized by decreased secretion of one or more of the pituitary hormones, which can affect the function of the target endocrine gland; for example, hypothyroidism can result from decreased secretion of thyroid-stimulating hormone by the pituitary gland)
hypothyroidism (*hī*-pō-THĪ-royd-izm)	state of deficient thyroid gland activity (characterized by decreased secretion of thyroid hormones. Signs and symptoms include fatigue, weight gain, and cold intolerance.)
panhypopituitarism (pan-*hī*-pō-pi-TŪ-i-ta-*rizm*)	state of total deficient pituitary gland activity (characterized by decreased secretion of all the anterior pituitary hormones; this is a more serious condition than hypopituitarism in that it affects the function of all the other endocrine glands) *(Note: two prefixes are contained in this term)*
parathyroidoma (*par*-a-*thī*-royd-Ō-ma)	tumor of a parathyroid gland
thyroiditis (*thī*-royd-Ī-tis)	inflammation of the thyroid gland

HYPOTHYROIDISM
is the state of deficient thyroid gland activity, resulting in the decreased production of the thyroid hormone called thyroxine. A severe form of hypothyroidism in adults is called **myxedema** and in infants is called **congenital hypothyroidism**.

EXERCISE 9

Practice saying aloud each of the Disease and Disorder Terms Built from Word Parts.

To hear the terms, go to Evolve Resources at evolve.elsevier.com and select:
Practice Student Resources > Student Resources > Chapter 16 > **Pronounce and Spell**

See Appendix B for instructions.

❑ Check the box when complete.

EXERCISE 10

Analyze and define the following terms.

1. adrenalitis
   ____
   ____
2. hypocalcemia
   ____
   ____
3. hyperthyroidism
   ____
   ____
4. hyperkalemia
   ____
   ____
5. hyperglycemia
   ____
   ____
6. adrenomegaly
   ____
   ____
7. hypothyroidism
   ____
   ____
8. hypokalemia
   ____
   ____
9. parathyroidoma
   ____
   ____
10. acromegaly
    ____
    ____
11. panhypopituitarism
    ____
    ____
12. hypoglycemia
    ____
    ____
13. hypercalcemia
    ____
    ____
14. hyperpituitarism
    ____
    ____

15. hyponatremia

____

____

16. hyperparathyroidism

____

____

17. thyroiditis

____

____

18. hypopituitarism

____

____

EXERCISE 11

Build disease and disorder terms for the following definitions with the word parts you have learned.

1. enlargement of (one or both of) the adrenal glands ______ / ______ / ______ (WR / CV / S)
2. state of deficient thyroid gland activity ______ / ______ / ______ (P / WR / S)
3. enlargement of the extremities ______ / ______ / ______ (WR / CV / S)
4. deficient sugar in the blood ______ / ______ / ______ (P / WR / S)
5. excessive potassium in the blood ______ / ______ / ______ (P / WR / S)
6. deficient calcium in the blood ______ / ______ / ______ (P / WR / S)
7. state of excessive thyroid gland activity ______ / ______ / ______ (P / WR / S)
8. state of deficient pituitary gland activity ______ / ______ / ______ (P / WR / S)
9. excessive calcium in the blood ______ / ______ / ______ (P / WR / S)
10. state of excessive pituitary gland activity ______ / ______ / ______ (P / WR / S)
11. tumor of a parathyroid gland ______ / ______ (WR / S)
12. excessive sugar in the blood ______ / ______ / ______ (P / WR / S)
13. deficient potassium in the blood ______ / ______ / ______ (P / WR / S)
14. inflammation of the adrenal glands ______ / ______ (WR / S)

15. deficient sodium in the blood ______ P / ______ WR / ______ S

16. state of excessive parathyroid gland activity ______ P / ______ WR / ______ S

17. inflammation of the thyroid gland ______ WR / ______ S

18. state of total deficient pituitary gland activity ______ P / ______ P / ______ WR / ______ S

EXERCISE 12

Spell each of the Disease and Disorder Terms Built from Word Parts by having someone dictate them to you. Use a separate sheet of paper.

To hear and spell the terms, go to Evolve Resources at evolve.elsevier.com and select:
Practice Student Resources > Student Resources > Chapter 16 > **Pronounce and Spell**

See Appendix B for instructions.

❑ Check the box when complete.

Disease and Disorder Terms
NOT BUILT FROM WORD PARTS

Word parts may be present in the following terms; however, their full meanings cannot be translated using definitions of word parts alone.

ADDISON DISEASE was named in **1855** for **Thomas Addison**, an English physician and pathologist. He described the disease as a "morbid state with feeble heart action, anemia, irritability of the stomach, and a peculiar change in the color of the skin."

CUSHING SYNDROME was named for an American neurosurgeon, **Harvey Williams Cushing** (1869-1939), after he described adrenocortical hyperfunction.

TERM	DEFINITION
Addison disease (AD-i-sun) (di-ZĒZ)	chronic syndrome resulting from a deficiency in the hormonal secretion of the adrenal cortex. Signs and symptoms may include weakness, weight loss, hypotension, darkening of skin, and loss of appetite.
congenital hypothyroidism (kon-JEN-i-tal) (hī-pō-THĪ-royd-izm)	condition caused by congenital absence or atrophy (wasting away) of the thyroid gland, resulting in hypothyroidism. The disease is characterized by puffy features, mental deficiency, large tongue, and dwarfism.
Cushing syndrome (KŪSH-ing) (SIN-drōm)	group of signs and symptoms attributed to the excessive production of cortisol by the adrenal cortices (pl. of cortex). This syndrome may be the result of a pituitary tumor that produces ACTH or a primary adrenal cortex hypersecretion. Signs include abnormally pigmented skin, "moon face," pads of fat on the chest and abdomen, "buffalo hump" (fat on the upper back), wasting away of muscle, and hypertension.
diabetes insipidus (DI) (*dī*-a-BĒ-tēz) (in-SIP-i-dus)	result of decreased secretion of antidiuretic hormone by the posterior lobe of the pituitary gland. Symptoms include excessive thirst (polydipsia), large amounts of urine (polyuria), and water being excreted from the body.

TERM	DEFINITION
diabetes mellitus (DM) (*dī*-a-BĒ-tēz) (MEL-li-tus)	chronic disease involving a disorder of carbohydrate metabolism caused by under-activity of the insulin-producing islets of Langerhans and characterized by elevated blood sugar (hyperglycemia). DM can cause chronic renal disease, retinopathy, and neuropathy. In extreme cases the patient may develop ketosis, acidosis, and finally coma. (Table 16.1)
gigantism (jī-GAN-tizm)	condition brought about by hypersecretion of growth hormone by the pituitary gland before puberty
goiter (GOY-ter)	enlargement of the thyroid gland. May be caused by autoimmune diseases of the thyroid (Graves disease or Hashimoto thyroiditis), iodine deficiency, or the presence of multiple nodules.
Graves disease (grāvz) (di-ZĒZ)	autoimmune disorder of the thyroid gland characterized by the production of more thyroid hormone than the body needs (hyperthyroidism), goiter, and exophthalmos (abnormal protrusion of the eyeballs)
ketoacidosis (*kē*-tō-*as*-i-DŌ-sis)	serious condition resulting from uncontrolled diabetes mellitus in which acid ketones accumulate from fat metabolism in the absence of adequate insulin. If not promptly controlled by adequate insulin and hydration, can progress to coma and death.
metabolic syndrome (*met*-a-BOL-ik) (SIN-drōm)	group of signs and symptoms including insulin resistance, obesity characterized by excessive fat around the area of the waist and abdomen, hypertension, hyperglycemia, elevated triglycerides, and low levels of the "good" cholesterol HDL. Risks include development of type 2 diabetes mellitus, coronary heart disease, or stroke (also called **syndrome X** and **insulin resistance syndrome**).
myxedema (*mik*-se-DĒ-ma)	condition resulting from an extreme deficiency of the thyroid hormone thyroxine; a severe form of hypothyroidism in an adult. Signs include puffiness of the face and hands, coarse and thickened skin, enlarged tongue, slow speech, and anemia.
pheochromocytoma (*fē*-ō-*krō*-mō-sī-TŌ-ma)	tumor of the adrenal medulla, which is usually non-malignant and characterized by hypertension, headaches, palpitations, diaphoresis, chest pain, and abdominal pain. Surgical removal of the tumor is the most common treatment. Though usually curable with early detection, it can be fatal if untreated.
tetany (TET-a-nē)	condition affecting nerves causing muscle spasms as a result of low amounts of calcium in the blood caused by a deficiency of the parathyroid hormone
thyrotoxicosis (*thī*-rō-*tok*-si-KŌ-sis)	condition caused by excessive thyroid hormones

GIGANTISM AND ACROMEGALY

are both caused by overproduction of growth hormone. **Gigantism** occurs before puberty and before the growing ends of the bones have closed. If untreated, an individual may reach 8 feet tall in adulthood. **Acromegaly** occurs after puberty. The body parts most affected are those in the hands, feet, and jaw.

EXERCISE 13

Practice saying aloud each of the Disease and Disorder Terms NOT Built from Word Parts.

> To hear the terms, go to Evolve Resources at evolve.elsevier.com and select:
> Practice Student Resources > Student Resources > Chapter 16 > **Pronounce and Spell**
>
> See Appendix B for instructions.

INTEGRATIVE MEDICINE TERM

Yoga is the practice of physical postures, conscious breathing, and meditation. Studies have revealed the regular practice of yoga demonstrates efficacy as an adjunct therapy for management of **type 2 diabetes mellitus**, may promote healthy aging by maintaining the basal levels of growth hormone and DHEA, supports regulation of several reproductive hormones, and contributes to the improvement of psycho-physical health when under stress.

TABLE 16.1 Diabetes Mellitus

Two major forms of diabetes mellitus are **type 1,** previously called insulin-dependent diabetes mellitus (IDDM) or juvenile-onset diabetes, and **type 2,** previously called noninsulin-dependent diabetes mellitus (NIDDM) or adult-onset diabetes (AODM). Type 2 diabetes mellitus has reached epidemic proportions and is a major cause of cardiovascular disease.

TYPE 1 DIABETES MELLITUS	
Cause	autoimmune disease in which the beta cells of the pancreas that produce insulin are destroyed and eventually no insulin is produced
Characteristics	abrupt onset, occurs primarily in childhood or adolescence; patients often are thin
Signs and Symptoms	polyuria, polydipsia, weight loss, and hyperglycemia; these are present if blood sugar is not controlled, and can progress to ketoacidosis if not promptly treated
Treatment	insulin injections and diet
TYPE 2 DIABETES MELLITUS	
Cause	resistance of body cells to the action of insulin, coupled with a decrease in the ability of the pancreas to make sufficient insulin to overcome this resistance
Characteristics	slow onset, usually occurs in middle-aged or elderly adults; most patients are obese
Signs and Symptoms	fatigue, blurred vision, thirst, and hyperglycemia; these may be present if blood sugar is not controlled
Treatment	diet, exercise, oral or injected medication, and sometimes insulin

LONG-TERM COMPLICATIONS OF DIABETES MELLITUS

MACROVASCULAR COMPLICATIONS

- coronary artery disease → myocardial infarction
- cerebrovascular disease → stroke
- peripheral artery disease → leg pain when walking (intermittent vascular claudication)

MICROVASCULAR COMPLICATIONS

- diabetic retinopathy → loss of vision
- diabetic nephropathy → chronic renal disease, kidney failure
- neuropathy → loss of feeling in the distal extremities (feet, hands), which can lead to amputation

EXERCISE 14

Match the terms in the first column with the correct definitions in the second column.

_____ 1. diabetes insipidus
_____ 2. tetany
_____ 3. pheochromocytoma
_____ 4. thyrotoxicosis
_____ 5. diabetes mellitus
_____ 6. ketoacidosis

a. serious condition resulting from uncontrolled diabetes mellitus in which acid ketones accumulate from fat metabolism in the absence of adequate insulin
b. tumor of the adrenal medulla, characterized by hypertension, headaches, palpitations, diaphoresis, chest pain, and abdominal pain
c. result of decreased secretion of antidiuretic hormone by the posterior lobe of the pituitary gland
d. condition caused by excessive thyroid hormones
e. condition affecting nerves causing muscle spasms as a result of low amounts of calcium in the blood
f. chronic disease involving a disorder of carbohydrate metabolism characterized by elevated blood sugar (hyperglycemia)

EXERCISE 15

Write the medical term pictured and defined.

1. ___________________________
condition brought about by hypersecretion of growth hormone by the pituitary gland before puberty

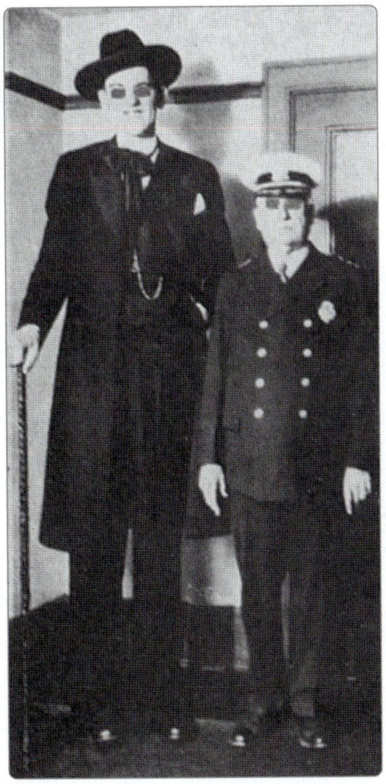

2. ___________________________
chronic syndrome resulting from a deficiency in the hormonal secretion of the adrenal cortex with symptoms of weight loss, hypotension, and skin darkening

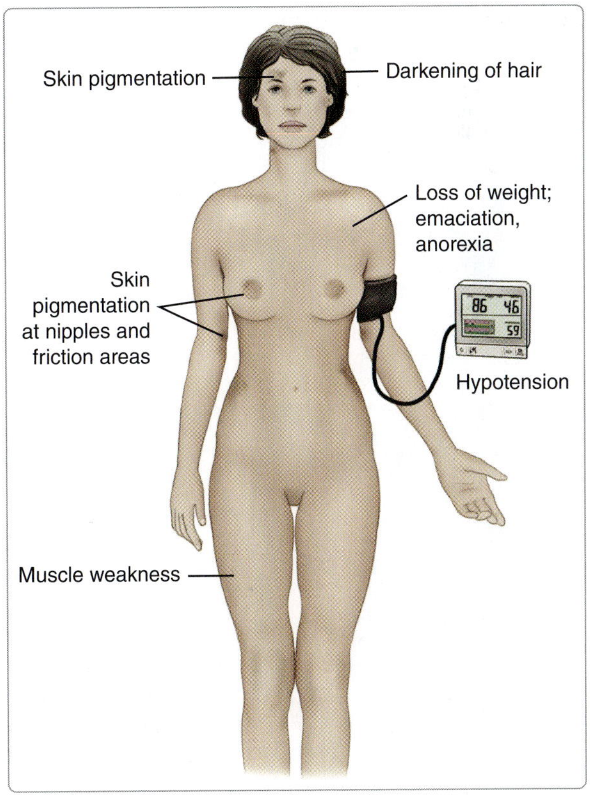

EXERCISE 15 *Pictured and Defined—cont'd*

3. ______________________________

A. condition caused by congenital absence or atrophy of the thyroid gland, resulting in hypothyroidism; characterized by puffy features, mental deficiency, large tongue, and dwarfism

B. same child after treatment for this condition

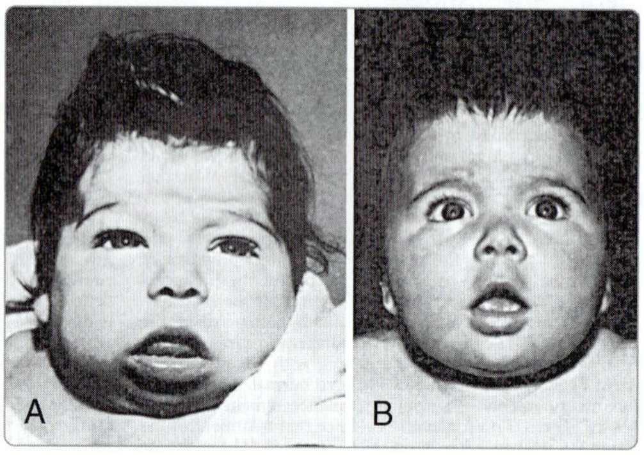

4. ______________________________

condition resulting from a deficiency of the thyroid hormone thyroxine; a severe form of hypothyroidism in an adult, characterized by puffiness of the face and hands, coarse and thickened skin, enlarged tongue, slow speech, and anemia

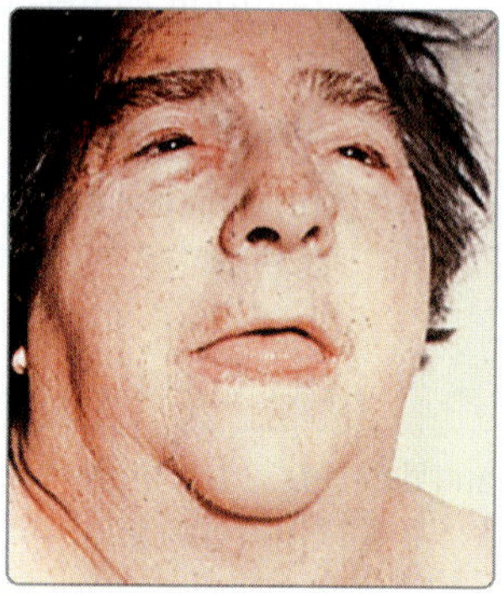

5. ______________________________

A. group of signs and symptoms attributed to the excessive production of cortisol by the adrenal cortices

B. same child after treatment for this condition

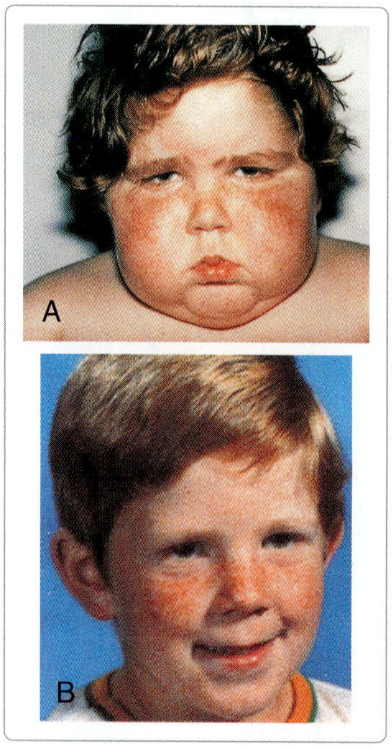

6. ______________________________

group of signs and symptoms including insulin resistance, obesity characterized by excessive fat around the area of the waist, hypertension, hyperglycemia, elevated triglycerides, and low levels of the "good" cholesterol HDL

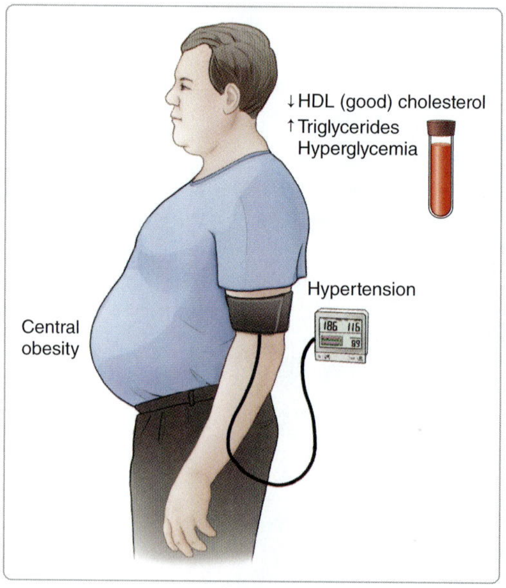

7. ______________________
enlargement of the thyroid gland

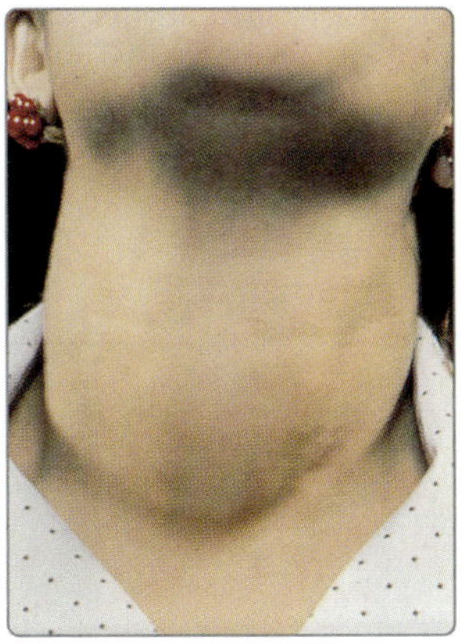

8. ______________________
autoimmune disorder of the thyroid gland characterized by hyperthyroidism, goiter, and protrusion of the eyeballs

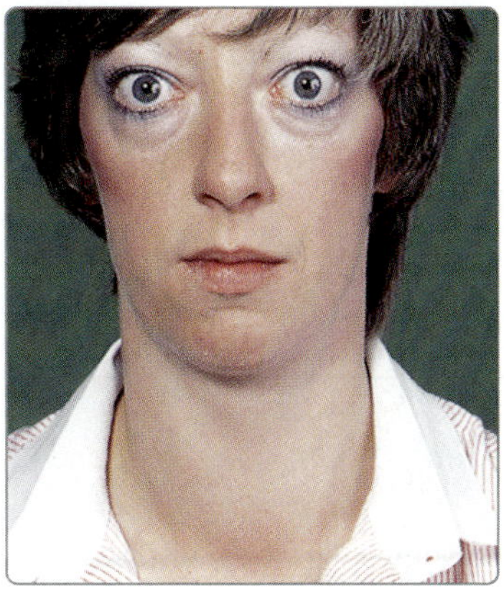

EXERCISE 16

Spell each of the Disease and Disorder Terms NOT Built from Word Parts by having someone dictate them to you. Use a separate sheet of paper.

To hear and spell the terms, go to Evolve Resources at evolve.elsevier.com and select:
Practice Student Resources > Student Resources > Chapter 16 > **Pronounce and Spell**

See Appendix B for instructions.

❑ Check the box when complete.

Surgical Terms

BUILT FROM WORD PARTS

The following terms can be translated using definitions of word parts. Further explanation is provided within parentheses as needed.

TERM	DEFINITION
adrenalectomy (ad-*rē*-nal-EK-to-mē)	excision of (one or both) adrenal glands
pancreatectomy (*pan*-crē-a-TEK-ta-mē)	excision of the pancreas
parathyroidectomy (*par*-a-*thī*-royd-EK-to-mē)	excision of (one or more) parathyroid glands
thyroidectomy (thī-royd-EK-to-mē)	excision of the thyroid gland

EXERCISE 17

Practice saying aloud each of the Surgical Terms Built from Word Parts.

To hear the terms, go to Evolve Resources at evolve.elsevier.com and select:
Practice Student Resources > Student Resources > Chapter 16 > **Pronounce and Spell**

See Appendix B for instructions.

❑ Check the box when complete.

EXERCISE 18

Analyze and define the following terms.

1. pancreatectomy

____

____

2. adrenalectomy

____

____

3. thyroidectomy

____

____

4. parathyroidectomy

____

____

EXERCISE 19

Build surgical terms for the following definitions by using the word parts you have learned.

1. excision of the thyroid gland _______ / _______ (WR / S)
2. excision of (one or both) adrenal glands _______ / _______ (WR / S)
3. excision of (one or more) parathyroid glands _______ / _______ (WR / S)
4. excision of the pancreas _______ / _______ (WR / S)

EXERCISE 20

Spell each of the Surgical Terms Built from Word Parts by having someone dictate them to you. Use a separate sheet of paper.

> To hear and spell the terms, go to Evolve Resources at evolve.elsevier.com and select:
> Practice Student Resources > Student Resources > Chapter 16 > **Pronounce and Spell**
>
> See Appendix B for instructions.

❑ Check the box when complete.

Diagnostic Terms

NOT BUILT FROM WORD PARTS

Word parts may be present in the following terms; however, their full meanings cannot be translated using definitions of word parts alone.

TERM	DEFINITION
DIAGNOSTIC IMAGING	
radioactive iodine uptake (RAIU) (*rā*-dē-ō-AK-tiv) (Ī-ō-dīn) (UP-tāk)	nuclear medicine scan that measures thyroid function, particularly when distinguishing different causes of hyperthyroidism. Radioactive iodine is given to the patient orally, after which the amount of its uptake into the thyroid gland is measured. Images of the gland can also be obtained using this procedure.

TERM	DEFINITION
sestamibi parathyroid scan (*ses*-ta-MIB-ē) (*par*-a-THĪ-royd) (skan)	nuclear medicine procedure used to localize hyperactive parathyroid glands. The glands that take up an abnormal amount of radioactive substance are identified and selected for surgical removal; the other parathyroid glands may be left in place.
thyroid sonography (THĪ-royd) (so-nog-ra-fē)	ultrasound test of the thyroid gland used to help determine whether a thyroid nodule is likely benign or possibly malignant, including whether it is cystic or solid. Also used to help guide a fine needle aspiration (FNA) biopsy.
LABORATORY	
fasting blood sugar (FBS) (FAST-ing) (blud) (SHOOG-er)	blood test to determine the amount of glucose (sugar) in the blood after fasting for 8–10 hours. Elevation may indicate diabetes mellitus.
fine needle aspiration (FNA) (FĪN) (NĒ-del) (*as*-pi-RĀ-shen)	biopsy technique that uses a narrow hollow needle to obtain tiny amounts of tissue for pathologic examination. Thyroid nodules are frequently biopsied using FNA.
glycosylated hemoglobin (HbA1C) (glī-KŌ-sa-*lāt*-ad) (HĒ-mō-*glō*-bin)	blood test used to diagnose diabetes and monitor its treatment by measuring the amount of glucose (sugar) bound to hemoglobin in the blood. HbA1C provides an indication of blood sugar level over the past three months, covering the 120-day lifespan of the red blood cell (also called **glycated hemoglobin, hemoglobin A1C, and A1C test**).
thyroid-stimulating hormone level (TSH) (THĪ-royd) (STIM-yuh-lāt-ing) (HŌR-mōn) (LEV-el)	blood test that measures the amount of thyroid-stimulating hormone in the blood; used to diagnose hypothyroidism and to monitor patients on thyroid replacement therapy
thyroxine level (T_4) (thī-ROK-sin) (LEV-el)	blood test that gives the direct measurement of the amount of thyroxine in the patient's blood. A greater-than-normal amount indicates hyperthyroidism; a less-than-normal amount indicates hypothyroidism.

EXERCISE 21

Practice saying aloud each of the Diagnostic Terms NOT Built from Word Parts.

To hear the terms, go to Evolve Resources at evolve.elsevier.com and select:
Practice Student Resources > Student Resources > Chapter 16 > **Pronounce and Spell**

See Appendix B for instructions.

❑ Check the box when complete.

EXERCISE 22

Match the terms in the first column with their correct definitions in the second column.

_____ 1. fasting blood sugar
_____ 2. sestamibi parathyroid scan
_____ 3. thyroxine level
_____ 4. radioactive iodine uptake
_____ 5. thyroid-stimulating hormone level
_____ 6. glycosylated hemoglobin
_____ 7. thyroid sonography
_____ 8. fine needle aspiration

a. nuclear medicine procedure used to localize hyperactive parathyroid glands
b. determines the amount of glucose in the blood after fasting for 8 to 10 hours
c. uses a hollow needle to obtain tiny amounts of tissue for pathologic examination
d. uses radioactive iodine to measure thyroid function
e. used to indicate whether a thyroid nodule is likely benign or possibly malignant
f. used to diagnose hypothyroidism and to monitor thyroid replacement therapy
g. measures the amount of thyroxine in the blood
h. provides an indication of blood sugar level over the past three months

EXERCISE 23

Write the name of the procedure that gives information about each of the following.

1. thyroid function _____
2. amount of glucose in the blood at the time of the test _____
3. amount of thyroid-stimulating hormone in the blood _____
4. amount of thyroxine in the blood _____
5. localize hyperactive parathyroid glands _____
6. amount of hemoglobin coated with sugar _____
7. thyroid nodules, likely benign or possibly malignant _____
8. examination of a tiny amount of tissue from a thyroid nodule _____

EXERCISE 24

Spell each of the Diagnostic Terms NOT Built from Word Parts by having someone dictate them to you. Use a separate sheet of paper.

To hear and spell the terms, go to Evolve Resources at evolve.elsevier.com and select:
Practice Student Resources > Student Resources > Chapter 16 > **Pronounce and Spell**

See Appendix B for instructions.

❑ Check the box when complete.

Complementary Terms
BUILT FROM WORD PARTS

The following terms can be translated using definitions of word parts. Further explanation is provided within parentheses as needed.

TERM	DEFINITION
adrenocorticohyperplasia (a-*drē*-nō-*kōr*-ti-kō-*hī*-per-PLĀ-zha)	excessive development of the adrenal cortex *(Note: hyper, a prefix, appears within this term.)*
adrenopathy (*ad*-ren-OP-a-thē)	disease of the adrenal gland

TERM	DEFINITION
cortical (KŌR-ti-kal)	pertaining to the cortex
corticoid (KŌR-ti-koyd)	resembling the cortex
endocrinologist (*en*-dō-kri-NOL-o-jist)	physician who studies and treats diseases of the endocrine (system)
endocrinology (*en*-dō-kri-NOL-o-jē)	study of the endocrine (system) (a branch of medicine dealing with diseases of the endocrine system)
endocrinopathy (*en*-dō-kri-NOP-a-thē)	(any) disease of the endocrine (system)
euglycemia (*ū*-glī-SĒ-mē-a)	normal (level of) sugar in the blood (within normal range)
euthyroid (ū-THĪ-royd)	resembling a normal thyroid gland (normal thyroid function)
glycemia (glī-SĒ-mē-a)	sugar in the blood
polydipsia (*pol*-ē-DIP-sē-a)	abnormal state of much thirst
syndrome (SIN-drōm)	run together (signs and symptoms occurring together that are characteristic of a specific disorder)

EXERCISE 25

Practice saying aloud each of the Complementary Terms Built from Word Parts.

> To hear the terms, go to Evolve Resources at evolve.elsevier.com and select:
> Practice Student Resources > Student Resources > Chapter 16 > **Pronounce and Spell**
>
> See Appendix B for instructions.

❑ Check the box when complete.

EXERCISE 26

Analyze and define the following terms.

1. corticoid

____

____

2. syndrome

____

____

3. adrenopathy

____

____

4. endocrinologist

____

____

5. polydipsia

____

____

6. euglycemia

____

____

7. endocrinopathy

____

____

8. adrenocorticohyperplasia

____

____

9. euthyroid

____

____

10. cortical

____

____

11. endocrinology

____

____

12. glycemia

____

____

EXERCISE 27

Build the complementary terms for the following definitions by using the word parts you have learned.

1. (any) disease of the endocrine (system) _______ / _______ / _______ (WR / CV / S)

2. resembling the cortex _______ / _______ (WR / S)

3. run together (signs and symptoms occurring together) _______ / _______ (P / S(WR))

4. excessive development of the adrenal cortex _______ / _______ / _______ / _______ / _______ / _______ (WR / CV / WR / CV / P / S)

5. study of the endocrine (system) _______ / _______ / _______ (WR / CV / S)

6. abnormal state of much thirst _______ / _______ / _______ (P / WR / S)

7. disease of the adrenal gland _______ / _______ / _______ (WR / CV / S)

8. normal (level of) sugar in the blood _______ / _______ / _______ (P / WR / S)

9. resembling a normal thyroid gland _______ / _______ / _______ (P / WR / S)

10. pertaining to the cortex _______ / _______ (WR / S)

11. physician who studies and treats diseases of the endocrine (system) ______ WR / CV / ______ S

12. sugar in the blood ______ WR / ______ S

EXERCISE 28

Spell each of the Complementary Terms Built from Word Parts by having someone dictate them to you. Use a separate sheet of paper.

To hear and spell the terms, go to Evolve Resources at evolve.elsevier.com and select:
Practice Student Resources > Student Resources > Chapter 16 > **Pronounce and Spell**

See Appendix B for instructions.

❑ Check the box when complete.

Complementary Terms
NOT BUILT FROM WORD PARTS

Word parts may be present in the following terms; however, their full meanings cannot be translated using definitions of word parts alone.

TERM	DEFINITION
exophthalmos (*ek*-sof-THAL-mos)	abnormal protrusion of the eyeball (Fig. 16.5)
hormone (HOR-mōn)	chemical substance secreted by an endocrine gland that is carried in the blood to a target tissue
incretins (in-KRĒ-tins)	a group of hormones produced by the gastrointestinal system that stimulate the release of insulin from the pancreas and help preserve the beta cells. *Incretin mimetics* are medications that copy this action and help control blood sugar in patients with type 2 diabetes mellitus.
isthmus (IS-mus)	narrow strip of tissue connecting two larger parts in the body, such as the isthmus that connects the two lobes of the thyroid gland (Fig. 16.3C)
metabolism (me-TAB-ō-*lizm*)	sum total of all the chemical processes that take place in a living organism

EXOPHTHALMOS is derived from the Greek **ex,** meaning **outward,** and **ophthalmos,** meaning **eye.** Protrusion of the eyeball is sometimes a symptom of Graves disease, first described by Dr. Robert Graves, an Irish physician, in 1835.

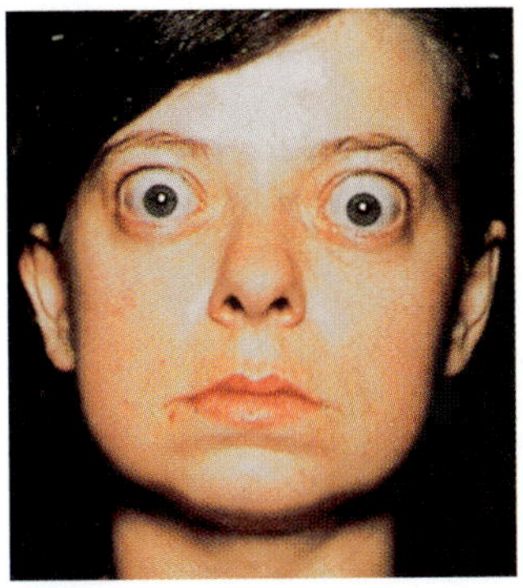

FIG. 16.5 Abnormal protrusion of eyeballs, exophthalmos, a characteristic of Graves disease.

EXERCISE 29

Practice saying aloud each of the Complementary Terms NOT Built from Word Parts.

To hear the terms, go to Evolve Resources at evolve.elsevier.com and select:
Practice Student Resources > Student Resources > Chapter 16 > **Pronounce and Spell**

See Appendix B for instructions.

❑ Check the box when complete.

EXERCISE 30

Fill in the blanks with the correct terms.

1. The sum total of all the chemical processes that take place in a living organism is called its ________________.
2. A chemical substance secreted by an endocrine gland is called a(n) ________________.
3. A narrow strip of tissue connecting larger parts in the body is called a(n) ________________.
4. Abnormal protrusion of the eyeball is called ________________.
5. Hormones produced by the gastrointestinal system that stimulate insulin release are called ________________.

EXERCISE 31

Write the definitions of the following terms.

1. isthmus ________________
2. metabolism ________________
3. hormone ________________
4. exophthalmos ________________
5. incretins ________________

EXERCISE 32

Spell each of the Complementary Terms NOT Built from Word Parts by having someone dictate them to you. Use a separate sheet of paper.

To hear and spell the terms, go to Evolve Resources at evolve.elsevier.com and select:
Practice Student Resources > Student Resources > Chapter 16 > **Pronounce and Spell**

See Appendix B for instructions.

❑ Check the box when complete.

Refer to **Appendix F** for pharmacology terms related to the endocrine system.

Abbreviations

ABBREVIATION	TERM
ACTH	adrenocorticotropic hormone
ADH	antidiuretic hormone
DI	diabetes insipidus
DKA	diabetic ketoacidosis
DM	diabetes mellitus
FBS	fasting blood sugar
FNA	fine needle aspiration
FSH	follicle-stimulating hormone
GH	growth hormone
HbA1C	glycosylated hemoglobin
LH	luteinizing hormone
PRL	prolactin
RAIU	radioactive iodine uptake

ABBREVIATION	TERM
TSH	thyroid-stimulating hormone
T2DM	type 2 diabetes mellitus (also abbreviated **T2D**)
T_4	thyroxine level

Refer to **Appendix E** for a complete list of abbreviations.

EXERCISE 33

Write the terms abbreviated.

1. RAIU ______
2. FBS ______
3. DM ______
4. DI ______
5. T_4 ______
6. HbA1C ______
7. TSH ______
8. PRL ______
9. LH ______
10. GH ______
11. FSH ______
12. ADH ______
13. ACTH ______
14. DKA ______
15. FNA ______
16. T2DM ______

For additional practice with Abbreviations, go to Evolve Resources at evolve.elsevier.com and select: Practice Student Resources > Student Resources > Chapter 16 > **Flashcards:** Abbreviations

See Appendix B for instructions.

PRACTICAL APPLICATION

EXERCISE 34 *Case Study: Translate Between Everyday Language and Medical Language*

CASE STUDY: Lily Macabal

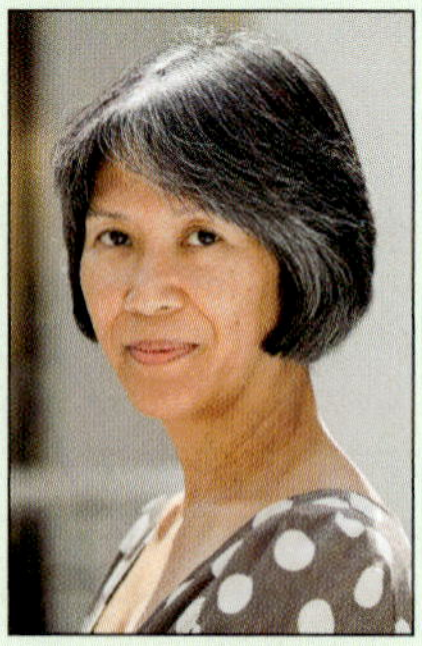

Lily Macabal has not been feeling well. She feels restless all the time, and feels more irritable. Her appetite is increased but she has been losing weight. She seems to always feel warm, and sometimes her heart races. Her hair seems thin and brittle. Recently she has noticed a lump in the front of her neck, and her husband says that her eyes seem to stick out more than they used to. She remembers her mother having a condition caused by too much thyroid hormone and she wonders if she is going through the same thing. She sees her family doctor, who recommends a referral to an endocrine specialist.

Now that you have worked through Chapter 16 on the endocrine system, consider the medical terms that might be used to describe Mrs. Macabal's experience. See the Review of Terms at the end of the chapter for a list of terms that might apply.

A. *Underline phrases in the case study that could be substituted with medical terms.*

B. *Write the medical term and its definition for three of the phrases you underlined.*

MEDICAL TERM	DEFINITION
1. ______________	______________
2. ______________	______________
3. ______________	______________

DOCUMENTATION: Excerpt from Emergency Department Visit

Mrs. Macabal saw an endocrinologist; an excerpt from her medical record is presented below.

This 56-year-old female was referred by her PCP for evaluation of a thyroid endocrinopathy. She has had multiple symptoms of hyperthyroidism and appears to be experiencing thyrotoxicosis. Her exophthalmos is suggestive of Graves disease. Thyroid sonography performed in our office showed no discrete nodules, with increased vascularity and diffuse hypoechoic tissue throughout. We have ordered a TSH and free T_4 level to assess her thyroid function. A radioactive iodine uptake test will be performed to assess her thyroid function. We will consider treatment with either radioiodine therapy or near-total thyroidectomy, with the understanding that either treatment may result in hypothyroidism and require thyroid hormone replacement therapy.

C. *Underline medical terms presented in Chapter 16 used in the previous excerpt from Mrs. Macabal's medical record. See the Review of Terms at the end of the chapter for a complete list.*

D. *Select and define three of the medical terms you underlined. To check your answers, go to Appendix A.*

MEDICAL TERM	DEFINITION
1. ______________	______________
2. ______________	______________
3. ______________	______________

EXERCISE 35 *Interact with Medical Documents and Electronic Health Records*

A. Read the report and complete it by writing medical terms on answer lines within the document. Definitions of terms to be written appear after the document.

021286 BLACKWATER, Josephina

File Patient Navigate Custom Fields Help

Chart Review | Encounters | Notes | Labs | Imaging | Procedures | Rx | Documents | Referrals | Scheduling | Billing

Name: BLACKWATER, Josephina MR#: 021286 DOB: 05/21/19xx Gender: F Allergies: NKDA PCP: Julius Netou, PA-C

DATE: 06/20/20XX
HISTORY AND PHYSICAL
CHIEF COMPLANT: Josephina Blackwater is a 51-year-old female complaining of excessive urination, excessive thirst, and fatigue for approximately 1 month.
HISTORY OF PRESENT ILLNESS: For the past 4 weeks she has been having polyuria and 1. ______________________, drinking 3 to 4 quarts of water daily for the past 10 days. This has also resulted in nocturia, getting up 2 to 3 times each night to void. She also reports fatigue which has been present for at least 4 weeks. She denies anorexia, nausea, vomiting, hematemesis, or any abdominal pain. She denies blurred vision.
MEDICAL HISTORY: No known allergies. No previous hospitalizations. She has had no recent illness.
FAMILY HISTORY: Her mother died of a stroke at age 63. Her father is still living at the age of 78, but has had 2. __________ ____________ for 20 years. She has two brothers, both in good health, and no sisters.
SOCIAL HISTORY: She is married with 3 children . She does not smoke and does not use alcohol or other drugs.
REVIEW OF SYSTEMS: She denies fever, chills, headache, palpitations, chest pain, or edema.
PHYSICAL EXAM: Temperature, 98.9°F. Pulse, 80. Respirations, 24. Her blood pressure is 125/80 mm Hg. Her height is 5 ft. 3 inches, weight is 186 pounds, and BMI is 33 (obese).
HEENT: Normal, no evidence of 3. ________________ . CHEST: Clear to auscultation and percussion. HEART: Regular rhythm. No murmurs or extra heart sounds. ABDOMEN: Soft, nontender, bowel sounds normal, without evidence of organomegaly. RECTAL: Unremarkable. EXTREMITIES: No clubbing, cyanosis, or edema. Pedal pulses are intact. NEUROLOGIC: Alert and oriented to time, person, and place. Cranial nerves 2 through 12 are grossly intact.
LABORATORY FINDINGS: 4. ____________ ________ ________ was discovered to be 200 mg/dL. Urinalysis showed moderate proteinuria. 5. _____________ ________________ was 9.2%.
ASSESSMENT: Newly diagnosed 6. _________ _________ ____________ ___________.
PLAN:
1. Since her fasting glucose and hemoglobin A1C are quite elevated, we will immediately institute a regimen of metformin 500 mg at bedtime, with increase to 500 mg bid as tolerated. She will be given a glucometer and test strips so that she can monitor her sugars at home. She is already familiar with this after caring for her diabetic father for many years.
2. The patient was educated about her diagnosis and the relationship between strict control of 7. ________________ and the reduction of diabetes-related complications. She was also educated about the risks of 8. ________________. She will schedule appointments with the diabetes educator and nutritionist for further management of her condition.
3. Consider a(n) 9.________________ consult if she does not respond to lifestyle changes and metformin.

Christina Kraemer, MD
CK/mcm

Start | Log On/Off | Print | Edit

Definitions of Medical Terms to Complete the Document

Write the medical terms defined on corresponding answer lines in the document.

1. excessive thirst
2. chronic disease involving a disorder of carbohydrate metabolism and characterized by elevated blood sugar
3. abnormal protrusion of the eyeball
4. blood test to determine the amount of glucose (sugar) in the blood after fasting for 8 to 10 hours
5. the test measuring the amount of hemoglobin coated in sugar over the lifespan of the red blood cell
6. T2DM
7. excessive sugar in the blood
8. deficient sugar in the blood
9. study of the endocrine (system)

EXERCISE 35 *Interact With Medical Documents and Electronic Health Records—cont'd*

B. Read the medical report and answer the questions below it.

029210 GOMEZ, RUTH

File Patient Navigate Custom Fields Help

Patient Chart | Lab | Rad | Notes | Documents | Rx | Scheduling | Images | Billing

Name: **GOMEZ, RUTH** MR#: **029210** DOB: **5/11/19XX** Gender: **Female** Age: **39** Allergies: **None known** PCP: **Anna Tang, MD**

DATE OF OPERATION: April 10, 20XX

SURGERY PERFORMED: Right laparoscopic adrenalectomy

PREOPERATIVE DIAGNOSIS: Primary hyperaldosteronism (Conn syndrome), adrenal adenoma.

INDICATIONS: The patient is a 39-year-old woman who has a history of hypertension and hypokalemia seen on referral from her endocrinologist. The patient complained of headache and muscle weakness. She underwent a 24-hour urine collection, a general metastatic workup, and evaluation for Cushing syndrome. Laboratory studies indicated elevated plasma and urinary aldosterone levels. CT scan revealed the presence of a 3.5-cm right adrenal mass, and adrenal biopsy confirmed that it was an aldosterone-producing adenoma.

PROCEDURE: The procedure was performed with the patient under general endotracheal anesthesia and with an arterial line, a Foley catheter, and a central venous pressure line in place. A Veress needle was inserted into the abdominal cavity between the midclavicular and anterior axillary lines. The abdominal cavity was then insufflated with CO_2. A 10- to 11-mm trocar was placed at the site of the Veress needle, and a 30-degree videotelescope was inserted. A third 10- to 11-mm port was placed 3 to 4 cm behind the posterior axillary line, and a fourth port inserted after mobilization of the right lobe of the liver. The superior pole and lateral border of the adrenal gland were mobilized first, with the dissection proceeding carefully along the lateral edge of the inferior vena cava. The right adrenal vein was ligated with endoscopic clips and divided, freeing the adrenal gland from its surrounding attachments. The gland was placed in an impermeable entrapment sac and removed from the most anterior port site. After evacuation of CO_2, all ports were removed, and the incisions were closed with absorbable sutures.

POSTOPERATIVE DIAGNOSIS: Aldosteronoma

Electronically signed by: Merriam Fitch, MD 4/11/20XX 11:24

Start | Log On/Off | Print | Edit

Use the medical report above to answer the questions.

1. Which procedure was performed during surgery:
   a. excision of a parathyroid gland
   b. surgical repair of the thyroid gland
   c. excision of an adrenal gland
   d. surgical repair of the thymus
2. The patient had a history of:
   a. excessive sugar in the blood
   b. deficient potassium in the blood
   c. deficient sodium in the blood
   d. deficient calcium in the blood
3. The patient was evaluated for a:
   a. group of symptoms from the excessive production of cortisol
   b. condition caused by congenital absence of the thyroid gland
   c. syndrome caused by deficient secretion from the adrenal cortex
   d. condition causing muscle spasms resulting from low amounts of calcium

C. Complete the three medical documents within the electronic health record (EHR) on Evolve.

Topic: Hyperparathyroidism
Documents: Pre-operative Note, Nuclear Medicine Report, Office Visit Report

To complete the three medical records, go to Evolve Resources at evolve.elsevier.com and select:
Practice Student Resources > Student Resources > Chapter 16 > **Electronic Health Records**

See Appendix B for instructions.

EXERCISE 36 *Pronounce Medical Terms in Use*

Practice pronunciation of terms by reading aloud the following paragraph. Use the phonetic spellings following medical terms from the chapter to assist with pronunciation. The script also contains medical terms not presented in the chapter. Treat them as information only or look for their meanings in a medical dictionary or a reliable online source.

A 65-year-old female patient presented to her doctor because of a 10-pound weight gain, fatigue, hair loss, dry skin, and cold intolerance. She was referred to an **endocrinologist** (*en*-dō -kri-NOL-o-jist) who established a diagnosis of **hypothyroidism** (*hī*-pō-THĪ -royd-izm) after test results indicated an elevated **thyroid-stimulating hormone level** (THĪ -royd) (STIM-yuh-lāt-ing) (HŌR-mōn) (LEV-el) and a low **thyroxine** (thī -ROK-sin) level. Approximately 20 years ago she had a painless thyroid nodule. At that time, **thyroid sonography** (THĪ -royd) (so-nog-ra-fē) and **fine needle aspiration** (FĪN) (NĒ-del) (*as*-pi-RĀ-shen) were performed; a diagnosis of thyroid cancer was confirmed, but it had not spread beyond the gland. She underwent a **thyroidectomy** (*thī*-royd-EK-to-mē) and received thyroid hormone replacement therapy thereafter. She remained in a **euthyroid** (ū-THĪ-royd) state until she stopped taking the medication 6 months ago. Consequently she became hypothyroid and could have easily developed **myxedema** (*mik*-se-DĒ-ma) if she had not sought treatment.

EXERCISE 37 *Chapter Content Quiz*

Test your understanding of terms and abbreviations introduced in this chapter. Circle the letter for the medical term or abbreviation related to the words in italics.

1. Inez Villalvazo was diagnosed with Hashimoto thyroiditis after she presented to her doctor with *enlargement of the thyroid gland.*
   a. myxedema
   b. tetany
   c. goiter
2. An episode of *serious condition resulting from uncontrolled diabetes mellitus in which acid ketones accumulate* resulted in admission to the intensive care unit for Mr. Khalile.
   a. ketoacidosis
   b. tetany
   c. euglycemia
3. Diana Worthington complained of weight loss and muscle aches, as well as darkening of her skin. She was diagnosed with *chronic syndrome resulting from a deficiency in hormonal secretion from the adrenal cortex.*
   a. Cushing syndrome
   b. Graves disease
   c. Addison disease
4. Malini Sobel noticed polydipsia and polyuria and found herself drinking a lot of water. This was related to *decreased secretion of antidiuretic hormone by the posterior lobe of the pituitary gland.*
   a. diabetes mellitus
   b. diabetes insipidus
   c. diabetic retinopathy

5. Ryan McAvoy had *condition brought about by hypersecretion of growth hormone by the pituitary gland before puberty* and was over 6-feet tall as an 11-year-old.
   a. gigantism
   b. acromegaly
   c. metabolic syndrome
6. *Deficient sodium in the blood* and *excessive potassium in the blood* are two laboratory findings in Addison disease.
   a. hypoglycemia and hypercalcemia
   b. hyponatremia and hyperkalemia
   c. hypocalcemia and hyperglycemia
7. A distal *excision of the pancreas was performed* on Mr. Rockov after a tumor was discovered.
   a. pancreatectomy
   b. adrenalectomy
   c. parathyroidectomy
8. Mrs. Lucio has been working hard to help control her diabetes mellitus with diet and exercise. Her recent *blood test used to diagnose diabetes and monitor its treatment by measuring the amount of glucose (sugar) bound to hemoglobin in the blood* showed marked improvement since the last test 3 months ago.
   a. FSH
   b. FBS
   c. HbA1C
9. Dr. Chen told Mrs. Onwubiko that weight loss, regular exercise, and healthy eating are central in the treatment and prevention of *a group of health problems including insulin resistance, obesity, hypertension, hyperglycemia, elevated triglycerides, and low levels of HDL.*
   a. metabolic syndrome
   b. Cushing syndrome
   c. irritable bowel syndrome
10. Congenital hypothyroidism is a(n) *any disease of the endocrine system* that is characterized by puffy features, mental deficiency, large tongue, and dwarfism.
    a. adrenopathy
    b. neuropathy
    c. endocrinopathy
11. Dr. Turecki performed a *biopsy technique that uses a narrow hollow needle to obtain tiny amounts of tissue for pathologic examination* on the patient who had been found to have a multinodular goiter on thyroid sonography.
    a. thyroid-stimulating hormone level (TSH)
    b. thyroxine level (T_4)
    c. fine needle aspiration (FNA)
12. *Excessive development of the adrenal cortex* was the cause of Cushing syndrome in Mr. Lim when he presented with "moon face," "buffalo hump," and hypertension.
    a. pheochromocytoma
    b. thyrotoxicosis
    c. adrenocorticohyperplasia
13. The pharmacist told Mrs. Tranh that her new diabetes medication acted in the same way as *a group of hormones produced by the gastrointestinal system that stimulate the release of insulin from the pancreas.*
    a. hormones
    b. incretins
    c. corticoids
14. Mrs. Webber had *nuclear medicine scan that measures thyroid function using radioactive iodine* and was diagnosed with Graves disease. Since she had her thyroid removed, she has been on thyroid hormone replacement therapy and had periodic measurements of her *blood test that measures the amount of thyroid-stimulating hormone in the blood.*
    a. thyroid scan and T_4
    b. RAIU and TSH
    c. thyroid sonography and LH
15. Dr. Nair performed a parathyroidectomy on Mrs. Chaugary to treat her *state of excessive parathyroid gland activity.*
    a. hyperpituitarism
    b. hyperthyroidism
    c. hyperparathyroidism

CHAPTER REVIEW

REVIEW OF CHAPTER CONTENT ON EVOLVE RESOURCES

Go to evolve.elsevier.com and click on Gradable Student Resources and Practice Student Resources. Online learning activities found there can be used to review chapter content and to assess your learning of word parts, medical terms, and abbreviations. Place check marks in the boxes next to activities used for review and assessment.

GRADABLE STUDENT RESOURCES

Chapter 16 >	Exercises >	☐ Word Parts ☐ Terms Built from Word Parts ☐ Terms Not Built from Word Parts ☐ Abbreviations
	Quizzes >	☐ Quiz 1: Disease and Disorder Terms ☐ Quiz 2: Surgical and Diagnostic Terms ☐ Quiz 3: Complementary Terms

PRACTICE STUDENT RESOURCES > STUDENT RESOURCES

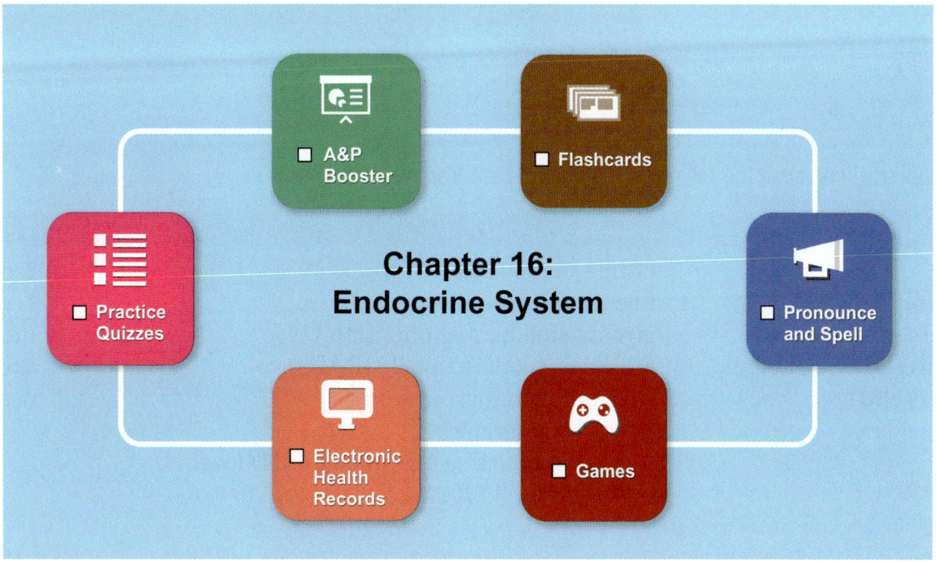

REVIEW OF WORD PARTS

Can you define and spell the following word parts?

COMBINING FORMS		SUFFIX
acr/o	endocrin/o	-drome
adren/o	kal/i	
adrenal/o	natr/o	
calc/i	parathyroid/o	
cortic/o	pituitar/o	
dips/o	thyr/o	
	thyroid/o	

REVIEW OF TERMS

Can you build, analyze, define, pronounce, and spell the following terms built from word parts?

DISEASES AND DISORDERS	SURGICAL	COMPLEMENTARY
acromegaly	adrenalectomy	adrenocorticohyperplasia
adrenalitis	pancreatectomy	adrenopathy
adrenomegaly	parathyroidectomy	cortical
hypercalcemia	thyroidectomy	corticoid
hyperglycemia		endocrinologist
hyperkalemia		endocrinology
hyperparathyroidism		endocrinopathy
hyperpituitarism		euglycemia
hyperthyroidism		euthyroid
hypocalcemia		glycemia
hypoglycemia		polydipsia
hypokalemia		syndrome
hyponatremia		
hypopituitarism		
hypothyroidism		
panhypopituitarism		
parathyroidoma		
thyroiditis		

Can you define, pronounce, and spell the following terms NOT built from word parts?

DISEASES AND DISORDERS	DIAGNOSTIC	COMPLEMENTARY
Addison disease	fasting blood sugar (FBS)	exophthalmos
congenital hypothyroidism	fine needle aspiration (FNA)	hormone
Cushing syndrome	glycosylated hemoglobin (HbA1C)	incretins
diabetes insipidus (DI)	radioactive iodine uptake (RAIU)	isthmus
diabetes mellitus (DM)	sestamibi parathyroid scan	metabolism
gigantism	thyroid sonography	
goiter	thyroid-stimulating hormone (TSH) level	
Graves disease	thyroxine level (T_4)	
ketoacidosis		
metabolic syndrome		
myxedema		
pheochromocytoma		
tetany		
thyrotoxicosis		

Appendix A

Answer Key

ANSWERS TO CHAPTER 1 EXERCISES

Exercise Figure A

A. oste/o/arthr/itis

Exercise 1

Online Activity

Exercise 2

1. b
2. a
3. c
4. d
5. a
6. d
7. c
8. b

Exercise 3

built from word parts; not built from word parts

Exercise 4

a word part that is the core of the word

Exercise 5

a word part attached to the end of the word root to modify its meaning

Exercise 6

a word part attached at the beginning of a word root to modify its meaning

Exercise 7

1. a word part, usually an o, used to ease pronunciation
2. used
3. vowel
4. word roots
5. not

Exercise 8

a word root with the combining vowel attached, separated by a slash

Exercise 9

1. b
2. a
3. d
4. e
5. c

Exercise 10

1. *F*, a medical term may begin with the word root and have no prefix.
2. *F*, if the suffix begins with a vowel, the combining vowel is usually not used.
3. *T*
4. *T*
5. *F*, *o* is the combining vowel most often used.
6. *T*
7. *F*, a combining vowel is used between two word roots or between a word root and a suffix to ease pronunciation.
8. *F*, a combining form is a word root with a combining vowel attached and is not one of the four word parts.
9. *T*

Exercise 11

WR CV S
oste/o/pathy
CF

Exercise 12

1. Divide the term into word parts.
2. Label each word part.
3. Label each combining form.

Exercise 13

disease of the bone and joint

Exercise 14

apply the meaning of each word part contained in the term

Exercise 15

1. WR S
   arthr/itis
   inflammation of a joint
2. WR S
   hepat/itis
   inflammation of the liver
3. P WR S
   sub/hepat/ic
   pertaining to under the liver
4. P WR S
   intra/ven/ous
   pertaining to within the vein
5. WR CV S
   arthr/o/pathy
   CF
   disease of a joint
6. WR S
   oste/itis
   inflammation of the bone
7. WR CV S
   hepat/o/megaly
   CF
   enlargement of the liver

Exercise 16

arthr/o/pathy

Exercise 17

to place word parts together to form terms

Exercise 18

1. arthr/itis
2. hepat/ic
3. sub/hepat/ic
4. intra/ven/ous
5. oste/itis
6. hepat/itis
7. oste/o/arthr/o/pathy
8. hepat/o/megaly

Exercise 19

Check marks for numbers 2, 3, 4, 5, 7, 8, 10

ANSWERS TO CHAPTER 2 EXERCISES

Exercise Figure A
1. carcin/oma
2. melan/oma
3. sarc/oma
4. rhabd/o/my/o/sarcoma

Exercise Figure B
erythr/o/cyte

Exercise Figure C
hyper/plasia

Exercise Figure D
leuk/o/cyte

Exercise 1
Pronunciation Exercise

Exercise 2
A. 1. tissue: hist/o
   2. cell: cyt/o
   3. nucleus: kary/o
   4. organ: organ/o
   5. system: system/o
   6. internal organs: viscer/o

B. 1. neur/o
   2. epitheli/o
   3. sarc/o
   4. my/o
   5. aden/o
   6. fibr/o

Exercise 3
1. f, flesh, connective tissue
2. e, fat
3. d, nucleus
4. c, internal organs
5. g, cell
6. b, tissue
7. a, muscle

Exercise 4
1. c, nerve
2. f, organ
3. d, system
4. a, epithelium
5. b, fiber
6. e, gland

Exercise 5
1. tumor, mass
2. cancer
3. cause (of disease)
4. disease
5. body
6. cancer
7. rod-shaped, striated
8. smooth
9. knowledge
10. physician, medicine

Exercise 6
1. path/o
2. onc/o
3. eti/o
4. a. cancer/o
   b. carcin/o
5. somat/o
6. lei/o
7. rhabd/o
8. gno/o
9. iatr/o

Exercise 7
1. blue
2. red
3. white
4. yellow
5. color
6. black
7. green

Exercise 8
1. cyan/o
2. erythr/o
3. leuk/o
4. melan/o
5. xanth/o
6. chrom/o
7. chlor/o

Exercise 9
1. new
2. above, excessive
3. after, beyond, change
4. below, incomplete, deficient, under
5. painful, abnormal, difficult, labored
6. through, complete
7. before

Exercise 10
1. neo-
2. hyper-
3. hypo-
4. meta-
5. dys-
6. dia-
7. pro-

Exercise 11
A. 1. g
   2. j
   3. b
   4. c
   5. e
   6. d
   7. f
   8. i
   9. a
   10. h

B. 1. -cyte
   2. -plasia
   3. -logist
   4. -logy
   5. -megaly
   6. -oma

Exercise 12
1. one who studies and treats (specialist, physician)
2. disease
3. study of
4. pertaining to
5. control, stop, standing
6. cell
7. abnormal condition
8. pertaining to
9. growth, substance, formation
10. pertaining to
11. condition of formation, development, growth
12. resembling
13. substance or agent that produces or causes
14. producing, originating, causing
15. tumor, swelling
16. malignant tumor
17. state of
18. enlargement

Exercise 13
Pronunciation Exercise

Exercise 14
1. WR S
   sarc/oma
   tumor composed of connective tissue
2. WR S
   melan/oma
   black tumor
3. WR S
   epitheli/oma
   tumor composed of epithelium
4. WR S
   lip/oma
   tumor composed of fat
5. P S(WR)
   neo/plasm
   new growth
6. WR S
   my/oma
   tumor composed of muscle
7. WR S
   neur/oma
   tumor composed of nerve
8. WR S
   carcin/oma
   cancerous tumor

9. WR CV WR S
melan/o/carcin/oma
CF
cancerous black tumor

10. WR CV WR CV S
rhabd/o/my/o/sarcoma
CF CF
malignant tumor of striated muscle

11. WRCVWR S
lei/o/my/oma
CF
tumor composed of smooth muscle

12. WR CV WR S
rhabd/o/my/oma
CF
tumor composed of striated muscle

13. WR S
fibr/oma
tumor composed of fiber (fibrous tissue)

14. WR CV S
lip/o/sarcoma
CF
malignant tumor of fat

15. WR CV S
fibr/o/sarcoma
CF
malignant tumor of fiber (fibrous tissue)

16. WR S
aden/oma
tumor composed of glandular tissue

17. WR CV WR S
aden/o/carcin/oma
CF
cancerous tumor composed of glandular tissue

18. WR S
chlor/oma
tumor of green color

Exercise 15

1. melan/oma
2. carcin/oma
3. neo/plasm
4. epitheli/oma
5. sarc/oma
6. melan/o/carcin/oma
7. neur/oma
8. my/oma
9. rhabd/o/my/o/sarcoma
10. lei/o/my/oma
11. rhabd/o/my/oma
12. lei/o/my/o/sarcoma
13. lip/o/sarcoma
14. fibr/oma
15. fibr/o/sarcoma
16. aden/oma
17. aden/o/carcin/oma
18. chlor/oma

Exercise 16

Spelling Exercise

Exercise 17

Pronunciation Exercise

Exercise 18

1. WR CV S
cyt/o/logy
CF
study of cells

2. WR CV S
hist/o/logy
CF
study of tissue

3. WR S
viscer/al
pertaining to internal organs

4. WR CV S
kary/o/cyte
CF
cell with a nucleus

5. WR CV S
kary/o/plasm
CF
substance of a nucleus

6. WR S
system/ic
pertaining to a (body) system

7. WR CV S
cyt/o/plasm
CF
cell substance

8. WR S
somat/ic
pertaining to the body

9. WR CV S
somat/o/genic
CF
originating in the body

10. WR CV S
somat/o/plasm
CF
body substance

11. WR CV S
somat/o/pathy
CF
disease of the body

12. WR S
neur/oid
resembling a nerve

13. WR CV S
my/o/pathy
CF
disease of the muscle

14. WR CV S
erythr/o/cyte
CF
red (blood) cell

15. WR CV S
leuk/o/cyte
CF
white (blood) cell

16. WR S
epitheli/al
pertaining to epithelium

17. WR S
lip/oid
resembling fat

18. P S(WR)
hyper/plasia
excessive development (number of cells)

19. WR CV WR S
erythr/o/cyt/osis
CF
increase in the number of red (blood) cells

20. WR CV WR S
leuk/o/cyt/osis
CF
increase in the number of white (blood) cells

21. P S(WR)
hypo/plasia
incomplete development (of an organ or tissue)

22. WR S
cyt/oid
resembling a cell

23. P S(WR)
dys/plasia
abnormal development

24. WR CV S
organ/o/megaly
CF
enlargement of an organ

Exercise 19

1. cyt/o/plasm
2. kary/o/plasm
3. somat/ic
4. my/o/pathy
5. somat/o/plasm
6. viscer/al
7. somat/o/genic
8. somat/o/pathy
9. erythr/o/cyte
10. neur/oid
11. system/ic
12. leuk/o/cyte
13. kary/o/cyte
14. lip/oid
15. cyt/o/logy
16. hyper/plasia
17. cyt/oid
18. epitheli/al
19. hist/o/logy
20. erythr/o/cyt/osis
21. hypo/plasia
22. leuk/o/cyt/osis
23. dys/plasia
24. organ/o/megaly

Exercise 20
Spelling Exercise

Exercise 21
Pronunciation Exercise

Exercise 22
1. WR CV S
   path/o/logy
   CF
   study of disease
2. WR CV S
   path/o/logist
   CF
   physician who studies diseases
3. P S(WR)
   meta/stasis
   beyond control (transfer of disease)
4. WR CV S
   onc/o/genic
   CF
   causing tumors
5. WR CV S
   onc/o/logy
   CF
   study of tumors
6. WR S
   cancer/ous
   pertaining to cancer
7. WR CV S
   carcin/o/genic
   CF
   producing cancer
8. WR S
   cyan/osis
   abnormal condition of blue (bluish discoloration of the skin)
9. WR CV S
   eti/o/logy
   CF
   study of causes (of disease)
10. WR S
    xanth/osis
    abnormal condition of yellow
11. WR CV WR S
    xanth/o/chrom/ic
    CF
    pertaining to yellow color
12. WR CV S
    carcin/o/gen
    CF
    substance that causes cancer
13. WR CV S
    onc/o/logist
    CF
    physician who studies and treats tumors
14. P WR S
    pro/gno/sis
    state of before knowledge
15. WR S
    organ/ic
    pertaining to an organ
16. P WR S
    dia/gno/sis
    state of complete knowledge
17. WR CV S
    iatr/o/genic
    CF
    produced by a physician
18. WR CV S
    iatr/o/logy
    CF
    study of medicine

Exercise 23
1. xanth/o/chrom/ic
2. meta/stasis
3. eti/o/logy
4. onc/o/logy
5. path/o/logy
6. path/o/logist
7. xanth/osis
8. onc/o/genic
9. cancer/ous
10. cyan/osis
11. carcin/o/genic
12. carcin/o/gen
13. onc/o/logist
14. iatr/o/logy
15. organ/ic
16. dia/gno/sis
17. iatr/o/genic
18. pro/gno/sis

Exercise 24
Spelling Exercise

Exercise 25
Pronunciation Exercise

Exercise 26
1. not malignant, nonrecurrent, favorable for recovery
2. tending to become progressively worse and to cause death, as in cancer
3. improvement or absence of signs of disease
4. pertaining to disease of unknown origin
5. localized protective response to injury or tissue destruction; signs are redness, swelling, heat, and pain
6. treatment of cancer with drugs
7. treatment of cancer with radioactive substance, such as x-ray or radiation
8. enclosed within a capsule, as in benign or malignant tumors that have not spread beyond the capsule
9. outside the body, in a lab setting
10. within the living body
11. cancer in the early stage before invading the surrounding tissue
12. increase in the severity of a disease or its symptoms
13. providing relief but not cure
14. state of being mortal (death); incidence of the number of deaths in a population
15. state of being diseased; incidence of illness in a population
16. provides palliative and supportive care for terminally ill patients and their families
17. without fever
18. treatment of cancer with biological response modifiers that work with the immune system
19. programmed cell death
20. having a fever

Exercise 27
1. f
2. i
3. a
4. g
5. b
6. c
7. d
8. j
9. e
10. h

Exercise 28
1. f
2. d
3. a
4. i
5. b
6. h
7. j
8. e
9. c
10. g

Exercise 29
Spelling Exercise

Exercise 30
1. etiologies
2. staphylococci
3. cyanoses
4. bacteria
5. nuclei
6. pharynges
7. sarcomata
8. carcinomata
9. anastomoses
10. pubes
11. prognoses
12. spermatozoa
13. fimbriae
14. thoraces
15. appendices

Exercise 31

1. diverticula
2. bronchus
3. testes
4. melanoma
5. emboli
6. diagnoses
7. metastases

Exercise 32

diagnosis; carcinoma; metastases; prognosis; red blood cell; white blood cell; chemotherapy; radiation therapy

Exercise 33

A. disease was identified; cancerous tumor; did not have a fever
B. diagnosis; carcinoma; afebrile
C. cytology, pathologist, diagnosis, carcinoma, dysplasia, inflammation
D. Answers may vary and may include cytology, pathologist, diagnosis, carcinoma, dysplasia, inflammation, along with their respective definitions.

Exercise 34

A. 1. chemotherapy
   2. adenocarcinoma
   3. pathology
   4. malignant
   5. radiation therapy
   6. organomegaly
   7. cyanosis
   8. metastases

B. 1. b
   2. b
   3. d
   4. a. prognoses
      b. lipomata
      c. histologies

Exercise 35

Pronunciation Exercise

Exercise 36

1. a
2. b
3. a
4. b
5. c
6. b
7. b
8. a
9. b
10. c
11. b
12. b
13. b
14. c
15. b
16. a
17. c
18. a
19. b
20. a

ANSWERS TO CHAPTER 3 EXERCISES

Exercise Figure A

1. head: cephal/o
2. back: dors/o
3. back, behind: poster/o
4. tail: caud/o
5. front: anter/o
6. belly (front): ventr/o
7. side: later/o
8. above: super/o
9. middle: medi/o
10. near: proxim/o
11. away: dist/o
12. below: infer/o

Exercise Figure B

1. poster/o/anter/ior
2. anter/o/poster/ior

Exercise Figure C

1. frontal or coronal plane
2. transverse plane
3. midsagittal plane

Exercise Figure D

1. right hypochondriac
2. right lumbar
3. right iliac
4. hypogastric
5. epigastric
6. left hypochondriac
7. umbilical
8. left lumbar
9. left iliac

Exercise Figure E

1. right upper quadrant (RUQ)
2. left upper quadrant (LUQ)
3. right lower quadrant (RLQ)
4. left lower quadrant (LLQ)

Exercise 1

1. belly (front)
2. head (upward)
3. side
4. middle
5. below
6. near (the point of attachment of a body part)
7. above
8. away (from the point of attachment of a body part)
9. back
10. tail (downward)
11. front
12. back, behind

Exercise 2

1. c
2. b
3. d
4. a

Exercise 3

1. pertaining to
2. toward
3. two
4. one

Exercise 4

Pronunciation Exercise

Exercise 5

1. WR S
   cephal/ad
   toward the head
2. WR S
   proxim/al
   pertaining to near
3. WR S
   later/al
   pertaining to a side
4. P WR S
   uni/later/al
   pertaining to one side
5. WR CV WR S
   anter/o/poster/ior
   CF
   pertaining to the front and to the back
6. WR S
   cephal/ic
   pertaining to the head
7. WR S
   super/ior
   pertaining to above
8. WR S
   anter/ior
   pertaining to the front
9. WR S
   caud/ad
   toward the tail

10. WR S
dist/al
pertaining to away
11. WR S
medi/al
pertaining to the middle
12. P WR S
bi/later/al
pertaining to two sides
13. WR CV WR S
poster/o/anter/ior
CF
pertaining to the back and to the front
14. WR S
caud/al
pertaining to the tail
15. WR S
infer/ior
pertaining to below
16. WR S
poster/ior
pertaining to the back
17. WR S
ventr/al
pertaining to the belly (front)
18. WR S
dors/al
pertaining to the back

Exercise 6
A. 1. cephal/ad
2. proxim/al
3. dist/al
4. later/al
5. medi/al
6. caud/ad
7. poster/o/anter/ior
8. medi/o/later/al
9. uni/later/al
10. anter/o/poster/ior
11. bi/later/al

B. 1. super/ior
2. cephal/ic
3. poster/ior, dors/al
4. infer/ior
5. caud/al
6. anter/ior
7. ventr/al

Exercise 7
Spelling Exercise

Exercise 8
Pronunciation Exercise

Exercise 9
1. transverse
2. midsagittal
3. frontal or coronal
4. sagittal
5. parasagittal

Exercise 10
Spelling Exercise

Exercise 11
Pronunciation Exercise

Exercise 12
A. 1. d
2. a
3. f
4. c
5. b
6. e

B. 1. supine
2. prone
3. orthopnea
4. Trendelenburg
5. lithotomy
6. Sims

Exercise 13
Spelling Exercise

Exercise 14
Pronunciation Exercise

Exercise 15
1. iliac
2. epigastric
3. hypogastric
4. hypochondriac
5. umbilical
6. lumbar

Exercise 16
1. b
2. d
3. a
4. e
5. c
6. f

Exercise 17
Spelling Exercise

Exercise 18
1. RLQ
2. RUQ
3. LLQ
4. LUQ
5. RLQ
6. RUQ
7. RLQ

Exercise 19
Spelling Exercise

Exercise 20
1. superior
2. anterior
3. inferior
4. posteroanterior
5. anteroposterior
6. medial
7. lateral

Exercise 21
A. near (her shoulder); belly near the navel; lower back near her waist; on her back facing upward
B. Answers will vary and may include proximal, ventral, umbilical region, lumbar region, supine, recumbent along with their respective definitions.
C. medial, lateral, proximal, AP
D. Answers will vary and may include medial, lateral, proximal, and AP along with their respective definitions.

Exercise 22
A. 1. anteroposterior
2. lateral
3. posterior (dorsal is used for head, trunk, and surfaces of hand and foot)
4. medial
5. anterior

B. 1. b
2. a
3. a
4. answers may vary: the upper surface of the foot; the surface opposite the sole

Exercise 23
Pronunciation Exercise

Exercise 24
1. c
2. a
3. c
4. a
5. c
6. a
7. c
8. a
9. b
10. c
11. a
12. b
13. c
14. a
15. b
16. c
17. a. superior
b. inferior
c. medial
d. lateral

ANSWERS TO CHAPTER 4 EXERCISES

Exercise Figure A
1. dermat/itis
2. kerat/osis

Exercise Figure B
1. onych/o/myc/osis
2. par/onych/ia

Exercise Figure C
1. leuk/o/derm/a
2. erythr/o/derm/a
3. xanth/o/derm/a

Exercise Figure D
1. intra/derm/al
2. sub/cutane/ous, hypo/derm/ic
3. trans/derm/al

Exercise Figure E
staphyl/o/cocci

Exercise Figure F
strept/o/cocci

Exercise 1
Pronunciation Exercise

Exercise 2
1. horny tissue: kerat/o
2. skin: cutane/o, dermat/o, derm/o
3. sebum: seb/o
4. sweat: hidr/o
5. nail: onych/o, ungu/o

Exercise 3
1. d, skin
2. b, sebum (oil)
3. c, nail
4. d, skin
5. e, horny tissue (keratin), hard
6. c, nail
7. a, sweat

Exercise 4
1. death
2. grapelike clusters
3. hidden
4. thick
5. dust
6. fungus
7. life
8. other
9. twisted chains
10. dry, dryness
11. self
12. wrinkles

Exercise 5
1. myc/o
2. necr/o
3. heter/o
4. xer/o
5. pachy/o
6. strept/o
7. rhytid/o
8. staphyl/o
9. aut/o
10. crypt/o
11. coni/o
12. bi/o

Exercise 6
1. under, below
2. beside, beyond, around, abnormal
3. on, upon, over
4. within
5. through
6. through, across, beyond

Exercise 7
1. intra-
2. sub-
3. epi-
4. para-
5. per-
6. trans-

Exercise 8
A. 1. e
   2. c
   3. a
   4. b
   5. d

B. 1. -coccus
   2. -opsy
   3. -tome
   4. -itis
   5. -plasty
   6. -ectomy

Exercise 9
1. surgical repair
2. excision or surgical removal
3. softening
4. inflammation
5. instrument used to cut
6. eating, swallowing
7. flow, discharge
8. berry-shaped
9. view of, viewing
10. diseased or abnormal state, condition of
11. noun suffix, no meaning

Exercise 10
Pronunciation Exercise

Exercise 11
1. WR CV WR S
   dermat/o/coni/osis (dermat/o = CF)
   abnormal condition of the skin caused by dust
2. WR WR S
   hidr/aden/itis
   inflammation of a sweat gland
3. WR S
   dermat/itis
   inflammation of the skin
4. WR WR S
   pachy/derm/a
   thickening of the skin
5. WR CV S
   onych/o/malacia (onych/o = CF)
   softening of the nails
6. WR S
   kerat/osis
   abnormal condition (growth) of horny tissue (keratin)
7. WR CV WR S
   dermat/o/fibr/oma (dermat/o = CF)
   fibrous tumor of the skin
8. P WR S
   par/onych/ia
   diseased state around the nail
9. WR CV WR S
   onych/o/crypt/osis (onych/o = CF)
   abnormal condition of a hidden nail
10. WR CV S
    seb/o/rrhea (seb/o = CF)
    discharge of sebum (excessive)
11. WR CV S
    onych/o/phagia (onych/o = CF)
    eating the nails, nail biting
12. WR CV WR S
    xer/o/derm/a (xer/o = CF)
    dry skin
13. WR CV WR S
    lei/o/derm/ia (lei/o = CF)
    condition of smooth skin
14. WR S
    xanth/oma
    yellow tumor

Exercise 12
1. pachy/derm/a
2. onych/o/myc/osis
3. seb/o/rrhea
4. dermat/itis
5. dermat/o/fibr/oma
6. onych/o/malacia
7. hidr/aden/itis
8. onych/o/crypt/osis
9. dermat/o/coni/osis
10. onych/o/phagia
11. par/onych/ia
12. xer/o/derm/a
13. lei/o/derm/ia
14. xanth/oma

Exercise 13
Spelling Exercise

Exercise 14
Pronunciation Exercise

Exercise 15

A.
1. systemic lupus erythematosus
2. abscess
3. abrasion
4. pediculosis
5. contusion
6. gangrene
7. lesion
8. carbuncle
9. acne
10. laceration
11. scleroderma
12. infection
13. albinism
14. MRSA infection

B.
1. a. fissure
   b. eczema
2. cellulitis
3. psoriasis
4. herpes
5. tinea
6. Kaposi sarcoma
7. actinic keratosis
8. furuncle
9. squamous cell carcinoma
10. basal cell carcinoma
11. impetigo
12. scabies
13. urticaria
14. candidiasis
15. vitiligo
16. rosacea

Exercise 16

1. d	9. e
2. j	10. i
3. h	11. g
4. l	12. a
5. k	13. f
6. c	14. m
7. n	15. o
8. b	

Exercise 17

1. d	9. n
2. b	10. e
3. f	11. i
4. p	12. g
5. m	13. k
6. l	14. c
7. o	15. j
8. a	16. h

Exercise 18

Spelling Exercise

Exercise 19

Pronunciation Exercise

Exercise 20

1. WR S
   rhytid/ectomy
   excision of wrinkles
2. WR S
   bi/opsy
   view of life (removal of living tissue)
3. WR CV WR CV S
   dermat/o/aut/o/plasty
   CF CF
   surgical repair using one's own skin (for the skin graft)
4. WR CV S
   rhytid/o/plasty
   CF
   surgical repair of wrinkles
5. WR CV WR CV S
   dermat/o/heter/o/plasty
   CF CF
   surgical repair using skin from others (for the skin graft)
6. WR S
   derma/tome
   instrument used to cut skin

Exercise 21

1. rhytid/ectomy
2. bi/opsy
3. dermat/o/heter/o/plasty
4. rhytid/o/plasty
5. dermat/o/plasty
6. derma/tome

Exercise 22

Spelling Exercise

Exercise 23

Pronunciation Exercise

Exercise 24

1. Mohs surgery
2. incision
3. cauterization
4. suturing
5. incision and drainage
6. debridement
7. excision
8. laser surgery
9. cryosurgery
10. dermabrasion

Exercise 25

1. i	6. e
2. h	7. b
3. g	8. f
4. d	9. j
5. a	10. c

Exercise 26

Spelling Exercise

Exercise 27

Pronunciation Exercise

Exercise 28

1. WR S
   ungu/al
   pertaining to the nail
2. P WR S
   trans/derm/al
   pertaining to through the skin
3. WR CV S
   strept/o/coccus
   CF
   berry-shaped (bacterium) in twisted chains
4. P WR S
   hypo/derm/ic
   pertaining to under the skin
5. WR CV S
   dermat/o/logy
   CF
   study of the skin
6. P WR S
   sub/cutane/ous
   pertaining to under the skin
7. WR CV S
   staphyl/o/coccus
   CF
   berry-shaped (bacterium) in grapelike clusters
8. WR CV S
   kerat/o/genic
   CF
   producing horny tissue
9. WR CV S
   dermat/o/logist
   CF
   physician who studies and treats skin (diseases)
10. WR S
    necr/osis
    abnormal condition of death (of cells and tissue)
11. P WR S
    epi/derm/al
    pertaining to upon the skin
12. WR CV WR S
    xanth/o/derm/a
    CF
    yellow skin
13. WR CV WR S
    erythr/o/derm/a
    CF
    red skin
14. P WR S
    per/cutane/ous
    pertaining to through the skin
15. WR S
    xer/osis
    abnormal condition of dryness
16. P WR S
    sub/ungu/al
    pertaining to under the nail

17. WR CV WR S
leuk/o/derm/a
CF
white skin

Exercise 29

1. dermat/o/logy
2. necr/osis
3. ungu/al
4. staphyl/o/coccus
5. dermat/o/logist
6. intra/derm/al
7. epi/derm/al
8. sub/cutane/ous, hypo/derm/ic
9. strept/o/coccus
10. kerat/o/genic
11. erythr/o/derm/a
12. xanth/o/derm/a
13. per/cutane/ous, trans/derm/al
14. sub/ungu/al
15. leuk/o/derm/a
16. xer/osis

Exercise 30

Spelling Exercise

Exercise 31

Pronunciation Exercise

Exercise 32

1. cicatrix
2. diaphoresis
3. verruca
4. macule
5. jaundice
6. leukoplakia
7. petechia
8. ulcer
9. keloid
10. pallor
11. ecchymosis
12. pressure injury
13. nodule
14. cyst
15. pruritus
16. erythema
17. purpura
18. nevus
19. bacteria
20. alopecia
21. papule
22. wheal
23. pustule
24. vesicle
25. fungus
26. virus
27. induration
28. edema
29. cytomegalovirus

Exercise 33

1. m
2. a
3. j
4. e
5. f
6. l
7. g
8. d
9. b
10. k
11. c
12. h
13. i

Exercise 34

1. g
2. d
3. j
4. a
5. l
6. k
7. n
8. b
9. e
10. f
11. o
12. c
13. h
14. i
15. m
16. p

Exercise 35

Spelling Exercise

Exercise 36

1. basal cell carcinoma
2. cytomegalovirus
3. systemic lupus erythematosus
4. squamous cell carcinoma
5. biopsy
6. subcutaneous
7. staphylococcus
8. streptococcus
9. incision and drainage
10. transdermal
11. intradermal
12. dermatology
13. methicillin-resistant *Staphylococcus aureus*, healthcare-associated MRSA infection, community-associated MRSA infection

Exercise 37

A. pale; very itchy; (lips beginning to) swell; red; tiny bumps
B. Answers will vary and may include pallor, pruritus, edema, erythema, urticaria.
C. pallor, pruritus, edema, urticaria
D. Answers will vary and may include pallor, pruritus, edema, urticaria along with their respective definitions.

Exercise 38

A.
1. dermatology
2. nodule
3. medial
4. actinic keratosis
5. eczema
6. lesion
7. excision
8. superior
9. pathology
10. cauterization
11. biopsy
12. basal cell carcinoma

B.
1. a. s
   b. p
   c. p
   d. s
   e. s
   f. p
   g. s
   h. p
2. b
3. dictionary exercise

Exercise 39

Pronunciation Exercise

Exercise 40

1. b
2. b
3. c
4. b
5. a
6. c
7. a
8. a
9. c
10. b
11. a
12. c
13. c
14. b
15. a
16. b
17. b

ANSWERS TO CHAPTER 5 EXERCISES

Exercise Figure A

bronchi/ectasis

Exercise Figure B

hem/o/thorax

Exercise Figure C

pneum/o/thorax

Exercise Figure D

sinus/itis

Exercise Figure E

adenoid/ectomy, aden/o/tome

Exercise Figure F

thorac/o/centesis

Exercise Figure G

endo/trache/al, laryng/o/scope

Exercise Figure H

1. ox/i/meter
2. capn/o/meter
3. spir/o/meter

Exercise 1
Pronunciation Exercise

Exercise 2
1. sinus: sinus/o
2. nose: nas/o, rhin/o
3. tonsil: tonsill/o
4. epiglottis: epiglott/o
5. larynx: laryng/o
6. trachea: trache/o
7. pleura: pleur/o
8. lobe: lob/o
9. diaphragm: diaphragmat/o, phren/o
10. adenoids: adenoid/o
11. pharynx: pharyng/o
12. lung: pneum/o, pneumat/o, pneumon/o, pulmon/o
13. thorax, chest, chest cavity: thorac/o
14. bronchus: bronch/o, bronchi/o
15. alveolus: alveol/o

Exercise 3
1. h, alveolus
2. a, bronchus
3. c, lung
4. g, larynx
5. d, pleura
6. i, thorax, chest, chest cavity
7. b, trachea
8. e, tonsil
9. f, sinus

Exercise 4
1. d, adenoids
2. h, diaphragm
3. e, epiglottis
4. b, lobe
5. a, nose
6. g, pharynx
7. c, lung, air
8. c, lung, air
9. a, nose
10. f, septum
11. h, diaphragm

Exercise 5
1. oxygen
2. breathe, breathing
3. mucus
4. imperfect, incomplete
5. straight
6. pus
7. blood
8. sleep
9. carbon dioxide
10. sound, voice
11. sound
12. x-rays, ionizing radiation
13. to cut, section, or slice

Exercise 6
1. spir/o
2. ox/i
3. atel/o
4. orth/o
5. py/o
6. muc/o
7. a. hem/o
   b. hemat/o
8. somn/o
9. phon/o
10. capn/o
11. son/o
12. radi/o
13. tom/o

Exercise 7
1. within
2. absence of, without
3. normal, good
4. many, much
5. fast, rapid

Exercise 8
1. endo-
2. eu-
3. a. a-
   b. an-
4. poly-
5. tachy-

Exercise 9
1. g
2. c
3. d
4. e
5. a
6. f
7. i
8. k
9. l
10. b
11. h
12. m
13. j

Exercise 10
1. -scope
2. -scopy
3. -tomy
4. -stomy
5. -meter
6. -metry
7. -graph
8. -graphy
9. -gram

Exercise 11
1. chest, chest cavity
2. pertaining to
3. constriction, narrowing
4. hernia, protrusion
5. creation of an artificial opening
6. surgical fixation, suspension
7. instrument used to measure
8. sudden, involuntary muscle contraction
9. pain
10. visual examination
11. surgical puncture to aspirate fluid
12. cut into, incision
13. instrument used for visual examination
14. rapid flow of blood, excessive bleeding
15. stretching out, dilation, expansion
16. process of recording, radiographic imaging
17. measurement
18. in the blood
19. pertaining to visual examination
20. breathing
21. instrument used to record; the record
22. the record, radiographic image

Exercise 12
Pronunciation Exercise

Exercise 13
1. WR S
   pleur/itis
   inflammation of the pleura
2. WR CV WR S
   naso/o/pharyng/itis
   CF
   inflammation of the nose and pharynx
3. WR CV S
   pneum/o/thorax
   CF
   air in the chest cavity
4. WR S
   sinus/itis
   inflammation of the sinuses
5. WR S
   atel/ectasis
   incomplete expansion (or collapsed lung)
6. WR CV WR S
   rhin/o/myc/osis
   CF
   abnormal condition of fungus in the nose
7. WR CV S
   trache/o/stenosis
   CF
   narrowing of the trachea
8. WR S
   epiglott/itis
   inflammation of the epiglottis
9. WR S
   thorac/algia
   pain in the chest
10. WR S P S(WR)
    pulmon/ary neo/plasm
    pertaining to (in) the lung new growth (tumor)
11. WR S
    bronchi/ectasis
    dilation of the bronchi
12. WR S
    tonsill/itis
    inflammation of the tonsils
13. WR CV WR S
    pneum/o/coni/osis
    CF
    abnormal condition of dust in the lungs

14. WR CV WR S
bronch/o/pneumon/ia
CF
diseased state of bronchi and lungs

15. WR S
pneumon/itis
inflammation of the lung

16. WR S
laryng/itis
inflammation of the larynx

17. WR CV S
py/o/thorax
CF
pus in the chest cavity

18. WR CV S
rhin/o/rrhagia
CF
rapid flow of blood from the nose

19. WR S
bronch/itis
inflammation of the bronchi

20. WR S
pharyng/itis
inflammation of the pharynx

21. WR S
trache/itis
inflammation of the trachea

22. WR CV WR CV WR S
laryng/o/trache/o/bronch/itis
CF CF
inflammation of the larynx, trachea, and bronchi

23. WR S
adenoid/itis
inflammation of the adenoids

24. WR CV S
hem/o/thorax
CF
blood in the chest cavity (pleural space)

25. WR S WR S
lob/ar pneumon/ia
pertaining to the lobe, diseased state of a lung

26. WR S
rhin/itis
inflammation of the nose

27. WR CV S WR S
bronch/o/genic carcin/oma
CF
cancerous tumor originating in a bronchus

28. WR S
alveol/itis
inflammation of the alveoli

29. WR S
pneumon/ia
diseased state of the lung

30. WR CV S
pneumat/o/cele
CF
hernia of the lung

Exercise 14

1. thorac/algia
2. rhin/o/myc/osis
3. pulmon/ary neo/plasm
4. laryng/itis
5. atel/ectasis
6. adenoid/itis
7. laryng/o/trache/o/bronch/itis
8. bronchi/ectasis
9. pleur/itis
10. pneum/o/coni/osis
11. pneumon/itis
12. sinus/itis
13. trache/o/stenosis
14. nas/o/pharyng/itis
15. py/o/thorax
16. epiglott/itis
17. diaphragmat/o/cele
18. pneum/o/thorax
19. bronch/o/pneumon/ia
20. rhin/o/rrhagia
21. pharyng/itis
22. hem/o/thorax
23. trache/itis
24. bronch/itis
25. lob/ar pneumon/ia
26. rhin/itis
27. bronch/o/genic carcin/oma
28. alveol/itis
29. pneumon/ia
30. pneumat/o/cele

Exercise 15

Spelling Exercise

Exercise 16

Pronunciation Exercise

Exercise 17

1. pulmonary emphysema
2. pleural effusion
3. coccidioidomycosis
4. cystic fibrosis
5. influenza
6. chronic obstructive pulmonary disease
7. pertussis
8. croup
9. asthma
10. pulmonary edema
11. upper respiratory infection
12. pulmonary embolism
13. epistaxis
14. idiopathic pulmonary fibrosis
15. deviated septum
16. obstructive sleep apnea
17. tuberculosis
18. acute respiratory distress syndrome

Exercise 18

1. i
2. d
3. g
4. f
5. c
6. a
7. e
8. b
9. h

Exercise 19

1. d
2. b
3. c
4. e
5. f
6. g
7. h
8. i
9. a

Exercise 20

Spelling Exercise

Exercise 21

Pronunciation Exercise

Exercise 22

1. WR CV S
trache/o/tomy
CF
incision into the trachea

2. WR CV S
laryng/o/stomy
CF
creation of an artificial opening into the larynx

3. WR S
adenoid/ectomy
excision of the adenoids

4. WR CV S
rhin/o/plasty
CF
surgical repair of the nose

5. WR CV S
aden/o/tome
CF
instrument used to cut the adenoids

6. WR CV S
trache/o/stomy
CF
creation of an artificial opening into the trachea

7. WR CV S
sinus/o/tomy
CF
incision into a sinus

8. WR CV S
laryng/o/plasty
CF
surgical repair of the larynx

9. WR CV S
bronch/o/plasty
CF
surgical repair of a bronchus

10. WR S
lob/ectomy
excision of a lobe (of the lung)

11. WR CV WR CV S
laryng/o/trache/o/tomy
CF CF
incision into larynx and trachea

12. WR CV S
trache/o/plasty
CF
surgical repair of the trachea

13. WR CV S
thorac/o/tomy
CF
incision into the chest cavity

14. WR S
laryng/ectomy
excision of the larynx

15. WR CV S
thorac/o/centesis
CF
surgical puncture to aspirate fluid from the chest cavity

16. WR S
tonsill/ectomy
excision of the tonsils

17. WR CV S
pleur/o/pexy
CF
surgical fixation of the pleura

18. WR CV S
sept/o/plasty
CF
surgical repair of the septum

19. WR CV S
sept/o/tomy
CF
incision into the septum

Exercise 23

1. trache/o/plasty
2. laryng/o/trache/o/tomy
3. aden/o/tome
4. thorac/o/tomy
5. trache/o/stomy
6. tonsill/ectomy
7. trache/o/tomy
8. bronch/o/plasty
9. laryng/ectomy
10. rhin/o/plasty
11. sinus/o/tomy
12. thorac/o/centesis
13. adenoid/ectomy
14. laryng/o/plasty
15. lob/ectomy
16. laryng/o/stomy
17. pneumon/ectomy
18. sept/o/tomy
19. sept/o/plasty

Exercise 24

Spelling Exercise

Exercise 25

Pronunciation Exercise

Exercise 26

1. WR CV S
spir/o/meter
CF
instrument used to measure breathing

2. WR CV S
laryng/o/scope
CF
instrument used for visual examination of the larynx

3. WR CV S
capn/o/meter
CF
instrument used to measure carbon dioxide

4. WR CV S
spir/o/metry
CF
measurement of breathing

5. WRCV S
ox/i/meter
CF
instrument used to measure oxygen

6. WR CV S
laryng/o/scopy
CF
visual examination of the larynx

7. WR CV S
bronch/o/scope
CF
instrument used for visual examination of the bronchi

8. WR CV S
thorac/o/scope
CF
instrument used for visual examination of the chest cavity

9. P S(WR)
endo/scope
instrument used for visual examination within (a hollow organ or body cavity)

10. WR CV S
thorac/o/scopy
CF
visual examination of the chest cavity

11. P S(WR)
endo/scopic
pertaining to visual examination within (a hollow organ or body cavity)

12. P S(WR)
endo/scopy
visual examination within (a hollow organ or body cavity)

13. P WR CV S
poly/somn/o/graphy
CF
process of recording many (tests) during sleep

14. WR CV S
son/o/gram
CF
record of sound

15. WR CV S
son/o/graphy
CF
process of recording sound

16. WR CV S
tom/o/graphy
CF
process of recording slices (anatomical cross sections)

17. WR CV S
radi/o/graph
CF
record of x-rays

18. WR CV S
radi/o/graphy
CF
process of recording x-rays

Exercise 27

1. laryng/o/scopy
2. spir/o/meter
3. capn/o/meter
4. laryng/o/scope
5. bronch/o/scopy
6. spir/o/metry
7. bronch/o/scope
8. endo/scopy
9. thorac/o/scope
10. endo/scope
11. thorac/o/scopy
12. endo/scopic
13. poly/somn/o/graphy
14. radi/o/graphy
15. radi/o/graph
16. son/o/graphy
17. son/o/gram
18. tom/o/graphy

Exercise 28

Spelling Exercise

Exercise 29

Pronunciation Exercise

Exercise 30

A. 1. acid-fast bacilli smear
2. pulmonary function tests

3. percussion
4. auscultation
5. sputum culture and sensitivity

B. 1. PPD (purified protein derivative) skin test
2. peak flow meter
3. arterial blood gasses
4. pulse oximetry
5. stethoscope
6. lung ventilation/profusion scan
7. chest radiograph
8. chest computed tomography (CT) scan

Exercise 31

1. f
2. e
3. a
4. d
5. b
6. c
7. h
8. i
9. l
10. j
11. k
12. m
13. g

Exercise 32

Spelling Exercise

Exercise 33

Pronunciation Exercise

Exercise 34

1. WR S
laryng/eal
pertaining to the larynx

2. P S(WR)
eu/pnea
normal breathing

3. WR S
muc/oid
resembling mucus

4. P S(WR)
a/pnea
absence of breathing

5. P WR S
hyp/ox/ia
condition of deficient oxygen (to tissues)

6. WR CV S
laryng/o/spasm
CF
spasmodic contraction of the larynx

7. P WR S
endo/trache/al
pertaining to within the trachea

8. P WR S
an/ox/ia
condition of absence of oxygen

9. P WR S
dys/phon/ia
condition of difficulty in speaking (voice)

10. WR CV WR S
bronch/o/alveol/ar
CF
pertaining to the bronchi and alveoli

11. P S(WR)
dys/pnea
difficult breathing

12. P WR S
hypo/capn/ia
condition of deficient in carbon dioxide (in the blood)

13. WR CV S
bronch/o/spasm
CF
spasmodic contraction of the bronchus

14. WR CV S
orth/o/pnea
CF
able to breathe easier in a straight (upright) position

15. P S(WR)
hyper/pnea
excessive breathing

16. P WR S
a/capn/ia
condition of absence of carbon dioxide (in the blood)

17. P S(WR)
hypo/pnea
deficient breathing

18. P WR S
hyp/ox/emia
deficient oxygen in the blood

19. P WR S
a/phon/ia
condition of absence of voice

20. WR CV S
rhin/o/rrhea
CF
discharge from the nose

21. WR S
thorac/ic
pertaining to the chest

22. WR S
muc/ous
pertaining to mucus

23. WR CV WR S
nas/o/pharyng/eal
CF
pertaining to the nose and pharynx

24. WR S
diaphragmat/ic
pertaining to the diaphragm

25. P WR S
intra/pleur/al
pertaining to within the pleura

26. WR S
pulmon/ary
pertaining to the lungs

27. WR S
phren/algia
pain in the diaphragm

28. P S(WR)
tachy/pnea
rapid breathing

29. WR CV S
phren/o/spasm
CF
spasm of the diaphragm

30. WR CV S
pulmon/o/logist
CF
a physician who studies and treats diseases of the lung

31. WR CV S
pulmon/o/logy
CF
study of the lung

32. WR S
alveol/ar
pertaining to the alveolus

33. WR CV S
radi/o/logy
CF
study of x-rays

34. WR CV S
radi/o/logist
CF
physician who specializes in using medical imaging

Exercise 35

1. hyp/ox/ia
2. muc/oid
3. orth/o/pnea
4. endo/trache/al
5. an/ox/ia
6. dys/pnea
7. laryng/eal
8. hyper/capn/ia
9. eu/pnea
10. a/phon/ia
11. laryng/o/spasm
12. hypo/capn/ia
13. nas/o/pharyng/eal
14. diaphragmat/ic
15. a/pnea
16. hyp/ox/emia
17. hyper/pnea
18. bronch/o/spasm
19. hypo/pnea
20. a/capn/ia
21. dys/phon/ia
22. rhin/o/rrhea
23. muc/ous
24. thorac/ic

25. intra/pleur/al
26. pulmon/ary
27. phren/o/spasm
28. tachy/pnea
29. phren/algia
30. alveol/ar
31. pulmon/o/logy
32. pulmon/o/logist
33. radi/o/logist
34. radi/o/logy

Exercise 36

Spelling Exercise

Exercise 37

Pronunciation Exercise

Exercise 38

1. hyperventilation
2. nebulizer
3. bronchodilator
4. ventilator
5. asphyxia
6. sputum
7. aspirate
8. airway
9. stridor
10. rhonchi
11. mucopurulent
12. hypoventilation
13. nosocomial
14. paroxysm
15. patent
16. bronchoconstrictor
17. mucus
18. crackles

Exercise 39

1. b
2. g
3. c
4. h
5. a
6. d
7. f
8. e
9. i

Exercise 40

1. e
2. g
3. h
4. c
5. i
6. a
7. b
8. d
9. f

Exercise 41

Spelling Exercise

Exercise 42

1. chronic obstructive pulmonary disease; pulmonary function tests, chest radiograph, arterial blood gases, computed tomography
2. shortness of breath
3. A. left upper lobe; left lower lobe
   B. right upper lobe, right middle lobe, right lower lobe
4. acid-fast bacilli; tuberculosis
5. polysomnography; obstructive sleep apnea
6. oxygen; carbon dioxide
7. peak flow meter
8. idiopathic pulmonary fibrosis
9. culture and sensitivity
10. hospital-acquired pneumonia
11. lung ventilation/perfusion scan; pulmonary embolism

Exercise 43

1. acute respiratory distress syndrome
2. cystic fibrosis
3. influenza
4. laryngotracheobronchitis
5. upper respiratory infection
6. continuous positive airway pressure
7. community-acquired pneumonia

Exercise 44

A. difficulty breathing; runny nose; her throat was very sore; thick yellow mucus; cold

B. Answer will vary and may include dyspnea, rhinorrhea, pharyngitis, sputum, and/or upper respiratory infection.

C. dyspnea, mucoid, sputum, rhinorrhea, auscultation, percussion, crackles, rhonchi

D. Answer will vary and may include dyspnea, mucoid, sputum, rhinorrhea, auscultation, percussion, crackles, and/or rhonchi along with their respective definitions.

Exercise 45

A. 1. dyspnea
   2. pulmonary
   3. rhonchi
   4. chest radiograph
   5. bronchoscopy
   6. arterial blood gases
   7. hypoxemia
   8. bronchogenic carcinoma
   9. pulmonary function tests
   10. thoracic

B. 1. a
   2. F
   3. F
   4. T

C. Online Exercise

Exercise 46

Pronunciation Exercise

Exercise 47

1. b
2. c
3. a
4. c
5. a
6. a
7. b
8. c
9. c
10. b
11. a
12. c
13. b
14. c
15. b
16. c

ANSWERS TO CHAPTER 6 EXERCISES

Exercise Figure A

cyst/o/lith

Exercise Figure B

cyst/o/stomy

Exercise Figure C

lith/o/tripsy

Exercise Figure D

nephr/o/stomy

Exercise Figure E

pyel/o/lith/o/tomy

Exercise Figure F

ur/o/gram

Exercise Figure G

urin/ary

Exercise 1

Pronunciation Exercise

Exercise 2

A. 1. kidney: nephr/o, ren/o
   2. meatus: meat/o
   3. ureter: ureter/o
   4. bladder: cyst/o, vesic/o
   5. urethra: urethr/o

B. 1. renal pelvis: pyel/o
   2. glomerulus: glomerul/o

Exercise 3

1. g, kidney
2. a, bladder
3. g, kidney
4. d, glomerulus
5. f, renal pelvis
6. c, ureter
7. a, bladder
8. b, meatus
9. e, urethra

Exercise 4

1. water
2. urea, nitrogen
3. night
4. stone, calculus
5. albumin
6. urine, urinary tract
7. sugar
8. developing cell, germ cell
9. scanty, few
10. urine, urinary tract
11. sugar

Exercise 5

1. a. glyc/o
   b. glycos/o
2. a. urin/o
   b. ur/o
3. hydr/o
4. blast/o
5. albumin/o
6. noct/i
7. azot/o
8. lith/o
9. olig/o

Exercise 6

A. 1. -lysis
   2. -ptosis
   3. -tripsy
   4. -rrhaphy

B. 1. -iasis, -esis
   2. -uria

Exercise 7

1. suturing, repairing
2. loosening, dissolution, separating
3. condition
4. urine, urination
5. drooping, sagging, prolapse
6. surgical crushing

Exercise 8

Pronunciation Exercise

Exercise 9

1. WR S
   nephr/oma
   tumor of the kidney
2. WR CV S
   cyst/o/lith
   CF
   stone(s) in the bladder
3. WR CV WR S
   nephr/o/lith/iasis
   CF
   condition of stone(s) in the kidney
4. WR S
   azot/emia
   urea in the blood
5. WR CV S
   nephr/o/ptosis
   CF
   drooping kidney
6. WR CV S
   cyst/o/cele
   CF
   protrusion of the bladder
7. WR S
   cyst/itis
   inflammation of the bladder
8. WR S
   pyel/itis
   inflammation of the renal pelvis
9. WR CV S
   ureter/o/cele
   CF
   protrusion of a ureter
10. WR CV WR S
    hydr/o/nephr/osis
    CF
    abnormal condition of water in the kidney
11. WR CV S
    nephr/o/megaly
    CF
    enlargement of a kidney
12. WR CV WR S
    ureter/o/lith/iasis
    CF
    condition of stone(s) in the ureter
13. WR CV WR S
    pyel/o/nephr/itis
    CF
    inflammation of the renal pelvis and the kidney
14. WR S
    ureter/itis
    inflammation of a ureter
15. WR S
    nephr/itis
    inflammation of a kidney
16. WR CV WR S
    urethr/o/cyst/itis
    CF
    inflammation of the urethra and bladder
17. WR CV S
    ureter/o/stenosis
    CF
    narrowing of the ureter
18. WR CV WR S
    nephr/o/blast/oma
    CF
    kidney tumor containing developing cells

Exercise 10

1. nephr/o/megaly
2. cyst/itis
3. urethr/o/cyst/itis
4. cyst/o/cele
5. hydr/o/nephr/osis
6. cyst/o/lith
7. glomerul/o/nephr/itis
8. nephr/oma
9. nephr/o/ptosis
10. nephr/itis
11. nephr/o/lith/iasis
12. ureter/o/cele
13. pyel/itis
14. azot/emia
15. ureter/o/stenosis
16. pyel/o/nephr/itis
17. ureter/o/lith/iasis
18. nephr/o/blast/oma

Exercise 11

Spelling Exercise

Exercise 12

Pronunciation Exercise

Exercise 13

1. renal calculus
2. urinary retention
3. polycystic kidney disease
4. hypospadias
5. renal hypertension
6. urinary suppression
7. epispadias
8. urinary tract infection
9. renal failure

Exercise 14

1. c
2. f
3. d
4. h
5. a
6. e
7. b
8. g
9. i

Exercise 15

Spelling Exercise

Exercise 16

Pronunciation Exercise

Exercise 17

1. WR CV S
   vesic/o/tomy
   CF
   incision into the bladder
2. WR CV S
   cyst/o/tomy
   CF
   incision into bladder
3. WR CV S
   nephr/o/stomy
   CF
   creation of an artificial opening into the kidney

4. WR CV S
nephr/o/lysis
CF
separating the kidney

5. WR S
cyst/ectomy
excision of the bladder

6. WR CV WR CV S
pyel/o/lith/o/tomy
CF CF
incision into the renal pelvis to remove stone(s)

7. WR CV S
nephr/o/pexy
CF
surgical fixation of the kidney

8. WR CV WR CV S
cyst/o/lith/o/tomy
CF CF
incision into the bladder to remove stone(s)

9. WR S
nephr/ectomy
excision of the kidney

10. WR S
ureter/ectomy
excision of the ureter

11. WR CV S
cyst/o/stomy
CF
creation of an artificial opening into the bladder

12. WR CV S
pyel/o/plasty
CF
surgical repair of the renal pelvis

13. WR CV S
cyst/o/rrhaphy
CF
suturing the bladder

14. WR CV S
meat/o/tomy
CF
incision into the meatus

15. WR CV S
lith/o/tripsy
CF
surgical crushing of stone(s)

16. WR CV S
urethr/o/plasty
CF
surgical repair of the urethra

17. WR CV WR S
vesic/o/urethr/al (suspension)
CF
suspension pertaining to the bladder and urethra

18. WR CV WR CV S
nephr/o/lith/o/tomy
CF CF
incision into the kidney to remove stone(s)

19. WR CV S
ureter/o/stomy
CF
creation of an artificial opening into the ureter

20. WR CV WR CV S
nephr/o/lith/o/tripsy
CF CF
surgical crushing of stone(s) in the kidney

Exercise 18

1. ureter/o/stomy
2. nephr/ectomy
3. nephr/o/lith/o/tomy
4. cyst/o/rrhaphy
5. nephr/o/lysis
6. nephr/o/stomy
7. urethr/o/plasty
8. cyst/ectomy
9. meat/o/tomy
10. a. cyst/o/tomy
    b. vesic/o/tomy
11. pyel/o/plasty
12. ureter/ectomy
13. nephr/o/pexy
14. cyst/o/lith/o/tomy
15. lith/o/tripsy
16. vesic/o/urethr/al (suspension)
17. cyst/o/stomy
18. pyel/o/lith/o/tomy
19. nephr/o/lith/o/tripsy

Exercise 19

Spelling Exercise

Exercise 20

Pronunciation Exercise

Exercise 21

1. renal transplant
2. fulguration
3. extracorporeal shock wave lithotripsy

Exercise 22

1. b
2. a
3. c

Exercise 23

Spelling Exercise

Exercise 24

Pronunciation Exercise

Exercise 25

1. WR CV WR CV S
(voiding) cyst/o/urethr/o/graphy
CF CF
radiographic imaging of the bladder and the urethra

2. WR CV S
cyst/o/graphy
CF
radiographic imaging of the bladder

3. WR CV WR CV S
nephr/o/son/o/graphy
CF CF
process of recording the kidney with sound

4. WR CV S
cyst/o/scope
CF
instrument used for visual examination of the bladder

5. WR CV S
cyst/o/gram
CF
radiographic image of the bladder

6. WR CV S
cyst/o/scopy
CF
visual examination of the bladder

7. WR CV S
nephr/o/graphy
CF
radiographic imaging of the kidney

8. WR CV S
ur/o/gram
CF
radiographic image of the urinary tract

9. WR CV S
(retrograde) ur/o/gram
CF
radiographic image of the urinary tract

10. WR CV S
ren/o/gram
CF
radiographic record of the kidney

11. WR CV S
nephr/o/scopy
CF
visual examination of the kidney

12. WR CV S
ureter/o/scopy
CF
visual examination of the ureter

Exercise 26
1. cyst/o/scopy
2. ur/o/gram
3. nephr/o/son/o/graphy
4. cyst/o/gram
5. cyst/o/scope
6. (voiding) cyst/o/urethr/o/graphy
7. cyst/o/graphy
8. ren/o/gram
9. nephr/o/graphy
10. (retrograde) ur/o/gram
11. nephr/o/scopy
12. ureter/o/scopy

Exercise 27
Spelling Exercise

Exercise 28
Pronunciation Exercise

Exercise 29
1. KUB
2. urinalysis
3. A. blood urea nitrogen
   B. creatinine
4. specific gravity

Exercise 30
1. c
2. b
3. d
4. a
5. e

Exercise 31
Spelling Exercise

Exercise 32
Pronunciation Exercise

Exercise 33
1. WR S
   noct/uria
   night urination
2. WR CV S
   ur/o/logist
   CF
   physician who studies and treats diseases of the urinary tract
3. WR S
   olig/uria
   condition of scanty urine (amount)
4. WR CV S
   nephr/o/logist
   CF
   physician who studies and treats diseases of the kidney
5. WR S
   hemat/uria
   blood in the urine
6. WR CV S
   ur/o/logy
   CF
   study of the urinary tract
7. P S(WR)
   poly/uria
   much (excessive) urine
8. WR S
   albumin/uria
   albumin in the urine
9. P S(WR)
   an/uria
   absence of urine
10. P WR S
    di/ur/esis
    condition of urine passing through (increased excretion of urine)
11. WR S
    py/uria
    pus in the urine
12. WR S
    urin/ary
    pertaining to urine
13. WR S
    glycos/uria
    sugar in the urine
14. P S(WR)
    dys/uria
    difficult or painful urination
15. WR CV S
    nephr/o/logy
    CF
    study of the kidney
16. WR CV S
    nephr/o/logist
    CF
    physician who studies and treats diseases of the kidney

Exercise 34
1. noct/uria
2. olig/uria
3. py/uria
4. ur/o/logist
5. poly/uria
6. nephr/o/logist
7. urin/ary
8. hemat/uria
9. ur/o/logy
10. di/ur/esis
11. an/uria
12. glycos/uria
13. dys/uria
14. albumin/uria
15. meat/al
16. nephr/o/logy

Exercise 35
Spelling Exercise

Exercise 36
Pronunciation Exercise

Exercise 37
1. urinal
2. hemodialysis
3. distended
4. catheter
5. incontinence
6. urinary catheterization
7. peritoneal dialysis
8. void
9. stricture
10. enuresis
11. micturate
12. urodynamics
13. electrolytes

Exercise 38
1. d
2. f
3. e
4. a
5. c
6. b

Exercise 39
1. a
2. d
3. g
4. b
5. f
6. c
7. e

Exercise 40
Spelling Exercise

Exercise 41
1. voiding cystourethrogram
2. specific gravity; urinalysis
3. blood urea nitrogen
4. extracorporeal shock wave lithotripsy
5. catheterization; urinary tract infection
6. hemodialysis
7. acute renal failure, chronic kidney disease, end-stage renal disease
8. overactive bladder

Exercise 42
A. blood when he urinated; infection of his bladder; difficulty urinating; physician who treats diseases of the urinary tract
B. Answers will vary and may include hematuria; cystitis; dysuria; urologist
C. and D. hematuria; renal calculi; UTI; renal failure; hemodialysis along with their respective definitions

Exercise 43
A. 1. nephrolithiasis
   2. hematuria
   3. urology
   4. KUB

5. calculi
6. cystoscopy
7. urogram
8. nephrolithotomy
9. catheter

B. 1. c
2. d
3. *F*, calculus is singular for stone
4. a. pertaining to the ureter
   b. instrument used for visual examination of the ureter

C. Online Exercise

Exercise 44

Pronunciation Exercise

Exercise 45

1. c
2. b
3. c
4. b
5. a
6. a
7. b
8. c
9. c
10. c
11. b
12. c
13. a
14. b
15. b

ANSWERS TO CHAPTER 7 EXERCISES

Exercise Figure A

balan/itis

Exercise Figure B

crypt/orchid/ism

Exercise Figure C

vas/ectomy

Exercise 1

Pronunciation Exercise

Exercise 2

1. male: andr/o
2. seminal vesicle: vesicul/o
3. prostate gland: prostat/o
4. epididymis: epididym/o
5. testis: orchid/o, orchi/o, orch/o
6. vas deferens or ductus deferens: vas/o
7. glans penis: balan/o
8. sperm, spermatozoon: sperm/o, spermat/o

Exercise 3

1. g, sperm, spermatozoon
2. a, vessel, duct
3. g, sperm, spermatozoon
4. b, glans penis
5. f, prostate gland
6. d, testis, testicle
7. c, seminal vesicle(s)
8. d, testis, testicle
9. e, epididymis
10. d, testis, testicle
11. male

Exercise 4

state of

Exercise 5

Pronunciation Exercise

Exercise 6

1. WR CV WR
   prostat/o /lith
   CF
   stone(s) in the prostate gland
2. WR S
   balan/itis
   inflammation of the glans penis
3. WR S
   orch/itis
   inflammation of the testis
4. WR CV WR S
   prostat/o /vesicul/itis
   CF
   inflammation of the prostate gland and the seminal vesicles
5. WR CV WR S
   prostat/o /cyst/itis
   CF
   inflammation of the prostate gland and the (urinary) bladder
6. WR WR S
   orchi/epididym/itis
   inflammation of the testis and the epididymis
7. WR CV S
   prostat/o /rrhea
   CF
   discharge from the prostate gland
8. WR S
   epididym/itis
   inflammation of the epididymis
9. WR S P S(WR)
   (benign) prostat/ic hyper/plasia
   excessive development pertaining to the prostate gland
10. WR WR S
    crypt/orchid/ism
    state of hidden testis
11. WR CV S
    balan/o /rrhea
    CF
    discharge from the glans penis
12. WR S
    prostat/itis
    inflammation of the prostate gland
13. P WR S
    an/orch/ism
    state of absence of testis

Exercise 7

1. prostat/o/cyst/itis
2. prostat/o/lith
3. orch/itis
4. benign prostat/ic hyper/plasia
5. crypt/orchid/ism
6. prostat/o/vesicul/itis
7. an/orch/ism
8. prostat/itis
9. orchi/epididym/itis
10. balan/o/rrhea
11. epididym/itis
12. balan/itis
13. prostat/o/rrhea

Exercise 8

Spelling Exercise

Exercise 9

Pronunciation Exercise

Exercise 10

A. 1. testicular cancer
2. erectile dysfunction
3. priapism
4. testicular torsion
5. spermatocele

B. 1. varicocele
2. phimosis
3. hydrocele
4. prostate cancer

Exercise 11

1. d
2. c
3. e
4. b
5. a
6. f
7. i
8. h
9. g

Exercise 12

Spelling Exercise

Exercise 13

Pronunciation Exercise

Exercise 14

1. WR S
   vas/ectomy
   excision of a duct

2. WR CV WR CV S
prostat/o/cyst/o/tomy
CF CF
incision into the prostate gland and (urinary) bladder
3. WR CV S
orchi/o/tomy
CF
incision into the testis
4. WR S
epdidym/ectomy
excision of the epididymis
5. WR CV S
orchi/o/pexy
CF
surgical fixation of the testicle
6. WR CV WR S
prostat/o/vesicul/ectomy
CF
excision of the prostate gland and the seminal vesicles
7. WR CV S
orchi/o/plasty
CF
surgical repair of the testis
8. WR S
vesicul/ectomy
excision of the seminal vesicle(s)
9. WR S
prostat/ectomy
excision of the prostate gland
10. WR CV S
balan/o/plasty
CF
surgical repair of the glans penis
11. WR CV WR CV S
vas/o/vas/o/stomy
CF CF
creation of artificial openings between ducts
12. WR S
orchi/ectomy
excision of the testis
13. WR CV WR CV S
prostat/o/lith/o/tomy
CF CF
incision into the prostate gland to remove stone(s)

Exercise 15

1. orchi/ectomy
2. balan/o/plasty
3. prostat/o/cyst/o/tomy
4. vesicul/ectomy
5. prostat/o/lith/o/tomy
6. orchi/o/tomy
7. epididym/ectomy
8. orchi/o/plasty
9. prostat/ectomy
10. vas/ectomy
11. prostat/o/vesicul/ectomy
12. orchi/o/pexy
13. vas/o/vas/o/stomy

Exercise 16

Spelling Exercise

Exercise 17

Pronunciation Exercise

Exercise 18

1. enucleation
2. circumcision
3. ablation
4. hydrocelectomy
5. transurethral microwave thermotherapy
6. transurethral incision of the prostate gland
7. transurethral resection of the prostate gland
8. laser surgery
9. robotic surgery
10. morcellation
11. MRI ultrasound fusion (biopsy)

Exercise 19

Spelling Exercise

Exercise 20

Pronunciation Exercise

Exercise 21

1. digital rectal examination
2. prostate-specific antigen
3. transrectal ultrasound
4. semen analysis
5. multiparametric MRI

Exercise 22

Spelling Exercise

Exercise 23

Pronunciation Exercise

Exercise 24

1. WR S
orchi/algia
pain in the testis
2. WR CV WR S
olig/o/sperm/ia
CF
condition of scanty sperm
3. WR CV S
andr/o/pathy
CF
disease of the male
4. WR CV S
spermat/o/lysis
CF
dissolution of sperm
5. P WR S
a/sperm/ia
condition of without sperm
6. P WR S
trans/urethr/al
pertaining to through the urethra

Exercise 25

1. spermat/o/lysis
2. a/sperm/ia
3. andr/o/pathy
4. olig/o/sperm/ia
5. orchi/algia
6. trans/urethr/al

Exercise 26

Spelling Exercise

Exercise 27

Pronunciation Exercise

Exercise 28

1. e
2. c
3. f
4. b
5. g
6. a
7. h
8. d
9. i

Exercise 29

1. a
2. g
3. d
4. i
5. b
6. h
7. e
8. f
9. c

Exercise 30

Spelling Exercise

Exercise 31

1. lower urinary tract symptoms; bladder outlet obstruction
2. digital rectal examination; benign prostatic hyperplasia
3. transurethral incision (of the prostate gland); transurethral resection (of the prostate gland); transurethral microwave thermotherapy; photoselective vaporization (of the prostate gland); holmium laser enucleation (of the prostate gland)
4. human immunodeficiency virus; acquired immunodeficiency syndrome
5. human papillomavirus
6. sexually transmitted infection; sexually transmitted disease
7. prostate-specific antigen
8. radical prostatectomy
9. erectile dysfunction
10. transrectal ultrasound

Exercise 32

A. pain in his testicle; twisting of the spermatic cord with decreased blood flow to the testis; surgical fixation of the testis; surgical removal of the testis; reduced or absent ability to achieve pregnancy

B. Answers will vary and may include orchialgia, testicular torsion, orchiopexy, orchiectomy, infertility, and their respective definitions.

C. orchialgia, orchiectomy, infertility, testicular torsion, orchiopexy

D. Answers will vary and may include orchialgia, orchiectomy, infertility, testicular torsion, orchiopexy, and their respective definitions.

Exercise 33

A. 1. nocturia
 2. hematuria
 3. BOO
 4. urinary
 5. benign prostatic hyperplasia
 6. urology

B. 1. c
 2. b
 3. c
 4. a

C. Online Exercise

Exercise 34

Pronunciation Exercise

Exercise 35

1. a
2. b
3. a
4. c
5. a
6. c
7. b
8. a
9. c
10. c
11. b
12. a
13. c
14. a
15. c
16. a

ANSWERS TO CHAPTER 8 EXERCISES

Exercise Figure A

salping/itis

Exercise Figure B

1. hyster/ectomy
2. salping/o/-oophor/ectomy
3. hyster/o/salping/o/-oophor/ectomy

Exercise Figure C

colp/o/rrhaphy, cyst/o/cele

Exercise Figure D

hyster/o/salping/o/gram, hydr/o/salpinx

Exercise 1

Pronunciation Exercise

Exercise 2

A. 1. ovary: oophor/o
 2. uterus: hyster/o, metr/o
 3. uterine (fallopian) tube: salping/o
 4. endometrium: endometri/o
 5. cervix: cervic/o, trachel/o
 6. vagina: colp/o, vagin/o
 7. hymen: hymen/o

B. 1. vulva: episi/o, vulv/o
 2. perineum: perine/o

C. 1. men/o
 2. gyn/o, gynec/o
 3. arche/o
 4. mamm/o, mast/o
 5. pelv/i

Exercise 3

1. f: uterine tube (fallopian tube)
2. e: uterus
3. a: perineum
4. c: cervix
5. b: vagina
6. c: cervix
7. d: breast
8. arche/o: first, beginning
9. pelv/i: pelvis, pelvic bones, pelvic cavity

Exercise 4

1. b: vagina
2. a: hymen
3. d: vulva
4. f: uterus
5. e: breast
6. g: ovary
7. d: vulva
8. c: endometrium
9. men/o: menstruation
10. gynec/o, gyn/o: woman

Exercise 5

1. -salpinx
2. peri-
3. -cleisis

Exercise 6

1. uterine tube
2. surrounding
3. surgical closure

Exercise 7

Pronunciation Exercise

Exercise 8

1. WR S
 endometri/osis
 abnormal condition of the endometrium (endometrial tissue grows outside of the uterus in various areas of the pelvic cavity)

2. WR S
 cervic/itis
 inflammation of the cervix

3. WR CV S
 hydr/o/salpinx
 CF
 water in the uterine tube

4. WR CV S
 hemat/o/salpinx
 CF
 blood in the uterine tube

5. WR CV S
 metr/o/rrhagia
 CF
 excessive bleeding from the uterus (irregular, out-of-cycle bleeding ranging from heavy to light, including spotting)

6. WR S
 oophor/itis
 inflammation of the ovary

7. WR S
 (Bartholin) aden/itis
 inflammation of (Bartholin) gland

8. WR CV WR S
 vulv/o/vagin/itis
 CF
 inflammation of the vulva and vagina

9. WR CV S
 salping/o/cele
 CF
 hernia of the uterine tube

10. WR CV WR CV S
 men/o/metr/o/rrhagia
 CF CF
 excessive bleeding from the uterus at menstruation (and between menstrual cycles; heavy and irregular bleeding)

11. P WR CV S
a/men/o/rrhea
CF
absence of menstrual flow

12. P WR CV S
dys/men/o/rrhea
CF
painful menstrual flow

13. WR S
mast/itis
inflammation of the breast

14. P WR S
peri/metr/itis
inflammation surrounding the uterus (outer layer)

15. WR CV WR S
my/o/metr/itis
CF
inflammation of the uterine muscle

16. WR S
endometr/itis
inflammation of the endometrium

17. WR CV S
py/o/salpinx
CF
pus in the uterine tube

18. WR S
vagin/osis
abnormal condition of the vagina (caused by a bacterial imbalance)

19. WR S
salping/itis
inflammation of the uterine tube

20. WR S
vagin/itis
inflammation of the vagina

21. WR CV S
men/o/rrhagia
CF
excessive bleeding at menstruation (heavy bleeding in regular, cyclical pattern)

22. WR CV WR CV S
olig/o/men/o/rrhea
CF CF
scanty menstrual flow (infrequent menstrual flow)

Exercise 9

1. mast/itis
2. metr/o/rrhagia
3. salping/itis
4. vulv/o/vagin/itis
5. a/men/o/rrhea
6. cervic/itis
7. (Bartholin) aden/itis
8. hydr/o/salpinx
9. dys/men/o/rrhea
10. hemat/o/salpinx
11. vagin/itis
12. men/o/metr/o/rrhagia
13. oophor/itis
14. salping/o/cele
15. peri/metr/itis
16. endometr/itis
17. vagin/osis
18. my/o/metr/itis
19. py/o/salpinx
20. endometri/osis
21. olig/o/men/o/rrhea
22. men/o/rrhagia

Exercise 10

Spelling Exercise

Exercise 11

Pronunciation Exercise

Exercise 12

1. downward displacement of the uterus into the vagina
2. inflammation of some or all of the female pelvic organs
3. abnormal opening between the vagina and another organ
4. benign fibroid tumor of the uterine muscle
5. condition typically characterized by hormonal imbalances, ovulatory dysfunction, and multiple ovarian cysts
6. growth of endometrium into the muscular portion of the uterus
7. severe illness characterized by high fever, vomiting, diarrhea, and myalgia
8. fibrosis, benign cysts, and a pain or tenderness in one or both breasts
9. malignant tumor of the ovary
10. malignant tumor of the breast
11. malignant tumor of the cervix
12. malignant tumor of the endometrium

Exercise 13

A. 1. adenomyosis
2. toxic shock syndrome
3. fibrocystic breast changes
4. polycystic ovary syndrome
5. ovarian cancer
6. cervical cancer

B. 1. uterine prolapse
2. uterine fibroid
3. endometrial cancer
4. breast cancer
5. pelvic inflammatory disease
6. vaginal fistula

Exercise 14

Spelling Exercise

Exercise 15

Pronunciation Exercise

Exercise 16

1. WR CV S
colp/o/rrhaphy
CF
suturing of the vagina

2. WR CV S
colp/o/plasty
CF
surgical repair of the vagina

3. WR CV S
episi/o/rrhaphy
CF
suturing of the vulva (tear)

4. WR CV S
hymen/o/tomy
CF
incision into the hymen

5. WR CV S
hyster/o/pexy
CF
surgical fixation of the uterus

6. WR S
vulv/ectomy
excision of the vulva

7. WR CV S
perine/o/rrhaphy
CF
suturing of the perineum (tear)

8. WR CV S
salping/o/stomy
CF
creation of an artificial opening in the uterine tube

9. WR CV WR S
salping/o/-oophor/ectomy
CF
excision of the uterine tube and the ovary

10. WR S
oophor/ectomy
excision of the ovary

11. WR S
mast/ectomy
surgical removal of the breast

12. WR S
salping/ectomy
excision of the uterine tube

13. WR S
trachel/ectomy
excision of the cervix

14. WR CV WR CV S
colp/o/perine/o/rrhaphy
CF CF
suturing of the vagina and the perineum

15. WR CV WR CV S
episi/o/perine/o/plasty
CF CF
surgical repair of the vulva and the perineum

16. WR S
hymen/ectomy
excision of the hymen

17. WR CV WR CV WR S
hyster/o/salping/o/-oophor/ectomy
CF CF
excision of the uterus, uterine tubes, and ovaries

18. WR S
hyster/ectomy
excision of the uterus

19. WR CV S
mamm/o/plasty
CF
surgical repair of the breast

20. WR CV S
mast/o/pexy
CF
surgical fixation of the breast

21. WR CV S
trachel/o/rrhaphy
CF
suturing of the cervix

22. WR CV S
colp/o/cleisis
CF
surgical closure of the vagina

Exercise 17

1. colp/o/rrhaphy
2. trachel/ectomy
3. episi/o/rrhaphy
4. episi/o/perine/o/plasty
5. colp/o/plasty
6. colp/o/perine/o/rrhaphy
7. hyster/o/salping/o/-oophor/ectomy
8. hyster/o/pexy
9. hymen/ectomy
10. hymen/o/tomy
11. hyster/ectomy
12. oophor/ectomy
13. mast/ectomy
14. salping/ectomy
15. perine/o/rrhaphy
16. salping/o/-oophor/ectomy
17. salping/o/stomy
18. vulv/ectomy
19. mamm/o/plasty
20. mast/o/pexy
21. trachel/o/rraphy
22. colp/o/cleisis

Exercise 18

Spelling Exercise

Exercise 19

Pronunciation Exercise

Exercise 20

1. tubal ligation
2. anterior and posterior colporrhaphy
3. dilation and curettage
4. stereotactic breast biopsy
5. myomectomy
6. endometrial ablation
7. uterine artery embolization
8. conization
9. sentinel lymph node biopsy
10. laparoscopy or laparoscopic surgery

Exercise 21

1. c	6. f
2. a	7. h
3. a	8. c
4. b	9. g
5. c	10. c

Exercise 22

Spelling Exercise

Exercise 23

Pronunciation Exercise

Exercise 24

1. WR CV S
colp/o/scopy
CF
visual examination of the vagina

2. WR CV S
mamm/o/gram
CF
radiographic image of the breast

3. WR CV S
colp/o/scope
CF
instrument used for visual examination of the vagina

4. WR CV S
hyster/o/scopy
CF
visual examination of the uterus

5. WR CV WR CV S
hyster/o/salping/o/gram
CF CF
radiographic image of the uterus and uterine tubes

6. WR CV S
pelv/i/scopic
CF
pertaining to visual examination of the pelvic cavity

7. WR CV S
pelv/i/scopy
CF
visual examination of the pelvic cavity

8. WR CV S
mamm/o/graphy
CF
radiographic imaging of the breast

9. WR CV S
hyster/o/scope
CF
instrument used for visual examination of the uterus

10. WR CV WR CV S
son/o/hyster/o/graphy
CF CF
process of recording the uterus with sound

Exercise 25

1. hyster/o/salping/o/gram
2. colp/o/scopy
3. colp/o/scope
4. hyster/o/scopy
5. mamm/o/gram
6. pelv/i/scopic
7. pelv/i/scopy
8. hyster/o/scope
9. mamm/o/graphy
10. son/o/hyster/o/graphy

Exercise 26

Spelling Exercise

Exercise 27

Pronunciation Exercise

Exercise 28

A. 1. cytological study of cervical and vaginal secretions to detect abnormal and cancerous cells
2. ultrasound procedure that obtains images of the ovaries, uterus, cervix, and uterine tubes
3. blood test primarily used to monitor treatment of ovarian cancer and to detect recurrence
4. cytological study of cervical and vaginal secretions to detect high-risk forms of the human papillomavirus (HPV) that can cause abnormal cervical cells and cervical cancer

B. 1. a. Pap test
b. HPV test
2. CA-125
3. transvaginal sonography

Exercise 29

Spelling Exercise

Exercise 30

Pronunciation Exercise

Exercise 31

1. WR CV S
gynec/o/logist
CF
physician who studies and treats (female reproductive system) women
2. WR CV S
gynec/o/logy
CF
study of women (branch of medicine dealing with health and diseases of the female reproductive system)
3. WR CV WR S
vulv/o/vagin/al
CF
pertaining to the vulva and vagina
4. WR S
mast/algia
pain in the breast
5. WR WR
men/arche
beginning of menstruation (first menstrual period)
6. WR CV S
leuk/o/rrhea
CF
white discharge (from the vagina)
7. WR CV WR S
gyn/o/path/ic
CF
pertaining to (reproductive system) diseases of women
8. WR CV WR S
vesic/o/vagin/al
CF
pertaining to the (urinary) bladder and the vagina
9. WR S
vagin/al
pertaining to the vagina
10. P WR S
endo/cervic/al
pertaining to within the cervix

Exercise 32

1. leuk/o/rrhea
2. men/arche
3. mast/algia
4. vulv/o/vagin/al
5. gynec/o/logist
6. gynec/o/logy
7. vesic/o/vagin/al
8. gyn/o/path/ic
9. vagin/al
10. endo/cervic/al

Exercise 33

Spelling Exercise

Exercise 34

Pronunciation Exercise

Exercise 35

1. cessation of menstruation
2. difficult or painful intercourse
3. abnormal passageway between two organs or between an internal organ and the body surface
4. syndrome involving physical and emotional symptoms occurring up to 10 days before menstruation
5. instrument for opening a body cavity to allow for visual inspection
6. replacement of hormones to treat symptoms associated with menopause
7. displacement of an organ or anatomic structure from its normal position
8. intentional prevention of conception
9. release of an ovum from a mature graafian follicle
10. infrequent ovulation
11. absence of ovulation

Exercise 36

1. fistula
2. ovulation
3. dyspareunia
4. menopause
5. premenstrual syndrome
6. speculum
7. hormone replacement therapy
8. contraception
9. prolapse
10. anovulation
11. oligoovulation

Exercise 37

Spelling Exercise

Exercise 38

1. anterior and posterior colporrhaphy
2. total abdominal hysterectomy and bilateral salpingo-oophorectomy; hormone replacement therapy
3. sonohysterography; transvaginal sonography
4. total vaginal hysterectomy; laparoscopically assisted vaginal hysterectomy; total laparoscopic hysterectomy
5. dilation and curettage; cervix
6. fibrocystic breast changes
7. pelvic inflammatory disease; gynecology
8. premenstrual syndrome
9. uterine artery embolization
10. intrauterine device; intrauterine system; birth control
11. polycystic ovary syndrome

Exercise 39

A. trying for over a year to get pregnant; menstruating is very painful; she bleeds a lot; may have given her a disease; only one of his testicles was down; surgery to fix the other one

B. Answers will vary and may include infertility, dysmenorrhea, menorrhagia, sexually transmitted disease (sexually transmitted infection), cryptorchidism, orchiopexy along with their respective definitions.

C. infertility, cryptorchidism, orchidopexy, menarche, dysmenorrhea, menorrhagia, Pap test, cervicitis, chlamydia, pelvic inflammatory disease, semen analysis, hysterosalpingogram

D. Answers will vary and may include infertility, cryptorchidism, orchidopexy, menarche, dysmenorrhea, menorrhagia, Pap test, cervicitis, chlamydia, pelvic inflammatory disease, semen analysis, hysterosalpingogram, along with their respective definitions

Exercise 40

A.
1. mammography
2. carcinoma
3. hysterectomy
4. adenomyosis
5. endometriosis
6. HRT
7. stereotactic breast biopsy
8. mediolateral
9. mastectomy
10. sentinel lymph node biopsy

B.
1. c
2. a
3. d

C. Online Exercise

Exercise 41

Pronunciation Exercise

Exercise 42

1. a
2. c
3. a
4. c
5. b
6. a
7. b
8. b
9. a
10. a
11. b
12. a
13. c
14. b
15. b
16. a

ANSWERS TO CHAPTER 9 EXERCISES

Exercise Figure A
omphal/o/cele

Exercise Figure B
neo/nat/e

Exercise 1
Pronunciation Exercise

Exercise 2
A. 1. umbilicus: omphal/o
2. fetus: fet/o, fet/i
3. amnion, amniotic fluid: amni/o, amnion/o
4. chorion: chori/o

B. 1. puerper/o
2. a. par/o
b. part/o
3. gravid/o
4. embry/o
5. nat/o
6. omphal/o

Exercise 3
A. 1. d: amnion, amniotic fluid
2. b: embry/o
3. e: umbilicus, navel
4. d: amnion, amniotic fluid
5. c: fetus, unborn offspring
6. a: chorion

B. 1. milk
2. bear, give birth to, labor, childbirth
3. childbirth
4. pregnancy
5. birth

Exercise 4
1. first
2. pylorus
3. head
4. esophagus
5. false
6. malformations

Exercise 5
1. cephal/o
2. pylor/o
3. pseud/o
4. esophag/o
5. prim/i
6. terat/o

Exercise 6
1. after
2. many
3. none
4. small
5. before
6. before

Exercise 7
1. nulli-
2. micro-
3. multi-
4. a. ante-
b. pre-
5. post-

Exercise 8
1. rupture
2. birth, labor
3. pregnancy
4. amnion, amniotic fluid

Exercise 9
1. -tocia
2. -rrhexis
3. -cyesis
4. -amnios

Exercise 10
1. -e
2. -is
3. -us
4. -um

Answers may be in any order.

Exercise 11
Pronunciation Exercise

Exercise 12
1. WR CV WR S
chori/o/amnion/itis
CF
inflammation of the chorion and amnion

2. WR CV WR S
chori/o/carcin/oma
CF
cancerous tumor of the chorion

3. P S(WR)
dys/tocia
difficult labor

4. WR S
amnion/itis
inflammation of the amnion

5. WR CV S
hyster/o/rrhexis
CF
rupture of the uterus

6. WR CV WR S
olig/o/hydr/amnios
CF
scanty amnion water (less than the normal amount of amniotic fluid)

7. P WR S
poly/hydr/amnios
much amnion water (more than the normal amount of amniotic fluid)

Exercise 13
1. chori/o/carcin/oma
2. amnion/itis
3. chori/o/amnion/itis
4. dys/tocia
5. hyster/o/rrhexis
6. olig/o/hydr/amnios
7. poly/hydr/amnios

Exercise 14
Spelling Exercise

Exercise 15
Pronunciation Exercise

Exercise 16
1. premature separation of the placenta from the uterine wall
2. termination of pregnancy by the expulsion from the uterus of an embryo or fetus
3. abnormally low implantation of the placenta on the uterine wall
4. severe complication and progression of preeclampsia
5. pregnancy occurring outside the uterus
6. abnormal condition, encountered during pregnancy or shortly after delivery, of high blood pressure and proteinuria

Exercise 17
1. abruptio placentae
2. eclampsia
3. abortion
4. ectopic pregnancy
5. placenta previa
6. preeclampsia

Exercise 18
Spelling Exercise

Exercise 19
Pronunciation Exercise

Exercise 20
1. WR S
pylor/ic (stenosis)
narrowing pertaining to the pyloric sphincter

2. WR CV S
omphal/o/cele
CF
herniation at the umbilicus

3. WR S
omphal/itis
inflammation of the umbilicus

4. P WR S
micro/cephal/us
(fetus with a very) small head

5. WR CV WR S
trache/o/esophag/eal (fistula)
CF
abnormal passageway pertaining to the trachea and the esophagus (between the trachea and esophagus)

Exercise 21

1. omphal/o/cele
2. micro/cephal/us
3. pylor/ic (stenosis)
4. trache/o/esophag/eal (fistula)
5. omphal/itis

Exercise 22

Spelling Exercise

Exercise 23

Pronunciation Exercise

Exercise 24

1. f	5. h
2. c	6. b
3. a	7. g
4. d	8. e

Exercise 25

Spelling Exercise

Exercise 26

Pronunciation Exercise

Exercise 27

1. WR CV S
episi/o/tomy
CF
incision into the vulva (perineum)

2. WR CV S
amni/o/tomy
CF
incision into the amnion (rupture of the fetal membrane to induce labor)

3. WR S WR CV S
pelv/ic son/o/graphy
CF
pertaining to the pelvis, process of recording sound

4. WR CV S
amni/o/centesis
CF
surgical puncture to aspirate amniotic fluid

Exercise 28

1. amni/o/tomy
2. episi/o/tomy
3. amni/o/centesis
4. pelv/ic son/o/graphy

Exercise 29

Spelling Exercise

Exercise 30

Pronunciation Exercise

Exercise 31

1. WR S
puerper/a
childbirth

2. WR CV S
amni/o/rrhexis
CF
rupture of the amnion

3. P WR S
ante/part/um
before childbirth

4. WR CV S
pseud/o/cyesis
CF
false pregnancy

5. P WR S
pre/nat/al
pertaining to before birth

6. WR S
lact/ic
pertaining to milk

7. WR CV S
lact/o/rrhea
CF
(spontaneous) discharge of milk

8. WR CV S
amni/o/rrhea
CF
discharge (escape) of amniotic fluid

9. P WR S
multi/par/a
many births

10. WR CV S
embry/o/genic
CF
producing an embryo

11. WR S
embry/oid
resembling an embryo

12. WR S
fet/al
pertaining to the fetus

13. WR S
gravid/a
pregnant (woman)

14. WR CV WR S
amni/o/chori/al
CF
pertaining to the amnion and chorion

15. P WR S
multi/gravid/a
many pregnancies

16. WR CV S
lact/o/genic
CF
producing milk (by stimulation)

17. WR S
nat/al
pertaining to birth

18. WR CV WR S
gravid/o/puerper/al
CF
pertaining to pregnancy and childbirth

19. P WR CV S
neo/nat/o/logy
CF
study of the newborn

20. P WR S
nulli/par/a
no births

21. WR S
par/a
birth

22. WR CV WR S
prim/i/gravid/a
CF
first pregnancy

23. P WR S
post/part/um
after childbirth

24. P WR S
neo/nat/e
new birth (an infant from birth to 4 weeks of age, synonymous with newborn)

25. WR CV WR S
prim/i/par/a
CF
first birth

26. WR S
puerper/al
pertaining to (immediately after) childbirth

27. P WR S
nulli/gravid/a
no pregnancies

28. P WR S
intra/part/um
within (during) labor and childbirth

29. WR CV S
terat/o/gen
CF
(any agent) producing malformations (in the developing embryo)

30. P WR S
post/nat/al
pertaining to after birth

31. WR CV S
terat/o/logy
CF
study of malformations (in the developing embryo)

32. P WR CV S
neo/nat/o/logist
CF
physician who studies and treats disorders of the newborn

33. WR CV S
terat/o/genic
CF
producing malformations

Exercise 32

1. amni/o/chori/al
2. ante/part/um
3. embry/o/genic
4. fet/al
5. pre/nat/al
6. lact/ic
7. lact/o/rrhea
8. amni/o/rrhea
9. pseud/o/cyesis
10. lact/o/genic
11. amni/o/rrhexis
12. embry/oid
13. gravid/a
14. gravid/o/puerper/al
15. multi/par/a
16. nat/al
17. neo/nat/e
18. neo/nat/o/logy
19. nulli/par/a
20. par/a
21. prim/i/gravid/a
22. post/part/um
23. prim/i/par/a
24. multi/gravid/a
25. puerper/al
26. nulli/gravid/a
27. terat/o/gen
28. puerper/a
29. intra/part/um
30. terat/o/genic
31. neo/nat/o/logist
32. post/nat/al
33. terat/o/logy

Exercise 33

Spelling Exercise

Exercise 34

Pronunciation Exercise

Exercise 35

1. a
2. e
3. i
4. g
5. f
6. b
7. j
8. d
9. c
10. h

Exercise 36

1. h
2. e
3. b
4. c
5. i
6. f
7. a
8. d
9. g

Exercise 37

1. first stool of the newborn
2. medical specialty dealing with pregnancy, childbirth, and puerperium
3. infant born before completing 37 weeks of gestation
4. vaginal discharge after childbirth
5. period after delivery until the reproductive organs return to normal
6. act of giving birth
7. physician who specializes in obstetrics
8. abnormality present at birth
9. birth position in which the buttocks, feet, or knees emerge first
10. birth of a fetus through an incision in the mother's abdomen and uterus
11. first feeling of movement of the fetus in utero by the pregnant woman
12. secretion of milk
13. birth position in which any part of the head emerges first
14. fluid secreted by the breast during pregnancy and after birth until lactation begins
15. individual who practices midwifery
16. born dead
17. practice of assisting in childbirth
18. method of fertilizing human ova outside the body
19. system for rapid neonatal assessment

Exercise 38

Spelling Exercise

Exercise 39

1. obstetrics
2. expected (estimated) date of delivery
3. last menstrual period
4. date of birth
5. newborn
6. multipara
7. cesarean section
8. vaginal birth after cesarean section
9. respiratory distress syndrome
10. primipara
11. fetal alcohol syndrome
12. in vitro fertilization
13. abortion
14. chorionic villus sampling

Exercise 40

A. pregnant for the third time, born dead, ultrasound test, genetic condition that causes physical and mental problems, needle to take fluid out

B. Answers will vary and may include multigravida, para, stillborn, pelvic sonography, Down syndrome, and amniocentesis

C. gravida, para, EDD, prenatal, Down syndrome, amniocentesis, abortion, congenital anomalies, tracheoesophageal fistula, neonatologist

D. Answers will vary and may include gravida, para, EDD, prenatal, Down syndrome, amniocentesis, abortion, congenital anomalies, tracheoesophageal fistula, neonatologist

Exercise 41

A. 1. gravida
2. para
3. EDD
4. prenatal
5. pelvic sonography
6. cephalic presentation

B. 1. c
2. T
3. F, sonography was used

C. Online Exercise

Exercise 42

Pronunciation Exercise

Exercise 43

1. b
2. b
3. a
4. a
5. c
6. b
7. a
8. c
9. b
10. b
11. b
12. a

ANSWERS TO CHAPTER 10 EXERCISES

Exercise Figure A
thromb/osis, ather/o/sclerosis

Exercise Figure B
hemat/oma

Exercise Figure C
end/arter/ectomy

Exercise Figure D
arteri/o/gram

Exercise Figure E
ven/o/gram

Exercise Figure F
electr/o/cardi/o/gram

Exercise Figure G
intra/ven/ous

Exercise 1
Pronunciation Exercise

Exercise 2
1. heart: cardi/o
2. blood vessel: angi/o
3. valve: valv/o, valvul/o
4. ventricle: ventricul/o
5. aorta: aort/o
6. artery: arteri/o
7. atrium: atri/o

Exercise 3
1. thymus gland: thym/o
2. lymph nodes: lymphaden/o
3. spleen: splen/o

Exercise 4
1. vein
   a. phleb/o
   b. ven/o
2. lymph, lymph tissue: lymph/o
3. vessel: angi/o
4. plasma: plasm/o
5. bone marrow: myel/o

Exercise 5
1. g, heart
2. f, bone marrow
3. a, valve
4. c, artery
5. b, lymph, lymph tissue
6. e, thymus gland
7. d, vein

Exercise 6
1. d, lymph node
2. e, aorta
3. c, ventricle
4. g, vein
5. f, vessel
6. h, valve
7. b, plasma
8. a, atrium

Exercise 7
1. sound
2. clot
3. deficiency, blockage
4. heat
5. yellowish, fatty plaque
6. electricity, electrical activity

Exercise 8
1. thromb/o
2. ech/o
3. isch/o
4. ather/o
5. therm/o
6. electr/o

Exercise 9
1. slow
2. all, total
3. abnormal reduction in number
4. hardening
5. removal
6. formation
7. pertaining to

Exercise 10
1. -poiesis
2. -ac
3. -sclerosis
4. pan-
5. -penia
6. brady-
7. -apheresis

Exercise 11
Pronunciation Exercise

Exercise 12
1. P WR S
   endo/card/itis
   inflammation of the inner (lining) of the heart
2. WP CV S
   brady/card/ia
   condition of slow heart (rate)
3. WR CV S
   cardi/o/megaly
   CF
   enlargement of the heart
4. WR CV S
   arteri/o/sclerosis
   CF
   hardening of the arteries
5. WR S
   valvul/itis
   inflammation of a valve (of the heart)
6. WR S
   (multiple) myel/oma
   tumors of the bone marrow
7. P WR S
   tachy/card/ia
   condition of a rapid heart (rate)
8. WR CV S
   angi/o/stenosis
   CF
   narrowing of a blood vessel
9. WR S
   thromb/us
   (blood) clot
10. P WR S
    peri/card/itis
    inflammation of the sac surrounding the heart
11. WR S
    aort/ic (stenosis)
    narrowing, pertaining to the aorta (narrowing of the aortic valve)
12. WR S
    thromb/osis
    abnormal condition of a (blood) clot
13. WR CV S
    ather/o/sclerosis
    CF
    hardening of fatty plaque (deposited on the arterial wall)
14. WR CV WR S
    my/o/card/itis
    CF
    inflammation of the muscle of the heart
15. WR S
    angi/oma
    tumor composed of blood vessels
16. WR S
    thym/oma
    tumor of the thymus gland
17. WR S
    lymph/oma
    tumor of lymphatic tissue
18. WR S
    lymphaden/itis
    inflammation of lymph nodes
19. WR CV S
    splen/o/megaly
    CF
    enlargement of the spleen

20. WR S
hemat/oma
tumor of blood

21. P WR S
poly/arter/itis
inflammation of many (sites in the) arteries

22. WR CV WR CV S
cardi/o/my/o/pathy
CF CF
disease of the heart muscle

23. WR CV S
lymphaden/o/pathy
CF
disease of lymph nodes

24. WR CV WR S
thromb/o/phleb/itis
CF
inflammation of a vein associated with a clot

25. WR S
phleb/itis
inflammation of a vein

26. P WR CV S
pan/cyt/o/penia
CF
abnormal reduction of all (blood) cells

27. WR CV WR CV S
erythr/o/cyt/o/penia
CF CF
abnormal reduction of red (blood) cells

28. WR CV WR CV S
leuk/o/cyt/o/penia
CF CF
abnormal reduction of white (blood) cells

29. WR CV WR CV S
thromb/o/cyt/o/penia
CF CF
abnormal reduction of (blood) clotting cells

30. WR S
isch/emia
deficiency in blood (flow); (caused by constriction or obstruction of a blood vessel)

Exercise 13

1. (multiple) myel/oma
2. cardi/o/megaly
3. endo/card/itis
4. brady/card/ia
5. arteri/o/sclerosis
6. thromb/osis
7. my/o/card/itis
8. angi/o/stenosis
9. tachy/card/ia
10. ather/o/sclerosis
11. angi/oma
12. valvul/itis
13. aort/ic (stenosis)
14. peri/card/itis
15. lymph/oma
16. isch/emia
17. thym/oma
18. splen/o/megaly
19. hemat/oma
20. lymphaden/itis
21. cardi/o/my/o/pathy
22. poly/arter/itis
23. lymphaden/o/pathy
24. thromb/o/phleb/itis
25. phleb/itis
26. thromb/us
27. pan/cyt/o/penia
28. erythr/o/cyt/o/penia
29. leuk/o/cyt/o/penia
30. thromb/o/cyt/o/penia

Exercise 14

Spelling Exercise

Exercise 15

Pronunciation Exercise

Exercise 16

1. coarctation
2. embolus
3. cardiac arrest
4. congenital
5. varicose veins
6. aneurysm
7. Hodgkin disease
8. coronary artery disease
9. angina pectoris
10. myocardial infarction
11. atrial fibrillation
12. arrhythmia
13. hypertensive
14. heart failure
15. peripheral artery disease
16. hemophilia
17. leukemia
18. anemia
19. infectious mononucleosis
20. intermittent claudication
21. cardiac tamponade
22. mitral valve stenosis and rheumatic heart disease
23. deep vein thrombosis
24. acute coronary syndrome
25. sepsis
26. cor pulmonale

Exercise 17

1. c
2. b
3. e
4. d
5. a
6. i
7. h
8. j
9. f
10. g
11. k
12. m
13. l

Exercise 18

1. i
2. e
3. a
4. h
5. j
6. b
7. d
8. k
9. l
10. g
11. c
12. m
13. f
14. n

Exercise 19

Spelling Exercise

Exercise 20

Pronunciation Exercise

Exercise 21

1. P WR CV S
peri/cardi/o/centesis
CF
surgical puncture to aspirate fluid from the sac surrounding the heart (pericardium)

2. WR S
thym/ectomy
excision of the thymus gland

3. WR CV S
angi/o/plasty
CF
surgical repair of a blood vessel

4. WR CV S
splen/o/rrhaphy
CF
suturing, repairing of the spleen

5. WR CV S
valvul/o/plasty
CF
surgical repair of a valve

6. P WR S
end/arter/ectomy
excision within an artery

7. WR CV S
phleb/o/tomy
CF
incision into a vein

8. WR S
splen/ectomy
excision of the spleen

9. WR S
phleb/ectomy
excision of a vein

10. WR S
ather/ectomy
excision of fatty plaque

Exercise 22

1. end/arter/ectomy
2. splen/o/rrhaphy
3. valvul/o/plasty
4. phleb/o/tomy
5. thym/ectomy
6. peri/cardi/o/centesis
7. angi/o/plasty
8. splen/ectomy
9. phleb/ectomy
10. ather/ectomy

Exercise 23

Spelling Exercise

Exercise 24

Pronunciation Exercise

Exercise 25

1. c
2. d
3. e
4. b
5. a

Exercise 26

1. bone marrow aspiration
2. bone marrow biopsy
3. coronary artery bypass graft
4. catheter ablation
5. coronary stent
6. percutaneous transluminal coronary angioplasty
7. automatic implantable cardiac defibrillator
8. femoropopliteal bypass

Exercise 27

Spelling Exercise

Exercise 28

Pronunciation Exercise

Exercise 29

1. WR CV WR CV S
electr/o/cardi/o/graph
CF CF
instrument used to record the electrical activity of the heart
2. WR CV S
ven/o/gram
CF
radiographic image of the veins (after an injection of contrast medium)
3. WR CV S
angi/o/graphy
CF
radiographic imaging of a blood vessel
4. WR CV WR CV S
ech/o/cardi/o/gram
CF CF
record of the heart (structure and motion) using sound (waves)
5. WR CV S
aort/o/gram
CF
radiographic image of the aorta (after an injection of contrast media)
6. WR CV WR CV S
electr/o/cardi/o/gram
CF CF
record of the electrical activity of the heart
7. WR CV S
arteri/o/gram
CF
radiographic image of an artery (after an injection of contrast media)
8. WR CV WR CV S
electr/o/cardi/o/graphy
CF CF
process of recording the electrical activity of the heart
9. WR CV S
angi/o/scopy
CF
visual examination (of the inside) of a blood vessel
10. WR CV S
angi/o/scope
CF
instrument used for visual examination (of the inside) of a blood vessel

Exercise 30

1. electr/o/cardi/o/graph
2. arteri/o/gram
3. ven/o/gram
4. angi/o/graphy
5. electr/o/cardi/o/gram
6. ech/o/cardi/o/gram
7. aort/o/gram
8. electr/o/cardi/o/graphy
9. angi/o/scopy
10. angi/o/scope

Exercise 31

Spelling Exercise

Exercise 32

Pronunciation Exercise

Exercise 33

A.
1. sphygmomanometer
2. coagulation time
3. prothrombin time
4. hemoglobin
5. transesophageal echocardiogram
6. activated partial thromboplastin time
7. single-photon emission computed tomography
8. creatine phosphokinase
9. C-reactive protein
10. pulse
11. troponin
12. lipid profile
13. hematocrit

B.
1. Doppler ultrasound
2. complete blood count and differential
3. exercise stress test
4. sestamibi test
5. digital subtraction angiography
6. blood pressure
7. cardiac catheterization

Exercise 34

1. d
2. h
3. k
4. g
5. j
6. c
7. a
8. e
9. b
10. f
11. i

Exercise 35

1. c
2. e
3. b
4. f
5. d
6. a
7. g
8. h
9. i

Exercise 36

Spelling Exercise

Exercise 37

Pronunciation Exercise

Exercise 38

1. P WR S
hypo/therm/ia
condition of (body) temperature that is below (normal)
2. WR CV S
hemat/o/poiesis
CF
formation of blood (cells)
3. WR CV S
cardi/o/logy
CF
study of the heart

4. WR CV S
cardi/o/logist
CF
physician who studies and treats diseases of the heart

5. WR CV S
hem/o/lysis
CF
dissolution of blood (cells)

6. WR CV S
hemat/o/logist
CF
physician who studies and treats diseases of the blood

7. WR S
cardi/ac
pertaining to the heart

8. WR CV S
hemat/o/logy
CF
study of the blood

9. WR S
plasm/apheresis
removal of plasma (from withdrawn blood)

10. WR CV S
hem/o/stasis
CF
stoppage of bleeding

11. WR CV S
cardi/o/genic
CF
originating in the heart

12. WR CV S
myel/o/poiesis
CF
formation of bone marrow

13. WR CV S
thromb/o/lysis
CF
dissolution of a clot

14. WR CV WR S
atri/o/ventricul/ar
CF
pertaining to the atrium and ventricle

15. P WR S
intra/ven/ous
pertaining to within the vein

Exercise 39

1. cardi/o/logy
2. hemat/o/poiesis
3. hypo/therm/ia
4. hem/o/lysis
5. plasm/apheresis
6. hemat/o/logist
7. cardi/ac
8. cardi/o/logist
9. hemat/o/logy
10. hem/o/stasis
11. myel/o/poiesis
12. cardi/o/genic
13. thromb/o/lysis
14. atri/o/ventricul/ar
15. intra/ven/ous

Exercise 40

Spelling Exercise

Exercise 41

Pronunciation Exercise

Exercise 42

1. vasoconstrictor
2. lumen
3. cardiopulmonary resuscitation
4. diastole
5. fibrillation
6. hypotension
7. extravasation
8. venipuncture
9. systole
10. vasodilator
11. hypertension
12. occlude
13. hypertriglyceridemia
14. hyperlipidemia
15. hemorrhage
16. hypercholesterolemia
17. blood dyscrasia
18. murmur
19. extracorporeal
20. lipids
21. defibrillation
22. anticoagulant
23. bruit
24. phlebotomist

Exercise 43

Spelling Exercise

Exercise 44

Pronunciation Exercise

Exercise 45

1. e
2. j
3. m
4. f
5. l
6. g
7. d
8. a
9. h
10. c
11. i
12. b
13. k

Exercise 46

Spelling Exercise

Exercise 47

1. coronary artery disease; electrocardiogram; single-photon emission computed tomography; echocardiogram
2. deep vein thrombosis
3. complete blood count, differential; red blood cell, white blood cell, hemoglobin, hematocrit
4. coronary artery bypass graft; percutaneous transluminal coronary angioplasty
5. myocardial infarction; coronary care unit
6. blood pressure
7. heart failure
8. cardiopulmonary resuscitation
9. hypertensive heart disease
10. prothrombin time
11. atrioventricular
12. acute coronary syndrome
13. peripheral artery disease
14. digital subtraction angiography
15. transesophageal echocardiogram
16. C-reactive protein, creatine phosphokinase
17. atrial fibrillation
18. automatic implantable cardiac defibrillator
19. intravenous
20. hypertension

Exercise 48

A. high blood pressure, pain in chest, heart was racing, breathing faster
B. answers will vary and may include hypertension, angina pectoris, tachycardia, tachypnea (from Chapter 5)
C. coronary artery disease, hypertension, hypercholesterolemia, varicose veins, cardiologist, coronary artery bypass grafts, abdominal aortic aneurysm
D. answers will vary and may include coronary artery disease, hypertension, hypercholesterolemia varicose veins, cardiologist, coronary artery bypass grafts. abdominal aortic aneurysm, along with their respective definitions

Exercise 49

A. 1. infectious mononucleosis
2. splenomegaly
3. splenectomy
4. lymphoma
5. vaccine
6. lymphadenopathy
7. arrhythmia
8. Hodgkin disease
9. leukemia

10. bone marrow biopsy
11. hematologist

B.
1. b
2. c
3. b
4. F, no indication of hemolysis
5. T

C. Online Exercise

Exercise 50

Pronunciation Exercise

Exercise 51

1. c
2. a
3. b
4. c
5. b
6. a
7. b
8. c
9. a
10. b
11. c
12. c
13. c
14. a
15. b
16. a
17. b
18. c
19. a
20. b

ANSWERS TO CHAPTER 11 EXERCISES

Exercise Figure A

1. Normal appendix
2. appendic/itis

Exercise Figure B

chol/e/lith/iasis, choledoch/o/lith/iasis

Exercise Figure C

gastr/ectomy

Exercise Figure D

per/cutane/ous
endo/scopic
gastr/o/stomy

Exercise Figure E

1. ile/o/stomy
2. col/o/stomy

Exercise Figure F

CT colon/o/graphy

Exercise Figure G

1. gastr/o/scopy
2. gastr/o/scope

Exercise 1

Pronunciation Exercise

Exercise 2

1. mouth: or/o, stomat/o
2. esophagus: esophag/o
3. duodenum: duoden/o
4. colon: col/o, colon/o
5. cecum: cec/o
6. anus: an/o
7. stomach: gastr/o
8. antrum: antr/o
9. jejunum: jejun/o
10. ileum: ile/o
11. sigmoid colon: sigmoid/o
12. rectum: proct/o, rect/o

Exercise 3

1. e, jejunum
2. g, anus
3. h, stomach
4. b, rectum
5. a, mouth
6. c, colon
7. f, sigmoid colon
8. d, intestine(s) (small intestine)

Exercise 4

1. d, ileum
2. g, mouth
3. h, rectum
4. e, esophagus
5. a, antrum
6. f, colon
7. b, duodenum
8. c, cecum

Exercise 5

1. palate: palat/o
2. uvula: uvul/o
3. tongue: gloss/o, lingu/o
4. gallbladder: chol/e (gall), cyst/o (bladder)
5. pyloric sphincter: pylor/o
6. appendix: append/o, appendic/o
7. gum(s): gingiv/o
8. lip(s): cheil/o
9. salivary glands: sial/o
10. liver: hepat/o
11. bile duct(s): cholangi/o
12. common bile duct: choledoch/o
13. pancreas: pancreat/o
14. abdomen, abdominal cavity: abdomin/o, celi/o, lapar/o

Exercise 6

1. peritone/o
2. chol/e
3. herni/o
4. diverticul/o
5. polyp/o
6. steat/o

Exercise 7

1. hernia
2. abdomen, abdominal cavity
3. saliva, salivary gland
4. gall, bile
5. diverticulum
6. gum(s)
7. appendix
8. tongue
9. liver
10. lip(s)
11. peritoneum
12. palate
13. pancreas
14. abdomen, abdominal cavity
15. tongue
16. common bile duct
17. pylorus, pyloric sphincter
18. uvula
19. bile duct(s)
20. polyp, small growth
21. abdomen
22. fat
23. appendix

Exercise 8

A.
1. digestion
2. half

B.
1. -pepsia
2. hemi-

Exercise 9

Pronunciation Exercise

Exercise 10

1. WR CV WR S
   chol/e/lith/iasis
   CF
   condition of gallstones
2. WR S
   diverticul/osis
   abnormal condition of having diverticula
3. WR CV WR
   sial/o/lith
   CF
   stone in the salivary gland
4. WR S
   hepat/oma
   tumor of the liver
5. WR S
   uvul/itis
   inflammation of the uvula
6. WR S
   pancreat/itis
   inflammation of the pancreas
7. WR S
   proct/itis
   inflammation of the rectum
8. WR S
   gingiv/itis
   inflammation of the gums

9. WR S
gastr/itis
inflammation of the stomach

10. WR CV S
rect/o/cele
CF
hernia of the rectum

11. WR S
palat/itis
inflammation of the palate

12. WR S
hepat/itis
inflammation of the liver

13. WR S
appendic/itis
inflammation of the appendix

14. WR CV WR S
chol/e/cyst/itis
CF
inflammation of the gallbladder

15. WR S
diverticul/itis
inflammation of a diverticulum

16. WR CV WR S
gastr/o/enter/itis
CF
inflammation of the stomach and intestines

17. WR S
enter/itis
inflammation of the intestines

18. WR CV WR S
choledoch/o/lith/iasis
CF
condition of stones in the common bile duct

19. WR S
cholangi/oma
tumor of the bile duct

20. WR S
polyp/osis
abnormal condition of (multiple) polyps

21. WR S
esophag/itis
inflammation of the esophagus

22. WR S
periton/itis
inflammation of the peritoneum

23. WR CV WR S
steat/o/hepat/itis
CF
inflammation of the liver associated with (excess) fat

24. WR S
gloss/itis
inflammation of the tongue

25. WR S
col/itis
inflammation of the colon

Exercise 11

1. hepat/oma
2. gastr/itis
3. sial/o/lith
4. appendic/itis
5. diverticul/itis
6. chol/e/cyst/itis
7. diverticul/osis
8. gastr/o/enter/itis
9. proct/itis
10. rect/o/cele
11. uvul/itis
12. gingiv/itis
13. hepat/itis
14. palat/itis
15. chol/e/lith/iasis
16. steat/o/hepat/itis
17. enter/itis
18. pancreat/itis
19. cholangi/oma
20. esophag/itis
21. choledoch/o/lith/iasis
22. polyp/osis
23. periton/itis
24. gloss/itis
25. col/itis

Exercise 12

Spelling Exercise

Exercise 13

Pronunciation Exercise

Exercise 14A

1. e
2. g
3. c
4. b
5. f
6. h
7. d
8. a

Exercise 14B

1. peptic ulcer
2. volvulus
3. polyp
4. gastroesophageal reflux disease
5. adhesions
6. intussusception
7. hemorrhoids

Exercise 15

Spelling Exercise

Exercise 16

Pronunciation Exercise

Exercise 17

1. WR S
gastr/ectomy
excision of the stomach

2. WR CV WR CV S
esophag/o/gastr/o/plasty
CF CF
surgical repair of the esophagus and the stomach

3. WR S
diverticul/ectomy
excision of a diverticulum

4. WR S
antr/ectomy
excision of the antrum

5. WR CV S
palat/o/plasty
CF
surgical repair of the palate

6. WR S
uvul/ectomy
excision of the uvula

7. WR CV WR CV S
gastr/o/jejun/o/stomy
CF CF
creation of an artificial opening between the stomach and the jejunum

8. WR CV WR S
chol/e/cyst/ectomy
CF
excision of the gallbladder

9. WR S
col/ectomy
excision of the colon

10. WR CV S
col/o/stomy
CF
creation of an artificial opening into the colon

11. WR CV S
pylor/o/plasty
CF
surgical repair of the pylorus

12. WR CV S
an/o/plasty
CF
surgical repair of the anus

13. WR S
append/ectomy
excision of the appendix

14. WR CV S
cheil/o/plasty
CF
surgical repair of the lip

15. WR S
gingiv/ectomy
surgical removal of gum (tissue)

16. WR CV S
lapar/o/tomy
CF
incision into the abdominal cavity

17. WR CV S
ile/o/stomy
CF
creation of an artificial opening into the ileum

18. WR CV S
gastr/o/stomy
CF
creation of an artificial opening into the stomach

19. WR CV S
herni/o/rrhaphy
CF
suturing of a hernia

20. WR CV S
gloss/o/rrhaphy
CF
suturing of the tongue

21. WR CV WR CV S
choledoch/o/lith/o/tomy
CF CF
incision into the common bile duct to remove a stone

22. P WR S
hemi/col/ectomy
excision of half of the colon

23. WR S
polyp/ectomy
excision of a polyp

24. WR CV S
enter/o/rrhaphy
CF
suturing of the intestine

25. WR CV S
abdomin/o/plasty
CF
surgical repair of the abdomen

26. WR CV WR CV S
pylor/o/my/o/tomy
CF CF
incision into the pylorus muscle

27. WR CV WR CV WR CV S
uvul/o/palat/o/pharyng/o/plasty
CF CF CF
surgical repair of the uvula, palate, and pharynx

28. WR CV S
gastr/o/plasty
CF
surgical repair of the stomach

29. WR CV S
abdomin/o/centesis
CF
surgical puncture to aspirate fluid from the abdominal cavity

Exercise 18

1. append/ectomy
2. gloss/o/rrhaphy
3. esophag/o/gastr/o/plasty
4. diverticul/ectomy
5. ile/o/stomy
6. gingiv/ectomy
7. lapar/o/tomy
8. an/o/plasty
9. antr/ectomy
10. chol/e/cyst/ectomy
11. col/ectomy
12. col/o/stomy
13. gastr/ectomy
14. gastr/o/stomy
15. gastr/o/jejun/o/stomy
16. uvul/ectomy
17. palat/o/plasty
18. pylor/o/plasty
19. herni/o/rrhaphy
20. cheil/o/plasty
21. hemi/col/ectomy
22. choledoch/o/lith/o/tomy
23. polyp/ectomy
24. enter/o/rrhaphy
25. abdomin/o/plasty
26. pylor/o/my/o/tomy
27. uvul/o/palat/o/pharyng/o/plasty
28. gastr/o/plasty
29. abdomin/o/centesis

Exercise 19

Spelling Exercise

Exercise 20

Pronunciation Exercise

Exercise 21

1. vagotomy
2. anastomosis
3. abdominoperitoneal resection
4. bariatric surgery
5. hemorrhoidectomy

Exercise 22

Spelling Exercise

Exercise 23

Pronunciation Exercise

Exercise 24

1. WR CV S
esophag/o/scopy
CF
visual examination of the esophagus

2. WR CV S
gastr/o/scope
CF
instrument used for visual examination of the stomach

3. WR CV S
gastr/o/scopy
CF
visual examination of the stomach

4. WR CV S
proct/o/scope
CF
instrument used for visual examination of the rectum

5. WR CV S
proct/o/scopy
CF
visual examination of the rectum

6. P S(WR)
(capsule) endo/scopy
procedure that uses a tiny wireless camera to take pictures of the digestive tract, especially the small intestine

7. WR CV S
sigmoid/o/scopy
CF
visual examination of the sigmoid colon

8. WR CV S
cholangi/o/gram
CF
radiographic image of bile ducts

9. WR CV WR CV WR CV S
esophag/o/gastr/o/duoden/o/scopy
CF CF CF
visual examination of the esophagus, stomach, and duodenum

10. WR CV S
colon/o/scope
CF
instrument used for visual examination of the colon

11. WR CV S
lapar/o/scope
CF
instrument used for visual examination of the abdominal cavity

12. WR CV S
colon/o/scopy
CF
visual examination of the colon

13. WR CV S
lapar/o/scopy
CF
visual examination of the abdominal cavity

14. WR CV S
(CT) colon/o/graphy
CF
radiographic imaging of the colon

15. WR CV S
esophag/o/gram
CF
radiographic image of the esophagus

16. WR CV S
cholangi/o/graphy
CF
radiographic imaging of the bile ducts

Exercise 25

1. (capsule) endo/scopy
2. gastr/o/scope
3. proct/o/scope
4. proct/o/scopy
5. esophag/o/scopy

6. sigmoid/o/scopy
7. cholangi/o/gram
8. gastr/o/scopy
9. lapar/o/scope
10. esophag/o/gastr/o/duoden/o/scopy
11. colon/o/scopy
12. lapar/o/scopy
13. colon/o/scope
14. (CT) colon/o/graphy
15. cholangi/o/graphy
16. esophag/o/gram

Exercise 26

Spelling Exercise

Exercise 27

Pronunciation Exercise

Exercise 28

1. d
2. f
3. a
4. b
5. e
6. g
7. c

Exercise 29

Spelling Exercise

Exercise 30

Pronunciation Exercise

Exercise 31

1. P S(WR)
   a/phagia
   without swallowing (inability to)
2. P S(WR)
   dys/pepsia
   difficult digestion
3. WR S
   an/al
   pertaining to the anus
4. P S(WR)
   dys/phagia
   difficult swallowing
5. WR CV S
   hepat/o/megaly
   CF
   enlargement of the liver
6. WR CV WR S
   ile/o/cec/al
   CF
   pertaining to the ileum and cecum
7. WR S
   or/al
   pertaining to the mouth
8. WR CV WR S
   or/o/gastr/ic
   CF
   pertaining to the mouth and stomach
9. WR CV S
   gastr/o/malacia
   CF
   softening of the stomach
10. WR S
    pancreat/ic
    pertaining to the pancreas
11. WR S
    peritone/al
    pertaining to the peritoneum
12. WR S
    steat/osis
    abnormal condition of fat
13. P WR S
    sub/lingu/al
    pertaining to under the tongue
14. WR CV S
    proct/o/logy
    CF
    study of the rectum
15. WR CV WR S
    nas/o/gastr/ic
    CF
    pertaining to the nose and stomach
16. WR S
    abdomin/al
    pertaining to the abdomen
17. WR CV WR CV S
    gastr/o/enter/o/logy
    CF CF
    study of the stomach and intestines
18. WR CV WR CV S
    gastr/o/enter/o/logist
    CF CF
    physician who studies and treats diseases of the stomach and intestines
19. WR CV WR S
    col/o/rect/al
    CF
    pertaining to the colon and rectum
20. WR S
    rect/al
    pertaining to the rectum
21. WR CV S
    steat/o/rrhea
    CF
    discharge of fat
22. WR S
    stomat/itis
    inflammation of the mouth (mucous membrane)
23. WR CV S
    enter/o/pathy
    CF
    disease of the intestine
24. WR S
    gastr/ic
    pertaining to the stomach
25. WR S
    duoden/al
    pertaining to the duodenum
26. WR S
    esophag/eal
    pertaining to the esophagus
27. WR S
    celi/ac
    pertaining to the abdomen

Exercise 32

1. hepat/o/megaly
2. a/phagia
3. sub/lingu/al
4. nas/o/gastr/ic
5. or/o/gastr/ic
6. an/al
7. peritone/al
8. abdomin/al, celi/ac
9. dys/phagia
10. ile/o/cec/al
11. gastr/o/malacia
12. dys/pepsia
13. pancreat/ic
14. proct/o/logy
15. steat/o/rrhea
16. or/al
17. gastr/o/enter/o/logist
18. gastr/o/enter/o/logy
19. col/o/rect/al
20. rect/al
21. steat/osis
22. esophag/eal
23. gastr/ic
24. duoden/al
25. enter/o/pathy
26. stomat/itis

Exercise 33

Spelling Exercise

Exercise 34

Pronunciation Exercise

Exercise 35

1. m
2. e
3. f
4. c
5. l
6. i
7. k
8. a
9. d
10. h
11. b
12. j
13. g
14. o
15. q
16. n
17. p

Exercise 36

1. abnormal collection of fluid in the peritoneal cavity
2. process of feeding a person through a nasogastric tube
3. washing out of the stomach

4. waste from the gastrointestinal tract expelled through the rectum
5. urge to vomit
6. disorder that involves inflammation of the intestine
7. frequent discharge of liquid stool
8. gas expelled through the anus
9. abnormal backward flow
10. vomiting of blood
11. involuntary wavelike contractions that propel food along the gastrointestinal tract
12. black, tarry stools that contain digested blood
13. surgical opening between an organ and the surface of the body
14. passage of visibly bloody feces
15. expelling matter from the stomach through the mouth
16. impaired digestion or intestinal absorption
17. to examine by hand

Exercise 37

Spelling Exercise

Exercise 38

1. UGI
2. *H. pylori*
3. N&V
4. ERCP
5. GI
6. UPPP
7. GERD
8. UC
9. BE
10. IBS
11. EGD
12. PEG
13. EUS
14. APR
15. FOBT

Exercise 39

A. felt sick to her stomach, throwing up, difficult to eat, stomach doctor
B. Answers will vary and may include nausea, emesis, dysphagia, and gastroenterologist, along with their respective definitions.
C. Esophagogastroduodenoscopy (EGD), gastroscope, gastric, *H. pylori*, peptic ulcer
D. Answers will vary and may include esophagogastroduodenoscopy (EGD), gastroscope, gastric, *Helicobacter pylori* antibodies test, peptic ulcer, along with their respective definitions.

Exercise 40

A. 1. hematochezia
   2. diarrhea
   3. nausea
   4. emesis
   5. gastroesophageal reflux disease (GERD)
   6. *Helicobacter pylori*
   7. peptic ulcer
   8. Crohn disease
   9. ulcerative colitis
   10. colorectal
   11. esophagitis
   12. abdominal
   13. ascites
   14. hepatomegaly
   15. hemorrhoids
   16. colonoscopy

B. 1. d
   2. b
   3. a
   4. d

C. Online Exercise

Exercise 41

Pronunciation Exercise

Exercise 42

1. a
2. b
3. a
4. a
5. c
6. a
7. c
8. a
9. b
10. c
11. c
12. a
13. a
14. b
15. c
16. a
17. c
18. b
19. b
20. c

ANSWERS TO CHAPTER 12 EXERCISES

Exercise Figure A

blephar/itis

Exercise Figure B

blephar/o/ptosis

Exercise Figure C

dacry/o/cyst/itis

Exercise Figure D

1. ophthalm/o/scopy
2. ophthalm/o/scope

Exercise 1

Pronunciation Exercise

Exercise 2

1. eye: ocul/o, ophthalm/o
2. eyelid: blephar/o
3. tear(s): dacry/o, lacrim/o
4. pupil: cor/o, core/o, pupill/o
5. sclera: scler/o
6. iris: ir/o, irid/o
7. vision: opt/o
8. conjunctiva: conjunctiv/o
9. cornea: corne/o, kerat/o
10. lens: phac/o, phak/o
11. retina: retin/o

Exercise 3

1. e, sclera
2. a, pupil
3. i, cornea
4. h, conjunctiva
5. f, tear(s)
6. g, retina
7. b, lens
8. c, eye
9. d, iris
10. a, pupil
11. i, cornea
12. c, eye
13. f, tear(s)
14. eyelid
15. vision

Exercise 4

1. tension, pressure
2. light
3. cold
4. two, double
5. equal
6. bladder, sac

Exercise 5

1. cry/o
2. ton/o
3. cyst/o
4. dipl/o
5. phot/o
6. is/o

Exercise 6

A. 1. vision (condition)
   2. two
   3. paralysis
   4. abnormal fear of or aversion to specific things
   5. two

B. 1. -plegia
   2. a. bi-
      b. bin-
   3. -phobia
   4. -opia

Exercise 7

Pronunciation Exercise

Exercise 8

1. WR S
   scler/itis
   inflammation of the sclera
2. WR S
   ophthalm/algia
   pain in the eye
3. WR CV S
   blephar/o/ptosis
   CF
   drooping of the eyelid
4. WR S
   dipl/opia
   double vision
5. WR S
   conjunctiv/itis
   inflammation of the conjunctiva
6. WR CV WR S
   leuk/o/cor/ia
   CF
   condition of white pupil
7. WR CV S
   irid/o/plegia
   CF
   paralysis of the iris
8. WR CV S
   scler/o/malacia
   CF
   softening of the sclera
9. WR CV S
   phot/o/phobia
   CF
   abnormal fear of (sensitivity to) light
10. WR S
    blephar/itis
    inflammation of the eyelid
11. WR CV WR S
    ocul/o/myc/osis
    CF
    abnormal condition of the eye caused by a fungus
12. WR CV WR S
    dacry/o/cyst/itis
    CF
    inflammation of the tear (lacrimal) sac
13. P WR S
    end/ophthalm/itis
    inflammation within the eye
14. WR S
    ir/itis
    inflammation of the iris
15. WR CV WR S
    retin/o/blast/oma
    CF
    tumor arising from a developing retinal cell
16. WR S
    kerat/itis
    inflammation of the cornea
17. WR CV S
    ophthalm/o/plegia
    CF
    paralysis of the eye (muscles)
18. WR CV S
    retin/o/pathy
    CF
    disease of the retina
19. WR WR S
    xer/ophthalm/ia
    condition of dry eye
20. WR CV S
    kerat/o/malacia
    CF
    softening of the cornea
21. WR CV S
    phac/o/malacia
    CF
    softening of the lens
22. P WR S
    a/phak/ia
    condition of without a lens

Exercise 9

1. conjunctiv/itis
2. ocul/o/myc/osis
3. ophthalm/algia
4. dipl/opia
5. blephar/itis
6. leuk/o/cor/ia
7. irid/o/plegia
8. blephar/o/ptosis
9. ir/itis
10. retin/o/blast/oma
11. scler/o/malacia
12. dacry/o/cyst/itis
13. scler/itis
14. phot/o/phobia
15. kerat/itis
16. retin/o/pathy
17. end/ophthalm/itis
18. ophthalm/o/plegia
19. xer/ophthalm/ia
20. kerat/o/malacia
21. a/phak/ia
22. phac/o/malacia

Exercise 10

Spelling Exercise

Exercise 11

Pronunciation Exercise

Exercise 12

1. myopia
2. presbyopia
3. anisometropia
4. astigmatism
5. nystagmus
6. glaucoma
7. hyperopia
8. retinitis pigmentosa
9. nyctalopia
10. amblyopia

Exercise 13

1. drusen
2. macular degeneration
3. pterygium
4. pinguecula
5. chalazion
6. sty
7. cataract
8. hyphema
9. strabismus
10. retinal detachment

Exercise 14

Spelling Exercise

Exercise 15

Pronunciation Exercise

Exercise 16

1. WR CV S
   kerat/o/plasty
   CF
   surgical repair of the cornea
2. WR CV S
   scler/o/tomy
   CF
   incision into the sclera
3. WR CV WR CV S
   dacry/o/cyst/o/tomy
   CF CF
   incision into the tear (lacrimal) sac
4. WR CV WR CV S
   cry/o/retin/o/pexy
   CF CF
   surgical fixation of the retina by using extreme cold
5. WR CV S
   blephar/o/plasty
   CF
   surgical repair of the eyelid
6. WR S
   irid/ectomy
   excision (part of) of the iris
7. WR CV WR CV WR CV S
   dacry/o/cyst/o/rhin/o/stomy
   CF CF CF
   creation of an artificial opening between the tear (lacrimal) sac and the nose
8. WR CV S
   irid/o/tomy
   CF
   incision into the iris

Exercise 17

1. dacry/o/cyst/o/rhin/o/stomy
2. irid/ectomy
3. kerat/o/plasty
4. scler/o/tomy
5. irid/o/tomy
6. blephar/o/plasty
7. cry/o/retin/o/pexy
8. dacry/o/cyst/o/tomy

Exercise 18

Spelling Exercise

Exercise 19

Pronunciation Exercise

Exercise 20

1. retinal photocoagulation
2. enucleation
3. phacoemulsification
4. LASIK
5. trabeculectomy
6. scleral buckling
7. vitrectomy
8. photorefractive keratectomy

Exercise 21

1. e
2. f
3. b
4. a
5. d
6. h
7. g
8. c

Exercise 22

Spelling Exercise

Exercise 23

Pronunciation Exercise

Exercise 24

1. WR CV S
pupill/o/scope
CF
instrument used for visual examination of the pupil

2. WR CV S
opt/o/metry
CF
measurement of vision

3. WR CV S
ophthalm/o/scope
CF
instrument used for visual examination of the eye

4. WR CV S
ton/o/metry
CF
measurement of pressure (within the eye)

5. WR CV S
pupill/o/meter
CF
instrument used to measure the pupil (diameter)

6. WR CV S
ton/o/meter
CF
instrument used to measure pressure (within the eye)

7. WR CV S
kerat/o/meter
CF
instrument used to measure (the curvature of) the cornea

8. WR CV S
ophthalm/o/scopy
CF
visual examination of the eye

9. WR CV S
(fluorescein) angi/o/graphy
CF
radiographic imaging of the blood vessels (of the eye with fluorescing dye)

10. WR CV S
retin/o/scopy
CF
visual examination of the retina

Exercise 25

1. ton/o/metry
2. pupill/o/meter
3. kerat/o/meter
4. opt/o/metry
5. ophthalm/o/scope
6. ton/o/meter
7. pupill/o/scope
8. ophthalm/o/scopy
9. fluorescein angi/o/graphy
10. retin/o/scopy

Exercise 26

Spelling Exercise

Exercise 27

Pronunciation Exercise

Exercise 28

1. WR CV S
ophthalm/o/logy
CF
study of the eye

2. P WR S
bin/ocul/ar
pertaining to two or both eyes

3. WR S
lacrim/al
pertaining to tears

4. WR S
pupill/ary
pertaining to the pupil

5. WR CV S
ophthalm/o/logist
CF
physician who studies and treats diseases of the eye

6. WR S
corne/al
pertaining to the cornea

7. WR S
ophthalm/ic
pertaining to the eye

8. WR CV WR S
nas/o/lacrim/al
CF
pertaining to the nose and tear (ducts)

9. WR S
opt/ic
pertaining to vision

10. P WR S
intra/ocul/ar
pertaining to within the eye

11. WR S
retin/al
pertaining to the retina

12. WR CV S
ophthalm/o/pathy
CF
disease of the eye

13. WRCVWR S
is/o/cor/ia
CF
condition of equal pupil (size)

14. P WRCVWR S
an/is/o/cor/ia
CF
condition of absence of equal pupil (size)

15. WR CV WR S
pseud/o/phak/ia
CF
condition of false lens

Exercise 29

1. ophthalm/o/logy
2. bin/ocul/ar
3. retin/al
4. intra/ocul/ar
5. ophthalm/o/logist
6. lacrim/al
7. opt/ic
8. ophthalm/ic
9. corne/al
10. nas/o/lacrim/al
11. ophthalm/o/pathy
12. pupill/ary

13. pseud/o/phak/ia
14. is/o/cor/ia
15. an/is/o/cor/ia

Exercise 30

Spelling Exercise

Exercise 31

Pronunciation Exercise

Exercise 32

1. health professional who diagnoses, treats, and manages diseases and disorders of the eyes and visual processing system
2. agent that dilates the pupil
3. sharpness of vision
4. agent that constricts the pupil
5. specialist who fills prescriptions for lenses
6. normal refractive condition of the eye
7. artificial lens implanted within the eye

Exercise 33

1. mydriatic
2. miotic
3. optometrist
4. visual acuity
5. optician
6. emmetropia
7. intraocular lens

Exercise 34

Spelling Exercise

Exercise 35

1. visual acuity
2. astigmatism
3. intraocular pressure
4. emmetropia
5. ophthalmology
6. age-related macular degeneration
7. phacoemulsification
8. intraocular lens
9. photorefractive keratectomy
10. laser-assisted in situ keratomileusis

Exercise 36

A. one of his eyes seemed to move more slowly and to look in a different direction; white part of the same eye seemed to be irritated and looked red and inflamed; pupil looked white; eye physician

B. Answers will vary and may include amblyopia, strabismus, scleritis, leukocoria, and ophthalmologist along with their respective definitions.

C. ophthalmologist; leukocoria; strabismus; amblyopia; scleritis; ophthalmoscopy; leukocoria; visual acuity; retinal; retinoblastoma

D. Answers will vary and may include ophthalmologist, leukocoria, strabismus, amblyopia, scleritis, ophthalmoscopy, visual acuity, retinal, and retinoblastoma along with their respective definitions.

Exercise 37

A. 1. ophthalmology
   2. glaucoma
   3. pterygium
   4. blepharoptosis
   5. astigmatism
   6. presbyopia
   7. retinopathy
   8. cataract

B. 1. b
   2. d
   3. b
   4. c

C. Online Exercise

Exercise 38

Pronunciation Exercise

Exercise 39

1. b
2. a
3. b
4. c
5. a
6. a
7. b
8. a
9. c
10. c
11. b
12. a
13. b
14. a
15. c
16. b

ANSWERS TO CHAPTER 13 EXERCISES

Exercise Figure A

myring/o/tomy

Exercise Figure B

ot/o/scopy, ot/o/scope

Exercise Figure C

tympan/o/meter

Exercise 1

Pronunciation Exercise

Exercise 2

A. 1. ear: aur/i, ot/o
   2. hearing: audi/o
   3. middle ear: tympan/o
   4. stapes: staped/o
   5. tympanic membrane: myring/o
   6. mastoid bone: mastoid/o

B. 1. labyrinth: labyrinth/o
   2. cochlea: cochle/o
   3. vestibule: vestibul/o

Exercise 3

1. g, stapes
2. d, vestibule
3. a, ear
4. f, cochlea
5. e, labyrinth
6. b, tympanic membrane (eardrum)
7. h, middle ear
8. a, ear
9. c, mastoid bone
10. hearing

Exercise 4

Pronunciation Exercise

Exercise 5

1. WR CV WR S
   ot/o/myc/osis
   CF
   abnormal condition of fungus in the ear
2. WR CV WR S
   ot/o/mastoid/itis
   CF
   inflammation of the ear and the mastoid bone
3. WR S
   ot/algia
   pain in the ear
4. WR S
   labyrinth/itis
   inflammation of the labyrinth
5. WR S
   myring/itis
   inflammation of the tympanic membrane
6. WR CV S
   ot/o/sclerosis
   CF
   hardening of the ear (stapes)
7. WR S
   mastoid/itis
   inflammation of the mastoid bone
8. WR CV WR CV S
   ot/o/py/o/rrhea
   CF CF
   discharge of pus from the ear
9. WR CV S
   ot/o/rrhea
   CF
   discharge from the ear

Exercise 6
1. myring/itis
2. ot/o/py/o/rrhea
3. mastoid/itis
4. ot/algia
5. ot/o/sclerosis
6. ot/o/myc/osis
7. ot/o/mastoid/itis
8. labyrinth/itis
9. ot/o/rrhea

Exercise 7
Spelling Exercise

Exercise 8
Pronunciation Exercise

Exercise 9
A. 1. vertigo; tinnitus
2. Ménière
3. presbycusis

B. 1. otitis externa
2. otitis media
3. cholesteatoma
4. acoustic neuroma

Exercise 10
1. d
2. e
3. b
4. f
5. c
6. a
7. g
8. h

Exercise 11
Spelling Exercise

Exercise 12
Pronunciation Exercise

Exercise 13
1. WR S
mastoid/ectomy
excision of the mastoid bone
2. WR CV S
myring/o/tomy
CF
incision into the tympanic membrane
3. WR S
labyrinth/ectomy
excision of the labyrinth
4. WR CV S
mastoid/o/tomy
CF
incision into the mastoid bone
5. WR CV S
tympan/o/plasty
CF
surgical repair of the middle ear
6. WR CV S
myring/o/plasty
CF
surgical repair of the tympanic membrane
7. WR S
staped/ectomy
excision of the stapes
8. WR S
cochle/ar (implant)
pertaining to the cochlea implant

Exercise 14
1. mastoid/o/tomy
2. labyrinth/ectomy
3. tympan/o/plasty
4. mastoid/ectomy
5. myring/o/tomy
6. myring/o/plasty
7. staped/ectomy
8. cochle/ar implant

Exercise 15
Spelling Exercise

Exercise 16
Pronunciation Exercise

Exercise 17
1. WR CV S
ot/o/scope
CF
instrument used for visual examination of the ear
2. WR CV S
audi/o/metry
CF
measurement of hearing
3. WR CV S
audi/o/gram
CF
(graphic) record of hearing
4. WR CV S
ot/o/scopy
CF
visual examination of the ear
5. WR CV S
audi/o/meter
CF
instrument used to measure hearing
6. WR CV S
tympan/o/metry
CF
measurement of middle ear (function)
7. WR CV S
tympan/o/meter
CF
instrument used to measure middle ear (function)
8. WR CV WR CV S
electr/o/cochle/o/graphy
CF CF
process of recording the electrical activity in the cochlea

Exercise 18
1. tympan/o/metry
2. audi/o/meter
3. ot/o/scopy
4. audi/o/gram
5. ot/o/scope
6. audi/o/metry
7. tympan/o/meter
8. electr/o/cochle/o/graphy

Exercise 19
Spelling Exercise

Exercise 20
Pronunciation Exercise

Exercise 21
1. WR CV S
ot/o/logy
CF
study of the ear
2. WR CV S
audi/o/logist
CF
one who studies and specializes in hearing
3. WR CV WR CV S
ot/o/laryng/o/logist
CF CF
physician who studies and treats diseases of the ear, (nose), and larynx (throat)
4. WR CV S
audi/o/logy
CF
study of hearing
5. WR CV S
ot/o/logist
CF
physician who studies and treats diseases of the ear
6. WR S
aur/al
pertaining to the ear
7. WR S
cochle/ar
pertaining to the cochlea
8. WR S
vestibul/ar
pertaining to the vestibule
9. WR CV WR S
vestibul/o/cochle/ar
CF
pertaining to the vestibule and the cochlea

Exercise 22
1. audi/o/logy
2. ot/o/laryng/o/logist
3. ot/o/logy
4. audi/o/logist

5. ot/o/logist
6. aur/al
7. vestibul/o/cochle/ar
8. vestibul/ar
9. cochle/ar

Exercise 23

Spelling Exercise

Exercise 24

1. ears, nose, throat; otolaryngologist
2. hard of hearing
3. otitis media
4. acute otitis media

Exercise 25

A. middle ear infections (inflammation); ear as if it is painful; pus-like liquid coming out of her left ear; redness and swelling on her skull behind Marisol's earlobe; ear, nose, and throat physician

B. Answers will vary and may include otitis media, otalgia, otopyorrhea, mastoiditis, and otolaryngologist along with their respective definitions.

C. mastoiditis, otitis media, otalgia, otopyorrhea, otoscopy, otitis externa, tympanometry, mastoiditis, myringotomies, and mastoidectomy

D. Answers will vary and may include mastoiditis, otitis media, otalgia, otopyorrhea, otoscopy, otitis externa, tympanometry, mastoiditis, myringotomies, and mastoidectomy along with their respective definitions.

Exercise 26

A. 1. ENT
   2. tinnitus
   3. vertigo
   4. otoscopy
   5. otitis media
   6. presbycusis
   7. audiologist
   8. audiometry

B. 1. a
   2. b
   3. d

C. Online Exercise

Exercise 27

Pronunciation Exercise

Exercise 28

1. c
2. a
3. b
4. a
5. c
6. a
7. b
8. a
9. c
10. a
11. c
12. a
13. c
14. a

ANSWERS TO CHAPTER 14 EXERCISES

Exercise Figure A

1. lord/osis
2. kyph/osis
3. scoli/osis

Exercise Figure B

arthr/o/scopy

Exercise Figure C

electr/o/my/o/gram

Exercise 1

Pronunciation Exercise

Exercise 2

1. mandible: mandibul/o
2. sternum: stern/o
3. phalanges: phalang/o
4. patella: patell/o
5. tarsals: tars/o
6. phalanges: phalang/o
7. cranium: crani/o
8. maxilla: maxill/o
9. clavicle: clavic/o, clavicul/o
10. ribs: cost/o
11. lumbar: lumb/o
12. femur: femor/o
13. fibula: fibul/o
14. tibia: tibi/o

Exercise 3

1. vertebra: rachi/o, spondyl/o, vertebr/o
2. pelvis: pelv/i
3. scapula: scapul/o
4. humerus: humer/o
5. ulna: uln/o
6. radius: radi/o
7. carpals: carp/o
8. ilium: ili/o
9. sacrum: sacr/o
10. pubis: pub/o
11. ischium: ischi/o

Exercise 4

1. f: vertebra, spine, vertebral column
2. d: patella (kneecap)
3. a: maxilla
4. b: phalanx
5. c: carpals (wrist)
6. g: clavicle (collarbone)
7. e: humerus (upper arm bone)

Exercise 5

1. d: loin, lumbar spine
2. e: ischium
3. a: pubis
4. b: vertebra, spine, vertebral column
5. f: scapula (shoulder blade)
6. c: tarsals (ankle bones)
7. g: pelvis, pelvic bones, pelvic cavity

Exercise 6

1. c: mandible
2. g: sacrum
3. a: femur (upper leg bone)
4. f: clavicle (collarbone)
5. b: ilium
6. d: vertebra, spine, vertebral column
7. e: sternum (breastbone)

Exercise 7

1. rib: cost/o
2. radius: radi/o
3. tibia: tibi/o
4. fibula: fibul/o
5. ulna: uln/o
6. cranium: crani/o

Exercise 8

1. synovial membrane: synovi/o
2. joint: arthr/o
3. meniscus: menisc/o
4. tendon: ten/o, tend/o, tendin/o
5. cartilage: chondr/o
6. bursa: burs/o

Exercise 9

1. c: intervertebral disk
2. d: synovial, synovial membrane
3. e: aponeurosis
4. a: tendon
5. b: joint

Exercise 10

1. b: tendon
2. c: bursa
3. b: tendon
4. d: meniscus
5. a: cartilage

Exercise 11

1. muscle
2. stone
3. movement, motion
4. bone
5. lamina
6. bone marrow
7. hump
8. stiff, bent
9. (lateral) curved (spine)
10. muscle
11. bent forward
12. flesh, connective tissue

Exercise 12

1. a. my/o
   b. myos/o
2. petr/o
3. kinesi/o
4. oste/o
5. lamin/o
6. myel/o
7. kyph/o
8. ankyl/o
9. scoli/o
10. lord/o
11. sarc/o

Exercise 13

1. above
2. together, joined
3. between

Exercise 14

1. a. syn-
   b. sym-
2. inter-
3. supra-

Exercise 15

1. growth
2. surgical fixation, fusion
3. split, fissure
4. weakness
5. nourishment, development

Exercise 16

1. -physis
2. -asthenia
3. -desis
4. -schisis
5. -trophy

Exercise 17

Pronunciation Exercise

Exercise 18

1. WR S
   oste/itis
   inflammation of the bone
2. WR CV WR S
   oste/o/myel/itis
   CF
   inflammation of the bone and bone marrow
3. WR CV WR S
   oste/o/petr/osis
   CF
   abnormal condition of stonelike bones (very dense bones caused by defective resorption of bone)
4. WR CV S
   oste/o/malacia
   CF
   softening of bone
5. WR CV WR S
   oste/o/chondr/itis
   CF
   inflammation of the bone and cartilage
6. WR CV WR S
   oste/o/fibr/oma
   CF
   tumor of the bone and fibrous tissue
7. WR S
   arthr/itis
   inflammation of a joint
8. WR CV WR CV S
   rhabd/o/my/o/lysis
   CF CF
   dissolution of striated muscle
9. WR S
   myel/oma
   tumor of the bone marrow
10. WR S
    tendin/itis
    inflammation of a tendon
11. WR CV S
    oste/o/penia
    CF
    abnormal reduction of bone (mass)
12. WR S
    spondyl/osis
    abnormal condition of the vertebrae
13. WR S
    burs/itis
    inflammation of the bursa
14. WR WR S
    spondyl/arthr/itis
    inflammation of the vertebral joints
15. WR S
    ankyl/osis
    abnormal condition of stiffness
16. WR S
    kyph/osis
    abnormal condition of a hump in the thoracic spine
17. WR S
    scoli/osis
    abnormal condition of (lateral) curved (spine)
18. WR CV S
    crani/o/schisis
    CF
    fissure (split) of the cranium
19. WR S
    maxill/itis
    inflammation of the maxilla
20. WR S
    menisc/itis
    inflammation of the meniscus
21. WR S
    rachi/schisis
    fissure (split) of the vertebral column
22. WR S
    my/asthenia
    muscle weakness
23. WR CV S
    oste/o/sarcoma
    CF
    malignant tumor of the bone
24. WR CV S
    chondr/o/malacia
    CF
    softening of cartilage
25. WR CV S
    synovi/o/sarcoma
    CF
    malignant tumor of the synovial membrane
26. WR CV WR S
    ten/o/synov/itis
    CF
    inflammation of the tendon and synovial membrane
27. P WR S
    poly/myos/itis
    inflammation of many muscles
28. WR S
    disk/itis
    inflammation of an intervertebral disk
29. WR S
    lord/osis
    abnormal condition of bending forward (in the lumbar spine)
30. WR CV WR S
    oste/o/arthr/itis
    CF
    inflammation of bone and joint
31. WR CV WR S
    fibr/o/my/algia
    CF
    pain in the fibrous tissues and muscles
32. WR CV S
    sarc/o/penia
    CF
    abnormal reduction of connective tissue

Exercise 19

1. oste/o/chondr/itis
2. oste/o/fibr/oma
3. arthr/itis
4. rhabd/o/my/o/lysis
5. myel/oma
6. tendin/itis
7. spondyl/osis
8. oste/o/penia
9. burs/itis
10. spondyl/arthr/itis
11. ankyl/osis
12. kyph/osis
13. scoli/osis
14. crani/o/schisis
15. maxill/itis
16. menisc/itis
17. rachi/schisis
18. my/asthenia
19. oste/itis
20. oste/o/myel/itis
21. oste/o/petr/osis
22. oste/o/malacia
23. ten/o/synov/itis
24. synovi/o/sarcoma

25. oste/o/sarcoma
26. chondr/o/malacia
27. disk/itis
28. poly/myos/itis
29. lord/osis
30. oste/o/arthr/itis
31. fibr/o/my/algia
32. sarc/o/penia

Exercise 20

Spelling Exercise

Exercise 21

Pronunciation Exercise

Exercise 22

1. c
2. a
3. b
4. d

Exercise 23

1. herniated disk
2. rheumatoid arthritis
3. carpal tunnel syndrome
4. spondylolisthesis
5. gout
6. osteoporosis
7. fracture
8. Lyme disease
9. bunion
10. spinal stenosis
11. plantar fasciitis
12. Colles fracture

Exercise 24

Spelling Exercise

Exercise 25

Pronunciation Exercise

Exercise 26

1. WR CV S
oste/o/tomy
CF
incision into a bone

2. WR S
ost/ectomy
excision of bone

3. WR CV S
arthr/o/desis
CF
surgical fixation of a joint

4. WR CV S
arthr/o/plasty
CF
surgical repair of a joint

5. WR S
chondr/ectomy
excision of a cartilage

6. WR CV S
chondr/o/plasty
CF
surgical repair of a cartilage

7. WR CV S
my/o/rrhaphy
CF
suturing of a muscle

8. WR CV WR CV S
ten/o/my/o/plasty
CF CF
surgical repair of the tendon and muscle

9. WR CV S
ten/o/rrhaphy
CF
suturing of a tendon

10. WR S
cost/ectomy
excision of a rib

11. WR S
patell/ectomy
excision of a patella

12. WR CV S
aponeur/o/rrhaphy
CF
suturing of an aponeurosis

13. WR S
carp/ectomy
excision of a carpal bone

14. WR S
phalang/ectomy
excision of a finger or toe bone

15. WR S
menisc/ectomy
excision of a meniscus

16. WR CV P S
spondyl/o/syn/desis
CF
fusing together of the vertebrae

17. WR S
lamin/ectomy
excision of a lamina

18. WR S
burs/ectomy
excision of a bursa

19. WR CV S
crani/o/tomy
CF
incision into the cranium

20. WR CV S
crani/o/plasty
CF
surgical repair of the skull

21. WR S
maxill/ectomy
excision of the maxilla

22. WR CV S
rachi/o/tomy
CF
incision into the vertebral column

23. WR S
tars/ectomy
excision of (one or more) tarsal bones

24. WR S
synov/ectomy
excision of the synovial membrane

25. WR S
disk/ectomy
excision of an intervertebral disk

26. WR CV S
vertebr/o/plasty
CF
surgical repair of a vertebra

27. WR CV S
arthr/o/centesis
CF
surgical puncture to aspirate fluid from a joint

Exercise 27

1. oste/o/tomy
2. ost/ectomy
3. arthr/o/desis
4. arthr/o/plasty
5. chondr/ectomy
6. chondr/o/plasty
7. my/o/rrhaphy
8. ten/o/my/o/plasty
9. ten/o/rrhaphy
10. cost/ectomy
11. patell/ectomy
12. aponeur/o/rrhaphy
13. carp/ectomy
14. phalang/ectomy
15. menisc/ectomy
16. spondyl/o/syn/desis
17. lamin/ectomy
18. burs/ectomy
19. crani/o/tomy
20. crani/o/plasty
21. maxill/ectomy
22. rachi/o/tomy
23. tars/ectomy
24. synov/ectomy
25. disk/ectomy
26. vertebr/o/plasty
27. arthr/o/centesis

Exercise 28

Spelling Exercise

Exercise 29

Pronunciation Exercise

Exercise 30

1. WR CV WR CV S
electr/o/my/o/gram
CF CF
record of the electrical activity in a muscle

2. WR CV S
arthr/o/graphy
CF
radiographic imaging of a joint

3. WR CV S
arthr/o/scopy
CF
visual examination of a joint

Exercise 31

1. arthr/o/graphy
2. arthr/o/scopy
3. electr/o/my/o/gram

Exercise 32

Spelling Exercise

Exercise 33

Pronunciation Exercise

Exercise 34

1. P S(WR)
sym/physis
growing together
2. WR S
femor/al
pertaining to the femur
3. WR S
humer/al
pertaining to the humerus
4. P WR S
inter/vertebr/al
pertaining to between the vertebrae
5. P WR S
hyper/kinesi/a
excessive movement (hyperactivity)
6. P WR S
dys/kinesi/a
difficult movement
7. P WR S
brady/kinesi/a
slow movement
8. P WR S
intra/crani/al
pertaining to within the cranium
9. WR CV WR S
stern/o/clavicul/ar
CF
pertaining to the sternum and clavicle
10. WR CV WR S
ili/o/femor/al
CF
pertaining to the ilium and femur
11. WR S
fibul/ar
pertaining to the fibula
12. P WR S
sub/maxill/ary
pertaining to below the maxilla
13. WR CV WR S
ischi/o/pub/ic
CF
pertaining to the ischium and pubis
14. P WR S
sub/mandibul/ar
pertaining to below the mandible
15. P WR S
supra/scapul/ar
pertaining to above the scapula
16. P WR S
sub/cost/al
pertaining to below the rib
17. WR CV WR S
vertebr/o/cost/al
CF
pertaining to the vertebrae and ribs
18. P WR S
sub/scapul/ar
pertaining to below the scapula
19. WR CV WR
oste/o/blast
CF
developing bone (cell)
20. WR CV S
oste/o/cyte
CF
bone cell
21. WR CV WR S
oste/o/necr/osis
CF
abnormal condition of bone death
22. WR S
stern/oid
resembling the sternum
23. WR S
arthr/algia
pain in the joint
24. WR S
carp/al
pertaining to the wrist
25. WR S
lumb/ar
pertaining to the loins
26. WR CV WR S
lumb/o/cost/al
CF
pertaining to the loins and ribs
27. WR CV WR S
lumb/o/sacr/al
CF
pertaining to the lumbar region (loin) and the sacrum
28. WR S
sacr/al
pertaining to the sacrum
29. WR S
pub/ic
pertaining to the pubis
30. P WR S
sub/stern/al
pertaining to under the sternum
31. P WR S
supra/patell/ar
pertaining to above the patella
32. P S(WR)
dys/trophy
abnormal development
33. P S(WR)
a/trophy
without development
34. P S(WR)
hyper/trophy
excessive development
35. P WR S
inter/cost/al
pertaining to between the ribs
36. WR S
crani/al
pertaining to the cranium
37. WR S
pelv/ic
pertaining to the pelvis
38. WR S
clavicul/ar
pertaining to the clavicle
39. WR S
tibi/al
pertaining to the tibia
40. WR S
radi/al
pertaining to the radius
41. WR CV WR S
uln/o/radi/al
CF
pertaining to the ulna and radius
42. WR CV WR S
cost/o/chondr/al
CF
pertaining to ribs and cartilage
43. WR S
my/algia
pain in muscle

Exercise 35

1. sym/physis
2. femor/al
3. humer/al
4. inter/vertebr/al
5. hyper/kinesi/a
6. dys/kinesi/a
7. brady/kinesi/a
8. intra/crani/al
9. stern/o/clavicul/ar
10. ili/o/femor/al
11. fibul/ar
12. sub/maxill/ary
13. ischi/o/pub/ic
14. sub/mandibul/ar
15. supra/scapul/ar
16. sub/cost/al
17. vertebr/o/cost/al
18. sub/scapul/ar

19. oste/o/blast
20. oste/o/cyte
21. oste/o/necr/osis
22. stern/oid
23. arthr/algia
24. carp/al
25. sacr/al
26. lumb/ar
27. pub/ic
28. lumb/o/sacr/al
29. lumb/o/cost/al
30. sub/stern/al
31. supra/patell/ar
32. dys/trophy
33. a/trophy
34. hyper/trophy
35. crani/al
36. inter/cost/al
37. pelv/ic
38. clavicul/ar
39. tibi/al
40. radi/al
41. uln/o/radi/al
42. cost/o/chondr/al
43. my/algia

Exercise 36
Spelling Exercise

Exercise 37
Pronunciation Exercise

Exercise 38

1. b	8. h
2. e	9. j
3. c	10. k
4. g	11. f
5. i	12. m
6. a	13. l
7. d	14. n

Exercise 39
1. specialist in chiropractic
2. system of treatment that consists of manipulation of the vertebral column
3. study and treatment of diseases and abnormalities of the musculoskeletal system
4. physician who specializes in the study and treatment of diseases and abnormalities of the musculoskeletal system
5. specialist in treating and diagnosing diseases and disorders of the foot
6. physician who specializes in osteopathy
7. system of medicine in which greater emphasis is on the relation between body organs and the musculoskeletal system
8. making and fitting of orthopedic appliances
9. artificial substitute for a missing body part
10. person who specializes in orthotics
11. crackling sensation heard or felt when two bones rub against each other or grating caused by rubbing together of dry surfaces
12. type of bone cell involved in absorption and removal of bone minerals
13. physician who specializes in the study and treatment of rheumatic diseases
14. study and treatment of rheumatic diseases

Exercise 40
Spelling Exercise

Exercise 41
Pronunciation Exercise

Exercise 42

1. h	6. a
2. d	7. g
3. i	8. f
4. e	9. b
5. c	

Exercise 43
Spelling Exercise

Exercise 44
1. cervical vertebrae; thoracic vertebrae; lumbar vertebrae
2. rheumatoid arthritis
3. osteoarthritis
4. myasthenia gravis
5. electromyogram
6. carpal tunnel syndrome
7. muscular dystrophy
8. herniated nucleus pulposus
9. total hip arthroplasty
10. Doctor of Osteopathy
11. total knee arthroplasty

Exercise 45
A. wrist bones, broken, musculoskeletal specialist, bones are not dense enough
B. Answers will vary and may include carpal, fracture, orthopedist, osteoporosis.
C. kyphosis, Colles fracture, fracture, osteoporosis, DEXA scan, radioulnar, carpal
D. Answers will vary and may include kyphosis, Colles fracture, fracture, osteoporosis, DEXA scan, radioulnar, and carpal, along with their respective definitions.

Exercise 46
A. 1. orthopedic
   2. arthroscopy
   3. arthritis
   4. medial
   5. suprapatellar
   6. chondromalacia
   7. pathology
B. 1. c
   2. b
C. Online Exercise

Exercise 47
Pronunciation Exercise

Exercise 48
1. epiphyses
2. phalanx
3. vertebrae
4. prosthesis
5. bursae

Exercise 49

1. b	11. a
2. c	12. c
3. a	13. b
4. b	14. a
5. c	15. b
6. b	16. c
7. c	17. b
8. b	18. c
9. a	19. a
10. c	20. c

ANSWERS TO CHAPTER 15 EXERCISES

Exercise Figure A
rhiz/o/tomy or radic/o/tomy

Exercise Figure B
CT myel/o/graphy

Exercise Figure C
1. hemi/plegia
2. paraplegia
3. quadr/i/plegia

Exercise 1
Pronunciation Exercise

Exercise 2
A. 1. brain: encephal/o
   2. spinal cord: myel/o

3. cerebrum: cerebr/o
4. cerebellum: cerebell/o
5. meninges: meningi/o, mening/o

B. 1. dura mater: dur/o
2. ganglion: gangli/o, ganglion/o
3. nerve root: radic/o, radicul/o, rhiz/o

C. 1. glia: gli/o
2. nerve: neur/o

Exercise 3

1. e, ganglion
2. d, dura mater
3. c, brain
4. a, cerebellum
5. f, meninges
6. b, nerve

Exercise 4

1. b, glia
2. d, ganglia
3. e, meninges
4. c, cerebrum
5. a, spinal cord

Exercise 5

1. radic/o, radicul/o, rhiz/o

Exercise 6

1. one, single
2. mind
3. four
4. mind
5. speech
6. sensation, sensitivity, feeling
7. gray matter

Exercise 7

1. quadr/i
2. mon/o
3. a. psych/o
b. ment/o
4. phas/o
5. poli/o
6. esthesi/o

Exercise 8

1. slight paralysis
2. treatment, specialty
3. seizure, attack
4. specialist, physician

Exercise 9

1. -paresis
2. -iatry
3. -ictal
4. -iatrist

Exercise 10

Pronunciation Exercise

Exercise 11

1. WR S
neur/itis
inflammation of a nerve

2. WR S
neur/algia
pain in a nerve

3. WR CV WR CV S
neur/o/arthr/o/pathy
CF CF
disease of nerves and joints

4. WR S
meningi/oma
tumor of the meninges

5. WR CV S
encephal/o/malacia
CF
softening of the brain

6. WR S
encephal/itis
inflammation of the brain

7. WR CV WR CV WR S
encephal/o/myel/o/radicul/itis
CF CF
inflammation of the brain, spinal cord, and nerve roots

8. WR S
mening/itis
inflammation of the meninges

9. WR CV S
mening/o/cele
CF
protrusion of the meninges

10. WR CV WR CV S
mening/o/myel/o/cele
CF CF
protrusion of the meninges and spinal cord

11. WR S
radicul/itis
inflammation of the nerve roots

12. WR S
cerebell/itis
inflammation of the cerebellum

13. WR S
gangli/itis
inflammation of a ganglion

14. WR S
dur/itis
inflammation of the dura mater

15. P WR S
poly/neur/itis
inflammation of many nerves

16. WR CV WR S
poli/o/myel/itis
CF
inflammation of the gray matter of the spinal cord

17. WR S WR S
cerebr/al thromb/osis
pertaining to the cerebrum, abnormal condition of a clot

18. P WR S WR S
sub/dur/al hemat/oma
pertaining to below the dura mater; tumor of blood

19. WR CV WR CV WR S
rhiz/o/mening/o/myel/itis
CF CF
inflammation of the nerve root, meninges, and spinal cord

20. WR CV WR CV S
mon/o/neur/o/pathy
CF CF
disease affecting a single nerve

21. WR CV S
neur/o/pathy
CF
disease of the nerves (peripheral)

22. WR CV S
radicul/o/pathy
CF
disease of the nerve roots

23. WR S
gli/oma
tumor composed of glia

24. WR CV WR S
gli/o/blast/oma
CF
tumor composed of developing glia

25. P WR CV S
poly/neur/o/pathy
CF
disease of many nerves

Exercise 12

1. neur/itis
2. neur/algia
3. neur/o/arthr/o/pathy
4. radicul/o/pathy
5. encephal/o/malacia
6. encephal/itis
7. encephal/o/myel/o/radicul/itis
8. mening/itis
9. mening/o/cele
10. mening/o/myel/o/cele
11. radicul/itis
12. cerebell/itis
13. gangli/itis
14. dur/itis
15. poly/neur/itis
16. poli/o/myel/itis
17. cerebr/al thromb/osis
18. sub/dur/al hemat/oma
19. rhiz/o/mening/o/myel/itis
20. meningi/oma
21. mon/o/neur/o/pathy
22. neur/o/pathy
23. gli/oma
24. gli/o/blast/oma
25. poly/neur/o/pathy

Exercise 13

Spelling Exercise

Exercise 14

Pronunciation Exercise

Exercise 15

A. 1. d
2. g
3. a
4. f
5. b
6. c
7. e

B. 1. transient ischemic attack
2. Bell palsy
3. sciatica
4. Alzheimer disease
5. shingles
6. cerebral aneurysm
7. intracerebral hemorrhage
8. cerebral embolism
9. subarachnoid hemorrhage
10. stroke

Exercise 16

Spelling Exercise

Exercise 17

Pronunciation Exercise

Exercise 18

1. WR CV S
radic/o/tomy
CF
incision into a nerve root
2. WR S
neur/ectomy
excision of a nerve
3. WR CV S
neur/o/rrhaphy
CF
suturing of a nerve
4. WR S
ganglion/ectomy
excision of a ganglion
5. WR CV S
neur/o/tomy
CF
incision into a nerve
6. WR CV S
neur/o/lysis
CF
loosening, separating a nerve (to release it from surrounding tissue)
7. WR CV S
neur/o/plasty
CF
surgical repair of a nerve
8. WR CV S
rhiz/o/tomy
CF
incision into a nerve root

Exercise 19

1. a. radic/o/tomy
b. rhiz/o/tomy
2. neur/ectomy
3. neur/o/rrhaphy
4. ganglion/ectomy
5. neur/o/tomy
6. neur/o/lysis
7. neur/o/plasty

Exercise 20

Spelling Exercise

Exercise 21

Pronunciation Exercise

Exercise 22

1. WR CV WR CV S
electr/o/encephal/o/gram
CF CF
record of the electrical activity of the brain
2. WR CV WR CV S
electr/o/encephal/o/graph
CF CF
instrument used to record the electrical activity of the brain
3. WR CV WR CV S
electr/o/encephal/o/graphy
CF CF
process of recording the electrical activity of the brain
4. WR CV S
CT myel/o/graphy
CF
process of recording (scan of) the spinal cord
5. WR S WR CV S
cerebr/al angi/o/graphy
CF
process of recording (scan of) the (blood) vessels of the cerebrum

Exercise 23

1. electr/o/encephal/o/gram
2. electr/o/encephal/o/graph
3. electr/o/encephal/o/graphy
4. CT myel/o/graphy
5. cerebr/al angi/o/graphy

Exercise 24

Spelling Exercise

Exercise 25

Pronunciation Exercise

Exercise 26

1. c
2. d
3. e
4. a
5. b

Exercise 27

1. evoked potential studies
2. positron emission tomography
3. computed tomography
4. magnetic resonance imaging
5. lumbar puncture

Exercise 28

Spelling Exercise

Exercise 29

Pronunciation Exercise

Exercise 30

1. P S(WR)
hemi/plegia
paralysis of half (left or right side of the body)
2. P WR S
par/esthesi/a
abnormal sensation
3. WR CV S
neur/o/logist
CF
physician who studies and treats diseases of the nervous system
4. WR CV S
neur/o/logy
CF
study of nerves (branch of medicine dealing with diseases of the nervous system)
5. WR S
neur/oid
resembling a nerve
6. WR CV S
quadr/i/plegia
CF
paralysis of four (limbs)
7. WR S
cerebr/al
pertaining to the cerebrum
8. WR CV S
mon/o/plegia
CF
paralysis of one (limb)
9. P WR S
a/phas/ia
condition of without speaking
10. P WR S
dys/phas/ia
condition of difficulty speaking
11. P S(WR)
hemi/paresis
slight paralysis of half (right or left side of the body)
12. P WR S
an/esthesi/a
without (loss of) feeling or sensation
13. P WR S
hyper/esthesi/a
excessive sensitivity (to stimuli)
14. P WR S
sub/dur/al
pertaining to below the dura mater
15. WR S
ceph/algia
pain in the head (headache)

16. WR CV WR S
crani/o/cerebr/al
CF
pertaining to the cranium and cerebrum
17. WR CV S
myel/o/malacia
CF
softening of the spinal cord
18. WR CV S
encephal/o/pathy
CF
disease of the brain
19. P S(WR)
post/ictal
(occurring) after a seizure or attack
20. P WR S
dys/esthesi/a
painful sensation
21. P S(WR)
inter/ictal
(occurring) between seizures or attacks
22. WR CV S
mon/o/paresis
CF
slight paralysis of one (limb)
23. P S(WR)
pre/ictal
(occurring) before a seizure or attack
24. P WR S
intra/cerebr/al
pertaining to within the cerebrum
25. WR CV S
gli/o/cyte
CF
glial cell
26. WR S
ment/al
pertaining to the mind

Exercise 31

1. hemi/paresis
2. an/esthesi/a
3. hyper/esthesi/a
4. sub/dur/al
5. ceph/algia
6. crani/o/cerebr/al
7. myel/o/malacia
8. encephal/o/pathy
9. hemi/plegia
10. neur/o/logist
11. neur/o/logy
12. neur/oid
13. quadr/i/plegia
14. cerebr/al
15. mon/o/plegia
16. a/phas/ia
17. dys/phas/ia
18. pre/ictal
19. mon/o/paresis
20. post/ictal
21. dys/esthesi/a
22. inter/ictal
23. intra/cerebr/al
24. gli/o/cyte
25. par/esthesi/a
26. ment/al

Exercise 32

Spelling Exercise

Exercise 33

Pronunciation Exercise

Exercise 34

1. concussion
2. unconsciousness
3. conscious
4. seizure
5. convulsion
6. shunt
7. paraplegia
8. coma
9. syncope
10. ataxia
11. gait
12. dysarthria
13. incoherent
14. disorientation
15. cognitive
16. afferent
17. efferent

Exercise 35

1. c
2. i
3. b
4. j
5. a
6. l
7. p
8. k
9. g
10. o
11. f
12. q
13. e
14. m
15. d
16. n
17. h

Exercise 36

Spelling Exercise

Exercise 37

Pronunciation Exercise

Exercise 38

1. WR CV WR S
psych/o/somat/ic
CF
pertaining to the mind and body
2. WR CV S
psych/o/pathy
CF
(any) disease of the mind
3. WR CV S
psych/o/logy
CF
study of the mind
4. WR S
psych/iatry
specialty of the mind (branch of medicine that deals with the treatment of mental disorders)
5. WR CV S
psych/o/logist
CF
specialist of the mind
6. WR CV S
psych/o/genic
CF
originating in the mind
7. WR S
psych/iatrist
physician who studies and treats disorders of the mind
8. WR S
psych/osis
abnormal condition of the mind

Exercise 39

1. psych/iatry
2. psych/osis
3. psych/o/logy
4. psych/o/genic
5. psych/iatrist
6. psych/o/logist
7. psych/o/somat/ic
8. psych/o/pathy

Exercise 40

Spelling Exercise

Exercise 41

Pronunciation Exercise

Exercise 42

1. i
2. m
3. b
4. c
5. j
6. a
7. g
8. d
9. h
10. f
11. e
12. n
13. l
14. k

Exercise 43

Spelling Exercise

Exercise 44

1. electroencephalogram, computed tomography, magnetic resonance imaging, positron emission tomography, evoked potential studies, lumbar puncture

2. Alzheimer disease, amyotrophic lateral sclerosis, cerebral palsy, multiple sclerosis, Parkinson disease
3. cerebrovascular accident, transient ischemic attack, subarachnoid hemorrhage
4. cerebrospinal fluid
5. obsessive-compulsive disorder, attention deficit/hyperactivity disorder
6. central nervous system, peripheral nervous system
7. posttraumatic stress disorder, chronic traumatic encephalopathy

Exercise 45

A. unable to speak, right arm was hanging limply by his side, left side of his face was also droopy, strokes
B. Answers will vary and may include aphasia, hemiplegia, Bell palsy, stroke or cerebrovascular accident, and their respective definitions.
C. aphasia, hemiplegia, dysphasia, hemiparesis, paresthesias, gait, CT, cerebral, subarachnoid hemorrhage, CVA
D. Answers will vary and may include aphasia, hemiplegia, dysphasia, hemiparesis, paresthesias, gait, CT, cerebral, subarachnoid hemorrhage, CVA

Exercise 46

A. 1. disorientation
2. cognitive
3. aphasia
4. conscious
5. neurology
6. magnetic resonance imaging
7. encephalitis
8. electroencephalogram
9. seizure
10. incoherent

B. 1. b
2. a

C. Online Exercise

Exercise 47

Pronunciation Exercise

Exercise 48

1. a
2. b
3. c
4. c
5. c
6. a
7. b
8. a
9. b
10. a
11. a
12. c
13. c
14. a
15. c
16. b
17. a
18. c

ANSWERS TO CHAPTER 16 EXERCISES

Exercise Figure A

acr/o/megaly

Exercise 1

Pronunciation Exercise

Exercise 2

1. parathyroid glands: parathyroid/o
2. adrenal glands: adren/o, adrenal/o
3. pituitary gland: pituitar/o
4. thyroid gland: thyr/o, thyroid/o
5. endocrine: endocrin/o

Exercise 3

cortex: cortic/o

Exercise 4

1. c, thyroid gland
2. d, adrenal glands
3. a, pituitary gland
4. e, cortex
5. b, parathyroid glands
6. d, adrenal glands
7. c, thyroid gland
8. endocrine

Exercise 5

1. thirst
2. potassium
3. calcium
4. extremities, height
5. sodium

Exercise 6

1. acr/o
2. calc/i
3. dips/o
4. kal/i
5. natr/o

Exercise 7

1. run, running

Exercise 8

1. -drome

Exercise 9

Pronunciation Exercise

Exercise 10

1. WR S
adrenal/itis
inflammation of the adrenal glands

2. P WR S
hypo/calc/emia
deficient calcium in the blood

3. P WR S
hyper/thyroid/ism
state of excessive thyroid gland activity

4. P WR S
hyper/kal/emia
excessive potassium in the blood

5. P WR S
hyper/glyc/emia
excessive sugar in the blood

6. WR CV S
adren/o/megaly
CF
enlargement of the adrenal glands

7. P WR S
hypo/thyroid/ism
state of deficient thyroid gland activity

8. P WR S
hypo/kal/emia
deficient potassium in the blood

9. WR S
parathyroid/oma
tumor of a parathyroid gland

10. WR CV S
acr/o/megaly
CF
enlargement of the extremities

11. P P WR S
pan/hypo/pituitar/ism
state of total deficient pituitary gland activity

12. P WR S
hypo/glyc/emia
deficient sugar in the blood

13. P WR S
hyper/calc/emia
excessive calcium in the blood

14. P WR S
hyper/pituitar/ism
state of excessive pituitary gland activity

15. P WR S
hypo/natr/emia
deficient sodium in the blood
16. P WR S
hyper/parathyroid/ism
state of excessive parathyroid gland activity
17. WR S
thyroid/itis
inflammation of the thyroid gland
18. P WR S
hypo/pituitar/ism
state of deficient pituitary gland activity

Exercise 11

1. adren/o/megaly
2. hypo/thyroid/ism
3. acr/o/megaly
4. hypo/glyc/emia
5. hyper/kal/emia
6. hypo/calc/emia
7. hyper/thyroid/ism
8. hypo/pituitar/ism
9. hyper/calc/emia
10. hyper/pituitar/ism
11. parathyroid/oma
12. hyper/glyc/emia
13. hypo/kal/emia
14. adrenal/itis
15. hypo/natr/emia
16. hyper/parathyroid/ism
17. thyroid/itis
18. pan/hypo/pituitar/ism

Exercise 12

Spelling Exercise

Exercise 13

Pronunciation Exercise

Exercise 14

1. c
2. e
3. b
4. d
5. f
6. a

Exercise 15

1. gigantism
2. Addison disease
3. congenital hypothyroidism
4. myxedema
5. Cushing syndrome
6. metabolic syndrome
7. goiter
8. Graves disease

Exercise 16

Spelling Exercise

Exercise 17

Pronunciation Exercise

Exercise 18

1. WR S
pancreat/ectomy
excision of the pancreas
2. WR S
adrenal/ectomy
excision of (one or both) adrenal glands
3. WR S
thyroid/ectomy
excision of the thyroid gland
4. WR S
parathyroid/ectomy
excision of (one or more) parathyroid glands

Exercise 19

1. thyroid/ectomy
2. adrenal/ectomy
3. parathyroid/ectomy
4. pancreat/ectomy

Exercise 20

Spelling Exercise

Exercise 21

Pronunciation Exercise

Exercise 22

1. b
2. a
3. g
4. d
5. f
6. h
7. e
8. c

Exercise 23

1. radioactive iodine uptake
2. fasting blood sugar
3. thyroid-stimulating hormone level
4. thyroxine level
5. sestamibi parathyroid scan
6. glycosylated hemoglobin
7. thyroid sonography
8. fine needle aspiration

Exercise 24

Spelling Exercise

Exercise 25

Pronunciation Exercise

Exercise 26

1. WR S
cortic/oid
resembling the cortex
2. P S(WR)
syn/drome
run together
3. WR CV S
adren/o/pathy
CF
disease of the adrenal glands
4. WR CV S
endocrin/o/logist
CF
physician who studies and treats diseases of the endocrine (system)
5. P WR S
poly/dips/ia
abnormal state of much thirst
6. P WR S
eu/glyc/emia
normal (level of) sugar in the blood
7. WR CV S
endocrin/o/pathy
CF
(any) disease of the endocrine (system)
8. WR CV WR CV P S
adren/o/cortic/o/hyper/plasia
CF CF
excessive development of the adrenal cortex
9. P WR S
eu/thyr/oid
resembling normal thyroid gland
10. WR S
cortic/al
pertaining to the cortex
11. WR CV S
endocrin/o/logy
CF
study of the endocrine (system)
12. WR S
glyc/emia
sugar in the blood

Exercise 27

1. endocrin/o/pathy
2. cortic/oid
3. syn/drome
4. adren/o/cortic/o/hyper/plasia
5. endocrin/o/logy
6. poly/dips/ia
7. adren/o/pathy
8. eu/glyc/emia
9. eu/thyr/oid
10. cortic/al
11. endocrin/o/logist
12. glyc/emia

Exercise 28

Spelling Exercise

Exercise 29

Pronunciation Exercise

Exercise 30

1. metabolism
2. hormone
3. isthmus
4. exophthalmos
5. incretins

Exercise 31

1. narrow strip of tissue connecting two larger parts in the body
2. total of all chemical processes that take place in living organisms
3. chemical substance secreted by an endocrine gland
4. abnormal protrusion of the eyeball
5. hormones produced by the gastrointestinal system that stimulate insulin release

Exercise 32

Spelling Exercise

Exercise 33

1. radioactive iodine uptake
2. fasting blood sugar
3. diabetes mellitus
4. diabetes insipidus
5. thyroxine level
6. glycosylated hemoglobin
7. thyroid-stimulating hormone
8. prolactin
9. luteinizing hormone
10. growth hormone
11. follicle-stimulating hormone
12. antidiuretic hormone
13. adrenocorticotropic hormone
14. diabetic ketoacidosis
15. fine needle aspiration
16. type 2 diabetes mellitus

Exercise 34

A. a lump in the front of her neck, eyes seem to stick out more, too much thyroid hormone, endocrine specialist

B. Answers will vary and may include goiter, exophthalmos, hyperthyroidism or thyrotoxicosis, endocrinologist, and their respective definitions.

C. endocrinopathy, hyperthyroidism, thyrotoxicosis, exophthalmos, Graves disease, thyroid sonography, TSH, T_4, radioactive iodine uptake, thyroidectomy, hypothyroidism

D. Answers will vary and may include endocrinopathy, hyperthyroidism, thyrotoxicosis, exophthalmos, Graves disease, thyroid sonography, TSH, T_4, radioactive iodine uptake, thyroidectomy, hypothyroidism, and their respective definitions.

Exercise 35

A.
1. polydipsia
2. diabetes mellitus
3. exophthalmos
4. fasting blood sugar
5. glycosylated hemoglobin
6. type 2 diabetes mellitus
7. hyperglycemia
8. hypoglycemia
9. endocrinology

B.
1. c
2. b
3. a

C. Online Exercise

Exercise 36

Pronunciation Exercise

Exercise 37

1. c
2. a
3. c
4. b
5. a
6. b
7. a
8. c
9. a
10. c
11. c
12. c
13. b
14. b
15. c

Appendix B

Evolve Resources

Evolve Resources for *Exploring Medical Language*, which are available free of charge, offer multiple ways to practice chapter content and extend learning. They can be used side by side with the textbook as you work through the exercises and as an exam preparation tool to review material. Evolve Resources provide the following:

Gradable Student Resources offer scored exercises and quizzes that may populate an electronic gradebook if your instructor elects to create one. Although there is some variation between chapters, generally, exercises and quizzes will be as follows:

Exercises
- Word Parts
- Terms Built from Word Parts
- Terms NOT Built from Word Parts
- Abbreviations

Quizzes
- Quiz 1: Disease and Disorder Terms
- Quiz 2: Surgical Terms
- Quiz 3: Diagnostic Terms
- Quiz 4: Complementary Terms

Practice Student Resources offer a variety of ways to practice chapter content:

From the Main Menu
- **A&P Booster** with tutorials
- **Flashcards** for word parts and abbreviations
- **Pronounce & Spell** corresponding with textbook exercises
- **Practice Quizzes**, multiple choice; results may be emailed to your instructor
- **Electronic Health Records**; modules with three related medical documents
- **Games**

Extra Content Tab
- **Career Videos**
- **Appendices**—Additional Word Parts, Health Care Delivery, Integrative Medicine, Behavioral Health, Clinical Research, Nutrition, Dental, and Health Information Technology

Mobile Resources may be accessed from portable devices:
- Word Part and Abbreviation Flashcards
- Practice Quizzes

Registering for Evolve Resources

The following is a general overview of how to register:
1. Go to the website at evolve.elsevier.com.
2. Type in *Exploring Medical Language* in the search box. If a search box does not appear on your screen, click on the Catalog tab near the top of the page.
3. Locate and click on the link for **Evolve Resources for Exploring Medical Language, 10th Edition**. You may need to scroll down. Look for a picture of the textbook cover next to the label **Resources**.
4. Click on the second button entitled **REGISTER FOR THIS NOW**. Registering for Evolve Resources is different from Enrolling in your instructor's course. Your instructor will give directions and provide a Course ID if it is offered for your class.
5. Click on **REDEEM/CHECKOUT**.
6. Log in or follow directions to create an account.

For assistance in registering for Evolve Resources, call **1-800-222-9570** or visit **evolvesupport.elsevier.com**.

7. Click to place a checkmark next to Registered User Agreement.

Accessing Gradable Student Resources Once Registered

1. Go to the website at evolve.elsevier.com and log in.
2. Click on **Evolve Resources for Exploring Medical Language, 10th Edition** (if the title does not appear, click on the tab entitled **My Evolve** near the top of the screen).
3. Click on **Gradable Student Resources** on the menu to the left of the screen.
4. Click on the chapter you are studying.
5. Click on Exercises or Quizzes.
6. Click on the specific exercise or quiz.
7. The Evolve Resources will open in a new window. Pop-up blockers may need to be removed. The browsers Google Chrome and FireFox best support the functionality of Evolve Resources.

Note: If your instructor has linked Gradable Student Resources to an electronic gradebook, your scores will automatically populate the gradebook. If your instructor has not linked to an electronic gradebook, using the Global Course available to all registered, your scores will be seen by you only.

Accessing Practice Student Resources Once Registered

1. Go to the website at evolve.elsevier.com and log in.
2. Click on **Evolve Resources for Exploring Medical Language, 10th Edition** (if the title does not appear, click on the tab entitled **My Evolve** near the top of the screen).
3. Click on **Practice Student Resources** on the menu to the left of the screen.
4. Click on **Student Resources.** The Evolve Resources will open in a new window. Pop-up blockers may need to be removed. The browsers Google Chrome and FireFox best support the functionality of Evolve Resources.

Accessing Mobile Resources

1. Go to the website at evolve.elsevier.com using your mobile device and log in.
2. Click on **Evolve Resources for Exploring Medical Language, 10th Edition** (if the title does not appear, click on the tab entitled **My Evolve** near the top of the screen).
3. Click on **Mobile Resources** in the menu on the left side of the screen.
4. Select the resource you would like to use, Flashcards or Practice Quizzes.

How to Find It

Once you have created an account, registered for Evolve Resources, and launched the program, access specific resources using the following steps:

A&P Booster With Tutorials

1. Click on Practice Student Resources on the menu to the left of the screen. Follow links to reach the main menu.
2. Select Chapter on pull-out tab to the left of the screen.
3. Click on the A&P Booster button on the main menu wheel.

Flashcards for Word Parts and Abbreviations

1. Click on Practice Student Resources on the menu to the left of the screen. Follow links to reach the main menu.
2. Select a Chapter on the pull-out tab to the left of the screen.
3. Click on Flashcards button on the main menu wheel.
4. Select Combining Forms, Prefixes, Suffixes, or Abbreviations.
5. Use buttons in lower left of the screen to flip the card and to move forward and backward through the stack.

Pronunciation & Spelling

1. Click on Practice Student Resources on the menu to the left of the screen. Follow links to reach the main menu.
2. Select a Chapter on the pull-out tab to the left of the screen.
3. Click on Pronounce and Spell button on the main menu wheel.
4. Select the Exercise and term list to practice.
5. Toggle between Pronunciation and Spelling using the tabs above the exercise.

Electronic Health Record Modules

1. Click on Practice Student Resources on the menu to the left of the screen. Follow links to reach the main menu.
2. Select a Chapter on the pull-out tab to the left of the screen.
3. Click on the Electronic Health Records button on the main menu wheel.
4. The first of three medical records appears.
5. Click on answer boxes to select the correct medical term.
6. Click on report tabs near the top of the electronic health record to access other medical documents, such as Chart Review, Imaging, Notes, etc.

Games

1. Click on Practice Student Resources on the menu to the left of the screen. Follow links to reach the main menu.
2. Select a Chapter on the pull-out tab to the left of the screen.
3. Click on the Games button on the main menu wheel.
4. Select a game: Medical Millionaire or Tournament of Terminology.

Practice Quizzes

1. Click on Practice Student Resources on the menu to the left of the screen. Follow links to reach the main menu.
2. Select a Chapter on the pull-out tab to the left of the screen.
3. Click on the Practice Quizzes button on the main menu wheel.
4. Select the quiz from the menu to the left.
5. Click the submit button when complete.
6. Click the Email Results button to send your scores to your instructor.

Additional Appendices With Term Lists

1. Click on Practice Student Resources on the menu to the left of the screen. Follow links to reach the main menu.
2. From the main menu, click on the Extra Content tab on the lower right of the screen.
3. Click on Appendices.
4. Select an appendix: Additional Word Parts, Health Care Delivery, Integrative Medicine, Behavioral Health, Clinical Research, Nutrition, Dental, and Health Information Technology.
5. Open PDF file.

Career Videos

1. Click on Practice Student Resources on the menu to the left of the screen. Follow links to reach the main menu.
2. From the main menu, click on the Extra Content tab on the lower right of the screen.
3. Click on Career Videos.
4. Select a video; scroll down if needed.

Exercises

1. Click on Gradable Student Resources on the menu to the left of the screen. *Note: If your instructor has linked to an electronic gradebook, scores may be recorded.*
2. Select Chapter.
3. Click on Exercises.
4. Select an Exercise: Word Parts, Terms Built from Word Parts, Terms NOT Built from Word Parts, or Abbreviations. Follow links to launch the exercise.

Quizzes

1. Click on Gradable Student Resources on the menu to the left of the screen. *Note: If your instructor has linked to an electronic gradebook, scores may be recorded.*
2. Select Chapter.
3. Click on Quizzes.
4. Select a Quiz: Disease and Disorder Terms, Surgical Terms, Diagnostic Terms, Complementary Terms, or other. Follow links to launch the quiz.

Appendix

C Combining Forms, Prefixes, and Suffixes Alphabetized by Word Part

COMBINING FORMS	DEFINITION	CHAPTER
A		
abdomin/o	abdomen, abdominal cavity	11
acr/o	extremities, height	16
aden/o	gland	2
adenoid/o	adenoids	5
adren/o	adrenal glands	16
adrenal/o	adrenal glands	16
albumin/o	albumin	6
alveol/o	alveolus	5
amni/o	amnion, amniotic fluid	9
amnion/o	amnion, amniotic fluid	9
andr/o	male	7
angi/o	vessel (usually refers to blood vessel)	10
ankyl/o	stiff, bent	14
an/o	anus	11
anter/o	front	3
antr/o	antrum	11
aort/o	aorta	10
aponeur/o	aponeurosis	14
appendic/o	appendix	11
append/o	appendix	11
arche/o	first, beginning	8
arteri/o	artery	10
arthr/o	joint	14
atel/o	imperfect, incomplete	5
ather/o	yellowish, fatty plaque	10
atri/o	atrium	10
audi/o	hearing	13
aur/i	ear	13
aut/o	self	4
azot/o	urea, nitrogen	6
B		
balan/o	glans penis	7
bi/o	life	4

COMBINING FORMS	DEFINITION	CHAPTER
blast/o	developing cell, germ cell	6
blephar/o	eyelid	12
bronch/o	bronchus	5
bronchi/o	bronchus	5
burs/o	bursa (cavity)	14
C		
calc/i	calcium	16
cancer/o	cancer	2
capn/o	carbon dioxide	5
carcin/o	cancer	2
cardi/o	heart	10
carp/o	carpals (wrist)	14
caud/o	tail (downward)	3
cec/o	cecum	11
celi/o	abdomen, abdominal cavity	11
cephal/o	head	3, 9
cerebell/o	cerebellum	15
cerebr/o	cerebrum, brain	15
cervic/o	cervix	8
cheil/o	lip(s)	11
chlor/o	green	2
cholangi/o	bile duct	11
chol/e	gall, bile	11
choledoch/o	common bile duct	11
chondr/o	cartilage	14
chori/o	chorion	9
chrom/o	color	2
clavic/o	clavicle (collarbone)	14
clavicul/o	clavicle (collarbone)	14
cochle/o	cochlea	13
col/o	colon (large intestine)	11
colon/o	colon (large intestine)	11
colp/o	vagina	8
coni/o	dust	4

COMBINING FORMS	DEFINITION	CHAPTER
conjunctiv/o	conjunctiva	12
cor/o	pupil	12
core/o	pupil	12
corne/o	cornea	12
cortic/o	cortex (outer layer of body organ)	16
cost/o	rib	14
crani/o	cranium (skull)	14
cry/o	cold	12
crypt/o	hidden	4
cutane/o	skin	4
cyan/o	blue	2
cyst/o	bladder, sac	6, 12
cyt/o	cell	2
D		
dacry/o	tear(s)	12
dermat/o	skin	4
derm/o	skin	4
diaphragmat/o	diaphragm	5
dipl/o	two, double	12
dips/o	thirst	16
disk/o	intervertebral disk	14
dist/o	away (from the point of attachment of a body part)	3
diverticul/o	diverticulum	11
dors/o	back	3
duoden/o	duodenum	11
dur/o	hard, dura mater	15
E		
ech/o	sound	10
electr/o	electricity, electrical activity	10
embry/o	embryo	9
encephal/o	brain	15
endocrin/o	endocrine	16
endometri/o	endometrium	8
enter/o	intestine(s) (small intestine)	11
epididym/o	epididymis	7
epiglott/o	epiglottis	5
episi/o	vulva	8
epitheli/o	epithelium	2

COMBINING FORMS	DEFINITION	CHAPTER
erythr/o	red	2
esophag/o	esophagus	9, 11
esthesi/o	sensation, sensitivity, feeling	15
eti/o	cause (of disease)	2
F		
femor/o	femur (upper leg bone)	14
fet/i	fetus, unborn offspring	9
fet/o	fetus, unborn offspring	9
fibr/o	fiber	2
fibul/o	fibula (lower leg bone)	14
G		
gangli/o	ganglion	15
ganglion/o	ganglion	15
gastr/o	stomach	11
gingiv/o	gum	11
gli/o	glia	15
glomerul/o	glomerulus	6
gloss/o	tongue	11
glyc/o	sugar	6
glycos/o	sugar	6
gno/o	knowledge	2
gravid/o	pregnancy	9
gynec/o	woman	8
gyn/o	woman	8
H		
hemat/o	blood	5
hem/o	blood	5
hepat/o	liver	11
herni/o	hernia (protrusion of an organ through a membrane or cavity wall)	11
heter/o	other	4
hidr/o	sweat	4
hist/o	tissue	2
humer/o	humerus (upper arm bone)	14
hydr/o	water	6
hymen/o	hymen	8
hyster/o	uterus	8
I		
iatr/o	physician, medicine (also means treatment)	2

COMBINING FORMS	DEFINITION	CHAPTER
ile/o	ileum	11
ili/o	ilium	14
infer/o	below	3
irid/o	iris	12
ir/o	iris	12
is/o	equal	12
ischi/o	ischium	14
isch/o	deficiency, blockage	10
J		
jejun/o	jejunum	11
K		
kal/i	potassium	16
kary/o	nucleus	2
kerat/o	cornea	12
kerat/o	horny tissue (keratin), hard	4
kinesi/o	movement, motion	14
kyph/o	hump (increased convexity of the spine)	14
L		
labyrinth/o	labyrinth	13
lacrim/o	tear(s)	12
lact/o	milk	9
lamin/o	lamina (thin, flat plate or layer)	14
lapar/o	abdomen, abdominal cavity	11
laryng/o	larynx	5
later/o	side	3
lei/o	smooth	2
leuk/o	white	2
lingu/o	tongue	11
lip/o	fat	2
lith/o	stone, calculus	6
lob/o	lobe	5
lord/o	bent forward (increased concavity of the spine)	14
lumb/o	loin, lumbar region of the spine	14
lymphaden/o	lymph node	10
lymph/o	lymph, lymph tissue	10
M		
mamm/o	breast	8
mandibul/o	mandible (lower jawbone)	14
mast/o	breast	8
mastoid/o	mastoid bone	13
maxill/o	maxilla (upper jawbone)	14
meat/o	meatus (opening)	6
medi/o	middle	3
melan/o	black	2
meningi/o	meninges	15
mening/o	meninges	15
menisc/o	meniscus (crescent)	14
men/o	menstruation	8
ment/o	mind	15
metr/o	uterus	8
mon/o	one, single	15
muc/o	mucus	5
myc/o	fungus	4
myel/o	bone marrow	10, 14
myel/o	spinal cord	15
my/o	muscle	2, 14
myos/o	muscle	14
myring/o	tympanic membrane (eardrum)	13
N		
nas/o	nose	5
nat/o	birth	9
natr/o	sodium	16
necr/o	death (cells, body)	4
nephr/o	kidney	6
neur/o	nerve	2, 15
noct/i	night	6
O		
ocul/o	eye	12
olig/o	scanty, few	6
omphal/o	umbilicus, navel	9
onc/o	tumor, mass	2
onych/o	nail	4
oophor/o	ovary	8
ophthalm/o	eye	12
opt/o	vision	12
orchid/o	testis, testicle	7
orchi/o	testis, testicle	7

COMBINING FORMS	DEFINITION	CHAPTER
orch/o	testis, testicle	7
organ/o	organ	2
or/o	mouth	11
orth/o	straight	5
oste/o	bone	14
ot/o	ear	13
ox/i	oxygen	5
P		
pachy/o	thick	4
palat/o	palate	11
pancreat/o	pancreas	11
parathyroid/o	parathyroid glands	16
par/o	bear, give birth to, labor, childbirth	9
part/o	bear, give birth to, labor, childbirth	9
patell/o	patella (kneecap)	14
path/o	disease	2
pelv/i	pelvis, pelvic bones, pelvic cavity	8, 14
perine/o	perineum	8
peritone/o	peritoneum	11
petr/o	stone	14
phac/o	lens	12
phak/o	lens	12
phalang/o	phalanx (pl. phalanges) (any bone of the fingers or toes)	14
pharyng/o	pharynx	5
phas/o	speech	15
phleb/o	vein	10
phon/o	sound, voice	5
phot/o	light	12
phren/o	diaphragm	5
pituitar/o	pituitary gland	16
plasm/o	plasma	10
pleur/o	pleura	5
pneumat/o	lung, air	5
pneum/o	lung, air	5
pneumon/o	lung, air	5
poli/o	gray matter	15
polyp/o	polyp, small growth	11
poster/o	back, behind	3

COMBINING FORMS	DEFINITION	CHAPTER
prim/i	first	9
proct/o	rectum	11
prostat/o	prostate gland	7
proxim/o	near (the point of attachment of a body part)	3
pseud/o	false	9
psych/o	mind	15
pub/o	pubis	14
puerper/o	childbirth	9
pulmon/o	lung	5
pupill/o	pupil	12
pyel/o	renal pelvis	6
pylor/o	pylorus, pyloric sphincter	9, 11
py/o	pus	5
Q		
quadr/i	four	15
R		
rachi/o	vertebra, spine, vertebral column	14
radic/o	nerve root	15
radicul/o	nerve root	15
radi/o	radius (lower arm bone)	14
radi/o	x-rays, ionizing radiation	5
rect/o	rectum	11
ren/o	kidney	6
retin/o	retina	12
rhabd/o	rod-shaped, striated	2
rhin/o	nose	5
rhiz/o	nerve root	15
rhytid/o	wrinkles	4
S		
sacr/o	sacrum	14
salping/o	uterine tube (fallopian tube)	8
sarc/o	flesh, connective tissue	2, 14
scapul/o	scapula (shoulder blade)	14
scler/o	sclera	12
scoli/o	(lateral) curved (spine)	14
seb/o	sebum (oil)	4

COMBINING FORMS	DEFINITION	CHAPTER
sept/o	septum	5
sial/o	saliva, salivary gland	11
sigmoid/o	sigmoid colon	11
sinus/o	sinus	5
somat/o	body	2
somn/o	sleep	5
son/o	sound	5
sperm/o	sperm, spermatozoon (pl. spermatozoa)	7
spermat/o	sperm, spermatozoon (pl. spermatozoa)	7
spir/o	breathe, breathing	5
splen/o	spleen	10
spondyl/o	vertebra, spine, vertebral column	14
staped/o	stapes	13
staphyl/o	grapelike clusters	4
steat/o	fat	11
stern/o	sternum (breastbone)	14
stomat/o	mouth	11
strept/o	twisted chains	4
super/o	above	3
synovi/o	synovia, synovial membrane	14
system/o	system	2
T		
tars/o	tarsals (ankle bones)	14
tendin/o	tendon	14
tend/o	tendon	14
ten/o	tendon	14
terat/o	malformations	9
therm/o	heat	10
thorac/o	thorax, chest, chest cavity	5
thromb/o	clot	10
thym/o	thymus gland	10
thyroid/o	thyroid gland	16
thyr/o	thyroid gland	16
tibi/o	tibia (lower leg bone)	14
tom/o	to cut, section, or slice	5
ton/o	tension, pressure	12
tonsill/o	tonsil	5
trachel/o	cervix	8
trache/o	trachea	5
tympan/o	middle ear	13
U		
uln/o	ulna (lower arm bone)	14
ungu/o	nail	4
ureter/o	ureter	6
urethr/o	urethra	6
ur/o	urine, urinary tract	6
urin/o	urine, urinary tract	6
uvul/o	uvula	11
V		
vagin/o	vagina	8
valv/o	valve	10
valvul/o	valve	10
vas/o	vessel, duct	7
ven/o	vein	10
ventricul/o	ventricle	10
ventr/o	belly (front)	3
vertebr/o	vertebra, spine, vertebral column	14
vesic/o	bladder, sac	6
vesicul/o	seminal vesicle(s)	7
vestibul/o	vestibule	13
viscer/o	internal organs	2
vulv/o	vulva	8
X		
xanth/o	yellow	2
xer/o	dry, dryness	4

PREFIX	DEFINITION	CHAPTER
a-	absence of, without	5
an-	absence of, without	5
ante-	before	9
bi-	two	3, 12
bin-	two	12
brady-	slow	10
dia-	through, complete	2
dys-	painful, abnormal, difficult, labored	2
endo-	within	5
epi-	on, upon, over	4
eu-	normal, good	5
hemi-	half	11
hyper-	above, excessive	2
hypo-	below, incomplete, deficient, under	2
inter-	between	14
intra-	within	4
meta-	after, beyond, change	2

PREFIX	DEFINITION	CHAPTER
micro-	small	9
multi-	many	9
neo-	new	2
nulli-	none	9
pan-	all, total	10
para-	beside, beyond, around, abnormal	4
per-	through	4
peri-	surrounding (outer)	8
poly-	many, much	5
post-	after	9
pre-	before	9
pro-	before	2
sub-	under, below	4
supra-	above	14
sym-	together, joined	14
syn-	together, joined	14
tachy-	fast, rapid	5
trans-	through, across, beyond	4
uni-	one	3

SUFFIX	DEFINITION	CHAPTER
-a	no meaning	4
-ac	pertaining to	10
-ad	toward	3
-al	pertaining to	2
-algia	pain	5
-amnios	amnion, amniotic fluid	9
-apheresis	removal	10
-ar	pertaining to	5
-ary	pertaining to	5
-asthenia	weakness	14
-cele	hernia or protrusion	5
-centesis	surgical puncture to aspirate fluid	5
-cleisis	surgical closure	8
-coccus (pl. -cocci)	berry-shaped (form of bacterium)	4
-cyesis	pregnancy	9
-cyte	cell	2
-desis	surgical fixation, fusion	14

SUFFIX	DEFINITION	CHAPTER
-drome	run, running	16
-e	no meaning	9
-eal	pertaining to	5
-ectasis	stretching out, dilation, expansion	5
-ectomy	excision or surgical removal	4
-emia	in the blood	5
-esis	condition	6
-gen	substance or agent that produces or causes	2
-genic	producing, originating, causing	2
-gram	the record, radiographic image	5
-graph	instrument used to record; the record	5
-graphy	process of recording, radiographic imaging	5
-ia	diseased or abnormal state, condition of	4
-iasis	condition	6

SUFFIX	DEFINITION	CHAPTER
-iatrist	specialist, physician	15
-iatry	treatment, specialty	15
-ic	pertaining to	2
-ictal	seizure, attack	15
-ior	pertaining to	3
-is	no meaning	9
-ism	state of	7
-itis	inflammation	4
-logist	one who studies and treats (specialist, physician)	2
-logy	study of	2
-lysis	loosening, dissolution, separating	6
-malacia	softening	4
-megaly	enlargement	2
-meter	instrument used to measure	5
-metry	measurement	5
-oid	resembling	2
-oma	tumor, swelling	2
-opia	vision (condition)	12
-opsy	view of, viewing	4
-osis	abnormal condition (means increase when used with blood cell word roots)	2
-ous	pertaining to	2
-paresis	slight paralysis	15
-pathy	disease	2
-penia	abnormal reduction in number	10
-pepsia	digestion	11
-pexy	surgical fixation, suspension	5
-phagia	eating or swallowing	4
-phobia	abnormal fear of or aversion to specific things	12
-physis	growth	14
-plasia	condition of formation, development, growth	2

SUFFIX	DEFINITION	CHAPTER
-plasm	growth, substance, formation	2
-plasty	surgical repair	4
-plegia	paralysis	12
-pnea	breathing	5
-poiesis	formation	10
-ptosis	drooping, sagging, prolapse	6
-rrhagia	rapid flow of blood, excessive bleeding	5
-rrhaphy	suturing, repairing	6
-rrhea	flow, discharge	4
-rrhexis	rupture	9
-salpinx	uterine tube (fallopian tube)	8
-sarcoma	malignant tumor	2
-schisis	split, fissure	14
-sclerosis	hardening	10
-scope	instrument used for visual examination	5
-scopic	pertaining to visual examination	5
-scopy	visual examination	5
-sis	state of	2
-spasm	sudden, involuntary muscle contraction	5
-stasis	control, stop, standing	2
-stenosis	constriction or narrowing	5
-stomy	creation of an artificial opening	5
-thorax	chest, chest cavity	5
-tocia	birth, labor	9
-tome	instrument used to cut	4
-tomy	cut into, incision	5
-tripsy	surgical crushing	6
-trophy	nourishment, development	14
-um	no meaning	9
-uria	urine, urination	6
-us	no meaning	9

Appendix D

Combining Forms, Prefixes, and Suffixes Alphabetized by Definition

DEFINITION	COMBINING FORM	CHAPTER
A		
abdomen, abdominal cavity	abdomin/o, lapar/o, celi/o	11
above	super/o	3
adenoids	adenoid/o	5
adrenal glands	adren/o, adrenal/o	16
albumin	albumin/o	6
alveolus	alveol/o	5
amnion, amniotic fluid	amni/o, amnion/o	9
antrum	antr/o	11
anus	an/o	11
aorta	aort/o	10
aponeurosis	aponeur/o	14
appendix	append/o, appendic/o	11
artery	arteri/o	10
atrium	atri/o	10
away (from the point of attachment of a body part)	dist/o	3
B		
back	dors/o	3
back, behind	poster/o	3
bear, give birth to, labor, childbirth	par/o, part/o	9
belly (front)	ventr/o	3
below	infer/o	3
bent forward (increased concavity of the spine)	lord/o	14
bile duct(s)	cholangi/o	11
birth	nat/o	9
black	melan/o	2
bladder, sac	cyst/o, vesic/o	6, 12
blood	hem/o, hemat/o	5
blue	cyan/o	2

DEFINITION	COMBINING FORM	CHAPTER
body	somat/o	2
bone	oste/o	14
bone marrow	myel/o	10
brain	encephal/o	15
breast	mamm/o, mast/o	8
breathe, breathing	spir/o	5
bronchus	bronch/o, bronchi/o	5
bursa (cavity)	burs/o	14
C		
calcium	calc/i	16
cancer	cancer/o, carcin/o	2
carbon dioxide	capn/o	5
carpals (wrist)	carp/o	14
cartilage	chondr/o	14
cause (of disease)	eti/o	2
cecum	cec/o	11
cell	cyt/o	2
cerebellum	cerebell/o	15
cerebrum, brain	cerebr/o	15
cervix	cervic/o, trachel/o	8
childbirth	puerper/o	9
chorion	chori/o	9
clavicle (collarbone)	clavic/o, clavicul/o	14
clot	thromb/o	10
cochlea	cochle/o	13
cold	cry/o	12
colon	col/o, colon/o	11
color	chrom/o	2
common bile duct	choledoch/o	11
conjunctiva	conjunctiv/o	12
cornea	corne/o, kerat/o	12
cortex	cortic/o	16
cranium (skull)	crani/o	14
(lateral) curved (spine)	scoli/o	14

DEFINITION	COMBINING FORM	CHAPTER
D		
death (cells, body)	necr/o	4
deficiency, blockage	isch/o	10
developing cell, germ cell	blast/o	6
diaphragm	diaphragmat/o, phren/o	5
disease	path/o	2
diverticulum	diverticul/o	11
dry, dryness	xer/o	4
duodenum	duoden/o	11
dust	coni/o	4
E		
ear	aur/i, ot/o	13
electricity, electrical activity	electr/o	10
embryo	embry/o	9
endocrine	endocrin/o	16
endometrium	endometri/o	8
epididymis	epididym/o	7
epiglottis	epiglott/o	5
epithelium	epitheli/o	2
equal	is/o	12
esophagus	esophag/o	9, 11
extremities, height	acr/o	16
eye	ocul/o, ophthalm/o	12
eyelid	blephar/o	12
F		
false	pseud/o	9
fat	lip/o	2
fat	steat/o	11
femur (upper leg bone)	femor/o	14
fetus, unborn offspring	fet/o, fet/i	9
fiber	fibr/o	2
fibula (lower leg bone)	fibul/o	14
first	prim/i	9
first, beginning	arche/o	8
flesh, connective tissue	sarc/o	2, 14
four	quadr/i	15
front	anter/o	3
fungus	myc/o	3

DEFINITION	COMBINING FORM	CHAPTER
G		
gall, bile	chol/e	11
ganglion	gangli/o, ganglion/o	15
gland	aden/o	2
glans penis	balan/o	7
glia	gli/o	15
glomerulus	glomerul/o	6
grapelike clusters	staphyl/o	4
gray matter	poli/o	15
green	chlor/o	2
gum(s)	gingiv/o	11
H		
hard, dura mater	dur/o	15
head	cephal/o	3, 9
hearing	audi/o	13
heart	cardi/o	10
heat	therm/o	10
hernia	herni/o	11
hidden	crypt/o	4
horny tissue (keratin), hard	kerat/o	4
humerus (upper arm bone)	humer/o	14
hump (increased convexity of the spine)	kyph/o	14
hymen	hymen/o	8
I		
ileum	ile/o	11
ilium	ili/o	14
imperfect, incomplete	atel/o	5
internal organs	viscer/o	2
intervertebral disk	disk/o	14
intestine(s) (small intestine)	enter/o	11
iris	ir/o, irid/o	12
ischium	ischi/o	14
J		
jejunum	jejun/o	11
joint	arthr/o	14
K		
kidney	nephr/o, ren/o	6
knowledge	gno/o	2

DEFINITION	COMBINING FORM	CHAPTER
L		
labyrinth	labyrinth/o	13
lamina (thin, flat plate or layer)	lamin/o	14
larynx	laryng/o	5
lens	phac/o, phak/o	12
life	bi/o	4
light	phot/o	12
lip(s)	cheil/o	11
liver	hepat/o	11
lobe	lob/o	5
loin, lumbar region of the spine	lumb/o	14
lung	pulmon/o	5
lung, air	pneum/o, pneumat/o, pneumon/o	5
lymph node	lymphaden/o	10
lymph, lymph tissue	lymph/o	10
M		
male	andr/o	7
malformations	terat/o	9
mandible (lower jawbone)	mandibul/o	14
mastoid bone	mastoid/o	13
maxilla (upper jawbone)	maxill/o	14
meatus (opening)	meat/o	6
meninges	mening/o, meningi/o	15
meniscus (crescent)	menisc/o	14
menstruation	men/o	8
middle	medi/o	3
middle ear	tympan/o	13
milk	lact/o	9
mind	ment/o, psych/o	15
mouth	or/o, stomat/o	11
movement, motion	kinesi/o	14
mucus	muc/o	5
muscle	my/o, myos/o	2, 14
N		
nail	onych/o, ungu/o	4
near (the point of attachment of a body part)	proxim/o	3
nerve	neur/o	2, 15
nerve root	radic/o, radicul/o, rhiz/o	15
night	noct/i	6
nose	nas/o, rhin/o	5
nucleus	kary/o	2
O		
one, single	mon/o	15
organ	organ/o	2
other	heter/o	4
ovary	oophor/o	8
oxygen	ox/i	5
P		
palate	palat/o	11
pancreas	pancreat/o	11
parathyroid glands	parathyroid/o	16
patella (kneecap)	patell/o	14
pelvis, pelvic bones, pelvic cavity	pelv/i	8, 14
perineum	perine/o	8
peritoneum	peritone/o	11
phalanx (any bone of the fingers or toes)	phalang/o	14
pharynx	pharyng/o	5
physician, medicine (also means treatment)	iatr/o	2
plasma	plasm/o	10
pleura	pleur/o	5
polyp, small growth	polyp/o	11
potassium	kal/i	16
pregnancy	gravid/o	9
prostate gland	prostat/o	7
pubis	pub/o	14
pupil	cor/o, core/o, pupill/o	12
pus	py/o	5
pylorus, pyloric sphincter	pylor/o	9, 11
R		
radius (lower arm bone)	radi/o	14
rectum	proct/o, rect/o	11
red	erythr/o	2

DEFINITION	COMBINING FORM	CHAPTER
renal pelvis	pyel/o	6
retina	retin/o	12
rib	cost/o	14
rod-shaped, striated	rhabd/o	2
S		
sacrum	sacr/o	14
saliva, salivary gland	sial/o	11
scanty, few	olig/o	6
scapula (shoulder blade)	scapul/o	14
sclera	scler/o	12
sebum (oil)	seb/o	4
self	aut/o	4
seminal vesicle(s)	vesicul/o	7
sensation, sensitivity, feeling	esthesi/o	15
septum	sept/o	5
side	later/o	3
sigmoid colon	sigmoid/o	11
sinus	sinus/o	5
skin	cutane/o, derm/o, dermat/o	4
sleep	somn/o	5
smooth	lei/o	2
sodium	natr/o	16
sound	son/o, ech/o	5, 10
sound, voice	phon/o	5
speech	phas/o	15
sperm, spermatozoon	sperm/o, spermat/o	7
spinal cord	myel/o	15
spleen	splen/o	10
stapes	staped/o	13
sternum (breastbone)	stern/o	14
stiff, bent	ankyl/o	14
stomach	gastr/o	11
stone	petr/o	14
stone, calculus	lith/o	6
straight	orth/o	5
sugar	glyc/o, glycos/o	6
sweat	hidr/o	4
synovia, synovial membrane	synovi/o	14
system	system/o	2
T		
tail (downward)	caud/o	3
tarsals (ankle bones)	tars/o	14
tear(s)	dacry/o, lacrim/o	12
tendon	ten/o, tend/o, tendin/o	14
tension, pressure	ton/o	12
testis, testicle	orch/o, orchi/o, orchid/o	7
thick	pachy/o	4
thirst	dips/o	16
thorax, chest, chest cavity	thorac/o	5
thymus gland	thym/o	10
thyroid gland	thyr/o, thyroid/o	16
tibia (lower leg bone)	tibi/o	14
tissue	hist/o	2
to cut, section, or slice	tom/o	5
tongue	gloss/o, lingu/o	11
tonsil	tonsill/o	5
trachea	trache/o	5
tumor, mass	onc/o	2
twisted chains	strept/o	4
two, double	dipl/o	12
tympanic membrane (eardrum)	myring/o	13
U		
ulna (lower arm bone)	uln/o	14
umbilicus, navel	omphal/o	9
urea, nitrogen	azot/o	6
ureter	ureter/o	6
urethra	urethr/o	6
urine, urinary tract	ur/o, urin/o	6
uterine tube (fallopian tube)	salping/o	8
uterus	hyster/o, metr/o	8
uvula	uvul/o	11

DEFINITION	COMBINING FORM	CHAPTER
V		
vagina	colp/o, vagin/o	8
valve	valv/o, valvul/o	10
vein	phleb/o, ven/o	10
ventricle	ventricul/o	10
vertebra, spine, vertebral column	rachi/o, spondyl/o, vertebr/o	14
vessel (usually refers to blood vessel)	angi/o	10
vessel, duct	vas/o	7
vestibule	vestibul/o	13
vision	opt/o	12
vulva	episi/o, vulv/o	8
W		
water	hydr/o	6
white	leuk/o	2
woman	gyn/o, gynec/o	8
wrinkles	rhytid/o	4
X		
x-rays, ionizing radiation	radi/o	5
Y		
yellow	xanth/o	2
yellowish, fatty plaque	ather/o	10

DEFINITION	PREFIX	CHAPTER
above	supra-	14
above, excessive	hyper-	2
absence of, without	a-, an-	5
after	post-	9
after, beyond, change	meta-	2
all, total	pan-	10
before	ante-, pre-	9
before	pro-	2
below, incomplete, deficient, under	hypo-	2
beside, beyond, around, abnormal	para-	4
between	inter-	14
fast, rapid	tachy-	5
half	hemi-	11
many	multi-	9
many, much	poly-	5
new	neo-	2
none	nulli-	9
normal, good	eu-	5
on, upon, over	epi-	4
one	uni-	3
painful, abnormal, difficult, labored	dys-	2
slow	brady-	10
small	micro-	9
surrounding (outer)	peri-	8
through	per-	4
through, across, beyond	trans-	4
through, complete	dia-	2
together, joined	sym-, syn-	14
two	bin-	12
two	bi-	3, 12
under, below	sub-	4
within	intra-	4
within	endo-	5

DEFINITION	SUFFIX	CHAPTER
abnormal condition (means increase when used with blood cell word roots)	-osis	2
abnormal fear of or aversion to specific things	-phobia	12
abnormal reduction in number	-penia	10
amnion, amniotic fluid	-amnios	9
berry-shaped (form of bacterium)	-coccus (pl. -cocci)	4
birth, labor	-tocia	9
breathing	-pnea	5
cell	-cyte	2
chest, chest cavity	-thorax	5
condition	-esis, -iasis	6
condition of formation, development, growth	-plasia	2
constriction or narrowing	-stenosis	5
control, stop, standing	-stasis	2
creation of an artificial opening	-stomy	5
cut into, incision	-tomy	5
digestion	-pepsia	11
disease	-pathy	2
diseased or abnormal state, condition of	-ia	4
drooping, sagging, prolapse	-ptosis	6
eating or swallowing	-phagia	4
enlargement	-megaly	2
excision or surgical removal	-ectomy	4
flow, discharge	-rrhea	4
formation	-poiesis	10
growth	-physis	14
growth, substance, formation	-plasm	2
hardening	-sclerosis	10
hernia or protrusion	-cele	5
in the blood	-emia	5
inflammation	-itis	4
instrument used for visual examination	-scope	5
instrument used to cut	-tome	4
instrument used to measure	-meter	5
instrument used to record; the record	-graph	5
loosening, dissolution, separating	-lysis	6
malignant tumor	-sarcoma	2
measurement	-metry	5
no meaning	-a, -e, -is, -um, -us	4, 9
nourishment, development	-trophy	14
one who studies and treats (specialist, physician)	-logist	2
pain	-algia	5
paralysis	-plegia	12
pertaining to	-ac	10
pertaining to	-ous	2, 6
pertaining to	-ar, -ary, -eal	5
pertaining to	-al, -ic	2
pertaining to	-ior	3
pertaining to visual examination	-scopic	5
pregnancy	-cyesis	9
process of recording, radiographic imaging	-graphy	5
producing, originating, causing	-genic	2
rapid flow of blood, excessive bleeding	-rrhagia	5
removal	-apheresis	10
resembling	-oid	2
run, running	-drome	16
rupture	-rrhexis	9
seizure, attack	-ictal	15
slight paralysis	-paresis	15
softening	-malacia	4
specialist, physician	-iatrist	15
split, fissure	-schisis	14

DEFINITION	SUFFIX	CHAPTER
state of	-ism	7
state of	-sis	2
stretching out, dilation, expansion	-ectasis	5
study of	-logy	2
substance or agent that produces or causes	-gen	2
sudden, involuntary muscle contraction	-spasm	5
surgical closure	-cleisis	8
surgical crushing	-tripsy	6
surgical fixation, fusion	-desis	14
surgical fixation, suspension	-pexy	5
surgical puncture to aspirate fluid	-centesis	5
surgical repair	-plasty	4
suturing, repairing	-rrhaphy	6
the record, radiographic image	-gram	5
toward	-ad	3
treatment, specialty	-iatry	15
tumor, swelling	-oma	2
urine, urination	-uria	6
uterine tube (fallopian tube)	-salpinx	8
view of, viewing	-opsy	4
vision (condition)	-opia	12
visual examination	-scopy	5
weakness	-asthenia	14

Appendix

E Abbreviations

Topics include:

Common Medical Abbreviations, p. 736

Institute for Safe Medication Practices' (ISMP) List of Error-Prone Abbreviations, Symbols and Dose Designations; includes The Joint Commission's "Do Not Use" list, p. 745

Abbreviations are written as they appear most commonly in the medical and healthcare environment. Some may also appear in both capital and small letters and with or without periods. To make a plural, add "s" to uppercase abbreviations (e.g., BPs for blood pressures) and apostrophe ('s) for lower case abbreviations (e.g., cm's for centimeters).

COMMON MEDICAL ABBREVIATIONS	DEFINITIONS
A1c	glycated hemoglobin
AAA	abdominal aortic aneurysm
AAD	antiobiotic-associated diarrhea
AB	abortion
ABD	abdomen
ABE	acute bacterial endocarditis
ABGs	arterial blood gases
ABX	antibiotics
AC	acromioclavicular
ac	acute
a.c.	before meals
ACS	acute coronary syndrome
ACTH	adrenocorticotropic hormone
AD	Alzheimer disease
ADC	AIDS dementia complex
ADH	antidiuretic hormone
ADHD	attention deficit/hyperactivity disorder
ADLs	activities of daily living
ad lib	as desired
Adm	admission
AER	auditory evoked response
AFB	acid-fast bacilli
AFib	atrial fibrillation
AFP	alpha-fetoprotein
AHD	arteriosclerotic heart disease
AI	aortic insufficiency
AICD	automatic implantable cardiac defibrillator
AIDS	acquired immunodeficiency syndrome
AKA	above-knee amputation
alk phos	alkaline phosphatase
ALL	acute lymphoblastic leukemia
ALS	amyotrophic lateral sclerosis
ALT	alanine aminotransferase
AM (or a.m.)	between midnight and noon
AMA	against medical advice; American Medical Association
AMB	ambulate, ambulatory
AMI	acute myocardial infarction
AML	acute myeloid leukemia
AMP (or amp)	ampule
amt	amount
angio	angiogram, angiography
ant	anterior
A&O	alert and oriented
AODM	adult-onset diabetes mellitus
AOM	acute otitis media
AP	anteroposterior; angina pectoris
A&P	anatomy and physiology; auscultation and percussion; anterior and posterior
A&P repair	anterior and posterior colporrhaphy

COMMON MEDICAL ABBREVIATIONS	DEFINITIONS
APR	abdominoperineal resection
aPTT	activated partial thromboplastin time
ARDS	acute respiratory distress syndrome
ARF	acute renal failure
ARM	artificial rupture of membranes
ARMD	age-related macular degeneration
ART	assisted reproductive technology
ASA	aspirin (acetylsalicylic acid)
ASCVD	arteriosclerotic cardiovascular disease
ASD	atrial septal defect; autism spectrum disorder
ASHD	arteriosclerotic heart disease
Ast (or AST)	astigmatism
as tol	as tolerated
AUB	abnormal uterine bleeding
AUL	acute undifferentiated leukemia
AV	atrioventricular, arteriovenous
AVM	arteriovenous malformation
AVR	aortic valve replacement
ax	axillary
BA	bronchial asthma
BBB	bundle branch block
BC	birth control
BCC	basal cell carcinoma
BE	barium enema
b.i.d.	twice a day
BK	below knee
BKA	below-knee amputation
BM	bowel movement
BMI	body mass index
BOM	bilateral otitis media
BOO	bladder outlet obstruction
BP	blood pressure
BPH	benign prostatic hyperplasia
BR	bedrest
BRBPR	bright red blood per rectum
BRM	biological response modifier
BRP	bathroom privileges
BS	blood sugar; bowel sounds; breath sounds

COMMON MEDICAL ABBREVIATIONS	DEFINITIONS
BSO	bilateral salpingo-oophorectomy
BUN	blood urea nitrogen
Bx or bx	biopsy
$\bar{c}$	with
C	Celsius
C1-C7 or C_1-C_7	cervical vertebrae
Ca (or Ca^{2+})	calcium
CA	cancer; carcinoma
CABG	coronary artery bypass graft
CAD	coronary artery disease
CAL (or cal)	calorie
CA-MRSA	community-associated MRSA (methicillin-resistant *Staphylococcus aureus*) infection
CAP	capsule (or cap); community-acquired pneumonia
CAPD	continuous ambulatory peritoneal dialysis
cath	catheterization, catheter
CBC and Diff	complete blood count and differential
CBR	complete bed rest
CBS	chronic brain syndrome
CC	chief complaint; colony count
CCU	coronary care unit
CDC	Centers for Disease Control and Prevention
CDH	congenital dislocation of the hip
CDI	*Clostridium difficile* infection
C. diff* or *C. difficile	*Clostridium difficile* (bacteria)
CEA	carcinoembryonic antigen
CF	cystic fibrosis
CHB	complete heart block
CHD	coronary heart disease
chemo	chemotherapy
CHF	congestive heart failure
CHO	carbohydrate
chol	cholesterol
CI	coronary insufficiency
circ	circumcision
CIS	carcinoma in situ

COMMON MEDICAL ABBREVIATIONS	DEFINITIONS
CJD	Creutzfeldt-Jakob disease
Cl (or Cl^-)	chloride
CKD	chronic kidney disease
CLBSI	central line bloodstream infection
CLD	chronic liver disease
CLL	chronic lymphocytic leukemia
cl liq	clear liquid
cm	centimeter
CML	chronic myelogenous leukemia
CMV	cytomegalovirus
CNS	central nervous system
c/o	complains of
CO	carbon monoxide
CO_2	carbon dioxide
COB	coordination of benefits
COLD	chronic obstructive lung disease
comp	compound
cond	condition
COPD	chronic obstructive pulmonary disease
CP	cerebral palsy
CPAP	continuous positive airway pressure
CPD	cephalopelvic disproportion
CPK	creatine phosphokinase
CPN	chronic pyelonephritis
CPR	cardiopulmonary resuscitation
CRD	chronic respiratory disease
creat	creatinine
CRF	chronic renal failure
crit	hematocrit (also HCT, Hct)
CRP	C-reactive protein
C&S	culture and sensitivity
C/S, CS, C-section	cesarean section
CSF	cerebrospinal fluid
CT	computed or computerized tomography
CTE	chronic traumatic encephalopathy
CTS	carpal tunnel syndrome
Cu	copper
CVA	cerebrovascular accident (stroke)
CVD	cardiovascular disease
CVP	central venous pressure

COMMON MEDICAL ABBREVIATIONS	DEFINITIONS
CVS	chorionic villus sampling
Cx	cervix
CXR	chest radiograph (x-ray)
DAT	diet as tolerated
D&C	dilation and curettage
DC	Doctor of Chiropractic
D&E	dilation and evacuation
DCIS	ductal carcinoma in situ
decub	pressure ulcer
del	delivery
derm	dermatology
DI	diabetes insipidus
DIC	diffuse intravascular coagulation
diff	differential (part of complete blood count)
disch	discharge
DISH	diffuse idiopathic skeletal hyperostosis
DKA	diabetic ketoacidosis
DLE	discoid lupus erythematosus
DM	diabetes mellitus
DNA	deoxyribonucleic acid
DND	died natural death
DO	Doctor of Osteopathy
DOA	dead on arrival
DOB	date of birth
DOD	date of death
Dr	dram
DRE	digital rectal examination
DRG	diagnosis-related group
DSA	digital subtraction angiography
DVT	deep vein thrombosis
DW	distilled water
D/W	dextrose in water
Dx	diagnosis
E	enema
EBL	estimated blood loss
ECG	electrocardiogram
ECHO	echocardiogram
ECT	electroconvulsive therapy
ED	erectile dysfunction, emergency department

COMMON MEDICAL ABBREVIATIONS	DEFINITIONS
EDD	expected (estimated) date of delivery
EEG	electroencephalogram
EGD	esophagogastroduodenoscopy
EKG	electrocardiogram
Elix (or elix)	elixir
Em	emmetropia
EMG	electromyogram
ENG	electronystagmography
ENT	ears, nose, throat; otolaryngologist
EP	ectopic pregnancy
EP studies	evoked potential studies
ER	emergency room
ERCP	endoscopic retrograde cholangiopancreatography
ERT	estrogen replacement therapy
ESR	erythrocyte sedimentation rate
ESRD	end-stage renal disease
ESWL	extracorporeal shock wave lithotripsy
etio	etiology
EUS	endoscopic ultrasound
exam	examination
ext	extract; external
F	Fahrenheit
FAS	fetal alcohol syndrome
FBD	fibrocystic breast disease
FBS	fasting blood sugar
FCC	fibrocystic breast changes
FDA	Food and Drug Administration
Fe	iron
FHT	fetal heart tones
flu	influenza
FNA	fine needle aspiration
FOBT	fecal occult blood test
Fr	French (catheter size)
FS	frozen section
FSH	follicle-stimulating hormone
FTD	frontotemporal dementia
FTT	failure to thrive
FUO	fever of undetermined origin
fx	fracture

COMMON MEDICAL ABBREVIATIONS	DEFINITIONS
g	gram
GC	gonorrhea
GERD	gastroesophageal reflux disease
GH	growth hormone
GI	gastrointestinal
GSW	gunshot wound
gtt	drops
GTT	glucose tolerance test
GU	genitourinary
GYN	gynecology; gynecologist
h	hour
H	hypodermic
HAART	highly active antiretroviral therapy
HAI	healthcare-associated infection
HA-MRSA	healthcare-associated MRSA infection
HAND	HIV-associated neurocognitive disorder
HAP	hospital-acquired pneumonia
HB	heart block
HbA1C (or HgbA1c)	glycosylated (or glycated) hemoglobin
HBV	hepatitis B virus
HCl	hydrochloric acid
HCO_3	bicarbonate
Hct	hematocrit
HCVD	hypertensive cardiovascular disease
HD	hemodialysis
HDL	high-density lipoprotein
HF	heart failure
Hg	mercury
Hgb	hemoglobin
H&H	hemoglobin and hematocrit
HHD	hypertensive heart disease
HIV	human immunodeficiency virus
HMD	hyaline membrane disease
HME	heat and moisture exchanger
HNP	herniated nucleus pulposus
H_2O	water
H_2O_2	hydrogen peroxide (hydrogen dioxide)
HOB	head of bed

COMMON MEDICAL ABBREVIATIONS	DEFINITIONS
HOH	hard of hearing
HoLEP	holmium laser enucleation of the prostate gland
H&P	history and physical examination
H. pylori	*Helicobacter pylori*
HPV	human papillomavirus
HRT	hormone replacement therapy
HSG	hysterosonography; hysterosalpingogram
ht	height
HTN	hypertension
Hx	history
hypo	hypodermic
IBD	inflammatory bowel disease
IBS	irritable bowel syndrome
ICD	implantable cardiac defibrillator
ICU	intensive care unit
ID	intradermal
I&D	incision and drainage
IDDM	insulin-dependent diabetes mellitus
IHD	ischemic heart disease
IM	intramuscular
inf	inferior
INR	international normalized ratio
I&O	intake and output
IOL	intraocular lens
IOP	intraocular pressure
IPF	idiopathic pulmonary fibrosis
IPPB	intermittent positive pressure breathing
IR	interventional radiology
irrig	irrigation
isol	isolation
IUD	intrauterine device
IUS	intrauterine system
IV	intravenous
IVC	intravenous cholangiogram
IVF	in vitro fertilization
IVP	intravenous pyelogram
IVU	intravenous urogram
K	potassium
KCl	potassium chloride
kg	kilogram
KO	keep open
KUB	kidney, ureter, bladder (radiograph)
KVO	keep vein open
L	liter
L1-L5 or L_1-L_5	lumbar vertebrae
lab	laboratory
LAC (or lac)	laceration
LAD	left anterior descending (coronary artery)
LAGB	laparoscopic adjustable gastric banding
LAP	laparotomy
LAR	low anterior resection
LARC	long-acting reversible contraception
LASIK	laser-assisted in situ keratomileusis
lat	lateral
LAVH	laparoscopically-assisted vaginal hysterectomy
L&D	labor and delivery
LDH	lactic dehydrogenase
LDL	low-density lipoprotein
LE	lupus erythematosus
LEEP	loop electrosurgical excision procedure
lg	large
LH	luteinizing hormone
LLL	left lower lobe (of lung)
LLQ	left lower quadrant
LMP	last menstrual period
LOC	loss of consciousness, level of consciousness
LP	lumbar puncture
LPM	liters per minute (oxygen)
LPN	licensed practical nurse
LPR	laryngopharyngeal reflux
LR	lactated Ringer (IV solution)
lt	left
LTB	laryngotracheobronchitis
LUL	left upper lobe (of lung)
LUQ	left upper quadrant

COMMON MEDICAL ABBREVIATIONS	DEFINITIONS
LUTS	lower urinary tract symptoms
lytes	electrolytes
mcg	microgram
MCH	mean corpuscular hemoglobin
MCV	mean corpuscular volume
MD	muscular dystrophy; medical doctor
med	medial
mEq	milliequivalent
MET (or met)	metastasis
METS (or mets)	metastases
mg	milligram
MG	myasthenia gravis
MI	myocardial infarction
mL	milliliter
mm	millimeter
MM	multiple myeloma
MOM	milk of magnesia
MR	magnetic resonance; mitral regurgitation
MRI	magnetic resonance imaging
MRCP	magnetic resonance cholangiopancreatography
MRSA	methicillin-resistant *Staphylococcus aureus*
MS	multiple sclerosis
multip	multipara
MVP	mitral valve prolapse
Na	sodium
NaCl	sodium chloride (salt)
NAS	no added salt
NB	newborn
NCD	neurocognitive disorder
neg	negative
neuro	neurology
NG	nasogastric
NICU	neonatal intensive care unit
NIDDM	non-insulin-dependent diabetes mellitus
NIH	National Institutes of Health
NIVA	noninvasive vascular assessment

COMMON MEDICAL ABBREVIATIONS	DEFINITIONS
NK	natural killer (immune system cells)
NKDA	no known drug allergies
noc, noct	night
NPH	normal pressure hydrocephalus
NPO	nothing by mouth
NPPV	noninvasive positive-pressure ventilator
NS	normal saline
NSAID	nonsteroidal antiinflammatory drug
NSR	normal sinus rhythm
N&V	nausea and vomiting
NVS	neurologic signs
OA	osteoarthritis
O_2	oxygen
OAB	overactive bladder
OB	obstetrics
OCD	obsessive-compulsive disorder
OD	Doctor of Optometry, overdose
OIC	opioid-induced constipation
oint	ointment
OM	otitis media
OOB	out of bed
OP	outpatient
Ophth	ophthalmic or ophthalmology
OR	operating room
Ortho or ortho	orthopedics
OSA	obstructive sleep apnea
OT	occupational therapy
OTC	over-the-counter drugs
oto	otology
oz	ounce
$\bar{p}$	after
P	phosphorus, pulse
PA	physician's assistant or posteroanterior
PAC	premature atrial complex
$PaCo_2$	carbon dioxide partial pressure (measure of amount of carbon dioxide in arterial blood)
PAD	peripheral artery disease

COMMON MEDICAL ABBREVIATIONS	DEFINITIONS
PAE	prostatic artery embolization
PAF	paroxysmal atrial fibrillation
PaO_2	oxygen partial pressure (measure of amount of oxygen in arterial blood)
PAT	paroxysmal atrial tachycardia
PBSCT	peripheral blood stem cell transplant
pc (or p.c.)	after meals
PCI	percutaneous coronary intervention
PCOS	polycystic ovary syndrome
PCP	primary care physician; *Pneumocystis* pneumonia
PCU	progressive care unit
PCV	packed cell volume
PD	Parkinson disease
PDA	patent ductus arteriosus
PDR	*Physicians' Desk Reference*
PE	pulmonary embolism; pulmonary edema
Peds (or peds)	pediatrics
PEEP	positive end-expiratory pressure
PEG	percutaneous endoscopic gastrostomy
PEP	positive expiratory pressure
per	by
PERRLA	pupils equal, round, reactive to light and accommodation
PET	positron emission tomography
PFM	peak flow meter
PFTs	pulmonary function tests
PHACO	phacoemulsification
PICC	peripherally inserted central catheter
PICU	pediatric intensive care unit
PID	pelvic inflammatory disease
PJP	*Pneumocystis jiroveci* pneumonia
PKU	phenylketonuria
PM	between noon and midnight
PMDD	premenstrual dysphoric disorder
PMS	premenstrual syndrome
PNS	peripheral nervous system

COMMON MEDICAL ABBREVIATIONS	DEFINITIONS
po (or PO)	orally; postoperative; phone order
post-op	postoperatively
PP	postpartum or postprandial (after meals)
PPD	purified protein derivative
pr	per rectum
PRBC	packed red blood cells
pre-op	preoperatively
PRH	prolactin-releasing hormone
primip	primipara
PRK	photorefractive keratectomy
PRL	prolactin
PRN	as needed (whenever necessary)
PSA	prostate-specific antigen
PSG	polysomnography
pt	patient; pint
PT	prothrombin time; physical therapy
PTCA	percutaneous transluminal coronary angioplasty
PT/INR	prothrombin time/international normalized ratio
PTSD	posttraumatic stress disorder
PTT	partial thromboplastin time
PUL	percutaneous ultrasound lithotripsy
PVC	premature ventricular complex
PVD	peripheral vascular disease
PVP	photoselective vaporization of the prostate gland
Px	prognosis
q	every
q_h	every (number) hour (e.g., q2h)
qt	quart
R	rectal
RA	rheumatoid arthritis
RAD	reactive airway disease
RAIU	radioactive iodine uptake
RALRP	robotic-assisted prostatectomy
RBC	red blood cell (erythrocyte)
RDS	respiratory distress syndrome
reg	regular
REM	rapid eye movement

COMMON MEDICAL ABBREVIATIONS	DEFINITIONS
resp	respirations
RHD	rheumatic heart disease
RLL	right lower lobe (of lung)
RLQ	right lower quadrant
RML	right middle lobe (of lung)
RN	registered nurse
R/O	rule out
ROM	range of motion, rupture of membranes
RP	radical prostatectomy
RR	recovery room
RSV	respiratory syncytial virus infection
rt	right; routine
RT	respiratory therapy
RUL	right upper lobe (of lung)
RUQ	right upper quadrant
Rx	prescription
RYGB	Roux-en-Y gastric bypass
$\bar{s}$	without
SAB	spontaneous abortion
SABA	short-acting beta agonist (relief of asthma symptoms)
SAH	subarachnoid hemorrhage
SARS	severe acute respiratory syndrome
SBE	subacute bacterial endocarditis; self-breast examination
SCC	squamous cell carcinoma
SCLC	small cell lung cancer
SG	specific gravity
SHG	sonohysterography
SI	sacroiliac
SICU	surgical intensive care unit
SIDS	sudden infant death syndrome
SLE	systemic lupus erythematosus
SMAC	Sequential Multiple Analyzer Computer
SMR	submucous resection
SNF	skilled nursing facility
SOB	shortness of breath
SPECT	single-photon emission computed tomography
SSE	soapsuds enema

COMMON MEDICAL ABBREVIATIONS	DEFINITIONS
SSER	somatosensory evoked response
STAPH or staph	staphylococcus
stat	immediately
STD	sexually transmitted disease
STI	sexually transmitted infection
STREP or strep	streptococcus
subcut	subcutaneous
subling	sublingual
sup	superior
supp	suppository
surg	surgical
SVD	spontaneous vaginal delivery
SVN	small-volume nebulizer
SWL	shock wave lithotripsy
T1-T12 or T_1-T_{12}	thoracic vertebrae
T2D	type 2 diabetes (mellitus)
T2DM	type 2 diabetes mellitus
T_3	triiodothyronine
T_4	thyroxine
tab	tablet
TAB	therapeutic abortion
T&A	tonsillectomy and adenoidectomy
TAH	total abdominal hysterectomy
TAH/BSO	total abdominal hysterectomy/ bilateral salpingo-oophorectomy
TAT	tetanus antitoxin
TB	tuberculosis
TCDB	turn, cough, deep breathe
TCT	thrombin clotting time
TD	transdermal
TEE	transesophageal echocardiogram
temp	temperature
TENS	transcutaneous electrical nerve stimulation
TGs	triglycerides
THA	total hip arthroplasty
THR	total hip replacement
TIA	transient ischemic attack
tid	three times per day
tinct	tincture
TKA	total knee arthroplasty

COMMON MEDICAL ABBREVIATIONS	DEFINITIONS
TLC	total lung capacity
TLH	total laparoscopic hysterectomy
TPN	total parenteral nutrition
tr	tincture
trach	tracheostomy
TRUS	transrectal ultrasound
TSH	thyroid-stimulating hormone
TSS	toxic shock syndrome
TUIP	transurethral incision of the prostate gland
TULIP	transurethral laser incision of the prostate gland
TUMT	transurethral microwave thermotherapy
TUNA	transurethral needle ablation
TURP	transurethral resection of the prostate gland
TVH	total vaginal hysterectomy
TVS	transvaginal sonography
TWE	tap water enema
Tx	treatment; traction
UA	urinalysis
UAE	uterine artery embolization
UC	ulcerative colitis
UGI	upper gastrointestinal
UGI-SBFT	upper gastrointestinal [series] with small bowel follow through [radiograph]
ung	ointment
UPPP	uvulopalatopharyngoplasty
URI	upper respiratory infection

COMMON MEDICAL ABBREVIATIONS	DEFINITIONS
US	ultrasound
UTI	urinary tract infection
UV	ultraviolet
UVR	ultraviolet radiation
V_1	tidal volume
VA	visual acuity
vag	vaginal
VATS	video-assisted thoracic surgery
VBAC	vaginal birth after cesarean section
VC	vital capacity
VCUG	voiding cystourethrogram
VD	venereal disease
VDRL	Venereal Disease Research Laboratory
vent	ventilator
VER	visual evoked response
VFib	ventricular fibrillation
VLAP	visual laser ablation of the prostate
VLDL	very-low-density lipoprotein
VQ scan	lung ventilation/perfusion scan
VRE	vancomycin-resistant enterococci
VS	vital signs
WA	while awake
WBC	white blood cell (leukocyte)
W/C	wheelchair
wt	weight
XRT	radiation therapy, x-ray radiotherapy, x-ray therapy

Institute for Safe Medication Practices' List of Error-Prone Abbreviations, Symbols, and Dose Designations

The abbreviations, symbols, and dose designations found in this table have been reported to ISMP through the ISMP National Medication Errors Reporting Program (ISMP MERP) as being frequently misinterpreted and involved in harmful medication errors. They should **NEVER** be used when communicating medical information. This includes internal communications, telephone/verbal prescriptions, computer-generated labels, labels for drug storage bins, medication administration records, as well as pharmacy and prescriber computer order entry screens.

ABBREVIATIONS	INTENDED MEANING	MISINTERPRETATION	CORRECTION
µg	Microgram	Mistaken as "mg"	Use "mcg"
AD, AS, AU	Right ear, left ear, each ear	Mistaken as OD, OS, OU (right eye, left eye, each eye)	Use "right ear," "left ear," or "each ear"
OD, OS, OU	Right eye, left eye, each eye	Mistaken as AD, AS, AU (right ear, left ear, each ear)	Use "right eye," "left eye," or "each eye"
BT	Bedtime	Mistaken as "BID" (twice daily)	Use "bedtime"
cc	Cubic centimeters	Mistaken as "u" (units)	Use "mL"
D/C	Discharge or discontinue	Premature discontinuation of medications if D/C (intended to mean "discharge") has been misinterpreted as "discontinued" when followed by a list of discharge medications	Use "discharge" and "discontinue"
IJ	Injection	Mistaken as "IV" or "intrajugular"	Use "injection"
IN	Intranasal	Mistaken as "IM" or "IV"	Use "intranasal" or "NAS"
HS	Half-strength	Mistaken as bedtime	Use "half-strength" or "bedtime"
hs	At bedtime, hours of sleep	Mistaken as half-strength	
IU**	International unit	Mistaken as IV (intravenous) or 10 (ten)	Use "units"
o.d. or OD	Once daily	Mistaken as "right eye" (OD-oculus dexter), leading to oral liquid medications administered in the eye	Use "daily"
OJ	Orange juice	Mistaken as OD or OS (right or left eye); drugs meant to be diluted in orange juice may be given in the eye	Use "orange juice"
Per os	By mouth, orally	The "os" can be mistaken as "left eye" (OS-oculus sinister)	Use "PO," "by mouth," or "orally"
q.d. or QD**	Every day	Mistaken as q.i.d., especially if the period after the "q" or the tail of the "q" is misunderstood as an "i"	Use "daily"
qhs	Nightly at bedtime	Mistaken as "qhr" or every hour	Use "nightly"
qn	Nightly or at bedtime	Mistaken as "qh" (every hour)	Use "nightly" or "at bedtime"
q.o.d. or QOD**	Every other day	Mistaken as "q.d." (daily) or "q.i.d." (four times daily) if the "o" is poorly written	Use "every other day"
q1d	Daily	Mistaken as q.i.d. (four times daily)	Use "daily"

ABBREVIATIONS	INTENDED MEANING	MISINTERPRETATION	CORRECTION
q6PM, etc.	Every evening at 6 PM	Mistaken as every 6 hours	Use "daily at 6 PM" or "6 PM daily"
SC, SQ, sub q	Subcutaneous	SC mistaken as SL (sublingual); SQ mistaken as "5 every;" the "q" in "sub q" has been mistaken as "every" (e.g., a heparin dose ordered "sub q 2 hours before surgery" misunderstood as every 2 hours before surgery)	Use "subcut" or "subcutaneously"
ss	Sliding scale (insulin) or ½ (apothecary)	Mistaken as "55"	Spell out "sliding scale;" use "one half" or "½"
SSRI	Sliding scale regular insulin	Mistaken as "selective-serotonin reuptake inhibitor"	Spell out "sliding scale (insulin)"
SSI	Sliding scale insulin	Mistaken as "Strong Solution of Iodine" (Lugol's)	
i/d	One daily	Mistaken as "tid"	Use "1 daily"
TIW or tiw	3 times a week	Mistaken as "3 times a day" or "twice in a week"	Use "3 times weekly"
U or u**	Unit	Mistaken as the number 0 or 4, causing a 10-fold overdose or greater (e.g., 4U seen as "40" or 4u seen as "44"); mistaken as "cc" so dose given in volume instead of units (e.g., 4u seen as 4cc)	Use "unit"
UD	As directed ("ut dictum")	Mistaken as unit dose (e.g., diltiazem 125 mg IV infusion "UD" misinterpreted as meaning to give the entire infusion as a unit [bolus] dose)	Use "as directed"
DOSE DESIGNATIONS AND OTHER INFORMATION	**INTENDED MEANING**	**MISINTERPRETATION**	**CORRECTION**
Trailing zero after decimal point (e.g., 1.0 mg)**	1 mg	Mistaken as 10 mg if the decimal point is not seen	Do not use trailing zeros for doses expressed in whole numbers
"Naked" decimal point (e.g., .5 mg)**	0.5 mg	Mistaken as 5 mg if the decimal point is not seen	Use zero before a decimal point when the dose is less than a whole unit
Abbreviations such as mg. or mL. with a period following the abbreviation	mg mL	The period is unnecessary and could be mistaken as the number 1 if written poorly	Use mg, mL, etc., without a terminal period
Drug name and dose run together (especially problematic for drug names that end in "l" such as Inderal40 mg; Tegretol300 mg)	Inderal 40 mg Tegretol 300 mg	Mistaken as Inderal 140 mg Mistaken as Tegretol 1300 mg	Place adequate space between the drug name, dose, and unit of measure

ABBREVIATIONS	INTENDED MEANING	MISINTERPRETATION	CORRECTION
Numerical dose and unit of measure run together (e.g., 10mg, 100mL)	10 mg 100 mL	The "m" is sometimes mistaken as a zero or two zeros, risking a 10- to 100-fold overdose	Place adequate space between the dose and unit of measure
Large doses without properly placed commas (e.g., 100000 units; 1000000 units)	100,000 units 1,000,000 units	100000 has been mistaken as 10,000 or 1,000,000; 1000000 has been mistaken as 100,000	Use commas for dosing units at or above 1,000, or use words such as 100 "thousand" or 1 "million" to improve readability
ABBREVIATIONS	**INTENDED MEANING**	**MISINTERPRETATION**	**CORRECTION**
To avoid confusion, do not abbreviate drug names when communicating medical information. Examples of drug name abbreviations involved in medication errors include:			
APAP	acetaminophen	Not recognized as acetaminophen	Use complete drug name
ARA A	vidarabine	Mistaken as cytarabine (ARA C)	Use complete drug name
AZT	zidovudine (Retrovir)	Mistaken as azathioprine or aztreonam	Use complete drug name
CPZ	Compazine (prochlorperazine)	Mistaken as chlorpromazine	Use complete drug name
DPT	Demerol-Phenergan-Thorazine	Mistaken as diphtheria-pertussis-tetanus (vaccine)	Use complete drug name
DTO	Diluted tincture of opium, or deodorized tincture of opium (Paregoric)	Mistaken as tincture of opium	Use complete drug name
HCl	hydrochloric acid or hydrochloride	Mistaken as potassium chloride (the "H" is misinterpreted as "K")	Use complete drug name unless expressed as a salt of a drug
HCT	hydrocortisone	Mistaken as hydrochlorothiazide	Use complete drug name
HCTZ	hydrochlorothiazide	Mistaken as hydrocortisone (seen as HCT250 mg)	Use complete drug name
MgSO4**	magnesium sulfate	Mistaken as morphine sulfate	Use complete drug name
MS, MSO4**	morphine sulfate	Mistaken as magnesium sulfate	Use complete drug name
MTX	methotrexate	Mistaken as mitoxantrone	Use complete drug name
NoAC	novel/new anticoagulant	No anticoagulant	Use complete drug name
PCA	procainamide	Mistaken as patient controlled analgesia	Use complete drug name

ABBREVIATIONS	INTENDED MEANING	MISINTERPRETATION	CORRECTION
PTU	propylthiouracil	Mistaken as mercaptopurine	Use complete drug name
T3	Tylenol with codeine No. 3	Mistaken as liothyronine	Use complete drug name
TAC	triamcinolone	Mistaken as tetracaine, Adrenalin, cocaine	Use complete drug name
TNK	TNKase	Mistaken as "TPA"	Use complete drug name
TPA or tPA	tissue plasminogen activator, Activase (alteplase)	Mistaken as TNKase (tenecteplase), or less often as another tissue plasminogen activator, Retavase (retaplase)	Use complete drug name
ZnSO4	zinc sulfate	Mistaken as morphine sulfate	Use complete drug name

STEMMED DRUG NAMES	INTENDED MEANING	MISINTERPRETATION	CORRECTION
"Nitro" drip	nitroglycerin infusion	Mistaken as sodium nitroprusside infusion	Use complete drug name
"Norflox"	norfloxacin	Mistaken as Norflex	Use complete drug name
"IV Vanc"	intravenous vancomycin	Mistaken as Invanz	Use complete drug name

SYMBOLS	INTENDED MEANING	MISINTERPRETATION	CORRECTION
ʒ	Dram	Symbol for dram mistaken as "3"	Use metric system
ɱ	Minim	Symbol for minim mistaken as "mL"	
x3d	For three days	Mistaken as "3 doses"	Use "for three days"
> and <	More than and less than	Mistaken as opposite of intended; mistakenly use incorrect symbol; "< 10" mistaken as "40"	Use "more than" or "less than"
/ (slash mark)	Separates two doses or indicates "per"	Mistaken as the number 1 (e.g., "25 units/10 units" misread as "25 units and 110" units)	Use "per" rather than a slash mark to separate doses
@	At	Mistaken as "2"	Use "at"
&	And	Mistaken as "2"	Use "and"
+	Plus or and	Mistaken as "4"	Use "and"
°	Hour	Mistaken as a zero (e.g., q2° seen as q 20)	Use "hr," "h," or "hour"
Φ or ∅	zero, null sign	Mistaken as numerals 4, 6, 8, and 9	Use 0 or zero, or describe intent using whole words

**These abbreviations are included on The Joint Commission's "minimum list" of dangerous abbreviations, acronyms, and symbols that must be included on an organization's "Do Not Use" list, effective Jan. 1, 2004. Visit www.jointcommission.org for more information about this Joint Commission requirement.

 Report actual or potential medication errors to the ISMP Medication Errors Reporting Program (MERP) via the Web at www.ismp.org or by calling 1-800-FAIL-SAFE.

Appendix F

Pharmacology Terms

Topics include:

General Pharmacy Terms, p. 749
Routes of Administration, p. 751
General Drug Categories, p. 751
Terms related to body systems introduced in Chapters 2, 4–16, p. 752

GENERAL PHARMACY TERMS	
absorption	process in which drug is taken up into the body, organ, tissue, or cell
adverse drug reaction (ADR)	any unintended harmful reaction to drug administered at a normal dose
ampule (or ampoule)	small, sterile glass or plastic container that usually holds a single dose of a liquid medication
aseptic technique	method used to minimize the microbial contamination of compounded sterile drugs
bioavailability	percentage of administered drug available to affect the body and target site(s) after absorption, metabolism, and other factors
capsule (cap)	small, digestible container (usually made of gelatin) used to hold a dose of medication for oral administration
chemotherapy (also called chemo)	treatment of cancer with medications
compounding	act of combining drug ingredients to prepare a customized prescription or drug order for a patient
contraindication	factor that prohibits administration of drug
controlled substance	drug that has been identified as having the potential for abuse or addiction; designated as schedule I, II, III, IV, or V under the Controlled Substance Act
cream	water-based, semisolid preparation that is applied topically to external parts of the body
dietary supplement	any vitamin, mineral, amino acid, botanical, herbal, or natural non-drug agent that may be taken orally for general well-being; these agents are not approved by the FDA to diagnose, cure, treat, or prevent any disease
distribution	uptake pattern of drug throughout the body to various tissues
dose	amount of drug or other substance to be administered at one time
drug	any substance taken by mouth; injected into a muscle, the skin, a blood vessel, or a cavity of the body; or applied topically to treat, cure, prevent, or diagnose a disease or condition
drug-drug interaction (DDI)	modification of the effect of drug when administered with another drug; food, diseases, and conditions can also interact with drug to cause a modification of the drug's effect
elimination	removal of a substance from the body by any route, including the kidneys, liver, lungs, and sweat glands
elixir	liquid containing sweeteners, flavorings, water, and/or alcohol in which an oral medication may be dispersed
emulsion	stable mixture that contains one component suspended within another component that it cannot normally dissolve in or mix with

Food and Drug Administration (FDA)	the U.S. federal agency responsible for the enforcement of federal regulations regarding the manufacturing and distribution of food, drugs, and cosmetics as protection against the sale of impure or dangerous substances
formulary	listing of drugs and drug information used by health practitioners within an institution to prescribe treatment that is medically appropriate
generic name	official, established nonproprietary name assigned to drug
inhaler	device containing drug to be breathed in nasally or by mouth
mechanism of action (MOA)	means by which drug exerts a desired effect
metabolism	chemical changes that drug or other substance undergoes in the body
ointment	oil-based, semisolid preparation that is applied topically to external parts of the body
over-the-counter (OTC) drug	drug that may be purchased without a prescription (also called **nonprescription drug**)
pharmaceutical	drug used for medicinal purposes
pharmacist	person formally trained to formulate and dispense medications and provide drug information
pharmacodynamics	study of the actions of drug on the body
pharmacogenomics	study of the correlation between genetics and response to drug
pharmacokinetics	study of the actions of the body on drug
pharmacology	study of the preparation, properties, uses, and actions of drugs
pharmacy	place for preparing and dispensing drugs
placebo	inactive substance, prescribed as if it were an effective dose of a needed medication
prescription (Rx)	order for a medication, therapy, or a therapeutic device given by a properly authorized person for a specified patient
preservative	substance included in some parenteral and topical medications used to prevent the growth of microorganisms in the product
route of administration	method in which drug or agent is given to a patient
side effect	any reaction or result from a medication other than what is the primary intended effect
solution	homogenous mixture of one or more substances dissolved into another substance
state board of pharmacy	agency responsible for regulating the practice of pharmacy within the state
suppository	topical form of drug that is inserted into the rectum, vagina, or penis
suspension	liquid in which particles of a solid are dispersed, but not dissolved, and in which the dispersal is maintained by stirring or shaking
tablet	small, solid dose form of a medication
toxicity	level at which drug's concentration within the body produces serious adverse effects
trade name	proprietary name assigned to drug by its manufacturer that is registered as part of the drug's identity (also called **brand name**)
United States Pharmacopeia (USP)	compendium, recognized officially by the federal Food and Drug Administration that contains descriptions, uses, strengths, and standards of purity for selected drugs and guidance for related standards of practice

ROUTES OF ADMINISTRATION	
buccal	administration of drug by absorption through the inner cheek tissue
enteral	administration of a medication through the digestive tract, including oral ingestion
epidural	injection of drug into the epidural space of the spinal cord
infusion	prolonged administration of a fluid substance directly into a vein, artery, or under the skin in which the flow rate is driven by gravity or a mechanical pump
inhalation	method of drug administration that involves the breathing in of a spray, vapor, or powder via the nose or mouth
injection	introduction of a liquid substance directly into the body bypassing natural routes of entry by using a needle
intramuscular (IM)	administration of a medication directly into a muscle
intrathecal	administration of drug into the subarachnoid space of the meninges in the spine
intravenous (IV)	administration of a medication directly into a vein
oral	administration of a medication by mouth
parenteral	drug or agent that is administered into the body via a route that bypasses the digestive tract
rectal	administration of drug by absorption through the rectum
subcutaneous	introduction of a medication into the tissue just beneath the skin
sublingual	administration of drug by absorption through tissue under the tongue
topical	administration of a medication to an external area of the body
transdermal	method of applying drug to unbroken skin so that it is continuously absorbed through the skin to produce a systemic effect; a transdermal patch is drug delivery system that controls the rate of absorption through the skin

GENERAL DRUG CATEGORIES	
antibacterial	drug that targets bacteria to kill or halt growth
antibiotic	drug that targets bacteria, fungi, or protozoa to kill or halt growth
antifungal	drug that targets fungi to kill or halt growth
antihistamine	drug that treats allergic and hypersensitivity reactions by blocking histamine-1 receptors
antiinflammatory	drug that reduces inflammation
antimicrobial	drug that targets microorganisms to kill or halt growth
antineoplastic agent	drug used to destroy or slow the rapid replication of cancer cells
antiretroviral	drug that suppresses the replication of the human immunodeficiency virus (HIV); highly active antiretroviral therapy (HAART) is the combination of three or more of these drugs to treat HIV infection
antiviral	drug that targets viruses to kill or halt growth
antiadrenergic agent	drug that blocks adrenergic receptors to reduce sympathetic nervous system activity in the body
bactericidal	designation for an antimicrobial agent that kills or destroys bacteria
bacteriostatic	the designation for an antimicrobial agent that halts the growth or replication of bacteria but does not kill them
cytotoxic	agent that causes cell death
dietary supplement	product that provides nutrients that may be missing from the diet; dietary supplements are not as strictly regulated as drugs for safety and efficacy

disinfectant	chemical agent that can be applied to inanimate objects to destroy microorganisms
herbal supplement	naturally derived, often plant-based, dietary supplement that is touted to improve health; herbal supplements are not as strictly regulated as drugs for safety and efficacy
immunosuppressant	drug that reduces the response of the immune system; used in autoimmune diseases and to prepare a patient for an organ transplant (also called **immunomodulator**)
narcotic	type of drug that has opium-like effects to cause drowsiness, pain relief, and sedation; can be habit-forming and is regulated as a controlled substance
nonsteroidal antiinflammatory drug (NSAID)	drug that reduces pain, inflammation, and fever
parasympatholytic	agent that blocks the actions of the parasympathetic nervous system
parasympathomimetic	agent that enhances the actions of the parasympathetic nervous system
radiopharmaceutical	drug with a radioactive component; used for diagnosis or treatment
smoking cessation agent	drug that helps a patient quit smoking; may be a behavioral deterrent or a nicotine substitute
sympatholytic	agent that blocks the actions of the sympathetic nervous system
sympathomimetic	agent that enhances the actions of the sympathetic nervous system
vaccine (also called immunization)	preparation of microbial antigen that will confer a degree of immunity to a future infection by that microbial
vitamin	organic compound essential in small quantities for normal physiologic and metabolic functioning
CHAPTER 2: BODY STRUCTURE, COLOR, AND ONCOLOGY	
alkylating agent	type of antineoplastic agent that binds to cellular DNA to interfere with replication
antimetabolite	type of antineoplastic agent that interferes with a cell's normal metabolism
antineoplastic agent	drug used to destroy or slow the replication of cancer cells
chemotherapeutic agent	drug used to destroy or slow the replication of cancer cells
kinase inhibitor	type of antineoplastic agent that interferes with protein phosphorylation
mitotic inhibitor	type of antineoplastic agent that interrupts cellular division
CHAPTER 4: INTEGUMENTARY SYSTEM	
antibacterial	drug used to combat an infection caused by bacteria
antifungal	drug used to combat an infection caused by fungi
antihistamine	drug used to minimize allergy symptoms by blocking histamine-1 receptors
antipruritic	agent that reduces itching
antipsoriatic	drug that treats psoriasis
antiseptic	chemical agent that can safely be applied to external tissues to kill or halt the growth of microorganisms
astringent	agent that reduces inflammation and irritation and provides a protective barrier on mucosa and skin by contracting the surface tissue
emollient	external agent that softens or soothes the skin
keratolytic	agent that augments the shedding of the top layer of dead skin
pediculicide	agent that kills lice
retinoid	derivative of vitamin A that regulates the growth of epithelial cells
rubefacient	topical agent that increases blood flow to the area to treat muscle aches
scabicide	agent that kills scabies

CHAPTER 5: RESPIRATORY SYSTEM	
antitussive	drug that suppresses coughing
bronchodilator	drug that expands the airways by relaxing smooth muscle in the lungs
decongestant	drug that relieves nasal congestion by reducing swelling of mucous membranes
expectorant	drug that promotes expulsion of mucus from the lungs
leukotriene receptor antagonist (LTRA)	drug that blocks late-stage regulators of allergic and hypersensitivity reactions to treat allergy-induced asthma
mucolytic	drug that thins out mucus in the lungs so that it can be expelled more easily
CHAPTER 6: URINARY SYSTEM	
aldosterone receptor antagonist (ARA)	drug that decreases reabsorption of water and sodium by the kidneys to treat edema or high blood pressure
alpha-1 blocker	drug that relaxes the muscles in the prostate and bladder neck to improve urination in men with an enlarged prostate
antispasmodic	drug that prevents or relieves bladder muscle spasms associated with incontinence
diuretic	drug that promotes the formation and excretion of urine to reduce the volume of extracellular fluid; used to reduce high blood pressure or edema; commonly referred to as a "water pill"
muscle relaxant	drug that reduces bladder muscle contractility to relieve spasm-induced pain or uncontrolled urination
urinary alkalinizer	agent that increases the urine pH
vasopressin	drug that increases water retention by the kidneys (also called ***antidiuretic hormone*** or ***ADH***)
CHAPTER 7: MALE REPRODUCTIVE SYSTEM	
androgen	natural or synthetic hormone involved in male reproduction and secondary gender attributes
antiandrogen	drug that blocks the effects of androgen hormones in the body
phosphodiesterase-5 inhibitor (PDE5 inhibitor)	drug that blocks the inactivation of cyclic guanosine monophosphate to increase vasodilation in the penis
spermicide	contact agent that kills sperm
CHAPTER 8: FEMALE REPRODUCTIVE SYSTEM	
antiestrogen	drug used to block the action of estrogen hormones in the body
contraceptive	agent (drug or barrier) used to prevent conception or pregnancy
estrogen	natural or synthetic hormone involved in female reproduction and secondary gender characteristics
fertility drugs	drugs that enhance a female's ability to conceive a child
hormone replacement therapy (HRT)	regimen that mimics the body's normal levels of female hormones when they are no longer produced; typically used during menopause
intrauterine device (IUD)	hormone-containing or metal-based device that is inserted directly in the uterus to prevent pregnancy long-term
oral contraceptive	exogenous hormones taken by mouth to prevent pregnancy
ovulation stimulant	drug that enhances the release of an egg from the ovary to promote pregnancy
progestin	synthetic or natural hormone involved in female reproduction and secondary sex characteristics
vaginal ring	device containing estrogen and progestin hormones that is inserted in the vagina to prevent pregnancy

CHAPTER 9: OBSTETRICS AND NEONATOLOGY	
abortifacient	drug that causes uterine muscles to contract with subsequent abortion of the fetus
oxytocic	hormone that stimulates the uterine muscles to contract, thereby inducing labor in pregnant woman
pregnancy category	level of risk the Food and Drug Administration assigns drug based on documented problems with the use of that drug during pregnancy
tocolytic	agent that suppresses labor contractions
CHAPTER 10: CARDIOVASCULAR, IMMUNE, AND LYMPHATIC SYSTEMS AND BLOOD	
angiotensin-converting enzyme inhibitor (ACE inhibitor)	drug that prevents the formation of angiotensin-II, which is a strong vasoconstrictor and major contributor to high blood pressure
angiotensin receptor blocker (ARB)	drug that blocks the angiotensin-II molecule from binding to its receptors throughout the body to prevent its effects and to reduce high blood pressure
antianginal	drug that relieves the chest pain paroxysms caused by lack of oxygen delivery to the heart; typically involves vasodilation
antiarrhythmic	drug that treats abnormal heart rhythm
anticoagulant	drug that prevents blood clotting and coagulation; commonly referred to as a blood thinner
antihypertensive	drug that lowers blood pressure
antiplatelet agent	drug that prevents platelet formation or aggregation or causes platelet destruction
beta-blocker (BB)	drug that inhibits beta-adrenergic receptors to decrease heart rate and force of contractility; used to treat arrhythmias, hypertension, heart failure, and more
calcium channel blocker (CCB)	drug that regulates the entry of calcium into muscle cells of the heart and blood vessels; used to treat heart failure, arrhythmias, angina, and hypertension
colony-stimulating factor (CSF)	agent that promotes the replication of blood cells in the bone marrow
direct thrombin inhibitor (DTI)	drug that blocks the action of thrombin, thereby reducing blood coagulation
erythropoiesis stimulating agent (ESA)	agent that stimulates red blood cell production in the bone marrow
hemostatic	drug that stops bleeding or hemorrhaging
inotropic agent	drug that strengthens or weakens the contraction of the heart muscles
nitrate	drug that dilates the blood vessels
platelet aggregation inhibitor	drug that stops platelets from adhering together
renin inhibitor	drug that blocks renin activity to reduce high blood pressure; renin is the first step in the renin-angiotensin-aldosterone system (RAAS), which is a common contributor to chronic high blood pressure
thrombolytic	drug that dissolves blood clots
vasodilator	drug that expands blood vessels to lower blood pressure
vasopressor	drug that contracts blood vessels to raise blood pressure (also called **vasoconstrictor**)
CHAPTER 11: DIGESTIVE SYSTEM	
antacid	drug that neutralizes acid in the stomach
antidiarrheal	drug that treats diarrhea by increasing water absorption, decreasing muscle contraction of the intestines, altering electrolyte exchange, or absorbing toxins or microorganisms
antiemetic	drug that reduces or prevents nausea and vomiting

antihyperlipidemic agent	drug used to reduce high levels of bad cholesterol and/or raise levels of good cholesterol by affecting levels of low-density lipoproteins, high-density lipoproteins, total cholesterol, and/or triglycerides, which are collectively called lipids (also called **hypolipidemic agent**)
bile acid sequestrant	type of antihyperlipidemic agent used to lower high cholesterol levels by increasing the excretion of bile acids
enema	liquid agent administered rectally to clear the contents of the bowel
fibrate	type of antihyperlipidemic agent that affects lipid levels by facilitating lipid metabolism
histamine-2 receptor antagonist (H2RA)	drug that reduces production of stomach acid (also called **H_2 blocker**)
laxative	drug that aids the evacuation of the bowel
proton pump inhibitor (PPI)	drug that reduces acid production in the stomach
statin	type of antihyperlipidemic agent that treats dyslipidemia by inhibiting 3-hydroxy-3-methylglutaryl coenzyme A reductase (also called **HMG-CoA reductase inhibitor**)
CHAPTER 12: EYE	
antiglaucoma agent	drug that treats glaucoma of the eye
miotic	agent that contracts the pupil
mydriatic	agent that dilates the pupil
ophthalmic	agent that is intended to be used in the eye
CHAPTER 13: EAR	
ceruminolytic	agent that breaks down ear wax
otic	agent intended to be used in the ear
CHAPTER 14: MUSCULOSKELETAL SYSTEM	
antiarthritic agent	drug used in the treatment of arthritis
antigout agent	drug that opposes the buildup of uric acid crystals in the joints to prevent and treat gout attacks
antispasmodic	drug that prevents or relieves muscle spasms
biologic	genetically-engineered protein that targets a specific hyper-functioning component of the immune system to treat diseases such as rheumatoid arthritis
bisphosphonate	drug that binds to bone matrix to treat osteoporosis
disease-modifying antirheumatic drug (DMARD)	drug that slows the progression of rheumatoid arthritis
muscle relaxant	drug that reduces muscle contractility to relieve tension- or spasm-induced pain
neuromuscular blocking agent (NMBA)	drug that blocks all nerve stimulation of the skeletal muscles to cause paralysis
CHAPTER 15: NERVOUS SYSTEM AND BEHAVIORAL HEALTH	
adrenergic agonist	drug that stimulates aspects of the sympathetic nervous system
amphetamine	drug that stimulates the central nervous system
anticonvulsant	drug that reduces the incidence and severity of seizures and convulsions (also called **antiepileptic drug**)
analgesic	drug that relieves pain
anesthetic	drug that causes numbness or a loss of feeling that can be used locally or systemically; often used systemically to put a patient "to sleep" during extensive procedures

anticholinergic	drug that blocks the action of acetylcholine and therefore suppresses the parasympathetic nervous system
anticholinesterase	drug that prevents the breakdown of acetylcholine to yield a cholinergic or parasympathetic effect
antidepressant	drug used to treat depression
antiparkinsonian agent	drug that treats Parkinson disease and parkinsonism by affecting levels of dopamine or acetylcholine in the brain
antipsychotic	drug that treats psychosis disorders by inducing a calming or tranquilizing effect or by adjusting neurotransmitter levels in the brain (also called **neuroleptic**)
antipyretic	drug that reduces fever
anxiolytic	drug that relieves anxiety
barbiturate	drug used to produce relaxation and sleep
benzodiazepine (BZD)	drug that binds to receptors in the brain to calm and sedate the central nervous system
central nervous system stimulant	drug that excites the central nervous system; can be used for many brain disorders
cholinergic	agent that acts like acetylcholine to activate the parasympathetic nervous system
dopaminergic	drug that acts like dopamine, a neurotransmitter in the brain
hypnotic	drug used to induce sleep; may also be used as a sedative
mood stabilizer	drug that balances neurotransmitters in the brain to prevent periods of mania or depression
monoamine oxidase inhibitor (MAOI)	type of antidepressant that prevents the breakdown of many active neurotransmitters in the brain
nonsteroidal antiinflammatory drug (NSAID)	drug that reduces pain, inflammation, and fever
opioid antagonist	drug that can treat opioid or narcotic overdose
sedative	drug that depresses the central nervous system to calm a patient
selective serotonin reuptake inhibitor (SSRI)	type of antidepressant that maintains a higher level of serotonin in the synapse
tranquilizer	drug that reduces anxiety or agitation
tricyclic antidepressant (TCA)	type of antidepressant that maintains a higher level of various neurotransmitters in the synapse
CHAPTER 16: ENDOCRINE SYSTEM	
antidiabetic agent	drug that treats diabetes by controlling blood sugar levels
antithyroid agent	drug that counters hyperthyroidism by reducing the production of thyroid hormones
corticosteroid	drug that mimics hormones produced by the adrenal glands and has antiinflammatory and immunosuppressive effects
hypoglycemic agent	drug that lowers blood sugar levels (also called **antihyperglycemic**)
thyroid hormone	replacement hormone to regulate metabolism and endocrine functions

Bibliography

2016 Conn's current therapy, Philadelphia, 2016, Elsevier.

American Journal of Nursing, 2008-2016, Wolters Kluwer.

AAFP, http://www.aafp.org, 2016, American Academy of Family Physicians.

Abbas A: *Basic immunology: functions and disorders of the immune system*, ed 4, Philadelphia, 2013, Saunders.

ACOG: The American congress of obstetricians and gynecologists, women's health care physicians, http://www.acog.org, 2016, American Congress of Obstetricians and Gynecologists.

Adams J: *Emergency medicine, clinical essentials*, ed 2, Philadelphia, 2014, Saunders.

American academy of dermatology, https://www.aad.org, 2016, American Academy of Dermatology.

American academy of ophthalmology: eyesmart, http://www.aao.org, 2016, American Academy of Ophthalmology.

American board of medical specialties, http://www.abms.org, 2016, American Board of Medical Specialties.

American cancer society, http://www.cancer.org, 2016, American Cancer Society, Inc.

American society for gastrointestinal endoscopy, www.asge.org, 2016, American Society for Gastrointestinal Endoscopy.

Aminoff M: *Neurology and general medicine*, ed 4, 2008, Elsevier.

Applegate EJ: *The anatomy and physiology learning system*, ed 4, St. Louis, 2011, Saunders.

Ballinger PW, Frank ED: *Merrill's atlas of radiographic positions and radiologic procedures*, ed 13, 2016, Elsevier.

Bontrager KL: *Textbook of radiographic positioning and related anatomy*, ed 8, St. Louis, 2013, Mosby.

Buchbinder R, et al: Percutaneous vertebroplasty for osteoporotic vertebral compression fracture, Cochrane Database Syst Rev (4):Art. No.: CD006349, 2015. doi:10.1002/14651858.CD006349.pub2.

Cancer.Net: http://www.cancer.net, 2005-2016, American Society of Clinical Oncology (ASCO).

CDC: *Centers for disease control and prevention*, https://www.cdc.gov, 2016, US Department of Health and Human Services.

Chabner D: *The language of medicine*, ed 11, Philadelphia, 2017, Saunders.

Chen Y, et al: The differences between blast-induced and sports-related brain injuries, Front Neurol 2013. http://dx.doi.org/10.3389/fneur.2013.00119. Frontiers Media, SA.

Christensen B, Kockrow E: *Foundations of nursing*, ed 6, St. Louis, 2011, Mosby.

Declerck A, et al: Closed-loop titration of propofol and remifentanil guided by Bispectral Index in a patient with extreme gigantism, J Clin Anesth 21(7):542–544, 2009. doi:10.1016/j.jclinane.2009.02.008.

DermNet NZ, www.dermnetnz.org, 2016, DermNet New Zealand Trust.

Diehl M: *Medical transcription guide: do's and don'ts*, ed 3, St. Louis, 2005, Saunders.

Diehl M: *Diehl and Fordney's medical transcription, techniques and procedures*, ed 5, 2002, Saunders.

Dorland's illustrated medical dictionary, ed 32, Philadelphia, 2011, Saunders.

Drazner M: The progression of hypertensive heart disease, Circulation 2011. http://dx.doi.org/10.1161/CIRCULATIONAHA.108.845792. The American Heart Association.

Ferri F: *Ferri's clinical advisor*, 2016, Elsevier.

First consult, https://www.clinicalkey.com, 2016, Elsevier.

Fitzpatrick JE, Aeling JL: *Dermatology secrets in color*, ed 4, Philadelphia, 2010, Mosby.

Frazier M, Drzymkowski JW: *Essentials of human diseases and conditions*, ed 5, Philadelphia, 2013, Saunders.

Gillingham EA, Seibel MW: *LaFleur Brooks' health unit coordinating*, ed 7, Philadelphia, 2014, Saunders.

Goldman L, Shafer AI: *Goldman-cecil medicine*, ed 25, Philadelphia, 2015, Saunders.

Goljan EF: *Rapid review pathology*, ed 4, Philadelphia, 2014, Saunders.

Gould B, Dyer R: *Pathophysiology for the health professions*, ed 4, Philadelphia, 2011, Saunders.

Habif T: *A color guide to diagnosis and therapy, clinical dermatology*, ed 5, Philadelphia, 2010, Mosby.

Haubrich WS: *Medical meanings: a glossary of word origins*, ed 2, Philadelphia, 2004, American College of Physicians.

Hein C, Batista EL: Obesity and cumulative inflammatory burden: a valuable risk assessment parameter in caring for dental patients, J Evid Based Dent Pract 14:17–26.e1, 2014. Elsevier.

Herlihy B, Maebius N: *The human body in health and illness*, ed 5, Philadelphia, 2015, Saunders.

Hockenberry MJ, Wilson D: *Wong's nursing care of infants and children*, ed 9, St. Louis, 2011, Mosby.

Huth EJ, Murray TJ: *Medicine in quotations: views of health and disease through the ages*, Philadelphia, 2006, American College of Physicians.

Ignatavicius DD, et al: *Medical-surgical nursing: patient-centered collaborative care*, ed 8, Philadelphia, 2015, Saunders.

Jameson JL, DeGroot LJ: *Endocrinology: adult and pediatric*, ed 7, Philadelphia, 2016, Saunders.

Jarvis C: *Physical examination & health assessment*, ed 7, Philadelphia, 2016, Saunders.

Johns Hopkins Medicine: www.hopkinsmedicine.org, 2016, The Johns Hopkins University, The Johns Hopkins Hospital, and Johns Hopkins Health System.

Lab tests online, https://labtestsonline.org, 2001-2016, American Association for Clinical Chemistry.

LaFleur Brooks M, LaFleur Brooks D: *Basic medical language*, ed 5, St. Louis, 2016, Mosby.

LaFranchi SH, Huang SA: *Nelson textbook of pediatrics*, ed 20, 2016, Elsevier.

Lewis SM, et al: *Medical-surgical nursing*, ed 8, St. Louis, 2011, Mosby.

Littleton LY, Engebretson JC: *Maternal, neonatal, and women's health nursing*, Albany, 2002, Delmar.

Lowdermilk DL, et al: *Maternity & women's health care*, ed 11, St. Louis, 2016, Mosby.
Marx J, et al: *Rosen's emergency medicine, concepts and clinical practice*, ed 8, Philadelphia, 2014, Saunders.
Mayo Clinic Health Letter, Rochester, 2008-2016, Mayo Foundation for Medical Education and Research.
Mayo Clinic: *Patient care and health information*, http://www.mayoclinic.org, 1998-2016, Mayo Foundation for Medical Education and Research.
Mayo Clinic Women's Health Source, Rochester, 2008-2016, Mayo Foundation for Medical Education and Research.
Medical dictionary, http://www.medical-dictionary.thefreedictionary.com, n.d., The Free Dictionary by Farlex.
Medline Plus, http://www.nlm.nih.gov/medlineplus, 2008-2016, National Library of Medicine and the National Institutes of Health.
Merck manuals, https://www.merckmanuals.com, 2016, Merck Sharp & Dohme Corp.
Medscape, http://www.medscape.com, 1994-2016, WebMD LLC.
Mosby's medical, nursing, & health professions dictionary, ed 9, St. Louis, 2013, Mosby.
National institute of diabetes and digestive and kidney diseases, www.niddk.nih.gov, 2016, National Institutes of Health.
New England Journal of Medicine, 2008-2016, Massachusetts Medical Society.
Novey D: *Clinicians' complete reference to complementary and alternative medicine*, St. Louis, 2000, Mosby.
Ontjes DA: Disorders of the adrenal cortex. In *Netter's internal medicine*, ed 2, Philadelphia, 2009, Saunders, pp 321–327. 44.
Pagana KD, Pagana TJ: *Mosby's manual of diagnostic and laboratory test reference*, ed 5, St. Louis, 2015, Mosby.
Patient care and health information, www.mayoclinic.org/patient-care-and-health-information, 1998-2016, Mayo Foundation for Medical Education and Research.
Phillips N: *Berry & Kohn's operating room technique*, ed 12, St. Louis, 2013, Mosby.
Powell J, et al: The Canadian arthroplasty society's experience with hip resurfacing arthroplasty. An analysis of 2773 hips, Canadian Arthroplasty Society, Bone Joint J 2013. doi:10.1302/0301-620X.95B8.31811.
Rakel D: *Integrative medicine*, ed 3, Philadelphia, 2012, Saunders.
Retinoblastoma, http://www.cancer.org/acs/groups/cid/documents/webcontent/003135-pdf.pdf, 2015, American Cancer Society.
Schoenwolf, et al: *Larsen's human embrology*, ed 5, 2015, Elsevier Churchill Livingstone.
Seckeler MD, Hoke TR: The worldwide epidemiology of acute rheumatic fever and rheumatic heart disease, Clin Epidemiol 2011. doi:10.2147/CLEP.S12977.
Spencer JW, Jacobs JJ: *Complementary and alternative medicine: an evidence-based approach*, St Louis, 2003, Mosby.
Stedman's abbreviations, acronyms, and symbols, ed 5, Baltimore, 2013, Lippincott Williams & Wilkins.
Stern T, et al: *Massachusetts general hospital comprehensive clinical psychiatry*, 2016, Elsevier.
The fecal transplant foundation, http://thefecaltransplantfoundation.org, 2016, The Fecal Transplant Foundation.
Thibodeau GA, Patton KT: *Anthony's textbook of anatomy and physiology*, ed 20, St. Louis, 2016, Mosby.
Torpy JM: The metabolic syndrome, JAMA 295(7):850, 2006.
UpToDate, http://www.uptodate.com, 2008-2016, Wolters Kluwer Health.
Wein AJ, et al: *Campbell-walsh urology*, ed 11, Philadelphia, 2016, Elsevier.
Whiteside MM, et al: Sensory impairment in older adults: part 2, vision loss, Consultant 106(11):52–62, 2006.
Wong CC, McGirt M: Vertebral compression fractures: a review of current management and multimodal therapy, J Multidiscip Healthc 2013.
Workman ML, LaCharity L: *Understanding pharmacology: essentials for medication safety*, ed 2, 2016, Elsevier.
World Health Organization, https://who.int/en, 2016, WHO.

Illustration Credits

Adam A et al: *Grainger and Allison's diagnostic radiology*, ed 5, London, 2008, Churchill Livingstone. **Fig. 15.8**

American Cancer Society. **Fig. 5.5**

Amplivox Limited, Eynsham, Oxfordshire, United Kingdom. **Ch 13 Ex Fig. C**

Anderson KN: *Mosby's medical, nursing and allied health dictionary*, St. Louis, 2003, Mosby. **Fig. 11.10A**

Apple DJ, Robb MF: *Ocular pathology*, ed 5, St. Louis, 1998, Mosby. **Fig. 12.7**

Ball J et al: *Seidel's guide to physical examination*, ed 8, St. Louis, 2014, Elsevier. **Unn Figs. 12.2, 12.4, 14.6**

Ballinger PW, Frank ED: *Merrill's atlas of radiographic positions and radiologic procedures*, ed 10, St. Louis, 2003, Mosby. **Figs. 2.9, 5.16, Unn Fig. 5.8B, 6.12, Unn Fig. 10.10, 10.15, Ch 10 Ex Figs. D, E, Fig. 14.11, Unn Fig. 15.16, Ch 15 Ex Fig. B, Unn Fig. 15.14**

Bedford MA: *Ophthalmological diagnosis*, London, 1986, Wolfe. **Unn Fig. 12.7**

Biopsys Medical, Inc, Irvine, Calif. **Fig. 8.13A**

Black J, Hawks J: *Medical-surgical nursing*, ed 8, St. Louis, 2009, Elsevier. **Figs. 8.9, 12.8**

Black M et al: *Obstetric and gynecologic dermatology*, ed 5, Edinburgh, 2008, Mosby Ltd. **Fig. 4.4**

Bolognia JL et al: *Dermatology*, ed 2, St. Louis, 2008, Mosby. **Ch 4 Ex Fig. B**

Bontrager KL, Lampignano JP: *Radiographic positioning and related anatomy*, ed 8, St. Louis, 2014, Mosby. **Unn Figs. 3.12, 3.13, 3.15, 5.14A, 5.15A, 6.15, 8.15, 9.12, Ch 11 Ex Fig. G, Fig. 14.10B**

Bontrager KL: *Radiographic positioning and related anatomy*, ed 5, St. Louis, 2002, Mosby. **Table 3.2 images, Ch 3 Ex Fig. B, unn 15.5**

Bork K, Brauninger W: *Skin diseases in clinical practice*, ed 2, Philadelphia, 1998, WB Saunders. **Ex Fig. B1, Figs. 4.3A, 4.10, 4.11, 4.12, 4.13, Ch 7 Ex Fig. A, Fig. 10.12B**

Buckingham Richard A, MD, University of Illinois, Chicago. **Fig. 13.3**

Bullough P: *Orthopaedic pathology*, ed 5, St. Louis, 2010, Elsevier. **Ch 2 Ex Fig. A3**

Canale S, Beaty J: *Campbell's operative orthopaedics*, ed 12, St. Louis, 2013, Elsevier. **Unn Fig. 14.19**

CDC. **Unn Figs. 5.11, 15.1, 15.2**

Christensen B, Kockrow E: *Adult health nursing*, ed 5, St. Louis, 2006, Elsevier Mosby. **Unn Figs. 4.10, 4.20**

Cohen BA: *Pediatric dermatology*, ed 3, St. Louis, 2005, Mosby. **Fig. 4.6**

Cohen J: *Infectious diseases*, ed 3, St. Louis, 2010, Mosby. **Unn Fig. 4.29**

Cummings N: *Perspectives in athletic training*, ed 1, St. Louis, 2009, Mosby. **Fig. 5.21**

Damjanov I: *Pathology, A color atlas*, ed 2, St. Louis, 2000, Mosby. **Fig. 2.5, Ch 2 Ex Fig. A4, Figs. 6.5A, 6.6**

Dickason EJ, Schultz MO, Silverman BL: *Maternal-infant nursing care*, ed 3, St. Louis, 1998, Mosby. **Fig. 9.2**

Dorland's illustrated medical dictionary, ed 31, Philadelphia, 2007, Saunders. **Fig. 4.5**

Dornier Medical Systems, Kennesaw, Ga. **Unn Fig. 6.5**

EDAP Technomed, Inc., Vaulx-en-Velin, France. **Fig. 7.6B**

Eisenberg RL, Johnson NM: *Comprehensive radiographic pathology*, ed 3, St. Louis, 2003, Mosby. **Fig. 5.3**

Forbes CD and Jackson WF: **Unn Fig. 16.9**

Frank, Julia MD. **Dermatology poem.**

Frazier M: *Essentials of human disease and conditions*, ed 3, St. Louis, 2004, Elsevier Mosby. **Unn Fig. 4.8**

Fucentese SF et al: Total shoulder arthroplasty with an uncemented soft-metal-backed glenoid component, *J Shoulder Elbow Surg* 19:624-631, 2010. **Unn Fig. 14.19**

Gawkrodger D, Ardern-Jones M: *Dermatology*, ed 5, Oxford, 2012, Churchill Livingstone. **Unn Fig. 4.15**

GE Medical Systems, Waukesha, Wis. **Fig. 5.17**

Goering R et al: *Mims' medical microbiology*, ed 4, Edinburgh, 2008, Mosby Ltd. **Unn Fig. 4.17**

Goldman L, Schafer A: *Goldman's Cecil medicine*, ed 24, Philadelphia, 2012, Saunders. **Fig. 4.3 (upper right), Unn Fig. 4.28, Fig. 7.7C**

Goljan E: *Rapid review pathology*, ed 1, St. Louis, 2004, Mosby. **Unn Fig. 16.3**

Habif TP: *Clinical dermatology*, ed 4, St. Louis, 2004, Elsevier Mosby. **Ch 2 Ex Fig. A2, Figs. 4.3 (right halftone), 4.8**

Hagen-Ansert S: *Textbook of diagnostic ultrasonography*, ed 5, St. Louis, 2001, Mosby. **Unn Fig. 11.13**

Haught JM, Patel S, and English JC: Xanthoderma: A clinical review, *J Amer Acad Derm* 57(6):1051-1058, 2007. **Ch 4 Ex Fig. C**

Hockenberry M et al: *Wong's nursing care of infants and children*, ed 9, St. Louis, 2011, Elsevier. **Figs. 9.9, 9.10, Ch 9 Ex Figs. A, B**

Ignatavicius DM, Workman L: *Medical-surgical nursing*, ed 6, St. Louis, 2010, Saunders. **Ch 11 Ex Fig. G**

iStock: **Unn Figs. 2.5, 2.6, 4.2, 4.3 to 4.7, 5.4, 5.9, 6.9, 7.12, 9.6, 12.12, 13.6, 14.9, 13.6**

James S, Ashwill J: *Nursing care of children*, ed 3, St. Louis, 2008, Saunders. **Fig. 6.19**
Jarvis C: *Physical examination and health assessment*, ed 5, Philadelphia, 2008, Saunders. **Ch 12 Ex Fig. D, Ch 13 Ex Fig. B**
Kamal A, Brockelhurst JC: *Color atlas of geriatric medicine*, ed 2, St. Louis, 1991, Mosby. **Fig. 2.3**
Kliegman R et al: *Nelson textbook of pediatrics*, ed 20, St. Louis, 2016, Elsevier. **Unn Fig. 16.5**
Kliegman R et al: *Nelson textbook of pediatrics*, ed 18, St. Louis, 2008, Saunders. **Fig. 13.6B**
Kowalczyk N: *Radiographic pathology for technologists*, ed 6, St. Louis, 2014, Elsevier. **Fig. 11.16**
Kumar V et al: *Robbins' basic pathology*, ed 7, Philadelphia, 2003, Saunders. **Fig. 5.7**
Ladenson Paul W, MD, The Johns Hopkins University and Hospital, Baltimore, Md. **Fig. 16.5**
Lewis SM: *Medical-surgical nursing*, ed 7, St. Louis, 2007, Mosby. **Fig. 11.18**
Long et al: *Merrill's atlas of radiographic positions and radiologic procedures*, ed 13, St. Louis, 2016, Elsevier. **Fig. 14.7A(right), Unn Fig. 14.17**
Lowdermilk DL et al: *Maternity and women's health care*, ed 10, St. Louis, 2012, Mosby. **Fig. 9.6**
Mace JD: *Radiography pathology*, ed 4, St. Louis, 2004, Elsevier Mosby. **Ch 2 Ex Fig. A1**
Magee D: *Orthopedic physical assessment*, ed 5, St. Louis, 2008, Saunders. **Fig. 14.7B(right)**
Mahon C et al: *Textbook of diagnostic microbiology*, ed 4, Philadelphia, 2011, Elsevier. **Fig. 7.7B**
Manaster BJ: *Musculoskeletal imaging*, ed 3, St. Louis, 2007, Mosby. **Fig. 14.7C(right)**
Marcdante K et al: *Nelson essentials of pediatrics*, ed 6, Philadelphia, 2011, Elsevier. **Unn Fig. 4.12**
Marks J, Miller J: *Lookingbill and Marks' principles of dermatology*, ed 5, Philadelphia, 2014, Elsevier. **Unn Fig. 4.13**
Mercier LR: *Practical orthopedics*, ed 4, St. Louis, 1995, Mosby. **Fig. 14.23 and Unn Fig. 14.11**
Murray P et al: *Medical microbiology*, ed 5, St. Louis, 2005, Mosby. **Fig. 7.7A**
National Cancer Institute (NCI). Courtesy Rhoda Baer (Photographer). **Fig. 2.8.**
Nelcor Puritan Bennett. **Fig. 5.22**
Newell FW: *Ophthalmology*, ed 7, St. Louis, 1992, Mosby. **Unn Fig. 12.6**
Nidek, Inc., Fremont, Calif. **Fig. 12.9**
Nonin Medical, Inc. Reprinted with permission of Nonin Medical, Inc. © 2013. **Ex Fig. G1, 2**
Pagana KD, Pagana TJ: *Mosby's manual of diagnostic and laboratory test reference*, ed 7, St. Louis, 2004, Elsevier Mosby. **Figs. 5.18, 5.19, Unn Fig. 14.16, Fig. 8.13B, C**
Patton KT, Thibodeau GA: *Anatomy and physiology*, ed 7, St. Louis, 2010, Mosby. **Unn Fig. 5.8A, Ch 10 Ex Fig. F, Unn Fig. 14.10**
Paulino A: *PET-CT in radiotherapy treatment planning*, ed 1, Philadelphia, 2008, Saunders/Elsevier. **Unn Fig. 5.18**
Perkin GD, Hotchberg FH, Miller D: *The atlas of clinical neurology*, St. Louis, 1986, Mosby. **Unn Fig. 15.4**
Perry A, Potter P, Elkin M: *Nursing interventions & clinical skills*, ed 4, St. Louis, 2008, Mosby/Elsevier. **Unn Figs. 3.14, 4.11, Unn Fig. G3**
Richardson M et al: *Cummings otolaryngology - head and neck surgery*, ed 5, St. Louis, 2010, Mosby. **Unn 13.4**
Ruppel GL: *Manual pulmonary function testing*, ed 7, St. Louis, 1998, Mosby. **Figs. 5.13, 5.14B, Unn Fig. 5.17**
Schwarzenberger K et al: *General dermatology*, ed 1, Philadelphia, 2009, Saunders. **Ch 4 Ex Fig. A2**
Seidel H et al: *Mosby's guide to physical examination*, ed 5, St. Louis, 2003, Mosby. **Fig. 12.4A, B, Unn 16.8**
Shiland BJ: *Mastering healthcare terminology*, ed 2, St. Louis, 2006, Elsevier Mosby. **Fig. 4.38, Ch 4 Ex Fig. D1, 2, Fig. 6.8, Fig. 11.9, Unn Figs. 11.3, Unn 15.6, Fig. 16.7, Ch 16 Ex A**
Siemens Medical Systems, Inc., New Jersey. **Fig. 5.15B**
Śliwa LS et al: A comparison of audiometric and objective methods in hearing screening of school children: A preliminary study, *Internat J Pediatr Otorhinol* 75(4):483-488, 2011. **Fig. 13.6A**
Stein HA, Slatt BJ, Stein RM: *The ophthalmic assistant: fundamentals and clinical practice*, ed 5, St. Louis, 1998, Mosby. **Ch 12 Ex Fig. C**
Swartz M: *Textbook of physical diagnosis*, ed 5, Philadelphia, 2006, Saunders. **Unn Figs. 2.8, 12.5, Fig. 12.9**
Taylor J, Resnick D: *Skeletal imaging: atlas of the spine and extremities*, ed 1, Philadelphia, 2000, Saunders. **Fig. 14.10A**
Thibodeau GA, Patton KT: *Anatomy and physiology*, ed 4, St. Louis, 2001, Mosby. **Figs. 10.12 (A), 14.5, Unn Fig. 16.10**
Turgeon M: *Linne & Ringsrud's clinical laboratory science*, ed 5, St. Louis, 2007, Mosby. **Unn Fig. 10.12**
Waldman S: *Atlas of common pain syndromes*, ed 2, Philadelphia, 2008, Saunders. **Fig. 15.5**
Wein A et al: *Campbell-Walsh urology*, ed 10, 2012, Saunders. **Figs. 6.13, 6.14, 6.18, Unn Fig. 6.18**
Weston W et al: *Color textbook of pediatric dermatology*, ed 4, St. Louis, 2007, Mosby. **Unn Fig. 4.18**
White RA, Klein SR: *Endoscopic surgery*, St. Louis, 1991, Mosby. **Fig. 11.13**
Wilson S, Giddens J: *Health assessment for nursing practice*, ed 4, St. Louis, 2009, Mosby. Courtesy Gary Monheit, MD, University of Alabama at Birmingham School of Medicine. **Fig. 4.3C**
Wilson SF, Thompson JM: *Respiratory disorders*, St. Louis, 1990, Mosby. **Unn 5.13**
Zitelli BJ, David HW: *Atlas of pediatric physical diagnosis*, ed 2, St. Louis, 1992, Mosby. **Ch 7 Ex Fig. B1, Figs. 9.7, 12.3, Ch 12 Ex Figs. A, C, Unn Fig. 13.2**

Index

Page numbers followed by "*f*" indicate figures, "*t*" indicate tables, and "*b*" indicate boxes.

B

C

M

NOTES

Tables

APPENDICES ON EVOLVE